DRUGS WITH ILLUSTRATED MECHANISMS OF ACTION	DRUGS WITH SIMILAR MECHANISMS OF ACTION
enoxacin	alatrofloxacin mesylate, cin... cin, lomefloxacin hydrochlo... acid, norfloxacin, ofloxacin, ...
etanercept	infliximab
exenatide	none
ezetimibe	none
famotidine	cimetidine, nizatidine, ranitidine hydrochloride
hydrochlorothiazide	chlorothiazide, chlorothiazide sodium, chlorthalidone, indapamide, metolazone
ipratropium bromide	none
isosorbide dinitrate, isosorbide mononitrate	nitroglycerin
lanthanum carbonate	sevelamer hydrochloride
levodopa	none
linezolid	none
memantine hydrochloride	none
milrinone lactate	inamrinone (formerly amrinone lactate)
nateglinide	repaglinide
olmesartan medoxomil	irbesartan, losartan potassium, valsartan
omeprazole	esomeprazole magnesium, lansoprazole, pantoprazole sodium, rabeprazole sodium
orlistat	none
palonosetron	alosetron, dolasetron, granisetron, ondansetron
pegvisomant	none
phenelzine sulfate	isocarboxazid, tranylcypromine sulfate

(continued)

DRUGS WITH ILLUSTRATED MECHANISMS OF ACTION	DRUGS WITH SIMILAR MECHANISMS OF ACTION
remifentanil hydrochloride	codeine phosphate, codeine sulfate, fentanyl citrate, fentanyl transdermal, fentanyl transmucosal, hydrocodone bitartrate and acetaminophen, hydrocodone and ibuprofen, hydromorphone hydrochloride, levomethadyl acetate hydrochloride, levorphanol tartrate, meperidine hydrochloride, methadone hydrochloride, morphine sulfate, oxycodone and acetaminophen, oxycodone hydrochloride, oxymorphone hydrochloride, propoxyphene hydrochloride
reserpine	guanadrel sulfate, guanethidine monosulfate
spironolactone	none
tacrine hydrochloride	donepezil hydrochloride, galantamine hydrobromide, rivastigmine tartrate
teriparatide	none
ticlopidine hydrochloride	clopidogrel bisulfate
tubocurarine chloride	atracurium besylate
vasopressin	desmopressin acetate, lypressin
ziconitide	none

2010
Nurse's Drug Handbook

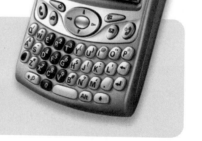
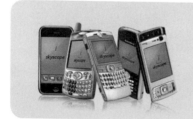

Jones and Bartlett Publishers

2010
Nurse's
Drug
Handbook

Ninth Edition

JONES AND BARTLETT PUBLISHERS
Sudbury, Massachusetts
BOSTON   TORONTO   LONDON   SINGAPORE

World Headquarters

Jones and Bartlett Publishers
40 Tall Pine Drive
Sudbury, MA 01776
978-443-5000
info@jbpub.com
www.jbpub.com

Jones and Bartlett Publishers Canada
6339 Ormindale Way
Mississauga, Ontario L5V 1J2
Canada

Jones and Bartlett Publishers
International
Barb House, Barb Mews
London W6 7PA
United Kingdom

Jones and Bartlett's books and products are available through most bookstores and online booksellers. To contact Jones and Bartlett Publishers directly, call 800-832-0034, fax 978-443-8000, or visit our website www.jbpub.com.

Substantial discounts on bulk quantities of Jones and Bartlett's publications are available to corporations, professional associations, and other qualified organizations. For details and specific discount information, contact the special sales department at Jones and Bartlett via the above contact information or send an email to specialsales@jbpub.com.

Production Credits

Publisher: Kevin Sullivan
Acquisitions Editor: Emily Ekle
Acquisitions Editor: Amy Sibley
Associate Editor: Patricia Donnelly
Editorial Assistant: Rachel Shuster
Senior Production Editor: Carolyn F. Rogers
Senior Marketing Manager: Barb Bartoszek
**V. P., Manufacturing and Inventory
   Control:** Therese Connell

Clinical Reviewer: Marlene Ciranowicz-
   Steenburg, RN, MSN, CDE
Composition: Catherine E. Harold
Interior Illustrations: Rolin Graphics, Inc.
Cover Design: Kristin E. Parker
Cover Image: © ajt/ShutterStock, Inc.
Printing and Binding: Malloy, Inc.
Cover Printing: Malloy, Inc.

6048

Printed in the United States of America
13 12 11 10 09   10 9 8 7 6 5 4 3 2 1

Contents

Jack E. Fincham, RPh, PhD
Dean and Professor of Pharmacy
Practice
School of Pharmacy
University of Kansas
Lawrence, KS

Martha Mitchell Funnell, RN, MS, CDE
Associate Director for Administration
Diabetes Research and Training Center
University of Michigan
Ann Arbor, MI

Mary E. MacCara, PharmD
Associate Professor
College of Pharmacy
Assistant Professor
Department of Family Medicine
Dalhousie University
Halifax, NS, Canada

S. Edet Ohia, PhD
Professor of Pharmaceutical Sciences
Associate Dean for Administration
School of Pharmacy and Allied Health
Professions
Creighton University
Omaha, NE

Kristine A. Quart, PharmD
Medical Education Consultant
Ôlivenhain, CA

Ruth Stanley, PharmD, FASHP
Consultant
Birmingham, AL

Joseph P. Zbilut, RN,C, DNSc, PhD, ANP
Professor
Adult Health Nursing
Rush University College of Nursing
Professor
Molecular Biophysics and Physiology
Rush Medical College
Chicago, IL

Patti Rager Zuzelo, RN,CS, MSN, EdD
Associate Professor
School of Nursing
La Salle University
Philadelphia, PA
Associate Director of Nursing for
Research
Albert Einstein Medical Center
Philadelphia, PA
Casual Pool Registered Nurse
Emergency Trauma Care
Abington Memorial Hospital
Abington, PA

Reviewers and Clinical Consultants

Reviewers

Peter J. Ambrose, PharmD
Associate Clinical Professor, Step III
Director
Los Angeles-Orange County Area
Clerkships
University of California, San Francisco
San Francisco, CA

Donna Barto, RN, MA, CCRN
Nurse Educator
Helene Fuld School of Nursing
Blackwood, NJ
Staff Nurse
Virtua Memorial Hospital
Mount Holly, NJ

Edward M. Bednarczyk, PharmD
Clinical Assistant Professor
Pharmacy Practice and Nuclear
Medicine
State University of New York at Buffalo
Buffalo, NY

Cristina E. Bello, PharmD
Assistant Professor of Pharmacy
Practice
College of Pharmacy
Nova Southeastern University
Fort Lauderdale, FL

Scott M. Bonnema, PharmD
Consultant Pharmacist
Emissary Pharmacy and Infusion
Casper, WY

Felesia R. Bowen, RN, MS, PNP,C
Clinical Nurse Specialist
Children's Hospital at Robert Wood
Johnson University Hospital
New Brunswick, NJ

Cynthia Burman, PharmD
Clinical Assistant Professor
School of Pharmacy
Temple University
Philadelphia, PA

Kimberly A. Couch, PharmD
Clinical Pharmacy Specialist, Infectious
Diseases
Department of Pharmacy
Christiana Care Health System
Newark, DE

Brenda S. Frymoyer, RN, MSN
Clinical Nurse Specialist
Berks Cardiologists, Inc.
Reading, PA

Kimberly A. Galt, PharmD, FASHP
Associate Professor of Pharmacy
Practice
Director
Drug Information Services
Co-Director
Center for Practice Improvement and
Outcomes Research
Creighton University
Omaha, NE

John Gatto, RPh.
Clinical Pharmacist
Eckerd Pharmacy
Owego, NY

Deborah L. Green, RN, MSN
Director
Medical Telemetry-CHF Program
Moses H. Cone Health System
Greensboro, NC

Ronald L. Greenberg, PharmD, BCPS
Clinical Pharmacy Coordinator
Fairview Ridges Hospital
Burnsville, MN

Jan K. Hastings, PharmD
Assistant Professor
College of Pharmacy
University of Arkansas for Medical
Science
Little Rock, AR

Michael D. Hogue, PharmD
Assistant Professor of Pharmacy
Practice
McWhorter School of Pharmacy
Samford University
Clinical Coordinator
Walgreen Drug Store
Birmingham, AL

Kimberly A. Hunter, PharmD
Assistant Professor of Pharmacy
Practice
Albany College of Pharmacy
Albany, NY

William A. Kehoe, Jr., PharmD, BCPS,
FCCP
Professor of Clinical Pharmacy and
Psychology
School of Pharmacy and Health
Sciences
University of the Pacific
Stockton, CA

Julienne K. Kirk, PharmD, BCPS, CDE
Assistant Professor
Department of Family Medicine
School of Medicine
Wake Forest University
Winston-Salem, NC

Peter G. Koval, PharmD, BCPS
Clinical Pharmacist
Moses H. Cone Family Practice
Greensboro, NC

Lisa M. Krupa, RN,C, CEN, FNP
Nurse Practitioner
Medical Specialists
Munster, IN

Amista A. Lone, PharmD
Clinical Assistant Professor
College of Pharmacy
University of Arizona
Tucson, AZ

Jennifer L. Lutz, PharmD
Pharmacy Resident
Samuel S. Stratton Veterans Affairs
Medical Center
Albany, NY

T. Donald Marsh, PharmD, FASCP,
FASHP
Director
Department of Pharmacotherapy
Mountain Area Health Education Center
Asheville, NC

Patrick McDonnell, PharmD
Assistant Professor of Clinical
Pharmacy
School of Pharmacy
Temple University
Philadelphia, PA

Kenyetta N. Nesbitt, PharmD
Assistant Professor
Wayne State University
Detroit, MI

Catherine M. Oliphant, PharmD
Assistant Professor of Pharmacy
Practice
School of Pharmacy
University of Wyoming
Laramie, WY

Michael A. Oszko, PharmD, BCPS
Associate Professor
Dept. of Pharmacy
University of Kansas
Kansas City, KS

Vinita B. Pai, PharmD
Assistant Professor of Pharmacy
Practice
College of Pharmacy
Idaho State University
Pocatello, ID

David J. Quan, PharmD
Clinical Pharmacist
University of California, San Francisco
San Francisco, CA

(continued)

Reviewers, *continued*

Susan M. Rao, RN, MSN
Staff Nurse
Intensive Care Unit
Saint Luke East
Fort Thomas, KY

Susan L. Ravnan, PharmD
Assistant Professor of Pharmacy
Practice
School of Pharmacy and Health
Sciences
University of the Pacific
Stockton, CA

Brenda M. Reap-Thompson, RN, MSN
Nurse Educator
Community College of Philadelphia
Philadelphia, PA
Nurse Consultant
Chauncey International, ETS
Princeton, NJ

Nancy Jex Sabin, RN, MSN, CFNP
Instructor
Hahn School of Nursing and Health
Science
Family Nurse Practitioner
Student Health Center
University of San Diego
San Diego, CA

Melissa L. Sanders, PharmD
Assistant Professor of Clinical
Pharmacy
School of Pharmacy
Temple University
Philadelphia, PA

Regina E. Silk, PharmD, RPh, BCPS
Assistant Clinical Professor
University of Connecticut Health Center
Farmington, CT

Elizabeth Sloand, RN, MSN, CPNP
Assistant Professor
School of Nursing
Johns Hopkins University
Baltimore, MD

Thomas F. Turco, PharmD
Clinical Pharmacist
Assistant Director of Pharmacy
Our Lady of Lourdes Medical Center
Camden, NJ

Lili Wang, PhD
Assistant Professor
School of Pharmacy
Memorial University of Newfoundland
St. Johns, NF, Canada

Craig Williams, PharmD
Clinical Specialist
Wishard Memorial Hospital
Assistant Professor of Clinical
Pharmacy
School of Pharmacy
Purdue University
Indianapolis, IN

Clinical Consultants

Madeline Albanese, RN, MSN
Nurse Educator
Hospital of the University of
Pennsylvania
Philadelphia, PA

Sheree M. Fitzgerald, RN,C, MSN, CNA
Program Coordinator
Ancora Psychiatric Hospital
Hammonton, NJ

Maryann Foley, RN, BSN
Independent Consultant
Flourtown, PA

Grace Hukushi, RN, BSN, LNC
Critical Care Nurse
Nursing Enterprises, Inc.
Brick, NJ

Sammie Justesen, RN, BSN
Independent Nurse Consultant
Providence, UT

Catherine T. Kelly, RN, PhD, CCRN, CEN, ANP
Faculty
School of Nursing
Mount Saint Mary College
Newburgh, NY

Sharon Kumm, RN, MN, CCRN
Assistant Professor
School of Nursing
University of Kansas
Kansas City, KS

Leanne McQuade, RN, BSN, CEN
Staff Nurse
Emergency Dept.
Doylestown Hospital
Case Manager
CAB Medical Consultant
Doylestown, PA

Pamela S. Ronning, RN, MPA
Program Coordinator
Kirkhof School of Nursing
Grand Valley State University
Allendale, MI

Maureen Ryan, RN,CS, MSN, FNP
Assistant Professor
Grand Valley State University
Allendale, MI
Nurse Practitioner
Emergency Dept.
St. Mary's Hospital
Grand Rapids, MI

Julie M. Smith, RN, BA
Staff Nurse
Radiology-Heart Station
Rancocas Hospital
Willingboro, NJ

Aaron J. Strehlow, RN,CS, FNP-C, NPNP
Administrator and Director of Clinical
Services
UCLA School of Nursing
Health Center at the Rescue Mission
Los Angeles, CA

Maria Wilson, RN, MSN, CCRN
Staff Nurse
Emergency Dept.
Chestnut Hill Hospital
Philadelphia, PA

Jones and Bartlett's 2010 Nurse's Drug Handbook gives you what today's nurses and nursing students need: accurate, concise, and reliable drug facts. This book emphasizes the vital information you need to know before, during, and after drug administration. The information is presented in easy-to-understand language and organized alphabetically, so you can find what you need quickly.

What's Special

In addition to the drug information you expect to find in each entry (see "Drug Entries" for details), the *2010 Nurse's Drug Handbook* boasts these special features:

•**Practical trim size** allows the book to open flat so you can find the information you need without wrestling with a book that wants to close. You can hold the book in one hand, see complete pages at a glance, and use your other hand to document or perform other activities.

•**Introductory material** reviews essential general information you need to know to administer drugs safely and effectively, including an overview of pharmacology and the principles of drug administration. In addition, the five steps of the nursing process are explained and related specifically to drug therapy.

•**Highly useful illustrations** throughout the text help you visualize selected mechanisms of action by showing how drugs work at the cellular, tissue, and organ levels. In addition, the inside front cover features a chart listing all the drugs whose mechanisms of action are illustrated as well as other drugs with the same mechanisms of action.

•**No-nonsense writing style** speaks everyday language and uses the terms and abbreviations you typically encounter in your practice and your studies. To avoid sexist language, we alternate between male and female pronouns throughout the book.

•**Up-to-date drug information** includes the latest FDA-approved drugs, new and changed indications, new warnings, and newly reported adverse reactions.

•**Dosage adjustment,** highlighted in color, alerts you to expected dosage changes for a patient with a specific condition or disorder, such as advanced age or renal impairment.

•**Warning,** highlighted in color, calls attention to important facts that you need to know before, during, and after drug administration. For example, in the alatrofloxacin entry, this feature informs you that the drug usually is reserved for hospitalized patients and is given for no more than 2 weeks because of the high risk of severe liver damage.

•**Easy-to-use tables** showing route, onset, peak, and duration (see page *xv* for more details) and other tables in the appendices provide a timesaving way to track and check information. The appendices give you an overview of the most important facts and nursing considerations for important drug groups, including insulin preparations, antihistamines, topical drugs, selected antivirals, antineoplastic drugs, interferons, and antihypertensive combination drugs. You'll also find such handy information as immunization schedules and instructions for calculating drug dosages and I.V. flow rates.

Drug Entries

2010 Nurse's Drug Handbook clearly and concisely presents all the vital facts on the drugs that you'll typically administer. To help you find the information you need quickly, drug entries are organized alphabetically by generic drug name—from abatacept to zonisamide. For ease of use, every drug entry follows a consistent format. However, if specific details are unknown or don't apply, the heading isn't included so you can go right to the next section.

GENERIC AND TRADE NAMES

First, each entry identifies the drug's main generic name as well as alternate generic names. (For drugs prescribed by trade name, you can quickly check the comprehensive index, which refers you to the appropriate generic name and page.)

Next, the entry lists the most common U.S. trade names for each drug. It also includes common trade names available only in Canada, marked (CAN).

CLASS, CATEGORY, AND SCHEDULE

Each entry lists the drug's chemical and therapeutic classes. With this information, you can compare drugs in the same chemical class but in different therapeutic classes and vice versa.

The entry also lists the FDA's pregnancy risk category, which categorizes drugs based on their potential to cause birth defects. (For details, see *FDA pregnancy risk categories*.)

Where appropriate, the entry also includes the drug's controlled substance schedule. (For details, see *Controlled substance schedules,* page *xvi*.)

INDICATIONS AND DOSAGES

This section lists FDA-approved therapeutic indications. For each indication, you'll find the applicable drug form or route, age-group (adults, adolescents, or children), and dosage (which includes amount per dose, timing, and duration, when known and appropriate).

ROUTE, ONSET, PEAK, AND DURATION

Quick-reference tables show the drug's onset, peak, and duration (when known) for each administration route. The *onset of action* is the time a drug takes to be absorbed, reach a therapeutic blood level, and elicit an initial therapeutic response. The *peak therapeutic effect* occurs when a drug reaches its highest blood concentration and the greatest amount of drug reaches the site of action to produce the

FDA pregnancy risk categories

Each drug may be placed in a pregnancy risk category based on the FDA's estimate of risk to the fetus. If the FDA hasn't provided a category, the *Drug Handbook* notes that the drug is "Not rated." The categories range from A to X, signifying least to greatest fetal risk.

A Controlled studies show no risk

Adequate, well-controlled studies with pregnant women have failed to demonstrate a risk to the fetus in any trimester of pregnancy.

B No evidence of risk in humans

Adequate, well-controlled studies with pregnant women haven't shown increased risk of fetal abnormalities despite adverse findings in animals, or, in the absence of adequate human studies, animal studies show no fetal risk. The chance of fetal harm is remote, but remains possible.

C Risk can't be ruled out

Adequate, well-controlled human studies are lacking, and animal studies have demonstrated a risk to the fetus or are lacking as well. A chance of fetal harm exists if the drug is administered during pregnancy, but the potential benefits may outweigh the potential risk.

D Positive evidence of risk

Studies in humans, or investigational or post-marketing data, have demonstrated fetal risk. Nevertheless, potential benefits from the drug's use may outweigh potential risks. For example, the drug may be acceptable if needed in a life-threatening situation or serious disease for which safer drugs can't be used or are ineffective.

X Contraindicated in pregnancy

Studies in animals or humans, or investigational or post-marketing reports, have demonstrated positive evidence of fetal abnormalities or risks that clearly outweigh any possible benefit to the patient.

maximum therapeutic response. The *duration of action* is the amount of time the drug remains at a blood level that produces a therapeutic response.

MECHANISM OF ACTION

Set off by a box, this section concisely describes how a drug achieves its therapeutic effects at cellular, tissue, organ levels, as appropriate. Illustrations of selected mechanisms of action lend exceptional clarity to sometimes complex processes.

INCOMPATIBILITIES

You'll be alerted to drugs or solutions that are incompatible with the topic drug when mixed in a syringe or solution or infused through the same I.V. line.

CONTRAINDICATIONS

An alphabetical list details the conditions and disorders that preclude administration of the topic drug.

INTERACTIONS

This section presents the drugs, foods, and activities (such as alcohol use and smoking) that can cause important, problematic, or life-threatening interactions with the topic drug. For each interacting drug, food, or activity, you'll learn the effects of the interaction.

ADVERSE REACTIONS

Organized by body system, this section highlights common, serious, and life-threatening adverse reactions in alphabetical order.

NURSING CONSIDERATIONS

Warnings, general precautions, and key information that you must know before, during, and after drug administration are detailed in this section. Examples include whether a pill can be crushed and how to properly reconstitute, dilute, store, handle, or dispose of a drug.

Patient teaching information is also included here. You'll find important guidelines for patients, such as how and when to take each prescribed drug, how to spot and manage adverse reactions, which cautions to observe, when to call the prescriber, and more. To save you time, however, this section doesn't repeat basic patient-teaching points. (For a summary of those, see *Teaching your patient about*

Teaching your patient about drug therapy

Your teaching about drug therapy will vary with your patient's needs and your practice setting. To help guide your teaching, each drug entry provides key information that you must teach your patient about that drug. For all patients, however, you also should:

✓ Teach the generic and trade name for each prescribed drug that he'll take after discharge—even if he took the drug before admission.

✓ Clearly explain why each drug was prescribed, how it works, and what it's supposed to do.
To help your patient understand the drug's therapeutic effects, relate its action to her disorder or condition.

✓ Review the drug form, dosage, and route with the patient. Tell him whether the drug is a tablet, suppository, spray, aerosol, or other form, and explain how to administer it correctly. Also, tell him how often to take the drug and for what length of time. Emphasize that he should take the drug exactly as prescribed.

✓ Describe the drug's appearance and explain that scored tablets can be broken in half for safe, accurate dosing. Warn the patient not to break unscored tablets because doing so may alter the drug dosage. If your patient has difficulty swallowing capsules, explain that she can open ones that contain sprinkles and take them with food or a drink but that she shouldn't do this with capsules that contain powder. Also, warn her not to crush or chew enteric-coated, extended-release, sustained-release, or similar drug forms.

✓ Teach the patient about common adverse reactions that may occur. Advise him to notify the prescriber at once if a dangerous adverse reaction, such as syncope, occurs.

✓ Warn her not to suddenly stop taking a drug if she's bothered by unpleasant adverse reactions, such as a rash and mild itching. Instead, encourage her to discuss the reactions with her prescriber, who may adjust the dosage or substitute a drug that causes fewer adverse reactions.

✓ Because many drugs cause some adverse reactions, such as dizziness and drowsiness, that can impair the patient's ability to perform activities that require alertness, help him develop a dosing schedule that prevents adverse reactions from interfering with such activities.

✓ Inform the patient which adverse reactions resolve with time.

✓ Teach the patient how to store the drug properly. Let him know if the drug is sensitive to light or temperature and how to protect it from these elements.

✓ Instruct the patient to store the drug in its original container, if possible, with the drug's name and dosage clearly printed on the label.

✓ Inform the patient which devices to use—and which ones to avoid—for drug storage or administration. For example, warn him not to take liquid cyclosporine with a plastic cup or utensils.

✓ Teach the patient what to do if she misses a dose. Generally, she should take a once-daily drug as soon as she remembers—provided that she remembers within the first 24 hours. If 24 hours have elapsed, she should take the next scheduled dose, but not double the dose. If she has questions or concerns about missed doses, tell her to contact the prescriber.

✓ Provide information that's specific to the prescribed drug. For example, if a patient takes a diuretic to manage heart failure, instruct him to weigh himself daily at the same time of day, using the same scale and wearing the same amount of clothing. Or if the patient takes digoxin or an antihypertensive drug, teach him how to measure his pulse and blood pressure and how to record the measurements. Then instruct him to bring the diary to his regular appointments so that the prescriber can monitor his response to the drug.

✓ Advise the patient to refill prescriptions promptly, unless she no longer needs the drug. Also instruct her to discard expired drugs because they may become ineffective or even dangerous over time.

✓ Warn the patient to keep all drugs out of the reach of children at all times.

drug therapy, page *xvii*, and *Federal guidelines for drug disposal*.)

In short, *Jones and Bartlett's 2010 Nurse's Drug Handbook* is designed expressly to give you more of what you need. It puts vital drug information at your fingertips and helps you stay ALWAYS CURRENT in this critical part of your practice or studies.

Federal guidelines for drug disposal

Give patients these important instructions for properly disposing of their unwanted prescription drugs:

✓ Take unused, unneeded, or outdated prescription drugs out of their original containers and throw them in the trash.

✓ Consider mixing discarded prescription drugs with a substance like coffee grounds or used cat litter and putting them in impermeable, nondescript containers, such as empty cans or sealable bags.

✓ Flush prescription drugs down the toilet only if the label or accompanying patient information specifically tells you to do so.

✓ See if your community has a pharmaceutical take-back program that allows citizens to bring unused drugs to a central location for proper disposal.

Safe, effective drug therapy is one of your most important responsibilities. Not infrequently, a patient's life will depend on your ability to give drugs accurately and safely. In addition, you must keep up with the latest drug information, including newly approved drugs and recently reported life-threatening adverse reactions, as well as those drugs withdrawn from the market after widespread use.

Despite all the drug information available, medication errors remain one of the greatest threats to patients' well-being and a leading cause of lawsuits against nurses, physicians, and hospitals.

Your Responsibilities in Drug Therapy

Your basic responsibilities in drug therapy include:

•administering the right drug in the right dose by the right route at the right time to the right patient

•knowing the therapeutic use, dosage, interactions, adverse reactions, and warnings of each administered drug

•being aware of newly approved drugs that may be prescribed

•knowing about changes to existing drugs, such as new indications and dosages and recently discovered adverse reactions and interactions

•concentrating fully when preparing and administering drugs

•responding promptly and appropriately to serious or life-threatening adverse reactions, interactions, and complications

•instructing each patient about the drug, how it's administered, which effects it causes or may cause, and which reactions to watch for and report.

Several factors may reduce your ability to meet these basic responsibilities—and contribute to medication errors. First, hospitals and other health care facilities have budget restraints that may result in the elimination of professional nursing posi-tions or the hiring of less qualified technicians to fill them. This forces the remaining nurses to care for more patients. Second, hospital patients are older and more acutely ill, and they typically receive more complex drug therapy than ever. Together, these factors place greater demands on you—increasing your stress level, reducing the time you have to concentrate on drug administration, and increasing your risk of making medication errors or overlooking serious adverse reactions or interactions.

The same factors reduce your time and energy for learning the latest drug facts—which you need to have at your command. You must have this information at your fingertips because your next patient may need a recently approved drug or a complex and unfamiliar drug regimen.

How can you balance your limited time, on the one hand, with your need to know the latest developments, on the other?

Meeting Your Needs

Nurses and students need a reliable, accurate, easy-to-use, quick-reference drug book. They need a book clearly written by and for nurses that has been reviewed by experts in nursing and pharmacology. You hold such a book in your hands: *Jones and Bartlett's 2010 Nurse's Drug Handbook*, with its ALWAYS CURRENT features.

The content of *2010 Nurse's Drug Handbook* was developed, written, and edited by experienced practicing nurses. Expert consultants, reviewers, and advisors—both nurses and pharmacists—help ensure the accuracy and reliability of the information covered in each entry and help target that information to your needs. What's more, every drug fact is checked against the most prominent drug references today, including the *American Hospital Formulary Service Drug Information, Drug Facts and Comparisons, The Physicians' Desk Reference,* the FDA's website of new drug approvals, and the USP DI's *Drug Information for the Health Care Professional.*

In addition, to help you quickly access much-needed information, the book is organized alphabetically by generic drug name, follows a consistent format, and is concise.

To ensure that you're always current, *Jones and Bartlett's Nurse's Drug Handbook* is updated every year. This newest edition contains:
•important new drug entries in the main part of the book and in the appendices
•new drug facts on hundreds of existing entries, including updated information on new indications and dosages, new incompatibilities and interactions, new adverse reactions, and new nursing considerations
•hundreds of patient-teaching guidelines and suggestions
•thoroughly updated appendices on insulin preparations, antiviral drugs, topical drugs, antihistamines, combination antihypertensive drugs, immunization schedules, interferons, ophthalmic drugs, and antineoplastic drugs
•a comprehensive new index.

And as always, you'll find the same color-coded, highly readable type that reduces eyestrain as you speed to the information you need.

Getting More from Your Drug Reference
Whether you work in or are preparing to work in acute care, home care, long-term care, or another health care setting, you'll want your own copy of *2010 Nurse's Drug Handbook.* That's because this book can help you:
•reduce your risk of medication errors because you'll have easy access to accurate, reliable drug information that's relevant to your practice
•stay current on the most up-to-date drug developments of the year

•improve your drug administration skills and patient care before, during, and after drug therapy
•quickly detect and manage serious or life-threatening adverse reactions and complications or prevent them from occurring
•save time because you won't have to sift through volumes of information to find what you need, search for a book that's up-to-date, or look through several drug handbooks to get enough information
•increase your confidence about drug administration and enhance your professional interactions with other health care team members
•ensure the delivery of safe, effective care
•improve the depth and quality of your patient teaching.

Reaping the Rewards
Your patients deserve the best and safest care possible—and you deserve to have the tools to deliver that care. Whether you're a student or an experienced clinician, *Jones and Bartlett's 2010 Nurse's Drug Handbook* will help you provide safe, effective drug therapy because of its practical, easy-to-understand, accurate, and reliable information on virtually all the drugs you're likely to administer.

This handbook has aided thousands of nurses in their patient care. Take it with you to the clinical setting, share it with your peers, and use it to enhance your present and future position in the nursing profession.

Kathleen Dracup, RN, FNP, DNSc, FAAN
Dean and Professor
School of Nursing
University of California, San Francisco
San Francisco, CA

Understanding the basics of pharmacology is an essential nursing responsibility. Pharmacology is the science that deals with the physical and chemical properties, and biochemical and physiologic effects, of drugs. It includes the areas of pharmacokinetics, pharmacodynamics, pharmacotherapeutics, pharmacognosy, and toxicodynamics.

The *2010 Nurse's Drug Handbook* deals primarily with pharmacokinetics, pharmacodynamics, and pharmacotherapeutics—the information you need to administer safe and effective drug therapy (discussed below). *Pharmacognosy* is the branch of pharmacology that deals with the biological, biochemical, and economic features of naturally occurring drugs. *Toxicodynamics* is the study of the harmful effects that excessive amounts of a drug produce in the body; in a drug overdose or drug poisoning, large drug doses may saturate or overwhelm normal mechanisms that control absorption, distribution, metabolism, and excretion.

Drug Nomenclature
Most drugs are known by several names—chemical, generic, trade, and official—each of which serves a specific function. (See *How drugs are named.*) However, multiple drug names can also contribute to medication errors. You may find a familiar drug packaged with an unfamiliar name if your institution changes suppliers or if a familiar drug is newly approved in a different dose or for a new indication.

Drug Classification
Drugs can be classified in various ways. Most pharmacology textbooks group drugs by their functional classification, such as psychotherapeutics, which is based on common characteristics. Drugs can also be classified according to their therapeutic use, such as antipanic or antiobsessional drugs. Drugs within a certain therapeutic class may be further divided into subgroups based on their mechanisms of action. For example, the therapeutic class antineoplastics can be further classified as alkylating agents, antibiotic antineoplastics, antimetabolites, antimitotics, biological response modifiers, antineoplastic enzymes, and hormonal antineoplastics.

How drugs are named

A drug's chemical, generic, trade, and official names are developed at different phases of the drug development process and serve different functions. For example, the various names of the commonly prescribed anticonvulsant divalproex sodium are:
- Chemical name: Pentanoic acid, 2-propyl-, sodium salt (2:1) or ($C_{16}H_{31}O_4Na$)
- Generic name: divalproex sodium
- Trade name: Depakote
- Official name: Divalproex Sodium Delayed-Release Tablets, USP

A drug's *chemical name* describes its atomic and molecular structure. The chemical name of divalproex sodium—pentanoic acid, 2-propyl-, sodium salt (2:1), or $C_{16}H_{31}O_4Na$ (pronounced valproate semisodium)—indicates that the drug is a combination of two valproic acid compounds with a sodium molecule attached to only one side.

Once a drug successfully completes several clinical trials, it receives a *generic name,* also known as the nonproprietary name. The generic name is usually derived from but shorter than the chemical name. The United States Adopted Names Council is responsible for selecting generic names, which are intended for unrestricted public use.

Before submitting the drug for FDA approval, the manufacturer creates and registers a *trade name* (or brand name) when the drug appears ready to be marketed. Trade names are copyrighted and followed by the symbol ® to indicate that they're registered and that their use is restricted to the drug manufacturer. Once the original patent on a drug has expired, any manufacturer may produce the drug and market it with its own trade name.

A drug's *official name* is the name under which it's listed in the United States Pharmacopoeia (USP) and the National Formulary (NF).

Pharmacokinetics

Pharmacokinetics is the study of a drug's actions—or fate—as it passes through the body during absorption, distribution, metabolism, and excretion.

ABSORPTION

Before a drug can begin working, it must be transformed from its pharmaceutical dosage form to a biologically available (bioavailable) substance that can pass through various biological cell membranes to reach its site of action. This process is known as absorption. A drug's absorption rate depends on its route of administration, its circulation through the tissue into which it's administered, and its solubility—that is, whether it's more water-soluble (*hydrophilic*) or fat-soluble (*lipophilic*).

Although drugs may penetrate cellular membranes either actively or passively, most drugs do so by *passive diffusion*, moving inertly from an area of higher concentration to an area of lower concentration. Passive diffusion may occur through water or fat. Passive diffusion through water—*aqueous diffusion*—occurs within large water-filled compartments, such as interstitial spaces, and across epithelial membrane tight junctions and pores in the epithelial lining of blood vessels. Aqueous diffusion is driven by concentration gradients. Drug molecules that are bound to large plasma proteins, such as albumin, are too large to pass through aqueous pores in this way. Passive diffusion through fat—*lipid diffusion*—plays an important role in drug metabolism because of the large number of lipid barriers that separate the aqueous compartments of the body. The tendency of a drug to move through lipid layers between aqueous compartments often depends on the pH of the medium—that is, the ability of the water-soluble or fat-soluble drug to form weak acid or weak base.

Drugs with molecules that are too large to readily diffuse may rely on *active diffusion,* in which special carriers on molecules, including peptides, amino acids, and glucose, transport the drug through the membranes. However, some molecules with selective membrane carriers can expel foreign drug molecules; this is why many drugs can't cross the blood-brain barrier.

Drug absorption begins at the administration route. The three main administration route categories are enteral, parenteral, and transcutaneous. Depending on its nature or chemical makeup, a drug may be better absorbed from one site than from another.

Enteral Administration

Enteral administration consists of the oral, nasogastric, and rectal routes.

Oral: Drugs administered orally are absorbed in the GI tract and then proceed by the hepatic portal vein to the liver and into the systemic circulation. Although generally considered the preferred route, oral drug administration has a number of disadvantages:

• The oral route doesn't always yield sufficiently high blood concentrations to be effective.

• Bioavailability may be less than optimal because of incomplete absorption and first-pass elimination (the part of metabolism that occurs during transit through the liver before the drug reaches the general circulation).

• Drug absorption may be incomplete if the drug is degraded by digestive enzymes or the acidic pH in the stomach or if it's excreted from the liver into the bile.

• Food in the GI tract, gastric emptying time, and intestinal motility may also impede drug absorption.

Nasogastric: Drugs administered through a nasogastric tube enter the stomach directly and are absorbed in the GI tract.

Rectal: Rectal drugs and suppositories also enter the GI tract directly after being inserted in the rectum and absorbed through the rectal mucosa. After being absorbed into the lower GI tract, rectal drugs enter the circulation through the inferior vena cava, bypassing the liver and thus avoiding first-pass metabolism. Suppositories, however, tend to travel upward into the rectum, where veins, such as the superior hemorrhoidal vein, lead to the liver. As a result, drug absorption by this route is often unreliable and difficult to predict.

Parenteral Administration

Parenteral routes may be used whenever enteral routes are contraindicated or inadequate. These routes include intramuscular (I.M.), intravenous (I.V.), subcutaneous (SubQ) and intradermal (I.D.) administration. Drug absorption is much faster and more predictable after parenteral administration than after enteral administration.

I.M.: Drugs administered by the I.M. route are injected deep into the muscle, where they're absorbed relatively quickly. The rate of drug absorption depends on the vascularity of the injection site, the physiochemical properties of the drug, and the solution in which the drug is contained.

I.V.: I.V. drug administration involves injecting or infusing the drug directly into the blood circulation, allowing for rapid distribution throughout the body. This route usually provides the greatest bioavailability.

SubQ: Drugs administered by the subcutaneous route are injected into the alveolar connective tissue just below the skin and are absorbed by simple diffusion from the injection site. The factors that affect I.M. absorption also affect subcutaneous absorption. Absorption by the subcutaneous route may be slower than

by the I.M. route.

I.D.: Drugs administered intradermally, such as purified protein derivative (PPD), are injected into the dermis, from which they diffuse slowly into the local microcapillary system.

Transcutaneous Administration

Transcutaneous drug administration allows drug absorption through the skin or soft-tissue surface. Drugs may be inhaled, inserted sublingually, applied topically, or administered by the eyes, ears, nose, or vagina.

Inhalation: Inhaled drugs may be given as a powder and aerosolized or mixed in solution and nebulized directly into the respiratory tract, where they're absorbed through the alveoli. Inhaled drugs are usually absorbed quickly because of the abundant blood flow in the lungs.

Sublingual: Sublingual drug administration involves placing a tablet, troche, or lozenge under the tongue. The drug is absorbed across the epithelial lining of the mouth, usually quickly. This route avoids first-pass metabolism.

Topical: Topical drugs—creams, ointments, lotions, and patches—are placed on the skin and then cross the epidermis into the capillary circulation. They may also be absorbed through sweat glands, hair follicles, and other skin structures. Absorption by the skin is enhanced if the drug is in a solution.

Ophthalmic: Ophthalmic drugs include solutions and ointments that are instilled or applied directly to the cornea or conjunctiva as well as small, elliptical disks that are placed directly on the eyeball behind the lower eyelid. The movements of the eyeball promote distribution of these drugs over the surface of the eye. Although ophthalmic drugs produce a local effect on the conjunctiva or anterior chamber, some preparations may be absorbed systemically and therefore produce systemic effects.

Otic: Drops administered into the external auditory canal, otic drugs are used to treat infection or inflammation and to soften and remove ear wax. Otic solutions exert a local effect and may result in minimal systemic absorption with no adverse effects.

Nasal: Nasal solutions and suspensions are applied directly to the nasal mucosa by instillation or inhalation to produce local effects, such as vasoconstriction to reduce nasal congestion. Some nasal solutions, such as vasopressin, are administered by this route specifically to produce systemic effects.

Vaginal: Vaginal drugs include creams, suppositories, and troches that are inserted into the vagina, sometimes using a special applicator. These drugs are absorbed locally to treat such conditions as bacterial and fungal infections.

DISTRIBUTION

Distribution is the process by which a drug is transported by the circulating fluids to various sites, including its sites of action. To ensure maximum therapeutic effectiveness, the drug must permeate all membranes that separate it from its intended site of action. Drug distribution is influenced by blood flow, tissue availability, and protein binding.

METABOLISM

Drug metabolism is the enzymatic conversion of a drug's structure into substrate molecules or polar compounds that are either less active or inactive and are readily excreted. Drugs can also be synthesized to larger molecules. Metabolism may also convert a drug to a more toxic compound. Because the primary site of drug metabolism is the liver, children, the elderly, and patients with impaired hepatic function are at risk for altered therapeutic effects.

Biotransformation is the process of changing a drug into its active metabolite. Compounds that require metabolic biotransformation for activation are known as *prodrugs*. During phase I of biotransformation, the parent drug is converted into an inactive or partially active metabolite. Much of the original drug may be eliminated during this phase. During phase II, the inactive or partially active metabolite binds with available substrates, such as acetic acid, glucuronic acid, sulfuric acid, or water, to form its active metabolite. When biotransformation leads to synthesis, larger molecules are produced to create a pharmacologic effect.

EXCRETION

The body eliminates drugs by both metabolism and excretion. Drug metabolites—and, in some cases, the active drug itself—are eventually excreted from the body, usually through bile, feces, and urine. The primary organ for drug elimination is the kidney. Impaired renal function may alter drug elimination, thereby altering the drug's therapeutic effect. Other excretion routes include evaporation through the skin, exhalation from the lungs, and secretion into saliva and breast milk.

A drug's elimination *half-life* is the amount of time required for half of the drug to be eliminated from the body. The half-life roughly correlates with the drug's duration of action and is based on normal renal and hepatic function. Typically, the longer the half-life, the less often the drug has to be given and the longer it remains in the body.

Pharmacodynamics

Pharmacodynamics is the study of the biochemical and physiologic effects of drugs and their mechanisms of action. A drug's actions may be structurally specific or nonspecific. Structurally specific drugs combine with cell receptors, such as proteins or glycoproteins, to enhance or inhibit cellular enzyme actions. Drug receptors are the cellular components affected at the site of action. Many drugs form chemical bonds with drug receptors, but a drug can bond with a receptor only if it has a similar shape—much the same way that a key fits into a lock. When a drug combines with a receptor, channels are either opened or closed and cellular biochemical messengers, such as cyclic adenosine monophosphate or calcium ions, are activated. Once activated, cellular functions can be turned either on or off by these messengers.

Structurally nonspecific drugs, such as biological response modifiers, don't combine with cell receptors; rather, they produce changes within the cell membrane or interior.

The mechanisms by which drugs interact with the body are not always known. Drugs may work by physical action (such as the protective effects of a topical ointment) or chemical reaction (such as an antacid's effect on the gastric mucosa), or by modifying the metabolic activity of invading pathogens (such as an antibiotic) or replacing a missing biochemical substance (such as insulin).

AGONISTS

Agonists are drugs that interact with a receptor to stimulate a response. They alter cell physiology by binding to plasma membranes or intracellular structures. *Partial agonists* can't achieve maximal effects even though they may occupy all available receptor sites on a cell. *Strong agonists* can cause maximal effects while occupying only a small number of receptor sites on a cell. *Weak agonists* must occupy many more receptor sites than strong agonists to produce the same effect.

ANTAGONISTS

Antagonists are drugs that attach to a receptor but don't stimulate a response; instead, they inhibit or block responses that would normally be caused by agonists. *Competitive antagonists* bind to receptor sites that are also compatible with an agonist, thus preventing the agonist from binding to the site. *Noncompetitive antagonists* bind to receptor sites that aren't occupied by an agonist; this changes the receptor site so that it's no longer recognized by the agonist. *Irreversible antagonists* work in much the same way that noncompetitive ones do, except that they permanently bind with the receptor.

Antagonism plays an important role in drug interactions. When two agonists that cause opposite therapeutic effects, such as a vasodilator and a vasoconstrictor, are combined, the effects cancel each other out. When two antagonists, such as morphine and naloxone, are combined, both drugs may become inactive.

Pharmacotherapeutics

Pharmacotherapeutics is the study of how drugs are used to prevent or treat disease. Understanding why a drug is prescribed for a certain disease can assist you in prioritizing drug administration with other patient care activities. Knowing a drug's desired and unwanted effects may help you uncover problems not readily apparent from the admitting diagnosis. This information may also help you prevent such problems as adverse reactions and drug interactions.

A drug's *desired effect* is the intended or expected clinical response to the drug. This is the response you start to evaluate as soon as a drug is given. Dosage adjustments and the continuation of therapy often depend on your accurate evaluation and documentation of the patient's response.

An *adverse reaction* is any noxious and unintended response to a drug that occurs at therapeutic doses used for prophylaxis, diagnosis, or therapy. Adverse reactions associated with excessive amounts of a drug are considered drug overdoses. Be prepared to follow your institution's policy for reporting adverse drug reactions.

An *idiosyncratic response* is a genetically determined abnormal or excessive response to a drug that occurs in a particular patient. The unusual response may indicate that the drug has saturated or overwhelmed mechanisms that normally control absorption, distribution, metabolism, or excretion, thus altering the expected response. You may be unsure whether a reaction is adverse or idiosyncratic. Once you report the reaction, the pharmacist usually determines the appropriate course of action.

An *allergic reaction* is an adverse response that results from previous exposure to the same drug or to one that's chemically similar to it. The patient's immune system reacts to the drug as if it were a foreign invader and may produce a mild hypersensitivity reaction, characterized by localized dermatitis, urticaria, angioedema, or photosensitivity. Allergic reactions should be reported to the prescriber immediately and the drug should be discontinued. Follow-up care may include giving drugs, including antihistamines and corticosteroids, to counteract the allergic response.

An *anaphylactic reaction* involves an immediate hypersensitivity response characterized by urticaria, pruritus, and angioedema. Left untreated, an anaphylactic reaction can lead to systemic involvement, resulting in shock. It's often associated with life-threatening hypotension and respiratory distress. Be prepared to assist with emergency life support measures, especially if the reaction occurs in response to I.V. drugs, which have the fastest rate of absorption.

A *drug interaction* occurs when one drug alters the pharmacokinetics of another drug—for example, when two or more drugs are given concurrently. Such concurrent administration can increase or decrease the therapeutic or adverse effects of either drug. Some drug interactions are beneficial. For example, when taken with penicillin, probenecid decreases the excretion rate of penicillin, resulting in higher blood levels of penicillin. Drug interactions also may occur when a drug's metabolism is altered, often owing to the induction of or competition for metabolizing enzymes. For example, H_2-receptor agonists, which reduce secretion of the enzyme gastrin, may alter the breakdown of enteric coatings on other drugs. Drug interactions due to carrier protein competition typically occur when a drug inhibits the kidneys' ability to reduce excretion of other drugs. For example, probenecid is completely reabsorbed by the renal tubules and is metabolized very slowly. It competes with the same carrier protein as sulfonamides for active tubular secretion and so decreases the renal excretion of sulfonamides. This particular competition can lead to an increased risk of sulfonamide toxicity.

Special Considerations

Although every drug has a usual dosage range, certain factors—such as a patient's age, weight, culture and ethnicity, gender, pregnancy status, and renal and hepatic function—may contribute to the need for dosage adjustments. When you encounter special considerations such as these, be prepared to reassess the prescribed dosage to make sure that it's safe and effective for your patient.

CULTURE AND ETHNICITY

Certain drugs are more effective or more likely to produce adverse effects in particular ethnic groups or races. For example, blacks with hypertension respond better to thiazide diuretics than do patients of other races; on the other hand, blacks also have an increased risk of developing angioedema with angiotensin-converting enzyme (ACE) inhibitors. A patient's religious or cultural background also may call for special consideration. For example, a drug made from porcine products may be unacceptable to a Jewish or Muslim patient.

ELDERLY PATIENTS

Because aging produces certain changes in body composition and organ function, elderly patients present unique therapeutic and dosing problems that require special attention. For example, the weight of the liver, the number of functioning hepatic cells, and hepatic blood flow all decrease as a person ages, resulting in slower drug metabolism. Renal function may also decrease with aging. These processes can lead to the accumulation of active drugs and metabolites as well as increased sensitivity to the effects of some drugs in elderly patients. Because they're also more likely to have multiple chronic illnesses, many elderly patients take multiple prescription drugs each day, thus increasing the risk of drug interactions.

CHILDREN

Because their bodily functions aren't fully developed, children—particularly those under age 12—may metabolize drugs differently than adults. In infants, immature renal and hepatic function delay metabolism and excretion of drugs. As a result, pediatric drug dosages are very different from adult dosages.

The FDA has provided drug manufacturers with guidelines that define pediatric age categories. Unless the manufacturer provides a specific age range, use these categories as a guide when administering drugs:
• neonates—birth up to age 1 month

• infants—ages 1 month to 2 years
• children—ages 2 to 12
• adolescents—ages 12 to 16.

PREGNANCY

The many physiologic changes that take place in the body during pregnancy may affect a drug's pharmacokinetics and alter its effectiveness. Additionally, exposure to drugs may pose risks for the developing fetus. Before administering a drug to a pregnant patient, be sure to check its assigned FDA pregnancy risk category and intervene appropriately.

Because there are thousands of drugs and hundreds of facts about each one, taking responsibility for drug administration can seem overwhelming. One way that you can enhance your understanding of the principles of drug administration is to *associate, ask,* and *predict* during the critical thinking process. For example, *associate* each drug with general information you may already know about the drug or drug class. *Ask* yourself why a drug is administered by a certain route and why it's given multiple times throughout the day rather than only once. Learn to *predict* a drug's actions, uses, adverse effects, and possible drug interactions based on your knowledge of the drug's mechanism of action. As you apply these principles to drug administration, you'll begin to intuitively know which facts you need to make rational clinical decisions.

Prescriptions for patients in hospitals and other institutions typically are written by a physician on a form called the *physician's order sheet* or they're directly input into a computerized system with an electronic signature. Drugs are prescribed based not only on their specific mechanisms of action but also on the patient's profile, which commonly includes age, ethnicity, gender, pregnancy status, smoking and drinking habits, and use of other drugs.

"Rights" of Drug Administration

Always keep in mind the following "rights" of drug administration: the right drug, right time, right dose, right patient, right route, and right preparation and administration.

RIGHT DRUG

Many drugs have similar spellings, different concentrations, and several generic forms. Before administering any drug, compare the exact spelling and concentration of the prescribed drug that ap-

pears on the label with the information contained in the medication administration record or drug profile. Regardless of which drug distribution system your facility uses, you should read the drug label and compare it to the medication administration record at least three times:

- before removing the drug from the dispensing unit or unit dose cart
- before preparing or measuring the prescribed dose
- before opening a unit dose package (just before administering the drug to the patient).

RIGHT TIME

Various factors can affect the time that a drug is administered, such as the timing of meals and other drugs, scheduled diagnostic tests, standardized times used by the institution, and factors that may alter the consistency of blood levels and drug absorption. Before administering any p.r.n. drug, check the patient's chart to ensure that no one else has already administered it and that the specified time interval has passed. Also, document administration of a p.r.n. drug immediately.

RIGHT DOSE

Whenever you're dispensing an unfamiliar drug or in doubt about a dosage, check the prescribed dose against the range specified in a reliable reference. Be sure to consider any reasons for a dosage adjustment that may apply to your particular patient. Also, make sure you're familiar with the standard abbreviations your institution uses for writing prescriptions.

RIGHT PATIENT

Always compare the name of the patient on the medication record with the name on the patient's identification bracelet. When using a unit dose system, compare the name on the drug profile with that on the identification bracelet.

RIGHT ROUTE

Each prescribed drug should specify the administration route. If the administration route is missing, consult the prescribing physician. Never substitute one route for another unless you obtain a prescription for the change.

RIGHT PREPARATION AND ADMINISTRATION

For drugs that need to be mixed, poured, or measured, be sure to maintain aseptic technique. Follow any specific directions included by the manufacturer regarding diluent type and amount and the use of filters, if needed. Clearly label any drug that you've reconstituted with the patient's name, the strength or dose, the date and time that you prepared the drug, the amount and type of diluent that you used, the expiration date, and your initials.

Administration Routes

Drugs may be administered by a variety of routes and dosage forms. A particular route may be chosen for convenience or to maximize drug concentration at the site of action, to minimize drug absorption elsewhere, to prolong drug absorption, or to avoid first-pass metabolism. Different dosage forms of the same drug may have different drug absorption rates, times of onset, and durations of action. For example, nitroglycerin is a coronary vasodilator that may be administered by the I.V., sublingual, oral, or buccal route, or as a topical ointment or disk. The I.V., sublingual, and buccal forms of nitroglycerin provide a rapid onset of action, whereas the oral, ointment, and disk forms have a slower onset and a prolonged duration of action.

Drug administration routes include the enteral, parenteral, and transcutaneous routes.

ENTERAL

The enteral route consists of oral, nasogastric, and rectal administration. Drugs administered enterally enter the blood circulation by way of the GI tract. This route is considered the most natural and convenient route as well as the safest. As a result, most drugs are taken enterally, usually to provide systemic effects.

Oral

• *Tablets:* Tablets, the most commonly used dosage form, come in a variety of colors, sizes, and shapes. Some tablets are specially coated for various purposes. Enteric coatings permit safe passage of a tablet through the stomach, where some drugs may be degraded or may produce unwanted effects, to the environment of the intestine. Some coatings protect the drug from the destructive influences of moisture, light, or air during storage; some coatings actually contain the drug, such as procainamide; still others conceal a bad taste. Coatings are also used to ensure appropriate drug release and absorption. Some tablets shouldn't be crushed or broken because doing so may alter drug release.

• *Capsules:* Capsules are solid dosage forms in which the drug and other ingredients are enclosed in a hard or soft shell of varying size and shape. Drugs typically are released faster from capsules than from tablets.

• *Solutions:* Drugs administered in solution are absorbed more rapidly than those administered in solid form; however, they don't always produce predictable drug levels in the blood. Some drugs in solution should be administered with meals or snacks to minimize their irritating effect on the gastric mucosa.

• *Suspensions:* Suspensions are preparations consisting of finely divided drugs in a suitable vehicle, usually water. Suspensions should be shaken before administration to ensure the uniformity of the preparation and administration of the proper dosage.

Nasogastric

Drugs administered through a nasogastric or gastrostomy tube enter the stomach directly, bypassing the mouth and esophagus. They're usually administered in liquid form because an intact tablet or capsule could cause an obstruction in a gastric tube. Sometimes a tablet may be crushed or a capsule opened for nasograstic administration; however, doing so will affect the drug's release. You may need to consult a pharmacist to determine which tablets can be crushed or capsules opened.

Rectal

Some enteral drugs are administered rectally—as suppositories, solutions, or ointments—to provide either local or systemic effects. When inserted into the rectum, suppositories soften, melt, or dissolve, releasing the drug contained inside them. The rectal route may be preferred for drugs that are destroyed or inactivated by the gastric or intestinal environment or that irritate the stomach. It also may be indicated when the oral route is contraindicated because of vomiting or difficulty swallowing. The drawbacks of rectal administration include inconvenience, noncompliance, and incomplete or irregular drug absorption.

PARENTERAL

In parenteral drug administration, a drug enters the circulatory system through an injection rather than through GI absorption. This administration route is chosen when rapid drug action is desired; when the patient is uncooperative, unconscious, or unable to accept medication by the oral route; or when a drug is ineffective by other routes. Drugs may be injected into the joints, spinal column, arteries, veins, and muscles. However, the most common parenteral routes are the intramuscular (I.M.), intravenous (I.V.), subcutaneous (SubQ), and intradermal (I.D.) routes.

Drugs administered parenterally may be mixed in either a solution or a suspension; those mixed in a solution typically act more rapidly than those mixed in a suspension. Parenteral administration has several disadvantages: The drug can't be removed or the dosage reduced once it has been injected, and injections typically are more expensive to administer than other dosage forms because they require strict sterility.

Intramuscular

I.M. injections are administered deep into the anterolateral aspect of the thigh (vastis lateralis), the dorsogluteal muscle (gluteus maximus), the upper arm (deltoid), or the ventrogluteal muscle (gluteus medius). I.M. injections typically provide sustained drug action. This route is commonly chosen for drugs that irritate the subcutaneous tissue. The drug should be injected as far as possible from major nerves and blood vessels.

Intravenous

In I.V. drug administration, an aqueous solution is injected directly into the vein—typically of the forearm. Drugs may be administered as a single, small-volume injection or as a slow, large-volume infusion. Because drugs injected I.V. don't encounter absorption barriers, this route produces the most rapid drug action, making it vital in emergency situations. Except for I.V. fat emulsions used as nutritional supplements, oleaginous preparations aren't usually administered by this route because of the risk of fat embolism.

Subcutaneous

The subcutaneous route may be used to inject small volumes of medication, usually 1 ml or less. Subcutaneous injections typically are given below the skin in the abdominal area, lateral area of the anterior thigh, posterior surface of the upper arm, or lateral lumbar area. Injection sites should be rotated to minimize tissue irritation if the patient receives frequent subcutaneous injections—as, for example, in a patient who takes insulin.

Intradermal
Common sites for I.D. injection are the arm and the back. Because only about 0.1 ml may be administered intradermally, this route is rarely used except in diagnostic and test procedures, such as screening for allergic reactions.

TRANSCUTANEOUS
In transcutaneous administration, a drug crosses the skin layers from either the outside (dermal) or the inside (mucocutaneous). This route includes sublingual (S.L.), inhalation, ophthalmic, otic, nasal, topical, and vaginal administration.

Sublingual
In S.L. administration, tablets are placed under the tongue and allowed to dissolve. Nitroglycerin is commonly administered by this route, which allows rapid drug absorption and action. The S.L. route also avoids first-pass metabolism.

Inhalation
Some drugs may be inhaled orally or nasally to produce a local effect on the respiratory tract or a systemic effect. Although drugs given by inhalation avoid first-pass hepatic metabolism, the lungs can also serve as an area of first-pass metabolism by providing respiratory conversion to more water-soluble compounds.

Ophthalmic
Ophthalmic solutions and ointments are applied directly to the cornea or conjunctiva for enhanced local penetration and decreased systemic absorption. These drugs usually are used in eye examinations and to treat glaucoma. Ophthalmic solutions pose a greater risk of drug loss through the nasolacrimal duct into the nasopharynx than ophthalmic ointments do.

Otic
Otic solutions are instilled directly into the external auditory canal for local penetration and decreased systemic absorption. These drugs, which include anesthetics, antibiotics, and anti-inflammatory drugs, usually require occlusion of the ear canal with cotton after instillation.

Nasal
Nasal solutions and suspensions are applied directly to the nasal mucosa for enhanced local penetration and decreased systemic absorption. These drugs are usually used to reduce the inflammation typically associated with seasonal or perennial rhinitis.

Topical
Topical drugs—including creams, ointments, lotions, and pastes—are applied directly to the skin. Transdermal delivery systems, usually in the form of an adhesive patch or a disk, are among the latest developments in topical drug administration. Because they provide slow drug release, these systems are typically used to avoid first-pass metabolism and ensure prolonged duration of action.

Vaginal
Vaginal troches, suppositories, and creams are inserted into the vagina for slow, localized absorption. Body pH that differs from blood pH causes drug trapping or reabsorption, which delays drug excretion through the renal tubules. Vaginal secretions are alkaline, with a pH of 3.4 to 4.2, whereas blood has a pH of 7.35 to 7.45.

A systematic approach to nursing care, the nursing process helps guide you as you develop, implement, and evaluate your care and ensures that you'll deliver safe, consistent, and effective drug therapy to your patients. The nursing process consists of five steps, including assessment, nursing diagnosis, planning, implementation, and evaluation. Even though documentation is not a step in the nursing process, you're legally and professionally responsible for documenting all aspects of your care before, during, and after drug administration.

Assessment

The first step in the nursing process, assessment involves gathering information that's essential to guide your patient's drug therapy. This information includes the patient's drug history, present drug use, allergies, medical history, and physical examination findings. Assessment is an ongoing process that serves as a baseline against which to compare any changes in your patient's condition; it's also the basis for developing and individualizing your patient's plan of care.

DRUG HISTORY

The patient's drug history is critical in your planning of drug-related care. Ask about his previous use of over-the-counter and prescription drugs as well as herbal remedies. For each drug, determine:
• the reason the patient took it
• the prescribed dosage
• the administration route
• the frequency of administration
• the duration of the drug therapy
• any adverse reactions the patient may have experienced and how he handled them.

Also determine if the patient has a history of drug abuse or addiction. Depending on his physical and emotional state,

you may need to obtain the drug history from other sources, such as family members, friends, other caregivers, and the medical record.

PRESENT DRUG USE

Ask about the patient's current use of over-the-counter and prescription drugs as well as herbal remedies. As you did in the drug history, find out the specific details for each drug (dosage, route, frequency, and reason for taking). Also ask the patient if he thinks the drug has been effective and when he took the last dose.

If the patient uses herbal remedies, similarly explore the use of these products because herbs may interact with certain drugs. Also ask about the patient's use of recreational drugs, such as alcohol and tobacco, as well as illegal drugs, such as marijuana and heroin. If the patient acknowledges use of these drugs, be alert for possible drug interactions. This information also may provide you with insight about the patient's response—or lack of response—to his current drug treatment plan.

Try to find out if the patient has any other problems that might affect his compliance with the drug treatment plan, and intervene appropriately. For instance, a patient who is unemployed and has no health insurance may fail to fill a needed prescription. In such a case, contact an appropriate individual in your facility who may be able to help the patient obtain financial assistance.

Be sure to ask the patient if his drug treatment plan requires special monitoring or follow-up laboratory tests. For example, patients who take antihypertensives need to have their blood pressure checked routinely, and those who take warfarin must have their prothrombin time tested regularly. Other patients must undergo periodic blood tests to assess their hepatic and renal function. Determine whether the patient has complied with this part of his treatment plan, and ask him if he knows the results of the latest monitoring or laboratory tests.

ALLERGIES

Find out if the patient is allergic to any drugs or foods. If he has an allergy, explore it further by determining the type of drug or food that triggers a reaction, the first time he experienced a reaction, the characteristics of the reaction, and other related information. Keep in mind that some patients consider annoying symptoms, such as indigestion, an allergic reaction. However, be sure to document a true allergy according to your facility's policy to ensure that the patient doesn't receive that drug or any related drug that may cause a similar reaction. Also, document allergies to foods because they may lead to drug interactions or adverse drug reactions. For example, sulfite is a food additive as well as a drug additive, so a patient with a known allergy to sulfite-containing foods is likely to react to sulfite-containing drugs.

MEDICAL HISTORY

While reviewing your patient's medical history, determine if he has any acute or chronic conditions that may interfere with his drug therapy. Certain disorders involving major body systems, such as the cardiovascular, GI, hepatic, and renal systems, may affect a drug's absorption, transport, metabolism, or excretion and interfere with its action; they also may increase the incidence of adverse reactions and lead to toxicity. For each disorder identified, try to determine when the condition was diagnosed, what drugs were prescribed, and who prescribed them. This information can help you determine whether the patient is receiving incompatible drugs and whether more than one prescriber is managing his drug therapy.

Ask a female patient if she is or may be pregnant or if she's breast-feeding. Many drugs are safe to use during pregnancy, but others may harm the fetus. Also, some drugs are distributed into breast milk. If your patient is or might be pregnant, check the FDA's pregnancy risk category for the prescribed drug and notify the prescriber if the drug may pose a risk to the fetus. If the patient is breast-feeding, find out if the drug is distributed in breast milk and intervene appropriately.

PHYSICAL EXAMINATION FINDINGS

As part of the physical examination, note the patient's age and weight. Be aware that age determines the dosage of certain drugs, such as sedatives and hypnotics, whereas weight determines the dosage of others, including some I.V. antibiotics and anticoagulants. As you perform the physical examination, note any abnormal findings that may point to body organ or system dysfunction. For example, if you detect liver enlargement and ascites, the patient may have impaired hepatic function, which can affect the metabolism of a drug he's taking and lead to harmful adverse or toxic effects. Also note whether a body organ or system appears to be responding to drug treatment. For example, if a patient has been taking an antibiotic to treat chronic bronchitis, thoroughly evaluate his respiratory status to measure his progress. And be sure to assess the patient for possible adverse reactions to the drugs he's taking.

Assess the patient's neurologic function to make sure that he can understand his drug regimen and carry out required tasks, such as performing a fingerstick to obtain blood for glucose measurement. If the patient can't understand essential drug information, you'll need to identify a family member or another person who is willing to become involved in the teaching process.

Nursing Diagnosis

Based on information derived from the assessment and physical examination findings, the nursing diagnoses are statements of actual or potential problems that a nurse is licensed to treat or manage alone or in collaboration with other members of the health care team. They're worded according to guidelines established by the North American Nursing Diagnosis Association (NANDA).

One of the most common nursing diagnoses related to drug therapy is *knowledge deficit,* which indicates that the patient doesn't have sufficient understanding of his drug regimen. However, adverse reactions are the basis for most nursing diagnoses related to drug administration. For example, a patient receiving an opioid analgesic might have a nursing diagnosis of *constipation* related to decreased intestinal motility or *ineffective breathing pattern* related to respiratory depression. A patient receiving long-term, high-dose corticosteroids may have a *risk for impaired skin integrity* related to cortisone acetate or *self-concept disturbance* related to physical changes from prednisone therapy. Many antiarrhythmics cause orthostatic hypotension and thus may place an elderly patient at *high risk for injury* related to possible syncope. Broad-spectrum antibiotics, especially penicillin, may lead to the overgrowth of *Clostridium difficile,* a bacterium that normally is present in the intestine. This overgrowth in turn may lead to pseudomembranous colitis, characterized by abdominal pain and severe diarrhea. The nursing diagnoses in such a case might include *potential for infection* related to bacterial overgrowth, *alteration in comfort* related to abdominal pain, and *fluid balance deficit* related to diarrhea.

Planning

During the planning phase, you'll establish expected outcomes—or goals—for the patient and then develop specific nursing interventions to achieve them. Expected outcomes are observable or measurable goals that should occur as a result of nursing interventions and sometimes in conjunction with medical interventions. Developed in collaboration with the patient, the outcomes should be realistic and objective and should clearly communicate the direction of the plan of care to other nurses. They should be written as behaviors or responses for the patient, not the nurse, to achieve and should include a time frame for measuring the patient's progress. An example of a typical expected outcome is, *The patient will accurately demonstrate self-administration of insulin before discharge.* Based on each outcome statement you establish, you'd then develop appropriate nursing interventions, which might include drug administration techniques, patient teaching, monitoring of vital signs, calculation of drug dosages based on weight, and recording of intake and output.

Implementation

As you implement the nursing interventions, be sure to stringently follow the classic rule of drug administration: administer the right dose of the right drug by the right route to the right patient at the right time. Also, keep in mind that you have a legal and professional responsibility to follow institutional policy regarding standing orders, prescription renewal, and the use of nursing judgment. During the implementation phase, you'll also begin to evaluate the patient's expected outcomes and nursing interventions and make necessary changes to the plan of care.

Evaluation

Evaluation is an ongoing process rather than a single step in the nursing process. During this phase, you evaluate each expected outcome to determine whether or not it has been achieved and whether the original plan of care is working or needs to be modified. In evaluating a patient's drug treatment plan, you should determine whether or not the drug is controlling the signs and symptoms for which it was prescribed. You also should evaluate the patient for psychological or physiologic responses to the drug, especially adverse reactions. This constant monitoring allows you to make appropriate and timely suggestions for changes to the plan of care, such as dosage adjustments or changes in delivery routes, until each expected outcome has been achieved.

Documentation

You're responsible for documenting all your actions related to the patient's drug therapy, from the assessment phase to evaluation. Each time you administer a drug, document the drug name, dose, time given, and your evaluation of its effect. When you administer drugs that require additional nursing judgment, such as those prescribed on an as-needed basis, document the rationale for administering the drug and follow-up assessment or interventions for each dose administered.

If you decide to withhold a prescribed drug based on your nursing judgment, document your action and the rationale for it, and notify the prescriber of your action in a timely manner. Whenever you notify a prescriber about a significant finding related to drug therapy, such as an adverse reaction, document the date and time, the person you contacted, what you discussed, and how you intervened.

abatacept

Orencia

Class and Category
Chemical class: Soluble fusion protein, human recombinant fusion protein
Therapeutic class: Antirheumatic
Pregnancy category: C

Indications and Dosages
➤ *To reduce signs and symptoms, induce major clinical response, inhibit progression of structural damage, and improve physical function in patients with moderate to severe active rheumatoid arthritis and an inadequate response to methotrexate or a tumor necrosis factor antagonist*

I.V. INFUSION

Adults weighing more than 100 kg (220 lb). *Initial:* 1,000 mg infused over 30 min, repeated in 2 to 4 wk. *Maintenance:* 1,000 mg infused over 30 min every 4 wk starting at wk 8.
Adults weighing 60 to 100 kg (132 to 220 lb). *Initial:* 750 mg infused over 30 min, repeated in 2 to 4 wk. *Maintenance:* 750 mg infused over 30 min every 4 wk starting at wk 8.
Adults weighing less than 60 kg. *Initial:* 500 mg infused over 30 min, repeated in 2 to 4 wk. *Maintenance:* 500 mg infused over 30 min every 4 wk starting at wk 8.
➤ *To reduce signs and symptoms of moderate to severe active polyarticular juvenile idiopathic arthritis*

I.V. INFUSION

Children ages 6 to 17 weighing more than 100 kg. *Initial:* 1,000 mg infused over 30 min, repeated in 2 to 4 wk. *Maintenance:* 1,000 mg infused over 30 min every 4 wk starting at wk 8.
Children ages 6 to 17 weighing 75 to 100 kg. *Initial:* 750 mg infused over 30 min, repeated in 2 to 4 wk. *Maintenance:* 750 mg infused over 30 min every 4 wk starting at wk 8.
Children ages 6 to 17 weighing less than

75 kg. *Initial:* 10 mg/kg infused over 30 min, repeated in 2 to 4 wk. *Maintenance:* 10 mg/kg infused over 30 min every 4 wk starting at wk 8.

Mechanism of Action
Inhibits T-cell activation by binding to CD80 and CD86 to block interaction with CD28. CD28 is part of the co-stimulatory signal needed for full activation of T cells. Activated T cells have been implicated in the pathogenesis of rheumatoid arthritis. With decreased proliferation of T cells, inflammation and other evidence of rheumatoid arthritis decrease.

Incompatiblities
Don't infuse abatacept solution with other drugs in the same intravenous line concomitantly because it is not known if the drugs may interact.

Contraindications
Hypersensitivity to abatacept or its components

Interactions
DRUGS
immunosuppressants: Possibly increased risk of serious infection
live-virus vaccines: Possibly decreased response to vaccine, and risk of infection with live virus
tumor necrosis factor antagonists: Increased risk of serious infection

Adverse Reactions
CNS: Dizziness, fever, headache
CV: Hypertension, hypotension
EENT: Nasopharyngitis, rhinitis, sinusitis
GI: Abdominal pain, diarrhea, diverticulitis, dyspepsia, nausea
GU: Acute pyelonephritis, UTI
MS: Back or limb pain
RESP: Bronchitis, COPD worsening, cough, dyspnea, pneumonia, upper respiratory tract infection, wheezing
SKIN: Cellulitis, flushing, pruritus, rash, urticaria
Other: Anaphylaxis, antibody formation, herpes simplex, herpes zoster infection, influenza, malignancies, varicella infection

Nursing Considerations
• Screen patient for latent tuberculosis with a tuberculin skin test before starting abatacept. If the test is positive, expect to provide treatment, as ordered, before starting abatacept. Also screen patient for hepatitis B. If present, expect abatacept to be withdrawn because anti-rheumatic therapies such as abatacept may reactivate hepatitis B.
• Review patient's immunization record and make sure all immunizations are current before therapy starts because drug may blunt effectiveness of some immunizations and increase the risk of infection with live viruses.
• Use cautiously in patients with a history of recurrent infections, underlying conditions that may predispose them to infection, or existing chronic, latent, or localized infection because they have an increased risk of infection with abatacept therapy.
• Use cautiously in patients with COPD and monitor respiratory status closely because abatacept may worsen COPD and increase the risk of adverse respiratory reactions.
• Tumor necrosis factor antagonists shouldn't be given with abatacept because of an increased of serious infection.
• Reconstitue each vial with 10 ml of sterile water for injection. Use only the silicone-free disposable syringe provided with each vial because a siliconized syringe may cause translucent particles to form in the solution. After injecting the sterile water into the vial, gently swirl the vial until contents are completely dissolved. To minimize foaming, don't shake. Vent the vial with a needle to dissipate any foam that may be present.
• Further dilute the reconstituted solution with 0.9% sodium chloride injection to achieve a final solution of 100 ml. Slowly add solution into the infusion bag or bottle using the same silicone-free disposable syringe provided with each vial. Gently mix. Do not shake the bag or bottle.
• Administer the entire dose of fully diluted drug over 30 minutes using an infusion set and a sterile, nonpyrogenic, low protein-binding filter with a pore size of 0.2 μm.
• Once fully diluted, the solution may be kept for 24 hours at room temperature or refrigerated. If reconstituted solution is not used within 24 hours, discard.
• After giving abatacept, monitor patient closely for evidence of a hypersensitivity re-

action such as rash, pruritus, urticaria, dyspnea, or wheezing. If present, stop drug immediately, notify prescriber, and provide supportive emergency care, as ordered.
• Monitor patient closely for evidence of infection or malignancy because abatacept inhibits T-cell activation, making the patient more susceptible to these disorders.

PATIENT TEACHING
• Instruct patient not to receive immunizations with live vaccines during abatacept therapy and for 3 months afterward.
• Stress the importance of reporting any signs and symptoms of infection or hypersensitivity to the prescriber.
• Alert the patient that abatacept may increase the risk of maligancy.
• Warn patient to avoid crowds and people with infections.

abciximab

ReoPro

Class and Category
Chemical class: Fab fragment of chimeric 7E3 antibody
Therapeutic class: Platelet aggregation inhibitor
Pregnancy category: C

Indications and Dosages
➤ *To prevent acute myocardial ischemic complications after percutaneous transluminal coronary angioplasty (PTCA) in patients at high risk for abrupt closure of treated coronary artery*

I.V. INFUSION OR INJECTION
Adults. 250-mcg/kg bolus 10 to 60 min before PTCA. *Maintenance:* 0.125 mcg/kg/min by continuous infusion for 12 hr. *Maximum:* 10 mcg/min.

➤ *To treat unstable angina in patients who haven't responded to conventional therapy and are scheduled for PTCA within 24 hr*

I.V. INFUSION OR INJECTION
Adults. 250-mcg/kg bolus, then 10 mcg/min by continuous infusion over 18 to 24 hr, concluding 1 hr after PTCA.

Route	Onset	Peak	Duration
I.V.	Unknown	Unknown	48 hr

Mechanism of Action
Binds to glycoprotein IIb/IIIa receptor sites on surface of activated platelets. Circulating fibrinogen can bind to these receptor sites and link platelets together, forming a clot that eventually blocks a coronary artery. By binding to receptor sites, abciximab prevents normal binding of fibrinogen and other factors and inhibits platelet aggregation.

Incompatibilities
•Don't mix abciximab with other drugs. Give through separate I.V. line when possible.

Contraindications
Active internal bleeding, arteriovenous malformation or aneurysm, bleeding disorders, stroke in past 2 years or that caused significant neurologic deficit at any time, GI or GU bleeding in past 6 weeks, hypersensitivity to abciximab, intracranial neoplasm, I.V. dextran therapy before or during PTCA, oral anticoagulant therapy in past 7 days unless PT is less than 1.2 times the control, severe uncontrolled hypertension, surgery in past 6 weeks, thrombocytopenia, vasculitis

Interactions
Drugs
dipyridamole, heparin, NSAIDs, oral anticoagulants, thrombolytic drugs, ticlopidine: Increased risk of bleeding

Adverse Reactions
CNS: Confusion, dizziness, hyperesthesia
CV: Atrial fibrillation or flutter, bradycardia, embolism, hypotension, peripheral edema, pseudoaneurysm, supraventricular tachycardia, third-degree AV block, thrombophlebitis, weak pulse
GI: Dysphagia, hematemesis, nausea, vomiting
GU: Dysuria, hematuria, renal dysfunction, urinary frequency, urinary incontinence, urine retention
HEME: Anemia, bleeding, leukocytosis, thrombocytopenia
RESP: Bronchitis, bronchospasm, crackles, dyspnea, pleural effusion, pneumonia, pulmonary edema, pulmonary embolism, wheezing
SKIN: Pruritus, rash, urticaria
Other: Development of human antichimeric antibodies

Nursing Considerations
•Know that abciximab may be used with heparin and aspirin therapy.
•Inspect abciximab for particles; don't use if opaque particles are present.
•For continuous I.V. infusion, withdraw 4.5 ml from 2-mg/ml solution and inject prescribed amount into 250-ml bag of normal saline solution or D_5W, using an in-line sterile, nonpyrogenic, low–protein-binding 0.2- to 0.22-micron filter. Discard unused portion.
•Give I.V. bolus with sterile, nonpyrogenic, low–protein-binding 0.2- to 0.22-micron filter.
•Avoid I.M. injections, venipunctures, and use of indwelling urinary catheters, NG tubes, and automatic blood pressure cuffs during abciximab therapy to prevent bleeding. If appropriate, insert an intermittent I.V. access device to obtain blood samples.
•Watch for GI, GU, and retroperitoneal bleeding and for bleeding at puncture sites.
•**WARNING** If hemorrhage occurs, prepare to stop infusion immediately. Expect to treat severe thrombocytopenia with platelet transfusions if needed.
•Monitor patient for hypersensitivity reactions, such as rash, pruritus, wheezing, and dysphagia from laryngeal edema. If such reactions occur, stop infusion and notify prescriber immediately. If anaphylaxis occurs, give epinephrine, antihistamines, and corticosteroids, as prescribed.
•Obtain platelet count 2 to 4 hours after initial bolus and every 24 hours thereafter during abciximab therapy as ordered. Expect platelet function to return to normal within 48 hours of conclusion of therapy.
•Monitor vital signs and continuous ECG tracings during treatment.
Patient Teaching
•Teach about possible adverse reactions, including bleeding and hypersensitivity reactions, such as rash, urticaria, and dyspnea.
•Tell patient to prevent injury from falls by maintaining bed rest and from bleeding by keeping limb immobile while catheter sheath is in place.

acamprosate calcium
Campral

Class and Category
Chemical class: Synthetic endogenous amino

Mechanism of Action

Chronic alcoholism may alter the balance between excitation and inhibition in neurons in the brain; acamprosate restores it.

When the neurotransmitter gamma-aminobutyric acid (GABA) binds to its receptors in the CNS, it *opens* the chloride ion channel and releases chloride (Cl^-) into the cell (below left), thereby reducing neuronal excitability by inhibiting depolarization. By interacting with GABA receptor sites, acamprosate prevents GABA from binding (below right).

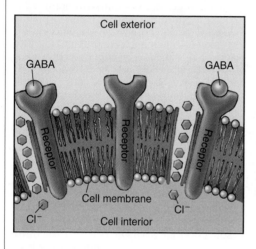

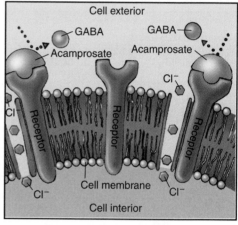

When glutamate binds to its receptors, it *closes* the chloride ion channel, increasing neuronal excitability by promoting depolarization (below left). This imbalance fosters a craving for alcohol. By interacting with glutamate receptor sites, acamprosate prevents glutamate from binding (below right).

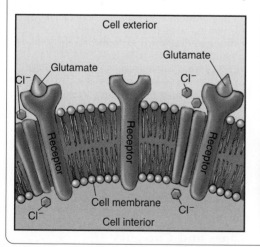

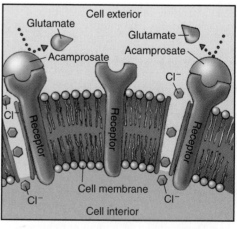

acid homotaurine, gamma-aminobutyric acid (GABA) analogue
Therapeutic class: Antialcoholic
Pregnancy category: C

Indications and Dosages
➤ *To maintain abstinence from alcohol for alcohol-dependent patients who are abstinent at the start of treatment*
E.R. TABLETS
Adults. 666 mg t.i.d.
DOSAGE ADJUSTMENT For patients with moderate renal impairment (creatinine clearance of 30 to 50 ml/min), 333 mg t.i.d.

Route	Onset	Peak	Duration
P.O.	Unknown	3 to 8 hr	Unknown

Contraindications
Hypersensitivity to acamprosate or its components, severe hepatic (Child-Pugh class C) or renal impairment

Interactions
DRUGS
antidepressants: Increased weight gain
tetracyclines: Decreased absorption of tetracyclines

Adverse Reactions
CNS: Abnormal thinking, amnesia, anxiety, asthenia, chills, depression, dizziness, headache, insomnia, paresthesia, somnolence, suicidal ideation, syncope, tremor
CV: Chest pain, hypertension, palpitations, peripheral edema, vasodilation
EENT: Abnormal vision, dry mouth, pharyngitis, rhinitis, taste perversion
GI: Abdominal pain, anorexia, constipation, diarrhea, flatulence, increased appetite, indigestion, nausea, vomiting
GU: Acute renal failure, decreased libido, impotence
HEME: Leukopenia, lymphocytosis, thrombocytopenia
MS: Arthralgia, back pain, myalgia
RESP: Bronchitis, cough, dyspnea
SKIN: Diaphoresis, pruritus, rash
Other: Flulike symptoms, infection, weight gain

Nursing Considerations
• Be aware that acamprosate therapy should start as soon as possible after the patient has undergone alcohol withdrawal and achieved abstinence.

• Continue to administer acamprosate even during periods of alcohol relapse.
PATIENT TEACHING
• Instruct patient to take acamprosate exactly as prescribed, even if a relapse occurs, and to seek help for a relapse.
• Warn the patient that acamprosate won't reduce the symptoms of alcohol withdrawal if relapse occurs followed by cessation.
• Urge caregivers to monitor patient for signs and symptoms of depression (lack of appetite or interest in life, fatigue, excessive sleeping, difficulty concentrating) or suicidal tendencies because a small number of patients taking acamprosate have attempted suicide.
• Advise patient to use caution when performing hazardous activities until adverse CNS effects of the drug are known.
• Tell female patient to notify prescriber if she is or intend to become pregnant while taking acamprosate; the drug may need to be stopped because fetal risks are unknown.

acarbose

Precose

Class and Category
Chemical class: Alpha-glucosidase inhibitor, oligosaccharide
Therapeutic class: Antidiabetic drug
Pregnancy category: B

Indications and Dosages
➤ *To control blood glucose level in patients with type 2 (non–insulin-dependent) diabetes mellitus when the level can't be controlled by diet alone*
TABLETS
Adults. *Initial:* 25 mg t.i.d. with first bite of each meal. *Maintenance:* Increased to maximum at 4- to 8-wk intervals p.r.n. *Maximum:* 50 mg t.i.d. for patients weighing 65 kg (143 lb) or less; 100 mg t.i.d. for patients weighing more than 65 kg.

Contraindications
Chronic intestinal disease, cirrhosis, colonic ulceration, conditions that may deteriorate because of increased gas formation in intestines, diabetic ketoacidosis, digestive or absorption disorders, history of bowel obstruction, hypersensitivity to acarbose, inflammatory bowel disease

Mechanism of Action

Inhibits action of alpha-amylase and alpha-glucoside enzymes. Normally, alpha-amylase hydrolyzes complex starches to oligosaccharides in the small intestine, and alpha-glucoside hydrolyzes oligosaccharides, trisaccharides, and disaccharides to glucose and other monosaccharides in brush border of the small intestine. In diabetic patients, acarbose inhibits these actions and delays glucose absorption, reducing the blood glucose level after meals.

Interactions

DRUGS

calcium channel blockers, digestive enzymes (such as pancreatin), diuretics, estrogen, intestinal adsorbents (such as activated charcoal), isoniazid, nicotinic acid, oral contraceptives, phenothiazines, phenytoin, sympathomimetics, thyroid hormones: Possibly decreased therapeutic effects of acarbose
digoxin: Decreased serum level and therapeutic effects of digoxin
insulin, sulfonylureas: Decreased insulin action, possibly increased risk of hypoglycemia

Adverse Reactions

CV: Edema
GI: Abdominal distention and pain, diarrhea, flatulence, hepatitis, hepatotoxicity, ileus, jaundice
SKIN: Erythema, exanthema, rash, urticaria

Nursing Considerations

•WARNING Be aware that acarbose isn't recommended for patients with significant renal dysfunction and a serum creatinine level above 2 mg/dl.
•If patient is receiving acarbose and a sulfonylurea or insulin to enhance glucose control, check blood glucose level often, as appropriate.
•Store drug in sealed container in cool environment.
•Expect to decrease dosage to control GI upset.
•Monitor glycosylated hemoglobin level as ordered every 3 months for first year to evaluate glucose control and patient compliance.
•Monitor hematocrit and serum AST level every 3 months during first year of therapy and periodically thereafter, as ordered, because acarbose may decrease hematocrit and increase serum AST level.

PATIENT TEACHING

•Explain importance of self-monitoring glucose levels during acarbose therapy.
•Teach patient to recognize signs and symptoms of hypoglycemia and hyperglycemia.
•Warn patient that noncompliance with prescribed regimen can increase risk of diabetic complications, including neuropathy, retinopathy, and renal insufficiency.
•Explain that temporary insulin therapy may be needed if fever, trauma, infection, illness, surgery, or other stress alters blood glucose control.
•Warn patient not to take other drugs within 2 hours of taking acarbose unless specifically instructed by prescriber.
•Tell him to consult prescriber before taking OTC drugs during acarbose therapy.
•Advise patient who also takes another antidiabetic drug to carry glucose with him at all times in case hypoglycemia occurs.

acebutolol hydrochloride

Monitan (CAN), Sectral

Class and Category

Chemical class: Beta$_1$-selective (cardioselective) adrenergic receptor blocker
Therapeutic class: Antihypertensive, class II antiarrhythmic
Pregnancy category: B

Indications and Dosages

➤ *To treat hypertension*

TABLETS

Adults. *Initial:* 400 mg daily or 200 mg b.i.d. *Usual:* 200 to 800 mg daily. Dosage increased to 1,200 mg daily in divided doses b.i.d. for severe hypertension or hypertension that isn't well controlled with usual dosage.

➤ *To treat premature ventricular arrhythmias*

TABLETS

Adults. *Initial:* 200 mg b.i.d. *Usual:* 600 to 1,200 mg daily.

DOSAGE ADJUSTMENT Maximum dosage of 800 mg daily for elderly patients. Dosage reduced by 50% for patients with creatinine

A

clearance of less than 50 ml/min/1.73 m^2. Dosage reduced by 75% for patients with creatinine clearance of less than 25 ml/min/1.73 m^2.

Route	Onset	Peak	Duration
P.O.	1 to 1.5 hr	2 to 8 hr	24 hr or longer

Mechanism of Action

Inhibits stimulation of $beta_1$ receptors in the heart, decreasing cardiac excitability, heart rate, cardiac output, and myocardial oxygen demand. Acebutolol also decreases kidneys' release of renin, which helps reduce blood pressure. Drug suppresses SA node automaticity and AV node conductivity, which suppresses atrial and ventricular ectopy. By decreasing myocardial oxygen demand, acebutolol decreases myocardial ischemia. At high doses, it inhibits stimulation of $beta_2$ receptors in the lungs and may cause bronchoconstriction.

Contraindications

Cardiogenic shock, heart failure unless caused by tachyarrhythmia, hypersensitivity to acebutolol, overt heart failure, second- and third-degree heart block, severe bradycardia

Interactions

DRUGS

alpha agonists, nasal decongestants: Increased risk of hypertension
aluminum salts, barbiturates, calcium salts, cholestyramine, colestipol, indomethacin, NSAIDs, penicillins, rifampin, salicylates, sulfinpyrazone: Decreased antihypertensive effects
anticholinergics, hydralazine, methyldopa, prazosin, reserpine: Increased risk of bradycardia and hypotension
beta$_2$ agonists, theophylline: Decreased bronchodilation
epinephrine: Increased risk of blocked sympathomimetic effects
ergot alkaloids: Increased risk of peripheral ischemia and gangrene
flecainide: Possibly increased effects of both drugs
lidocaine: Possibly increased serum lidocaine level, causing toxicity
oral contraceptives, quinidine: Possibly increased serum acebutolol level

sulfonylureas: Possibly decreased hypoglycemic effects
verapamil: Increased cardiac effects, leading to bradycardia and hypotension

Adverse Reactions

CNS: Abnormal dreams, anxiety, confusion, depression, dizziness, fatigue, fever, headache, insomnia
CV: Bradycardia, chest pain, edema, heart block, heart failure, hypotension
EENT: Abnormal vision, conjunctivitis, dry eyes, eye pain, pharyngitis, rhinitis
GI: Constipation, diarrhea, flatulence, hepatotoxicity, indigestion, nausea
GU: Dysuria, impotence, polyuria
MS: Arthralgia, myalgia
RESP: Bronchospasm, cough, dyspnea, wheezing
SKIN: Rash

Nursing Considerations

• Before therapy begins, obtain baseline renal function tests, as ordered.
• Check apical and radial pulses before giving acebutolol. Also, frequently monitor blood pressure and pulse rate, rhythm, and quality during treatment.
• Give drug with food to prevent GI upset.
• Acebutolol may elevate uric acid, potassium, triglyceride, lipoprotein, and antinuclear antibody levels; it also may interfere with accuracy of glucose tolerance tests.
• Monitor diabetic patient's blood glucose level to spot alterations.
• Notify prescriber if you detect a heart rate below 50 beats/min or signs of heart failure, such as dyspnea, crackles, unexplained weight gain, and jugular vein distention.
• Monitor patient for peripheral edema and evaluate fluid intake and output.

PATIENT TEACHING

• Tell patient that tablets may be crushed or swallowed whole.
• Warn him against discontinuing acebutolol abruptly, which could cause angina or dangerously high blood pressure.
• Instruct patient to take a missed dose as soon as possible up to 6 hours before next scheduled dose but not to double the next dose.
• Advise patient to consult prescriber before taking OTC drugs that contain alpha agonists, such as nasal decongestants and cold preparations.

•Instruct patient to report dizziness, confusion, and fever immediately.
•Urge patient to maintain diet and lifestyle changes to help control blood pressure.

acetaminophen

Abenol (CAN), Acephen, Aceta Elixir, Acetaminophen Uniserts, Aceta Tablets, Apacet Capsules, Apacet Elixir, Apacet Extra Strength Tablets, Apacet Regular Strength Tablets, Aspirin Free Pain Relief, Exdol (CAN), Feverall, Feverall Sprinkle Caps, Genapap Infants' Drops, Genebs Extra Strength, Halenol Children's Junior Strength, Liquiprin Elixir, Liquiprin Infants' Drops, Meda Cap, Neopap, Oraphen-PD, Panadol, Panadol Infants' Drops, Pediaphen, Redutemp, Robigesic (CAN), St. Joseph Aspirin-Free Infant Drops, Tapanol Extra Strength, Tempra, Tempra Drops, Tylenol, Tylenol Caplets, Tylenol Children's Chewable Tablets, Tylenol Extra Strength, Tylenol Gelcaps, Tylenol Infants' Drops

Class and Category

Chemical class: Nonsalicylate, para-aminophenol derivative
Therapeutic class: Antipyretic, nonnarcotic analgesic
Pregnancy category: B

Indications and Dosages

➤ *To relieve mild to moderate pain associated with headache, muscle ache, backache, minor arthritis, common cold, toothache, and menstrual cramps; to reduce fever*

CAPLETS, CAPSULES, CHEWABLE TABLETS, ELIXIR, E.R. CAPLETS, GELCAPS, LIQUID, SOLUTION, SPRINKLES, SUSPENSION, TABLETS

Adults. 325 to 650 mg every 4 to 6 hr, or 1,000 mg t.i.d. or q.i.d., or 2 E.R. caplets every 8 hr. *Maximum:* 4,000 mg daily.
Children over age 14. 650 mg every 4 hr. *Maximum:* 5 doses in 24 hr.
Children ages 12 to 14. 640 mg every 4 hr. *Maximum:* 5 doses in 24 hr.
Children age 11. 480 mg every 4 hr. *Maximum:* 5 doses in 24 hr.
Children ages 9 to 10. 400 mg every 4 hr. *Maximum:* 5 doses in 24 hr.
Children ages 6 to 8. 320 mg every 4 hr. *Maximum:* 5 doses in 24 hr.

Children ages 4 to 5. 240 mg every 4 hr. *Maximum:* 5 doses in 24 hr.
Children ages 2 to 3. 160 mg every 4 hr. *Maximum:* 5 doses in 24 hr.
Children age 1. 120 mg every 4 hr. *Maximum:* 5 doses in 24 hr.
Children ages 4 to 11 months. 80 mg every 4 hr. *Maximum:* 5 doses in 24 hr.
Children ages 0 to 3 months. 40 mg every 4 hr. *Maximum:* 5 doses in 24 hr.

SUPPOSITORIES

Adults and adolescents. 650 mg every 4 to 6 hr. *Maximum:* 4,000 mg daily.
Children ages 6 to 12. 325 mg every 4 to 6 hr. *Maximum:* 2,600 mg daily.
Children ages 3 to 6. 120 to 125 mg every 4 to 6 hr. *Maximum:* 720 mg daily.
Children ages 1 to 3. 80 mg every 4 hr.
Children ages 3 to 11 months. 80 mg every 6 hr.

Route	Onset	Peak	Duration
P.O., P.R.	Varies	1 to 3 hr	3 to 4 hr

Mechanism of Action

Inhibits the enzyme cyclooxygenase, blocking prostaglandin production and interfering with pain impulse generation in the peripheral nervous system. Acetaminophen also acts directly on temperature-regulating center in the hypothalamus by inhibiting synthesis of prostaglandin E_2.

Contraindications

Hypersensitivity to acetaminophen or its components

Interactions

DRUGS

anticholinergics: Decreased onset of action of acetaminophen
barbiturates, carbamazepine, hydantoins, isoniazid, rifampin, sulfinpyrazone: Decreased therapeutic effects and increased hepatotoxic effects of acetaminophen
lamotrigine, loop diuretics: Possibly decreased therapeutic effects of these drugs
oral contraceptives: Decreased effectiveness of acetaminophen
probenecid: Possibly increased therapeutic effects of acetaminophen
propranolol: Possibly increased action of acetaminophen

A

zidovudine: Possibly decreased effects of zidovudine
ACTIVITIES
alcohol use: Increased risk of hepatotoxicity

Adverse Reactions

GI: Abdominal pain, hepatotoxicity, nausea, vomiting
HEME: Hemolytic anemia (with long-term use), leukopenia, neutropenia, pancytopenia, thrombocytopenia
SKIN: Jaundice, rash, urticaria
Other: Angioedema, hypoglycemic coma

Nursing Considerations

•Before and during long-term therapy, monitor liver function test results, including AST, ALT, bilirubin, and creatinine levels, as ordered.
•Monitor renal function in patient on long-term therapy. Keep in mind that blood or albumin in urine may indicate nephritis; decreased urine output, renal failure; and dark brown urine, presence of the metabolite phenacetin.
•Expect to reduce dosage for patients with renal dysfunction.
•Store suppositories under 80° F (26.6° C).
•**WARNING** Be aware that Pediaphen is a concentrated form of acetaminophen containing 80 mg/0.8 ml (standard liquid forms contain 32 mg/ml). Make sure to use correct concentration and correct dosage of liquid acetaminophen because serious adverse reactions can result from confusing concentrated form with regular liquid form.
PATIENT TEACHING
•Tell patient that tablets may be crushed or swallowed whole.
•Instruct patient to read manufacturer's label and follow dosage guidelines precisely. Explain that infants' and children's acetaminophen liquid aren't equal in drug concentration and aren't interchangeable.
•Advise patient to use manufacturer's dropper or dosage cup for measuring liquid acetaminophen.
•Advise him to contact prescriber before taking other prescription or OTC products because they may contain acetaminophen.
•Teach patient to recognize signs of hepatotoxicity, such as bleeding, easy bruising, and malaise, which commonly occurs with chronic overdose.

acetazolamide

Acetazolam (CAN), Ak-Zol, Apo-Acetazolamide (CAN), Dazamide, Diamox, Diamox Sequels, Storzolamide

Class and Category

Chemical class: Sulfonamide derivative
Therapeutic class: Anticonvulsant, antiglaucoma, diuretic
Pregnancy category: C

Indications and Dosages

➤ *To treat chronic simple (open-angle) glaucoma*
S.R. CAPSULES, TABLETS, I.V. OR I.M. INJECTION
Adults. 250 to 1,000 mg daily (divided for doses exceeding 250 mg).

➤ *As short-term therapy to treat secondary glaucoma and preoperatively to treat acute congestive (closed-angle) glaucoma*
S.R. CAPSULES, TABLETS, I.V. OR I.M. INJECTION
Adults. 250 mg b.i.d. or every 4 hr; or 1 S.R. capsule (500 mg) b.i.d.; or 500 mg initially, followed by 125 to 250 mg every 4 to 6 hr for severe acute glaucoma. To initially lower intraocular pressure rapidly, 500 mg I.V.; may repeat in 2 to 4 hr in acute cases, depending on patient response. Oral therapy usually initiated after initial I.V. dose.
S.R. CAPSULES, TABLETS
Children. 10 to 15 mg/kg daily in divided doses every 6 to 8 hr.
I.V. OR I.M. INJECTION
Children. 5 to 10 mg/kg/dose every 6 hr.

➤ *To induce diuresis in heart failure*
TABLETS, I.V. OR I.M. INJECTION
Adults. *Initial:* 250 to 375 mg or 5 mg/kg daily in morning. *Maintenance:* 250 to 375 mg or 5 mg/kg on alternate days or for 2 days followed by a drug-free day.

➤ *To treat drug-induced edema*
TABLETS, I.V. OR I.M. INJECTION
Adults. 250 to 375 mg daily for 1 to 2 days.
TABLETS, I.V. INJECTION
Children. 5 mg/kg/dose daily in morning.

➤ *To treat seizures, including generalized tonic-clonic, absence, and mixed seizures, and myoclonic jerk patterns*
TABLETS, I.V. OR I.M. INJECTION
Adults and children. 8 to 30 mg/kg daily in divided doses. *Optimal:* 375 to 1,000 mg

daily. When used with other anticonvulsants, 250 mg daily.

➤ *To prevent or relieve symptoms of acute mountain sickness*

S.R. CAPSULES, TABLETS

Adults. 500 to 1,000 mg daily in divided doses, given 24 to 48 hr before ascent and continued for 48 hr or longer while at high altitude p.r.n. to control symptoms.

Contraindications

Chronic noncongestive closed-angle glaucoma; cirrhosis; hyperchloremic acidosis; hypersensitivity to acetazolamide; hypokalemia; hyponatremia; severe pulmonary obstruction; severe renal, hepatic, or adrenocortical impairment

Route	Onset	Peak	Duration
P.O.	60 to 90 min	2 to 4 hr	8 to 12 hr
P.O. (S.R.)	2 hr	8 to 12 hr	18 to 24 hr
I.V.	2 min	15 min	4 to 5 hr

Mechanism of Action

Inhibits the enyzme carbonic anhydrase, which normally appears in the eyes' ciliary processes, brain's choroid plexes, and kidneys' proximal tubule cells. In the eyes, enzyme inhibition decreases aqueous humor secretion, which lowers intraocular pressure. In the brain, inhibition may delay abnormal, intermittent, and excessive discharge from neurons that cause seizures. In the kidneys, it increases bicarbonate excretion, which carries out water, potassium, and sodium, thus inducing diuresis and metabolic acidosis. This acidosis counteracts respiratory alkalosis and reduces symptoms of mountain sickness, including headache, dizziness, nausea, and dyspnea.

Interactions

DRUGS

amphetamines, methenamine, phenobarbital, procainamide, quinidine: Decreased excretion and possibly toxicity of these drugs
corticosteroids: Increased risk of hypokalemia
cyclosporine: Increased cyclosporine level, possibly nephrotoxicity or neurotoxicity

diflunisal: Possibly significantly decreased intraocular pressure
lithium: Increased excretion and decreased effectiveness of lithium
primidone: Decreased serum and urine primidone levels
salicylates: Increased risk of salicylate toxicity

Adverse Reactions

CNS: Ataxia, confusion, depression, disorientation, dizziness, drowsiness, fatigue, fever, flaccid paralysis, headache, lassitude, malaise, nervousness, paresthesia, seizures, tremor, weakness
EENT: Altered taste, tinnitus, transient myopia
GI: Anorexia, constipation, diarrhea, hepatic dysfunction, melena, nausea, vomiting
GU: Crystalluria, decreased libido, glycosuria, hematuria, impotence, nephrotoxicity, phosphaturia, polyuria, renal calculi, renal colic, urinary frequency
HEME: Agranulocytosis, hemolytic anemia, leukopenia, pancytopenia, thrombocytopenia, thrombocytopenic purpura
SKIN: Photosensitivity, pruritus, rash, Stevens-Johnson syndrome, urticaria
Other: Acidosis, hyperuricemia, hypokalemia, weight loss

Nursing Considerations

• Use acetazolamide cautiously in patients with calcium-based renal calculi, diabetes mellitus, gout, or respiratory impairment.
• Know that acetazolamide may increase risk of hepatic encephalopathy in patients with hepatic cirrhosis.
• To avoid painful I.M. injections (caused by alkaline solution), administer acetazolamide by mouth or I.V. injection if possible.
• Reconstitute each 500-mg vial with at least 5 ml of sterile water for injection. Use within 24 hours because drug has no preservative.
• Monitor blood tests during acetazolamide therapy to detect electrolyte imbalances.
• Monitor fluid intake and output every 8 hours and body weight daily to detect excessive fluid and weight loss.

PATIENT TEACHING

• Inform patient that acetazolamide tablets may be crushed and suspended in chocolate or another sweet syrup. Or, one tablet may be dissolved in 10 ml of hot water and added to 10 ml of honey or syrup.
• Advise patient to avoid hazardous activities

A

if dizziness or drowsiness occurs.
•Instruct patient who takes high doses of salicylates to notify prescriber immediately if signs of salicylate toxicity, such as anorexia, tachypnea, and lethargy, occur.
•If patient plans to mountain climb, urge her to descend mountain gradually and to seek immediate medical care if symptoms of mountain sickness occur.

acetohexamide

Dimelor (CAN), Dymelor

Class and Category
Chemical class: Sulfonylurea
Therapeutic class: Antidiabetic
Pregnancy category: C

Indications and Dosages
➤ *To treat stable type 2 (non–insulin-dependent) diabetes mellitus*
TABLETS
Adults. *Initial:* 250 to 1,500 mg daily. Dosages of 1,000 mg or more daily may be divided and given b.i.d. before morning and evening meals.
DOSAGE ADJUSTMENT For patient being switched from another antidiabetic drug, acetohexamide dosage reduced to half the usual tolbutamide dosage or twice the usual chlorpropamide dosage. For patient being switched from insulin to acetohexamide monotherapy, dosages adjusted as follows: if insulin dosage is less than 20 units daily, acetohexamide begins at 250 mg daily and insulin is discontinued; if insulin dosage exceeds 20 units daily, acetohexamide begins at 250 mg daily and insulin is tapered by 25% to 30% before being reduced further according to patient response.

Route	Onset	Peak	Duration
P.O.	1 hr	Unknown	12 to 24 hr

Mechanism of Action
Stimulates insulin release from active beta cells in the pancreas, resulting in decreased blood glucose level. Improves insulin binding to insulin receptors. Increases the number of insulin receptors (with long-term administration). May reduce basal hepatic glucose secretion.

Contraindications
Diabetes mellitus complicated by ketoacidosis or pregnancy, hypersensitivity to acetohexamide, renal failure, sole therapy for type 1 (insulin-dependent) diabetes mellitus

Interactions
DRUGS
activated charcoal: Possibly reduced absorption and effectiveness of acetohexamide
androgens, anticoagulants, azole antifungals, chloramphenicol, clofibrate, fluconazole, gemfibrozil, H_2-receptor antagonists, magnesium salts, MAO inhibitors, methyldopa, probenecid, salicylates, sulfinpyrazone, sulfonamides, tricyclic antidepressants, urinary acidifiers: Enhanced hypoglycemic effect of acetohexamide
beta blockers, calcium channel blockers, cholestyramine, corticosteroids, diazoxide, estrogens, hydantoins, isoniazid, nicotinic acid, oral contraceptives, phenothiazines, rifampin, sympathomimetics, thiazide diuretics, thyroid drugs, urinary alkalizers: Decreased hypoglycemic effect
digitalis glycosides: Possibly increased serum digitalis level

Adverse Reactions
CNS: Anxiety, chills, confusion, depression, dizziness, drowsiness, fatigue, headache, hyperesthesia, insomnia, malaise, nervousness, paresthesia, somnolence, syncope, tremor, vertigo, weakness
CV: Arrhythmias, edema, hypertension, vasculitis
EENT: Blurred vision, conjunctivitis, eye pain, pharyngitis, retinal hemorrhage, rhinitis, tinnitus
ENDO: Hypoglycemia
GI: Abdominal pain, anorexia, constipation, diarrhea, epigastric fullness, flatulence, heartburn, hepatitis, hepatotoxicity, indigestion, nausea, proctocolitis, vomiting
GU: Decreased libido, dysuria, polyuria
HEME: Agranulocytosis, aplastic anemia, eosinophilia, hemolytic anemia, leukopenia, pancytopenia, thrombocytopenia
MS: Abnormal gait, arthralgia, hypertonia, leg cramps
RESP: Dyspnea
SKIN: Diaphoresis, eczema, erythema multiforme, exfoliative dermatitis, flushing, jaundice, lichenoid reaction (skin thickening,

accentuated lesions), maculopapular rash, photosensitivity, pruritus, rash, urticaria
Other: Disulfiram-like reaction (flushing, head throbbing, hypotension, nausea, tachycardia, vomiting), hyponatremia

Nursing Considerations
•Use acetohexamide cautiously in elderly patients and in those with cardiac, hepatic, or renal disease or thyroid dysfunction. The drug's duration of action is prolonged in patients with renal disease.
•Give acetohexamide 30 minutes before meals, crushing tablets if desired. If GI upset occurs, give in divided doses, as prescribed.
•Monitor for signs of hypoglycemia and hyperglycemia, especially after meals.
•Monitor blood glucose level frequently, as ordered. Provide additional insulin if needed during stressful periods, as prescribed.
•Monitor liver enzyme levels during therapy; acetohexamide may increase AST, ALT, and alkaline phosphatase levels.
•Store acetohexamide in tightly sealed container in a cool environment.
PATIENT TEACHING
•Stress need to adhere to prescribed drug regimen, diet, and exercise program.
•Advise patient to take acetohexamide with food to avoid GI upset.
•Teach patient how to self-monitor blood glucose level and check urine for glucose and ketones, as appropriate.
•Teach patient to recognize and report signs of hypoglycemia and hyperglycemia.

acetohydroxamic acid

Lithostat

Class and Category
Chemical class: Synthetic hydroxylamine and ethylacetate derivative
Therapeutic class: Urease inhibitor
Pregnancy category: X

Indications and Dosages
➤ *As an adjunct to antimicrobial therapy to treat chronic UTI caused by urea-splitting bacteria*
TABLETS
Adults. *Initial:* 12 mg/kg daily in divided

doses every 6 to 8 hr. *Usual:* 250 mg t.i.d. or q.i.d. for a total daily dose of 10 to 15 mg/kg. *Maximum:* 1,500 mg daily.
Children. 10 mg/kg daily.
DOSAGE ADJUSTMENT Maximum dosage reduced to 1,000 mg daily or 500 mg every 12 hr for patients with serum creatinine level that exceeds 1.8 mg/dl.

> ### Mechanism of Action
> Inhibits urease, the enzyme that catalyzes urea's hydrolysis to carbon dioxide and ammonia in urine infected with urea-splitting bacteria. This action reduces the urine ammonia level and pH, enhancing antimicrobial drug effectiveness.

Contraindications
Contributing disorder that's treatable by surgery or appropriate antimicrobial therapy, hypersensitivity to acetohydroxamic acid, inadequate renal function (serum creatinine level above 2.5 mg/dl or creatinine clearance below 20 ml/min/1.73 m^2), risk of pregnancy, UTI caused by non–urease-producing organisms, UTI that can be controlled by appropriate antimicrobial therapy

Interactions
DRUGS
iron: Decreased intestinal absorption of iron, decreased effects of iron and acetohydroxamic acid
ACTIVITIES
alcohol use: Increased risk of severe rash 30 to 45 minutes after drinking alcohol

Adverse Reactions
CNS: Anxiety, depression, fever, lack of coordination, malaise, headache, nervousness, slurred speech, tiredness, tremor
CV: Calf pain (deep vein blood clot), palpitations, sudden chest pain
EENT: Pharyngitis, sudden change in vision
GI: Anorexia, nausea, vomiting
HEME: Reticulocytosis, unusual bleeding
RESP: Dyspnea
SKIN: Ecchymosis, hair loss, nonpruritic macular rash

Nursing Considerations
•Use acetohydroxamic acid cautiously in patients with severe chronic renal disease or

A

anemia and those who've had phlebitis or thrombophlebitis.
•Be aware that risk of adverse psychomotor effects increases if patient drinks alcohol or takes drugs that affect alertness and reflexes, such as antihistamines, tranquilizers, sedatives, analgesics, and narcotics.
•Administer tablets with food or liquid, crushing them if needed.
•WARNING Acetohydroxamic acid chelates with dietary iron. If patient has iron deficiency anemia, expect to administer I.M. iron as needed during acetohydroxamic acid therapy.
•Monitor follow-up laboratory tests to check renal and hepatic function and urine pH, as ordered.

PATIENT TEACHING
•Instruct patient to take drug at same time each day, as prescribed.
•Tell patient to take a missed dose up to 2 hours after scheduled time. If more than 2 hours have passed, he should wait for next scheduled dose and shouldn't double that dose.
•Warn patient not to take drug with alcohol or iron and to consult prescriber before taking it with any other drug.
•Instruct patient to avoid hazardous activities during therapy.

acetylcysteine

Acetadote, Mucomyst, Mucosil

Class and Category
Chemical class: N-acetyl derivative of cysteine
Therapeutic class: Antidote (for acetaminophen overdose), mucolytic
Pregnancy category: B

Indications and Dosages
➤ *To liquefy abnormal, viscid, or thickened mucus secretions in chronic pulmonary disorders (including emphysema, bronchitis, tuberculosis, bronchiectasis, and cystic fibrosis) and in pneumonia, pulmonary complications of thoracic or cardiovascular surgery, and tracheostomy care*
SOLUTION BY DIRECT INSTILLATION INTO TRACHEOSTOMY (MUCOMYST, MUCOSIL)
Adults and children. 1 to 2 ml of 10% or 20% solution instilled every 1 to 4 hr, p.r.n.

SOLUTION BY INHALATION
Adults and children. 1 to 10 ml of 20% solution or 2 to 20 ml of 10% solution nebulized through face mask, mouthpiece, or tracheostomy every 2 to 6 hr. *Usual:* 3 to 5 ml of 20% solution or 6 to 10 ml of 10% solution t.i.d. or q.i.d.
➤ *To treat acetaminophen overdose*
SOLUTION P.O. (MUCOMYST, MUCOSIL)
Adults and children. *Loading dose:* 140 mg/kg. *Maintenance:* 70 mg/kg 4 hr after loading dose and then every 4 hr to a total of 17 doses.
I.V. INFUSION (ACETADOTE)
Adults and children weighing 40 kg (88 lb) or more. 150 mg/kg in 200 ml of diluent infused over 60 min, followed by 50 mg/kg in 500 ml of diluent infused over 4 hr, followed by 100 mg/kg in 1,000 ml of diluent infused over 16 hr.
Adults and children weighing more than 20 kg (44 lb) but less than 40 kg. 150 mg/kg in 100 ml of diluent infused over 60 min, followed by 50 mg/kg in 250 ml of diluent infused over 4 hr, followed by 100 mg/kg in 500 ml of diluent infused over 16 hr.
Children weighing 20 kg or less. 150 mg/kg in 3 ml/kg of diluent infused over 60 min, followed by 50 mg/kg in 7 ml/kg of diluent infused over 4 hr, followed by 100 mg/kg in 14 ml/kg of diluent infused over 16 hr.

Mechanism of Action
Decreases viscosity of pulmonary secretions by breaking disulfide links that bind glycoproteins in mucus. Reduces liver damage from acetaminophen overdose. Usually, acetaminophen's toxic metabolites bind with glutathione in the liver, which detoxifies them. When acetaminophen overdose depletes glutathione stores, toxic metabolites bind with protein in liver cells, killing them. Acetylcysteine maintains or restores levels of glutathione or acts as its substitute, which reduces liver damage from acetaminophen overdose.

Incompatibilities
Don't administer acetylcysteine with nebulization equipment if drug can contact iron, copper, or rubber. Don't administer drug with amphotericin B, ampicillin sodium,

chlortetracycline, chymotrypsin, erythromycin, hydrogen peroxide, iodized oil, oxytetracycline, tetracycline, or trypsin.

Contraindications
Hypersensitivity to acetylcysteine, no contraindications when used as antidote

Interactions
DRUGS
activated charcoal: Possibly adsorption and decreased effectiveness of oral acetylcysteine
nitroglycerin: Increased effects of nitroglycerin and possibly significant hypotension and headache

Adverse Reactions
CNS: Chills, dizziness, drowsiness, fever, headache
CV: Edema, hypertension, hypotension, tachycardia
EENT: Rhinorrhea, stomatitis, tooth damage
GI: Anorexia, constipation, hepatotoxicity, nausea, vomiting
RESP: Bronchospasm, chest tightness, cough, hemoptysis, respiratory distress, shortness of breath, stridor, wheezing
SKIN: Clammy skin, facial flushing, pruritus, rash, urticaria
Other: Anaphylaxis, angioedema

Nursing Considerations
•Be aware that acetylcysteine should be used cautiously in patients with asthma or a history of bronchospasm because drug may adversely affect respiratory function.
•**WARNING** To avoid fluid overload and possibly fatal hyponatremia or seizures, adjust total administered volume, as ordered, for patients weighing less than 40 kg (88 lb) and for those who need fluid restriction.
•If needed, dilute 20% instillation or inhalation solution with normal saline solution or sterile water. The 10% solution may be used undiluted.
•When treating acetaminophen overdose, dilute 20% oral solution with cola or other soft drink to a concentration of 5%, and use within 1 hour. Dilute parenteral solution with D_5W or half-normal saline (0.45% sodium chloride) solution for injection following manufacturer guidelines because dilution is based on dosage to be administered. Acetadote may turn from colorless to slight pink or purple once the stopper is punctured,

but the color change has no effect on product quality.
•Acetylcysteine is most effective if administered within 24 hours of acetaminophen ingestion. For specific instructions, contact a regional poison center at 1-800-222-1222 or a special health professional assistance hotline at 1-800-525-6115.
•If patient vomits loading dose or any maintenance dose within 1 hour of administration, repeat dose as prescribed.
•Keep in mind that suicidal patient may not provide reliable information about vomiting. Watch such a patient to ensure that he ingests all of prescribed dosage.
•During treatment for acetaminophen overdose, monitor for signs of hepatotoxicity, such as prolonged bleeding time, altered coagulation, and easy bruising.
•Be aware that acetylcysteine may have a disagreeable odor, which disappears as treatment progresses.
•Because nebulization causes sticky residue on face and in mouth, have patient wash his face and rinse his mouth at the end of each treatment.
•Be aware that an open vial of solution may turn light purple but that this doesn't alter its effectiveness.
•Refrigerate opened vials and discard after 96 hours.
•Assess type, frequency, and characteristics of patient's cough. Particularly note sputum. If cough doesn't clear secretions, prepare to perform mechanical suctioning.
•Monitor patient for tachycardia.
PATIENT TEACHING
•Instruct patient to notify prescriber immediately about nausea, rash, or vomiting.
•Warn patient about acetylcysteine's unpleasant smell; reassure him that it subsides as treatment progresses.
•To decrease mucus viscosity, encourage patient to consume 2 to 3 L of fluid daily unless contraindicated by another condition.

acitretin

Soriatane

Class and Category
Chemical class: Synthetic retinoid
Therapeutic class: Antipsoriatic
Pregnancy category: X

A

Indications and Dosages
➤ *To treat severe psoriasis*
CAPSULES
Adults. 25 to 50 mg once daily with a meal.

Route	Onset	Peak	Duration
P.O.	Unknown	2 to 5 hr	Unknown

Mechanism of Action
Binds to several retinoid receptors to regulate gene transcription. Exactly how the action of this second-generation retinoid allows normal growth and development of skin is unknown.

Contraindications
Alcohol consumption; blood donation; breast-feeding; chronic hyperlipidemia; concurrent use of etretinate, methotrexate, or tetracycline; hypersensitivity to acitretin, other retinoids, or their components; pregnancy; severe hepatic or renal impairment

Interactions
DRUGS
methotrexate: Increased risk of hepatitis
oral contraceptives containing only progestin: Possibly decreased effectiveness of oral contraceptive
phenytoin: Possibly decreased protein binding of phenytoin
sulfonylureas: Possibly increased risk for hypoglycemia
tetracyclines: Increased intracranial pressure
vitamin A and other oral retinoids: Increased risk of hypervitaminosis A
ACTIVITIES
alcohol use: Increased risk of adverse reactions and acitretin toxicity

Adverse Reactions
CNS: Aggression, depression, fatigue, headache, hyperesthesia, hypotonia, insomnia, intracranial hypertension, paresthesia, peripheral neuropathy, rigors, somnolence, stroke, suicidal ideation, thirst
CV: Chest pain, decreased high-density lipoproteins, edema, elevated cholesterol or triglyceride levels, MI, thromboembolism
EENT: Abnormal or blurred vision, blepharitis, conjunctivitis, corneal epithelial abnormality, decreased night vision, deafness, dry eyes or mouth, earache, epistaxis, eye pain, gingival bleeding, gingivitis, increased saliva, photophobia, sinusitis, stomatitis, taste perversion, tinnitus, ulcerative stomatitits
ENDO: Hot flashes, hyperglycemia
GI: Anorexia, abdominal pain, diarrhea, elevated liver enzymes, hepatitis, hepatotoxicity, nausea, pancreatitis
GU: Vulvovaginitis
HEME: Hemorrhage, increased bleeding time
MS: Arthralgia, arthrosis, back pain, hyperostosis, myalgia, myopathy
SKIN: Abnormal skin or hair texture, alopecia, bullous eruption, cold or clammy skin, dermatitis, diaphoresis, dry or peeling skin, erythematous rash, flushing, fragility or thinning of skin, photosensitivity, pruritus, purpura, pyogenic granuloma, rash, scaling, seborrhea, skin fissure or ulceration
Other: Hypervitaminosis A, increased appetite

Nursing Considerations
•**WARNING** Do not give acitretin to a pregnant woman, a woman contemplating pregnancy, or a woman who may not use reliable contraception during drug therapy and for at least 3 years afterward because acitretin causes major fetal abnormalities.
•Make sure patient has had two negative urine or serum pregnancy tests with a sensitivity of at least 25 mIU/ml before receiving acitretin. The first test should be obtained when the decision is made to use acitretin and the second test during the first 5 days of the menstrual period just before acitretin therapy starts. For patients with amenorrhea, the second test should be done at least 11 days after the last act of unprotected sexual intercourse (which means without using two effective forms of contraception simultaneously).
•Check to make sure a female patient of childbearing age has signed the patient agreement and informed consent form before starting acitretin therapy.
•Obtain a lipid profile, as ordered, before acitretin therapy starts and every 1 to 2 weeks for up to 8 weeks or until lipid effects are known. In high-risk patients, such as those with diabetes, obesity, or a history of alcohol abuse and those taking acitretin long-term, check lipid profile periodically throughout therapy.

•Monitor liver function test results, as ordered. If hepatotoxicity is suspected, expect to stop drug and investigate cause.

•If patient takes acitretin long-term or she develops a skeletal disorder, prepare her for periodic bone radiography because ossification abnormalities can occur, especially of the vertebral column, knees, and ankles.

•Monitor the patient's eyes for abnormalities throughout therapy. Expect patient to stop drug and have an ophthalmologic examination if eye abnormalities occur.

•Monitor patient for evidence of increased intracranial pressure, such as papilledema, headache, nausea, vomiting, and visual disturbances. If papilledema occurs, stop drug therapy immediately and obtain a neurological evaluation, as ordered. Patient should never receive a tetracycline while taking acitretin because combined use can increase intracranial pressure.

•Assess patient for suidical ideation because depression and other psychiatric symptoms, including thoughts of self-harm, may occur with acitretin use. Expect drug to be discontinued if psychiatric symptoms develop.

•Significantly lower doses of phototherapy are needed during acitretin therapy because drug increases the risk of erythema.

PATIENT TEACHING

•**WARNING** Warn women of childbearing age that acitretin causes major fetal abnormalities.

•Inform woman of childbearing age that she must have a pregnancy test before acitretin therapy starts, every month during acitretin therapy, and every 3 months for 3 years after therapy stops.

•Stress to woman of childbearing age that she must use two effective forms of contraception simultaneously unless she has chosen absolute abstinence or has had a hysterectomy. This must begin at least 1 month before acitretin therapy starts and continue throughout therapy and for at least 3 years after therapy ends.

•Caution women taking oral contraceptives that some prescribed and OTC drugs, including herbal supplements such as St. John's wort, may interfere with oral contraceptives, and urge her to tell prescriber about all drugs she takes.

•Caution patient not to consume alcohol or products that contain alcohol during ac-

itretin therapy and for 2 months after therapy ends.

•Warn patient, male or female of any age, nopt to donate blood during acitretin therapy and for at least 3 years after it ends.

•Review the acitretin medication guide with patient, and answer the patient's questions.

•Inform patient that psoriasis may worsen during initial treatment and that tull effects of drug may not be seen for up to 3 months.

•Caution patient to avoid hazardous activities until drug's CNS and ophthalmic effects are known.

•Inform patient that tolerance to contact lenses may decrease during therapy and for a period of time after treatment ends.

•Advise patient not to take more than the minimum recommended daily allowance of vitamin A during acetretin therapy because of the risk of vitamin A toxicity.

•Caution patient not to use sun lamps and to avoid excessive exposure to sunlight because the effects of UV light are enhanced by retinoids such as acitretin.

adalimumab

HUMIRA

Class and Category

Chemical class: Recombinant human IgG1 monoclonal antibody
Therapeutic class: Disease-modifying antirheumatic
Pregnancy category: B

Indications and Dosages

➤ *To reduce signs and symptoms, induce major clinical response, inhibit progression of structural damage, and improve physical function in patients with moderately to severely active rheumatoid arthritis; to reduce signs and symptoms, inhibit progression of structural damage, and improve physical function in patients with psoriatic arthritis; to reduce signs and symptoms in patients with active ankylosing spondylitis*

SUBCUTANEOUS INJECTION

Adults. 40 mg every other wk.

DOSAGE ADJUSTMENT Dosage may be adjusted to 40 mg every wk, as needed and prescribed, for patients not taking methotrexate.

➤ *To reduce signs and symptoms and induce and maintain clinical remission in patients with moderately to severely active Crohn's disease who have had an inadequate response to conventional therapy or who have stopped responding to or have become intolerant of infliximab*

SUBCUTANEOUS INJECTION

Adults. *Initial:* 40 mg q.i.d. for 1 day or 40 mg b.i.d. for 2 consecutive days, followed by 80 mg 2 wk later. *Maintenance:* 40 mg every other wk starting at week 4.

➤ *To reduce signs and symptoms of moderately to severely active polyarticular juvenile idiopathic arthritis*

SUBCUTANEOUS INJECTION

Children age 4 and over who weigh 30 kg (66 lb) or more. 40 mg every other wk.
Children age 4 and over who weigh less than 30 kg but at least 15 kg (33 lb). 20 mg every other wk.

➤ *To treat moderate to severe chronic plaque psoriasis in patients who are candidates for systemic therapy or phototherapy, and when other systemic therapies are less appropriate*

SUBCUTANEOUS INJECTION

Adults. *Initial:* 80 mg followed 1 wk later with 40 mg. *Maintenance:* 40 mg every other wk.

Mechanism of Action

Binds to tumor necrosis factor (TNF) to block interaction with p55 and p75 cell-surface TNF receptors and lyses surface TNF-expressing cells in the presence of complement. TNF may be a major component of rheumatoid arthritis inflammation and joint destruction. Reduced TNF level in synovial fluid improves signs and symptoms and prevent further structural damage in rheumatoid arthritis.

Contraindications

Active infection, breast-feeding, hypersensitivity to adalimumab or its components

Interactions

DRUGS

anakinra: Possibly increased risk of serious

infection and neutropenia
live vaccines: Increased risk of adverse vaccine effects

Adverse Reactions

CNS: Confusion, fever, headache, hypertensive encephalopathy, multiple sclerosis, paresthesia, subdural hematoma, syncope, tremor
CV: Arrhythmias, atrial fibrillation, cardiac arrest, chest pain, coronary artery disease, congestive heart failure, hypercholesterolemia, hyperlipidemia, hypertension, MI, palpitations, pericardial effusion, pericarditis, peripheral edema, tachycardia
EENT: Cataracts, sinusitis
ENDO: Ketosis, parathyroid disorder
GI: Abdominal pain, cholecystitis, cholelithiasis, diverticulitis, elevated alkaline phosphatase level, elevated liver enzyme levels, esophagitis, gastroenteritis, hemorrhage, hepatic necrosis, nausea, vomiting
GU: Hematuria, paraproteinemia, pyelonephritis, UTI
HEME: Agranulocytosis, aplastic anemia, granulocytopenia, leukopenia, lymphocytosis, pancytopenia, polycythemia, thrombocytopenia
MS: Arthritis (including pyogenic or septic arthritis); back, extremity, pelvic, or thorax pain; bone disorder, fracture, or necrosis; muscle spasms; myasthenia; prosthetic infections; synovitis
RESP: Asthma, bronchitis, bronchospasm, decreased pulmonary function, dyspnea, pleural effusion, pneumonia, pulmonary tuberculosis, upper respiratory tract infection
SKIN: Cellulitis, erysipelas, erythema multiforme, herpes zoster, rash, urticaria
Other: Anaphylaxis; antibody formation against adalimumab; dehydration; erythema multiforme; flare-up of disease process; flu-like symptoms; healing abnormalities; injection site erythema, hemorrhage, itching, pain, or swelling; invasive fungal infection; lupus-like symptoms; lymphomas; malignancies; opportunistic infection; postsurgical infections; sepsis; tuberculosis (miliary, lymphatic, or peritoneal)

Nursing Considerations

•Use adalimumab cautiously in patients with recurrent infection or increased risk of infection, patients who live in regions where tuberculosis and mycoses are endemic, and patients with a history of CNS demyelinating disorders because they occur, rarely, during adalimumab therapy.

• **WARNING** If patient has evidence of an active infection when drug is prescribed, therapy shouldn't begin until infection has been treated. Monitor all patients for infection during therapy, especially those receiving immunosuppressants. If a serious infection develops, expect prescriber to stop drug.

• Make sure patient has a tuberculin skin test before therapy starts. If skin test is positive, treatment of latent tuberculosis will start before adalimumab, as prescribed.

• Be aware that the needle cover of the syringe contains dry rubber. Don't handle if you're allergic to latex.

• To activate the protection device on the needles of prefilled syringes delivered to institutions, hold the syringe in one hand and, with the other hand, slide the outer protective shield over the exposed needle until it locks into place.

• **WARNING** Stop adalimumab immediately and tell prescriber if patient has an allergic reaction. Expect to provide supportive care.

• Monitor patient closely for signs and symptoms of congestive heart failure (sudden, unexplained weight gain; dyspnea; crackles; anxiety), and notify prescriber if they occur.

• Monitor patient's CBC, as ordered, because adalimumab may have adverse hematologic effects. Notify prescriber about persistent fever, bruising, bleeding, or pallor.

PATIENT TEACHING

• Inform patient that the first injection of adalimumab must be administered with a health care professional present.

• Teach patient or caregiver how to give adalimumab as a subcutaneous injection at home, if applicable. Emphasize importance of injecting the full amount in the syringe (0.8 ml) to obtain the correct dose of 40 mg.

• If patient is allergic to latex, explain that the needle cover contains rubber.

• Caution patient against reusing needles and syringes. Provide patient or caregiver with a puncture resistant container for disposal of needles and syringes at home.

• Instruct patient or caregiver to rotate injection sites and to avoid injecting in any area that is tender, bruised, red, or hard.

• Inform patient that prefilled syringes must be refrigerated (not frozen), protected from light, and stored in the original container.

• Urge patient to check expiration dates and not to use outdated drug.

• Review signs and symptoms of an allergic reaction (rash, swollen face, difficulty breathing), and tell patient to seek emergency care immediately if these occur.

• Inform patient that injection site reactions (such as redness, rash, swelling, itching, and bruising) may occur but are usually mild and transient. Instruct him to apply a towel soaked with cold water on the injection site if it hurts or remains swollen. If reaction does not disappear or seems to worsen, tell patient to call prescriber immediately.

• Inform patient that tuberculosis may occur during adalimumab therapy. Instruct him to report persistent cough, wasting or weight loss, and low-grade fever to prescriber.

• Teach patient to recognize evidence of infection and bleeding disorders and to tell prescriber if they occur; drug may need to be stopped. Advise patient to avoid people with infections and to have all prescribed laboratory tests.

• Inform patient that the risk of developing certain kinds of cancer, especially lymphomas, is higher in patients taking adalimumab but is still rare. Emphasize the importance of follow-up visits and reporting an unusual or sudden onset of signs or symptoms.

• Caution patient against receiving live-virus vaccines while taking adalimumab because doing so may adversely effect the immune system.

• Inform patient that blood samples may be required periodically, but especially around week 24 of therapy, to check for autoantibody development. Tell him that drug will need to be discontinued if autoantibodies are detected.

• Instruct patient to report lupus-like signs and symptoms that, although rare, may occur during therapy, such as chest pain that does not go away, shortness of breath, joint pain, or a rash on his cheeks or arms that's sensitive to the sun. Tell him that drug may need to be discontinued if these occur.

• Advise patient to inform all health care providers about adalimumab use and to inform prescriber about any OTC medications being taken, including herbal remedies and vitamin and mineral supplements.

adenosine

Adenocard, Adenoscan

Class and Category

Chemical class: Monophosphorylated adenine riboside
Therapeutic class: Antiarrhythmic
Pregnancy category: C

Indications and Dosages

➤ *To convert paroxysmal supraventricular tachycardia (PSVT) to normal sinus rhythm*

I.V. INJECTION
Adults and children weighing 50 kg (110 lb) or more. *Initial:* 6 mg by rapid peripheral I.V. bolus over 1 to 2 sec. If PSVT continues after 1 to 2 min, 12 mg given as rapid bolus and repeated in 1 to 2 min if needed.
WARNING Don't give single doses of more than 12 mg.
Children weighing less than 50 kg. *Initial:* 0.05 to 0.1 mg/kg as rapid central or peripheral I.V. bolus followed by saline flush. If PSVT continues after 1 to 2 min, additional bolus injections are given, incrementally increasing dose by 0.05 to 0.1 mg/kg. Follow each bolus with saline flush. Injections continue until PSVT converts to normal sinus rhythm or until patient reaches maximum single dose of 0.3 mg/kg.

Route	Onset	Peak	Duration
I.V.	Immediate	Immediate	Unknown

Mechanism of Action
Slows conduction time through the AV node and can interrupt AV node reentry pathways to restore normal sinus rhythm.

Incompatibilities
Don't mix adenosine with other drugs.

Contraindications
Atrial fibrillation or flutter; hypersensitivity to adenosine; second- or third-degree heart block or sick sinus syndrome, except in patients with a functioning artificial pacemaker; ventricular tachycardia

Interactions
DRUGS
carbamazepine: Increased heart block
digoxin, verapamil: Possibly increased depressant effect on SA or AV node
dipyridamole: Increased effects of adenosine
methylxanthines, such as theophylline: Antagonized effects of adenosine
FOODS
caffeine: Antagonized effects of adenosine

Adverse Reactions
CNS: Apprehension, dizziness, headache, heaviness in arms, light-headedness, nervousness, paresthesia, seizures
CV: Atrial fibrillation, bradycardia, chest pain or pressure, heart block, hypertension, hypotension, MI, palpitations, prolonged asystole, sinus exit block or pause, torsades de pointes, transient hypertension, ventricular fibrillation, ventricular tachycardia
EENT: Blurred vision, metallic taste, throat tightness
GI: Nausea, vomiting
MS: Jaw, neck, and back pain
RESP: Bronchoconstriction, bronchospasm, dyspnea, hyperventilation, respiratory arrest
SKIN: Diaphoresis, facial flushing
Other: Injection site reaction

Nursing Considerations
•Before use, inspect adenosine for crystals. If solution isn't clear, don't give it.
•Give adenosine by rapid I.V. bolus over 1 to 2 seconds only. Slower delivery can cause systemic vasodilation and reflex tachycardia.
•Expect prescriber to inject adenosine directly into a vein to make sure drug reaches systemic circulation. If given into an I.V. line, give as close to insertion site as possible and follow with rapid saline flush.
•Monitor heart rate and rhythm, blood pressure, and respiratory status often during adenosine therapy.
•Be aware that at the time of conversion to normal sinus rhythm, arrhythmias (such as PVCs, premature atrial contractions, sinus bradycardia, sinus tachycardia, and AV block) may occur for a few seconds but don't require intervention.
•**WARNING** Stop drug use and notify prescriber immediately if severe respiratory difficulties develop.
•Store adenosine at room temperature. Discard unused portion.
PATIENT TEACHING
•Instruct patient to report chest pain, palpi-

tations, difficulty breathing, or severe headache during adenosine therapy.
•Warn patient that mild, temporary reactions
may occur, such as flushing, nausea, and
dizziness.

alatrofloxacin mesylate
Trovan I.V.

trovafloxacin mesylate
Trovan

Class and Category
Chemical class: Fluoroquinolone
Therapeutic class: Antibacterial
Pregnancy category: C

Indications and Dosages
➤ *To treat life-threatening nosocomial
pneumonia*
TABLETS, I.V. INFUSION
Adults. 300 mg I.V. every 24 hr followed by
200 mg P.O. every 24 hr when patient is stabi-
lized for total of 10 to 14 days.
➤ *To treat life-threatening community-
acquired pneumonia*
TABLETS, I.V. INFUSION
Adults. 200 mg I.V. every 24 hr followed by
200 mg P.O. every 24 hr when patient is stabilized for total of 7 to 14 days; or 200 mg
P.O. every 24 hr for total of 7 to 14 days.
➤ *To treat complicated, life-threatening
intra-abdominal infections, including
postsurgical, gynecologic, and pelvic
infections*
TABLETS, I.V. INFUSION
Adults. 300 mg I.V. every 24 hr followed by
200 mg P.O. every 24 hr when patient is stabilized for total of 7 to 14 days.
➤ *To treat complicated, life-threatening or
limb-threatening skin and soft-tissue infections, including diabetic foot infections*
TABLETS, I.V. INFUSION
Adults. 200 mg P.O. every 24 hr—or 200 mg
I.V. every 24 hr followed by 200 mg P.O. every
24 hr when patient is stabilized—for total of
10 to 14 days.
DOSAGE ADJUSTMENT For patients with mild
to moderate cirrhosis, 300-mg I.V. dosage reduced to 200 mg and 200-mg I.V. and P.O.
dosage reduced to 100 mg.

Mechanism of Action
Interferes with DNA gyrase, the enzyme
needed for DNA replication in aerobic and
anaerobic bacteria. May be active against
pathogens resistant to such antibiotics as
penicillins, cephalosporins, aminoglycosides, macrolides, and tetracyclines.

Incompatibilities
Don't mix alatrofloxacin with or infuse it simultaneously through same I.V. line as other
drugs. Don't dilute it with normal saline solution or lactated Ringer's solution.

Contraindications
Hypersensitivity to alatrofloxacin, quinolone
antimicrobials, trovafloxacin, or their components

Interactions
DRUGS
*antacids that contain aluminum, citric acid,
magnesium, or sodium citrate; iron; morphine sulfate; sucralfate:* Reduced absorption
of trovafloxacin

Adverse Reactions
CNS: Dizziness, headache, light-headedness,
seizures
CV: Hypotension
EENT: Hoarseness, throat tightness
GI: Abdominal pain, acute hepatic failure
(anorexia, dark urine, dysphagia, fatigue,
jaundice, pale stool, and vomiting)
GU: Vaginitis
RESP: Dyspnea
SKIN: Photosensitivity, rash, urticaria or
other skin reactions
Other: Angioedema

Nursing Considerations
•Infuse alatrofloxacin over 60 minutes; rapid
or bolus I.V. delivery may cause hypotension.
•Periodically assess patient's liver function
test results. Results may be elevated for up
to 21 days after alatrofloxacin administration.
•WARNING Be aware that alatrofloxacin may
cause severe liver damage, requiring liver
transplantation or leading to death. Expect
therapy to last no longer than 2 weeks to reduce risk of liver damage. Alatrofloxacin is
reserved for hospitalized patients with life-
or limb-threatening infections.

A

PATIENT TEACHING
•Instruct patient to report rash; urticaria; difficulty swallowing; swelling of the lips, face, or tongue; hoarseness; or throat tightness.

albuterol
(salbutamol)

Proventil

albuterol sulfate
(salbutamol sulphate)

AccuNeb, Airet, Gen-Salbutamol (CAN), Novo-Salmol (CAN), Proair HFA, Proventil, Proventil HFA, Proventil Repetabs, Proventil Syrup, Ventolin HFA, Ventolin Syrup, Volmax

Class and Category
Chemical class: Selective beta$_2$-adrenergic agonist, sympathomimetic
Therapeutic class: Bronchodilator
Pregnancy category: C

Indications and Dosages
➤ *To prevent exercise-induced asthma*
INHALATION AEROSOL
Adults and children over age 4. 2 inhalations 15 to 30 min before exercise.

➤ *To treat bronchospasm in patients with reversible obstructive airway disease or acute bronchospastic attack*
E.R. TABLETS
Adults and children over age 12. *Initial:* 4 or 8 mg every 12 hr. *Maximum:* 32 mg daily in divided doses every 12 hr.
Children ages 6 to 12. *Initial:* 4 mg every 12 hr. *Maximum:* 24 mg daily in divided doses every 12 hr.
REPETABS
Adults and children over age 12. *Initial:* 4 to 8 mg every 12 hr. *Maximum:* 32 mg daily in divided doses every 12 hr.
Children ages 6 to 11. *Initial:* 4 mg every 12 hr.
Maximum: 24 mg daily in divided doses every 12 hr.
SYRUP
Adults and children over age 14. *Initial:* 2 to 4 mg (1 to 2 tsp) t.i.d. or q.i.d. *Maximum:* 32 mg daily in divided doses.
Children ages 6 to 14. *Initial:* 2 mg (1 tsp) t.i.d. or q.i.d. *Maximum:* 24 mg daily in divided doses.

Children ages 2 to 6. *Initial:* 0.1 mg/kg t.i.d. (not to exceed 2 mg t.i.d.), increased to 0.2 mg/kg t.i.d. (not to exceed 4 mg t.i.d.).
TABLETS
Adults and children over age 12. *Initial:* 2 or 4 mg t.i.d. or q.i.d. *Maximum:* 32 mg daily in divided doses.
Children ages 6 to 12. *Initial:* 2 mg t.i.d. or q.i.d. *Maximum:* 24 mg daily in divided doses.
DOSAGE ADJUSTMENT For elderly patients, initial dosage reduced to 2 mg (1 tsp) of syrup t.i.d. or q.i.d. or 2 mg of tablets t.i.d. or q.i.d. (up to 32 mg daily).
INHALATION AEROSOL
Adults and children age 4 and over. 1 inhalation every 4 hr to 2 inhalations every 4 to 6 hr.
INHALATION CAPSULES (ROTOCAPS)
Adults and children age 4 and over. 200 mcg inhaled every 4 to 6 hr using inhalation device. *Maximum:* 400 mcg every 4 to 6 hr.
INHALATION SOLUTION
Adults and children age 12 and over. 2.5 mg t.i.d. or q.i.d. by nebulization over 5 to 15 min.
Children ages 2 to 12. *Initial:* 0.1 to 0.15 mg/kg t.i.d. or q.i.d. *Maximum:* 2.5 mg t.i.d. or q.i.d.

Route	Onset	Peak	Duration
P.O. (E.R. tab)	30 min	2 to 3 hr	12 hr
P.O. (syrup)	Rapid	2 hr	Unknown
P.O. (tab)	30 min	2 to 3 hr	4 to 8 hr
Inhalation (aerosol)	5 to 15 min	50 to 55 min	3 to 6 hr
Inhalation (rotocap)	5 to 15 min	0.5 to 3 hr	2 to 6 hr
Inhalation (solution)	5 to 15 min	1 to 2 hr	3 to 6 hr

Contraindications
Hypersensitivity to albuterol or its components

Interactions
DRUGS
beta blockers: Inhibited effects of albuterol
bronchodilators (sympathomimetics), such as theophylline: Possibly adverse CV effects
digoxin: Decreased serum digoxin level
MAO inhibitors, tricyclic antidepressants:

Mechanism of Action

Albuterol attaches to beta$_2$ receptors on bronchial cell membranes, which stimulates the intracellular enzyme adenylate cyclase to convert adenosine triphosphate (ATP) to cyclic adenosine monophosphate (cAMP). This reaction decreases intracellular calcium levels. It also increases intracellular levels of cAMP, as shown. Together, these effects relax bronchial smooth-muscle cells and inhibit histamine release.

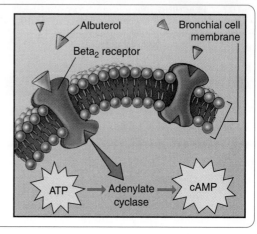

Increased vascular effects of albuterol
methyldopa: Increased vasopressor effect of methyldopa
potassium-lowering drugs: Possibly hypokalemia
potassium-wasting diuretics: Possibly increased hypokalemia

Adverse Reactions

CNS: Anxiety, dizziness, drowsiness, headache, hyperkinesia, insomnia, irritability, nervousness, tremor, vertigo, weakness
CV: Angina; arrhythmias, including atrial fibrillation, extrasystoles, supraventricular tachycardia, and tachycardia; chest pain; hypertension; hypotension; palpitations
EENT: Altered taste, dry mouth and throat, ear pain, glossitis, hoarseness, oropharyngeal edema, pharyngitis, rhinitis, taste perversion
ENDO: Hyperglycemia
GI: Anorexia, diarrhea, dysphagia, heartburn, nausea, vomiting
GU: UTI
MS: Muscle cramps
RESP: Bronchospasm, cough, dyspnea, paradoxical bronchospasm, pulmonary edema
SKIN: Diaphoresis, flushing, pallor, pruritus, rash, urticaria
Other: Angioedema, hypokalemia, infection, metabolic acidosis

Nursing Considerations

•Administer pressurized inhalations of albuterol during second half of inspiration, when airways are open wider and aerosol distribution is more effective.

•**WARNING** Use cautiously in patients with cardiac disorders, diabetes mellitus, digitalis intoxication, hypertension, hyperthyroidism, or history of seizures. Albuterol can worsen these conditions.
•Monitor serum potassium level because albuterol may cause transient hypokalemia.
•Be aware that drug tolerance can develop with prolonged use.

PATIENT TEACHING
•Teach patient to use inhaler. Tell him to shake canister before use and to check that a new canister is working by spraying it the appropriate number of times (once to four times based on manufacturer instructions) into the air while looking for a fine mist.
•Instruct patient to wash mouthpiece with water once a week and let it air-dry.
•Advise patient to wait at least 1 minute between inhalations.
•Tell patient to check with his prescriber before using other inhaled drugs.
•Warn patient not to exceed prescribed dose or frequency. If doses become less effective, tell him to contact his prescriber.
•Tell patient to immediately report signs and symptoms of allergic reaction, such as difficulty swallowing, itching, and rash.

alefacept

Amevive

Class and Category

Chemical class: Recombinant leukocyte func-

tion-associated antigen-3 immunoglobulin GI fusion protein
Therapeutic class: Immunosuppresant
Pregnancy category: B

Indications and Dosages

➤ *To treat moderate to severe chronic plaque psoriasis in patients who are candidates for systemic therapy or phototherapy*

I.V. INJECTION

Adults. *Initial:* 7.5 mg every wk for 12 wk. After at least 12 wk in which drug isn't given, a second 12-wk course may be given, if needed and if patient's CD4 and T-lymphocyte counts are within normal ranges.

I.M. INJECTION

Adults. 15 mg every week for 12 wk. After at least 12 wk in which drug isn't given, a second 12-wk course may be given, if needed and if patient's CD4 and T-lymphocyte counts are within normal ranges.

Mechanism of Action

Binds to the lymphocyte antigen and CD2 and inhibits LFA-3/CD2 interaction to interfere with T-lymphocyte activation. Alefacept also reduces the subsets of CD2+ T lymphocytes. Because activation of T lymphocytes plays a role in the pathophysiology of chronic plaque psoriasis, interference with lymphocytic activity helps to prevent plaque formation.

Incompatibilities

Don't add other drugs to solutions containing alefacept.

Contraindications

Breast-feeding, hypersensitivity to alefacept or its components

Adverse Reactions

CNS: Chills, dizziness, headache
CV: Coronary artery disease, MI
EENT: Pharyngitis
GI: Nausea
HEME: Lymphopenia
MS: Myalgia
RESP: Increased cough
SKIN: Pruritus, urticaria
Other: Angioedema, injection site pain or inflammation, infection, malignancies

Nursing Considerations

• Use alefacept cautiously in patients at high risk for malignancy because the drug increases risk of malignancy development. Know that drug isn't recommended for use in patients with a history of a systemic malignancy.
• Also use cautiously in patients with chronic infections or history of recurrent infection. Drug may increase risk of infection because of its immunosuppressive action.
• Obtain a CD4+ and T-lymphocyte count before initiating drug therapy, as ordered. If counts are below normal, be aware that therapy shouldn't be started. After therapy starts, monitor patient's CD4+ and T-lymphocyte counts weekly throughout therapy. If levels drop below 250 cells/microliter, notify prescriber because drug will need to be withheld. If counts remain below 250 cells/microliter for 1 month, know that drug should be discontinued.
• Reconstitute drug with 0.6 ml using only the supplied diluent (sterile water for injection) before administration. With the needle pointed at the sidewall of the vial, slowly inject the diluent into the vial of alefacept. Be aware that some foaming will occur. To prevent excessive foaming, don't shake or vigorously agitate vial. Instead, gently swirl vial during dissolution, which usually takes less than 2 minutes.
• Administer drug as soon as possible after reconstitution. Discard solution if not used within 4 hours.
• Don't filter reconstituted solution during preparation or administration.
• For I.M. administration, inject the full 0.5 ml of solution. Use a different injection site for each subsequent injection, injecting at least 1 inch away from previous sites. Never inject the drug into tender, bruised, red, or hard areas.
• For I.V. administration, prepare two syringes with 3 ml normal saline solution for preadministration and postadministration flush. Then prime the winged infusion set with 3 ml normal saline solution and insert into vein. Attach filled syringe to infusion set and administer solution over no more than 5 seconds. Finish by flushing set with 3 ml of normal saline solution.
• Be aware that drug therapy shouldn't be initiated in a patient with a concurrent seri-

ous infection. Monitor patient closely during and after therapy for signs and symptoms of infection. If these occur, report them to the prescriber immediately and initiate treatment, as prescribed, to reduce risk of serious infection. If infection becomes serious, expect drug to be discontinued.

•Monitor patient for allergic reactions. If these occur, discontinue drug and notify prescriber immediately.

PATIENT TEACHING

•Advise patient that weekly blood tests will be required to monitor his WBC during alefacept therapy.

•Teach patient signs and symptoms of infection and common warning signs of malignancy. Emphasize importance of complying with follow-up visits and promptly reporting any unusual or sudden signs or symptoms suggesting malignancy or infection.

•Inform female patient to notify prescriber if she becomes pregnant while taking alefacept or within 8 weeks after discontinuing drug.

alendronate sodium

Fosamax

Class and Category

Chemical class: Aminobisphosphonate
Therapeutic class: Bone resorption inhibitor
Pregnancy category: C

Indications and Dosages

➤ *To prevent postmenopausal osteoporosis*
TABLETS
Adults. 5 mg daily or 35 mg once weekly in the morning with a full glass of water at least 30 min before first food, drink, or drug.

➤ *To treat postmenopausal osteoporosis*
TABLETS
Adults. 10 mg daily or 70 mg once weekly in the morning with a full glass of water at least 30 min before first food, drink, or drug.

➤ *To treat Paget's disease of the bone in patients whose alkaline phosphatase level is twice the upper limit of normal or higher and who are symptomatic and at risk for further complications*
TABLETS
Adults. 40 mg daily with a full glass of water for 6 mo.

DOSAGE ADJUSTMENT Dosage increased to

10 mg daily for postmenopausal women not receiving estrogen.

➤ *To increase bone mass in men with osteoporosis*
TABLETS
Adults. 10 mg daily or 70 mg once weekly in the morning with a full glass of water at least 30 min before first food, drink, or drug.

➤ *To treat glucocorticoid-induced osteoporosis in men and women who receive a daily glucocorticoid dosage equal to or greater than 7.5 mg of prednisone and who have low bone mineral density*
TABLETS
Adults. 5 mg daily in the morning with a full glass of water at least 30 min before first food, drink, or drug.

Route	Onset	Peak	Duration
P.O.	Unknown	Unknown	6 wk*

Mechanism of Action

Reduces the activity of cells that cause bone loss, slows the rate of bone loss after menopause, and increases the amount of bone mass. May act by inhibiting osteoclast activity on newly formed bone resorption surfaces, which reduces the number of sites where bone is remodeled. Bone formation then exceeds bone resorption at these remodeling sites, which gradually increases bone mass. May also inhibit bone dissolution by binding to hydroxyapatite crystals, which are composed of calcium, phosphate, and hydroxide and give bone its rigid structure.

Contraindications

Esophageal abnormalities that delay esophageal emptying, such as stricture or achalasia; hypersensitivity to alendronate; hypocalcemia; inability to stand or sit upright for at least 30 minutes

Interactions

DRUGS

antacids, calcium, iron, multivalent cations:

---

* After single 5-mg dose for osteoporosis; 6 mo after single 5-mg dose for Paget's disease.

Decreased absorption of alendronate
aspirin: Increased risk of GI distress
FOODS
any food: Delayed absorption and decreased
serum level of alendronate

Adverse Reactions
CNS: Asthenia, dizziness, headache, vertigo
CV: Peripheral edema
GI: Abdominal distention and pain, constipation, diarrhea, dysphagia, esophageal perforation or ulceration, esophagitis, flatulence, gastritis, gastroesophageal reflux disease, heartburn, indigestion, melena, nausea,
vomiting
MS: Arthralgia, bone pain, focal osteomalacia, joint swelling, muscle spasms, myalgia
SKIN: Photosensitivity, pruritus, rash,
Stevens-Johnson syndrome, toxic epidermal
necrolysis
Other: Hypocalcemia

Nursing Considerations
•Monitor patient's serum calcium level before, during, and after treatment. Expect
hypocalcemia to be treated before alendronate therapy. If hypocalcemia occurs during therapy, expect prescriber to order a calcium supplement.
•Ensure adequate dietary intake of calcium
and vitamin D before, during, and after
treatment.
•**WARNING** Alendronate may irritate upper GI
mucosa, causing such adverse reactions as
esophageal ulceration. To help minimize
these reactions, have patient take it with a
full glass of water and remain upright for at
least 30 minutes.
PATIENT TEACHING
•Advise patient to take alendronate in the
morning with a full glass of water. Explain
that such beverages as orange juice, coffee,
and mineral water reduce alendronate's effects.
•To help reduce esophageal irritation, tell
patient not to chew or suck on tablet.
•Instruct patient to wait at least 30 minutes
after taking alendronate before eating,
drinking, or taking other drugs. Teach patient to remain upright for 30 minutes after
taking alendronate *and* until she has eaten
the first food of the day.
•Encourage patient to consume adequate
daily amounts of calcium and vitamin D.

alfuzosin hydrochloride
Uroxatral

A

Class and Category
Chemical class: Tetrahydro-2-
furancarboxamide hydrochloride
Therapeutic class: Selective alpha$_1$-
adrenergic antagonist
Pregnancy category: B

Indications and Dosages
➤ *To treat signs and symptoms of benign
    prostatic hyperplasia*
E.R. TABLETS
Adults. 10 mg daily taken immediately after
same meal each day.

Mechanism of Action
Selectively blocks alpha$_1$-adrenergic receptors in smooth muscle of the bladder
neck and prostate, causing relaxation, and
blocks postsynaptic alpha$_1$ adrenorecep-
tors in the bladder base and neck, prostate, prostatic capsule, and urethra, preventing further action at these sites. These
actions improve urine flow and bladder
emptying and reduce urinary hesitancy,
frequency, and nocturia.

Contraindications
Hypersensitivity to alfuzosin or its components, moderate or severe hepatic insufficiency, use with CYP3A4 inhibitors, such as
itraconazole, ketoconazole, and ritonavir

Interactions
DRUGS
alpha blockers: May potentiate action of alfuzosin
antihypertensives, nitrates: Possibly synergistic lowering of blood pressure and syncope
*CYP3A4 inhibitors (such as itraconazole, ke-
toconazole, and ritonavir):* Increased effects
of alfuzosin

Adverse Reactions
CNS: Dizziness, fatigue, headache
CV: Angina, chest pain, edema, orthostatic
hypotension, QT-interval prolongation,
tachycardia
EENT: Pharyngitis, rhinitis, sinusitis
GI: Abdominal pain, constipation, diarrhea,
indigestion, jaundice, hepatotoxicity, nausea

GU: Impotence, priapism
RESP: Bronchitis, upper respiratory tract infection
SKIN: Flushing, pruritus, rash, urticaria
Other: Angioedema, generalized pain

Nursing Considerations
•Use alfuzosin cautiously in patients who have symptomatic hypotension or who have had a hypotensive response to other drugs. Orthostatic hypotension (with or without symptoms such as dizziness) may occur within hours after alfuzosin administration.
•Use cautiously in patients with severe renal insufficiency; decreased drug clearance may increase risk of adverse reactions.
•Be aware that alfuzosin shouldn't be used to treat bladder symptoms in women.
•Know that alpha$_1$ blockers such as alfuzosin may predispose patients to intraoperative floppy iris syndrome during cataract surgery that may require surgical repair.
•Monitor patient for chest pain. If symptoms of angina pectoris occur or worsen, notify prescriber immediately and expect drug to be discontinued.

PATIENT TEACHING
•Stress need to take alfuzosin immediately after a meal because absorption is decreased by 50% if taken on an empty stomach.
•Tell patient not to crush or chew tablets but to swallow them whole.
•Caution patient to avoid hazardous activities until drug's CNS effects are known and also for several hours after taking dose; blood pressure may drop suddenly after use.

alglucerase

Ceredase

Class and Category
Chemical class: Glucocerebrosidase beta-glucosidase
Therapeutic class: Enzyme replacement
Pregnancy category: C

Indications and Dosages
➤ *To treat chronic nonneuropathic Gaucher's disease in patients with moderate to severe anemia, thrombocytopenia with bleeding tendencies, bone disease, or significant hepatomegaly or splenomegaly*

I.V. INFUSION
Adults and children age 2 and over. Highly individualized. 2.5 units/kg to 60 units/kg infused over 1 to 2 hr, usually every 2 wk.
DOSAGE ADJUSTMENT Highly individualized based on body size and disease severity. Some patients may need infusion once every other day; others may need it once every 4 wk. Maintenance dosage progressively reduced every 3 to 6 mo to as low as 1 unit/kg.

Route	Onset	Peak	Duration
I.V.	Up to 60 min	Unknown	Variable

Mechanism of Action
Catalyzes hydrolysis of glucocerebroside to glucose and ceramide in membrane lipids. Gaucher's disease results from deficiency of the enzyme beta-glucocerebrosidase and causes the lipid glucocerebroside to accumulate in tissue macrophages.

Contraindications
Hypersensitivity to alglucerase

Adverse Reactions
CNS: Chills, dizziness, fatigue, fever, headache
CV: Transient peripheral edema, vasomotor irritability
EENT: Oral ulcerations
GI: Abdominal discomfort, diarrhea, nausea, vomiting
MS: Backache
Other: I.V. site burning, itching, or swelling

Nursing Considerations
•Before starting therapy, expect to give antihistamines if patient is hypersensitive to drug.
•On day of dose, use aseptic technique to dilute alglucerase with normal saline solution to final volume of no more than 200 ml.
•Don't shake drug, which could inactivate it.
•Don't use alglucerase if it's discolored or contains precipitate.
•Be aware that drug doesn't contain preservatives. Discard unused portion.
•Infuse drug with in-line I.V. particle filter.

PATIENT TEACHING
•Tell patient that he may experience flulike symptoms with each dose of alglucerase.
•Instruct patient to report headache, hot flashes, nausea, and other adverse reactions.

•Inform patient that alglucerase is derived from pooled human placental tissue and poses a slight risk of viral contamination.
•Advise patient to keep appointments for scheduled doses of alglucerase.

aliskiren

Tekturna

Class and Category

Chemical class: Hemifumarate salt
Therapeutic class: Antihypertensive (direct renin inhibitor)
Pregnancy category: C (first trimester), D (second and third trimester)

Indications and Dosages

➤ *To treat hypertension*

TABLETS

Adults. 150 mg once daily, increased to 300 mg once daily, as needed.

Route	Onset	Peak	Duration
P.O.	Unknown	1 to 3 hr	Unknown

Mechanism of Action

Inhibits renin secreted by the kidneys in response to decreased blood volume and renal perfusion. Renin cleaves angiotensinogen to form angiotensin I, which is converted to angiotensin II by ACE and non-ACE pathways. Angiotensin II is a powerful vasoconstrictor that induces release of catecholamines from the adrenal medulla and prejunctional nerve endings. It also promotes aldosterone secretion and sodium reabsorption. Together, these actions increase blood pressure. By inhibiting renin release, aliskiren impairs the renin-angiotensin-aldosterone system. Without the vasoconstrictive effect of angiotension II, blood pressure decreases.

Contraindications

Hypersensitivity to aliskiren or its components; pregnancy; renal impairment, disease, or failure

Interactions

DRUGS

ACE inhibitors (diabetics): Increased risk of hyperkalemia
atorvastatin, cyclosporin, ketoconazole: Increased aliskiren blood level
furosemide: Decreased blood furosemide levels
irbesartan: Decreased blood aliskiren level

Adverse Reactions

CNS: Dizziness, fatigue, headache, seizures
CV: Hypotension
EENT: Nasopharyngitis
GI: Abdominal pain, diarrhea, dyspepsia, gastroesophageal reflux
GU: Renal calculi
HEME: Decreased hemoglobin and hematocrit
MS: Back pain
RESP: Increased cough, upper respiratory tract infection
SKIN: Rash
Other: Angioedema of head and neck, elevated creatine kinase or uric acid level, gout, hyperkalemia

Nursing Considerations

•Use cautiously in patients who have a history of dialysis or who have moderate to severe renal dysfunction; it isn't known whether nephritic syndrome and renovascular hypertension are adverse effects of aliskiren therapy.
•To prevent hypotension, take measures to correct volume or salt depletion from high-dose diuretic therapy before starting aliskiren therapy. If hypotension occurs during aliskiren therapy, place patient in a supine position and administer normal saline solution intravenously, as needed and prescribed.
•**WARNING** Watch closely for angioedema of the head or neck, especially if patient is black, which increases risk. If angioedema occurs, discontinue aliskiren, notify prescriber, and provide supportive therapy until swelling has ceased. If swelling of the tongue, glottis or larynx is involved, be prepared to administer epinephrine solution 1:1,000 (0.3 ml to 0.5 ml), as prescribed, and provide measures to ensure a patent airway.
•Monitor serum potassium levels as ordered in patients who are diabetic and are also receiving ACE inhibitor therapy because hyperkalemia may occur.

PATIENT TEACHING

•Advise patient to avoid high-fat meals

while taking aliskiren because fat decreases drug absorption significantly.

•Instruct patient how to monitor blood pressure to determine effectivenss of aliskiren therapy.

•If patient is diabetic and takes an ACE inhibitor, tell her to avoid using potassium supplements or potassium salt substitutes and to inform all prescribers about her aliskiren and ACE inhibitor therapy.

•Stress importance of stopping aliskiren and seeking immediate medical attention if patient has swelling of face, extremities, eyes, lips, or tongue or if patient has trouble swallowing or breathing.

•Instruct female patient to notify prescriber immediately if she is or could be pregnant because drug will need to be discontinued and another antihypertensive chosen.

allopurinol

Apo-Allopurinol (CAN), Lopurin, Purinol (CAN), Zyloprim

allopurinol sodium

Aloprim

Class and Category

Chemical class: Hypoxanthine derivative, xanthine oxidase inhibitor
Therapeutic class: Antigout
Pregnancy category: C

Indications and Dosages

➤ *To treat gout and hyperuricemia*
TABLETS
Adults. 200 to 600 mg daily in divided doses, depending on disease severity. *Usual:* 200 to 300 mg daily. *Maximum:* 800 mg daily.

➤ *To treat secondary hyperuricemia caused by neoplastic disease*
TABLETS
Children ages 6 to 10. 300 mg daily, adjusted after 48 hr, depending on response to treatment.
Children under age 6. 150 mg daily, adjusted after 48 hr, depending on response to treatment.

➤ *To prevent gout attack*
TABLETS
Adults. 100 mg daily increased by 100 mg/ wk until serum uric acid level is 6 mg/dl or less.

➤ *To prevent uric acid nephropathy during vigorous treatment of neoplastic disease*
TABLETS
Adults. 600 to 800 mg daily for 2 to 3 days, then adjusted to keep serum uric acid level within normal limits.

➤ *To treat recurrent calcium oxalate calculi*
TABLETS
Adults. 200 to 300 mg daily as a single dose or in divided doses, adjusted based on 24-hr urine urate level.

DOSAGE ADJUSTMENT For patient with impaired renal function, dosage adjusted to 200 mg daily if creatinine clearance is 10 to 20 ml/min/1.73 m^2, 100 mg daily if creatinine clearance is 3 to 10 ml/min/1.73 m^2, or 100 mg every other day if creatinine clearance falls below 3 ml/min/1.73 m^2.

➤ *To treat increased serum and urine uric acid levels in patients with leukemia, lymphoma, and solid tumors whose cancer chemotherapy has increased those levels and who can't tolerate oral therapy*

I.V. INFUSION
Adults. 200 to 400 mg/m^2 daily as a single infusion or in equally divided infusions every 6, 8, or 12 hr. *Maximum:* 600 mg daily.
Children. 200 mg/m^2 daily as a single infusion or in equally divided infusions every 6, 8, or 12 hr.

Route	Onset	Peak	Duration
P.O.	2 to 3 days	1 to 3 wk*	1 to 2 wk

Mechanism of Action

Inhibits uric acid production by inhibiting xanthine oxidase, the enzyme responsible for converting hypoxanthine and xanthine to uric acid. Allopurinol is metabolized to oxipurinol, which also inhibits xanthine oxidase.

Incompatibilities

Don't combine I.V. allopurinol in solution with amikacin, amphotericin B, carmustine, cefotaxime sodium, chlorpromazine hydrochloride, cimetidine hydrochloride, clinda-

---

* For hyperuricemia; several months for gout attack prevention.

mycin phosphate, cytarabine, dacarbazine, daunorubicin hydrochloride, diphenhydramine hydrochloride, doxorubicin hydrochloride, doxycycline hyclate, droperidol, floxuridine, gentamicin sulfate, haloperidol lactate, hydroxyzine hydrochloride, idarubicin hydrochloride, imipenem-cilastatin sodium, mechlorethamine hydrochloride, meperidine hydrochloride, metoclopramide hydrochloride, methylprednisolone sodium succinate, minocycline hydrochloride, nalbuphine hydrochloride, netilmicin sulfate, ondansetron hydrochloride, prochlorperazine edisylate, promethazine hydrochloride, sodium bicarbonate, streptozocin, tobramycin sulfate, vinorelbine tartrate.

Contraindications
Hypersensitivity to allopurinol

Interactions
DRUGS
ACE inhibitors: Increased risk of hypersensitivity reactions
amoxicillin, ampicillin: Increased risk of rash
azathioprine, mercaptopurine: Inactivation of these drugs
chlorpropamide: Increased risk of hypoglycemia in patients with renal insufficiency
cyclophosphamide, other cytotoxic drugs: Enhanced bone marrow suppression
dicumarol: Increased half-life and anticoagulant action of dicumarol
thiazide diuretics: Possibly increased risk of allopurinol toxicity
uricosuric agents: Increased urinary excretion of uric acid
vitamin C (large doses): Possibly urine acidification and increased risk of renal calculus formation

Adverse Reactions
CNS: Chills, drowsiness, fever, headache, neuritis, paresthesia, peripheral neuropathy, somnolence
CV: Vasculitis
EENT: Epistaxis, loss of taste
GI: Abdominal pain, diarrhea, dysphagia, elevated liver function test results, gastritis, granulomatous hepatitis, hepatic necrosis, hepatomegaly, nausea, vomiting
GU: Exacerbation of renal calculi, renal failure
HEME: Agranulocytosis, aplastic anemia, bone marrow depression, eosinophilia, leuko-

cytosis, leukopenia, thrombocytopenia
MS: Arthralgia, exacerbation of gout, myopathy
SKIN: Alopecia; ecchymosis; jaundice; maculopapular, scaly, or exfoliative rash (sometimes fatal); pruritus; urticaria

Nursing Considerations
• As ordered, obtain baseline CBC and uric acid level and review results of renal and liver function tests before and during allopurinol therapy.
• Reconstitute and dilute I.V. preparation to a concentration of 6 mg/ml or less.
• **WARNING** Discontinue allopurinol and notify prescriber immediately at first sign of hypersensitivity reaction, such as rash, which may precede more severe reactions.
• To decrease risk of calculus formation, maintain fluid intake of up to 3 L daily and monitor patient for output of 2 L daily. Also, don't give vitamin C.
PATIENT TEACHING
• Advise patient to take allopurinol after meals and to drink at least 10 large glasses of water daily.
• Instruct patient to report unusual bleeding or bruising, fever, chills, gout attack, numbness, and tingling.
• Inform patient that acute gout attacks may occur more frequently early in allopurinol treatment and that results may not be noticeable for 2 weeks or longer.
• Instruct patient not to drive or perform potentially hazardous tasks if drug causes drowsiness.

almotriptan malate
Axert

Class and Category
Chemical class: Selective 5-hydroxytryptamine₁ (5-HT₁) receptor agonist
Therapeutic class: Antimigraine drug
Pregnancy category: C

Indications and Dosages
➤ *To treat acute migraine*
TABLETS
Adults. *Initial:* 6.25 to 12.5 mg as a single dose, repeated in 2 hr p.r.n. *Maximum:* 2 doses/24 hr or 4 migraine treatments/mo.
DOSAGE ADJUSTMENT For patient with impaired renal or hepatic function, initial

dose reduced to 6.25 mg with maximum daily dose of 12.5 mg.

Mechanism of Action
May stimulate 5-HT$_1$ receptors on intracranial blood vessels and sensory nerves in the trigeminal vascular system. By activating these receptors, almotriptan selectively constricts inflamed and dilated cranial blood vessels and inhibits the production of proinflammatory neuropeptides. The drug also interrupts the transmission of pain signals to the brain.

Contraindications
Basilar or hemiplegic migraine; cerebrovascular, peripheral vascular, or ischemic or vasospastic coronary artery disease (CAD); hypersensitivity to almotriptan or its components; hypertension (uncontrolled); use within 24 hours of other serotonin-receptor agonists or ergotamine-containing or ergot-type drugs

Interactions
DRUGS
ergotamine-containing drugs: Prolonged vasospastic reactions
erythromycin, itraconazole, ketoconazole, ritonavir: Possibly increased blood almotriptan level
MAO inhibitors, verapamil: Increased blood almotriptan level
selective serotonin reuptake inhibitors: Increased risk of hyperreflexia, lack of coordination, and weakness

Adverse Reactions
CNS: Dizziness, headache, paresthesia, somnolence, syncope
CV: Coronary artery vasospasm, hypertension, ischemia, MI, palpitations, vasodilation, ventricular fibrillation, ventricular tachycardia
EENT: Dry mouth
GI: Nausea

Nursing Considerations
•**WARNING** Because almotriptan can cause coronary artery vasospasm, monitor patient with CAD for angina. Because drug also may cause peripheral vasospastic reactions, such as ischemic bowel disease, watch for abdom-

inal pain and bloody diarrhea.
•Be prepared to administer the first dose of almotriptan in a medical facility for patients who have risk factors for CAD but no known cardiovascular abnormalities.
•Obtain an ECG reading immediately after the first dose of almotriptan, as ordered, in patients who have risk factors for CAD because cardiac ischemia can occur without the patient having clinical symptoms.
•Expect to give a lower dosage to patients with hepatic or renal dysfunction because of impaired drug metabolism or excretion.
•Monitor blood pressure regularly during therapy in patients with hypertension because almotriptan may produce a transient increase in blood pressure.

PATIENT TEACHING
•Inform patient that almotriptan is used to treat acute migraine and that he shouldn't take it to treat nonmigraine headaches.
•Advise patient to consult prescriber before taking any OTC or prescription drugs.
•Advise patient not to take more than maximum prescribed.
•Caution patient that drug may cause adverse CNS reactions, and advise him to avoid hazardous activities until he knows how drug affects him.
•Instruct patient to seek emergency care immediately if he experiences cardiac symptoms—such as heaviness, pain, pressure, or tightness in the chest, jaw, neck, or throat—after taking drug.

alosetron hydrochloride
Lotronex

Class and Category
Chemical class: Selective serotonin 5-HT$_3$ receptor antagonist
Therapeutic class: Antidiarrheal
Pregnancy category: B

Indications and Dosages
➤ *To treat women with severe diarrhea-predominant irritable bowel syndrome (IBS) who have failed to respond to conventional therapy*
TABLETS
Adults. *Initial:* 1 mg daily for 4 wk, increased to 1 mg b.i.d., if needed, or discontinued if no response seen in first 4 wk of

therapy or if drug doesn't adequately control symptoms after 4 wk of b.i.d. regimen.

Mechanism of Action
Inhibits activation of 5-HT$_3$ nonselective cation channels found in enteric neurons in the GI tract, thereby decreasing visceral sensations, colonic transit, and secretions in the GI tract. These changes reduce GI pain and hyperactivity, symptoms that are prominent in diarrhea-predominant IBS.

Contraindications
Administration with fluvoxamine, history of chronic or severe constipation or sequelae from constipation, Crohn's disease, diverticulitis, GI perforation or adhesions, hypercoagulable state, impaired intestinal circulation, intestinal obstruction or stricture, ischemic colitis, thrombophlebitis, toxic megacolon, or ulcerative colitis; hypersensitivity to alosetron or its components; severe hepatic impairment

Interactions
DRUGS
fluvoxamine, ketoconazole: Increased blood alosetron level
cimetidine, clarithromycin, itraconazole, protease inhibitors, quinolones, telithromycin, voriconazole: Possibly increased alosetron level

Adverse Reactions
CNS: Anxiety, fatigue, headache, hypnagogic effects, malaise, temperature regulation disturbances
CV: Tachyarrhythmias
GI: Abdominal or GI discomfort and pain, abdominal distention, constipation (may be severe), diarrhea, dyspepsia, flatulence, GI spasms or lesions, hemorrhoids, hemorrhoidal hemorrhage, hyposalivation, ileus, impaction, ischemic colitis, nausea, obstruction, perforation, regurgitation and reflux, small-bowel mesenteric ischemia, ulceration
GU: Urinary frequency
RESP: Breathing disorders
SKIN: Diaphoresis, rash, urticaria
Other: Nonspecific cramps or pain

Nursing Considerations
• Be aware that only physicians enrolled in GlaxoSmithKline's prescribing program for alosetron should prescribe the drug and only patients who have read and signed the patient-physician agreement can receive the drug. Confirm that the agreement has been signed before therapy starts.
• Use alosetron cautiously in patients with mild to moderate liver dysfunction because alosetron is extensively metabolized in the liver.
• Report all adverse reactions to alosetron to the prescriber and to Prometheus at 1-888-423-5227.
• **WARNING** Monitor patient for constipation, especially if she's elderly or debilitated or she takes drugs that decrease GI motility. Also watch for evidence of ischemic colitis, such as rectal bleeding, bloody diarrhea, or new or worsening abdominal pain. These serious adverse GI reactions may occur without warning. If they do, be prepared to discontinue alosetron therapy immediately. Once alosetron is discontinued for ischemic colitis, it should not be resumed later; however, a patient who no longer has constipation can resume the drug, if needed.
• Ensure that program stickers required by the drug company are affixed to all prescriptions, including refills, before giving them to the patient.

PATIENT TEACHING
• Inform patient that alosetron therapy can't begin until she has read the medication guide that outlines drug's risks and benefits and has signed the permission form.
• Instruct patient not to start alosetron if constipated and to notify prescriber.
• Advise patient that serious adverse GI effects may occur without warning and that, if evidence of ischemic colitis or constipation arises, she should stop taking alosetron immediately and notify prescriber. Also advise her to notify prescriber if constipation doesn't resolve after drug is stopped.
• Inform patient that alosetron therapy will be stopped after 4 weeks of 1 mg b.i.d. if the drug isn't effective in controlling symptoms of IBS.

alpha₁-proteinase inhibitor (human)

Prolastin, Zemaira

Class and Category
Chemical class: Plasma protein
Therapeutic class: Enzyme replacement
Pregnancy category: C

Indications and Dosages
➤ *To treat congenital alpha₁-antitrypsin deficiency in patients with signs of panacinar emphysema (Prolastin); to augment and maintain patients with emphysema who are deficient in alpha₁-proteinase inhibitor*

I.V. INFUSION
Adults. 60 mg/kg infused over 30 min for Prolastin and 15 min for Zemaira at a rate of at least 0.08 ml/kg/min once weekly.

Mechanism of Action
Replaces the enzyme alpha₁-antitrypsin, which normally inhibits the proteolytic enzyme elastase in patients with alpha₁-antitrypsin deficiency. Without alpha₁-proteinase inhibitor, elastase attacks and destroys alveolar membranes and causes emphysema.

Contraindications
Hypersensitivity to alpha₁-proteinase inhibitor, its components, or other alpha₁-proteinase products; selective immunoglobulin A (IgA) deficiency in patients with anti-IgA antibodies

Interactions
ACTIVITIES
smoking: Inactivation of alpha₁-proteinase inhibitor

Adverse Reactions
CNS: Asthenia, dizziness, fever, headache, paresthesia
EENT: Sinusitis
HEME: Mild, transient leukocytosis
RESP: Exacerbation of existing COPD, upper respiratory tract infection
SKIN: Pruritus
Other: Flulike symptoms, infusion site pain

Nursing Considerations
• Use alpha₁-proteinase inhibitor cautiously in patients at risk for circulatory overload because drug is a colloid solution that increases plasma volume.

• Before reconstituting alpha₁-proteinase inhibitor, remove drug and diluent from refrigerator and let it warm to room temperature.

• To reconstitute, remove caps from vials and cleanse rubber stoppers with antiseptic solution. After stoppers are dry, remove protective cover from diluent end of transfer device and insert into center of upright diluent vial. Then remove protective cover from drug end of transfer device, invert the diluent vial with attached transfer device, and using minimal force, insert drug end of transfer device into center of rubber stopper of upright drug vial. Make sure flange of transfer device rests on stopper surface so that diluent flows into drug vial.

• During diluent transfer, wet lyophilized cake completely by gently tilting drug vial. Don't allow air inlet filter to face downward. (Take care not to lose the vacuum because this will prolong drug reconstitution.) Once diluent transfer is complete, pull transfer device along with attached diluent vial out of drug vial and discard. Gently swirl drug vial until powder is completely dissolved. Avoid shaking because this may cause drug to foam and degrade.

• If more than one vial of alpha₁-proteinase inhibitor is required, use aseptic technique to transfer reconstituted solution from each vial into a sterile I.V. administration container.

• Administer at room temperature within 3 hours of reconstitution as an I.V. infusion, using the large-volume 5-micron conical filter provided. Place filter between distal end of I.V. administration set and infusion set, and then infuse at a rate of 0.08 ml/kg/min or as determined by patient response and comfort. Expect the infusion to take about 15 minutes per vial.

• **WARNING** Alpha₁-proteinase inhibitor is made from human plasma and may contain infectious agents, such as viruses. Ensure that patient is immunized against hepatitis B before giving drug. If time doesn't allow for antibody formation, give a single dose of hepatitis B immune globulin with hepatitis B vaccine, as prescribed.

• Monitor patient for delayed fever, which may occur up to 12 hours after therapy. Fever usually resolves within 24 hours.

PATIENT TEACHING
• Tell patient to report immediately early evidence of allergic reaction, such as chest

tightness, trouble breathing, faintness, hives, wheezing, and any other unusual symptoms.
• Advise patient to notify prescriber if signs or symptoms of viral infection (chills, drowsiness, fever, and runny nose, followed 2 weeks later by joint pain and a rash) occur after receiving drug.
• Stress the importance of receiving weekly doses to maintain an adequate antielastase barrier in the lungs. Explain that treatment must continue for life.
• Warn patient not to smoke.

alprazolam

Apo-Alpraz (CAN), Novo-Alprazol (CAN), Nu-Alpraz, Xanax, Xanax XR

Class, Category, and Schedule

Chemical class: Benzodiazepine
Therapeutic class: Antianxiety drug
Pregnancy category: D
Controlled substance schedule: IV

Indications and Dosages

➤ *To control anxiety disorders, relieve anxiety (short-term therapy), or treat anxiety associated with depression*

TABLETS

Adults. *Initial:* 0.25 to 0.5 mg t.i.d., adjusted to patient's needs. *Maximum:* 4 mg daily in divided doses.

DOSAGE ADJUSTMENT In elderly or debilitate patients or patients with advanced hepatic disease, initial dosage adjusted to 0.25 mg b.i.d. or t.i.d. and increased gradually, as needed and tolerated.

➤ *To treat panic attack*

ORALLY DISINTEGRATING TABLETS, TABLETS

Adults. *Initial:* 0.5 mg t.i.d., increased every 3 to 4 days by no more than 1 mg daily, based on patient response. *Maximum:* 10 mg daily in divided doses.

E.R. TABLETS

Adults. *Initial:* 0.5 to 1 mg daily in morning, increased every 3 to 4 days by no more than 1 mg/day, based on patient response. *Maximum:* 10 mg daily as single dose in morning.

Contraindications

Acute angle-closure glaucoma; hypersensitivity to alprazolam, its components, or other benzodiazepines; itraconazole or ketoconazole therapy

Mechanism of Action

May increase the effects of gamma-aminobutyric acid (GABA) and other inhibitory neurotransmitters by binding to specific benzodiazepine receptors in the limbic and cortical areas of the CNS. GABA inhibits excitatory stimulation, which helps control emotional behavior. The limbic system contains many benzodiazepine receptors, which may help explain the drug's antianxiety effects.

Interactions

DRUGS

antacids: Altered rate of alprazolam absorption
cimetidine, disulfiram, fluoxetine, isoniazid, metoprolol, oral contraceptives, propoxyphene, propranolol, valproic acid: Decreased elimination and increased effects of alprazolam
CNS depressants: Possibly increased CNS effects of both drugs
digoxin: Possibly increased serum digoxin level, causing digitalis toxicity
itraconazole, ketoconazole: Possibly profoundly inhibited metabolism of alprazolam
levodopa: Decreased effects of levodopa
neuromuscular blockers: Possibly potentiated or antagonized effects of these drugs
phenytoin: Possibly increased serum phenytoin level, causing phenytoin toxicity
probenecid: Possibly faster onset or prolonged effects of alprazolam
ranitidine: Possibly reduced absorption of alprazolam

ACTIVITIES

alcohol use: Enhanced adverse CNS effects of alprazolam

Adverse Reactions

CNS: Agitation, akathisia, confusion, depression, dizziness, drowsiness, fatigue, hallucinations, headache, insomnia, irritability, lack of coordination, light-headedness, memory loss, nervousness, paresthesia, rigidity, speech problems, syncope, tremor, weakness
CV: Chest pain, edema, hypotension, nonspecific ECG changes, palpitations, tachycardia
EENT: Blurred vision, altered salivation, dry mouth, nasal congestion, tinnitus
ENDO: Galactorrhea, gynecomastia, hyperprolactinemia

GI: Abdominal discomfort, anorexia, constipation, diarrhea, elevated liver function test results, hepatitis, hepatic failure, nausea, vomiting
GU: Altered libido, urinary hesitancy
MS: Dysarthria, muscle rigidity and spasms
RESP: Hyperventilation, upper respiratory tract infection
SKIN: Dermatitis, diaphoresis, pruritus, rash, Stevens-Johnson syndrome
Other: Weight gain or loss

Nursing Considerations
•Expect to give a higher dosage if patient's panic attacks occur unexpectedly or during such activities as driving.
•Because alprazolam use can lead to dependency, expect to reduce dosage gradually when stopping drug. To prevent withdrawal symptoms, don't discontinue drug abruptly.

PATIENT TEACHING
•Warn against stopping alprazolam abruptly because withdrawal symptoms may occur.
•Instruct patient never to increase the prescribed dosage because of the increased risk of dependency.
•Urge patient to avoid drinking alcohol during alprazolam therapy.
•Advise patient to avoid driving and activities that require alertness until alprazolam's effects are known.
•Instruct female patient of childbearing age to notify prescriber immediately if she becomes or might be pregnant because drug isn't recommended during pregnancy.

alprostadil

Caverject, Edex, Muse

Class and Category
Chemical class: Prostaglandin E_1
Therapeutic class: Anti-impotence drug
Pregnancy category: C

Indications and Dosages
➤ *To treat erectile dysfunction due to vascular or psychogenic causes or both*
INTRACAVERNOUS INJECTION (CAVERJECT, EDEX)
Adults. *Initial:* 2.5 mcg. Dosage increased to 5 mcg if partial response is apparent or 7.5 mcg if no response is apparent, followed by incremental increases of 5 to 10 mcg until erection suitable for intercourse (not exceeding 1-hr duration) is achieved. No more than

2 doses, separated by 1 hr, should be given on a single day during initial titration phase. *Maximum:* 3 doses/week; each dose separated by 24 hr.
URETHRAL SUPPOSITORY (MUSE)
Adults. *Initial:* 125 to 250 mcg. If no response, dosage increased in increments to 500 or 1,000 mcg until erection suitable for intercourse (not exceeding 1-hr duration) is achieved. *Maximum:* 2 doses/24 hr.
➤ *To treat erectile dysfunction due to spinal cord injury*
INTRACAVERNOUS INJECTION (CAVERJECT, EDEX)
Adults. *Initial:* 1.25 mcg. Dosage increased to 2.5 mcg if partial response is apparent, then to 5 mcg, and increased in 5-mcg increments until erection suitable for intercourse (not exceeding 1-hr duration) is achieved. No more than 2 doses, separated by 1 hr, should be given on a single day during initial titration phase. *Maximum:* 3 doses/week; each dose separated by 24 hr.

Route	Onset	Peak	Duration
Intra-cavernous	5 to 20 min	Unknown	60 min
Intra-urethral	5 to 10 min	Unknown	30 to 60 min

Contraindications
Anuria, balanitis (inflammation of head of penis), cavernosal fibrosis, hypersensitivity to alprostadil or its components, hyperviscosity syndrome, indwelling urethral catheter, leukemia, men for whom sexual activity is contraindicated, multiple myeloma, penile angulation, penile implants, Peyronie's disease, polycythemia, severe hypospadius (urethral opening on underside of penis), sickle cell anemia or trait, tendency to develop venous thrombosis, thrombocythemia, urethral obstruction or stricture, urethritis

Interactions
DRUGS
anticoagulants: Possibly increased risk of bleeding
cyclosporine: Possibly decreased blood cyclosporine level

Adverse Reactions
CNS: Dizziness, headache, syncope
CV: Hypertension, hypotension, tachycardia, vasodilation

Mechanism of Action

Alprostadil causes penile erection by increasing blood flow to the penis through relaxation of trabecular smooth muscles and dilation of cavernosal arteries. A naturally occurring prostaglandin, alprostadil interacts with specific membrane-bound receptors in the corpora cavernosa cells of the penis. This action activates intracellular adenyl cyclase, which in turn converts adenosine triphosphate (ATP) into cyclic adenosine monophosphate (cAMP). In-creased intracellular levels of cAMP activate protein kinase, an enzyme that activates other enzymes to initiate a cascade of chemical reactions. These chemical reactions cause the trabecular smooth muscles to relax and the cavernosal arteries to dilate. Blood flow to the penis is then increased, which distends the penile lacunar spaces and compresses the veins, trapping blood in the penis and causing it to become enlarged and rigid.

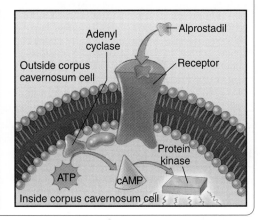

Transverse section of penis

Inside corpus cavernosum cell

EENT: Nasal congestion, sinusitis
GU: Pelvic pain; penile disorders, including edema, fibrosis, pain, and rash; priapism; prolonged erection; prostatic pain or enlargement; urethral abrasions; urethral bleeding
MS: Back pain
RESP: Cough, upper respiratory tract infection
Other: Flulike symptoms, injection site bruising or hematoma, needle breakage

Nursing Considerations

•Reconstitute solution with 1 ml diluent, for a concentration of 5, 10, 20, or 40 mcg/ml, depending on vial strength. Gently swirl contents of reconstituted vial. Use reconstituted solution within 24 hours when stored at room temperature. Don't use vials that contain precipitate or discolored solution. Discard unused reconstituted solution.
•Using a ½-inch 27G to 30G needle, inject drug at a 90-degree angle into the proximal third of the spongy tissue that runs the length of the dorsolateral aspect of the penis, avoiding any visible veins. Rotate injection sites by alternating sides of the penis.
•Carefully examine the penis for signs and symptoms of penile fibrosis. Expect to discontinue treatment if patient develops cavernosal fibrosis, penile angulation, or Peyronie's disease (hardening of the corpora cavernosa, which causes the penis to become distorted when erect) during therapy.
•WARNING Assess patient for prolonged erection after drug administration. Notify prescriber and be prepared to treat patient for priapism if erection lasts longer than 4 hours.
•If patient is receiving an anticoagulant, such as warfarin or heparin, monitor him for bleeding at injection site because alprostadil may inhibit platelet aggregation.
PATIENT TEACHING
•Inform patient that initial therapy must be performed in the office setting. Teach him how to correctly administer intracavernous injections or urethral suppositories. Inform

him that the goal of treatment is to produce an erection that lasts no longer than 1 hour.
•Advise patient to use alprostadil for injection no more than three times/week and to separate doses by 24 hours. Inform patient using urethral suppositories not to use more than two doses in a 24-hour period.
•Instruct patient to inform prescriber immediately of the development of nodules or hard tissue in the penis; an erection that persists for more than 4 hours; new or worsened penile pain; or persistent curvature, redness, swelling, or tenderness of the erect penis.
•Inform patient that common adverse reactions include mild to moderate pain immediately after injection and burning after suppository insertion. Also, needle may break. Advise patient to avoid it by following prescriber's instructions exactly and by handling injection device properly. If needle breaks during injection and he can see and grasp broken end, he should remove it and contact prescriber. If he can't see or grasp broken end, he should seek medical care.
•Instruct patient using suppository form to urinate just before inserting suppository and to insert suppository with the applicator supplied with drug. Tell patient to hold the penis upright after insertion and to roll it firmly between his hands to distribute drug.
•Tell patient to sit, stand, or walk for 10 minutes after inserting suppository to increase blood flow, which enhances erection.
•Inform patient that he can expect an erection 5 to 20 minutes after injecting drug or about 10 minutes after inserting suppository.
•Advise patient not to change dosage without consulting prescriber and to keep scheduled follow-up appointments.
•Warn patient that alprostadil offers no protection from sexually transmitted diseases. Urge him to use a condom to decrease risk of blood-borne disease, because injection can cause minor bleeding at injection site.
•Instruct patient not to reuse or share needles or syringes. Inform him of proper procedure for sharps disposal.
•Warn patient taking suppository form not to engage in sexual intercourse with a pregnant woman unless a condom is used because drug's effect on pregnancy is unknown.
•Advise patient who plans to travel not to check drug with airline baggage or store it in a closed car.

alteplase
(tissue plasminogen activator, recombinant)

Activase, Activase rt-PA (CAN)

Class and Category

Chemical class: Purified glycoprotein
Therapeutic class: Thrombolytic
Pregnancy category: C

Indications and Dosages

➤ *To treat acute MI*
ACCELERATED I.V. INFUSION
Adults weighing more than 67 kg (148 lb).
15-mg bolus followed by 50 mg infused over next 30 min and then by 35 mg infused over next 60 min.
Adults weighing 67 kg or less. 15-mg bolus followed by 0.75 mg/kg (up to 50 mg) infused over next 30 min and then 0.5 mg/kg (up to 35 mg) infused over next 60 min.
I.V. INFUSION
Adults weighing more than 65 kg (143 lb).
100 mg infused over 3 hr as follows: 6 to 10 mg by bolus over first 1 to 2 min, 50 to 54 mg over remainder of first hr, 20 mg over second hr, and 20 mg over third hr.
Adults weighing 65 kg or less. 1.25 mg/kg infused over 3 hr on similar administration schedule for those weighing more than 65 kg.
➤ *To treat acute ischemic stroke*
I.V. INFUSION
Adults. 0.9 mg/kg infused over 60 min, with 10% of total dose given as bolus over first min. *Maximum:* 90 mg.

WARNING To avoid acute bleeding complications, treatment for acute ischemic stroke must begin within 3 hr after onset of stroke symptoms and only after computed tomography or other diagnostic imaging method excludes intracranial hemorrhage.

➤ *To treat pulmonary embolism*
I.V. INFUSION
Adults. 100 mg infused over 2 hr.

Route	Onset	Peak	Duration
I.V.	Immediate	20 to 120 min	4 hr

Incompatibilities

Don't add other drugs to solution that contains alteplase.

> **Mechanism of Action**
> Binds to fibrin in a thrombus and converts trapped plasminogen to plasmin. Plasmin breaks down fibrin, fibrinogen, and other clotting factors, which dissolves the thrombus.

Contraindications
For all indications: Active internal bleeding, arteriovenous malformation or aneurysm, bleeding diathesis, intracranial neoplasm, severe uncontrolled hypertension
For acute MI and pulmonary embolism only: History of stroke, intracranial or intraspinal surgery or trauma in past 2 months
For acute ischemic stroke only: Recent head trauma, recent intracranial surgery, recent previous stroke, seizure activity at onset of stroke, subarachnoid hemorrhage, suspicion or history of intracranial hemorrhage

Interactions
DRUGS
drugs that alter platelet function, such as abciximab, acetylsalicylic acid, and dipyridamole; heparin; vitamin K antagonists: Increased risk of bleeding

Adverse Reactions
CNS: Cerebral edema, cerebral herniation, fever, seizure, stroke
CV: Arrhythmias (including bradycardia and electromechanical dissociation), cardiac arrest, cardiac tamponade, cardiogenic shock, cholesterol embolism, coronary thrombolysis, heart failure, hypotension, mitral insufficiency, myocardial reinfarction or rupture, pericardial effusion, pericarditis, venous thrombosis and embolism
EENT: Epistaxis, gingival bleeding, laryngeal edema
GI: GI bleeding, nausea, retroperitoneal bleeding, vomiting
GU: GU bleeding
RESP: Pleural effusion, pulmonary edema, pulmonary reembolization
SKIN: Bleeding at puncture sites, ecchymosis, rash, urticaria
Other: Anaphylaxis

Nursing Considerations
•Immediately before use, reconstitute alteplase with sterile water for injection only.

Swirl gently to dissolve powder; don't shake.
•Monitor for bleeding, especially at arterial puncture sites.
•Monitor blood pressure and heart rate and rhythm frequently during and after therapy.
•**WARNING** Alteplase therapy may cause arrhythmias from sudden reperfusion of the myocardium. Monitor continuous ECG for arrhythmias during drug therapy.
•Minimize bleeding from noncompressible sites by avoiding internal jugular and subclavian venous puncture sites.
•Discontinue alteplase immediately if serious bleeding occurs.
•After administering alteplase, apply pressure for at least 30 minutes, followed by a pressure dressing.
•Store reconstituted solution at room temperature (about 86° F [30° C]) or refrigerated (36° to 46° F [2.2° to 7.7° C]).
PATIENT TEACHING
•Tell patient to immediately report bleeding, including from the nose or gums.
•Advise patient to limit physical activity during alteplase administration to reduce risk of injury and bleeding.

aluminum carbonate

Basaljel

aluminum hydroxide

AlternaGEL, Alu-Cap, Alugel (CAN), Alu-Tab, Amphojel, Dialume

Class and Category
Chemical: Aluminum salt
Therapeutic: Antacid, phosphate binder
Pregnancy category: Not rated

Indications and Dosages
➤ *To treat hyperacidity associated with gastric hyperacidity, gastritis, hiatal hernia, peptic esophagitis, and peptic ulcers; to prevent phosphate renal calculus formation; to reduce hyperphosphatemia in chronic renal failure*
ALUMINUM CARBONATE CAPSULES, SUSPENSION, OR TABLETS
Adults. 2 capsules or tablets or 10 ml of suspension every 2 hr up to 12 times daily p.r.n.
ALUMINUM HYDROXIDE CAPSULES, SUSPENSION, OR TABLETS
Adults. 500 to 1,500 mg as capsules or tablets

in divided doses 3 to 6 times daily, taken between meals and at bedtime; 5 to 30 ml as suspension p.r.n., taken between meals and at bedtime.

Route	Onset	Peak	Duration
P.O.	Varies	Unknown	20 to 40 min*

Mechanism of Action
Neutralizes or reduces gastric acidity, resulting in increased stomach and duodenal alkalinity. Protects stomach and duodenum lining by inhibiting pepsin's proteolytic activity. Binds with phosphate ions in the intestine to form insoluble aluminum-phosphate compounds, which lower the blood phosphate level.

Contraindications
Hypersensitivity to aluminum

Interactions
DRUGS
allopurinol, chloroquine, corticosteroids, diflunisal, digoxin, ethambutol, H₂-receptor blockers, iron, isoniazid, penicillamine, phenothiazines, ranitidine, tetracyclines, thyroid hormones, ticlopidine: Decreased effects of these drugs
benzodiazepines: Increased effects of benzodiazepines

Adverse Reactions
CNS: Encephalopathy
GI: Constipation, intestinal obstruction, white-speckled stool
MS: Osteomalacia, osteoporosis
Other: Aluminum accumulation in serum, bone, and CNS; aluminum intoxication; electrolyte imbalances

Nursing Considerations
•Don't administer aluminum hydroxide within 1 to 2 hours of other oral drugs.
•Be aware that two 0.6-g aluminum hydroxide tablets can neutralize 16 mEq of acid.
•Monitor patient's serum levels of sodium, phosphate, and other electrolytes, as appropriate.
PATIENT TEACHING
•Instruct patient to chew tablets thoroughly

---

* If fasting; at least 3 hr if given 1 hr after meals.

before swallowing and then to drink a full glass of water.
•Warn patient not to take maximum dosage for more than 2 weeks unless prescribed because doing so may cause stomach to secrete excess hydrochloric acid.
•Teach patient to prevent constipation with a high-fiber diet and increased fluid intake (2 to 3 L daily), if appropriate.
•If patient takes other prescription drugs, advise him to notify prescriber about them before taking aluminum because of risk of interactions.
•Advise patient to notify prescriber if symptoms worsen or don't subside.

alvimopan
Entereg

Class and Category
Chemical class: Single stereoisomer
Therapeutic class: Mu opioid receptor antagonist
Pregnancy category: B

Indications and Dosages
➤ *To accelerate GI recovery in hospitalized patients after a partial large- or small-bowel resection with primary anastomosis*
CAPSULES
Adults. *Initial:* 12 mg started 30 min to 5 hr before surgery, followed by 12 mg b.i.d. starting the day after surgery for up to 7 days or until discharge. *Maximum:* 24 mg/day with a maximum of 15 doses total.

Route	Onset	Peak	Duration
P.O.	Unknown	2 hr	Unknown

Mechanism of Action
Competitively binds to selective mu opioid receptors in the GI tract, antagonizing the peripheral effects of opioids on GI motility and secretion without reversing the central analgesic effects of opioid agonists. This action alleviates postoperative ileus by causing bowel function to return more quickly after part of the bowel has been removed and an end-to-end anastomosis performed.

Contraindications

Hypersensitivity to alvimopan or its components, severe hepatic or renal impairment, use of opioids for more than 7 consecutive days immediately before alvimopan starts

Interactions

DRUGS

opioids given within previous 7 days at therapeutic doses: Increased sensitivity to alvimopan

Adverse Reactions

GI: Abdominal pain, constipation, dyspepsia, flatulence
GU: Urine retention
HEME: Anemia
MS: Back pain
Other: Hypokalemia

Nursing Considerations

•Don't give alvimopan to patients with severe hepatic or renal impairment or to patients having surgery to correct a complete bowel obstruction.
•Alvimopan is prescribed only for short-term use with maximum of 15 doses and is only dispensed in hospitals enrolled in Entereg Access Support and Education (E.A.S.E.) program. Closely monitor number of doses given, and expect to stop drug when patient has received 15 doses or is discharged from hospital.
•Monitor patient's serum potassium level closely, as ordered, because drug may cause hypokalemia. Also check patient's hemoglobin level and hematocrit because drug has been associated with anemia.
•Monitor patient with mild to moderate hepatic or renal failure for evidence of high alvimopan levels, such as abdominal pain or cramping, diarrhea, nausea, and vomiting. If present, alert prescriber.

PATIENT TEACHING

•Explain the need to accurately describe long-term or intermittent use of opioid pain therapy, including any use of opioids in the week before receiving alvimopan. Taking almivopan after such use may cause serious adverse GI reactions.
•Inform patient that the most common adverse effects of alvimopan are constipation, dyspepsia, and flatulence.
•Tell patient that drug is for in-hospital use only and will not be taken at home.

amantadine hydrochloride
(adamantanamine hydrochloride)

Endantadine (CAN), Gen-Amantadine (CAN), Symmetrel

Class and Category

Chemical class: Adamantane derivative
Therapeutic class: Antidyskinetic, antiviral
Pregnancy category: C

Indications and Dosages

➤ *To manage symptoms of primary Parkinson's disease, postencephalitic parkinsonism, arteriosclerotic parkinsonism, and parkinsonism caused by CNS injury from carbon monoxide intoxication*

CAPSULES, SYRUP, TABLETS

Adults. *Initial:* 100 mg b.i.d. *Maximum:* 400 mg daily in divided doses.

➤ *To treat drug-induced extrapyramidal reactions*

CAPSULES, SYRUP, TABLETS

Adults. *Initial:* 100 mg b.i.d. *Maximum:* 300 mg daily in divided doses.

DOSAGE ADJUSTMENT For elderly patients, patients taking high doses of other antidyskinetics, and patients who have a serious medical condition (such as heart failure, epilepsy, or psychosis), initial dosage reduced to 100 mg daily, with gradual titration to 100 mg b.i.d. after 1 to several wk. For patients with impaired renal function, dosage adjusted to 200 mg on day 1; and then to 100 mg daily if creatinine clearance is 30 to 50 ml/min/1.73 m^2; to 200 mg on day 1 and then to 100 mg every other day if creatinine clearance is 15 to 29 ml/min/1.73 m^2; and to 200 mg every wk if creatinine clearance is less than 15 ml/min/1.73 m^2 or if patient is receiving hemodialysis.

➤ *To prevent and treat respiratory tract infection caused by influenza A*

CAPSULES, SYRUP, TABLETS

Adults and children age 12 and over. *Initial:* 200 mg daily or 100 mg b.i.d. *Maximum:* 200 mg daily.

DOSAGE ADJUSTMENT For patients with impaired renal function, dosage adjusted to 200 mg on day 1 and then to 100 mg daily if creatinine clearance is 30 to 50 ml/min/ 1.73 m^2; to 200 mg on day 1 and then to 100 mg every other day if creatinine clearance is 15 to 29 ml/min/1.73 m^2; and to 200 mg every wk if creatinine clearance is less than 15 ml/min/1.73 m^2 or if patient is having hemodialysis.

Children ages 9 to 12. 100 mg every 12 hr. *Maximum:* 200 mg daily.

Children ages 1 to 9. 1.5 to 3 mg/kg every 8 hr or 2.2 to 4.4 mg/kg every 12 hr. *Maximum:* 150 mg/day.

Route	Onset	Peak	Duration
P.O.	In 48 hr*	Unknown	Unknown

Mechanism of Action

Affects dopamine, a neurotransmitter that is synthesized and released by neurons leading from substantia nigra to basal ganglia and is essential for normal motor function. In Parkinson's disease, progressive degeneration of these neurons reduces intrasynaptic dopamine. Amantadine may cause dopamine to accumulate in the basal ganglia by increasing dopamine release or by blocking dopamine reuptake into the presynaptic neurons of the CNS. Amantadine also may stimulate dopamine receptors or cause postsynaptic receptors to be more sensitive to dopamine. These actions help control alterations in involuntary muscle movements, such as tremors and rigidity, that are associated with Parkinson's disease.

Amantadine may inhibit influenza A viral replication by blocking uncoating of virus and release of viral nucleic acid into respiratory epithelial cells. It also may interfere with early replication of viruses that have already penetrated cells.

Contraindications

Angle-closure glaucoma, hypersensitivity to amantadine or its components

Interactions

DRUGS

anticholinergics or other drugs with anticho-linergic activity, other antidyskinetics, antihistamines, phenothiazines, tricyclic antidepressants: Possibly increased anticholinergic effects and risk of paralytic ileus

carbidopa-levodopa, levodopa: Increased effectiveness of these drugs

CNS stimulants: Excessive CNS stimulation, possibly causing arrhythmias, insomnia, irritability, nervousness, or seizures

hydrochlorothiazide, triamterene: Possibly decreased amantadine clearance and increased risk of toxicity

live-virus vaccines: Possibly interference with vaccine effectiveness

quinidine, quinine, trimethoprim-sulfamethoxazole: Increased blood amantadine level

ACTIVITIES

alcohol use: Possibly increased risk of CNS effects—including confusion, dizziness, and light-headedness—and orthostatic hypotension

Adverse Reactions

CNS: Agitation, anxiety, confusion, dizziness, drowsiness, fatigue, hallucinations, insomnia, irritability, light-headedness, mental impairment, nervousness, nightmares, suicidal ideation, syncope

CV: Orthostatic hypotension, peripheral edema

EENT: Blurred vision; dry mouth, nose, or throat

GI: Constipation, diarrhea, nausea

GU: Dysuria

HEME: Agranulocytosis, leukopenia, neutropenia

SKIN: Livedo reticularis (purplish, netlike rash)

Nursing Considerations

•Be aware that prophylactic therapy with amantadine should begin as soon as possible after exposure to persons infected with the influenza A virus and should continue for 10 days. During an influenza epidemic, expect drug to be given daily throughout the epidemic, which typically lasts 6 to 8 weeks. If patient has previously received the inactivated influenza A vaccine, prescriber may discontinue it when sure that patient has developed active immunity against the virus. If patient receives the inactivated influenza A vaccine at the same time amantadine therapy starts, expect amantadine to be given for 2 to 3 weeks.

---

* Antidyskinetic action; antiviral action unknown.

•Expect amantadine therapy to start 24 to 48 hours after the onset of influenza A symptoms and to continue for 48 hours after their disappearance.

•Monitor patients who have a history of psychiatric illness or substance abuse because amantadine may worsen these conditions. Be aware that some patients taking amantadine have attempted suicide or had suicidal ideations.

•If patient has a history of heart failure or peripheral edema, monitor for weight gain and edema because drug may cause redistribution of body fluid.

•Be aware that amantadine may increase seizure activity in patients with a history of seizures.

•**WARNING** Monitor patient for signs and symptoms of neuroleptic malignant syndrome during dosage reduction or discontinuation of therapy. These include fever, hypertension or hypotension, involuntary motor activity, mental changes, muscle rigidity, tachycardia, and tachypnea. Be prepared to provide supportive treatment and additional drug therapy, as prescribed.

•Be aware that patients receiving more than 200 mg daily are more likely to experience adverse or toxic reactions.

•Monitor patient for decreased drug effectiveness over time. If therapeutic response declines, expect to increase dosage or discontinue drug temporarily, as ordered.

PATIENT TEACHING

•Instruct patient to take amantadine exactly as prescribed and not to stop taking it abruptly. Advise patient to notify prescriber if drug becomes less effective.

•Advise patient to notify prescriber if influenza symptoms don't improve after 2 to 3 days.

•**WARNING** Advise patient or family member to notify prescriber immediately if patient reveals thoughts of suicide.

•Encourage patient to avoid consuming alcohol during amantadine therapy because alcohol may increase the risk of confusion, dizziness, light-headedness, or orthostatic hypotension.

•Advise patient to avoid driving and other activities that require a high level of alertness until he knows how the drug affects him because it may cause blurred vision and mental impairment.

•Advise patient to change positions slowly to minimize effects of orthostatic hypotension.

•Tell patient to use ice chips or sugarless candy or gum to relieve dry mouth.

•Caution patient to resume physical activities gradually as signs and symptoms improve.

ambenonium chloride

Mytelase

Class and Category

Chemical class: Synthetic quaternary ammonium compound
Therapeutic class: Antimyasthenic, cholinergic
Pregnancy category: C

Indications and Dosages

➤ *To improve muscle strength in patients with myasthenia gravis in whom pyridostigmine or neostigmine are contraindicated*

TABLETS

Adults and adolescents. *Initial:* 5 mg t.i.d. or q.i.d., increased at 1- to 2-day intervals to optimum dosage based on patient response. *Usual:* Highly individualized but usually 5 to 50 mg t.i.d. or q.i.d.

Children. *Initial:* 0.3 mg/kg or 10 mg/m^2 daily in divided doses t.i.d. or q.i.d. *Maintenance:* Up to 1.5 mg/kg or 50 mg/m^2 daily in divided doses t.i.d. or q.i.d.

Route	Onset	Peak	Duration
P.O.	20 to 30 min	Unknown	3 to 8 hr

Mechanism of Action

Attaches to acetylcholinesterase and blocks acetylcholine's breakdown. This action prolongs and exaggerates acetylcholine's effects, producing cholinergic responses, such as miosis, increased intestinal and skeletal muscle tone, bronchoconstriction, bradycardia, and increased salivary and sweat gland secretions.

Contraindications

Hypersensitivity to ambenonium, its components, or anticholinesterases; mechanical intestinal or urinary tract obstruction

Interactions

DRUGS

anesthetics, antiarrhythmics, corticosteroids, magnesium, methocarbamol: Decreased effects of ambenonium

aminoglycosides, anticholinesterase muscle stimulants, depolarizing muscle relaxants, ganglionic blockers, mecamylamine: Increased effects of ambenonium

Adverse Reactions

CNS: Dizziness, drowsiness, headache, loss of consciousness, seizures, syncope
CV: AV block, bradycardia, decreased cardiac output, hypotension
EENT: Dysphonia, increased salivation, laryngospasm
GI: Abdominal cramps, dysphagia, flatulence, increased gastric and intestinal secretions, increased peristalsis, mild diarrhea, nausea, vomiting
GU: Incontinence, urinary frequency or urgency
MS: Arthralgia, dysarthria, fasciculations, muscle spasms, muscle weakness
RESP: Bronchoconstriction, bronchospasm, dyspnea, increased tracheobronchial secretions, lung congestion, respiratory arrest or depression, respiratory muscle paralysis
SKIN: Diaphoresis, flushing, rash, urticaria

Nursing Considerations

• Increase dosage gradually as prescribed to avoid ambenonium buildup and overdose.
• When increasing dosage to optimum level, note when no further increase in muscle strength is observed. Then expect to reduce dosage to previous effective level and to use this as maintenance dosage.
• Expect prescriber to order ephedrine (25 mg per ambenonium dose) or potassium chloride (1 to 2 g per ambenonium dose) to further improve muscle strength.
• WARNING Drug has a narrow margin between effectiveness and overdose. If patient receives more than 200 mg daily, monitor closely for signs of overdose (cholinergic crisis), such as abdominal cramps, diarrhea, nausea, vomiting, increased salivation, diaphoresis, difficulty swallowing, blurred vision, miosis, hypertension, fasciculations, and voluntary muscle paralysis.
• Assess neuromuscular status to detect progressive or recurrent muscle weakness in patient on long-term ambenonium therapy.

• If patient develops drug resistance during long-term therapy, expect to restore responsiveness by decreasing dosage or briefly stopping drug with close supervision.

PATIENT TEACHING

• Instruct patient to swallow tablet with liquid or food to minimize GI irritation.
• Advise patient to consult prescriber before discontinuing drug—even if symptoms diminish or disappear.

ambrisentan

Letairis

Class and Category

Chemical class: Autocrine and paracrine peptide
Therapeutic class: Endothelin receptor antagonist
Pregnancy category: X

Indications and Dosages

➤ *To treat pulmonary arterial hypertension, improve exercise capacity, and delay worsening in patients with World Health Organization (WHO) class II or III symptoms*

TABLETS

Adults. *Initial:* 5 mg once daily, increased to 10 mg once daily as needed and tolerated.

Route	Onset	Peak	Duration
P.O.	Unknown	2 hr	Unknown

Mechanism of Action

Blocks the action of endothelin-1 (ET-1), a potent autocrine and paracrine peptide in vascular smooth muscle and endothelium of lung tissue. ET-1 levels increase in patients with pulmonary arterial hypertension, suggesting that ET-1 affects development and progression of pulmonary arterial hypertension. Ambrisentan blocks an ET-1 receptor subtype, ETA, that causes vasoconstriction and cell proliferation, decreasing pulmonary artery pressure and cell proliferation and possibly delaying disease progression.

Contraindications

Hypersensitivity to ambrisentan or its components, pregnancy, breast-feeding, moderate to severe hepatic disease

Interactions

DRUGS

cyclosporine A: Possibly increased exposure to ambrisentan

strong CYP3A inhibitors (such as ketoconazole) and CYP2C19 inhibitors (such as omeprazole): Possibly increased plasma ambrisentan level and increased risk of toxicity

FOODS

grapefruit juice: Possibly increased blood ambrisentan level

Adverse Reactions

CNS: Headache
CV: Palpitations, peripheral edema
EENT: Nasal congestion, nasopharyngitis, sinusitis
GI: Abdominal pain, constipation, elevated liver enzymes
RESP: Dyspnea
SKIN: Flushing

Nursing Considerations

•Be aware that ambrisentan isn't recommended for patients with moderate to severe hepatic impairment. Use it cautiously in patients with mild hepatic impairment.
•Ambrisentan is available only through a restricted distribution program. Patients must be enrolled and meet all conditions of the program.
•Before administering ambrisentan for the first time, make sure patient understands its risks, has signed the agreement form, and knows that he'll need to be re-enrolled after 6 months of therapy and then yearly.
•If patient is a woman of childbearing age, obtain a negative pregnancy test before giving ambrisentan and then monthly throughout therapy. A positive result requires immediate discontinuation of the drug because of the risk of serious birth defects.
•Obtain liver enzyme levels, as ordered, before starting ambrisentan therapy and monthly during therapy because drug may significantly increase liver aminotransferase (ALT and AST) levels. If liver enzymes are more than 3 times the upper limit of normal, expect to not start ambrisentan therapy. If they're somewhat elevated, expect to monitor bilirubin level before and monthly during therapy. If liver enzymes become elevated

during therapy and evidence of hepatic dysfunction (abdominal pain, fever, jaundice, nausea, vomiting, unusual lethargy or fatigue) develops or patient's bilirubin level exceeds twice the upper limit of normal, notify prescriber and expect to stop ambrisentan therapy.
•Monitor patient's hemoglobin level before starting ambrisentan, again after 1 month of therapy, and periodically thereafter. If level declines significantly, notify prescriber and expect to discontinue drug.
•Assess patient closely for peripheral edema, especially if elderly. If edema becomes pronounced, notify prescriber. Further evaluation will reveal whether it results from ambrisentan therapy or another condition, such as heart failure.
•If patient takes ambrisentan for longer than 12 months, watch for hepatic cirrhosis (abdominal pain, fever, jaundice, nausea, vomiting, or unusual lethargy or fatigue). A similar drug, bosentan, rarely has caused unexplained hepatic cirrhosis after being taken longer than 12 months.

PATIENT TEACHING

•Caution patient not to split, crush, or chew ambrisentan tablets.
•Instruct female patient of childbearing age to use two reliable forms of birth control during ambrisentan therapy unless she has had a tubal ligation or a Copper T 380A or LNg 20 intrauterine device inserted. Explain that she'll need monthly pregnancy test.
•Advise patient to promptly report any signs of liver dysfunction to the prescriber.
•Instruct patient to notify prescriber about fluid retention because further treatment may be needed.

amikacin sulfate

Amikin

Class and Category

Chemical class: Aminoglycoside
Therapeutic class: Antibiotic
Pregnancy category: D

Indications and Dosages

➤ *To treat serious gram-negative bacterial infections (including septicemia; neonatal sepsis; respiratory tract, bone, joint, CNS, skin, soft-tissue, intra-abdominal,* burn, and postoperative infections; and serious, complicated, and recurrent UTI) caused by Acinetobacter, Enterobacter, Escherichia coli, Klebsiella, Proteus, Providencia, Pseudomonas, and Serratia; and staphylococcal infections when penicillin is contraindicated

I.V. INFUSION, I.M. INJECTION

Adults and children. 15 mg/kg daily in equal doses at equally spaced intervals (7.5 mg/kg every 12 hr or 5 mg/kg every 8 hr) for 7 to 10 days. *Maximum:* 1,500 mg daily.

DOSAGE ADJUSTMENT For patients with impaired renal function, loading dose of 7.5 mg/ kg daily; then maintenance dosage based on creatinine clearance and serum creatinine level and given every 12 hr. For morbidly obese patients, dosage not to exceed 1.5 g daily.

Neonates. *Loading dose:* 10 mg/kg. *Maintenance:* 7.5 mg/kg every 12 hr for 7 to 10 days.

➤ *To treat uncomplicated UTI*

I.V. INFUSION, I.M. INJECTION

Adults. 250 mg b.i.d. for 7 to 10 days.

Route	Onset	Peak	Duration
I.V.	Immediate	Unknown	Unknown
I.M.	Rapid	Unknown	Unknown

Mechanism of Action

Binds to negatively charged sites on bacteria's outer cell membrane, disrupting cell integrity. Also binds to bacterial ribosomal subunits and inhibits protein synthesis. Both actions lead to cell death.

Incompatibilties

Don't mix or infuse amikacin with other drugs.

Contraindications

Hypersensitivity to amikacin or other aminoglycosides

Interactions

DRUGS

cephalosporins, enflurane, methoxyflurane, vancomycin: Increased nephrotoxic effects
general anesthetics: Increased risk of neuromuscular blockade
loop diuretics: Increased risk of ototoxicity

neuromuscular blockers: Possibly increased neuromuscular blockade and prolonged respiratory depression
penicillins: Possibly inactivation of or synergistic effects with amikacin

Adverse Reactions

CNS: Drowsiness, headache, loss of balance, neuromuscular blockade, tremor, vertigo
EENT: Hearing loss, ototoxicity, tinnitus
GI: Nausea, vomiting
GU: Azotemia, dysuria, nephrotoxicity, oliguria or polyuria, proteinuria
MS: Acute muscle paralysis; arthralgia; muscle fatigue, spasms, and weakness
RESP: Apnea
Other: Hyperkalemia

Nursing Considerations

•Expect to obtain results of culture and sensitivity testing before therapy begins.
•Prepare amikacin I.V. solution by adding contents of 500-mg vial to 100 to 200 ml of sterile diluent. Then infuse drug over 30 to 60 minutes.
•Give I.M. injection in large muscle mass.
•Monitor for signs of ototoxicity, such as tinnitus and vertigo, especially during high-dosage or prolonged amikacin therapy.
•WARNING Because amikacin may produce nephrotoxic effects, assess renal function before and daily during therapy, as ordered. To minimize renal tubule irritation, maintain hydration during therapy.
•Be aware that amikacin may exacerbate muscle weakness in such conditions as myasthenia gravis and Parkinson's disease.
•Measure serum amikacin concentrations as ordered, usually 30 to 90 minutes after injection (for peak concentration) and just before administering next dose (for trough concentration).

PATIENT TEACHING

•Tell patient that daily laboratory tests are necessary during treatment.
•Instruct patient to report ringing in ears, hearing changes, headache, nausea, vomiting, and changes in urination.

amiloride hydrochloride

Midamor

Class and Category

Chemical class: Pyrazine-carbonyl-guanidine

A

Therapeutic class: Potassium-sparing diuretic
Pregnancy category: B

Indications and Dosages

➤ *As adjunct to thiazide or loop diuretic in patient with heart failure or hypertension to correct diuretic-induced hypokalemia or to prevent diuretic-induced hypokalemia that increases the risk of arrhythmias or other complications*

TABLETS

Adults. 5 to 10 mg daily as single dose; if hypokalemia persists, increased to 15 mg daily and then 20 mg daily.

Route	Onset	Peak	Duration
P.O.	2 hr	6 to 10 hr	24 hr

Mechanism of Action

Inhibits sodium reabsorption in distal convoluted tubules and cortical collecting ducts, causing sodium and water loss and enhancing potassium retention.

Contraindications

Hypersensitivity to amiloride; impaired renal function; serum potassium level above 5.5 mEq/L; therapy with another potassium-sparing diuretic, such as spironolactone or triamterene, or a potassium supplement

Interactions

DRUGS

angiotensin II receptor antagonists, captopril, enalapril, lisinopril, potassium products, spironolactone: Increased risk of hyperkalemia
digoxin: Decreased effectiveness of digoxin
lithium: Reduced renal clearance of lithium and increased risk of lithium toxicity
NSAIDs: Reduced diuretic effect of amiloride
sympathomimetics: Possibly reduced antihypertensive effects of amiloride

FOODS

high-potassium food: Increased risk of hyperkalemia

Adverse Reactions

CNS: Confusion, depression, dizziness, drowsiness, encephalopathy, fatigue, headache, insomnia, nervousness, paresthesia, somnolence, tremor, vertigo
CV: Angina, arrhythmias, orthostatic hypotension, palpitations
EENT: Dry mouth, increased intraocular pressure, nasal congestion, tinnitus, vision disturbances
GI: Abdominal pain or fullness, anorexia, appetite changes, constipation, diarrhea, GI bleeding, heartburn, indigestion, nausea, thirst, vomiting
GU: Bladder spasms, dysuria, impotence, loss of libido, polyuria
HEME: Aplastic anemia, neutropenia
MS: Arthralgia, muscle spasms or weakness
RESP: Cough, dyspnea
SKIN: Alopecia, jaundice, pruritus, rash
Other: Dehydration, hyperchloremia, hyperkalemia, hypernatremia, metabolic acidosis

Nursing Considerations

• Administer amiloride with food to reduce GI upset and early in the day to minimize sleep interference from polyuria.
• Monitor renal function test results, fluid intake and output, and weight. Also monitor serum potassium level to detect hyperkalemia.
• **WARNING** Don't administer amiloride with other potassium-sparing diuretics.

PATIENT TEACHING

• Warn patient to avoid high-potassium food and salt substitutes that contain potassium.
• Advise patient to consult prescriber before taking other drugs, including OTC remedies, especially sympathomimetics.
• Tell patient to report dizziness, trembling, numbness, and muscle weakness or spasms.
• Advise patient to increase fluid and fiber intake to prevent constipation.
• Warn patient to expect reversible hair loss and impotence.

aminocaproic acid

Amicar

Class and Category

Chemical class: Aminohexanoic acid
Therapeutic class: Antifibrinolytic, antihemorrhagic
Pregnancy category: C

Indications and Dosages

➤ *To treat excessive bleeding caused by fibrinolysis*

SYRUP, TABLETS
Adults. *Initial:* 5 g during first hour followed by 1 to 1.25 g/hr to sustain drug plasma level of 0.13 mg/ml. *Maximum:* 30 g daily.
I.V. INJECTION
Adults. 4 to 5 g in 250 ml of diluent over 1 hr followed by continuous infusion of 1 g/hr in 50 ml of diluent. Continue for 8 hr or until bleeding stops.

Route	Onset	Peak	Duration
P.O.	Rapid	Unknown	Unknown
I.V.	Immediate	Unknown	Under 3 hr

Mechanism of Action
Inhibits the breakdown of blood clots by interfering with plasminogen activator substances and producing antiplasmin activity.

Contraindications
Hypersensitivity to aminocaproic acid; signs of active intravascular clotting, as in disseminated intravascular coagulation; upper urinary tract bleeding

Interactions
DRUGS
activated prothrombin, prothrombin complex concentrates: Increased risk of thrombosis
estrogens, oral contraceptives: Increased risk of hypercoagulation

Adverse Reactions
CNS: Delirium, dizziness, hallucinations, headache, malaise, stroke, weakness
CV: Bradycardia, cardiomyopathy, elevated serum CK level, hypotension, ischemia, thrombophlebitis
EENT: Nasal congestion, tinnitus
GI: Abdominal cramps and pain, diarrhea, elevated AST level, nausea, vomiting
GU: Elevated BUN level, intrarenal obstruction, renal failure
HEME: Agranulocytosis, leukopenia, thrombocytopenia
MS: Myopathy
RESP: Dyspnea, pulmonary embolism
SKIN: Pruritus, rash
Other: Elevated serum aldolase and potassium levels

Nursing Considerations
•Be aware that patients on oral therapy may need up to 10 tablets during the first hour of treatment and tablets around the clock during continued treatment.
•Mix aminocaproic acid solution with sterile water for injection, normal saline solution, D₅W, or Ringer's solution.
•**WARNING** Avoid rapid I.V. delivery because of increased risk of hypotension and bradycardia.
•Monitor neurologic status for drug-induced changes. Note that increased clotting may lead to stroke.
PATIENT TEACHING
•Tell patient that he'll be closely monitored during I.V. therapy and will have blood drawn for laboratory tests before, during, and after treatment.
•Advise patient who takes aminocaproic acid at home to report adverse reactions, take drug exactly as prescribed, and keep follow-up appointments with prescriber.

aminoglutethimide

Cytadren

Class and Category
Chemical class: Hormone
Therapeutic class: Adrenal steroid inhibitor
Pregnancy category: D

Indications and Dosages
➤ *To suppress adrenal function in patients with Cushing's syndrome who are waiting for surgery or for whom other treatment can't be used*
TABLETS
Adults. *Initial:* 250 mg every 6 hr. Increased as needed by 250 mg daily every 1 to 2 wk. *Maximum:* 2,000 mg daily.

Route	Onset	Peak	Duration
P.O.	3 to 5 days	Unknown	72 hr

Mechanism of Action
Inhibits the conversion of cholesterol to delta-5-pregnenolone, which is needed to produce certain hormones, including adrenal glucocorticoids, mineralocorticoids, estrogens, and androgens.

Contraindications
Hypersensitivity to aminoglutethimide or glutethimide

Interactions
DRUGS
antidiabetic drugs, dexamethasone, digoxin, medroxyprogesterone, synthetic glucocorticoids, theophylline, warfarin and other oral anticoagulants: Decreased effects of these drugs

Adverse Reactions
CNS: Dizziness, drowsiness, fever, headache
CV: Hypotension, orthostatic hypotension, tachycardia
ENDO: Adrenal insufficiency, hypothyroidism, masculinization
GI: Anorexia, nausea
SKIN: Hair growth, morbiliform rash, pruritus, urticaria

Nursing Considerations
•Expect to reduce aminoglutethimide dosage or discontinue treatment if extreme drowsiness, severe rash, or excessively low cortisol level occurs.
•**WARNING** Monitor for signs of hypothyroidism, including lethargy, dry skin, and slow pulse. If prescribed, administer thyroid hormone supplement.
•Monitor blood pressure for orthostatic or persistent hypotension.
PATIENT TEACHING
•Teach patient to recognize signs and symptoms of orthostatic hypotension, including dizziness and weakness when moving from sitting to standing position, and how to avoid this condition, such as by rising slowly from a supine to an upright position. dizziness and weakness when moving from sitting to standing position, and how to avoid this condition, such as by rising slowly from a supine to an upright position.
•Tell patient to report dizziness, appetite loss, nausea, headache, or severe drowsiness. Warn him to avoid driving if drowsiness occurs.
•Instruct patient to take a missed dose as soon as remembered and to evenly space out the day's remaining doses.
•Advise patient that rash, sometimes accompanied by fever, may appear on day 10 of treatment and should subside by day 15 or 16. Tell him to report severe rash or one that doesn't disappear.

aminophylline
(theophylline ethylenediamine)
Phyllocontin, Truphylline

Class and Category
Chemical class: Xanthine
Therapeutic class: Bronchodilator
Pregnancy category: C

Indications and Dosages
➤ *To relieve acute bronchospasm*
I.V. INFUSION
Adults (nonsmokers) not currently receiving theophylline products. *Initial:* 6 mg/kg (equal to 4.7 mg/kg anhydrous theophylline), not to exceed 25 mg/min. *Maintenance:* 0.7 mg/kg/hr for first 12 hr, then 0.5 mg/kg/hr.
Children ages 9 to 16 not currently receiving theophylline products. *Initial:* 6 mg/kg (equal to 4.7 mg/kg anhydrous theophylline), not to exceed 25 mg/min. *Maintenance:* 1 mg/kg/hr for first 12 hr, then 0.8 mg/kg/hr.
Children ages 6 months to 9 years and young adult smokers not currently receiving theophylline products. *Initial:* 6 mg/kg (equal to 4.7 mg/kg anhydrous theophylline), not to exceed 25 mg/min. *Maintenance:* 1.2 mg/kg/hr for first 12 hr, then 1 mg/kg/hr.
Adults and children currently receiving theophylline products. *Initial:* If possible, determine the time, amount, administration route, and form of last dose. The loading dose is based on the principle that each 0.63 mg/kg (0.5 mg/kg anhydrous theophylline) administered as a loading dose raises the serum theophylline level by 1 mcg/ml. Defer loading dose if serum theophylline level can be readily obtained. If this isn't possible and patient isn't exhibiting obvious signs of theophylline toxicity, prescriber may order 3.1 mg/kg (2.5 mg/kg anhydrous theophylline), which may increase the serum theophylline level by about 5 mcg/ml. *Maintenance:* For adults (nonsmokers), 0.7 mg/kg/hr for first 12 hr, then 0.5 mg/kg/hr. For children ages 9 to 16, 1 mg/kg/hr for first 12 hr, then 0.8 mg/kg/hr. For children ages 6 months to 9 years and young adult smokers, 1.2 mg/kg/hr for first 12 hr, then 1 mg/kg/hr.
DOSAGE ADJUSTMENT For elderly patients and those with cor pulmonale, dosage reduced to 0.6 mg/kg for 12 hr, then 0.3 mg/kg.

For patients with heart failure and hepatic disease, dosage reduced to 0.5 mg/kg for 12 hr, then 0.1 to 0.2 mg/kg.

➤ *To prevent or treat reversible bronchospasm from asthma, chronic bronchitis, and emphysema and to maintain patent airways*

E.R. TABLETS, ORAL LIQUID, TABLETS, SUPPOSITORIES
Adults and children. *Initial (rapidly absorbed forms):* 16 mg/kg daily or 400 mg daily (whichever is less) in divided doses every 6 to 8 hr. *Maintenance:* Daily dosage increased in increments of 25% every 3 days, as tolerated, until response achieved or maximum dose reached. When maximum dose is reached, dosage adjusted according to peak serum theophylline level. *Initial (E.R. forms):* 12 mg/kg daily or 400 mg daily (whichever is less) in divided doses every 8 to 12 hr. *Maintenance:* Daily dosage increased in increments of 2 to 3 mg/kg every 3 days. When maximum dose is reached, dosage adjusted according to peak serum theophylline level.

Route	Onset	Peak	Duration
P.O. (E.R.)	Unknown	Unknown	8 to 12 hr
P.O. (tab)	Unknown	Unknown	6 to 8 hr
I.V.	Immediate	Unknown	4 to 8 hr

Mechanism of Action
Inhibits phosphodiesterase enzymes, causing bronchodilation. Normally, these enzymes inactivate cyclic adenosine monophosphate (cAMP) and cyclic guanosine monophosphate (cGMP), which are responsible for bronchial smooth-muscle relaxation. Other mechanisms of action may include translocation of calcium, prostaglandin antagonism, stimulation of catecholamines, inhibition of cGMP metabolism, and adenosine receptor antagonism.

Incompatibilities
Don't add other drugs to prepared bag or bottle of aminophylline. Don't mix aminophylline in same syringe with doxapram. Also avoid administering amiodarone, ciprofloxacin, diltiazem, dobutamine, hydralazine, or ondansetron into the Y-port of a continuous infusion of aminophylline.

Contraindications
Active peptic ulcer disease, hypersensitivity to aminophylline, rectal or lower intestine irritation or infection (suppository form), underlying seizure disorder

Interactions
DRUGS
activated charcoal, aminoglutethimide, barbiturates, ketoconazole, rifampin, sulfinpyrazone, sympathomimetics: Decreased serum theophylline level
allopurinol, calcium channel blockers, cimetidine, corticosteroids, disulfiram, ephedrine, influenza virus vaccine, interferon, macrolides, mexiletine, nonselective beta blockers, oral contraceptives, quinolones, thiabendazole: Increased serum theophylline level
benzodiazepines: Antagonized sedative effects of benzodiazepines
beta agonists: Increased effects of aminophylline and beta agonist
carbamazepine, isoniazid, loop diuretics: Altered serum theophylline level
halothane: Increased risk of cardiotoxicity
hydantoins: Decreased serum hydantoin level
ketamine: Increased risk of seizures
lithium: Decreased serum lithium level
nondepolarizing muscle relaxants: Reversed neuromuscular blockade
propofol: Antagonized sedative effects of propofol
tetracyclines: Enhanced adverse effects of theophylline
FOODS
all foods: Altered bioavailability and absorption of E.R. aminophylline, leading to toxicity
high-carbohydrate, low-protein diet: Decreased theophylline elimination and prolonged aminophylline half-life
low-carbohydrate, high-protein diet; charcoalbroiled beef: Increased theophylline elimination and shortened aminophylline half-life
ACTIVITIES
alcohol abuse: Increased effects of aminophylline
smoking (1 or more packs daily): Decreased effects of aminophylline

Adverse Reactions
CNS: Dizziness, fever, headache, insomnia, irritability, restlessness, seizures
CV: Arrhythmias (including sinus tachycardia and life-threatening ventricular arrhythmias), hypotension, palpitations

EENT: Bitter aftertaste
ENDO: Hyperglycemia, syndrome of inappropriate ADH secretion
GI: Anorexia, diarrhea, epigastric pain, heavy feeling in stomach, hematemesis, indigestion, nausea, rectal bleeding or irritation (suppositories), vomiting
GU: Diuresis, proteinuria, urine retention in men with prostate enlargement
MS: Muscle twitching
RESP: Respiratory arrest, tachypnea
SKIN: Alopecia, exfoliative dermatitis, flushing, rash, urticaria

Nursing Considerations

•**WARNING** Because aminophylline has a narrow therapeutic window (10 to 20 mcg/ml), closely monitor serum theophylline level and watch for evidence of toxicity (tachycardia, tachypnea, nausea, vomiting, restlessness, seizures). Keep in mind that acetaminophen, furosemide, phenylbutazone, probenecid, theobromine, coffee, tea, soft drinks, and chocolate can alter serum theophylline result.
•To determine peak serum theophylline level, draw blood sample 15 to 30 minutes after administering I.V. loading dose.
•Give immediate-release and liquid forms with food to reduce GI upset. Give E.R. form 1 hour before or 2 hours after meals because food can alter drug absorption.

PATIENT TEACHING
•Advise patient to avoid excessive intake of caffeine (in coffee, tea, soft drinks, and chocolate), which can falsely elevate theophylline level.
•Inform patient that blood tests may be needed to monitor drug's therapeutic effect.

aminosalicylate sodium
(para-aminosalicylate, PAS)

Nemasol Sodium (CAN), PAS

Class and Category

Chemical class: Para-aminobenzoic acid analogue
Therapeutic class: Antitubercular
Pregnancy category: C

Indications and Dosages

➤ *To treat tuberculosis as adjunct to isoniazid, streptomycin, or both and in patients with multidrug-resistant tubercu-*

losis or when therapy with rifampin and isoniazid isn't possible because of resistance or intolerance

TABLETS
Adults. 14 to 16 g daily in 2 or 3 divided doses.
Children. 275 to 420 mg/kg daily in 3 or 4 divided doses.

> ### Mechanism of Action
> Inhibits the incorporation of para-aminobenzoic acid into folic acid and prevents the synthesis of folic acid, a compound necessary for bacterial growth. Aminosalicylate sodium is bacteriostatic against *Mycobacterium tuberculosis,* and it delays bacterial resistance to streptomycin and isoniazid.

Contraindications

Hypersensitivity to aminosalicylate sodium, severe renal disease

Interactions

DRUGS
digoxin: Decreased serum digoxin level
probenecid: Increased serum aminosalicylate level
rifampin: Decreased serum rifampin level

Adverse Reactions

CNS: Encephalopathy, fever
CV: Vasculitis
ENDO: Goiter with or without myxedema
GI: Abdominal pain, diarrhea, hepatitis, nausea, vomiting
HEME: Agranulocytosis, hemolytic anemia, leukopenia, thrombocytopenia
SKIN: Jaundice, various types of eruptions
Other: Infectious mononucleosis-like syndrome, Loeffler's syndrome (anorexia, breathlessness, fever, and weight loss)

Nursing Considerations
•Administer aminosalicylate with food to reduce GI upset.
•**WARNING** Protect drug from water, heat, and sunlight to prevent rapid deterioration. Don't administer tablets that have brown or purple discoloration—a sign of deterioration.

PATIENT TEACHING
•Teach patient to discard aminosalicylate that appears brown or purple.
•Instruct patient to take drug with food.

amiodarone hydrochloride

Cordarone, Nexterone, Pacerone

Class and Category

Chemical class: Iodinated benzofuran derivative
Therapeutic class: Class III antiarrhythmic
Pregnancy category: D

Indications and Dosages

➤ *To treat life-threatening, recurrent ventricular fibrillation and hemodynamically unstable ventricular tachycardia when these arrhythmias don't respond to other drugs or when patient can't tolerate other drugs*

TABLETS
Adults. *Loading:* 800 to 1,600 mg daily in divided doses for 1 to 3 wk. *Maintenance:* 600 to 800 mg daily in divided doses for 1 mo; then if cardiac rhythm is stable, 400 mg daily in one or two doses. Use lowest possible dose.

I.V. INFUSION
Adults. *Loading:* 150 mg over 10 min (15 mg/min) followed by 360 mg infused over 6 hr (1 mg/min). *Maintenance:* 540 mg infused over 18 hr (0.5 mg/min); then after the first 24 hr, 720 mg infused over 24 hr (0.5 mg/min), continued up to 2 to 3 wk, as needed. Rate may be increased in first 24 hr, if neded, but initial infusion rate should not exceed 30 mg/min. Change to oral form as soon as possible.

➤ *To treat breakthrough episodes of ventricular fibrillation or hemodynamically unstable ventricular tachycardia*

I.V. INFUSION (NEXTERONE)
Adults. 150 mg mixed in 100 ml D$_5$W and infused over 10 min (15 mg/min).

Route	Onset	Peak	Duration
P.O.	2 days to 3 wk	1 to 5 mo	Weeks to months
I.V.	Hours to 3 days	1 to 3 wk	Weeks to months

Incompatibilities

Amiodarone is incompatible with heparin. To prevent precipitation, don't add amiodarone admixed with D$_5$W to aminophylline 4 mg/ml, cefamandole nafate, cefazolin sodium, or mezlocillin sodium, and don't mix amiodarone 3 mg/ml with sodium bicarbonate. Also, don't use evacuated glass containers for admixing because precipitation may occur.

Mechanism of Action

Acts on cardiac cell membranes, prolonging repolarization and the refractory period and raising ventricular fibrillation threshold. Drug relaxes vascular smooth muscles, mainly in coronary circulation, and improves myocardial blood flow. It relaxes peripheral vascular smooth muscles, decreasing peripheral vascular resistance and myocardial oxygen consumption.

Contraindications

Bradycardia that causes syncope (unless pacemaker is present), cardiogenic shock, hypersensitivity to amiodarone or its components, hypokalemia, hypomagnesemia, SA node dysfunction, second- and third-degree AV block (unless pacemaker is present)

Interactions

DRUGS
anticoagulants: Increased anticoagulant response, which can result in serious bleeding
azole antifungals, fluoroquinolones, macrolide antibiotics: Increased risk of prolonged QT interval and life-threatening arrhythmias
beta blockers: Increased serum levels of beta blockers with increased risk of AV block, hypotension, and bradycardia
calcium channel blockers: Increased serum levels of these drugs and increased risk of AV block, bradycardia, and hypotension
cholestyramine, phenytoin, rifampin, St. John's wort: Decreased serum amiodarone level
cimetidine: Increased serum amiodarone level
clopidogrel: Increased risk of ineffective inhibition of platelet aggregation
cyclosporine: Increased serum cyclosporine level
dextromethorphan, methotrexate, phenytoin: Increased serum levels of these drugs and increased risk of toxicity if amiodarone is taken orally for more than 2 weeks
digoxin: Increased serum digoxin level and risk of digitalis toxicity

diltiazem, propranolol, verapamil: Increased risk of hemodynamic and electrophysiologic abnormalities
disopyramide: Increased serum disopyramide level with QT prolongation and increased risk of arrhythmias
fentanyl: Increased serum fentanyl level with increased risk of bradycardia, decreased cardiac output, and hypotension
flecainide: Increased serum flecainide level
HMG-CoA reductase inhibitors such as atorvastatin and simvastatin: Increased risk of myopathy and rhabdomyolysis
hydantoins: Increased serum hydantoin level with long-term use and reduced serum amiodarone level
lidocaine: Increased serum lidocaine level and risk of seizures and bradycardia
loratadine, trazodone: Increased risk of QT-interval prolongation and torsades de pointes
potassium- and magnesium-depleting drugs: Increased risk of hypokalemia and hypomagnesemia
procainamide: Increased serum procainamide or N-acetylprocainamide level
quinidine: Increased serum quinidine level with risk of life-threatening arrhythmias
ritonavir: Increased serum amiodarone level with increased risk of cardiotoxicity
theophylline: Increased serum theophylline level; increased risk of theophylline toxicity
warfarin: Increased PT and risk of bleeding

Foods
grapefruit juice: Increased serum amiodarone level

Adverse Reactions

CNS: Abnormal gait, ataxia, confusion, delirium, disorientation, dizziness, fatigue, fever, hallucinations, headache, insomnia, involuntary motor activity, lack of coordination, malaise, paresthesia, parkinsonian symptoms, peripheral neuropathy, pseudotumor cerebri, sleep disturbances, tremor
CV: Arrhythmias (including bradycardia, electromechanical dissociation, torsades de pointes, and ventricular tachycardia or fibrillation), cardiac arrest, cardiogenic shock, edema, heart failure, hypotension, vasculitis
EENT: Abnormal salivation, abnormal taste and smell, blurred vision, corneal microdeposits, dry eyes, halo vision, lens opacities, macular degeneration, optic neuritis, optic neuropathy, papilledema, permanent blindness, photophobia, scotoma

ENDO: Hyperthyroidism, hypothyroidism, syndrome of inappropriate antidiuretic hormone secretion, thyroid cancer
GI: Abdominal pain, anorexia, cirrhosis, constipation, diarrhea, elevated liver function test results, hepatitis, nausea, pancreatitis, vomiting
GU: Acute renal failure, decreased libido, epididymitis, impotence
HEME: Agranulocytosis, aplastic or hemolytic anemia, coagulation abnormalities, neutropenia, pancytopenia, spontaneous bruising, thrombocytopenia
MS: Muscle weakness, myopathy, rhabdomyolysis
RESP: Acute respiratory distress syndrome; bronchospasm; infiltrates that lead to dyspnea, cough, hemoptysis, hypoxia, pulmonary fibrosis, pulmonary alveolar hemorrhage, pulmonary interstitial pneumonitis, crackles, and wheezing; pleuritis; pneumonia; respiratory arrest or failure
SKIN: Alopecia, bluish gray pigmentation, erythema multiforme, exfoliative dermatitis, flushing, photosensitivity, pruritus, rash, skin cancer, Stevens-Johnson syndrome, toxic epidermal necrolysis
Other: Anaphylactic shock, angioedema

Nursing Considerations
•If patient has an implantable cardiac device checked, have it checked, as ordered, at the start of and during amiodarone therapy because drug may affect pacing or defibrillating thresholds.
•Parenteral amiodarone may be diluted in D₅W or normal saline solution and given in polyvinyl chloride (PVC), polyolefin, or glass containers.
•Use an in-line filter during I.V. administration of amiodarone. Also use a central venous catheter whenever possible. A central venous catheter is required when infusion rate exceeds 2 mg/ml because drug may cause peripheral vein phlebitis at higher rates. Cordarone I.V. must be administered with a volumetric infusion pump.
•Monitor amiodarone I.V. infusion closely because loading doses at higher concentrations and rates may cause hepatocellular necrosis, acute renal failure, and death.
•Although maintenance therapy usually is needed for only up to 96 hours, infusion of up to 0.5 mg/minute may be continued for 2 to 3 weeks regardless of patient's age, renal function, or left ventricular function.

•WARNING Be aware that amiodarone may cause or worsen pulmonary disorders that may develop days to weeks after therapy and progress to respiratory failure or even death.
•Monitor vital signs and oxygen levels often during and after giving amiodarone. Keep emergency equipment and drugs nearby.
•WARNING Monitor continuous ECG; check for increased PR and QRS intervals, arrhythmias, and heart rate below 60 beats/min because amiodarone toxicity may cause or worsen arrhythmias.
•Monitor serum amiodarone level, which normally ranges from 1.0 to 2.5 mcg/ml.
•Assess liver enzyme and thyroid hormone levels; drug inhibits conversion of T_4 to T_3 and may cause drug-induced hyperthyroidism, thyrotoxicosis, and new or worsened arrhythmias. If any new signs of arrhythmia occur, notify prescriber at once.

PATIENT TEACHING
•Explain that patient will need frequent monitoring and laboratory tests during treatment.
•Advise patient to report swollen hands and feet, wheezing, dyspnea, cough, nausea, vomiting, dark urine, fatigue, yellow skin or sclerae, stomach pain, light-headedness, fainting, or a rapid, slow, pounding, or irregular heartbeat.
•Instruct patient to report abnormal bleeding or bruising.
•Advise patient to avoid corneal refractive laser surgery while taking drug.

amitriptyline hydrochloride

Apo-amitriptyline (CAN), Endep, Levate (CAN), Novotriptyn (CAN)

Class and Category
Chemical class: Tertiary amine
Therapeutic class: Tricyclic antidepressant
Pregnancy category: D

Indications and Dosages
➤ *To relieve depression, especially when accompanied by anxiety and insomnia*
TABLETS
Adults and children over age 12. *Outpatient:* 75 mg daily in divided doses, increased to 150 mg daily, if needed. *Inpatient:* 100 mg daily, gradually increased to 300 mg daily, if needed. *Maintenance:* 40 to 100 mg daily at bedtime.
DOSAGE ADJUSTMENT Maintenance dosage reduced to 10 mg t.i.d. plus 20 mg at bedtime for adolescent and elderly patients.

Route	Onset	Peak	Duration
P.O.	14 to 21 days	Unknown	Unknown

Contraindications
During acute recovery phase after MI, hypersensitivity to amitriptyline, MAO inhibitor therapy within 14 days

Interactions
DRUGS
anticholinergics, epinephrine, norepinephrine: Increased effects of these drugs
barbiturates: Decreased serum amitriptyline level
carbamazepine: Decreased serum amitriptyline level and increased serum carbamazepine level, which increases therapeutic and toxic effects of carbamazepine
cimetidine, disulfiram, fluoxetine, fluvoxamine, haloperidol, H_2-receptor antagonists, methylphenidate, oral contraceptives, paroxetine, phenothiazines, sertraline: Increased serum amitriptyline level
cisapride: Possibly prolonged QT interval and increased risk for arrhythmias
clonidine, guanethidine, and other antihypertensives: Decreased antihypertensive effects
dicumarol: Increased anticoagulant effect
levodopa: Decreased levodopa absorption; sympathetic hyperactivity, sinus tachycardia, hypertension, agitation
MAO inhibitors: Possibly seizures and death
thyroid replacement drugs: Arrhythmias and increased antidepressant effects
ACTIVITIES
alcohol use: Enhanced CNS depression
smoking: Decreased amitriptyline effects

Adverse Reactions
CNS: Anxiety, ataxia, coma, chills, delusions, disorientation, drowsiness, extrapyramidal reactions, fatigue, fever, headache, insomnia, nightmares, peripheral neuropathy, suicidal ideation, tremor
CV: Arrhythmias (including prolonged AV conduction, heart block, and tachycardia), cardiomyopathy, hypertension, MI, nonspecific ECG changes, orthostatic hypotension,

Mechanism of Action

Normally, when an impulse reaches adrenergic nerves, the nerves release serotonin and norepinephrine from their storage sites. Some serotonin and norepinephrine reaches receptor sites on target tissues. Most is taken back into the nerves and stored by the reuptake mechanism, as shown below on the left.

Amitriptyline blocks serotonin and norepinephrine reuptake by adrenergic nerves. By doing so, it raises serotonin and norepinephrine levels at nerve synapses. This action may elevate mood and reduce depression.

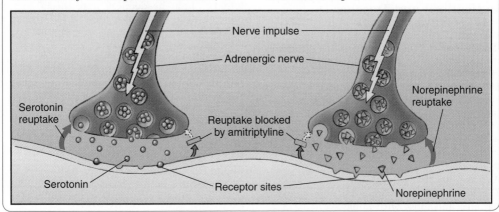

palpitations
EENT: Abnormal taste, black tongue, blurred vision, dry mouth, increased salivation, nasal congestion, tinnitus
ENDO: Gynecomastia, increased or decreased blood glucose level, increased prolactin level, syndrome of inappropriate ADH secretion
GI: Abdominal cramps, constipation, diarrhea, flatulence, ileus, increased appetite, nausea, vomiting
GU: Impotence, libido changes, menstrual irregularities, testicular swelling, urinary hesitancy, urine retention
HEME: Agranulocytosis, bone marrow depression, eosinophilia, leukopenia, thrombocytopenia
SKIN: Alopecia, flushing, purpura
Other: Weight gain

Nursing Considerations

• Because of amitriptyline's atropine-like effects, use caution if patient has a history of seizures, urine retention, or angle-closure glaucoma.
• **WARNING** Don't give an MAO inhibitor within 14 days of amitriptyline therapy because of the risk of seizures and death.
• Closely monitor patient with CV disorder because amitriptyline may cause arrhythmias, such as sinus tachycardia.
• Watch patients closely (especially children, adolescents, and young adults), for suicidal tendencies, particularly when therapy starts and dosage changes, because depression may worsen temporarily during these times.
• Monitor blood pressure for hypotension or hypertension.
• Stay alert for behavior changes, such as hallucinations and decreased interest in personal appearance. Be aware that psychosis may develop in schizophrenic patients, and symptoms may increase in paranoid patients.
• Abrupt withdrawal after long use may cause nausea, headache, vertigo, and nightmares.
PATIENT TEACHING
• Instruct patient to take amitriptyline at bedtime to avoid daytime drowsiness.
• Instruct patient to avoid using alcohol or OTC drugs that contain alcohol during amitriptyline therapy because alcohol enhances CNS depressant effects.
• Urge family or caregiver to watch patient closely for suicidal tendencies, especially when therapy starts or dosage changes and particularly if patient is a child, teenager, or young adult.

amlodipine besylate

Norvasc

Class and Category
Chemical class: Dihydropyridine
Therapeutic class: Antianginal, anti-hypertensive
Pregnancy category: C

Indications and Dosages
➤ *To control hypertension*
TABLETS
Adults. *Initial:* 5 mg daily, increased gradually over 10 to 14 days, as needed. *Maximum:* 10 mg daily.
DOSAGE ADJUSTMENT Initially 2.5 mg daily for elderly patients or patients with impaired hepatic function. Dosage increased gradually over 7 to 14 days based on response.

➤ *To treat chronic stable angina and Prinzmetal's (variant) angina*
TABLETS
Adults. 5 to 10 mg daily.
DOSAGE ADJUSTMENT 5 mg daily for elderly patients and those with impaired hepatic function.

Route	Onset	Peak	Duration
P.O.	Unknown	6 to 12 hr	24 hr

Mechanism of Action
Binds to dihydropyridine and nondihydro-pyridine cell membrane receptor sites on myocardial and vascular smooth-muscle cells and inhibits influx of extracellular calcium ions across slow calcium channels. This decreases intracellular calcium level, inhibiting smooth-muscle cell contractions and relaxing coronary and vascular smooth muscles, decreasing peripheral vascular resistance, and reducing systolic and diastolic blood pressure. Decreased peripheral vascular resistance also decreases myocardial workload, oxygen demand, and possibly angina. Also, by inhibiting coronary artery muscle cell contractions and restoring blood flow, drug may relieve Prinzmetal's angina.

Contraindications
Hypersensitivity to amlodipine or components

Interactions
DRUGS
beta blockers: Possibly excessive hypotension
fentanyl: Increased risk of severe hypotension and increased fluid volume requirements during surgery

Adverse Reactions
CNS: Anxiety, dizziness, fatigue, headache, lethargy, light-headedness, paresthesia, somnolence, syncope, tremor
CV: Arrhythmias, hypotension, palpitations, peripheral edema
EENT: Dry mouth, pharyngitis
ENDO: Hot flashes
GI: Abdominal cramps, abdominal pain, constipation, diarrhea, esophagitis, indigestion, nausea
GU: Decreased libido, impotence, urinary frequency
MS: Myalgia
RESP: Dyspnea
SKIN: Dermatitis, flushing, rash
Other: Weight loss

Nursing Considerations
•Use amlodipine cautiously in patients with heart block, heart failure, impaired renal function, hepatic disorder, or severe aortic stenosis.
•Monitor blood pressure while adjusting dosage, especially in patients with heart failure or severe aortic stenosis.
PATIENT TEACHING
•Tell patient to take missed dose as soon as it's remembered and next dose in 24 hours.
•Tell patient to immediately notify prescriber of dizziness, arm or leg swelling, difficulty breathing, hives, or rash.
•Suggest taking amlodipine with food to reduce GI upset.
•Advise patient to routinely have blood pressure checked for possible hypotension.

ammonium chloride

Class and Category
Chemical class: Ammonium ion
Therapeutic class: Acidifier
Pregnancy category: C

Indications and Dosages
➤ *To treat hypochloremia and metabolic alkalosis*

I.V. INFUSION
Adults. Individualized, based on serum bicarbonate level. *Usual:* 100 to 200 mEq added to 500 or 1,000 ml of normal saline solution, infused at 5 ml/min or less (about 3 hr for an infusion of 1,000 ml).

Route	Onset	Peak	Duration
I.V.	1 to 3 min	3 to 6 hr	Unknown

Mechanism of Action
Is converted to urea and hydrochloric acid in the liver. During conversion, the drug breaks into ammonium and chloride ions, and hydrogen ions are released. They enter the blood and extracellular fluid, where hydrogen reacts with bicarbonate ions to form water and carbon dioxide. This process decreases bicarbonate ions and increases chloride ions in blood and extracellular fluid, which decreases blood and urine pH and corrects alkalosis.

Incompatibilities
Don't mix I.V. ammonium chloride with codeine, levorphanol, or methadone.

Contraindications
Hypersensitivity to ammonium chloride or its components, markedly impaired renal or hepatic function, metabolic alkalosis caused by vomiting of hydrochloric acid and accompanied by sodium loss caused by sodium bicarbonate excretion in urine

Interactions
DRUGS
amphetamines, salicylates, sulfonylureas, tricyclic antidepressants: Decreased therapeutic blood level of ammonium
chlorpropamide: Increased ammonium effects

Adverse Reactions
CNS: Fever, headache
CV: Phlebitis or thrombosis extending from injection site
GI: Indigestion, nausea, severe hepatic dysfunction, vomiting
RESP: Hyperventilation
SKIN: Extravasation
Other: Injection site infection, irritation, or pain; hypovolemia; severe metabolic acidosis (with large doses)

Nursing Considerations
• Before use, warm ammonium chloride solution to room temperature to dissolve crystals by placing infusion in warm water.
• During I.V. use, keep sodium bicarbonate or sodium lactate nearby to treat overdose.
• Infuse ammonium chloride slowly to avoid I.V. site pain and irritation.
• **WARNING** Monitor patient for ammonia toxicity (arrhythmias, such as bradycardia; coma; irregular breathing; pallor; retching; seizures; diaphoresis; and twitching).
• Watch for signs of metabolic acidosis, such as increased respirations, increased serum pH, restlessness, and diaphoresis.
• Monitor serum bicarbonate level, the results of urinalysis, and the results of renal and liver function tests as appropriate.
PATIENT TEACHING
• Tell patient to eat potassium-rich foods, such as bananas, oranges, cantaloupe, spinach, dried fruit, and potatoes, during therapy.

amobarbital sodium
Amytal, Novamobarb (CAN)

Class, Category, and Schedule
Chemical class: Barbiturate
Therapeutic class: Anticonvulsant, sedative-hypnotic
Pregnancy category: D
Controlled substance schedule: II

Indications and Dosages
➤ *To produce preanesthesia sedation*
CAPSULES, ELIXIR, TABLETS
Adults. 200 mg 1 to 2 hr before surgery.
Children. 2 to 6 mg/kg up to a maximum of 100 mg/dose.
➤ *To produce sedation*
CAPSULES, ELIXIR, TABLETS, I.V. OR I.M. INJECTION
Adults. 30 to 50 mg (may range from 15 to 120 mg) b.i.d. or t.i.d. *Maximum I.V.:* 1,000 mg/dose. *Maximum I.M.:* 500 mg/dose.
Children over age 6. 2 mg/kg daily in four divided doses.
➤ *To treat insomnia*
CAPSULES, ELIXIR, TABLETS
Adults. 65 to 200 mg at bedtime for up to 2 wk.
➤ *To induce a hypnotic state*
CAPSULES, ELIXIR, TABLETS, I.V. OR I.M. INJECTION

Adults. 65 to 200 mg/dose. *Maximum I.V.:* 1,000 mg/dose. *Maximum I.M.:* 500 mg/dose
Children up to age 6. 2 to 3 mg/kg I.M. per dose.

➤ *To manage seizures*
I.V. OR I.M. INJECTION
Adults. *Usual:* 65 to 500 mg to a maximum of 1,000 mg. Dosage for acute seizures is determined by response; 200- to 500-mg doses are typically needed to control seizures.
Children age 6 and over. 65 to 500 mg I.V.
Children up to age 6. 3 to 5 mg/kg/dose.
WARNING Use I.V. route only when other routes aren't appropriate. For I.V. injection, use I.M. dose and inject slowly at a rate of 50 mg/min or less to prevent sudden respiratory depression, apnea, laryngospasm, or hypotension.

Route	Onset	Peak	Duration
P.O.*	60 min	Unknown	10 to 12 hr
I.V.	Unknown	Unknown	10 to 12 hr
I.M.	Unknown	Unknown	10 to 12 hr

Mechanism of Action
Nonselectively acts on the CNS to depress the sensory cortex, decrease motor activity, alter cerebellar function, and produce drowsiness, sedation, and hypnosis. Appears to reduce wakefulness and alertness by acting in the thalamus, where it depresses the reticular activating system and interferes with impulse transmission from the periphery to the cortex. Produces CNS depressant effects ranging from mild sedation and anxiety reduction to anesthesia and coma, depending on the dose, route, and individual patient's response.

Incompatibilities
Don't mix amobarbital in solution with other drugs.

Contraindications
Alcoholism, history of porphyria, history of sedative or barbiturate addiction, hypersensitivity to barbiturates, renal or hepatic disease, severe respiratory disease, sleep apnea, suicidal tendency, uncontrolled pain

---

* For capsules, elixir, and tablets.

Interactions
DRUGS
acetaminophen: Increased blood acetaminophen level and risk of hepatotoxicity
antihistamines, CNS depressants, phenothiazines, tranquilizers: Increased CNS depression
beta blockers, carbamazepine, clonazepam, corticosteroids, digitoxin, doxycycline, estrogens, griseofulvin, metronidazole, oral anticoagulants, oral contraceptives, phenylbutazones, quinidine, theophyllines, tricyclic antidepressants: Decreased blood levels and effects of these drugs
chloramphenicol: Inhibited amobarbital metabolism; enhanced chloramphenicol metabolism
MAO inhibitors: Increased serum level and sedative effects of amobarbital
methoxyflurane: Increased nephrotoxicity
phenytoin: Altered effects of phenytoin
rifampin: Decreased serum level and effects of amobarbital
valproic acid: Increased amobarbital effects
ACTIVITIES
alcohol use: Increased serum level of amobarbital and additive CNS depressant effects

Adverse Reactions
CNS: Agitation, anxiety, ataxia, CNS depression, confusion, dizziness, hallucinations, hangover, headache, hyperkinesia, insomnia, nightmares, nervousness, paradoxical stimulation, permanent neurologic deficit (with injection near nerve), psychiatric disturbance, somnolence, syncope, vertigo
CV: Bradycardia, hypotension, shock
EENT: Laryngospasm
GI: Constipation, diarrhea, epigastric pain, nausea, vomiting
RESP: Apnea, bronchospasm, hypoventilation, respiratory depression
SKIN: Exfoliative dermatitis, rash, Stevens-Johnson syndrome, urticaria
Other: Angioedema, gangrene of arm or leg from accidental injection into artery, injection site tissue damage and necrosis, physical and psychological dependence, potentially fatal withdrawal syndrome, tolerance

Nursing Considerations
•Use amobarbital cautiously in patients with cardiac disease, debilitation, diabetes mellitus, fever, hyperthyroidism, severe anemia, shock, status asthmaticus, or uremia.

A

• Administer by deep I.M. injection, preferably in large muscle.
• During I.V. administration, closely monitor blood pressure, pulse, and respirations. Keep emergency equipment and drugs nearby in case respiratory depression occurs.
• WARNING Don't administer solution after 30 minutes of exposure to air. Solution quickly becomes unstable because amobarbital sodium hydrolyzes in solution.
• To prevent withdrawal symptoms, such as diaphoresis, insomnia, irritability, nightmares, and tremors, expect to taper amobarbital dosage gradually after long-term use, especially for epileptic patients.
• WARNING To prevent tissue damage and necrosis at I.M. injection site, don't give more than 5 ml of this highly alkaline drug at any one site. Know that accidental arterial injection may cause gangrene of the arm or leg.

PATIENT TEACHING
• Advise patient to use caution when driving or performing tasks that require alertness.
• Instruct patient not to use alcohol or other CNS depressants (unless prescribed) because they increase amobarbital's effects.
• Warn patient not to stop taking drug abruptly; withdrawal symptoms can occur.
• Instruct patient to report severe dizziness, persistent drowsiness, rash, or skin lesions.
• Explain that drug effects, such as drowsiness, may become less pronounced after a few days and when drug is taken with food.

amoxapine

Asendin

Class and Category
Chemical class: Dibenzoxazepine derivative
Therapeutic class: Tricyclic antidepressant
Pregnancy category: C

Indications and Dosages
➤ *To relieve depression, including endogenous (long-term) depression and depression associated with anxiety and agitation*

TABLETS
Adults and children age 16 and over. *Initial:* 50 mg b.i.d. or t.i.d., increased to 100 mg b.i.d. or t.i.d. by end of first wk, if tolerated. *Maintenance:* If 300-mg daily dose is ineffective after 2-wk trial period, dosage increased

to a maximum of 400 mg daily in divided doses. Inpatients may receive up to a maximum of 600 mg daily in divided doses. When effective dose is achieved, a single dose may be given at bedtime, not to exceed 300 mg.
DOSAGE ADJUSTMENT For elderly patients: *Initial:* 25 mg b.i.d. or t.i.d., increased to 50 mg b.i.d. or t.i.d. by end of first wk. *Maintenance:* 100 to 150 mg daily in divided doses, carefully increased to 300 mg daily as tolerated. When effective dose is achieved, a single dose may be given at bedtime, not to exceed 300 mg.

Route	Onset	Peak	Duration
P.O.	2 to 3 wk	Unknown	Unknown

Mechanism of Action
Blocks serotonin and norepinephrine reuptake by adrenergic nerves. By doing this, it raises serotonin and norepinephrine levels at nerve synapses. This action may elevate mood and reduce depression.
    Normally, when an impulse reaches adrenergic nerves, they release serotonin and norepinephrine from their storage sites. Some serotonin and norepinephrine reach receptor sites on target tissues. The majority is taken back into the nerves and stored by the reuptake mechanism.

Contraindications
Acute recovery phase after MI, hypersensitivity to amoxapine or its components, MAO inhibitor therapy within 14 days

Interactions
DRUGS
anticholinergics, epinephrine, norepinephrine: Increased effects of these drugs
barbiturates: Decreased serum amoxapine level
carbamazepine: Decreased serum amoxapine level; increased serum carbamazepine level, increasing its therapeutic and toxic effects
cimetidine, disulfiram, fluoxetine, fluvoxamine, haloperidol, H_2-receptor antagonists, methylphenidate, oral contraceptives, paroxetine, phenothiazines, sertraline: Increased blood amoxapine level
clonidine, guanethidine, other antihypertensives: Decreased antihypertensive effects

dicumarol: Increased anticoagulant effect
levodopa: Decreased levodopa absorption;
agitation, hypertension, sinus tachycardia,
sympathetic hyperactivity
MAO inhibitors: Possibly seizures and death
thyroid replacement drugs: Arrhythmias and
increased antidepressant effects
ACTIVITIES
alcohol use: Increased CNS depression
smoking: Decreased amoxapine effects

Adverse Reactions

CNS: Agitation, anxiety, ataxia, chills, confusion, dizziness, drowsiness, excitement, extrapyramidal reactions, fatigue, fever, headache, insomnia, nervousness, nightmares,
paresthesia, restlessness, sedation, seizures,
stroke, syncope, tremor, weakness
CV: Atrial arrhythmias, heart block, heart
failure, hypertension, hypotension, MI, palpitations, tachycardia
EENT: Blurred vision, dry mouth, increased
salivation, nasal congestion, taste perversion,
tinnitus
ENDO: Gynecomastia, increased or decreased blood glucose level, increased prolactin level, syndrome of inappropriate ADH
secretion
GI: Anorexia, constipation, diarrhea, elevated liver function test results, flatulence,
increased appetite, nausea, vomiting
GU: Impotence, libido changes, menstrual irregularities, testicular swelling, urinary hesitancy, urine retention
HEME: Agranulocytosis, leukopenia
SKIN: Diaphoresis, flushing, photosensitivity,
pruritus, rash
Other: Weight gain or loss; withdrawal symptoms, such as headache, nausea, nightmares,
and vertigo

Nursing Considerations

• **WARNING** Don't administer an MAO inhibitor within 14 days of administering amoxapine therapy.
• To avoid withdrawal, don't stop drug
abruptly.
• Watch patients closely (especially children,
adolescents, and young adults), for suicidal
tendencies, particularly when therapy starts
and dosage changes, because depression may
worsen temporarily during these times.
PATIENT TEACHING
• Advise patient to take amoxapine at bedtime if daytime sedation occurs.

• Caution patient that stopping amoxapine
therapy abruptly may cause withdrawal
symptoms.
• Encourage patient to avoid alcohol because
it can potentiate amoxapine's effects.
• Tell patient to report adverse effects of
amoxapine.
• Instruct patient to take drug with food to
prevent GI upset.
• Urge family or caregiver to watch patient
closely for suicidal tendencies, especially
when therapy starts or dosage changes and
particularly if patient is a child, teenager, or
young adult.

amoxicillin trihydrate
(amoxycillin)

Amoxil, Apo-Amoxi (CAN), DisperMox,
Moxatag, Novamoxin (CAN), Nu-Amoxi (CAN),
Polymox, Trimox, Wymox

Class and Category

Chemical class: Aminopenicillin
Therapeutic class: Antibiotic
Pregnancy category: B

Indications and Dosages

➤ *To treat ear, nose, throat, GU tract, skin,*
and soft-tissue infections caused by sus-
ceptible gram-positive and gram-
negative organisms
CAPSULES, CHEWABLE TABLETS, ORAL SUSPENSION,
PEDIATRIC DROPS, POWDER OR TABLETS FOR ORAL
SUSPENSION, TABLETS
Adults and children weighing 20 kg (44 lb)
or more. 250 mg every 8 hr; for severe infections, 500 mg every 8 hr or 875 mg every
12 hr.
Children age 12 wk and over weighing less
than 20 kg. 20 mg/kg daily in divided doses
every 8 hr; for severe infections, 40 to 45 mg/
kg/day in divided doses every 8 hr.
Children under age 12 wk. 30 mg/kg/ day in
divided doses every 12 hr.

➤ *To treat tonsillitis or pharyngitis caused*
by Streptococcus pyogenes
E.R. TABLETS (MOXATAG)
Adults and children age 12 and over. 775 mg
once dailyfor 10 days, taken within 1 hr of
finishing a meal.

➤ *To treat lower respiratory tract infec-*
tions caused by susceptible gram-

positive and gram-negative organisms
CAPSULES, CHEWABLE TABLETS, ORAL SUSPENSION, PEDIATRIC DROPS, POWDER OR TABLETS FOR ORAL SUSPENSION, TABLETS

Adults and children weighing 20 kg or more. 875 mg every 12 hr; for severe infections, 500 mg every 8 hr.

Children age 12 wk and over weighing less than 20 kg. 40 to 45 mg/kg daily in divided doses every 8 hr.

Children under age 12 wk. 30 mg/kg daily in divided doses every 12 hr.

➤ *To treat gonorrhea and acute uncomplicated anogenital and urethral infections caused by susceptible strains of gram-positive and gram-negative organisms*
CAPSULES, CHEWABLE TABLETS, ORAL SUSPENSION, POWDER OR TABLETS FOR ORAL SUSPENSION, TABLETS

Adults and postpubertal children. 3 g as a single dose.

Prepubertal children age 2 and over. 50 mg/kg of amoxicillin plus 25 mg/kg of probenecid as a single dose.

➤ *As adjunct to eradicate* Helicobacter pylori *to reduce risk of duodenal ulcer recurrence*
CAPSULES, CHEWABLE TABLETS, ORAL SUSPENSION, POWDER OR TABLETS FOR ORAL SUSPENSION, TABLETS

Adults. 1 g every 12 hr with 500 mg of clarithromycin every 12 hr and 30 mg of lansoprazole every 12 hr for 14 days. Or, 1 g every 8 hr with 30 mg of lansoprazole every 8 hr for 14 days.

➤ *To prevent bacterial endocarditis before dental, oral, or upper respiratory tract procedures*
CAPSULES, CHEWABLE TABLETS, ORAL SUSPENSION, POWDER OR TABLETS FOR ORAL SUSPENSION, TABLETS

Adults and children weighing 20 kg or more. 2 g 1 hr before procedure.

Children weighing less than 20 kg. 50 mg/kg 1 hr before procedure.

Route	Onset	Peak	Duration
P.O.	Unknown	Unknown	6 to 8 hr

Mechanism of Action

Kills bacteria by binding to and inactivating penicillin-binding proteins on the inner bacterial cell wall, weakening the bacterial cell wall and causing lysis.

Contraindications

Hypersensitivity to amoxicillin or its components

Interactions

DRUGS

allopurinol: Increased risk of rash
chloramphenicol, erythromycins, sulfonamides, tetracyclines: Reduced bactericidal effect of amoxicillin
methotrexate: Increased risk of methotrexate toxicity
oral contraceptives with estrogen: Possibly reduced effectiveness of contraceptive
probenecid: Increased amoxicillin effects

Adverse Reactions

CNS: Agitation, anxiety, behavior changes, confusion, dizziness, insomnia, reversible hyperactivity, seizures
CV: Hypersensitivity vasculitis
EENT: Black, hairy tongue; mucocutaneous candididasis; tooth discoloration
GI: Diarrhea, diarrhea related to *Clostridium difficile,* elevated liver enzymes, hemorrhagic or pseudomembranous colitis, jaundice, hepatic dysfunction, nausea, vomiting
GU: Crystalluria, vaginal mycosis
HEME: Agranulocytosis, anemia (including hemolytic anemia), eosinophilia, granulocytosis, leukopenia, thrombocytopenia, thrombocytopenic purpura
SKIN: Erythema multiforme, erythematous maculopapular rash, generalized exanthematous pustulosis, Stevens-Johnson syndrome, toxic epidermal necrolysis, urticaria
Other: Allergic reaction, anaphylaxis, serum sicknesslike reaction (such as arthralgia, arthritis, fever, myalgia, rash, and urticaria)

Nursing Considerations

•Patients with mononucleosis shouldn't receive amoxicillin because this class of antibiotics may cause an erythematous rash.
•Use drug cautiously in patients with hepatic impairment. Monitor hepatic and renal function and CBC, as ordered, in patients on prolonged therapy. Also use cautiously in breast-feeding and elderly patients.
•Expect to start therapy before culture and sensitivity test results are known.
•Be aware that chewable tablets and tablets for oral suspension contain phenylalanine.
•Don't confuse amoxicillin tablets with amoxicillin tablets for oral suspension

(DisperMox). They're not interchangeable.
•**WARNING** If allergic reaction occurs, stop amoxicillin immediately and provide emergency care as indicated and ordered.
•Monitor patient closely for diarrhea, which may indicate pseudomembranous colitis caused by *Clostridium difficile.* If diarrhea occurs, notify prescriber, expect to withhold amoxicillin, and treat with fluids, electrolytes, protein, and an antibiotic effective against *C. difficile.*
•Expect treatment to last at least 10 days for infections caused by hemolytic streptococci.
•Monitor patient for superinfection. If it occurs, expect to discontinue drug and provide treatment as ordered.

PATIENT TEACHING
•Tell patient to refrigerate reconstituted suspension and to shake well before each use.
•When amoxicillin suspension is prescribed for a child, instruct parents to place it directly on child's tongue for him to swallow. If this doesn't work, tell parents to mix dose of suspension with formula or cold drink (milk, fruit juice, ginger ale, water) and then have child drink all of it immediately.
•Instruct patient using DisperMox tablets to place one tablet and about 2 teaspoonfuls of water in a glass, drink entire mixture, add more water to the glass, and drink again to ensure delivery of full dose.
•Tell patient to chew or crush chewable tablets and not to swallow them whole.
•To prevent infection from recurring, urge patient to take amoxicillin for full length of time prescribed, even if he feels better.
•Teach patient to report adverse reactions and notify prescriber if infection worsens or doesn't improve after 72 hours of therapy.
•Urge patient to tell prescriber about diarrhea that's severe or lasts longer than 3 days. Remind patient that watery or bloody stools can occur 2 or more months after antibiotic therapy and may be serious, requiring prompt treatment.

amphetamine sulfate

dexamphetamine sulfate

Liquadd

Class, Category, and Schedule

Chemical class: Sympathomimetic amine
Therapeutic class: CNS stimulant
Pregnancy category: C
Controlled substance schedule: II

Indications and Dosages

➤ *To treat attention deficit hyperactivity disorder (ADHD)*

ORAL SOLUTION (LIQUADD)
Children ages 3 to 6. *Initial:* 2.5 mg daily. Increased by 2.5 mg daily at 1-wk intervals until desired response occurs.
Children age 6 and over. *Initial:* 5 mg daily or b.i.d. Increased by 5 mg daily at 1-wk intervals until desired response occurs.

TABLETS
Children age 6 and over. *Initial:* 5 mg daily or b.i.d. Increased by 5 mg daily at 1-wk intervals until desired response occurs. *Usual:* 0.1 to 0.5 mg/kg daily.
Children ages 3 to 5. *Initial:* 2.5 mg daily. Increased by 2.5 mg daily at 1-wk intervals until desired response occurs. *Usual:* 0.1 to 0.5 mg/kg daily.

➤ *To treat narcolepsy*

ORAL SOLUTION (LIQUADD)
Adults and children age 12 and over. *Initial:* 10 mg daily. Increased by 10 mg daily at 1-wk intervals until desired response occurs.
Children ages 6 to 12. *Initial:* 2.5 mg b.i.d. Increased by 5 mg daily at 1-wk intervals until desired response occurs.

TABLETS
Adults and children age 12 and over. *Initial:* 10 mg daily. Increased by 10 mg daily at 1-wk intervals until desired response occurs.
Children ages 6 to 12. *Initial:* 2.5 mg b.i.d. Increased by 5 mg daily at 1-wk intervals until desired response occurs or adult dosage is reached to a maximum of 60 mg daily.

Contraindications

Advanced arteriosclerosis, agitation (for narcolepsy treatment), glaucoma, history of drug abuse, hypersensitivity or idiosyncratic reaction to sympathomimetic amines, hyperthyroidism, MAO inhibitor therapy within 14 days, moderate to severe hypertension, symptomatic cardiovascular disease

Interactions

DRUGS
adrenergic blockers: Inhibited adrenergic blockade
acetazolamide, alkalinizers (such as sodium bicarbonate), some thiazides: Increased blood

level and effects of amphetamine
antihistamines: Possibly reduced sedation from antihistamine
antihypertensives: Possibly decreased antihypertensive effects
chlorpromazine: Inhibited CNS stimulant effects of amphetamine
ethosuximide: Possibly delayed ethosuximide absorption
GI acidifiers (such as ascorbic acid), reserpine: Decreased amphetamine absorption
guanethidine: Decreased antihypertensive effect and decreased amphetamine absorption
haloperidol: Decreased CNS stimulation
lithium carbonate: Possibly decreased anorectic and stimulant effects of amphetamine
MAO inhibitors: Potentiated effects of amphetamine; possibly hypertensive crisis
meperidine: Increased analgesia
methenamine: Increased urine excretion and decreased effects of amphetamine
norepinephrine: Possibly increased adrenergic effect of norepinephrine
phenobarbital, phenytoin: Synergistic anticonvulsant action
propoxyphene: Increased CNS stimulation, potentially fatal seizures
tricyclic antidepressants: Possibly enhanced antidepressant effects and decreased effects of amphetamine
urinary acidifiers (such as ammonium chloride and sodium acid phosphate): Increased amphetamine excretion and decreased amphetamine blood level and effects
Veratrum *alkaloids:* Decreased hypotensive effect
FOODS
acidic fruit juices: Decreased amphetamine absorption

Adverse Reactions
CNS: Anxiety, dizziness, dyskinesia, dysphoria, euphoria, exacerbation of motor and phonic tics and Tourette's syndrome, hallucinations, headache, insomnia, overstimulation, paranoia, psychotic episodes, restlessness, tremor
CV: Cardiomyopathy, hypertension, palpitations, tachycardia
EENT: Dry mouth, unpleasant taste
GI: Anorexia, constipation, diarrhea
GU: Impotence, libido changes
SKIN: Urticaria
Other: Weight loss

Mechanism of Action
May produce its CNS stimulant effects by facilitating the release and blocking the reuptake of norepinephrine at the adrenergic nerve terminals and by direct stimulation of alpha and beta receptors in the peripheral nervous system. It also releases and blocks the reuptake of dopamine in limbic regions of the brain. The drug's main action appears to be in the cerebral cortex and, possibly, the reticular activating system. These actions cause decreased motor restlessness, increased alertness, and diminished drowsiness and fatigue. Its peripheral actions include increased blood pressure and mild bronchodilation and respiratory stimulation.

Nursing Considerations
•Keep in mind that when symptoms of ADHD occur with acute stress reactions, treatment with amphetamines usually isn't indicated.
•**WARNING** To prevent hypertensive crisis, don't administer amphetamine during or for up to 14 days after MAO therapy.
•Administer first dose when patient awakens and additional doses at 4- to 6-hour intervals.
•Be aware that 5 ml of oral solution contains 5 mg of dexamphetamine.
•If patient experiences bothersome adverse reactions, such as insomnia and anorexia, expect to decrease dosage. To minimize insomnia, administer drug earlier in day.
•Be alert for signs of long-term amphetamine abuse, such as severe dermatoses, marked insomnia, irritability, hyperactivity, and personality changes. If patient suddenly stops drug after long-term, high-dose regimen, watch for extreme fatigue and depression.

PATIENT TEACHING
•Instruct breast-feeding patient to avoid breast-feeding during amphetamine therapy because drug is excreted in breast milk.
•Teach patient to take first dose on awakening and subsequent doses at 4- to 6-hour intervals. Tell him not to take last dose late in evening because insomnia may occur.
•Inform patient or caregiver that each 5 ml

of oral solution contains 5 mg of dexamphet-amine. Advise patient to use a calibrated measuring device to ensure accurate dose.
•Urge patient to avoid potentially hazardous activities until drug's effects are known.
•Advise patient not to take amphetamine with acidic fruit juice because it decreases drug absorption.
•Explain drug's abuse potential, and caution against altering dosage unless prescribed.

amphotericin B
Amphocin, Fungizone Intravenous

amphotericin B cholesteryl sulfate complex
Amphotec

amphotericin B lipid complex
Abelcet

amphotericin B liposomal complex
AmBisome

Class and Category
Chemical class: Amphoteric polyene macrolide
Therapeutic class: Antifungal
Pregnancy category: B (I.V.); C (oral suspension)

Indications and Dosages
➤ *To treat severe fungal infections, using amphotericin B*
I.V. INFUSION
Adults and adolescents. *Initial:* 1-mg test dose in 20 ml of D_5W infused over 20 to 30 min; if test dose is tolerated, then 0.25 to 0.3 mg/kg daily prepared as a 0.1 mg/ml infusion, given over 2 to 6 hr. Increased in 5- to 10-mg increments up to 50 mg daily, based on patient tolerance and infection severity, not to exceed a total daily dose of 1.5 mg/kg. *Maximum:* 50 mg daily infused over 2 to 6 hr.
Children. *Initial:* 0.25 mg/kg daily in D_5W infused over 6 hr; then increased in 0.125- to 0.25-mg/kg increments daily or every other day as tolerated. *Maximum:* 1 mg/kg or 30 mg/m^2 of body surface daily.

➤ *To treat oral candidiasis, using amphotericin B*
ORAL SUSPENSION
Adults and children. 1 ml (100 mg) q.i.d. for 14 days.

➤ *To treat aspergillosis, using amphotericin B cholesteryl sulfate complex*
I.V. INFUSION
Adults and children. Test dose of 1.6 to 8.3 mg in 10 ml of D_5W infused over 15 to 30 min; if test dose is tolerated, then 3 to 4 mg/kg once daily infused at 1 mg/kg/hr.

➤ *To treat invasive amphotericin B-resistant fungal infections, using amphotericin B lipid complex*
I.V. INFUSION
Adults and children. 5 mg/kg daily infused at 2.5 mg/kg/hr.

➤ *To treat severe aspergillosis, candidiasis, or cryptococcosis, using amphotericin B liposomal complex*
I.V. INFUSION
Adults and children. 3 to 5 mg/kg daily infused over 2 hr. Infusion time may be decreased to 1 hr if tolerated or increased if patient experiences discomfort.

➤ *To treat leishmaniasis, using amphotericin B liposomal complex*
I.V. INFUSION
Immunocompetent adults and children. 3 mg/kg daily on days 1 through 5 and on days 14 and 21 infused over 2 hr. Infusion time may be decreased to 1 hr if tolerated or increased if patient has discomfort.
Immunocompromised adults and children. 4 mg/kg daily on days 1 through 5 and on days 10, 17, 24, 31, and 38 infused over 2 hr. Infusion time may be decreased to 1 hr if tolerated or increased if patient has discomfort.

➤ *To treat presumed fungal infections in patients with febrile neutropenia, using amphotericin B lipid complex*
I.V. INFUSION
Adults and children. 3 mg/kg daily infused over 2 hr. Infusion time may be decreased to 1 hr if tolerated or increased if patient has discomfort.

Incompatibilities
Don't reconstitute amphotericin B with diluents other than those recommended because solutions with sodium chloride or bacterio-

static agents (such as benzyl alcohol) may cause drug precipitation.

Route	Onset	Peak	Duration
I.V.	Immediate	Unknown	Unknown

Mechanism of Action

Binds to sterols in fungal cell plasma membranes, which changes membrane permeability and allows loss of potassium and small molecules from cells. This action results in cell impairment or death.

Contraindications

Hypersensitivity to amphotericin B or its components

Interactions

DRUGS

antineoplastics: Increased risk of bronchospasm, hypotension, and nephrotoxicity
corticosteroids, corticotropin: Increased risk of hypokalemia and cardiac dysfunction
cyclosporine, nephrotoxic drugs: Increased risk of nephrotoxicity
digitalis glycosides: Possibly hypokalemia and more severe digitalis toxicity
flucytosine: Possibly increased flucytosine toxicity
leukocyte transfusion: Possibly dyspnea, hypoxemia, and pulmonary infiltrates
skeletal muscle relaxants: Possibly hypokalemia and increased muscle relaxation
zidovudine: Possibly myelotoxicity and nephrotoxicity

Adverse Reactions

CNS: Fever, headache, shaking chills, tiredness, weakness
CV: Chest pain, hypotension, irregular heartbeat
EENT: Difficulty swallowing, pharyngitis
GI: Abdominal pain, anorexia, diarrhea, hepatic failure, indigestion, nausea, vomiting
GU: Decreased or increased urine output, impaired renal function
HEME: Anemia, leukopenia, thrombocytopenia, unusual bleeding or bruising
MS: Arthralgia, muscle spasms, myalgia
RESP: Apnea, dyspnea, hypoxia, pulmonary edema, tachypnea
SKIN: Flushing, jaundice, maculopapular rash, pruritus and redness especially around ears, urticaria
Other: Anaphylaxis, hypocalcemia, hypokalemia, hypomagnesemia, infusion site pain and thrombophlebitis

Nursing Considerations

•To prepare amphotericin B, add 10 ml of sterile water for injection without a bacteriostatic agent to vial containing 50 mg of amphotericin B. For I.V. infusion, dilute the solution containing 5 mg/ml to 0.1 mg/ml by adding 1 ml (5 mg) of solution to 49 ml of D_5W with a pH above 4.2.
•Before using D_5W to dilute amphotericin B solution, determine the injection's pH aseptically. If the pH is below 4.2, follow the manufacturer's instructions for buffering it.
•Because reconstituted amphotericin B is a colloidal suspension, avoid using an in-line membrane filter or use one with a mean pore diameter of more than 1 micron to prevent significant drug removal.
•To prepare amphotericin B cholesteryl sulfate complex, reconstitute it with sterile water for injection. Using a sterile syringe and a 20G needle, rapidly add 10 or 20 ml of sterile water for injection to a 50- or 100-mg vial, respectively, to obtain a solution containing 5 mg of amphotericin B per milliliter. Shake gently by hand, rotating vial until solids are dissolved; fluid may be clear or opalescent. For infusion, further dilute reconstituted solution to about 0.6 mg/ml. Don't filter the solution or use an in-line filter. Flush existing line with D_5W or use a separate line.
•To prepare amphotericin B lipid complex, shake vial gently until you see no yellow sediment. Using an 18G needle, withdraw prescribed dose from required number of vials into one or more 20-ml syringes. Replace needle with 5-micron filter needle that's supplied with each vial. Empty syringe contents into bag of D_5W so that final concentration is 1 mg/ml. Expect to use a concentration of 2 mg/ml for children and patients with cardiovascular disease. Before infusion, shake bag until contents are mixed thoroughly. Flush existing line with D_5W or use a separate line. Don't use an in-line filter. If infusion exceeds 2 hours, shake infusion bag every 2 hours.
•To prepare amphotericin B liposomal complex, add 12 ml sterile water for injection

(without bacteriostatic agent) to each 50-mg vial to achieve a concentration of 4 mg amphotericin B per milliliter. Immediately shake vial vigorously for at least 30 seconds until all particles completely disperse. Withdraw prescribed dose of amphotericin B liposomal complex suspension. Then use a 5-micron filter to inject it into D_5W to provide a final concentration of 1 to 2 mg/ml. Expect to use a lower concentration (0.2 to 0.5 mg/ml) for infants and young children. Flush existing line with D_5W or use a separate line. You may use an in-line filter with a mean pore diameter of at least 1 micron.

•To help minimize fever and shaking chills, expect to administer an antipyretic, antihistamine, meperidine, or corticosteroid just before infusing amphotericin B.

•Before giving amphotericin B oral suspension, shake well. Drop suspension on tongue with calibrated dropper. Then tell patient to swish suspension in mouth for as long as possible before swallowing. If drug must be swabbed on, use a nonabsorbent swab.

•Administer amphotericin B oral suspension between meals to permit prolonged contact with oral lesions.

•Assess I.V. insertion site regularly to detect extravasation of amphotericin B, which may cause severe local irritation. To minimize local thrombophlebitis, plan to add heparin to infusion or expect to administer amphotericin on alternate days, which also may help prevent anorexia. Alternate-day dose shouldn't exceed 1.5 mg/kg.

•Monitor renal function because of the risk of renal impairment. Plan to obtain serum creatinine level every other day while amphotericin B dosage is increasing and then at least twice weekly during therapy. If serum creatinine or BUN level increases significantly, expect to stop amphotericin B until renal function improves. Know that a cumulative dose of more than 4 g may cause irreversible renal dysfunction.

•Expect to monitor CBC and platelet count weekly throughout therapy to detect adverse hematologic effects. Also monitor serum calcium, magnesium, and potassium levels twice weekly to detect abnormalities.

•Use reconstituted amphotericin B within 24 hours if stored at room temperature or within 1 week if refrigerated. Use reconstituted amphotericin B cholesteryl sulfate complex within 24 hours. Use amphotericin B lipid complex within 6 hours if stored at room temperature or within 48 hours if refrigerated. Use diluted amphotericin B liposomal complex within 24 hours if refrigerated, but begin infusion within 6 hours.

•Because reconstituted amphotericin B is a colloidal suspension, avoid using an in-line membrane filter or use one with a mean pore diameter of more than 1 micron to prevent significant drug removal.

PATIENT TEACHING

•Instruct patient to shake bottle of oral suspension well before each dose; to drop suspension directly on his tongue, using calibrated dropper; and then to swish suspension in his mouth for as long as possible before swallowing. If prescriber orders drug swabbing onto oral lesions, tell patient to use nonabsorbent swab. Instruct him to take drug four times a day—between meals and at bedtime.

•Tell patient to notify prescriber if he develops local irritation, if existing symptoms worsen or return, or if new symptoms arise.

ampicillin

Apo-Ampi (CAN), Novo-Ampicillin (CAN), Nu-Ampi (CAN), Omnipen

ampicillin sodium

Ampicin (CAN), Omnipen-N, Polycillin-N, Totacillin-N

ampicillin trihydrate

D-Amp, Omnipen, Penbritin (CAN), Polycillin, Principen-250, Principen-500, Totacillin

Class and Category
Chemical class: Semisynthetic aminopenicillin
Therapeutic class: Antibiotic
Pregnancy category: B

Indications and Dosages
➤ *To treat GI infections and genitourinary infections (other than gonorrhea) caused by susceptible strains of* Shigella, Salmonella typhi *and other species,* Escherichia coli, Proteus mirabilis, *and enterococci*

CAPSULES, ORAL SUSPENSION, I.V. INFUSION, I.M. INJECTION
Adults and children weighing 20 kg (44 lb)

or more. 500 mg P.O. every 6 hr or 250 to 500 mg I.V. or I.M. every 6 hr.
Children weighing less than 20 kg. 50 to 100 mg/kg daily in divided doses P.O. every 6 hr or 12.5 mg/kg I.V. or I.M. every 6 hr.

➤ *To treat gonorrhea caused by susceptible strains of non–penicillinase-producing* Neisseria gonorrhoeae

CAPSULES, ORAL SUSPENSION
Adults and children. 3.5 g as a single dose with 1 g of probenecid.

I.V. INFUSION, I.M. INJECTION
Adults and children weighing 45 kg (99 lb) or more. 500 mg every 6 hr.
Children weighing less than 40 kg (88 lb). 50 mg/kg daily in divided doses every 6 to 8 hr.

➤ *To treat respiratory tract infections caused by susceptible strains of non-penicillinase–producing* Haemophilus influenzae, *staphylococci, and strepto-cocci, including* Streptococcus pneumoniae

CAPSULES, ORAL SUSPENSION, I.V. INFUSION, I.M. INJECTION
Adults and children weighing 40 kg or more. 250 to 500 mg I.V. or I.M. every 6 to 8 hr.
Adults and children weighing 20 kg or more. 250 mg P.O. every 6 hr.
Children weighing less than 40 kg. 25 to 50 mg/kg daily I.V. or I.M. in divided doses every 6 to 8 hr.
Children weighing less than 20 kg. 50 mg/kg daily P.O. in divided doses every 6 or 8 hr or 12.5 mg/kg I.V. or I.M. every 6 hr.

➤ *To treat septicemia*

I.V. INFUSION, I.M. INJECTION
Adults. 8 to 14 g I.V. daily in divided doses every 3 to 4 hr for at least 3 days; then I.M.
Children. 150 to 200 mg/kg daily I.V. in divided doses every 3 to 4 hr for at least 3 days; then I.M.

➤ *To prevent bacterial endocarditis from dental, oral, or upper respiratory tract procedures*

I.V. INFUSION, I.M. INJECTION
Adults. 2 g within 30 min of procedure
Children. 50 mg/kg within 30 min of procedure

➤ *To treat bacterial meningitis caused by susceptible strains of* Neisseria meningitidis

I.V. INFUSION, I.M. INJECTION
Adults. 8 to 14 g daily or 150 to 200 mg/kg daily I.V. in equally divided doses every 3 to 4 hr for at least 3 days; then I.M. at same dosage and schedule.
Children. 100 to 200 mg/kg daily I.V. in equally divided doses every 3 to 4 hr for at least 3 days; then I.M. at same dosage and schedule.

➤ *To treat listeriosis*

I.V. INFUSION, I.M. INJECTION
Adults and children weighing 20 kg or more. 50 mg/kg every 6 hr.
Children weighing less than 20 kg. 12.5 mg/kg every 6 hr.

Route	Onset	Peak	Duration
I.V.	Immediate	Unknown	Unknown

Mechanism of Action

Inhibits bacterial cell wall synthesis. The rigid, cross-linked cell wall is assembled in several steps. Ampicillin exerts its effects on susceptible bacteria in the final stage of the cross-linking process by binding with and inactivating penicillin-binding proteins (enzymes responsible for linking the cell wall strands). This action causes bacterial cell lysis and death.

Incompatibilities

Don't mix ampicillin and any aminoglycoside in the same I.V. bag, bottle, or tubing; otherwise, both drugs will be inactivated. If patient must receive both drugs, administer them in separate sites at least 1 hour apart.

Contraindications

Hypersensitivity to any penicillin, infection caused by penicillinase-producing organism

Interactions
DRUGS
allopurinol: Increased risk of rash, particularly in hyperuricemic patient
aminoglycosides: Possibly inactivated action of aminoglycoside and ampicillin when given together
heparin, oral anticoagulants: Increased risk of bleeding
oral contraceptives: Possibly reduced contraceptive effectiveness and breakthrough bleeding
probenecid: Possibly increased serum ampi-

cillin level and ampicillin toxicity
tetracyclines: Possibly impaired action of
ampicillin

Adverse Reactions
CNS: Chills, fatigue, fever, headache, malaise
CV: Chest pain, edema, thrombophlebitis
EENT: Epistaxis, glossitis, laryngeal stridor,
mucocutaneous candidiasis, stomatitis,
throat tightness
GI: Abdominal distention, diarrhea, diarrhea
related to *Clostridium difficile,* enterocolitis,
flatulence, gastritis, nausea, pseudomembranous colitis, vomiting
GU: Dysuria, urine retention, vaginal candidiasis
HEME: Agranulocytosis, anemia, eosinophilia, leukopenia, thrombocytopenia, thrombocytopenic purpura
SKIN: Erythema multiforme; erythematous,
mildly pruritic maculopapular rash or other
types of rash; exfoliative dermatitis; pruritus; urticaria
Other: Anaphylaxis, facial edema, injection
site pain

Nursing Considerations
•Avoid giving ampicillin to patients with mononucleosis because of increased risk of rash.
•Expect to give ampicillin for 48 to 72 hours
after patient becomes asymptomatic. For
streptococcal infection, expect to give ampicillin for at least 10 days after cultures show
streptococcal eradication to reduce risk of
rheumatic fever or glomerulonephritis.
•To dilute ampicillin for I.M. use, add (depending on manufacturer) 1.2 ml of sterile
water or bacteriostatic water for injection to
each 125-mg vial, 1 ml of diluent to each
250-mg vial, 1.8 ml of diluent to each 500-
mg vial, 3.5 ml of diluent to each 1-g vial, or
6.8 ml of diluent to each 2-g vial.
•To dilute ampicillin for intermittent infusion, add 5 ml of sterile water or bacteriostatic water for injection to each 125-, 250-,
or 500-mg vial or 7.4 to 10 ml of diluent to
each 1- or 2-g vial. Infuse in suitable diluent
at less than 30 mg/ml.
•**WARNING** Infuse I.V. solution for 3 to 5 minutes for each 125 or 500 mg or 10 to 15 minutes for each 1 or 2 g. More rapid infusion
may cause seizures.
•Monitor patient closely for anaphylaxis,
which may be life-threatening. Patients at
greatest risk are those with a history of multi-

ple allergies, hypersensitivity to cephalosporins,
or a history of asthma, hay fever, or urticaria.
•Notify prescriber if patient has evidence of
superinfection; expect to stop drug and provide appropriate treatment.
•**WARNING** In an anaphylactic reaction, stop
drug, notify prescriber immediately, and provide immediate treatment with epinephrine,
airway management, oxygen, and I.V. corticosteroids, as needed.
•If long-term or high-dose ampicillin therapy is required, closely monitor results of
renal and liver function tests and CBCs.
•Monitor patient closely for diarrhea, which
may be pseudomembranous colitis caused by
Clostridium difficile. If diarrhea occurs, notify prescriber and expect to withhold ampicillin and administer fluids, electrolytes, protein, and an antibiotic effective against *C.
difficile.*

PATIENT TEACHING
•Stress the importance of taking the full
course of ampicillin exactly as prescribed.
•Tell patient to take ampicillin with 8 oz of
water 30 minutes before or 2 hours after meals.
•Instruct patient to shake suspension well
before each use, keep bottle tightly closed
between uses, and discard unused portion
after 14 days if refrigerated or 7 days if
stored at room temperature.
•Review signs of allergic reaction; if they
occur, tell patient to hold next ampicillin
dose and contact prescriber immediately.
•Urge patient to tell prescriber about diarrhea that's severe or lasts longer than 3 days.
Remind patient that watery or bloody stools
may occur 2 or more months after antibiotic
therapy and may be serious, requiring
prompt treatment.

amyl nitrite

Class and Category
Chemical class: Nitrite ester
Therapeutic class: Antianginal
Pregnancy category: C

Indications and Dosages
➤ *To treat acute attacks of angina
pectoris*
CRUSHABLE AMPULES
Adults. 1 ampule (0.18 or 0.3 ml) inhaled and
repeated in 3 to 5 min, if needed.

Route	Onset	Peak	Duration
Inhalation	10 to 30 sec	Unknown	3 to 5 min

Mechanism of Action
After inhalation, is absorbed by pulmonary alveoli, which causes relaxation of vascular smooth-muscle cells, dilation of large coronary blood vessels, decreased systemic vascular resistance, decreased venous return to the heart, reduced afterload, decreased cardiac ouput, and subsequent relief of angina.

Contraindications
Hypersensitivity to amyl nitrite, its components, or nitrates

Interactions
DRUGS
aspirin: Increased serum level and action of amyl nitrite
calcium channel blockers: Possibly severe symptomatic hypotension
sildenafil: Increased risk of hypotension
sympathomimetics: Possibly decreased antianginal effects and severe hypotension and tachycardia
ACTIVITIES
alcohol use: Increased risk of severe hypotension and cardiovascular collapse

Adverse Reactions
CNS: Dizziness, headache, restlessness, syncope, weakness
CV: Orthostatic hypotension, tachycardia
GI: Fecal incontinence, nausea, vomiting
GU: Urinary incontinence
HEME: Hemolytic anemia, methemoglobinemia
SKIN: Face and neck flushing, pallor, rash

Nursing Considerations
•Use amyl nitrite cautiously in elderly patients and patients with cerebral hemorrhage, glaucoma, hyperthyroidism, recent head trauma or MI, or severe anemia.
•Monitor blood pressure during and after drug administration. Also monitor cardiac function periodically in patients who use amyl nitrite regularly.
•**WARNING** Stop drug and notify prescriber if you detect signs of overdose, such as bluish lips, fingernails, or palms; dizziness; fainting;

extreme pressure in head; dyspnea; unusual tiredness or weakness; a weak or fast heartbeat; or increased methemoglobin level. Cyanosis may occur when methemoglobin level reaches 1.5 g/dl. More pronounced signs occur at 20 to 50 g/dl.
•Expect to treat overdose with high-flow oxygen and I.V. methylene blue. If hypotension is severe, place patient head down. If he needs a vasopressor, avoid epinephrine because it may cause severe hypotension.

PATIENT TEACHING
•Advise patient to store amyl nitrate in a tight container, protected from light.
•Tell patient to crush ampule between finger and thumb, hold it to nostrils, and inhale 1 to 6 times.
•Instruct patient to remain seated or supine during administration and to rise slowly afterward to prevent dizziness.
•Inform patient that relief usually occurs in 1 to 5 minutes. If pain continues, he should repeat dose. If pain continues after another 5 minutes, he should seek emergency help.
•Remind patient not to use any more amyl nitrite than prescribed because of possible overdose.
•**WARNING** Caution patient that drug is flammable and must be kept from flame and heat.
•Inform patient that amyl nitrite commonly causes headaches. Tell him to notify prescriber if they become severe or bothersome.

anagrelide hydrochloride
Agrylin

Class and Category
Chemical class: Imidazoquinazolinone
Therapeutic class: Platelet count–reducing agent
Pregnancy category: C

Indications and Dosages
➤ *To treat essential thrombocythemia*
CAPSULES
Adults. 0.5 mg q.i.d. or 1 mg b.i.d. for 1 wk; then adjusted to the lowest dose that keeps platelet count below 600,000/mm^3 or within normal range. Dosage shouldn't be increased by more than 0.5 mg daily in any 1 wk. *Maximum:* 10 mg daily or 2.5 mg in a single

dose.

DOSAGE ADJUSTMENT For patients with moderate hepatic impairment, 0.5 mg daily for at least 1 wk, increased as needed by no more than 0.5 mg daily in any 1-wk period.

Route	Onset	Peak	Duration
P.O.	7 to 14 days	Unknown	Up to 4 days

Mechanism of Action
May decrease megakaryocyte hypermaturation (bone marrow cells from which platelets form), reducing platelet count. Higher doses may inhibit platelet aggregation.

Contraindications
Hypersensitivity to anagrelide, severe hepatic impairment

Interactions
DRUGS
amrinone, cilostazol, enoximone, milrinone, olprinone: Increased effects of these drugs; possible risk of increased adverse effects
sucralfate: Possibly interference with anagrelide absorption

Adverse Reactions
CNS: Amnesia, asthenia, chills, confusion, depression, dizziness, fever, headache, insomnia, malaise, nervousness, paresthesia, seizures, somnolence, stroke, syncope, weakness
CV: Angina, arrhythmias, edema, heart failure, hypertension, MI, orthostatic hypotension, palpitations, tachycardia, vasodilation
EENT: Amoblyopia, diplopia, epistaxis, rhinitis, sinusitis, stomatitis, tinnitus, vision or visual field abnormality
GI: Abdominal pain, anorexia, constipation, diarrhea, elevated liver function test results, eructation, flatulence, gastric and duodenal ulceration, gastritis, GI hemorrhage, hepatotoxicity, indigestion, melena, nausea, pancreatitis, vomiting
GU: Dysuria, hematuria, renal failure
HEME: Anemia, hemorrhage, thrombocytopenia
MS: Arthralgia, back pain, leg cramps, myalgia, neck pain
RESP: Allergic alveolitis, asthma, bronchitis, dyspnea, eosinophilic pneumonia, interstitial pneumonitis, lung infiltrations, pneumonia
SKIN: Alopecia, ecchymosis, photosensitivity, pruritus, rash, urticaria
Other: Dehydration, flulike symptoms, generalized body pain, lymphadenoma

Nursing Considerations
• Use anagrelide cautiously in patients with heart disease because it may cause cardiovascular problems, such as heart failure. Use drug cautiously in patients with renal insufficiency (serum creatinine level 2 mg/dl or more) or hepatic dysfunction (liver function tests more than 1.5 times normal) because of the increased risk of nephrotoxicity and hepatotoxicity.
• To assess efficacy and prevent thrombocytopenia, expect to monitor platelet count every 2 days for first week and then at least weekly until lowest effective dose is reached.
• While platelet count is declining (usually during first 2 weeks of therapy), assess WBC count and hemoglobin, AST, ALT, creatinine, and BUN levels to detect abnormalities.
• Monitor blood pressure to detect orthostatic hypotension.

PATIENT TEACHING
• Stress need to return for laboratory tests, such as platelet counts, to monitor anagrelide's effectiveness and adjust its dosage.
• Tell patient to keep bottle tightly capped between uses and to protect drug from light.

anakinra

Kineret

Class and Category
Chemical class: Recombinant human interleukin-1 receptor antagonist
Therapeutic class: Antirheumatic
Pregnancy category: B

Indications and Dosages
➤ *To reduce signs and symptoms and slow structural damage in moderate to severe active rheumatoid arthritis in patients who have not responded to disease-modifying antirheumatics*
SUBCUTANEOUS INJECTION
Adults. 100 mg daily.
DOSAGE ADJUSTMENT Dosage interval reduced to every other day in severe renal insuffi-

ciency or end-stage renal disease (creatinine clearance less than 30 ml/min/1.73 m²).

Mechanism of Action

Inhibits the binding of interleukin-1 (IL-1) to its type 1 receptor, blocking its activity. Inflammatory stimuli prompt T cells to release IL-1, a mediator of inflammation, pain, and stiffness in rheumatoid arthritis.

Contraindications

Active infection; hypersensitivity to anakinra, its components, or *Escherichia coli*–derived proteins

Interactions

DRUGS

etanercept, infliximab, and other drugs that block tumor necrosis factor: Increased risk of serious infection
vaccines, live virus: Possibly decreased antibody response to vaccine, potential for infection with live virus

Adverse Reactions

CNS: Headache
EENT: Sinusitis
GI: Abdominal pain, diarrhea, nausea
HEME: Neutropenia
MS: Bone and joint infections
RESP: Pneumonia, upper respiratory tract infection
Skin: Cellulitis
Other: Flulike symptoms; hypersensitivity reaction; injection site ecchymosis, erythema, inflammation, pain, and pruritus; malignancies; positive results for anti-anakinra antibodies; serious infections

Nursing Considerations

• Obtain baseline neutrophil count before administration, as ordered. Expect to monitor neutrophil count every month for 3 months and then every 3 months for up to 1 year.
• Discard solution if it contains particles or is discolored. Use prefilled syringe and needles to administer drug. Don't shake syringe; allow time for solution to clear if it becomes foamy.
• Administer drug at about the same time each day.
• WARNING Anakinra isn't recommended for patients with active infections. Monitor patient for evidence of infection, such as fever,

chills, sore throat, and mouth sores, before and during therapy because drug increases the risk of infections, such as cellulitis, pneumonia, and bone and joint infections. Notify prescriber if signs are present. Patients with asthma and those receiving etanercept or infliximab are at increased risk for serious infections. Expect anakinra to be stopped if serious infection develops.
• Be aware that live-virus vaccines shouldn't be given to patients receiving anakinra because drug decreases the immune response.
• Monitor patients with impaired renal function for signs of anakinra toxicity; they're at increased risk because drug is excreted primarily by the kidneys.
• Store anakinra at 2° to 8° C (36° to 46° F). Protect from freezing and light.

PATIENT TEACHING

• Teach proper injection technique if patient will self-administer anakinra. Verify that patient understands the process and can correctly prepare and inject first few doses.
• Instruct patient to rotate injection sites among thighs, stomach, and upper arms and to avoid areas that are tender, hard, red, or bruised. Advise him to make sure that each injection site is at least 1″ away from the previous site.
• Urge patient to discard used needles and syringes in a puncture-resistant container and not to reuse them. Instruct him to return container to prescriber for proper disposal.
• Review evidence of allergic reaction, including rash and shortness of breath.
• Urge patient to immediately report signs of infection, such as cough, fever, chills, dyspnea, or headache, to prescriber.

anastrozole

Arimidex

Class and Category

Chemical class: Nonsteroidal selective aromatase inhibitor
Therapeutic class: Antineoplastic
Pregnancy category: D

Indications and Dosages

➤ *To treat postmenopausal women with unknown or positive hormone receptor and locally advanced or metastatic breast cancer, and those with advanced*

Mechanism of Action

Anastrozole treats certain breast cancers in postmenopausal women by inhibiting the enzyme aromatase, which prevents production of estrone and estradiol. Thus, in women with breast tumors that contain estrogen receptors, anastrozole prevents the stimulatory effects of estrogen on tumor growth.

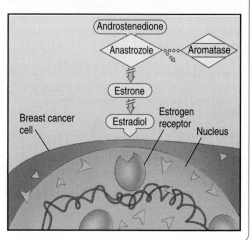

breast cancer that progresses after tamoxifen therapy; as adjunct to treat early breast cancer in postmenopausal women with positive hormone receptor

TABLETS

Adult women. 1 mg daily.

Adverse Reactions

CNS: Asthenia, depression, dizziness, headache, hypertonia, insomnia, lethargy, paresthesia

EENT: Dry mouth, pharyngitis

ENDO: Hot flashes, weight gain

CV: Chest pain, hypertension, peripheral edema, thromboembolic disease, vasodilation

GI: Abdominal or pelvic pain, anorexia, increased appetite, constipation, diarrhea, nausea, vomiting

GU: Leukorrhea; vaginal bleeding, dryness, or hemorrhage

MS: Back or bone pain

RESP: Increased cough, dyspnea

SKIN: Diaphoresis, rash, urticaria

Other: Anaphylaxis, angioedema, flulike symptoms, pain, tumor flare

Nursing Considerations

• Be aware that anastrozole is not recommended for premenopausal women. For these patients, obtain results of pregnancy test before giving first dose. Expect to withhold drug if results are positive.

• Assess patient for evidence of thromboembolic events during anastrozole therapy, such as shortness of breath, leg pain, and altered mental status.

• Store drug in a tightly closed container at room temperature.

PATIENT TEACHING

• Advise patient to notify prescriber immediately about known or suspected pregnancy because risks to the fetus will need to be evaluated.

• Inform patient about possible dizziness and lethargy, and advise her to avoid potentially hazardous activities until drug's CNS effects are known.

• Urge patient to tell prescriber about leg pain or calf swelling, which may indicate a blood clot.

• Advise patient to consume adequate calcium and to follow an exercise program because drug may reduce bone mineral density.

• Urge patient taking anastrozole to comply with follow-up appointments.

anisindione

Miradon

Class and Category

Chemical class: Indanedione derivative
Therapeutic class: Anticoagulant
Pregnancy category: X

Indications and Dosages

➤ *To prevent and treat venous thrombosis, atrial fibrillation with embolization, and pulmonary embolism; as adjunct to treat coronary artery occlusion, usually in patients who can't tolerate coumarin anticoagulants*

TABLETS

Adults. *Initial:* 300 mg on day 1; then 200 mg on day 2, and 100 mg on day 3. *Maintenance:* 25 to 250 mg daily.

Route	Onset	Peak	Duration
P.O.	In 6 hr	48 to 72 hr	1 to 3 days

Mechanism of Action

Interferes with the liver's ability to synthesize vitamin K-dependent clotting factors, which results in the depletion of clotting factors II (prothrombin), VII, IX, and X. By depleting levels of vitamin K–dependent clotting factors that are needed to form a stable fibrin clot, anisindione interferes with the clotting cascade and prevents coagulation.

Contraindications

Ascorbic acid deficiency; blood dyscrasias; continuous small-intestine drainage tube; diverticulitis; emaciation; GI, GU, or respiratory tract bleeding; hemophilia; hemorrhagic tendency; history of warfarin-induced necrosis; hypersensitivity to anisindione or its components; leukemia; major recent surgery; malnutrition; pericardial effusion; pericarditis; polyarthritis; pregnancy; prostatectomy; recent spinal puncture, percutaneous invasive procedure, diagnostic testing, or insertion of intrauterine device; recent or possible CNS or eye surgery; severe renal or hepatic disease; severe uncontrolled diabetes; severe uncontrolled malignant hypertension; subacute bacterial endocarditis; thrombocytopenic purpura; visceral carcinomas; ulcerative colitis

Interactions

DRUGS

abciximab, acetaminophen, allopurinol, alteplase, amiodarone, amitriptyline, amoxapine, androgens, aspirin, beta blockers, cephalosporins, chloral hydrate, chloramphenicol, chlorpropamide, cimetidine, cisapride, clofibrate, clomipramine, corticosteroids, cotrimoxazole, cyclophosphamide, danazol, desipramine, dextrothyroxine, diclofenac, diflunisal, disulfiram, doxepin, erythromycin, etodolac, fluconazole, fluoxymesterone, fosphenytoin, gemfibrozil, glucagon, hydantoins, ifosfamide, influenza virus vaccines, imipramine, indomethacin, isoniazid, itraconazole, ketoconazole, ketolorac, lepirudin, loop diuretics, lovastatin, low–molecular-weight heparins, meclofenamate, mefenamic acid, methyltestosterone, metronidazole, miconazole, moricizine, nabumetone, naproxen, nalidixic acid, neomycin, nortriptyline, NSAIDs, omeprazole, oxandrolone, penicillins, phenylbutazones, phenytoin, piroxicam, propafenone, propoxyphene, protriptyline, quinidine, quinine, quinolones, reteplase, salicylates, stanazolol, streptokinase, sulfamethoxazole, sulfinpyrazone, sulindac, tamoxifen, testosterone, thioamines, thyroid hormones, tomentin, urokinase: Increased anticoagulant effects

aminoglutethimide, ascorbic acid, barbiturates, carbamazepine, cholestyramine, corticosteroids, dicloxacillin, estrogen, ethanol, ethchlorvynol, etretinate, glutethimide, griseofulvin, nafcillin, oral contraceptives, rifampin, spironolactone, sucralfate, thiazide diuretics, thiopurines, trazodone, vitamin K: Decreased anticoagulant effects

aminoglycosides, mineral oil, tetracycline, vitamin E: Interference with vitamin K, leading to increased anticoagulant effects

FOODS

enteral products and foods high in vitamin K, such as dark green leafy vegetables: Interference with anticoagulant effects

ACTIVITIES

alcohol use: Possibly increased or decreased anticoagulation

Adverse Reactions

CNS: Fever, headache
EENT: Blurred vision, mouth ulcers, pharyngitis
GI: Abdominal cramps, diarrhea, hepatic

dysfunction, hepatitis, nausea, steatorrhea
GU: Albuminuria, anuria, priaprism, red-orange urine, renal tubular necrosis
HEME: Agranulocytosis, anemia, atypical mononuclear cells, eosinophilia, hemorrhage, leukocytosis, leukopenia, RBC aplasia, thrombocytopenia
SKIN: Alopecia, exfoliative dermatitis, jaundice, necrosis of the skin and tissues evidenced by gangrene and purple toes, urticaria

Nursing Considerations
•Watch for PT to become prolonged 6 hours after anisindione administration, although maximum therapeutic effects may take 48 to 72 hours to appear.
•WARNING Watch for signs of overanticoagulation, such as microscopic hematuria, excessive menstrual bleeding, melena, petechiae, and bleeding from superficial trauma, such as tooth brushing or shaving.
•Monitor INR, CBC, fecal occult blood test, and urinalysis results for signs of overanticoagulation.

PATIENT TEACHING
•Advise patient to avoid alcohol, salicylates, and drastic changes in his intake of vitamin K–rich food.
•Instruct patient to promptly report pregnancy to prescriber.
•Provide patient with a list of foods rich in vitamin K. Advise him to eat consistent daily amounts of vitamin K.
•Counsel patient to consult prescriber before undergoing dental work or elective surgery.
•Urge patient to immediately report unusual bleeding, bruising, red or red-orange urine, red or tarry black stools, diarrhea, bleeding from gums or nose, or excessive bleeding from minor cuts or scratches.

anistreplase
(anisoylated plasminogen-streptokinase activator complex)
Eminase

Class and Category
Chemical class: p-Anisoylated derivative of the Lys-plasminogen-streptokinase activator complex
Therapeutic class: Thrombolytic enzyme

Pregnancy category: C

Indications and Dosages
➤ *To treat acute MI, lyse thrombi that are obstructing coronary arteries, reduce infarct size, improve ventricular function after acute MI, reduce mortality from acute MI*

I.V. INFUSION
Adults. 30 units injected over 2 to 5 min.

Route	Onset	Peak	Duration
I.V.	Immediate	20 min to 2 hr	4 to 6 hr

Mechanism of Action
Indirectly promotes the conversion of plasminogen to plasmin, an enzyme that breaks down fibrin clots, fibrinogen, and other plasma proteins, including procoagulant factors V and VIII.

Incompatibilities
Don't add other drugs to anistreplase solution or infuse other drugs through same I.V. line.

Contraindications
Active internal bleeding, arteriovenous malformation or aneurysm, bleeding diathesis, history of stroke, hypersensitivity to anistreplase or streptokinase, intracranial neoplasm, intracranial or intraspinal surgery or trauma within past 2 months, severe uncontrolled hypertension

Interactions
DRUGS
aspirin, dipyridamole, and other drugs that alter platelet function; heparin; vitamin K antagonists: Possibly increased risk of bleeding if administered before anistreplase

Adverse Reactions
CNS: Dizziness, fever, headache, intracranial hemorrhage
CV: Ankle edema, arrhythmias (especially accelerated idioventricular rhythm, conduction disorders, premature ventricular beats, sinus bradycardia, ventricular fibrillation, ventricular tachycardia), hypotension, vasculitis
EENT: Epistaxis
GI: Abdominal pain or swelling, constipa-

tion, GI bleeding, nausea, vomiting
GU: Hematuria, proteinuria, vaginal bleeding
HEME: Bleeding tendency, eosinophilia, mild to severe hemorrhage
MS: Arthralgia, back pain, joint stiffness, myalgia
RESP: Bronchospasm, dyspnea, hemoptysis
SKIN: Flushing, pruritus, rash, urticaria
Other: Anaphylaxis (rare), angioedema

Nursing Considerations

•Use anistreplase cautiously in patients with acute pericarditis; cerebrovascular disease; hemorrhagic ophthalmic conditions; history of major surgery, GI or GU bleeding, or trauma within past 10 days; hypertension; mitral stenosis with atrial fibrillation; pregnancy; septic thrombophlebitis; severe hepatic or renal disease; or subacute bacterial endocarditis.
•Reconstitute anistreplase by slowly directing 5 ml of sterile water for injection USP or sodium chloride for injection against side of vial. Then gently roll vial to mix dry powder and fluid and minimize foaming. Don't shake vial. The resulting solution should be colorless to pale yellow and transparent.
•Before administering, inspect solution for particles and discoloration. If present, discard and reconstitute drug from a new vial. Then withdraw entire contents of vial. Don't dilute reconstituted solution further before administration or add it to I.V. fluid. Don't add other drugs to vial or syringe that contains anistreplase. Discard drug if it isn't administered within 30 minutes after reconstitution.
•For maximum effectiveness, expect to administer anistreplase as soon as possible after onset of MI symptoms.
•Closely monitor all puncture sites, such as catheter insertion and needle puncture sites, for bleeding.
•Don't give I.M. injections, and avoid handling patient unnecessarily during anistreplase therapy. Perform venipuncture only when necessary.
•If an arterial puncture is needed after anistreplase administration, use an arm vessel that allows easy manual compression. Apply a pressure dressing afterward, and check puncture site frequently for bleeding.
•Use continuous cardiac monitoring because arrhythmias may occur during reperfusion.

Keep antiarrhythmics on hand during anistreplase therapy, and manage arrhythmias according to facility policy.
•Keep epinephrine nearby to treat anaphylaxis.
•Know that anistreplase may be less effective if it's given more than 5 days after anistreplase or streptokinase administration. This occurs because patient may have developed antistreptokinase antibodies, which makes him more resistant to the drug and drug therapy less effective. Elevated serum antistreptokinase antibody levels and reduced drug effectiveness can persist for 5 days to 12 months.
•Closely monitor blood coagulation test results. The drug markedly decreases plasminogen and fibrinogen levels and increases thrombin time, APTT, and PT.

PATIENT TEACHING
•Instruct patient to report adverse reactions immediately, especially bleeding, dizziness, and chest pain.

antihemophilic factor (recombinant), plasma/albumin-free method (rAHF-PFM)

Advate, Kogenate FS, Xyntha

antihemophilic factor (human)

Alphanate

antihemophilic factor– von Willebrand factor complex (human, dried, pasteurized)

Humate-P

Class and Category

Chemical class: Recombinant protein
Therapeutic class: Antihemophilic factor
Pregnancy category: C

Indications and Dosages

➤ *To prevent and control bleeding episodes in patients with hemophilia A and factor VIII inhibitors not exceeding 10 Bethesda Units/ml*

I.V. INJECTION

Adults and children. Highly individualized. *For early hemarthrosis, muscle bleeding episode, or mild oral bleeding episode:* Dose administered to achieve peak post-infusion factor VIII activity in blood (determined by multiplying dose administered/kg body weight by 2) 20% to 40% of normal with infusions every 12 to 24 hr for 1 to 3 days until bleeding episode resolved. *For more extensive hemarthrosis, muscle bleeding episode, or hematoma:* Dose administered to achieve peak post-infusion factor VIII activity in blood 30% to 60% of normal with infusions every 12 to 24 hr for 3 or more days until pain and disability are resolved. *For life-threatening bleeding episodes:* Dose administered to achieve peak postinfusion factor VIII activity in blood 60% to 100% with infusions every 8 to 24 hr until bleeding episode stops.

➤ *To prevent and control perioperative bleeding in patients with hemophilia A*

I.V. INJECTION

Adults and children. Highly individualized. *For minor surgery, including tooth extraction:* Dose administered to achieve peak postinfusion factor VIII activity in blood (determined by multiplying dose administered/ kg body weight by 2) between 60% and 100% of normal, given as a single bolus infusion within 1 hr of operation, with optional additional dose every 12 to 24 hr, as needed. *For major surgery:* Dose administered to achieve peak postinfusion factor VIII activity in blood 80% to 100% before and after surgery with infusions every 8 to 24 hr.

I.V. INJECTION (KOGENATE FS)

Adults and children. Highly individualized and based on this formula: Body weight (kg) x Desired factor VIII rise (international units/dL or % of normal) x 0.5 (international units/kg per international units/dL). *For minor surgery, including tooth extraction:* 15 to 30 international units/kg to achieve a desired Factor VIII rise to 30% to 60% of normal with injections repeated every 12 to 24 hr until bleeding has resolved. *For major surgery:* 50 international units/kg preoperatively to achieve a desired Factor VIII rise to 100% of normal with dosage repeated 6 to 12 hr after initial dose as needed, and for 10 to 14 days thereafter, as needed, until

healing is complete.

I.V. INFUSION (XYNTHA)

Adults and children. Highly individualized and based on this formula: Body weight (kg) x Desired factor VIII rise (IU/dL or % of normal) x 0.5 (IU/kg per IU/dL). *For minor surgery, including tooth extraction:* The desired Factor VIII rise is 30% to 60% of normal with infusions every 12 to 24 hr for 3 to 4 days or until adequate local hemostasis is achieved (for tooth extraction, a single infusion plus oral antifibrinolytic therapy within 1 hr may be sufficient). *For major surgery:* The desired Factor VIII rise is 60% to 100% of normal with infusions every 8 to 24 hr until adequate local hemostasis and wound healing are achieved.

➤ *To prevent or treat bleeding in hemophilia A*

I.V. INJECTION (HUMATE-P)

Adults. Highly individualized. *For mild hemorrhage, such as early joint or muscle bleed or severe epistaxis:* Loading dose of 15 international units/kg to achieve factor VIII:C plasma level about 30% of normal, with half the loading dose repeated once or twice daily for 1 to 2 days as needed. *For moderate hemorrhage, such as advanced joint or muscle bleed; neck, tongue, or pharyngeal hematoma without airway compromise; tooth extraction; or severe abdominal pain:* Loading dose of 25 international units/kg to achieve factor VIII:C plasma level about 50% of normal, followed by 15 international units/kg every 8 to 12 hr for first 1 to 2 days to maintain factor VIII:C plasma level at 30% of normal, and then 15 international units/kg once or twice daily for total of up to 7 days or until adequate wound healing. *For life-threatening hemorrhage, as may occur in major surgery; GI bleeding; neck, tongue, or pharyngeal hematoma with potential for airway compromise; intracranial, intra-abdominal, or intrathoracic bleeding; or fractures:* Loading dose of 40 to 50 international units/kg, followed by 20 to 25 international units/kg every 8 hr to maintain factor VIII:C plasma level at 80% to 100% of normal for 7 days, followed by 20 to 25 international units/kg once or twice daily for another 7 days to maintain factor VIII:C level at 30% to 50% of normal.

I.V. INJECTION (KOGENATE FS)

Adults and children. Highly individualized

and based on this formula: Body weight (kg) x desired Factor VIII rise (international units/dL or % of normal) x 0.5 (international units/kg per international units/dL). *For early hemarthrosis or minor muscle or oral bleeds:* 10 to 20 international units/kg to achieve a desired Factor VIII rise of 20% to 40% of normal with dosage repeated, if needed. *For moderate bleeding into muscles, mild head trauma, or bleeding into the oral cavity:* 15 to 30 international units/kg to achieve a desired Factor VIII rise of 30% to 60% of normal with injections every 12 to 24 hr until bleeding has resolved. *For major GI bleeding; intracranial, intra-abdominal or intrathoracic bleeding; or fractures:* Initial dose of 40 to 50 international units/kg followed by a repeat dose of 20 to 25 international units/kg to achieve the desired Factor VIII rise of 60% to 100% of normal with injections of 20 to 25 international units/kg repeated every 8 to 24 hr until bleeding has resolved.

I.V. INFUSION (XYNTHA)
Adults and children. Highly individualized and based on this formula: Body weight (kg) x desired Factor VIII rise (international units/dL or % of normal) x 0.5 (international units/kg per international units/dL). *For early hemarthrosis or minor muscle or oral bleeds:* The desired Factor VIII rise is 20% to 40% of normal with infusions every 12 to 24 hr for at least 1 day, depending on the severity of the bleeding episode. *For moderate bleeding into muscles, mild head trauma, or bleeding into the oral cavity:* The desired Factor VIII rise is 30% to 60% of normal with infusions every 12 to 24 hr for 3 to 4 days or until adequate local hemostasis is achieved. *For major GI bleeding; intracranial, intra-abdominal, or intrathoracic bleeding; or fractures:* The desired Factor VIII rise is 60% to 100% of normal with infusions every 8 to 24 hr until bleeding has resolved.

➤ *To treat spontaneous and trauma-induced bleeding episodes and prevent excessive bleeding during and after surgery in patients with von Willebrand disease when use of desmopressin is inadequate*
I.V. INJECTION (HUMATE-P)
Adults and children. 40 to 80 international units/kg every 8 to 12 hr as needed.

➤ *To prevent excessive bleeding during and after surgery in patients with von Willebrand disease*
I.V. INJECTION (HUMATE-P)
Adults and children. Highly individualized. *For emergency surgery:* Loading dose of 50 to 60 international uits/kg, followed by half the loading dose every 6 to 12 hr as needed. *For preplanned surgery:* Individualized loading dose based on patient's need 1 to 2 hr before surgery, followed by half the loading dose every 6 to 12 hr for at least 12 hr (oral surgery), 48 hr (minor surgery), or 72 hr (major surgery).

Route	Onset	Peak	Duration
I.V.	Immediate	5 min	Unknown

Mechanism of Action
Provides supplemental factor VIII, the coagulation factor required for blood to clot that's missing in patients with hemophilia A and diminished in patients with factor VIII inhibitors. After blood clots, bleeding stops.

Contraindications
Life-threatening, immediate hypersensitivity reactions, including anaphylaxis, experienced with prior administration of drug or exposure to mouse or hamster proteins

Adverse Reactions
CNS: Dizziness, fever, headache, rigidity
CV: Chest pain, hypotension
EENT: Taste perversion
ENDO: Hot flashes
GI: Abdominal pain, diarrhea, nausea, vomiting
HEME: Bleeding tendency, decreased coagulation factor VIII, decreased hematocrit, hematoma, hemolytic anemia
MS: Joint swelling, lower limb edema
RESP: Dyspnea, shortness of breath
SKIN: Diaphoresis, pruritus, rash, urticaria
Other: Anaphylaxis, angioedema, catheter-related infection, injection site reactions

Nursing Considerations
•Check to confirm that clotting defect is factor VIII deficiency (Kogenate FS or Xyntha only) or von Willebrand disease (Humate-P

only) before administering antihemophilic factor (recombinant) because drug isn't effective in treating other coagulation factor deficiencies.

•Reconstitute Advate or Alphanate using sterile water for injection. Bring both drug and diluent to room temperature, then clean stoppers with antiseptic solution and allow to dry. Remove protective covering from one end of double-ended needle and insert through center of diluent stopper. Remove protective covering from other end of double-ended needle. Invert diluent bottle over upright drug bottle, then rapidly insert free end of needle through drug stopper at center. The vacuum in bottle will draw in the diluent. Then disconnect the two bottles by removing needle from diluent bottle stopper and remove the needle from drug bottle. Swirl gently until all of drug is dissolved. Avoid shaking to prevent foaming and degradation of drug. Administer in a separate line within 3 hours of reconstitution.

•Reconstitute Humate-P, Kogenate FS, and Xyntha according to manufacturer instructions in package insert.

•Take patient's pulse before and periodically during drug administration. If pulse rate increases significantly during administration, reduce administration rate or temporarily halt the injection to allow pulse rate to return to preadministration level before resuming administration.

•To administer Advate or Alphanate, use only plastic material because protein in drug will adhere to glass. Attach filter needle to syringe and draw back plunger to draw air into syringe. Insert needle into reconstituted drug vial. Inject air into bottle and then withdraw drug from vial. Remove and discard filter needle from syringe, attach a suitable needle, and inject I.V. bolus at no more than 10 ml/min over no more than 5 minutes.

•To administer Humate-P, slowly inject I.V. bolus at no more than 4 ml/min using a venipuncture or other suitable I.V. injection set.

•To administer Kogenate FS, check patient's pulse then slowly inject intravenously over 1 to 15 minutes, checking pulse rate throughout administration. If pulse rate rises significantly, slow administration or temporarily stop delivery to let pulse rate to return to normal; then continue administration.

•To administer Xyntha, slowly infuse intravenously over several minutes at a rate that's comfortable for the patient. Don't infuse in tubing or container that contains other drugs.

•Monitor patient's plasma factor VIII levels (and von Willebrand factor: Ristocetin cofactor if patient has von Willebrand disease) during and after treatment to ensure adequate levels have been reached and are being maintained, as ordered.

•Monitor patient for anaphylaxis, and have emergency equipment nearby.

•After giving drug, monitor patient for the formation of neutralizing antibodies to factor VIII, a known complication in the treatment of hemophilia A that may be exhibited by continued bleeding. Obtain laboratory analysis to detect the neutralizing antibodies, as ordered.

•Monitor patients with blood types A, B, and AB for hemolysis when giving large doses.

PATIENT TEACHING

•Teach patient and caregivers how to administer antihemophilic factor (recombinant) at home in an emergency situation.

•Explain that drug may be stored in the refrigerator or at room temperature but that it shouldn't be exposed to temperatures above 77° F (25° C) or below freezing because they may affect drug's effectiveness.

•Instruct patient to discontinue drug and seek emergency help immediately if he has an acute allergic reaction, such as hives, chest tightness, wheezing, low blood pressure, or fainting during or after drug administration.

antithrombin III, human
(AT-III, heparin co-factor I)
ATnativ, Thrombate III

Class and Category
Chemical class: Alpha₂-globulin
Therapeutic class: Anticoagulant, antithrombotic
Pregnancy category: C

Indications and Dosages
➤ *To treat patients with hereditary antithrombin III (AT-III) deficiency who are undergoing surgery or obstetric procedures or who have thromboembolism*

I.V. INJECTION

Adults and children. *Initial:* Individualized dosage (based on weight, degree of AT-III deficiency, and desired level of AT-III to be achieved) sufficient to increase AT-III activity to 120% of normal, administered at 50 to 100 international units/min. *Maintenance:* Individualized dosage sufficient to keep AT-III activity at 80% or more of normal, administered every 24 hr, continued for 2 to 8 days, depending on the patient's condition and history and prescriber's judgment. A pregnant, immobilized, or postsurgical patient may need more prolonged therapy.

Route	Onset	Peak	Duration
I.V.	Immediate	Unknown	4 days

Mechanism of Action

Inhibits blood coagulation by inactivating thrombin; activated forms of factors IX, X, XI, and XII; and plasmin.

Interactions

DRUGS

heparin: Enhanced anticoagulant effect

Adverse Reactions

CNS: Chills, dizziness, fever, light-headedness
CV: Chest pain or tightness, hypotension, vasodilation
EENT: Unpleasant taste
GI: Abdominal cramps, bowel fullness, nausea
GU: Diuresis
HEME: Hematoma
RESP: Dyspnea
SKIN: Oozing lesions, urticaria

Nursing Considerations

• Reconstitute AT-III with 10 ml of sterile water for injection (provided by manufacturer) or alternate solution, such as normal saline solution or D₅W injection. Don't shake vial during reconstitution. Let solution come to room temperature before administration. If desired, dilute reconstituted solution further, using same diluent.

• WARNING Don't use diluent that contains benzyl alcohol to reconstitute drug for a neonate. It can cause a fatal toxic syndrome with metabolic acidosis, CNS depression, respiratory problems, renal failure, hypotension, seizures, and intracranial hemorrhage.

• Don't refrigerate reconstituted solution. Use it within 3 hours; discard unused solution.

• Administer AT-III alone. Don't mix it with other drugs or solutions.

• If after 30 minutes the initial dose doesn't increase AT-III activity to 120% of normal, expect the prescriber to increase the dosage.

• If patient requires a dosage increase, monitor AT-III activity more frequently and expect to adjust dosage accordingly.

• To avoid bleeding, anticipate a reduction in heparin dosage during AT-III therapy.

• If mild adverse reactions occur, decrease infusion rate, as prescribed. If severe reactions occur, discontinue infusion, as prescribed, until they subside.

• Evaluate serum AT-III level twice daily until dosage is stabilized. After that, evaluate level once daily, just before a dose.

PATIENT TEACHING

• Tell patient that blood will be drawn periodically to guide AT-III dosage adjustments.

apomorphine hydrochloride

Apokyn

Class and Category

Chemical class: Nonergoline dopamine agonist
Therapeutic class: Hypomobilic antiparkinsonian
Pregnancy category: C

Indications and Dosages

➤ *To treat hypomobility "off" episodes (end-of-dose wearing off and unpredictable on/off episodes) in advanced Parkinson's disease*

SUBCUTANEOUS INJECTION

Adults. *Initial:* 0.2 ml (2 mg) p.r.n. Dosage adjusted as needed in 0.1-ml (1-mg) increments every few days. *Maximum:* 0.6 ml (6 mg).

DOSAGE ADJUSTMENT For patients who tolerate 0.2 ml (2 mg) but have no response, a 0.4-ml (4-mg) dose may be given under medical supervision, with standing and supine blood pressure checked every 20 min for 1 hr at the next observed "off" period, as long as it is at least 2 hr after the initial 0.2-ml (2-mg) test dose. If tolerated, a dose 0.1 ml (1 mg) lower may be given p.r.n. and increased in 0.1-ml (1-mg) increments every few days as needed to a maximum dose of 0.6 ml (6 mg).

If patient doesn't tolerate a 0.4-ml (4-mg) test dose, a 0.3-ml (3-mg) test dose may be given under medical supervision, with standing and supine blood pressure checked every 20 min for 1 hr at the next observed "off" period, as long as it is at least 2 hr after the initial 0.4-ml (4-mg) test dose. If tolerated, a 0.2-ml (2-mg) dose can be started p.r.n. and increased to no more than 0.3 ml (3 mg) if needed after a few days.

For patients with mild to moderate renal impairment, the initial dose should be reduced to 0.1 ml (1 mg).

Route	Onset	Peak	Duration
SubQ	10 to 60 min	Unknown	Unknown

Mechanism of Action

May stimulate postsynaptic dopamine D_2 receptors in the caudate-putamen of the brain. As a result, apomorphine improves motor function and activity levels in patients with Parkinson's disease.

Contraindications

Concurrent therapy with 5-HT$_3$ antagonists, such as alosetron, dolasetron, granisetron, ondansetron, and palonosetron; hypersensitivity to apomorphine or its components, including sodium metabisulfite

Interactions

DRUGS

5-HT$_3$ antagonists: Increased risk of profound hypotension and loss of consciousness
antihypertensives, vasodilators: Increased risk of serious adverse reactions, such as hypotension, MI, and bone or joint injuries
dopamine antagonists (such as butyrophenones, metoclopramide, phenothiazines, thioxanthenes): Decreased apomorphine effectiveness
drugs that prolong QT interval: Increased risk of torsades de pointes
entacapone, tolcapone: Increased risk of tachycardia, hypertension, and arrhythmias

ACTIVITIES

alcohol use: Increased risk of hypotension

Adverse Reactions

CNS: Aggravated Parkinson's disease, anxiety, confusion, depression, dizziness, drowsiness, dyskinesia, euphoria, fatigue, hallucinations, headache, insomnia, somnolence, weakness, yawning
CV: Angina, chest pain, congestive heart failure, edema, MI, orthostatic hypotension, prolonged QT interval
EENT: Rhinorrhea
GI: Constipation, diarrhea, nausea, vomiting
GU: UTI
MS: Arthralgia, back or limb pain
RESP: Dyspnea, pneumonia, tachypnea
SKIN: Contact dermatitis, diaphoresis, ecchymosis, flushing, pallor
Other: Dehydration; injection site bruising, granuloma, or pruritus

Nursing Considerations

•Use apomorphine cautiously in patients with hepatic or renal insufficiency.
•Be aware that an antiemetic, such as trimethobenzamide 300 mg t.i.d., should be started 3 days before apomorphine therapy starts and continue for at least the first 2 months of therapy. Apomorphine may cause severe nausea and vomiting, even with an antiemetic.
•Monitor patient's blood pressure closely because drug can cause severe orthostatic hypotension.
•Administer a 0.2-ml (2-mg) test dose of apomorphine, as prescribed, and then monitor patient's supine and standing blood pressure 20, 40, and 60 minutes later.
•Monitor patient closely if he has an increased risk of prolonged QT interval, as from hypokalemia, hypomagnesemia, bradycardia, use of certain drugs, or genetic predisposition. QT-interval prolongation may lead to torsades de pointes.
•Monitor patient for evidence of abuse. Although rare, drug may cause psychosexual stimulation and increased libido, which may cause patient to use it more often than needed for reducing Parkinson's disease symptoms.

PATIENT TEACHING

•Tell patient that an antiemetic will be prescribed starting three days before first apomorphine dose. Instruct patient to take the antiemetic exactly as prescribed. Explain that it will be needed for 2 months or longer

during apomorphine therapy.
•Explain that a test dose will be needed to determine response and drug's effects on blood pressure before patient can go home with drug.
•Teach patient how to use dosing pen and how to give drug subcutaneously.
•Emphasize that apomorphine doses are expressed as milliliters, not milligrams. Tell patient to draw up each dose carefully to reduce the chance of dosage error.
•Instruct patient to rotate injection sites in a systematic manner.
•Stress importance of taking apomorphine only as prescribed because serious adverse reactions may occur.
•Advise patient to avoid hazardous activities until drug's CNS effects are known. In particular, caution patient that apomorphine increases the risk of falling asleep suddenly, without feeling sleepy.

aprepitant

Emend

fosaprepitant dimeglumine

Emend for Injection

Class and Category

Chemical class: Substance P/neurokinin 1 (NK1) receptor antagonist
Therapeutic class: Antiemetic
Pregnancy category: B

Indications and Dosages

➤ *To prevent acute and delayed nausea and vomiting associated with highly emetogenic chemotherapy, including high-dose cisplatin*

CAPSULES

Adults. 125 mg 1 hr before chemotherapy treatment, followed by 80 mg daily in morning on next 2 days.

I.V. INFUSION

Adults. 115 mg 30 min before chemotherapy begins (day 1 only).

➤ *To prevent postoperative nausea and vomiting*

CAPSULES

Adults. 40 mg within 3 hr before induction of anesthesia

Route	Onset	Peak	Duration
P.O., I.V.	Unknown	4 hr	Unknown

Mechanism of Action

Crosses the blood–brain barrier to occupy brain NK1 receptors, which prevents nerve transmission of signals that cause nausea and vomiting.

Contraindications

Hypersensitivity to aprepitant, polysorbate 80, or their components; use of astemizole, cisapride, pimozide, or terfenadine

Interactions

DRUGS

carbamazepine, phenytoin, rifampin: Possibly decreased blood aprepitant level
corticosteroids: Increased blood corticosteroid level
CYP2C9 metabolizers (such as phenytoin, tolbutamide, and warfarin): Decreased blood level and effectiveness of CYP2C9 metabolizers
CYP3A4 inhibitors (such as clarithromycin, diltiazem, itraconazole, ketoconazole, nefazodone, nelfinavir, and troleandomycin): Increased blood aprepitant level
CYP3A4 substrates (such as astemizole, benzodiazepines, cisapride, docetaxel, etoposide, ifosfamide, imatinib, irinotecan, paclitaxel, pimozide, terfenadine, vinblastine, vincristine, and vinorelbine): Increased blood level of CYP3A4 substrates, resulting in possibly serious or life-threatening adverse reactions
oral contraceptives: Possibly decreased effectiveness of oral contraceptives
paroxetine: Possibly decreased blood level of both drugs

Adverse Reactions

CNS: Anxiety, asthenia, confusion, depression, dizziness, fatigue, fever, headache, insomnia, malaise, peripheral or sensory neuropathy, somnolence
CV: Deep vein thrombosis, edema, hypertension, hypotension, tachycardia
EENT: Increased salivation, mucous membrane alteration, nasal discharge, pharyngitis, stomatitis, taste perversion, tinnitus, vocal disturbance
ENDO: Hot flashes, hyperglycemia

GI: Abdominal pain, anorexia, constipation, diarrhea, dysphagia, elevated liver function test results, epigastric discomfort, flatulence, gastritis, gastroesophageal reflux, heartburn, hiccups, nausea, obstipation, vomiting
GU: Dysuria, elevated BUN and serum creatinine levels, hematuria, leukocyturia, renal insufficiency
HEME: Anemia, febrile neutropenia, leukocytosis, thrombocytopenia
MS: Muscle weakness, myalgia, pelvic pain
RESP: Cough, dyspnea, non–small-cell lung carcinoma, pneumonitis, pulmonary embolism, respiratory insufficiency, respiratory tract infection
SKIN: Alopecia, diaphoresis, flushing, pruritus, rash, urticaria
Other: Anaphylaxis, angioedema, dehydration, hypokalemia, hyponatremia, infusion site pain or induration, malignant neoplasm, septic shock, weight loss

Nursing Considerations
•Use caution when giving aprepitant to patients with severe hepatic insufficiency because drug's effects on such patients aren't known.
•For maximum antiemetic effects, expect to administer aprepitant with dexamethasone and a 5-HT$_3$ antagonist, such as dolasetron, granisetron, or ondansetron.
•Drug is given intravenously only as the first dose 30 minutes before chemotherapy. Later doses are given orally.
•To reconstitute parental aprepitant, inject 5 ml of normal saline for injection along the vial wall to prevent foaming. Swirl the vial gently. Withdraw contents from the vial and add to an infusion bag containing 110 ml of normal saline solution. Gently invert the bag two or three times. Administer over 15 minutes. Reconstituted solution may be stored at room temperature for 24 hours.
PATIENT TEACHING
•Instruct patient to take 125-mg oral dose of aprepitant 1 hour before chemotherapy, 80-mg dose in the morning for 2 days after chemotherapy, or 40-mg dose within 3 hours before induction of anesthesia.
•Tell female patients taking oral contraceptives to use an alternative or backup method of contraception during aprepitant therapy and for 1 month after last dose because drug reduces effectiveness of oral contraceptives.

•Tell patient taking warfarin regularly to have his clotting status monitored closely for 2 weeks after the first dose of aprepitant, especially every 7 to 10 days during each chemotherapy cycle in which the drug is used.
•Caution patient to inform prescriber of any drugs he's taking, including OTC drugs and herbal preparations, because they may interact with aprepitant.

arformoterol

Brovana

Class and Category
Chemical class: Selective beta$_2$-adrenergic agonist, sympathomimetic
Therapeutic class: Bronchodilator
Pregnancy category: C

Indications and Dosages
➤ *To provide maintenance treatment of bronchoconstriction in patients with COPD, including chronic bronchitis and emphysema*
INHALATION SOLUTION
Adults. 15 mcg (contents of one 2-ml vial) b.i.d. (morning and evening) via nebulization. Do not exceed 30 mcg daily.

Mechanism of Action
Attaches to beta$_2$ receptors on bronchial cell membranes, stimulating the intracellular enzyme adenylate cyclase to convert adenosine triphosphate to cyclic adenosine monophosphate (cAMP). The resulting increase in intracellular cAMP level relaxes bronchial smooth-muscle cells, stabilizes mast cells, and inhibits histamine release.

Contraindications
Hypersensitivity to arformoterol, racemic formoterol, or its components; acute bronchospasm; symptoms of COPD

Interactions
DRUGS
beta blockers: Decreased effectiveness of either drug
corticosteroids, methylxanthines such as aminophylline or theophylline, non–potassium-

A

sparing (such as loop and thiazide) diuretics: Increased risk of hypokalmia
drugs known to prolong the QT interval, MAO inhibitors, tricyclic antidepressants: Increased risk of life-threatening ventricular arrhythmias
thyroid hormones: Increased risk of coronary insufficiency

Adverse Reactions

CNS: Agitation, asthenia, circumoral paresthesia, fatigue, fever, headache, hypokinesia, insomnia, malaise, nervousness, paralysis, somnolence, stroke, tremor
CV: Angina, arrhythmias, atrial flutter, chest pain, congestive heart failure, dizziness, heart block, hyperlipemia, hypertension, hypertension, MI, palpitations, peripheral edema, prolonged QT interval
EENT: Abnormal vision, dry mouth, glaucoma, herpes simplex or zoster, oral moniliasis, rectal hemorrhage, sinusitis, voice alteration
ENDO: Hyperglycemia, hypoglycemia
GI: Constipation, diarrhea, gastritis, melena, nausea, pelvic pain, retroperitoneal hemorrhage, vomiting
GU: Cystitis, hematuria, nocturia, PSA elevation, pyuria, renal calculi
HEME: Leukocytosis
MS: Arthralgia, arthritis, back pain, leg or muscle cramps, neck rigidity
RESP: Bronchitis, bronchospasm, COPD, pulmonary congestion
SKIN: Discoloration, dryness, hypertrophy, photosensitivity, rash, urticaria
Other: Anaphylaxis, angioedema, dehyrdation, flulike syndrome, gout, hyperkalemia, hypokalemia, metabolic acidosis

Nursing Considerations

• Use cautiously in patients with cardiovascular disorders, especially insufficiency, cardiac arrhythmias, and hypertension; convulsive disorders; thyrotoxicosis; and unusual sensitivity to sympathomimetic amines because arformoterol may cause significant adverse effects.
• Be aware that arformoterol shouldn't be used to relieve bronchospasm quickly because of its prolonged onset of action and that patients already taking the drug twice daily shouldn't take additional doses for exercise-induced bronchospasm.
• Arformoterol shouldn't be used with other inhaled, long-acting beta₂-agonists or with other medications containing long-acting beta₂-agonists.
• **WARNING** Be aware that asthma-related deaths may increase in patients receiving salmeterol, a drug in the same class as arformoterol. Monitor patient closely and notify prescriber immediately of any changes in patient's respiratory status.
• Watch for arrhythmias and changes in heart rate or blood pressure after use in patients with cardiovascular disorders because of drug's beta-adrengeric effects.
• **WARNING** Stop arformoterol immediately and notify prescriber if patient develops paradoxical bronchospasm or an allergic reaction.
• Monitor patient's blood glucose level, especially if diabetic, and plasma potassium level, as ordered, because arformoterol may cause significant changes.

PATIENT TEACHING
• Advise patient to take doses 12 hours apart, morning and evening, for optimum effect. Caution against using drug more than every 12 hours.
• Teach patient to self-administer drug with a standard jet nebulizer connected to an air compressor and to use vial immediately after removing from foil package.
• Caution patient not to swallow solution.
• Tell patient to return unused vials to pouch and store arformoterol in the refrigerator.
• Inform patient taking inhaled, short-acting beta₂-agonists on a regular basis to discontinue regular use of these drugs and to use them only for symptomatic relief of acute respiratory symptoms.
• Instruct patient to notify prescriber if he needs four or more oral inhalations of rapid-acting inhaled bronchodilator a day for 2 or more consecutive days, or if he uses more than one canister of rapid-acting bronchodilator in an 8-week period.

argatroban

Acova

Class and Category

Chemical class: N2-substituted derivative of arginine
Therapeutic class: Anticoagulant
Pregnancy category: B

Indications and Dosages

➤ *To prevent or treat thrombosis in patients with heparin-induced thrombocytopenia (HIT)*

I.V. INFUSION

Adults. 2 mcg/kg/min as a continuous infusion. *Maximum:* 10 mcg/kg/min.

DOSAGE ADJUSTMENT Dosage adjusted as prescribed to maintain patient's APTT at 1.5 to 3 times the initial baseline value, not to exceed 100 sec. Initial dosage reduced to 0.5 mcg/kg/min for patients with moderate hepatic impairment.

➤ *To prevent or treat thrombosis in patients with or at risk for HIT when undergoing percutaneous coronary intervention (PCI)*

I.V. INFUSION

Adults. *Initial:* 350 mcg/kg over 3 to 5 min followed by a continuous infusion of 25 mcg/kg/min.

DOSAGE ADJUSTMENT Dosage adjusted as prescribed to keep activated clotting time (ACT) at 300 to 450 sec. If ACT is less than 300 sec, give additional I.V. bolus dose of 150 mcg/kg and increase infusion to 30 mcg/kg/min; if ACT exceeds 450 sec, reduce dosage to 15 mcg/kg/min. For dissection, impending abrupt closure, thrombus formation during PCI, or inability to reach or keep ACT above 300 sec, give additional bolus dose of 150 mcg/kg and increase infusion to 40 mcg/kg/min.

Route	Onset	Peak	Duration
I.V.	Immediate	3 to 4 hr	Unknown

Mechanism of Action

Forms a tight bond with thrombin, neutralizing this enzyme's actions, even when the enzyme is trapped within clots. Thrombin causes fibrinogen to convert to fibrin, which is essential for clot formation.

Contraindications

Active major bleeding, hypersensitivity to argatroban or its components

Interactions

DRUGS

alteplase, antineoplastic drugs, antiplatelets, antithymocyte globulin, heparin, NSAIDs, reteplase, salicylates, streptokinase, strontium chloride Sr 89, warfarin: Increased risk of bleeding

porfimer: Possibly decreased efficacy of porfimer photodynamic therapy

Adverse Reactions

CNS: Cerebrovascular bleeding, fever, headache
CV: Atrial fibrillation, cardiac arrest, hypotension, unstable angina, ventricular tachycardia
GI: Abdominal pain, anorexia, diarrhea, elevated liver function test results, GI bleeding, melena, nausea, vomiting
GU: Elevated BUN and serum creatinine levels, hematuria (microscopic), UTI
HEME: Hypoprothrombinemia, unusual bleeding or bruising
RESP: Cough, dyspnea, hemoptysis, pneumonia
SKIN: Bleeding at puncture site, rash
Other: Sepsis

Nursing Considerations

• **WARNING** Be aware that argatroban isn't recommended for PCI patients with significant hepatic disease or AST/ALT levels greater than or equal to three times the upper limits of normal.

• Reconstitute drug to 1 mg/ml before giving.

• Protect solution from direct sunlight.

• **WARNING** Monitor patients with thrombocytopenia or those receiving daily doses of salicylates greater than 6 g for signs and symptoms of bleeding because they're at increased risk of bleeding from hypoprothrombinemia.

• **WARNING** Expect to perform blood coagulation tests before and 2 hours after start of therapy because of the major risk of bleeding associated with argatroban. Be aware that coagulopathy must be ruled out before therapy is initiated. When giving drug to a patient undergoing PCI, expect to check ACT 5 to 10 minutes after each bolus and each infusion rate change and every 20 to 30 minutes during the PCI.

• Monitor the following patients for signs and symptoms of bleeding because they're at increased risk during argatroban therapy: females with active menstruation; patients with vascular or organ abnormalities, such as severe uncontrolled hypertension, advanced renal disease, infective endocarditis, dissecting aortic aneurysm, hemophilia, hepatic disease (especially if associated with a deficiency of vitamin K–dependent clotting factors), inflammatory bowel disease, or peptic ulcer disease; and those who have recently had a stroke, major surgery (including eye, brain, or spinal cord surgery), large vessel puncture or organ biopsy, lumbar puncture, spinal anesthesia, or major bleeding (including intracranial, GI, intraocular, retroperitoneal, or pulmonary bleeding).

•Whenever possible, avoid I.M. injections in patients receiving argatroban to decrease the risk of bleeding.

•Be aware that thrombin times may not be helpful for monitoring argatroban activity because the drug affects all thrombin-dependent coagulation tests.

•Expect dosage to be tapered before discontinuation to prevent the risk of rebound hypercoagulopathy; drug's effects last for only a short time once drug is discontinued.

PATIENT TEACHING

•Inform patient that argatroban is a blood thinner that's administered in the hospital by infusion into a vein. If he requires long-term anticoagulation, he'll be switched to another drug before discharge.

•Advise patient to immediately report unusual or unexplained bleeding, such as blood in urine, easy bruising, nosebleeds, tarry stools, and vaginal bleeding.

•Instruct patient to avoid injury while receiving argatroban. For example, suggest that he brush his teeth gently, using a soft-bristled toothbrush, and take special care when flossing.

aripiprazole

Abilify, Abilify Discmelt

Class and Category

Chemical class: Dihydrocarbostyril
Therapeutic class: Atypical antipsychotic
Pregnancy category: C

Indications and Dosages

➤ To treat acute schizophrenia; to maintain stability in patients with schizophrenia

ORAL SOLUTION, ORALLY DISINTEGRATING TABLETS, TABLETS

Adults. *Initial:* 10 or 15 mg daily. Increased to 30 mg daily, as needed, with dosage adjustments at 2-wk intervals. *Maintenance:* 15 mg daily.

➤ To treat acute manic and mixed epi-

sodes in bipolar I disorder with or without psychotic features; to maintain stability in patients with bipolar I disorder; as adjunct with lithium or valproate in patients with bipolar I disorder

ORAL SOLUTION, ORALLY DISINTEGRATING TABLETS, TABLETS

Adults. *Initial:* 15 mg daily, increased to 30 mg daily, as needed. *Maintenance:* 15 to 30 mg daily. *Maximum:* 30 mg daily.

Children ages 10 to 17. *Initial:* 2 mg daily, increased after 2 days to 5 mg daily and then after 2 days to 10 mg daily. Increased in 5-mg increments, as needed, at 2-wk intervals. *Maintenance:* Lowest dose possible to maintain remission. *Maximum:* 30 mg daily.

➤ As adjunct to treat depression in patients already taking an antidepressant

ORAL SOLUTION, ORALLY DISINTEGRATING TABLETS, TABLETS

Adults. *Initial:* 2 to 5 mg daily, with dosage increased to 5 mg daily at 1-wk intervals.

➤ To treat agitation in schizophrenia or bipolar mania

I.M. INJECTION

Adults. *Initial:* Depending on severity of agitation, 5.25 to 15 mg. May be repeated 2 or more hr later, as needed. *Maximum:* 30 mg daily.

DOSAGE ADJUSTMENT Dosage reduced to half normal amount when given with clarithromycin, fluoxetine, itraconazole, ketoconazole, paroxetine, or quinidine. Dosage doubled when administered with carbamazepine.

Mechanism of Action

May produce antipsychotic effects through partial agonist and antagonist actions. Aripiprazole acts as a partial agonist at dopamine—especially D_2—receptors and serotonin—especially 5-HT_{1A}—receptors. The drug acts as an antagonist at 5-HT_{2A} serotonin receptor sites.

Contraindications

Breast-feeding, hypersensitivity to aripiprazole or its components

Interactions

DRUGS
anticholingerics: Increased risk for poten-

tially fatal elevation of body temperature
carbamazepine and other CYP3A4 inducers:
Possibly increased clearance and decreased
blood level of aripiprazole
clarithromycin, fluoxetine, paroxetine, quinidine, and other CYP2D6 inhibitors; ketoconazole and other CYP3A4 inhibitors: Possibly inhibited aripiprazole elimination and
increased blood level
CNS depressants: Increased CNS depression
*fluoxetine, paroxetine, quinidine, and other
CYP2D6 inhibitors; ketoconazole and other
CYP3A4 inhibitors:* Possibly inhibited elimination and increased blood aripiprazole level
ACTIVITIES
alcohol use: Increased CNS depression

Adverse Reactions

CNS: Abnormal gait, agitation, akathisia,
anxiety, asthenia, cognitive and motor
impairment, confusion, delusions, depression,
dizziness, dream disturbances, dystonia, extrapyramidal reactions, fatigue, fever, hallucinations, headache, hostility, insomnia, intracranial hemorrhage, lethargy, light-headedness, mania, nervousness, neuroleptic malignant syndrome, paranoia, restlessness,
schizophrenic reaction, seizures, somnolence,
stroke (elderly), suicidal ideation, tardive
dyskinesia, transient ischemic attack (elderly), tremor
CV: Arrhythmias, bradycardia, cardiopulmonary arrest, chest pain, circulatory collapse, deep vein thrombosis, elevated serum
CK levels, heart failure, hypertension, MI,
orthostatic hypotension, peripheral edema,
prolonged QT interval, tachycardia
EENT: Blurred vision, conjunctivitis, dry
mouth, hepatitis, increased salivation, laryngospasm, nasopharyngitis, oropharyngeal
spasm, pharyngitis, rhinitis, sinusitis
ENDO: Hyperglycemia
GI: Abdominal discomfort, constipation, decreased appetite, diarrhea, difficulty swallowing, GI bleeding, indigestion, jaundice,
nausea, vomiting
GU: Renal failure, urinary incontinence
HEME: Anemia, leukopenia, thrombocytopenia
MS: Arthralgia, elevated blood CK level,
muscle spasms, muscleskeletal pain, myalgia,
neck and limb rigidity, rhabdomyolysis
RESP: Apnea, aspiration, asthma, cough,
dyspnea, pneumonia, pulmonary edema or
embolism, respiratory failure

SKIN: Diaphoresis, dry skin, ecchymosis,
pruritus, rash, ulceration, urticaria
Other: Anaphylaxis, angioedema, dehydration, flulike symptoms, heat stroke, weight
gain

Nursing Considerations

• Aripiprazole shouldn't be used to treat dementia related psychosis in the elderly because of an increased risk of death.
• Use cautiously in patients with CV disease,
cerebrovascular disease, or conditions that
would predispose them to hypotension. Also
use cautiously in those with a history of
seizures or with conditions that lower seizure
threshold, such as Alzheimer's disease.
• Also use cautiously in elderly patients because of increased risk of serious adverse
cerebrovascular effects, such as stroke and
transient ischemic attack.
• Be aware that oral solution may be given on
a milligram-per-milligram basis in place of
tablets up to 25 mg. For example, if patient
needs 30 mg of tablet and is switched to oral
solution, expect to give 25 mg of solution.
• Inject parenteral form slowly, deep into the
muscle, and never I.V. or subcutaneously.
• Monitor patient for difficulty swallowing or
excessive somnolence, which could predispose him to accidental injury or aspiration.
• **WARNING** Be aware that aripiprazole rarely
may cause neuroleptic malignant syndrome,
tardive dyskinesia, and seizures. Monitor patient closely throughout therapy, and take
safety precautions as needed.
• Monitor patient's blood glucose level routinely; risk of hyperglycemia may increase.
• Watch patients closely (especially children,
adolescents, and young adults) for suicidal
tendencies, particularly when therapy starts
and dosage changes, because depression may
worsen temporarily during these times.
PATIENT TEACHING
• Instruct patient prescribed orally disintegrating tablets to open the blister pack only
when ready to take the tablet. Tell him to
peel back the foil and not to push tablet
through the foil because doing so could damage the tablet. Tell him to place the tablet on
his tongue without breaking it and let it dissolve. If needed, he may take a drink.
• Advise patient to get up slowly from a lying
or sitting position to minimize orthostatic
hypotension during aripiprazole therapy.

A

•Urge patient to avoid alcohol during aripiprazole therapy.
•Instruct patient to avoid hazardous activities until drug's effects are known.
•Urge patient to avoid activities that raise body temperature suddenly, such as strenuous exercise and exposure to extreme heat, and to compensate for situations that cause dehydration, such as vomiting or diarrhea.
•Instruct patient to inform all prescribers of any drugs he's taking, including OTC drugs, because of a potential for interactions.
•Advise female patient of childbearing age to notify prescriber if she intends to become or suspects that she is pregnant during therapy.
•Instruct diabetic patient taking the oral solution to monitor blood glucose levels closely because each milliliter of solution contains 400 mg of sucrose and 200 mg of fructose.
•Urge family or caregiver to watch patient closely for suicidal tendencies, especially when therapy starts or dosage changes and particularly if patient is a child, teenager, or young adult.

armodafinil

Nuvigil

Class and Category
Chemical class: Diphenylmethyl sulfinylacetamide
Therapeutic class: CNS stimulant
Pregnancy category: C

Indications and Dosages
➤ *To treat narcolepsy or as adjunct to standard therapy for excessive daytime sleepiness in obstructive sleep apnea/hypopnea syndrome*
TABLETS
Adults. 150 or 250 mg once daily in the morning.

➤ *To improve daytime wakefulness in patients with excessive sleepiness from circadian rhythm disruption (shift-work sleep disorder)*
TABLETS
Adults. 150 mg once daily about 1 hr before start of work shift.
DOSAGE ADJUSTMENT Decreased dosage recommended for patients who are elderly, have severe hepatic impairment, or take steroidal contraceptives.

Route	Onset	Peak	Duration
P.O.	Unknown	2 hr (fasting) 4 to 6 hr (with food)	Unknown

Mechanism of Action
May produce CNS-stimulant effects by binding to the dopamine transporter in the brain and inhibiting dopamine reuptake in the limbic regions. These actions increase alertness and reduce drowsiness and fatigue.

Contraindications
Hypersensitivity to armodafinil, modafinil, or their components

Interactions
DRUGS
amitriptyline, citalopram, clomipramine, diazepam, imipramine, propranolol, tolbutamide, topiramate: Possibly prolonged elimination time and increased blood levels of these drugs
barbiturates (such as phenobarbital, primidone), dexamethasone, rifabutin, rifampin: Possibly decreased blood level and effectiveness of armodafinil
carbamazepine: Possibly decreased armodafinil effectiveness and decreased blood carbamazepine level
cimetidine, clarithromycin, erythromycin, fluconazole, fluoxetine, fluvoxamine, itraconazole, ketoconazole, nefazodone, sertraline: Possibly inhibited metabolism, decreased clearance, and increased blood level of armodafinil
clozapine: Possibly increased levels of clozapine caused by decreased secondary hepatic metabolism
contraceptive-containing implants or devices: Possibly contraceptive failure
cyclosporine: Possibly decreased blood cyclosporine level and increased risk of organ transplant rejection
dextroamphetamine, methylphenidate: Possibly 1-hr delay in armodafinil absorption when these drugs are given together
fosphenytoin, mephenytoin, phenytoin: Possibly decreased effectiveness of armodafinil, increased blood phenytoin level, and in-

creased risk of phenytoin toxicity
midazolam, triazolam: Possibly decreased effectiveness of triazolam or midazolam
oral contraceptives: Possibly decreased effectiveness of oral contraceptive
theophylline: Possibly decreased blood level and effectiveness of theophylline
warfarin: Possibly decreased warfarin metabolism and increased risk of bleeding

Foods
all foods: 2- to 4-hr delay for armodafinil to reach peak levels and possibly delayed onset of action
alcohol: Possibly adverse CNS effects
caffeine: Increased CNS stimulation
grapefruit juice: Possibly decreased armodafinil metabolism

Adverse Reactions

CNS: Agitation, anxiety, attention disturbance, depression, dizziness, fatigue, fever, headache (including migraine), insomnia, nervousness, paresthesia, suicidal ideation, thirst, tremor
CV: Increased heart rate, palpitations
EENT: Dry mouth
GI: Abdominal pain (upper), anorexia, constipation, decreased appetite, diarrhea, dyspepsia, loose stools, nausea, vomiting
GU: Polyuria
RESP: Dyspnea
SKIN: Contact dermatitis, hyperhydrosis, rash
Other: Angioedema, flulike illness

Nursing Considerations

•Be aware that armodafinil shouldn't be given to patients with mitral valve prolapse syndrome or a history of left ventricular hypertrophy because drug may cause ischemic changes.
•WARNING If patient has a history of alcoholism, stimulant abuse, or other substance abuse, monitor him for compliance with armodafinil therapy. Watch for signs of misuse or abuse, including frequent prescription refill requests, increased frequency of dosing, and drug-seeking behavior. Also watch for evidence of excessive armodafinil use, including agitation, anxiety, diarrhea, nausea, nervousness, palpitations, sleep disturbances, and tremor.
•Be aware that armodafinil, like other CNS stimulants, may alter mood, perception, thinking, judgment, feelings, and motor skills and may produce signs that patient needs sleep.
•If giving drug to patient with a history of psychosis, emotional instability, or psychological illness with psychotic features, be prepared to perform baseline behavioral assessments or frequent clinical observation.

Patient Teaching
•Inform patient that armodafinil can help, but not cure, narcolepsy and that drug's full effects may not be seen right away.
•Advise patient to avoid taking armodafinil within 2 hours of eating because food may delay the time to peak drug effect and onset of action. If patient drinks grapefruit juice, encourage him to drink a consistent amount daily.
•Inform patient that drug can affect his concentration and function and can hide signs of fatigue. Urge him not to drive or perform activities that require mental alertness until drug's full CNS effects are known.
•Because alcohol may decrease alertness, advise patient to avoid it with armodafinil.
•Encourage a regular sleeping pattern.
•Caution patient to avoid excessive intake of foods, beverages, and over-the-counter drugs that contain caffeine because caffeine may lead to increased CNS stimulation.
•Inform female patient that armodafinil can decrease the effectiveness of certain contraceptives, including birth control pills and implantable hormonal contraceptives. If she uses such contraceptives, urge her to use an alternate birth control method during armodafinil therapy and for up to 1 month after she stops taking the drug.
•Advise patient to keep follow-up appointments with prescriber so that her progress can be monitored.

aspirin
(acetylsalicylic acid, ASA)

Ancasal (CAN), Apo-As (CAN), Apo-ASEN (CAN), Arthrinol (CAN), Arthrisin (CAN), Aspergum, Aspirin, Atria S.R. (CAN), Bayer, Easprin, Ecotrin, Ecotrin Maximum Strength, 8-Hour Bayer Time Release, Empirin, Genprin, Maximum Bayer, Norwich Extra-Strength, Novasen (CAN), Sal-Adult (CAN), Sal-Infant (CAN), St. Joseph Children's, Supasa (CAN), Therapy Bayer, ZORprin

A

Class and Category
Chemical class: Salicylate
Therapeutic class: Anti-inflammatory, antiplatelet, antipyretic, nonopioid analgesic
Pregnancy category: D

Indications and Dosages
➤ *To relieve mild pain or fever*
CHEWABLE TABLETS, CHEWING GUM, CONTROLLED-RELEASE TABLETS, ENTERIC-COATED TABLETS, SOLUTION, TABLETS, TIMED-RELEASE TABLETS, SUPPOSITORIES
Adults and adolescents. 325 to 650 mg every 4 hr, p.r.n., or 500 mg every 3 hr, p.r.n., or 1,000 mg every 6 hr, p.r.n.
Children ages 2 to 14. 10 to 15 mg/kg/dose every 4 hr, p.r.n., up to 80 mg/kg daily.

➤ *To relieve mild to moderate pain from inflammation, as in rheumatoid arthritis and osteoarthritis*
CHEWABLE TABLETS, CHEWING GUM, CONTROLLED-RELEASE TABLETS, ENTERIC-COATED TABLETS, SOLUTION, TABLETS, TIMED-RELEASE TABLETS, SUPPOSITORIES
Adults and adolescents. 3.2 to 6 g daily in divided doses. *Maximum:* 6 g daily.
Children. 10 to 15 mg/kg daily, up to 80 mg/kg daily, in divided doses every 4 to 6 hr.

➤ *To treat juvenile rheumatoid arthritis*
CHEWABLE TABLETS, CHEWING GUM, CONTROLLED-RELEASE TABLETS, ENTERIC-COATED TABLETS, SOLUTION, TABLETS, TIMED-RELEASE TABLETS, SUPPOSITORIES
Children. 60 to 110 mg/kg daily in divided doses every 6 to 8 hr.

➤ *To treat acute rheumatic fever*
CHEWABLE TABLETS, CHEWING GUM, CONTROLLED-RELEASE TABLETS, ENTERIC-COATED TABLETS, SOLUTION, TABLETS, TIMED-RELEASE TABLETS, SUPPOSITORIES
Adults and adolescents. 5 to 8 g daily in divided doses.
Children. *Initial:* 100 mg/kg daily in divided doses for first 2 wk. *Maintenance:* 75 mg/kg/day in divided doses for next 4 to 6 wk.

➤ *To reduce the risk of recurrent transient ischemic attacks or stroke in men*
CHEWABLE TABLETS, CHEWING GUM, CONTROLLED-RELEASE TABLETS, ENTERIC-COATED TABLETS, SOLUTION, TABLETS, TIMED-RELEASE TABLETS, SUPPOSITORIES
Adults. 650 mg b.i.d. or 325 mg q.i.d.

➤ *To reduce the severity of or prevent acute MI*
CHEWABLE TABLETS, CHEWING GUM, CONTROLLED-RELEASE TABLETS, ENTERIC-COATED TABLETS, SOLUTION, TABLETS, TIMED-RELEASE TABLETS, SUPPOSITORIES

Adults. *Initial:* 160 to 162.5 mg (one-half of a 325-mg tablet or two 80- or 81-mg tablets) as soon as MI is suspected. *Maintenance:* 160 to 162.5 mg daily for 30 days.

➤ *To reduce risk of MI in patients with previous MI or unstable angina*
CHEWABLE TABLETS, CHEWING GUM, CONTROLLED-RELEASE TABLETS, ENTERIC-COATED TABLETS, SOLUTION, TABLETS, TIMED-RELEASE TABLETS, SUPPOSITORIES
Adults. 325 mg daily.

Contraindications
Allergy to tartrazine dye, asthma, bleeding problems (such as hemophilia), hypersensitivity to aspirin or its components, peptic ulcer disease

Route	Onset	Peak	Duration
P.O. (chewable tablets)	Rapid	Unknown	1 to 4 hr
P.O. (controlled-release)	5 to 30 min	1 to 4 hr	4 to 6 hr
P.O. (enteric-coated)	5 to 30 min	Unknown	1 to 4 hr
P.O. (solution)	5 to 30 min	15 to 40 min	1 to 4 hr
P.O. (tablets)	15 to 30 min	1 to 2 hr	4 to 6 hr
P.O. (timed-release)	5 to 30 min	1 to 4 hr	4 to 6 hr
P.R.	Unknown	Unknown	4 to 6 hr

Interactions
DRUGS
ACE inhibitors: Decreased antihypertensive effect
activated charcoal: Decreased aspirin absorption
antacids, urine alkalinizers: Decreased aspirin effectiveness
anticoagulants: Increased risk of bleeding; prolonged bleeding time
carbonic anhydrase inhibitors: Salicylism
corticosteroids: Increased excretion and decreased blood level of aspirin
heparin: Increased risk of bleeding
ibuprofen: Possibly reduced cardioprotective and stroke preventive effects of aspirin

methotrexate: Increased blood level and decreased excretion of methotrexate, causing toxicity
nizatidine: Increased blood aspirin level
NSAIDs: Possibly decreased blood NSAID level and increased risk of adverse GI effects
sulfonylureas: Possibly enhanced effect of sulfonylureas with large doses of aspirin
urine acidifiers, such as ammonium chloride and ascorbic acid: Decreased aspirin excretion
vancomycin: Increased risk of ototoxicity

ACTIVITIES
alcohol use: Increased risk of ulcers

Mechanism of Action

Blocks the activity of cyclooxygenase, the enzyme necessary for prostaglandin synthesis. Prostaglandins, important mediators in the inflammatory response, cause local vasodilation with swelling and pain. With the blocking of cyclooxygenase and the inhibition of prostaglandins, inflammatory symptoms subside. Pain relief is also achieved by inhibiting prostaglandins because they play a role in pain transmission from the periphery to the spinal cord. Aspirin inhibits platelet aggregation by interfering with the production of thromboxane A_2, a substance that stimulates platelet aggregation. Aspirin acts on the heat-regulating center in the hypothalamus and causes peripheral vasodilation, diaphoresis, and heat loss.

Adverse Reactions

CNS: Confusion, CNS depression
EENT: Hearing loss, tinnitus
GI: Diarrhea, GI bleeding, heartburn, hepatotoxicity, nausea, stomach pain, vomiting
HEME: Decreased blood iron level, leukopenia, prolonged bleeding time, shortened life span of RBCs, thrombocytopenia
SKIN: Ecchymosis, rash, urticaria
Other: Angioedema, Reye's syndrome, salicylism (dizziness, tinnitus, difficulty hearing, vomiting, diarrhea, confusion, CNS depression, diaphoresis, headache, hyperventilation, and lassitude) with regular use of large doses

Nursing Considerations

• Don't crush timed-release or controlled-release aspirin tablets unless directed.
• Ask about tinnitus. This reaction usually occurs when blood aspirin level reaches or exceeds maximum for therapeutic effect.

PATIENT TEACHING
• WARNING Advise parents not to give aspirin to a child or adolescent with chickenpox or flu symptoms because of risk of Reye's syndrome (rare life-threatening reaction characterized by vomiting, lethargy, belligerence, delirium, and coma). Tell them to consult prescriber about alternative drugs.
• Also advise adult patient taking low-dose aspirin not to take ibuprofen because it may reduce the cardioprotective and stroke preventive effects of aspirin.
• Instruct patient to take aspirin with food or after meals because it may cause GI upset if taken on an empty stomach.
• Advise patient with tartrazine allergy not to take aspirin.
• Tell patient to consult prescriber before taking aspirin with any prescription drug for blood disorder, diabetes, gout, or arthritis.
• Tell patient not to use aspirin if it has a strong vinegar-like odor.

atenolol

Apo-Atenol (CAN), Novo-Atenol (CAN), Tenormin

Class and Category

Chemical class: Beta-adrenergic blocker (beta$_1$ and at high doses beta$_2$)
Therapeutic class: Antianginal, antihypertensive
Pregnancy category: D

Indications and Dosages

➤ *To treat angina pectoris and control hypertension*

TABLETS
Adults. 50 mg daily increased, p.r.n., after 1 to 2 wk to 100 mg daily.

➤ *To treat acute MI*

TABLETS, I.V. INFUSION
Adults. *Initial:* 5 mg I.V. over 5 min followed by 5 mg I.V. 10 min later. After an additional 10 min, 50 mg given and followed by another 50 mg in 12 hr. *Maintenance:* 50 mg P.O. b.i.d. or 100 mg P.O. daily for 6 to 9 days or until discharged from hospital.
DOSAGE ADJUSTMENT Dosage reduced to 50 mg daily P.O. for renally impaired patients

and elderly, renally impaired patients with creatinine clearance of 15 to 35 ml/min/ 1.73 m². Dosage reduced to 25 mg daily P.O. for renally impaired patients and elderly, renally impaired patients with creatinine clearance of less than 15 ml/min/1.73 m².

Route	Onset	Peak	Duration
P.O.	1 hr	2 to 4 hr	24 hr
I.V.	Immediate	5 min	12 hr

Mechanism of Action
Inhibits stimulation of beta₁-receptor sites, located primarily in the heart, causing a decrease in cardiac excitability, cardiac output, and myocardial oxygen demand. Atenolol also acts to decrease the release of renin from the kidneys, aiding in reducing blood pressure. At high doses, it inhibits stimulation of beta₂ receptors in the lungs, which may cause bronchoconstriction.

Contraindications
Cardiogenic shock, heart block greater than first degree, hypersensitivity to beta blockers, overt heart failure, sinus bradycardia

Interactions
DRUGS
amiodarone: Additive atenolol effects
calcium channel blockers, such as verapamil and diltiazem: Possibly symptomatic bradycardia and conduction abnormalities
catecholamine-depleting drugs, such as reserpine: Additive antihypertensive effect
clonidine: Rebound hypertension
disopyramide: Increased risk of severe bradycardia, asystole, and heart failure

Adverse Reactions
CNS: Depression, disorientation, dizziness, drowsiness, emotional lability, fatigue, fever, lethargy, light-headedness, short-term memory loss, vertigo
CV: Arrhythmias, including bradycardia and heart block; cardiogenic shock; cold arms and legs; heart failure; mesenteric artery thrombosis; mitral insufficiency; myocardial reinfarction; orthostatic hypotension; Raynaud's phenomenon
EENT: Dry eyes, laryngospasm, pharyngitis
GI: Diarrhea, ischemic colitis, nausea

GU: Renal failure
HEME: Agranulocytosis
MS: Leg pain
RESP: Bronchospasm, dyspnea, pulmonary emboli, respiratory distress, wheezing
SKIN: Erythematous rash
Other: Allergic reaction

Nursing Considerations
• Use atenolol cautiously in patients with heart failure controlled by digitalis glycosides or diuretics, patients with conduction abnormalities or left ventricular dysfunction who take verapamil or diltiazem, patients with arterial circulatory disorders, and patients with impaired renal function.
• Use atenolol cautiously in diabetic patients because it may mask tachycardia caused by hypoglycemia. Unlike other beta-adrenergic blockers, it doesn't mask other signs of hypoglycemia, cause hypoglycemia, or delay the return of blood glucose to a normal level.
• At first sign of heart failure, expect patient to receive a digitalis glycoside, a diuretic, or both and to be monitored closely. If failure continues, expect to discontinue atenolol.
• Closely monitor patient with hyperthyroidism because atenolol may mask some signs of thyrotoxicosis. Abrupt withdrawal of atenolol may precipitate thyrotoxicosis.
• If patient also receives clonidine, expect to discontinue atenolol several days before gradually withdrawing clonidine. Then expect to restart atenolol therapy several days after clonidine has been discontinued.
• During I.V. atenolol therapy, monitor vital signs and cardiac rhythm closely.
• Discard parenteral mixture with atenolol if it isn't used within 48 hours.
• Stop atenolol therapy and notify prescriber if patient develops bradycardia, hypotension, or other serious adverse reaction.

PATIENT TEACHING
• Instruct patient not to stop taking atenolol abruptly. Otherwise, angina may worsen and an MI or arrhythmia may occur.
• While patient is being weaned from atenolol, tell him to perform minimal physical activity to prevent chest pain.
• Instruct patient to take a missed dose as soon as possible. However, if it's within 8 hours of the next scheduled dose, tell him to skip the missed dose and return to his regular schedule.

•Explain that atenolol may alter serum glucose level and mask hypoglycemia.
•Inform the patient that he may experience fatigue and reduced tolerance to exercise and that he should notify his prescriber if this interferes with his normal lifestyle.

atomoxetine hydrochloride

Strattera

Class and Catgegory

Chemical class: Selective norepinephrine reuptake inhibitor
Therapeutic class: Anti–attention deficit hyperactivity agent
Pregnancy category: C

Indications and Dosages

➤ *To treat attention deficit hyperactivity disorder (ADHD)*

CAPSULES

Adults and children weighing 70 kg (154 lb) or less. *Initial:* 0.5 mg/kg daily, increased after at least 3 days to 1.2 mg/kg daily given either as a single dose in the morning or in evenly divided doses morning and late afternoon or early evening, as needed. *Maximum:* 1.4 mg/kg or 100 mg daily, whichever is less.

Adults and children weighing more than 70 kg. *Initial:* 40 mg daily, increased after a minimum of 3 days to 80 mg daily given either as a single dose in the morning or in evenly divided doses morning and late afternoon or early evening. After 2 to 4 additional wk, dosage may be increased to 100 mg daily if optimal response hasn't been achieved. *Maximum:* 100 mg daily.

DOSAGE ADJUSTMENT For patients with moderate (Child-Pugh Class B) hepatic impairment, dosage reduced by 50%. For patients with severe (Child-Pugh Class C) hepatic impairment, dosage reduced by 75%. For patients weighing 70 kg or less and taking strong CYP2D6 inhibitors, such as paroxetine, fluoxetine, or quinidine, initial dosage of 0.5 mg/kg daily should be increased to 1.2 mg/kg daily only if symptoms fail to improve after 4 wk. For patients weighing more than 70 kg and taking strong CYP2D6 inhibitors, initial dosage of 40 mg daily should be increased to 80 mg daily only if symptoms fail to improve after 4 wk.

Mechanism of Action

Selectively inhibits presynaptic norepinephrine transport in the nervous system to increase attention span and produce a calming effect.

Contraindications

Angle-closure glaucoma, hypersensitivity to atomoxetine or its components, use within 14 days of MAO inhibitor therapy

Interactions

DRUGS

albuterol and other beta$_2$ agonists: May potentiate action of albuterol and other beta$_2$ agonists on cardiovascular system
CYP2D6 inhibitors (such as fluoxetine, paroxetine, and quinidine): Increased blood atomoxetine level
MAO inhibitors: Possibly induced hypertensive crisis
pressor agents: Possibly altered blood pressure

Adverse Reactions

CNS: Aggressiveness, anxiety, chills, crying, depression, dizziness, early morning awakening, fatigue, headache, hostility, insomnia, irritability, lethargy, mood changes, paresthesia, peripheral coldness, pyrexia, rigors, sedation, seizures, sleep disturbance, somnolence, stroke, suicidal ideation (children and adolescents), syncope, tremor, unusual dreams
CV: Chest pain, hypertension, orthostatic hypotension, MI, palpitations, QT-interval prolongation, Raynaud's phenomenon, tachycardia
EENT: Conjunctivitis, dry mouth, ear infection, mydriasis, nasal congestion, nasopharyngitis, pharyngitis, rhinorrhea, sinus congestion
ENDO: Hot flashes
GI: Abdominal pain (upper), anorexia, constipation, diarrhea, elevated liver function test results, flatulence, gastroenteritis (viral), indigestion, nausea, severe hepatic dysfunction, vomiting
GU: Decreased libido, dysmenorrhea, dysuria, ejaculation disorders, erectile dysfunction, impotence, male pelvic pain, menstrual irregularities, orgasm abnormality, priapism, prostatitis, urinary hesitancy, urine retention

MS: Arthralgia, back pain, myalgia
RESP: Cough, upper respiratory tract infection
SKIN: Dermatitis, diaphoresis, pruritus, rash, urticaria
Other: Angioedema, influenza, weight loss

Nursing Considerations
•Use atomoxetine cautiously in patients with cerebrovascular or CV disease (especially hypertension or tachycardia) because drug may cause an increase in blood pressure and heart rate. Also use cautiously in those who are prone to orthostatic hypotension and in those with serious structural cardiac abnormlities, cardiomyopathy, serious heart rhythm abnormalities, or other serious cardiac problems because drug may increase risk of sudden death from these conditions.
•**WARNING** Monitor children and adolescents closely for evidence of suicidal thinking and behavior as well as for psychotic or manic symptoms such as hallucinations, delusional thinking, or mania because atomoxetine increases the risk of suicidal ideation and the onset of psychotic or manic symptoms in these age-groups.
•Obtain baseline blood pressure and heart rate before starting therapy. Monitor patient's vital signs after dosage increases and periodically during therapy.
•Monitor patient closely for allergic reactions. If these occur, notify prescriber.
•Monitor child's or adolescent's growth and weight. Expect to interrupt therapy, as prescribed, if patient isn't growing or gaining weight appropriately.
•Monitor patient's liver function studies, as ordered. Notify prescriber immediately if enzyme levels are elevated or patient has evidence of hepatic dysfunction (jaundice, dark urine, pruritus, right-upper-quadrant tenderness, or unexplained flulike symptoms). Expect to stop atomoxetine permanently.

PATIENT TEACHING
•Caution patient not to open capsules. If a capsule opens, urge patient to promptly wash his hands and any surface drug touches. If drug gets in his eyes, tell him to flush immediately with water and seek medical care.
•Instruct patient or parent to immediately report to prescriber any adverse reactions to atomoxetine therapy, such as facial swelling, itching, or rash.

•**WARNING** Urge parents to watch their child or adolescent closely for evidence of abnormal thinking, abnormal behavior, or increased aggression or hostility. If unusual changes occur, stress need to notify prescriber.
•Urge patient to tell prescriber immediately about yellowing of his skin or eyes, itchiness, right upper abdominal pain, dark urine, or flulike symptoms. Also tell patient to notify prescriber immediately if he experiences exertional chest pain, unexplained syncope, or other symptoms suggestive of heart disease.
•Caution patient to assume sitting or standing position slowly because of drug's potential effect on blood pressure.
•Urge male patient to seek immediate medical attention for a penile erection that becomes prolonged or painful.
•Advise patient to report urinary hesitancy or urine retention to prescriber.
•Remind patient of the importance of alerting all prescribers to any OTC drugs, dietary supplements, or herbal remedies he's taking.
•Caution patient to avoid hazardous activities until drug's CNS effects are known.
•Reassure patient or parent that drug doesn't cause physical or psychological dependence.
•Instruct patient or parent to monitor weight during therapy.

atorvastatin calcium
Lipitor

Class and Category
Chemical class: Synthetically derived fermentation product
Therapeutic class: Antihyperlipidemic, HMG-CoA reductase inhibitor
Pregnancy category: X

Indications and Dosages
➤ *To control lipid levels as adjunct to diet in primary (heterozygous familial and nonfamilial) hypercholesterolemia and mixed dyslipidemia*
TABLETS
Adults. *Initial:* 10 or 20 mg once daily, then increased according to lipid level. *Maintenance:* 10 to 80 mg once daily.
DOSAGE ADJUSTMENT Initial dose may be increased to 40 mg once daily for patients who need cholesterol level reduced more than 45%.

➤ *To control lipid levels in homozygous familial hypercholesterolemia*
TABLETS
Adults. 10 to 80 mg daily.

➤ *To control lipid levels in pediatric heterozygous familial hypercholesterolemia*
TABLETS
Adolescents and children ages 10 to 17. *Initial:* 10 mg daily, adjusted at intervals of 4 wk or more, as needed. *Maximum:* 20 mg daily.

➤ *To reduce debilitating cardiovascular events such as stroke and MI in patients with multiple risk factors but without known coronary artery disease*
TABLETS
Adults. 10 mg once daily.

Mechanism of Action
Reduces plasma cholesterol and lipoprotein levels by inhibiting HMG-CoA reductase and cholesterol synthesis in the liver and by increasing the number of LDL receptors on liver cells to enhance LDL uptake and breakdown.

Contraindications
Active hepatic disease, hypersensitivity to atorvastatin or its components, unexplained persistent rise in serum transaminase level

Interactions
DRUGS
amlodipine, cimetidine, clarithromycin, diltiazem, erythromycin, itraconazole, ritonavir with saquinavir: Increased atorvastatin level
antacid, colestipol, efavirenz, rifampin: Possibly decreased blood atorvastatin level
azole antifungals, clarithromycin, cyclosporine, erythromycin, fibric acid derivatives, lopinavir with ritonavir, niacin (at dosage used for lipid modification), nicotinic acid, ritonavir with saquinavir: Increased risk of severe myopathy or rhabdomyolysis
cyclosporine: Increased atorvastatin bioavailability and risk of adverse reactions
digoxin: Possibly increased blood digoxin level, causing toxicity
oral contraceptives (such as ethinyl estradiol and norethindrone): Increased hormone level
FOODS
grapefruit juice (more than 1.2 L daily): Increased blood atorvastatin level

Adverse Reactions
CNS: Abnormal dreams, amnesia, asthenia, emotional lability, facial paralysis, fever, headache, hyperkinesia, lack of coordination, malaise, paresthesia, peripheral neuropathy, somnolence, syncope, weakness
CV: Arrhythmias, elevated serum CK level, orthostatic hypotension, palpitations, phlebitis, vasodilation
EENT: Amblyopia, altered refraction, dry eyes, dry mouth, epistaxis, eye hemorrhage, gingival hemorrhage, glaucoma, glossitis, hearing loss, lip swelling, loss of taste, pharyngitis, sinusitis, stomatitis, taste perversion, tinnitus
ENDO: Hyperglycemia or hypoglycemia
GI: Abdominal or biliary pain, anorexia, colitis, constipation, diarrhea, duodenal or stomach ulcers, dysphagia, eructation, esophagitis, flatulence, gastroenteritis, hepatitis, increased appetite, indigestion, melena, pancreatitis, rectal hemorrhage, tenesmus, vomiting
GU: Abnormal ejaculation; cystitis; decreased libido; dysuria; epididymitis; hematuria; impotence; nephritis; nocturia; renal calculi; urinary frequency, incontinence, or urgency; urine retention; vaginal hemorrhage
HEME: Anemia, thrombocytopenia
MS: Arthralgia, back pain, bursitis, gout, leg cramps, myalgia, myasthenia gravis, myositis, neck rigidity, tendon contracture, tenosynovitis, torticollis
RESP: Dyspnea, pneumonia
SKIN: Acne, alopecia, contact dermatitis, diaphoresis, dry skin, ecchymosis, eczema, jaundice, petechiae, photosensitivity, pruritus, rash, seborrhea, ulceration, urticaria
Other: Allergic reaction, facial or generalized edema, flulike symptoms, infection, lymphadenopathy, weight gain

Nursing Considerations
•Be aware that atorvastatin is used in patients with homozygous familial hypercholesterolemia as an adjunct to other lipid-lowering treatments or alone only if other treatments aren't available.
•Atorvastatin may be used with colestipol or cholestyramine for additive antihyperlipidemic effects.
•Expect atorvastatin to be used in patients without obvious coronary artery disease (CAD) but with multiple risk factors (such as age 55 or over, smoker, history of hypertension or low HDL level, or family history of

early CAD). Drug is used to reduce risk of MI, angina, and adverse effects of revascularization procedures.
•Also expect drug to be used in patients with type 2 diabetes who have no obvious CAD but multiple risk factors, such as retinopathy, albuminuria, smoking, or hypertension. Drug is used in these patients to reduce the risk of MI and stroke.
•Expect liver function tests to be performed before atorvastatin therapy starts, after 6 and 12 weeks of therapy, with each dosage increase, and every 6 months thereafter.
•Expect to measure lipid levels 2 to 4 weeks after therapy starts, to adjust dosage as directed, and to repeat periodically until lipid levels are within desired range.

PATIENT TEACHING
•Stress that atorvastatin is an adjunct to—not a substitute for—a low-cholesterol diet.
•Tell patient to take drug at the same time each day to maintain its effects.
•Instruct patient to take a missed dose as soon as possible. If it's almost time for his next dose, he should skip the missed dose. Tell him not to double the dose.
•Instruct patient to consult prescriber before taking OTC niacin preparations because of increased risk of rhabdomyolysis.
•Advise patient to notify prescriber immediately if he develops unexplained muscle pain, tenderness, or weakness, especially if accompanied by fatigue or fever.
•Be aware that atorvastatin is expensive. Reinforce the benefits of therapy, and encourage the patient to comply if possible.

atovaquone

Mepron

Class and Category

Chemical class: Hydroxy-1,4-naphtho-quinone
Therapeutic class: Antiprotozoal
Pregnancy category: C

Indications and Dosages

➤ *To prevent* Pneumocystis jiroveci *(formerly* carinii*) pneumonia in patients who can't tolerate co-trimoxazole*
SUSPENSION, TABLETS
Adults and adolescents. 750 mg (5 ml) b.i.d. with meals for 21 days.

➤ *To treat mild to moderate* P. jiroveci *pneumonia in patients who can't tolerate co-trimoxazole*
SUSPENSION, TABLETS
Adults and adolescents. 750 mg (5 ml) b.i.d. with meals for 21 days. *Maximum:* 1,500 mg/day.

Mechanism of Action
May destroy *P. jiroveci* organisms by inhibiting the enzymes needed to synthesize nucleic acid and adenosine triphosphate.

Contraindications

Hypersensitivity to atovaquone or its components

Interactions

DRUGS
rifabutin, rifampin: Possibly decreased blood atovaquone level

Adverse Reactions

CNS: Fever, headache, insomnia
EENT: Rhinitis, throat tightness, vortex keratopathy
GI: Abdominal pain, diarrhea, elevated liver enzyme levels, hepatitis, hepatic failure, nausea, pancreatitis, vomiting
GU: Acute renal dysfunction
HEME: Anemia, thrombocytopenia
RESP: Bronchospasm, cough, dyspnea
SKIN: Desquamation, erythema multiforme, Stevens-Johnson syndrome, rash, urticaria
Other: Allergic reaction, angioedema, methemoglobinemia

Nursing Considerations

•Use atovaquone cautiously in patient with severe hepatic impairment because, although rare, serious adverse reactions affecting liver function may occur.
•Monitor blood test results because atovaquone may decrease serum sodium and hemoglobin levels and neutrophil count and may increase AST, ALT, alkaline phosphatase, and serum amylase levels.
•Crush atovaquone tablets, if needed.
•Don't use tablets and oral suspension interchangeably; they aren't bio-equivalent.

PATIENT TEACHING
•Instruct patient to take atovaquone with meals for maximum effectiveness.

•Instruct patient to take a missed dose as soon as possible after he remembers. If it's almost time for the next dose, tell him to skip the missed dose. Tell him not to double the dose.

•Tell patient to notify prescriber if his condition doesn't improve in a few days or if he develops signs of an allergic reaction, such as fever or rash.

atracurium besylate

Tracrium

Class and Category

Chemical class: Biquaternary ammonium ester
Therapeutic class: Skeletal muscle relaxant
Pregnancy category: C

Indications and Dosages

➤ *To facilitate endotracheal intubation and induce skeletal muscle relaxation for surgery or mechanical ventilation as adjunct to anesthesia*

I.V. INFUSION OR INJECTION

Adults and children age 2 or over. *Initial:* 0.4 to 0.5 mg/kg by I.V. bolus for nearly complete neuromuscular blockade. *Maintenance:* 0.08 to 0.10 mg/kg 20 to 45 min after initial dose during prolonged surgery. Maintenance doses may be given every 15 to 25 min for patients under balanced anesthesia. For patients having extended surgical procedures, after an initial I.V. bolus, an infusion of 9 to 10 mcg/kg/min may be needed to counteract the spontaneous return of neuromuscular function and thereafter 5 to 10 mcg/kg/min as a constant infusion.

Children ages 1 month to 2 years having halothane anesthesia. *Initial:* 0.3 to 0.4 mg/kg. Frequent maintenance doses may be needed.

Route	Onset	Peak	Duration
I.V.	2 to 2.5 min	3 to 5 min	35 to 70 min

Incompatibilities

Don't mix atracurium in same syringe or administer it through same I.V. needle as an alkaline solution, such as a barbiturate injection. Don't mix atracurium with lactated Ringer's injection.

Mechanism of Action

Inhibits nerve impulse transmission by competing with acetylcholine for cholinergic receptors on motor end plate.

Contraindications

Hypersensitivity to atracurium, its components, or benzyl alcohol

Interactions

DRUGS

aminoglycosides, enflurane, furosemide, halothane, isoflurane, lithium, magnesium salts, polymyxin antibiotics, procainamide, quinidine, thiazide diuretics: Possibly enhanced or prolonged effects of atracurium

opioid analgesics: Possibly additive histamine release and increased risk and severity of bradycardia and hypotension

Adverse Reactions

CNS: Seizures
CV: Bradycardia, hypertension, hypotension, tachycardia
MS: Inadequate or prolonged neuromuscular blockade
RESP: Apnea, bronchospasm, dyspnea, laryngospasm, wheezing
SKIN: Flushing, rash, urticaria
Other: Anaphylaxis, injection site reaction

Nursing Considerations

•Use atracurium cautiously in patients with hypotension, and monitor blood pressure closely.

•Monitor closely for adverse reactions, especially those associated with histamine release. Be aware that atracurium is more likely than other neuromuscular blockers to cause skin flushing.

•Anticipate using lower doses for patients with neuromuscular disease, severe electrolyte disorders, or carcinomatosis because of risk of enhanced neuromuscular blockade and difficulties with reversal.

•Keep atropine nearby to treat atracurium-induced bradycardia.

•For I.V. infusion, dilute atracurium with normal saline solution, D₅W, or dextrose 5% in normal saline solution. To prepare a solution that yields 200 mcg of atracurium per milliliter, add 2 ml of atracurium to 98 ml of diluent. To prepare a solution that yields 500 mcg per milliliter, add 5 ml of atracurium to 95 ml of diluent.

• Refrigerate solution or store at room temperature for up to 24 hours.

PATIENT TEACHING

• Explain atracurium's purpose and administration during anesthesia. Keep in mind that the patient can still hear.

atropine

AtroPen

atropine sulfate

Class and Category

Chemical class: Belladonna alkaloid
Therapeutic class: Anticholinergic, antimuscarinic
Pregnancy category: C

Indications and Dosages

➤ *To reduce respiratory tract secretions related to anesthesia*

TABLETS (ATROPINE SULFATE)

Adults. 0.4 to 0.6 mg preoperatively.
Children. 0.01 mg/kg up to total of 0.4 mg preoperatively and repeated every 4 to 6 hr, p.r.n.

I.V., I.M., OR SUBCUTANEOUS INJECTION

Adults. 0.4 to 0.6 mg preoperatively.
Children. 0.01 mg/kg up to total of 0.4 mg preoperatively and repeated every 4 to 6 hr, p.r.n.

➤ *To correct bradycardia*

I.V. INJECTION (ATROPINE SULFATE)

Adults. 0.4 to 1 mg. If no response to first dose, repeat once after 5 min.
Children. 0.01 to 0.02 mg/kg with a minimum dose of 0.1 mg and a maximum dose of 0.5 mg. If no response to first dose, repeat once after 5 min.

➤ *To treat cholinesterase inhibitor (such as neostigmine, pilocarpine, and methacholine) toxicity*

I.V. INJECTION (ATROPINE SULFATE)

Adults. 2 to 4 mg. Then 2 mg every 5 to 10 min until muscarinic signs (bradycardia, vasodilation, and pupil dilation) disappear or signs of atropine intoxication develop.

I.V. OR I.M. INJECTION (ATROPINE SULFATE)

Children. 1 mg. Then 0.5 to 1 mg every 5 to 10 min until muscarinic signs disappear or signs of atropine intoxication develop.

➤ *To treat mushroom (muscarine) toxicity*

I.V. OR I.M. INJECTION (ATROPINE SULFATE)

Adults. 1 to 2 mg every hr until respiratory signs and symptoms subside.

➤ *To treat pesticide (organophosphate) toxicity*

I.V. OR I.M. INJECTION (ATROPINE SULFATE)

Adults. 1 to 2 mg, repeated in 20 to 30 min as soon as cyanosis has cleared. Then dosage continued until definite improvement is maintained, possibly for 2 or more days.

➤ *To treat known or suspected exposure to chemical nerve agent or insecticide*

I.M. INJECTION (ATROPEN)

Adults and children weighing over 41 kg (90 lb) with two or more mild symptoms. 2 mg. If severe symptoms develop after injection, two or more 2-mg injections given in rapid succession 10 min after initial injection.

Adults and children weighing over 41 kg who are unconscious or have other severe symptoms. 2 mg given immediately 3 times in rapid succession.

Children weighing 18 to 41 kg (40 to 90 lb) with two or more mild symptoms. 1 mg. If severe symptoms develop after injection, two more 1-mg injections given in rapid succession 10 min after initial injection.

Children weighing 18 to 41 kg who are unconscious or exhibit any other severe symptoms. 1 mg given immediately 3 times in rapid succession.

Children weighing 7 to 18 kg (15 to 40 lb) with two or more mild symptoms. 0.5 mg. If severe symptoms develop after injection, two more 0.5-mg injections given in rapid succession 10 min after initial injection.

Children weighing 7 to 18 kg who are unconscious or exhibit any other severe symptoms. 0.5 mg given immediately 3 times in rapid succession.

Route	Onset	Peak	Duration
P.O.	30 to 120 min	1 to 2 hr	4 to 6 hr
I.V.	Immediate	2 to 4 min	Brief
I.M.	5 to 40 min	20 to 60 min	Brief Brief
SubQ	Unknown	Unknown	Brief

Mechanism of Action

Inhibits acetylcholine's muscarinic action at the neuroeffector junctions of smooth muscles, cardiac muscles, exocrine glands, SA and AV nodes, and the urinary bladder. In small doses, atropine inhibits salivary and bronchial secretions and diaphoresis. In moderate doses, it increases impulse conduction through the AV node and increases heart rate. In large doses, it decreases GI and urinary tract motility and gastric acid secretion.

Contraindications

Angle-closure glaucoma, asthma, GI obstructive disease (achalasia, pyloric obstruction, pyloroduodenal stenosis), hepatic disease, hypersensitivity to atropine or its components, ileus, intestinal atony, myasthenia gravis, myocardial ischemia, obstructive uropathy, renal disease, severe ulcerative colitis, tachycardia, toxic megacolon, unstable cardiovascular status in acute hemorrhage

Interactions

Drugs

adsorbent antidiarrheals, antacids: Decreased atropine absorption
amantadine, anticholinergics, antidyskinetics, glutethimide, meperidine, muscle relaxants, phenothiazines, tricyclic antidepressants and other drugs with anticholinergic properties, including antiarrhythmics (disopyramide, procainamide, quinidine), antihistamines, buclizine, meclizine: Increased atropine effects
antimyasthenics: Reduced intestinal motility
cyclopropane: Risk of ventricular arrhythmias
haloperidol: Decreased antipsychotic effect
ketoconazole: Decreased ketoconazole absorption
metoclopramide: Decreased effect on GI motility
opioid analgesics: Increased risk of ileus, severe constipation, and urine retention
potassium chloride, especially wax-matrix forms: Possibly GI ulcers
urinary alkalizers (calcium or magnesium antacids, carbonic anhydrase inhibitors, citrates, sodium bicarbonate): Delayed excretion and increased risk of adverse atropine effects

Adverse Reactions

CNS: Agitation, amnesia, anxiety, ataxia, Babinski's or Chaddock's reflex, behavioral changes, CNS stimulation (with high doses), coma, confusion, decreased concentration, decreased tendon reflexes, delirium, dizziness, drowsiness, fever, hallucinations, headache, hyperreflexia, insomnia, lethargy, mania, mental disorders, nervousness, paranoia, restlessness, seizures, somnolence, stupor, syncope, vertigo, weakness
CV: Arrhythmias, bradycardia (with low doses), cardiac dilation, chest pain, hypertension, hypotension, left ventricular failure, MI, palpitations, tachycardia (with high doses), weak or impalpable peripheral pulses
EENT: Acute angle-closure glaucoma, altered taste, blepharitis, blindness, blurred vision, conjunctivitis, cyclophoria, cycloplegia, decreased visual acuity or accommodation, dry eyes or conjunctiva, dry mucous membranes, dry mouth, eye irritation, eyelid crusting, heterophoria, increased intraocular pressure, keratoconjunctivitis, lacrimation, laryngitis, laryngospasm, mydriasis, nasal congestion, oral lesions, photophobia, pupils poorly reactive to light, strabismus, tongue chewing
GI: Abdominal distention, abdominal pain, bloating, constipation, decreased bowel sounds or food absorption, delayed gastric emptying, dysphagia, heartburn, ileus, nausea, vomiting
GU: Bladder distention, enuresis, impotence, urinary hesitancy, urinary urgency, urine retention
MS: Dysarthria, hypertonia, muscle twitching
RESP: Bradypnea, dyspnea, inspiratory stridor, pulmonary edema, respiratory failure, shallow breathing, subcostal recession, tachypnea
SKIN: Cold skin, cyanosis, decreased sweating, dermatitis, flushing, rash, urticaria
Other: Anaphylaxis, dehydration, injection site reaction, polydipsia, sensations of warmth

Nursing Considerations

•**WARNING** For patient prescribed AtroPen for suspected nerve gas or insecticide exposure, dosage is determined by severity of symptoms. Mild symptoms include blurred vision, miosis, excessive unexplained teary eyes or runny nose, increased salivation, chest tightness, difficulty breathing, tremors, muscle twitching, nausea, vomiting, unexplained wheezing or coughing, acute onset of stomach cramps, tachycardia, and bradycardia. Severe symptoms include confusion or other strange behavior, severe difficulty breathing, extreme secretions from airway or lungs, severe muscle twitching and general weakness, involuntary urination and defecation, seizures, and unconsciousness.

•Avoid using high-dose atropine sulfate therapy in patients with ulcerative colitis because of risk of toxic megacolon or in patients with hiatal hernia and reflux esophagitis because of risk of esophagitis
•Be aware that AtroPen has no absolute contraindications when used to treat life-threatening nerve gas or insecticide exposure.
•**WARNING** Assess for symptoms of toxic doses of atropine, such as excitement, agitation, drowsiness, and confusion, which are likely to affect elderly patients even with low doses. If these symptoms occur, take safety precautions to prevent patient injury.
•Assess bowel and bladder elimination. Notify prescriber if diarrhea, constipation, urinary hesitancy, or urine retention develop.

PATIENT TEACHING
•Instruct patient at increased risk for exposure to nerve gas or insecticides who is prescribed to carry AtroPen when and how to self-administer the drug.
•Instruct patient to take atropine sulfate 30 to 60 minutes before meals.
•Advise patient to notify prescriber if he has persistent or severe diarrhea, constipation, or difficulty urinating.

auranofin

Ridaura

Class and Category
Chemical class: Gold salt
Therapeutic class: Anti-inflammatory
Pregnancy category: C

Indications and Dosages
➤ *To treat active rheumatoid arthritis that's unresponsive to NSAIDs*
CAPSULES
Adults. *Initial:* 6 mg daily or 3 mg b.i.d. *Maintenance:* Up to 9 mg daily after 3 mo of

treatment, if needed.
Children age 6 and over. *Initial:* 0.1 mg/kg/day. *Maintenance:* 0.15 mg/kg daily. *Maximum:* 0.2 mg/kg daily.
DOSAGE ADJUSTMENT Drug discontinued if therapeutic response isn't adequate after 3 mo at 9 mg daily.

Route	Onset	Peak	Duration
P.O.	3 to 6 mo	1 to 2 hr	Up to 26 days

Mechanism of Action
Decreases rheumatoid factor and humoral antibody (immunoglobulin) levels. Although its exact anti-inflammatory action is unknown, the drug may suppress the increased phagocytic activity of macrophages and polymorphonuclear leukocytes that occurs with rheumatoid arthritis and thereby inhibit release of the destructive enzymes that cause joint inflammation.

Contraindications
Agranulocytosis, blood dyscrasias, bone marrow aplasia, colitis, eczema, exfoliative dermatitis, hepatic disease, history of gold or heavy metal toxicity, hypersensitivity to auranofin, marked hypertension, necrotizing enterocolitis, pulmonary fibrosis, recent radiation therapy, renal disease, severe debilitation, systemic lupus erythematosus, uncontrolled diabetes mellitus, uncontrolled heart failure, urticaria, youth (under age 6)

Interactions
DRUGS
phenytoin: Possibly increased phenytoin level

Adverse Reactions
CNS: Confusion, dizziness, EEG abnormalities, hallucinations, seizures
EENT: Gingivitis, glossitis, iritis or corneal ulcers from gold deposits in ocular tissue, metallic taste, stomatitis
GI: Abdominal cramps, anorexia, constipation, diarrhea, enterocolitis, flatulence, indigestion, melena, nausea, vomiting
GU: Hematuria, elevated BUN and serum creatinine levels, proteinuria, vaginitis
HEME: Agranulocytosis, aplastic anemia, eosinophilia, leukopenia, neutropenia, thrombocytopenia

RESP: Cough, dyspnea, fibrosis, interstitial pneumonitis
SKIN: Alopecia, dermatitis, exfoliative dermatitis, jaundice, photosensitivity, pruritus, rash, urticaria

Nursing Considerations

• Monitor blood and urine tests for signs of gold toxicity during auranofin therapy.
• **WARNING** Gold toxicity may occur during treatment or several months after its discontinuation. Toxicity, which usually occurs with a cumulative dose of 400 to 800 mg, may cause a decreased hemoglobin level, WBC count of less than $4,000/mm^3$, granulocyte count of less than $1,500/mm^3$, platelet count of less than $150,000/mm^3$, severe diarrhea, stomatitis, hematuria, proteinuria, rash, and pruritus.
• Monitor fluid intake and output for signs of imbalance. If urine output decreases, assess BUN and serum creatinine levels for signs of renal impairment.
• Notify prescriber about evidence of allergic reaction, such as dermatitis, rash, and pruritus. The drug may need to be discontinued.

PATIENT TEACHING
• Advise patient that diarrhea commonly occurs, but that he should notify prescriber immediately if diarrhea becomes severe.
• Instruct patient to take drug exactly as prescribed and to return monthly for blood tests.
• Inform patient that drug may take 3 to 4 months to reach a therapeutic level.
• Advise patient to report skin problems, fatigue, or stomatitis, which may signal blood dyscrasias.
• Tell patient to notify prescriber if he sees blood in his stool or urine, he bruises easily, or his gums bleed.

azathioprine

Imuran

azathioprine sodium

Imuran

Class and Category

Chemical class: Purine analogue
Therapeutic class: Antimetabolite, immunosuppressant
Pregnancy category: D

Indications and Dosages

➤ *To prevent kidney rejection after transplantation*
TABLETS, I.V. INFUSION
Adults and children. *Initial:* 3 to 5 mg/kg/day P.O. or I.V. as a single dose on, or 1 to 3 days before, day of transplantation, followed by 3 to 5 mg/kg daily I.V. after surgery until P.O. dose is tolerated. *Maintenance:* 1 to 3 mg/kg daily P.O.
DOSAGE ADJUSTMENT Dosage reduced for patients with oliguria (as from tubular necrosis) after transplantation because drug or metabolite excretion may be delayed.

➤ *To treat refractory rheumatoid arthritis*
TABLETS
Adults. *Initial:* 1 mg/kg (50 to 100 mg) daily as a single dose or b.i.d. for 6 to 8 wk. *Maintenance:* If initial therapy doesn't produce therapeutic effects or serious adverse effects, dosage increased every 4 wk by 0.5 mg/kg up to 2.5 mg/kg. Optimal dosage is 2 to 2.5 mg/kg/day.
DOSAGE ADJUSTMENT Dosage reduced to 25% to 33% of usual dosage for patients who also take allopurinol.

Route	Onset	Peak	Duration
P.O., I.V.	4 to 8 wk	Unknown	Several days

Mechanism of Action
May prevent proliferation and differentiation of activated B and T cells by interfering with purine (protein) and nucleic acid (DNA and RNA) synthesis.

Contraindications
Hypersensitivity to azathioprine

Interactions
DRUGS
ACE inhibitors and drugs that affect bone marrow and cell development in bone marrow, such as co-trimoxazole: Possibly severe leukopenia
allopurinol: Possibly increased therapeutic and adverse effects of azathioprine
anticoagulants: Possibly decreased anticoagulant action
cyclosporine: Possibly decreased plasma cyclosporine level
methotrexate: Possibly increased plasma level of azathioprine's metabolite, 6-mercap-

topurine, which can lead to cell death
nondepolarizing neuromuscular blockers:
Possibly decreased or reversed action of neuromuscular blocker

Adverse Reactions
CNS: Fever, malaise
GI: Abdominal pain, diarrhea, hepatoxicity (elevated liver function test results), nausea, pancreatitis, steatorrhea, vomiting
HEME: Leukopenia, macrocytic anemia, pancytopenia, thrombocytopenia
MS: Arthralgia, myalgia
SKIN: Alopecia, rash
RESP: Reversible interstitial pneumonitis
Other: Infection, lymphomas and other neoplasms, negative nitrogen balance

Nursing Considerations
•Before I.V. administration, add 20 ml of sterile water for injection to azathioprine vial and swirl it until clear solution forms. The resulting drug concentration is 100 mg and can be diluted further as prescribed. Calculate infusion rate based on final volume to be infused. Then administer over 30 to 60 minutes or as prescribed (from 5 minutes to 8 hours).
•Obtain results of baseline laboratory tests, including WBC, RBC, and platelet counts. Then expect to monitor results once a week during first month of therapy, twice a month during second and third months of therapy, and once a month or more frequently thereafter.
•Be aware that hematologic reactions typically are dose related and may occur late in therapy, especially in patients with transplant rejection.
•**WARNING** If WBC count decreases rapidly or remains significantly and consistently low, expect to reduce dosage or discontinue use of azathioprine.
•Periodically monitor liver function test results to detect early signs of hepatotoxicity.
•If patient develops thrombocytopenia, take bleeding precautions, such as avoiding I.M. injections and venipunctures, applying ice to areas of trauma, and checking I.V. infusion sites every 2 hours for bleeding.
•If patient also receives an oral anticoagulant, monitor his PT.
•Know that azathioprine therapy increases risk of viral, fungal, bacterial, and protozoal infections. Monitor for signs of infection,

such as fever, chills, sore throat, and mouth sores. Expect to administer aggressive antibiotic, antiviral, or other drug therapy and reduce azathioprine dosage.
•Minimize the risk of infection. If patient has severe leukopenia, take neutropenic precautions, such as placing him in a private room and limiting visitors.
•Be aware that rheumatoid arthritis requires at least 12 weeks of azathioprine therapy. During this time, continue other pain-relief measures, such as rest, physical therapy, and other drugs, such as salicylates and corticosteroids.
•If oral azathioprine causes GI upset, administer it in divided doses or with meals.
•Plan to use lowest possible maintenance dosage for rheumatoid arthritis. Expect to reduce dosage gradually in 0.5-mg/kg (about 25-mg) increments at 4-week intervals.
•Know that drug can be stopped abruptly, but its effects may persist several days.

PATIENT TEACHING
•Advise patient to take oral drug with food or meals to minimize GI upset.
•**WARNING** Teach patient to recognize and report signs of infection, such as sore throat and fever.
•Teach patient how to reduce the risk of bleeding and falling.

azelastine hydrochloride

Astelin

Class and Category
Chemical class: Phthalazinone derivative
Therapeutic class: Antihistamine, H$_1$-receptor antagonist
Pregnancy category: C

Indications and Dosages
➤ *To treat symptoms of seasonal rhinitis (rhinorrhea, sneezing, and nasal itching)*
NASAL SPRAY
Adults and children age 12 and over.
2 sprays in each nostril b.i.d.

Route	Onset	Peak	Duration
Nasal	In 3 hr	Unknown	12 hr

Contraindications
Hypersensitivity to azelastine or its components

Mechanism of Action

Binds nonselectively to central and peripheral H$_1$ receptors, preventing histamine from reaching its site of action, which reduces or prevents most of histamine's physiologic effects. By blocking histamine at its site of action, azelastine inhibits respiratory, vascular, and GI smooth-muscle contraction; decreases capillary permeability, which reduces wheals, flares, and itching; and decreases salivary and lacrimal gland secretions.

Interactions

DRUGS
cimetidine, ketoconazole: Possibly increased blood azelastine level
CNS depressants: Possibly increased sedative effects and reduced mental alertness
ACTIVITIES
alcohol use: Possibly increased sedative effects and reduced mental alertness

Adverse Reactions

CNS: Dizziness, fatigue, headache, somnolence
CV: Atrial fibrillation, palpitations
EENT: Bitter taste, dry mouth, epistaxis, nasal burning, paroxysmal sneezing, pharyngitis, rhinitis
GI: Nausea
Other: Weight gain

Nursing Considerations

•Assess for changes in alertness and take safety precautions, if needed.
PATIENT TEACHING
•Teach patient how to use azelastine nasal spray properly to achieve maximum therapeutic effects.
•Before patient's first use of nasal spray, instruct him to prime pump by placing his thumb on base and his index and middle fingers on shoulder area of bottle and then pressing thumb firmly and quickly against bottle four times or until fine mist appears.
•If patient hasn't used spray in more than 3 days, instruct him to reprime pump with two sprays or until fine mist appears.
•Advise patient to clear nostrils gently, if needed, before using spray.
•Teach patient to inhale deeply after each spray and then exhale through his mouth and tilt his head back so drug can spread over nasopharynx.
•Advise patient to store bottle upright and tightly closed.
•**WARNING** Emphasize that patient must consult prescriber before taking any OTC drug, such as cough syrup or a cold remedy, because of the risk of extreme CNS depression.
•Inform patient that decreased alertness may occur. Advise him to avoid hazardous activities or those that require alertness, such as driving or operating machinery, until drug's effects are known.

azithromycin

Zithromax, Zmax

Class and Category

Chemical class: Azalide (subclass of macrolide)
Therapeutic class: Antibiotic
Pregnancy category: B

Indications and Dosages

➤ *To treat mild community-acquired pneumonia, otitis media, pharyngitis, tonsillitis, and uncomplicated skin and soft-tissue infections*
CAPSULES, ORAL SUSPENSION, TABLETS
Adults. 500 mg as a single dose on day 1, followed by 250 mg daily on days 2 through 5.
Children age 6 months or over with acute otitis media or community-acquired pneumonia. 10 mg/kg as a single dose (not to exceed 500 mg daily) on day 1, followed by 5 mg/kg (not to exceed 250 mg daily) daily on days 2 through 5. Or, for acute otitis media, 30 mg/kg of oral suspension as a single dose or 10 mg/kg daily for 3 days.
Children age 12 or over with pharyngitis or tonsillitis. 12 mg/kg (not to exceed 500 mg daily) as a single dose daily for 5 days.

➤ *To treat mild to moderate acute bacterial exacerbations of COPD*
CAPSULES, ORAL SUSPENSION, TABLETS
Adults. 500 mg daily for 3 days. Alternatively, 500 mg as single dose on day 1, followed by 250 mg daily on days 2 through 5.

➤ *To treat community-acquired pneumonia*
CAPSULES, ORAL SUSPENSION, TABLETS, I.V. INFUSION
Adults and adolescents age 16 or over.

500 mg I.V. as a single dose daily for at least 2 days, followed by 500 mg P.O. as a single dose daily until patient completes 7 to 10 days of therapy.

➤ *To treat community-acquired pneumonia caused by* Chlamydophila pneumoniae, Haemophilus influenzae, Mycoplasma pneumoniae, *or* Streptococcus pneumoniae

E.R. ORAL SOLUTION (ZMAX)
Adults. 2 g as a single dose on an empty stomach.

➤ *To treat chancroid caused by* Haemophilus ducreyi; *gonococcal pharyngitis; urethritis, cervicitis, or other infections caused by* Chlamydia trachomatis

CAPSULES, ORAL SUSPENSION, TABLETS
Adults. 1 g as a one-time dose.
Children age 8 or over and children under age 8 weighing 45 kg (99 lb) or more (with infections caused by *C. trachomatis*). 1 g as a one-time dose.

➤ *To treat urethritis or cervicitis caused by* Neisseria gonorrhoeae

CAPSULES, ORAL SUSPENSION, TABLETS
Adults. 2 g as a one-time dose.

➤ *To prevent* Mycobacterium avium *complex in patients with advanced HIV infection*

CAPSULES, ORAL SUSPENSION, TABLETS, I.V. INFUSION
Adults. 1.2 g once weekly, as indicated.

➤ *To treat pelvic inflammatory disease*

CAPSULES, ORAL SUSPENSION, TABLETS, I.V. INFUSION
Adults. 500 mg I.V. as a single dose daily for 1 to 2 days, followed by 250 mg P.O. as a single dose daily until patient completes 7 days of therapy.

➤ *To treat acute bacterial sinusitis*

ORAL SUSPENSION, TABLETS
Adults. 500 mg daily for 3 days.
Children. 10 mg/kg daily for 3 days.

➤ *To treat acute bacterial sinusitis caused by* Haemophilus influenzae, Moraxella catarrhalis, *or* S. pneumoniae

E.R. ORAL SOLUTION (ZMAX)
Adults. 2 g as a single dose on an empty stomach.

Incompatibilities

Don't add I.V. substances, additives, or drugs to azithromycin I.V. solution, and don't infuse through the same I.V. line.

Route	Onset	Peak	Duration
P.O.	Varies	Unknown	Unknown

Mechanism of Action

Binds to a ribosomal subunit of susceptible bacteria, blocking peptide translocation and inhibiting RNA-dependent protein synthesis. Drug concentrates in phagocytes, macrophages, and fibroblasts, which release it slowly and may help move it to infection sites.

Contraindications

Hypersensitivity to azithromycin, erythromycin, ketolide antibiotics, or other macrolide antibiotics

Interactions

DRUGS
antacids that contain aluminum or magnesium: Possibly decreased peak blood azithromycin level, but extent of absorption is unchanged
carbamazepine, cyclosporine, phenytoin, terfenadine (drugs metabolized by P-450 cytochrome system): Possibly increased blood levels of these drugs
digoxin: Possibly increased blood digoxin level
dihydroergotamine, ergotamine: Possibly severe peripheral vasospasm and abnormal sensations (acute ergot toxicity)
HMG-CoA reductase inhibitors: Increased risk of severe myopathy or rhabdomyolysis
pimozide: Possibly sudden death
theophylline: Possibly increased blood theophylline level
triazolam: Possibly decreased excretion and increased therapeutic effects of triazolam
warfarin: Possibly increased anticoagulation
FOODS
food: Dramatically increased absorption rate of azithromycin

Adverse Reactions

CNS: Aggressiveness, agitation, anxiety, asthenia, dizziness, fatigue, headache, hyperactivity, malaise, nervousness, paresthesia, seizures, somnolence, syncope, vertigo
CV: Chest pain, edema, elevated serum CK level, hypotension, palpitations, prolonged QT interval, torsades de pointes, ventricular tachycardia
EENT: Hearing loss, mucocutaneous candidi-

asis, perversion or loss of taste or smell, tinnitus

ENDO: Hyperglycemia

GI: Abdominal pain, anorexia, cholestatic jaundice, constipation, diarrhea, dyspepsia, elevated liver function test results, flatulence, hepatic necrosis or failure, hepatitis, nausea, pancreatitis, pseudomembranous colitis, vomiting

GU: Acute renal failure, elevated BUN and serum creatinine levels, nephritis, vaginal candidiasis

HEME: Leukopenia, neutropenia, thrombocytopenia

MS: Arthralgia

SKIN: Erythema multiforme, photosensitivity, pruritus, rash, Stevens-Johnson syndrome, toxic epidermal necrolysis, urticaria

Other: Allergic reaction, anaphylaxis, angioedema, elevated serum phosphorus level, hyperkalemia, infusion site reaction (such as pain and redness), superinfection

Nursing Considerations
•Obtain culture and sensitivity test results, if possible, before starting therapy.
•Use azithromycin cautiously in patients with hepatic dysfunction (because drug is metabolized in the liver) or renal dysfunction (because drug's effects are unknown in this group).
•Administer azithromycin capsules 1 hour before or 2 to 3 hours after food. Give tablets or suspension without regard to food.
•**WARNING** Don't give azithromycin by I.V. bolus or I.M. injection because it may cause erythema, pain, swelling, tenderness, or other reaction at the site. Infuse it over 60 minutes or longer, as prescribed (typically 1 mg/ml over 3 hours or 2 mg/ml over 1 hour.)
•If hepatic function is impaired, monitor liver function studies because azithromycin is eliminated mainly by the liver.
•Assess patient for bacterial or fungal superinfection, which may occur with prolonged or repeated therapy. If it occurs, expect to give another antibiotic or antifungal.
•Monitor bowel elimination; if needed, obtain stool culture to rule out pseudomembranous colitis. If it occurs, expect to stop azithromycin and give fluid, electrolytes, and antibiotics effective with *Clostridium difficile*.

PATIENT TEACHING
•Tell patient to take azithromycin capsules 1 hour before or 2 to 3 hours after food. Instruct patient to take tablets or suspension without regard to food.
•**WARNING** Urge patient to ask prescriber before taking OTC drugs, including antacids. If they're prescribed, tell patient to take drug 1 hour before or 2 to 3 hours after taking antacids.
•Tell patient to immediately report signs and symptoms of allergic reaction (such as rash, itching, hives, chest tightness, and trouble breathing).
•Warn patient that abdominal pain and loose, watery stools may occur. If diarrhea persists or becomes severe, urge him to contact prescriber and replace fluids.
•Because azithromycin may destroy normal flora, teach patient to watch for and immediately report signs of superinfection, such as white patches in the mouth.

aztreonam

Azactam

Class and Category
Chemical class: Monobactam
Therapeutic class: Antibiotic
Pregnancy category: B

Indications and Dosages
➤ *To treat infections of the urinary tract, lower respiratory tract, skin, soft tissue, female reproductive tract; intra-abdominal infections; septicemia; and surgical abscesses caused by susceptible strains of gram-negative bacteria*

I.V. INFUSION, I.V. OR I.M. INJECTION

Adults. 0.5 to 2 g every 8 to 12 hr up to a maximum of 8 g daily. For life-threatening systemic infection, 2 g every 6 to 8 hr up to a maximum of 8 g daily.

Children ages 9 months to 16 years. 30 mg/kg every 6 to 8 hr up to 120 mg/kg daily; 50 mg/kg every 4 to 6 hr (for *Pseudomonas aeruginosa*).

DOSAGE ADJUSTMENT If creatinine clearance is 10 to 30 ml/min/1.73 m^2, initial dose is 1 to 2 g; then 50% of usual dose at usual interval. If creatinine clearance less than 10 ml/ min/1.73 m^2, initial dose is 500 mg to 2 g; then 25% of the usual dose every 6, 8, or 12 hr.

Route	Onset	Peak	Duration
I.V. infusion	Immediate	Immediate	Unknown
I.V. injection	Immediate	Immediate	Unknown
I.M.	Variable	60 min	Unknown

Mechanism of Action

Inhibits bacterial cell wall synthesis in susceptible aerobic gram-negative bacteria. These bacteria assemble rigid, cross-linked cell walls in several steps. Aztreonam affects the final cross-linking step by inactivating penicillin-binding protein 3 (the enzyme that links cell wall strands), which causes cell lysis and death.

Incompatibilities

Don't mix aztreonam in same I.V. solution as cephradine, metronidazole, or nafcillin sodium. Don't mix it in same I.M. injection solution as local anesthetic.

Contraindications

Hypersensitivity to aztreonam or its components

Interactions

DRUGS
aminoglycosides (prolonged or high-dose therapy): Increased risk of nephrotoxicity and ototoxicity
cefoxitin, imipenem: Possibly antagonized action of aztreonam
furosemide, probenecid: Possibly increased blood aztreonam level

Adverse Reactions

CNS: Confusion, dizziness, fever, headache, insomnia, malaise, paresthesia, seizures, vertigo
CV: Chest pain, hypotension, transient ECG changes
EENT: Altered taste, diplopia, halitosis, mouth ulcers, mucocutaneous candidiasis, nasal congestion, sneezing, tinnitus, tongue numbness
GI: Abdominal cramps, diarrhea, elevated liver function test results, GI bleeding, hepatitis, nausea, pseudomembranous colitis, vomiting
GU: Breast tenderness, elevated serum creatinine level, vaginal candidiasis
HEME: Anemia, eosinophilia, leukocytosis, neutropenia, pancytopenia, positive Coombs' test, prolonged PT and APTT, thrombocytopenia, thrombocytosis
MS: Myalgia
RESP: Bronchospasm, dyspnea, wheezing
SKIN: Diaphoresis, erythema multiforme, exfoliative dermatitis, flushing, jaundice, petechiae, pruritus, purpura, rash, toxic epidermal necrolysis, urticaria
Other: Allergic reaction; injection site pain, phlebitis, swelling, or thrombophlebitis

Nursing Considerations

•Obtain culture and sensitivity test results, if possible, before initiating therapy. If patient is acutely ill, expect to begin therapy before results are available.
•Keep in mind that other antimicrobials may be used with aztreonam in seriously ill patients at risk for gram-positive infection.
•Expect to use I.V. route for patients who need single doses over 1 g and those with life-threatening systemic infections, such as septicemia or peritonitis.
•To reconstitute aztreonam for I.V. bolus injection, use sterile water for injection.
•Immediately after adding diluent to vial, shake it vigorously to mix. After obtaining correct dose, discard unused solution.
•Be aware that reconstituted solution may turn light pink on standing at room temperature. This doesn't affect drug potency.
•Administer I.V. bolus injection directly into I.V. tubing over 3 to 5 minutes.
•**WARNING** When preparing aztreonam for I.V. infusion, use at least 50 ml of appropriate infusion solution per gram of aztreonam. Further dilute drug in I.V. solution, such as normal saline solution, D_5W, dextrose 5% in normal saline solution, lactated Ringer's solution, or Ringer's solution.
•Know that I.V. infusion may be administered over 20 to 60 minutes.
•Flush I.V. tubing with solution, such as normal saline solution, before and after administering I.V. infusion to reduce risk of incompatibilities.
•If prescribed, mix aztreonam in same I.V. solution with other antibiotics (such as ampicillin sodium, cefazolin sodium, clindamycin phosphate, gentamicin sulfate, or

tobramycin sulfate), or mix it with cloxacillin sodium and vancomycin hydrochloride in peritoneal dialysis solution.

•Prepare solution for I.M. injection using sterile or bacteriostatic water or sodium chloride for injection. Administer injection deep into large muscle, such as in dorsogluteal or ventrogluteal area.

•Assess for signs of bacterial or fungal superinfection, which may occur with prolonged or repeated therapy. If superinfection occurs, treat it as prescribed.

•Monitor bowel elimination; if needed, obtain stool culture to rule out pseudomembranous colitis. If it occurs, expect to discontinue aztreonam and administer fluid, electrolytes, and antibiotics that are effective against *Clostridium difficile*.

•Evaluate patient's renal and liver function test results, as ordered, if the patient has renal or hepatic impairment.

•Monitor renal function if patient is receiving an aminoglycoside because of the increased risk of nephrotoxicity.

PATIENT TEACHING

•Stress the need to take the full course of aztreonam exactly as prescribed, even if the patient feels better before finishing it.

•Teach patient to recognize and immediately report signs and symptoms of allergic reactions, such as chest tightness, difficulty breathing, hives, itching, and rash.

•Warn patient that abdominal pain and loose, watery stools may occur 2 months or more after aztreonam therapy stops. If diarrhea persists or becomes severe, urge him to contact prescriber and replace fluids.

•Because aztreonam may destroy normal flora, teach patient to watch for and immediately report signs of superinfection, such as white patches in mouth.

B

bacampicillin hydrochloride

Penglobe (CAN), Spectrobid

Class and Category
Chemical class: Aminopenicillin
Therapeutic class: Antibiotic
Pregnancy category: B

Indications and Dosages
➤ *To treat upper respiratory tract infections (including otitis media) caused by* streptococci, pneumococci, non–penicillinase-producing staphylococci, *and* Haemophilus influenzae; *UTI caused by* Escherichia coli, Proteus mirabilis, *and* Streptococcus faecalis; *skin and soft-tissue infections caused by streptococci and susceptible staphylococci*

TABLETS
Adults. 400 mg every 12 hr; 800 mg every 12 hr for severe infections and those caused by less susceptible organisms.
Children weighing 25 kg (55 lb) or more. 25 mg/kg daily in divided doses every 12 hr; 50 mg/kg daily in divided doses every 12 hr for severe infections and those caused by less susceptible organisms.

➤ *To treat lower respiratory tract infections caused by* streptococci, pneumococci, non–penicillinase-producing staphylococci, *and* H. influenzae

TABLETS
Adults. 800 mg every 12 hr.
Children weighing 25 kg or more. 50 mg/kg/day in divided doses every 12 hr.

➤ *To treat uncomplicated gonorrhea caused by* Neisseria gonorrhoeae

TABLETS
Adults. 1.6 g plus 1 g of probenecid as a single dose.

Route	Onset	Peak	Duration
P.O.	Variable	Unknown	12 hr

Contraindications
Cholestatic jaundice and hepatic dysfunction associated with amoxicillin and clavulanate potassium; hypersensitivity to penicillins, cephalosporins, imipenem and cilastatin, or beta-lactamase inhibitors, such as piperacillin and tazobactam

Mechanism of Action
Inhibits bacterial cell wall synthesis in susceptible bacteria. These bacteria assemble rigid, cross-linked cell walls in several steps. Bacampicillin, which undergoes hydrolysis to ampicillin, affects final stage of cross-linking by binding with and inactivating penicillin-binding protein (enzyme responsible for linking cell wall strands). This action inhibits bacterial cell wall synthesis and causes cell lysis and death.

Interactions
DRUGS
allopurinol: Increased risk of rash from bacampicillin use
beta-adrenergic blockers: Increased risk of anaphylaxis
disulfiram: Possibly disulfiram reaction when administered together
oral contraceptives: Possibly reduced effectiveness of oral contraceptives, contraceptive failure, and breakthrough bleeding
tetracyclines: Possibly impaired bactericidal effects of bacampicillin

Adverse Reactions
CNS: Anxiety, confusion, depression, fatigue, fever, hallucinations, lethargy, malaise, neuromuscular irritability, seizures, stroke, syncope
CV: Hypotension, palpitations, periarteritis nodosa, pulmonary hypertension, tachycardia, vascular collapse
EENT: Altered taste, black "hairy" tongue, blurred vision, glossitis, laryngospasm, mouth soreness, mucocutaneous candidiasis, stomatitis, taste disorders
GI: Abdominal cramps or pain, anorexia, diarrhea, enterocolitis, epigastric distress, elevated liver function test results, gastritis, nausea, pseudomembranous colitis, vomiting
GU: Elevated BUN and serum creatinine levels, hematuria, impotence, interstitial nephritis, neurogenic bladder, priapism, renal failure, vaginal candidiasis
HEME: Agranulocytosis, anemia, bone marrow depression, decreased hemoglobin level

and hematocrit, eosinophilia, leukopenia, neutropenia, prolonged PT, thrombocytopenia, thrombocytopenic purpura
MS: Arthralgia, arthritis exacerbation
RESP: Bronchospasm
SKIN: Exfoliative dermatitis, rash, urticaria
Other: Allergic reaction, lymphadenopathy, serum sickness

Nursing Considerations

•Obtain culture and sensitivity test results, if possible, before initiating therapy. Be prepared to start bacampicillin therapy before results are available.
•Expect to continue treatment for at least 48 hours after symptoms resolve or culture detects no signs of infection.
•**WARNING** Expect to administer bacampicillin for 10 days to treat infection caused by group A beta-hemolytic streptococci to prevent development of acute rheumatic fever or acute glomerulonephritis.
•Assess for bacterial or fungal superinfection, which may occur with prolonged or repeated therapy. If it occurs, expect to administer another antibiotic or antifungal drug.
•Monitor bowel elimination; if needed, obtain stool culture to rule out pseudomembranous colitis. If this adverse reaction occurs, expect to discontinue bacampicillin and administer fluid, electrolytes, and antibiotics that are effective against *Clostridium difficile.*

PATIENT TEACHING

•Teach patient to recognize and immediately report signs of allergic reaction, including rash, itching, hives, chest tightness, and difficulty breathing.
•Warn patient that abdominal pain and loose, watery stools may occur. If diarrhea persists or becomes severe, urge him to contact prescriber and drink plenty of fluids.
•Because bacampicillin may destroy normal flora, teach patient to watch for and immediately report signs of superinfection, such as white patches in mouth and vaginal itching and discharge.

bacitracin

Baci-IM

Class and Category

Chemical class: Bacillus subtilis derivative (polypeptide)

Therapeutic class: Antibiotic
Pregnancy category: C

Indications and Dosages

➤ *To treat pneumonia and empyema caused by susceptible staphylococci*
I.M. INJECTION
Infants weighing more than 2.5 kg (5.5 lb). 1,000 units/kg daily in 2 or 3 divided doses.
Infants weighing less than 2.5 kg. 900 units/kg daily in 2 or 3 divided doses.

Route	Onset	Peak	Duration
I.M.	Rapid	Unknown	About 6 hr

Mechanism of Action

Interferes with bacterial cell wall synthesis by binding with isoprenyl pyrophosphate (a lipid-carrying molecule that transports substances out of bacterial cells to help build new cell walls), forming an unusable complex in bacterial cells. This weakens cell walls and causes lysis and death. Bacitracin is considered a bacteriostatic and bactericidal drug.

Incompatibilities

Don't dilute bacitracin with a solution that contains parabens.

Contraindications

Hypersensitivity or toxic reaction to bacitracin

Interactions

DRUGS
aminoglycosides: Increased risk of respiratory paralysis and renal dysfunction
nondepolarizing neuromuscular blockers: Possibly increased neuromuscular blockade

Adverse Reactions

GI: Nausea, vomiting
GU: Albuminuria, azotemia, cylindrical mucus casts in urine, nephrotoxicity
SKIN: Rash
Other: Injection site pain, superinfection

Nursing Considerations

•Obtain culture and sensitivity test results before therapy begins, if possible. However, be prepared to start bacitracin therapy before results are available.

•**WARNING** Use parenteral bacitracin for I.M. injection only.

•For an I.M. solution of 5,000 units/ml, reconstitute 50,000 units of bacitracin powder with 9.8 ml of sodium chloride for injection that contains 2% procaine hydrochloride.

•Administer I.M. injection into upper outer quadrant of buttocks, alternating between right and left sides. To prevent pain at injection site, avoid giving multiple injections in same site.

•During therapy, compare daily results of renal function tests with baseline results, as appropriate.

•Assess urine output often (hourly, if needed), and replace fluids orally and parenterally to maintain adequate renal function.

•**WARNING** Because of increased risk of nephrotoxicity, avoid concurrent use of other nephrotoxic drugs, such as streptomycin, kanamycin, polymyxin B, and neomycin.

•Assess infant for signs of superinfection, especially white patches in mouth and perineal area. If superinfection develops, plan to treat it with appropriate antibiotics.

PATIENT TEACHING

•Advise parents that daily blood tests are needed to assess infant's renal function.

•Encourage parents to provide oral fluids to promote renal function. Teach them how to record infant's fluid intake.

•Instruct parents to report signs or symptoms of superinfection, such as white patches in mouth or perineal area and bright red diaper rash.

baclofen

Apo-Baclofen (CAN), Lioresal, Lioresal Intrathecal, Novo-Baclofen (CAN)

Class and Category

Chemical class: Gamma-aminobutyric acid (GABA) chlorophenyl derivative
Therapeutic class: Skeletal muscle relaxant, spasmolytic
Pregnancy category: C

Indications and Dosages

➤ *To relieve symptoms of spasticity caused by multiple sclerosis (particularly flexor spasms and pain, clonus, and muscle rigidity) and spasticity from spinal cord injury or disease and brain injury*

TABLETS

Adults and children age 12 and over. 5 mg t.i.d. for 3 days, then 10 mg t.i.d. for 3 days, then 15 mg t.i.d. for 3 days, then 20 mg t.i.d. for 3 days, then increased if needed up to 80 mg daily. Usual dosage ranges from 40 to 80 mg daily.

➤ *To relieve severe symptoms of spasticity of spinal cord origin when symptoms don't respond to oral drug or when oral drug causes severe adverse CNS effects*

INTRATHECAL BOLUS, INTRATHECAL INFUSION

Adults. *For screening before implantable pump insertion:* 50 mcg in 1 ml of sterile preservative-free sodium chloride for injection as bolus injection into intrathecal space over 1 min or more. After 4 to 8 hr, if symptoms don't improve as much as desired, second bolus of 75 mcg in 1.5 ml of sterile preservative-free sodium chloride for injection injected after 24 hr followed by third bolus of 100-mcg/2 ml dilution injected after another 24 hr, if needed.

After implantable pump insertion: Effective screening dose doubled and infused over 24 hr. Or effective screening dose (if it provided desired effects for more than 12 hr) infused over 24 hr.

For spasticity of spinal cord origin after implantable pump insertion: After first 24 hr, daily dose increased by 10% to 30% once every 24 hr until desired effects achieved.

For spasticity of cerebral origin after implantable pump insertion: Daily dose increased by 5% to 15% once every 24 hr until desired effects achieved.

For long-term maintenance therapy in spasticity of spinal cord origin: 12 to 2,003 mcg/day (usual dose 300 to 800 mcg daily). Lowest possible therapeutic dose should be used. If adverse effects occur, daily dose may be decreased by 10% to 20%. During periodic pump refills, daily dose may be increased by 10% up to 40% to control symptoms adequately.

For long-term maintenance therapy in spasticity of cerebral origin: 90 to 703 mcg daily (usual) but ranging from 22 to 1,400 mcg/day. If adverse effects occur, daily dose may be decreased by 10% to 20%. During periodic pump refills, daily dose may be in-

B

creased by 5% to 20% to control symptoms adequately.

Children. *For screening before implantable pump insertion:* 1 ml of a 50-mcg/ml dilution or 1 ml of a 25-mcg/ml dilution (if child is very young) as bolus injection into intrathecal space over 1 min or more. After 4 to 8 hr, if symptoms don't improve as desired, second bolus of 75 mcg in 1.5 ml of sterile preservative-free sodium chloride for injection injected after 24 hr followed by third bolus of 100-mcg/2 ml dilution injected after another 24 hr, if needed.

After implantable pump insertion: Daily dose increased by 5% to 15% once every 24 hr until the desired effect is achieved.

For maintenance therapy: In children over age 12: 90 to 703 mcg daily (usual) but ranging from 22 to 1,400 mcg daily. In children under age 12: 274 mcg daily (average) but ranging from 24 to 1,199 mcg daily.

DOSAGE ADJUSTMENT Dosage reduced for patients with renal impairment because drug is excreted primarily unchanged by kidneys.

Route	Onset	Peak	Duration
P.O.	Hours to weeks	Unknown	Unknown
Intrathecal bolus injection	30 to 60 min	About 4 hr	4 to 8 hr
Intrathecal infusion	6 to 8 hr	24 to 48 hr	Unknown

Mechanism of Action

May inhibit transmission of monosynaptic and polysynaptic impulses, similar to effects of gamma-aminobutyric acid (GABA). Baclofen may work in the spinal cord at the afferent spinal end of upper motor neurons, where it hyperpolarizes nerve fibers and inhibits impulse transmission. This reduces excess muscle activity caused by muscle hypertonia, spasms, and spasticity.

Contraindications

Hypersensitivity to baclofen; treatment of skeletal muscle spasm resulting from rheumatic disorders, cerebral palsy, Parkinson's disease, or stroke (oral form only)

Interactions

DRUGS

CNS depressants: Possibly increased CNS depression

epidural morphine: Possibly hypotension and dyspnea

ACTIVITIES

alcohol use: Possibly increased CNS depression

Adverse Reactions

CNS: Abnormal gait, anxiety, ataxia, chills, coma, confusion, depression, dizziness, drowsiness, dystonia, emotional lability, euphoria, excitement, fatigue, fever, hallucinations, headache, hypertonia, hypothermia, hypotonia, impaired concentration, insomnia, lack of coordination, lethargy, memory loss, paresthesia, personality disorder, seizures, somnolence, stroke, syncope, tremor, weakness

CV: Bradycardia, chest pain, chest tightness, deep vein thrombosis, hypertension, orthostatic hypotension, palpitations, peripheral edema

EENT: Amblyopia, blurred vision, diplopia, dry mouth, miosis, mydriasis, nasal congestion, nystagmus, photophobia, ptosis, rhinitis, slurred speech, strabismus, taste loss, tinnitus

ENDO: Hyperglycemia

GI: Abdominal pain, anorexia, constipation, dysphagia, elevated liver function test results, flatulence, ileus, indigestion, nausea, vomiting

GU: Albuminuria, bladder spasms, dysuria, enuresis, hematuria, impotence, renal failure, sexual dysfunction, urinary frequency, urinary incontinence, urine retention

HEME: Anemia

MS: Muscle twitching

RESP: Aspiration pneumonia, pulmonary embolism, respiratory depression

SKIN: Alopecia, diaphoresis, facial edema, flushing, pruritus, rash, urticaria, wound dehiscence

Other: Dehydration, infection at pump implantation site, weight loss

Nursing Considerations

•Expect to start baclofen therapy at a low dose and gradually increase it until desired effects are achieved.

•WARNING Before screening dose is administered, expect prescriber to ensure that pa-

tient is free of infection to prevent systemic infection from interfering with patient's response. Before implantable pump insertion, also expect prescriber to ensure that patient is free of infection to reduce risk of complications and interference with determining most appropriate dose.
• Use baclofen cautiously in patients who have a history of autonomic dysreflexia. Nociceptor stimulation may precipitate autonomic dysreflexia. Be aware that abrupt withdrawal of intrathecal infusion may produce symptoms similar to autonomic dysreflexia, high fever, life-threatening complications such as multiple organ-system failure, and death.
• **WARNING** Never give the intrathecal form of baclofen by I.V., I.M., or subcutaneous routes.
• Assess patient for signs of effectiveness, such as relief of spasms, pain, and muscle rigidity.
• Because CNS depression can occur, take safety precautions to help prevent injury. Also take precautions for patients who use spasticity to maintain locomotion or upright posture and balance. Relief of spasticity may increase risk of falls and injury.
• **WARNING** Because continuous intrathecal infusion increases risk of life-threatening CNS depression, keep emergency equipment nearby.
• Expect baclofen to be discontinued slowly; hallucinations and seizures may occur with abrupt withdrawal.

PATIENT TEACHING
• Teach patient how to care for and operate programmable implanted pump. Have her demonstrate all procedures.
• Advise patient not to stop taking baclofen abruptly. Stress the importance of keeping follow-up appointments for intrathecal infusion.
• Instruct patient to avoid driving and other activities that require mental alertness, coordination, or physical dexterity until baclofen's effects are known.
• Urge patient to contact prescriber before taking OTC drugs, such as cough syrups and cold remedies, which may increase risk of sedation.
• Advise patient to notify prescriber if spasticity increases or baclofen is no longer effective.

balsalazide disodium
Colazal

Class and Category
Chemical class: Prodrug of 5-aminosalicylic acid (5-ASA)
Therapeutic class: Anti-inflammatory
Pregnancy category: B

Indications and Dosages
➤ *To treat mildly to moderately active ulcerative colitis*
CAPSULES
Adults. 2.25 g t.i.d. for 8 wk. *Maximum:* 6.75 g daily for 12 wk.
Children ages 5 to 17. 750 mg or 2.25 g t.i.d. for up to 8 wk.

Mechanism of Action
After it has been metabolized to 5-ASA, balsalazide may reduce inflammation by inhibiting the enzyme cyclooxygenase and decreasing the production of arachidonic acid metabolites, which may be increased in patients with inflammatory bowel disease. Cyclooxygenase is needed to form prostaglandin from arachidonic acid. Prostaglandin mediates inflammatory activity and produces signs and symptoms of inflammation. By inhibiting prostaglandin synthesis, balsalazide may reduce signs and symptoms of inflammation in inflammatory bowel disease. Balsalazide also interferes with leukotrine synthesis and inhibits the enzyme lipoxygenase. These substances are involved in the inflammatory response.

Contraindications
Hypersensitivity to balsalazide, salicylates, or their components

Adverse Reactions
CNS: Fatigue, fever, headache, insomnia
CV: Myocarditis, pericarditis, vasculitis
EENT Dry mouth, nasopharyngitis, pharyngitis, rhinitis, stomatitis
GI: Abdominal cramps or pain, anorexia, cirrhosis, constipation, diarrhea, dyspepsia, elevated liver enzyme levels, exacerbation of colitis, flatulence, hepatotoxicity, jaundice, nausea, pancreatitis, vomiting

GU: Dysmenorrhea, interstitial nephritis, renal failure, UTI
MS: Arthralgia, myalgia
RESP: Alveolitis, cough, flulike syndrome, pleural effusion, pneumonia, respiratory tract infection
SKIN: Alopecia, pruritus

Nursing Considerations
•**WARNING** Monitor patients who are sensitive to sulfasalazine or olsalazine for possible cross-sensitivity to balsalazide.
•Monitor patients with pyloric stenosis for decreased or delayed drug effects due to prolonged gastric retention of balsalazide capsules.
•Monitor patient for possible exacerbation of colitis symptoms.
PATIENT TEACHING
•Inform patient that balsalazide is used to reduce bowel inflammation and pain associated with ulcerative colitis and to minimize recurring inflammation.
•Instruct patient to swallow capsules whole, with a full glass of water, and not to crush or chew them.
•Advise patient to notify prescriber of any other drugs she may be taking, including OTC drugs, nutritional supplements, and herbal products, because they may interact with balsalazide.
•Instruct patient to notify prescriber immediately if her colitis symptoms worsen.
•Inform patient that she can expect some improvement in symptoms in 3 to 21 days but that she may need up to 6 weeks of treatment before she achieves optimal results.

basiliximab

Simulect

Class and Category
Chemical class: Chimeric (murine or human) monoclonal antibody
Therapeutic class: Immunosuppressant
Pregnancy category: B

Indications and Dosages
➤ *To prevent acute rejection in kidney transplantation*
I.V. INFUSION OR INJECTION
Adults and adolescents over age 15. 20 mg within 2 hr before transplantation; then 20 mg 4 days after transplantation.
Children and adolescents ages 2 to 15.
12 mg/m² within 2 hr before transplantation; then 12 mg/m² 4 days after transplantation. *Maximum:* 20 mg/dose.

Route	Onset	Peak	Duration
I.V.	Unknown	Unknown	22 to 50 days

Mechanism of Action
Initiates immunosuppression by blocking interleukin-2 receptors located on the surface of activated T cells. Normally, interleukin-2 is released by stimulated T lymphocytes, causing activation and differentiation of other T lymphocytes responsible for cell-mediated immunity.

Incompatibilities
Don't add or infuse any other drugs simultaneously through same I.V. line.

Contraindications
Hypersensitivity to basiliximab or its components

Adverse Reactions
CNS: Asthenia, dizziness, fever, headache, insomnia, tremor
CV: Hypertension, peripheral edema
EENT: Oral candidiasis, pharyngitis, rhinitis
ENDO: Hyperglycemia
GI: Abdominal pain, constipation, diarrhea, indigestion, nausea, vomiting
GU: Dysuria, increased urinary nitrogen level, UTI
HEME: Anemia
MS: Back pain, leg pain
RESP: Cough, dyspnea, upper respiratory tract infection
SKIN: Acne
Other: Hypercholesterolemia, hyperkalemia, hyperuricemia, hypocalcemia, hypokalemia, hypophosphatemia, impaired wound healing, injection site reaction, metabolic acidosis, weight gain

Nursing Considerations
•To reconstitute basiliximab, add 5 ml of sterile water for injection to powder and shake vial gently to dissolve. Further dilute with normal saline solution or D₅W for infusion to a volume of 50 ml. Gently invert in-

fusion bag to avoid foaming; don't shake. Drug should appear clear to opalescent and colorless.

• Administer reconstituted drug I.V. over 20 to 30 minutes or as a bolus dose directly through a central or peripheral I.V. line. Be aware that bolus dose may cause nausea, vomiting, and a localized injection site reaction, including pain.

• Expect drug to be given as adjunct to cyclosporine and corticosteroids.

• Don't store drug at room temperature for longer than 4 hours; don't refrigerate for longer than 24 hours.

• **WARNING** Be aware that patient may develop hypersensitivity reactions, including anaphylaxis, bronchospasm, dyspnea, hypotension, pruritus, rash, respiratory failure, sneezing, tachycardia, urticaria, and wheezing, on initial exposure or following re-exposure after several months. Notify prescriber immediately if such reactions occur.

PATIENT TEACHING

• Inform patient that second dose of basiliximab will be given 4 days after transplantation and that she may also receive cyclosporine and corticosteroid therapy.

• Inform patient that because of drug's immunosuppressant effects, she may experience slower wound healing and be more susceptible to upper respiratory tract infections.

beclomethasone dipropionate

Beclodisk (CAN), Beclovent Rotacaps (CAN), Beconase, Beconase AQ, QVAR, Vancenase, Vanceril

Class and Category

Chemical class: Synthetic glucocorticoid
Therapeutic class: Antiasthmatic, anti-inflammatory
Pregnancy category: C

Indications and Dosages

➤ *To control and prevent symptoms in patients with chronic asthma and those who also require oral corticosteroids*

INHALATION AEROSOL (84 MCG)

Adults and children age 12 and over. *Initial:* 2 inhalations (168 mcg) b.i.d. For patients with severe asthma, 6 to 8 inhalations (504 to 672 mcg) daily with dosage reduced based on patient response. *Maximum:* 10 inhalations (840 mcg) daily.

Children ages 6 to 12. *Initial:* 2 inhalations (168 mcg) b.i.d. *Maximum:* 5 inhalations (420 mcg) daily.

INHALATION AEROSOL (42 MCG)

Adults and children age 12 and over. *Initial:* 2 inhalations (84 mcg) t.i.d. or q.i.d. or 4 inhalations (168 mcg) b.i.d. For patients with severe asthma, 12 to 16 (504 to 672 mcg) inhalations daily with dosage reduced based on patient response. *Maximum:* 20 inhalations (840 mcg) daily.

Children ages 6 to 12. *Initial:* 1 or 2 inhalations (42 mcg or 84 mcg) t.i.d. or q.i.d. or 4 inhalations (168 mcg) b.i.d. with dosage reduced based on patient response. *Maximum:* 10 inhalations (420 mcg) daily.

INHALATION AEROSOL (40 MCG, 80 MCG [QVAR])

Adults and adolescents. *Initial for patients previously taking bronchodilators alone:* 1 to 2 inhalations (40 to 80 mcg) b.i.d., depending on strength used. *Maximum:* 4 to 8 inhalations (320 mcg) b.i.d., depending on strength used. *Initial for patients previously taking inhaled corticosteroids:* 1 to 4 inhalations (160 mcg) b.i.d., depending on strength used. *Maximum:* 4 to 8 inhalations (320 mcg) b.i.d., depending on strength used.

Children ages 5 to 11. 1 inhalation (40 mcg) b.i.d. *Maximum:* 1 to 2 inhalations (80 mcg) b.i.d., depending on strength used.

➤ *To relieve symptoms of seasonal or perennial allergic and nonallergic (vasomotor) rhinitis and prevent nasal polyps from recurring after surgical removal*

NASAL INHALATION AEROSOL

Adults and children age 12 and over. *Initial:* 1 inhalation (42 mcg) in each nostril b.i.d. to q.i.d. for total dose of 168 to 336 mcg daily. *Maintenance:* 1 inhalation (42 mcg) in each nostril t.i.d. for total dose of 252 mcg daily.

Children ages 6 to 12. 1 inhalation (42 mcg) in each nostril t.i.d. for total dose of 252 mcg daily.

NASAL SPRAY

Adults and children age 12 and over. 1 or 2 inhalations (42 or 84 mcg) in each nostril b.i.d. for total dose of 168 or 336 mcg daily.

Contraindications

Hypersensitivity to beclomethasone's ingredients, infrequent oral corticosteroid treatment, primary treatment of status asthmaticus or other acute asthma attack, relief of acute bronchospasm or of asthma controlled by bronchodilators or other nonsteroidal drugs, treatment of nonasthmatic bronchitis

Mechanism of Action

May decrease number and activity of cells involved in the inflammatory response of asthma, allergies, and rhinitis, such as mast cells, eosinophils, basophils, lymphocytes, macrophages, and neutrophils. Also may inhibit production or secretion of chemical mediators, such as histamine, eicosanoids, leukotrienes, and cytokines. May produce direct smooth-muscle cell relaxation and decrease airway hyperresponsiveness.

Adverse Reactions

CNS: Depression, fatigue, fever, headache, insomnia, light-headedness
CV: Chest pain, tachycardia
EENT: Cataracts, dry mouth, dysphonia, earache, epistaxis, glaucoma, hoarseness, lacrimation, nasal congestion, nose and throat dryness and irritation, oral candidiasis, pharyngitis, rhinorrhea, sinusitis, sneezing, unpleasant smell and taste
ENDO: Adrenal insufficiency, cushingoid symptoms
GI: Diarrhea, indigestion, nausea, rectal hemorrhage
GU: Dysmenorrhea, UTI
MS: Arthralgia, growth suppression in children (nasal aerosol)
RESP: Bronchitis, bronchospasm, chest congestion, cough, pulmonary infiltrates, upper respiratory tract infection, wheezing
SKIN: Acne, eczema, pruritus, rash, skin discoloration, urticaria
Other: Angioedema, flulike symptoms, lymphadenopathy, weight gain

Nursing Considerations

• If patient also receives an oral corticosteroid, expect to taper its dosage slowly (by decreasing the daily dosage or using the drug every other day) about 1 week after beclomethasone therapy begins. Expect dosage reductions of more than 2.5 mg daily.
• **WARNING** When gradually switching patient from an oral corticosteroid to inhaled beclomethasone, assess her for signs of life-threatening adrenal insufficiency, such as fatigue, lassitude, weakness, nausea, vomiting, and hypotension, during transition period and when exposed to trauma, surgery, infection, or other stressor. If signs occur, notify prescriber immediately.
• Expect to resume oral corticosteroid during a stressful period or severe asthma attack.
• Because beclomethasone may be absorbed systemically, monitor for signs of adrenal insufficiency during periods of stress.
• If patient experiences an acute asthma attack or increased wheezing after administering beclomethasone, administer a fast-acting bronchodilator, as prescribed. Expect to discontinue beclomethasone.
• Assess for signs of candidiasis, such as thick white plaques or coating on tongue and sides of mouth. If present, notify prescriber and expect to reduce drug dose or frequency or discontinue beclomethasone. Also anticipate treatment with antifungal drug.
• When administering beclomethasone nasal spray, periodically assess nasal discharge for color or consistency changes, which may indicate infection.
• Monitor the growth of children receiving beclomethasone nasally.

PATIENT TEACHING
• Advise patient not to abruptly stop taking beclomethasone because adrenal insufficiency may occur. Urge her to notify prescriber if she develops signs of adrenal insufficiency, such as nausea, fatigue, anorexia, dyspnea, hypotension, fever, malaise, dizziness, and fainting.
• Before patient uses nasal spray for first time, instruct her to prime the pump by placing her thumb on its base and index and middle fingers on its shoulder area and then pressing her thumb firmly and quickly against bottle several times or until fine mist appears. Before patient uses nasal inhalation canister for first time, instruct her to shake it and check that it's working properly by spraying it once in the air while looking for fine mist.
• Teach patient to inhale deeply after each nasal spray or inhalation, exhaling through mouth and tilting head back to let drug spread over the nasopharynx.
• Teach patient how to properly use oral inhalation aerosol, shaking canister well before

using. If patient has difficulty using device and coordinating inhalation with it, suggest using a spacer device.
• If two inhalations are prescribed, advise patient to wait a minute between them.
• If patient uses an inhaled bronchodilator with beclomethasone oral inhalation, instruct her to use bronchodilator first, wait 5 minutes, and then use beclomethasone.
• WARNING Warn patient that beclomethasone isn't intended to relieve acute bronchospasm. Urge patient to notify prescriber if asthma symptoms don't respond to drug.
• Advise patient to wear medical identification that states need for supplemental oral corticosteroids during stress or severe asthma attack. Inform patient that prescriber may order high-dose oral corticosteroid therapy.
• WARNING Caution patient to avoid exposure to chickenpox and measles because beclomethasone may cause immunosuppression. If she's exposed to these disorders, urge her to notify prescriber immediately.

belladonna alkaloids

Class and Category
Chemical class: Tertiary amine
Therapeutic class: GI anticholinergic
Pregnancy category: C

Indications and Dosages
➤ *To treat peptic ulcer disease, functional digestive disorders (including spastic, mucous, and ulcerative colitis), diarrhea, diverticulitis, pancreatitis, dysmenorrhea, nocturnal enuresis, idiopathic and postencephalitic parkinsonism, motion sickness, and nausea and vomiting of pregnancy*
TABLETS
Adults. 0.25 to 0.5 mg t.i.d.
Children over age 6. 0.125 to 0.25 mg t.i.d.
TINCTURE
Adults. 0.6 to 1 ml t.i.d. or q.i.d.
Children. 0.03 ml/kg (0.8 ml/m²) t.i.d.

Route	Onset	Peak	Duration
P.O.	1 to 2 hr	Unknown	4 hr

Contraindications
Hepatic disease, hypersensitivity to anticholinergic drugs or scopolamine, ileus, myasthe-

nia gravis, myocardial ischemia, narrow-angle glaucoma, obstructive condition of GI or GU tract, renal disease, severe ulcerative colitis, tachycardia, toxic megacolon, unstable cardiovascular status in acute hemorrhage

Mechanism of Action
Inhibits acetylcholine's muscarinic actions at postganglionic parasympathetic receptor sites, including smooth muscles, secretory glands, and CNS. These actions relax smooth muscles and diminish GI, GU, and biliary tract secretions.

Interactions
DRUGS
amantadine: Increased adverse anticholinergic effects
atenolol, digoxin: Possibly increased therapeutic and adverse effects of these drugs
phenothiazines: Possibly decreased phenothiazine effectiveness and increased adverse effects of belladonna alkaloids
tricyclic antidepressants: Possibly increased adverse anticholinergic effects

Adverse Reactions
CNS: CNS stimulation (with high doses), confusion, dizziness, drowsiness, headache, insomnia, nervousness, weakness
CV: Bradycardia, palpitations, tachycardia
EENT: Altered taste, blurred vision, dry mouth, increased intraocular pressure, mydriasis, nasal congestion, photophobia
GI: Bloating, constipation, dysphagia, heartburn, ileus, nausea, vomiting
GU: Impotence, urinary hesitancy, urine retention
SKIN: Decreased sweating, flushing, urticaria
Other: Anaphylaxis

Nursing Considerations
• Avoid using high doses of belladonna alkaloids in patients with ulcerative colitis because they may inhibit intestinal motility and precipitate or aggravate toxic megacolon. Also avoid using high doses in patients with hiatal hernia and reflux esophagitis because they may aggravate esophagitis.
• Use belladonna alkaloids cautiously in patients with allergies, arrhythmias, asthma, autonomic neuropathy, coronary artery disease, debilitating chronic lung disease, heart

failure, hypertension, hyperthyroidism, and prostatic hypertrophy.
• Give drug 30 to 60 minutes before a meal.
• **WARNING** Monitor patient for excitement, agitation, drowsiness, and confusion. Elderly patients are more sensitive to the effects of the drug even with small doses and are more likely to develop these adverse reactions. Dosage may need to be decreased.
• Take safety precautions to protect patient from injury from falling.

PATIENT TEACHING
• Instruct patient to take belladonna alkaloids 30 to 60 minutes before eating.
• Tell patient to notify prescriber if she has persistent or severe diarrhea, constipation, or difficulty urinating.
• Caution patient to avoid driving and similar activities until the effects of belladonna alkaloids are known.
• **WARNING** Urge patient to avoid extreme heat and humidity because heatstroke could occur.

benazepril hydrochloride

Lotensin

Class and Category
Chemical class: Ethylester of benazeprilat
Therapeutic class: Antihypertensive
Pregnancy category: D

Indications and Dosages
➤ *To control hypertension alone or with a thiazide diuretic*

TABLETS
Adults who don't receive a diuretic. *Initial:* 10 mg daily. *Maintenance:* 20 to 40 mg daily as a single dose or in two divided doses.
Adults who receive a diuretic. 5 mg daily.
DOSAGE ADJUSTMENT Initial dosage of 5 mg/day for patients with impaired renal function and creatinine clearance of less than 30 ml/min/1.73 m^2, then increased gradually until blood pressure is controlled or dosage reaches maximum of 40 mg daily.

TABLETS, SUSPENSION
Children age 6 and over with glomerular filtration rate of 30 ml/min/1.73 m^2 or higher. *Initial:* 0.2 mg/kg daily. *Maximum:* 0.6 mg/kg daily or 40 mg daily.

Route	Onset	Peak	Duration
P.O.	1 hr	2 to 4 hr	24 hr

Mechanism of Action
May reduce blood pressure by affecting renin-angiotensin-aldosterone system. By inhibiting angiotensin-converting enzyme, benazepril:
• prevents conversion of angiotensin I to angiotensin II, a potent vasoconstrictor that also stimulates aldosterone release.
• may inhibit renal and vascular production of angiotensin II.
• decreases serum angiotensin II level and increases serum renin activity. This decreases aldosterone secretion, slightly increasing serum potassium level and fluid loss.
• decreases vascular tone and blood pressure.
• inhibits aldosterone release, which reduces sodium and water resorption, increases their excretion, and reduces blood pressure.

Contraindications
Hypersensitivity to benazepril or other ACE inhibitor

Interactions
DRUGS
antacids: Possibly decreased bioavailability of benazepril; separate doses by 2 hours
antidiabetics (oral): Possibly increased risk of hypoglycemia
capsaicin: Possibly induction or exacerbation of ACE cough caused by benazepril
digoxin: Increased serum digoxin level
diuretics: Possibly excessive hypotension
indomethacin: Reduced hypotensive effects of benazepril
lithium: Increased serum lithium level and risk of lithium toxicity
phenothiazines: Possibly increased therapeutic and adverse effects of benazepril
potassium preparations, potassium-sparing diuretics: Possibly increased serum potassium level

Adverse Reactions
CNS: Anxiety, asthenia, dizziness, drowsiness, fatigue, headache, hypertonia, insomnia, nervousness, paresthesia, sleep disturbance, somnolence, syncope, weakness
CV: Angina, ECG changes, hypotension, orthostatic hypotension, palpitations, peri-

pheral edema
EENT: Sinusitis
ENDO: Hyperglycemia
GI: Abdominal pain, constipation, elevated liver function test results, gastritis, melena, nausea, pancreatitis, small bowel angio-edema, vomiting
GU: Decreased libido, elevated BUN and serum creatinine levels, impotence, nephrotic syndrome, proteinuria, renal insufficiency, UTI
HEME: Agranulocytosis, decreased hemoglobin level, leukopenia, neutropenia, thrombocytopenia
MS: Arthralgia, arthritis, myalgia
RESP: ACE cough, asthma, bronchitis, bronchospasm, dyspnea
SKIN: Dermatitis, diaphoresis, flushing, photosensitivity, pruritus, rash
Other: Anaphylaxis, angioedema, hyperkalemia, hyponatremia

Nursing Considerations
•Evaluate blood pressure with patient lying down, sitting, and standing before initiating benazepril and then every 4 to 8 hours, as appropriate, to monitor drug's effectiveness.
•Monitor urine output and BUN and serum creatinine levels, as needed, before therapy.
•**WARNING** Be alert for angioedema, especially after first dose. If it extends to larynx and patient has laryngeal stridor or signs of airway obstruction, prepare to give epinephrine subcutaneously immediately, as prescribed, and discontinue benazepril.
•Monitor WBC count periodically to detect neutropenia and agranulocytosis.
•Monitor serum potassium and other electrolyte levels to detect electrolyte imbalances.
•To prevent injury caused by orthostatic hypotension, take safety precautions, such as having patient change position slowly and sit on edge of bed before arising.

PATIENT TEACHING
•Teach patient how to monitor blood pressure, if appropriate, and how to recognize signs of hypertension and hypotension.
•**WARNING** Strongly urge patient to contact prescriber before using any OTC salt substitutes, which may contain potassium, or potassium supplements. These substances increase the risk of hyperkalemia.
•Inform patient that a persistent dry cough

may develop and may not subside unless benazepril is discontinued. If cough becomes bothersome or interferes with her sleep or activities, instruct her to notify prescriber.
•**WARNING** Instruct patient to contact prescriber immediately if she experiences signs of angioedema, such as swelling of the face, eyes, lips, or tongue.
•Caution patient to avoid sudden position changes and to rise slowly from sitting or lying to minimize orthostatic hypotension.
•**WARNING** Advise patient to stop benazepril and notify prescriber as soon as possible if she experiences syncope.
•**WARNING** Caution women of childbearing age to use a reliable form of contraception and to notify prescriber immediately if pregnancy is suspected because benazepril may cause fetal harm and should be discontinued.

benzonatate

Benzonatate Softgels, Tessalon Perles

Class and Category
Chemical class: Para-aminobenzoic acid (tetracaine-like)
Therapeutic class: Nonnarcotic antitussive
Pregnancy category: C

Indications and Dosages
➤ *To relieve cough*
CAPSULES
Adults and children over age 10. 100 mg t.i.d. up to 600 mg daily.

Route	Onset	Peak	Duration
P.O.	15 to 20 min	Unknown	3 to 8 hr

Mechanism of Action
Anesthetizes stretch receptors in respiratory tract, lung tissue, and pleura, interfering with their activity and reducing cough reflex at its source. In usual doses, benzonatate doesn't inhibit respiratory center.

Contraindications
Hypersensitivity to benzonatate or related compounds

Adverse Reactions
CNS: Confusion, hallucinations, headache,

mild dizziness, sedation
CV: Cardiogenic shock, chest numbness
EENT: Burning eyes, laryngospasm, nasal congestion
GI: Constipation, GI upset, nausea
RESP: Bronchospasm
SKIN: Pruritus, rash

Nursing Considerations

•Assess the type and frequency of patient's cough. Don't attempt to suppress cough with benzonatate if cough has therapeutic benefit, such as to move secretions and improve airflow.

•**WARNING** Don't break or crush capsules or let patient chew or dissolve them in her mouth. This may cause release of drug in patient's mouth, which can anesthetize mouth and throat, causing risk of choking. Also don't let patient suck or chew capsule to prevent severe hypersensitivity reaction.

PATIENT TEACHING

•Instruct patient to swallow capsules whole and not to chew, suck, or open them.
•Warn patient that mild dizziness and sedation may occur. Teach her to take safety measures, and encourage her to avoid activities that require mental alertness until benzonatate's effects are known.

benzquinamide hydrochloride

Emete-Con

Class and Category

Chemical class: Benzoquinolizine amide
Therapeutic class: Antiemetic
Pregnancy category: Not rated

Indications and Dosages

➤ *To treat nausea and vomiting related to anesthesia or surgery*

I.V. OR I.M. INJECTION

Adults. 50 mg or 0.5 to 1 mg/kg I.M., repeated in 1 hr, then every 3 to 4 hr, p.r.n. Or 25 mg or 0.2 to 0.4 mg/kg by slow infusion (1 ml every 0.5 to 1 min) as a single dose. Then, I.M. doses begin.

➤ *To prevent nausea and vomiting related to anesthesia and surgery*

I.M. INJECTION

Adults. 50 mg or 0.5 to 1 mg/kg 15 min before emergence from anesthesia.

Route	Onset	Peak	Duration
I.V., I.M.	15 min	Unknown	Unknown

Mechanism of Action

Exhibits antiemetic, antihistaminic, mild cholinergic, and sedative effects by unknown mechanism.

Contraindications

Hypersensitivity to benzquinamide or its components

Interactions

DRUGS

vasopressors: Increased hypertensive effects

Adverse Reactions

CNS: Chills, dizziness, drowsiness, excitement, fatigue, fever, headache, insomnia, nervousness, restlessness, tremor, weakness
CV: Atrial fibrillation, hypertension, hypotension, premature atrial or ventricular contractions
EENT: Blurred vision, dry mouth, increased salivation
GI: Anorexia, hiccups, nausea
MS: Muscle twitching
SKIN: Diaphoresis, flushing, rash, urticaria

Nursing Considerations

•**WARNING** Avoid I.V. route in patients with cardiovascular disease because sudden blood pressure increases and transient arrhythmias may occur. Use I.V. route only for patients without cardiovascular disease who aren't receiving a preanesthetic or cardiovascular drug.

•Administer benzquinamide I.M. into large, well-developed muscle. Avoid using deltoid muscle unless it's well developed.

•Take safety precautions to reduce the risk of injury from CNS depression.

PATIENT TEACHING

•Advise patient to stay in bed and call for assistance to reduce risk of injury.
•Tell patient to report whether nausea and vomiting have been relieved.

benztropine mesylate

Apo-Benztropine (CAN), Cogentin, PMS Benztropine (CAN)

Class and Category
Chemical class: Tertiary amine
Therapeutic class: Antiparkinsonian, central-acting anticholinergic
Pregnancy category: C

Indications and Dosages
➤ *As adjunct, to treat all forms of Parkinson's disease*
TABLETS, I.M. OR I.V. INJECTION
Adults with Parkinson's disease. 1 to 2 mg daily (usual dose) with a range of 0.5 to 6 mg daily.
Adults with idiopathic Parkinson's disease. *Initial:* 0.5 to 1 mg at bedtime. *Maximum:* 4 to 6 mg daily.
Adults with postencephalitic Parkinson's disease. 2 mg daily in one or more doses; may begin with 0.5 mg at bedtime and increase as needed.

➤ *To control extrapyramidal symptoms (except tardive dyskinesia) caused by phenothiazines and other neuroleptic drugs*
TABLETS, I.M. OR I.V. INJECTION
Adults. 1 to 4 mg once or twice daily.

➤ *To treat acute dystonic reactions*
TABLETS, I.M. OR I.V. INJECTION
Adults. *Initial:* 1 to 2 ml (1 to 2 mg total dose) I.V. or I.M. *Maintenance:* 1 to 2 mg P.O. b.i.d. to prevent recurrence.

Route	Onset	Peak	Duration
P.O.	1 to 2 hr	Unknown	24 hr
I.V., I.M	15 min	Unknown	24 hr

Mechanism of Action
Blocks acetylcholine's action at cholinergic receptor sites. This restores the brain's normal dopamine and acetylcholine balance, which relaxes muscle movement and decreases drooling, rigidity, and tremor. Benztropine also may inhibit dopamine reuptake and storage, which prolongs dopamine's action.

Contraindications
Achalasia, bladder neck obstruction, glaucoma, hypersensitivity to benztropine mesylate or its components, megacolon, myasthenia gravis, prostatic hypertrophy, pyloric or duodenal obstruction, stenosing peptic ulcer

Interactions
DRUGS
amantadine: Possibly increased adverse anticholinergic effects
digoxin: Possibly increased digoxin level
haloperidol: Possibly increased schizophrenic symptoms, decreased serum haloperidol level, and development of tardive dyskinesia
levodopa: Possibly decreased levodopa effectiveness
phenothiazines: Possibly reduced phenothiazine effects and increased psychiatric symptoms

Adverse Reactions
CNS: Agitation, confusion, delirium, delusions, depression, disorientation, dizziness, drowsiness, euphoria, excitement, fever, hallucinations, headache, light-headedness, listlessness, memory loss, nervousness, paranoia, psychosis, weakness
CV: Hypotension, mild bradycardia, orthostatic hypotension, palpitations, tachycardia
EENT: Blurred vision, diplopia, dry mouth, increased intraocular pressure, mydriasis, narrow-angle glaucoma, suppurative parotitis
GI: Constipation, duodenal ulcer, epigastric distress, ileus, nausea, vomiting
GU: Dysuria, urinary hesitancy, urine retention
MS: Muscle spasms, muscle weakness
SKIN: Decreased sweating, dermatoses, flushing, rash, urticaria

Nursing Considerations
•Expect to administer I.V. or I.M. benztropine when patient needs more rapid response than oral drug can provide. Be aware that I.M. route is commonly used because it provides effects in about the same time as I.V. route. Watch for improvement a few minutes after administration. If Parkinsonian symptoms reappear, expect to repeat dose.
•Know that therapy generally begins with a low dose followed by gradual increases of 0.5 mg every 5 or 6 days because benztropine has a cumulative action.
•Assess muscle rigidity and tremor at baseline. Then monitor them often for improvement, which indicates drug's effectiveness.
•Administer drug before or after meals

based on patient's need and response. If patient has increased salivary secretions, expect to administer benztropine after meals. If patient has dry mouth, plan to give drug before meals unless nausea develops.

•**WARNING** When giving drug to patient with drug-induced extrapyramidal reactions, watch for worsening psychiatric symptoms.

•Know that high-dose benztropine therapy may cause weakness and inability to move specific muscle groups. If this occurs, expect to reduce benztropine dosage.

PATIENT TEACHING

•Warn patient that benztropine has a cumulative effect, increasing risk of adverse reactions and overdose.

•Caution patient to avoid driving and similar activities until benztropine's effects are known because drug may cause blurred vision, dizziness, or drowsiness.

•**WARNING** Because benztropine decreases sweating, urge patient to avoid extremely hot or humid conditions to reduce risk of heatstroke and severe hyperthermia. This is especially important for elderly patients and those who abuse alcohol or have chronic illness or CNS disease.

•Stress need for periodic eye examinations and intraocular pressure measurements because benztropine may cause narrow-angle glaucoma and increase intraocular pressure.

bepridil hydrochloride

Vascor

Class and Category

Chemical class: Calcium channel blocker, diarylammopropylamine derivative
Therapeutic class: Antianginal
Pregnancy category: C

Indications and Dosages

➤ *To treat chronic stable angina in patients who don't respond to or can't tolerate other antianginal drugs*

TABLETS

Adults. *Initial:* 200 mg daily for 10 days followed by dosage increases, depending on patient's response (ability to perform daily activities, length of QT interval, heart rate, and frequency and severity of angina attacks). *Maintenance:* 300 to 400 mg daily (maximum).

Route	Onset	Peak	Duration
P.O.	Unknown	8 days	Unknown

Mechanism of Action

Inhibits calcium movement into coronary and vascular smooth-muscle cells by blocking slow calcium channels in their membranes. This decreases intracellular calcium level, which inhibits smooth-muscle cell contractions and causes:
• relaxation of coronary and vascular smooth muscles, decreased peripheral vascular resistance, and reduced systolic and diastolic blood pressure, which decrease myocardial oxygen demand
• depression of impulse formation (automaticity) and conduction velocity.
  Bepridil also inhibits fast inward sodium channels, reducing speed and degree of action potential and increasing its duration in cardiac muscle.

Contraindications

Congenital prolonged QT interval, history of serious ventricular arrhythmias, hypersensitivity to bepridil, hypotension (systolic pressure below 90 mm Hg), sick sinus syndrome and second- or third-degree AV block unless artificial pacemaker in place, uncompensated cardiac insufficiency, use of other drugs that prolong QT interval

Interactions

DRUGS

antiarrhythmics, such as quinidine and procainamide, with actions similar to bepridil's: Exaggerated and prolonged QT interval
beta blockers: Possibly increased depression of myocardial contractility and AV conduction
digoxin: Possibly increased serum digoxin level
fentanyl: Severe hypotension and increased need for fluid
nitrates: Additive hypotensive effect
tricyclic antidepressants: Exaggerated and prolonged QT interval

Adverse Reactions

CNS: Amnesia, anxiety, asthenia, depression, dizziness, drowsiness, fever, hallucinations, headache, insomnia, nervousness, paranoia,

paresthesia, psychosis, syncope, tremor, vertigo
CV: Edema, hypertension, palpitations, premature ventricular contractions, prolonged QT interval, sinus bradycardia or tachycardia, torsades de pointes, vasodilation, ventricular fibrillation, ventricular tachycardia
EENT: Altered taste, blurred vision, dry mouth, pharyngitis, rhinitis, tinnitus
GI: Abdominal cramps or discomfort, anorexia, appetite increase, constipation, diarrhea, flatulence, gastritis, nausea
GU: Decreased libido, impotence
HEME: Agranulocytosis, leukopenia, neutropenia
MS: Arthritis, myalgia
RESP: Cough, dyspnea, respiratory tract infection
SKIN: Dermatitis, diaphoresis, rash
Other: Flulike symptoms

Nursing Considerations

•Use bepridil cautiously in patients with heart failure because it can induce new arrhythmias and may worsen heart failure.
•Because bepridil is metabolized by the liver and its metabolites are excreted in urine, monitor results of liver function studies as well as BUN and serum electrolyte and creatinine levels as appropriate.
•Assess heart rate and rhythm to obtain baseline. Then monitor frequently during therapy. Also, monitor serial 12-lead ECG tracings. Be aware that bepridil can induce new arrhythmias, including ventricular tachycardia and fibrillation (which are more difficult to convert), torsades de pointes, and prolonged QT intervals.
•WARNING Be alert for QT intervals that exceed 0.52 second. If this occurs, expect to reduce bepridil dose or discontinue drug.
•Monitor WBC count to detect agranulocytosis, which may warrant stopping therapy.
•WARNING Be aware that bepridil shouldn't be discontinued abruptly. Instead, gradually taper its dosage as prescribed to prevent increased frequency and duration of chest pain as increased calcium moves into cells, causing coronary artery spasm.
•Monitor blood pressure often if patient takes a nitrate or beta blocker. Assess for hypotension.
•Monitor serum electrolyte levels. Especially note decreased potassium level, which may worsen existing arrhythmias or induce new ones.

PATIENT TEACHING
•Advise patient to avoid driving and other activities that require alertness and coordination until bepridil's CNS effects are known.

betamethasone

Celestone

betamethasone acetate-betamethasone sodium phosphate

Celestone Soluspan

betamethasone sodium phosphate

Betnesol (CAN), Celestone Phosphate, Selestoject

Class and Category

Chemical class: Synthetic glucocorticoid
Therapeutic class: Anti-inflammatory
Pregnancy category: C

Indications and Dosages

➤ *To treat conditions with severe inflammation and conditions requiring immunosuppression*
SYRUP, TABLETS (BETAMETHASONE)
Adults. 0.6 to 7.2 mg daily.
I.M. INJECTION (BETAMETHASONE ACETATE-BETAMETHASONE SODIUM PHOSPHATE)
Adults. 0.5 to 9 mg I.M. daily, or ⅓ to ½ of P.O. dose every 12 hr.
I.M OR I.V. INJECTION (BETAMETHASONE SODIUM PHOSPHATE)
Adults. *Initial:* Variable (given in emergency situations or when oral therapy isn't possible). *Maximum:* 9 mg daily.
➤ *To treat bursitis, gouty arthritis, osteoarthritis, periostitis of cuboid, peritendinitis, rheumatoid arthritis, skin lesions, tenosynovitis*
INTRA-ARTICULAR, INTRABURSAL, OR INTRADERMAL INJECTION (BETAMETHASONE ACETATE-BETAMETHASONE SODIUM PHOSPHATE)
Adults with bursitis, peritendinitis, or tenosynovitis. 1 ml by intrabursal or intra-articular injection. Three or four injections given every 1 to 2 wk.
Adults with osteoarthritis or rheumatoid arthritis. 0.5 to 2 ml, depending on joint size.

B

Adults with foot bursitis. 0.25 to 0.5 ml every 3 to 7 days.
Adults with foot tenosynovitis or periostitis of cuboid. 0.5 ml every 3 to 7 days.
Adults with acute gouty arthritis. 0.5 to 1 ml every 3 to 7 days.
Adults with skin lesions. 0.2 ml/cm² intradermally, up to 1 ml weekly.
DOSAGE ADJUSTMENT Dosage reduced for elderly patients and accompanied by periodic monitoring of blood pressure and blood glucose and electrolyte levels.

Route	Onset	Peak	Duration
P.O.	Unknown	1 to 2 hr	3.25 days
I.V., I.M. (sodium phosphate)	Rapid	Unknown	Unknown
I.M. (acetate-sodium phosphate)	1 to 3 hr	Unknown	1 wk
Other (acetate-sodium phosphate)	Unknown	Unknown	1 to 2 wk*

Mechanism of Action

Binds to intracellular glucocorticoid receptors and suppresses inflammatory and immune responses by:
• inhibiting neutrophil and monocyte accumulation at inflammation site and suppressing their phagocytic and bactericidal activity
• stabilizing lysosomal membranes
• suppressing antigen response of macrophages and helper T cells
• inhibiting synthesis of inflammatory response mediators, such as cytokines, interleukins, and prostaglandins.

Contraindications

Idiopathic thrombocytopenic purpura (I.M. injection), live virus vaccination, systemic fungal infection

* For intra-arterial or intrasynovial injection; 1 week for intralesional injection in soft tissue.

Interactions
DRUGS
anticholinesterase drugs: Possibly antagonized anticholinesterase effects in myasthenia gravis
barbiturates: Possibly decreased effects of betamethasone
cyclosporine: Possibly increased risk of cyclosporine toxicity
digitalis glycosides: Possibly increased risk of digitalis toxicity
estrogens: Possibly decreased excretion of betamethasone
hydantoins, rifampin: Possibly increased excretion and decreased therapeutic effects of betamethasone
isoniazid: Possibly decreased serum isoniazid level
ketoconazole: Possibly decreased excretion of betamethasone
oral anticoagulants: Possibly increased or decreased action of anticoagulants, requiring adjusted anticoagulant dosage
oral contraceptives: Possibly increased half-life and concentration and decreased excretion of betamethasone
potassium-wasting diuretics: Increased risk of hypokalemia
salicylates: Possibly decreased serum level and therapeutic effects of salicylates
somatrem: Possibly inhibition of somatrem's growth-promoting effects
theophyllines: Possibly changes in both drugs' effects

Adverse Reactions
CNS: Fatigue, headache, increased intracranial pressure with papilledema, insomnia, malaise, neuritis, paresthesia, seizures, steroid psychosis, syncope, vertigo
CV: Arrhythmias, ECG changes, fat embolism, heart failure, hypertension, thromboembolism, thrombophlebitis
EENT: Cataracts, exophthalmos, glaucoma, increased intraocular pressure
ENDO: Cushingoid symptoms (buffalo hump, central obesity, decreased carbohydrate tolerance, fat pad enlargement, moon face), fluid retention, growth suppression in children, hyperglycemia, masked signs of infection, negative nitrogen balance, secondary adrenocortical and pituitary unresponsiveness (in times of stress)
GI: Abdominal distention, increased appetite,

nausea, pancreatitis, peptic ulcer possibly with perforation, ulcerative esophagitis, vomiting
GU: Amenorrhea, glycosuria, menstrual irregularities
HEME: Leukocytosis
MS: Aseptic necrosis of femoral and humeral heads, loss of muscle mass, muscle weakness, osteoporosis, spontaneous pathologic and vertebral compression fractures, tendon rupture
SKIN: Acneiform lesions, allergic dermatitis, ecchymosis, facial erythema, hirsutism, impaired wound healing, increased sweating, petechiae, lupuslike lesions, purpura, subcutaneous fat atrophy, thin and fragile skin, urticaria
Other: Angioedema, hypocalcemia, hypokalemia, sodium retention, suppressed reaction to skin tests, weight gain

Nursing Considerations

•Expect prescriber to order baseline ophthalmologic examination before initiating therapy because prolonged betamethasone use may lead to increased intraocular pressure, glaucoma, and subsequent optic nerve damage. Use betamethasone cautiously in patients with ocular herpes simplex because corneal perforation may occur.
•Determine if latent or active amebiasis has been ruled out in patients who have spent time in the tropics or who have unexplained diarrhea before betamethasone therapy starts because drug may worsen it.
•**WARNING** Give betamethasone with extreme care in patients with known or suspected *Strongyloides* (threadworm) infestation because corticosteroids such as betamethasone may result in immunosuppression, *Strongyloides* hyperinfection and dissemination, and widespread larval migration, resulting in severe enterocolitis and potentially life-threatening gram-negative septicemia.
•Assess for signs of infection before administering betamethasone because drug may mask those signs. Because drug may cause immunosuppression, new infection may develop during therapy. If so, expect to administer appropriate antibiotic.
•Review serum electrolyte levels, as ordered, before initiating therapy. Monitor these levels frequently during therapy to detect imbalances. Sodium and water retention and

potassium and calcium depletion may occur with high-dose betamethasone therapy. If so, expect to restrict sodium intake and provide potassium and calcium supplements.
•Because betamethasone is linked to peptic ulcer formation, expect to administer it with an antacid or H_2-receptor blocker.
•**WARNING** Monitor ECG tracings for arrhythmias, and evaluate patient for anaphylactic reactions, such as angioedema and seizures, which have been associated with rapid I.V. administration of high-dose corticosteroids.
•**WARNING** During long-term betamethasone therapy, assess for signs of adrenal suppression and insufficiency (fatigue, hypotension, lassitude, nausea, vomiting, and weakness) when patient is exposed to stress. If she exhibits these signs, notify prescriber at once.
•Watch for signs of steroid psychosis, such as delirium, clouded sensorium, euphoria, insomnia, mood swings, personality changes, and severe depression, which may develop 15 to 30 days after therapy begins. Be prepared to discontinue therapy. If this isn't possible, expect to administer psychotropic drugs.
•Rotate I.M. injection sites. To prevent muscle atrophy, avoid subcutaneous injection, injection in deltoid site, and repeated I.M. injections into same site.
•Administer oral betamethasone before 9 a.m., if appropriate, to mimic body's natural release of corticosteroids.
•After intra-articular injection, assess joint for marked increase in pain, local swelling, and more restricted movement. If patient also develops fever and malaise, suspect septic arthritis and notify prescriber immediately. Expect to assist with joint fluid aspiration to confirm septic arthritis.
•Monitor patient for cushingoid signs and symptoms, such as moon face, buffalo hump, central obesity, striae, acne, ecchymosis, and weight gain. Notify prescriber if you detect these symptoms.
•Expect to slowly taper oral betamethasone dosage to prevent adrenal insufficiency.
PATIENT TEACHING
•Instruct patient to take betamethasone with food if GI upset occurs.
•Reinforce signs of adrenal insufficiency and possible need for dosage increases during stress. Advise patient to notify prescriber immediately if signs of insufficiency occur or if

she's exposed to stress.
•Instruct patient to avoid exposure to infections because drug can cause immunosuppression. Also teach patient to recognize and immediately report signs of infection.
•After intra-articular injection, advise patient not to overuse joint and to continue other treatments such as physical therapy.

betaxolol hydrochloride

Kerlone

Class and Category
Chemical class: Selective beta₁-adrenergic blocker
Therapeutic class: Antihypertensive
Pregnancy category: C

Indications and Dosages
➤ *To treat hypertension alone or with other antihypertensives*
TABLETS
Adults. *Initial:* 10 mg daily. If no response in 7 to 14 days, then 20 mg daily.
DOSAGE ADJUSTMENT For elderly patients and patients who have renal failure or are undergoing hemodialysis, initial dosage reduced to 5 mg daily. If desired response isn't achieved, dosage increased by 5-mg increments every 2 wk up to 20 mg daily.

Route	Onset	Peak	Duration
P.O.	Unknown	3 to 4 hr	Unknown

Mechanism of Action
Inhibits stimulation of beta₁-adrenergic receptor sites, primarily in the heart. This decreases myocardial excitability, cardiac output, and myocardial oxygen demand. It also decreases renin release from the kidneys, which helps reduce blood pressure.

Contraindications
Cardiogenic shock, heart failure unless caused by tachyarrhythmia or overt heart failure, hypersensitivity to betaxolol, second- or third-degree heart block, sinus bradycardia

Interactions
DRUGS
aluminum salts, barbiturates, calcium salts,

cholestyramine, colestipol, NSAIDs, penicillins, rifampin, salicylates, sulfinpyrazone: Decreased therapeutic and adverse effects of betaxolol
beta blockers, digoxin: Increased risk of additive systemic beta blockade, especially bradycardia
calcium channel blockers: Possibly increased therapeutic and adverse effects of betaxolol
ciprofloxacin, other quinolones: Possibly increased bioavailability of betaxolol, increasing the drug's pharmacologic effect
clonidine: Possibly severe hypertension when both drugs (or just clonidine) are simultaneously withdrawn
epinephrine: Possibly severe hypertension followed by bradycardia
ergot alkaloids: Possibly peripheral ischemia and gangrene
flecainide: Possibly increased therapeutic and adverse effects of both drugs
lidocaine: Possibly increased risk of lidocaine toxicity
nondepolarizing neuromuscular blockers: Possibly increased or decreased neuromuscular blockade
oral contraceptives: Possibly increased bioavailability and plasma level of betaxolol, increasing the drug's pharmacologic effect
prazosin: Possibly increased orthostatic hypotension
quinidine: Possibly increased effects of betaxolol
sulfonylureas: Possibly masking of hypoglycemic symptoms

Adverse Reactions
CNS: Amnesia, anxiety, behavior changes, confusion, depression, dizziness, emotional lability, fatigue, fever, hallucinations, headache, insomnia, lethargy, malaise, mood changes, nightmares, paresthesia, peripheral neuropathy, sedation, stroke, syncope, tremor, vertigo
CV: Arrhythmias, including asystole, bradycardia, heart block, and torsades de pointes; cardiogenic shock; chest pain; claudication; heart failure; hypercholesterolemia; hyperlipidemia; hypotension; mitral insufficiency; MI; orthostatic hypotension; peripheral vascular insufficiency; Raynaud's phenomenon; renal and mesenteric artery thrombosis
EENT: Altered taste, blurred vision, burning eyes, conjunctivitis, dry eyes, dry mouth, ear-

ache, eye irritation, eye pain or pressure, increased salivation, laryngospasm, mouth ulcers, nasal stuffiness, pharyngitis, ptosis, rhinitis, sinusitis, tinnitus
ENDO: Breast pain (in women), hyperglycemia, hypoglycemia
GI: Acute pancreatitis, anorexia, bloating, constipation, diarrhea, elevated liver function test results, epigastric pain, flatulence, gastritis, heartburn, hepatomegaly, increased appetite, indigestion, nausea, vomiting
GU: Decreased libido, dysuria, impotence, nocturia, Peyronie's disease, prostatitis, renal colic, renal failure, urinary frequency, urine retention, UTI
HEME: Agranulocytosis, eosinophilia, leukopenia, thrombocytopenia
MS: Arthralgia, arthritis, gout, muscle spasms or twitching, myalgia, neck pain, tendinitis
RESP: Bronchial obstruction, bronchitis, bronchospasm, cough, pulmonary embolus, respiratory distress, upper respiratory tract infection, wheezing
SKIN: Acne, diaphoresis, dry skin, eczema, erythema, exfoliative dermatitis, flushing, increased pigmentation, pallor, photophobia, pruritus, rash
Other: Acidosis, facial edema, hyperkalemia, hyperuricemia, lymphadenopathy, positive ANA titer, weight gain

Nursing Considerations
•Use betaxolol cautiously in patients with peripheral vascular disease. Assess color, temperature, and pulses of patient's arms and legs and ask about numbness or tingling and pain.
•Check blood pressure with patient lying, sitting, and standing before starting betaxolol therapy and periodically throughout day to detect changes.
•Review renal function test results before and during therapy.
•Closely monitor diabetic patient's blood glucose level for hypoglycemia because betaxolol may mask tachycardia, but not dizziness and diaphoresis. Be aware that betaxolol may mask tachycardia and blood pressure changes associated with hyperthyroidism.
•WARNING Avoid abrupt withdrawal of betaxolol, which can exacerbate or precipitate thyroid storm. Instead, expect to withdraw drug gradually and monitor patient closely.
•Expect to taper betaxolol over 2 weeks to prevent MI, ventricular arrhythmias, and,

possibly, death from catecholamine hypersensitivity caused by beta blocker therapy.
•If systolic pressure falls below 90 mm Hg, expect to discontinue drug and prepare for hemodynamic monitoring.
•Take safety precautions to prevent injury from falls caused by orthostatic hypotension.
PATIENT TEACHING
•Teach patient how to check her blood pressure, if appropriate. Also discuss signs and symptoms of hypertension and hypotension.
•Advise patient to avoid sudden position changes and to rise slowly from a sitting or lying position to minimize the effects of orthostatic hypotension.
•Advise patient to avoid driving and activities that require mental alertness until drug's CNS effects are known.
•Counsel patient to consult prescriber before using an OTC product, such as a cold remedy or nasal decongestant.

bethanechol chloride
Duvoid, PMS-Bethanechol chloride (CAN), Urabeth, Urecholine

Class and Category
Chemical class: Synthetic choline ester
Therapeutic class: Cholinergic, parasympathomimetic
Pregnancy category: C

Indications and Dosages
➤ *To treat postoperative and postpartal urine retention and retention caused by neurogenic atony of bladder*
TABLETS
Adults. 10 to 50 mg t.i.d. or q.i.d. *To determine minimum effective dose:* 5 to 10 mg repeated every hr until response is obtained or maximum of 50 mg is reached.
SUBCUTANEOUS INJECTION
Adults. 2.5 to 5 mg t.i.d. or q.i.d. *To determine minimum effective dose:* 2.5 mg repeated every 15 to 30 min until response is obtained or maximum of four doses is reached. Minimum effective dose may be repeated t.i.d. or q.i.d., p.r.n.

Route	Onset	Peak	Duration
P.O.	30 to 90 min	60 min	6 hr
SubQ	5 to 15 min	15 to 30 min	2 hr

Mechanism of Action
Acts directly on muscarinic receptors of the parasympathetic nervous system, increasing detrusor muscle tone in the bladder and allowing contraction strong enough to start voiding. Like natural neurotransmitter acetylcholine, bethanechol stimulates gastric motility, increases gastric tone, and enhances peristalsis.

Contraindications
Acute inflammatory lesions of GI tract, atrioventricular conduction defects, bronchial asthma, coronary artery disease, epilepsy, hypersensitivity to bethanecol or its components, hypertension, hyperthyroidism, hypotension, marked vagotonia, mechanical obstruction of GI or GU tract, Parkinson's disease, peptic ulcer disease, peritonitis, pronounced bradycardia, questionable integrity of GI or GU mucosa, spastic GI disorders, vasomotor instability

Interactions
DRUGS
cholinergic drugs: Possibly increased effects of bethanechol
ganglionic blockers: Possibly severe hypotension, usually first manifested by severe adverse GI reactions
procainamide, quinidine: Possibly decreased effects of bethanechol

Adverse Reactions
CNS: Headache, malaise
CV: Hypotension with reflex tachycardia, vasomotor response
EENT: Excessive salivation, lacrimation, miosis
GI: Abdominal cramps, colicky pain, diarrhea, eructation, nausea, vomiting
GU: Urinary urgency
RESP: Asthma attack, bronchoconstriction

Nursing Considerations
•Assess urine elimination before initiating bethanechol therapy.
•**WARNING** Be aware that patient must have functioning urinary sphincter because a sphincter that doesn't relax when bladder contracts can push urine up into renal pelvis and cause reflux infection.
•Give oral bethanechol 1 hour before or 2 hours after meals to reduce risk of nausea

and vomiting.
•**WARNING** Don't give bethanechol by I.M. or I.V. route because of risk of cholinergic overstimulation, which can cause abdominal cramps, bloody diarrhea, hypotension, shock, or sudden cardiac arrest. Always keep atropine nearby during subcutaneous administration.
PATIENT TEACHING
•Advise patient to take bethanechol on an empty stomach 1 hour before or 2 hours after meals to reduce risk of nausea and vomiting.

biperiden hydrochloride
Akineton

biperiden lactate
Akineton Lactate

Class and Category
Chemical class: Tertiary amine
Therapeutic class: Anticholinergic, antidyskinetic
Pregnancy category: C

Indications and Dosages
➤ *As adjunct to treat all forms of Parkinson's disease*
TABLETS
Adults. 2 mg t.i.d. or q.i.d up to 16 mg daily.
➤ *To control extrapyramidal symptoms (except tardive dyskinesia) caused by phenothiazines and other neuroleptic drugs*
TABLETS
Adults. 2 mg one to three times daily.
I.V. OR I.M. INJECTION
Adults. 2 mg repeated every 30 min until symptoms resolve or maximum of four consecutive doses in 24 hr is reached.

Route	Onset	Peak	Duration
I.V.	15 min	Unknown	1 to 8 hr
I.M.	10 to 30 min	Unknown	Unknown

Contraindications
Achalasia, bladder neck obstruction, hypersensitivity to biperiden, myasthenia gravis, narrow-angle glaucoma, prostatic hypertrophy, pyloric or duodenal obstruction, stenosing peptic ulcer, toxic megacolon

Mechanism of Action
Blocks acetylcholine's action at cholinergic receptor sites. This action restores the brain's normal dopamine and acetylcholine balance, which relaxes muscle movement and decreases rigidity and tremors. Biperiden also may inhibit dopamine reuptake and storage, which prolongs dopamine's action.

Interactions
DRUGS
amantadine: Possibly increased adverse anticholinergic effects
digoxin: Possibly increased serum digoxin level
haloperidol: Possibly increased schizophrenic symptoms, decreased serum haloperidol level, and development of tardive dyskinesia
levodopa: Possibly decreased levodopa effectiveness
phenothiazines: Possibly reduced phenothiazine effects and increased psychiatric symptoms

Adverse Reactions
CNS: Agitation, confusion, delirium, delusions, depression, disorientation, dizziness, drowsiness, euphoria, excitement, fever, hallucinations, headache, light-headedness, listlessness, memory loss, nervousness, paranoia, psychosis, weakness
CV: Hypotension, mild bradycardia, orthostatic hypotension, palpitations, tachycardia
EENT: Blurred vision, diplopia, dry mouth, increased intraocular pressure, mydriasis, narrow-angle glaucoma, suppurative parotitis
GI: Constipation, duodenal ulcer, epigastric distress, ileus, nausea, vomiting
GU: Dysuria, urinary hesitancy, urine retention
MS: Muscle spasms, muscle weakness
SKIN: Decreased sweating, dermatosis, flushing, rash, urticaria

Nursing Considerations
•Expect to administer I.V. or I.M. biperiden when patient needs more rapid response than oral drug can provide.
•Assess muscle rigidity and tremor as baseline. Then monitor them frequently for improvement, which indicates biperiden's effectiveness.
•**WARNING** When administering biperiden to patient with drug-induced extrapyramidal reactions, be alert for exacerbation of psychiatric symptoms.
PATIENT TEACHING
•Caution patient to avoid driving and other activities that require alertness until biperiden's CNS effects are known.
•**WARNING** Because biperiden decreases sweating, urge patient to avoid extremely hot and humid conditions to reduce risk of heatstroke and severe hyperthermia. This is especially important for elderly patients and those who abuse alcohol or have chronic illness or CNS disease.
•Emphasize the need for periodic eye examinations and intraocular pressure measurements because biperiden may cause narrow-angle glaucoma and increase intraocular pressure.

bisoprolol fumarate
Zebeta

Class and Category
Chemical class: Selective beta$_1$-adrenergic blocker
Therapeutic class: Antihypertensive
Pregnancy category: C

Indications and Dosages
➤ *To treat hypertension, alone or with other antihypertensives*
TABLETS
Adults. 5 mg daily, increased to 10 to 20 mg daily if blood pressure doesn't respond to lower dosage.
DOSAGE ADJUSTMENT Dosage reduced to 2.5 mg daily initially and increased gradually for patients who have impaired renal function and creatinine clearance of less than 40 ml/min/1.73 m^2 or who have impaired hepatic function, such as from cirrhosis or hepatitis.

Mechanism of Action
Inhibits stimulation of beta$_1$-receptors primarily in the heart, which decreases cardiac excitability, cardiac output, and myocardial oxygen demand. Bisoprolol also decreases renin release from kidneys, which helps reduce blood pressure.

Contraindications

Cardiogenic shock, heart failure unless caused by tachyarrhythmia, overt heart failure, second- or third-degree heart block, sinus bradycardia

Interactions

DRUGS

aluminum salts, barbiturates, calcium salts, cholestyramine, colestipol, NSAIDs, penicillins, rifampin, salicylates, sulfinpyrazone: Possibly decreased therapeutic and adverse effects of bisoprolol
beta blockers, digoxin: Increased risk of bradycardia
calcium channel blockers: Possibly increased therapeutic and adverse effects of bisoprolol
ciprofloxacin, quinolones: Possibly increased bioavailability of bisoprolol
clonidine: Possibly severe hypertension caused by withdrawal of clonidine or both drugs
epinephrine: Possibly hypertension followed by bradycardia
ergot alkaloids: Possibly peripheral ischemia and gangrene
flecainide: Possibly increased therapeutic and adverse effects of either drug
lidocaine: Possibly increased risk of lidocaine toxicity
oral contraceptives: Possibly increased bioavailability and plasma level of bisoprolol
prazosin: Possibly increased orthostatic hypotension
quinidine: Possibly increased effects of bisoprolol
sulfonylureas: Possibly masking of hypoglycemic symptoms

Adverse Reactions

CNS: Anxiety, confusion, depression, dizziness, emotional lability, fatigue, fever, hallucinations, headache, insomnia, malaise, nightmares, paresthesia, sleep disturbances, syncope, tremor, unsteadiness, vertigo
CV: Bradycardia, heart block, and other arrhythmias; chest pain; claudication; cold arms and legs; edema; heart failure; hypercholesterolemia; hyperlipidemia; hypotension; MI; orthostatic hypotension; palpitations; peripheral vascular insufficiency; renal and mesenteric artery thrombosis
EENT: Altered taste, blurred vision, dry mouth, eye pain or pressure, hearing loss, increased salivation, laryngospasm, pharyngitis, rhinitis, sinusitis, tinnitus
GI: Constipation, diarrhea, epigastric pain, gastritis, indigestion, ischemic colitis, nausea, vomiting
GU: Cystitis, decreased libido, impotence, Peyronie's disease, renal colic
HEME: Agranulocytosis, eosinophilia, leukopenia, thrombocytopenia, thrombocytopenic purpura
MS: Arthralgia, gout, muscle twitching, neck pain
RESP: Asthma, bronchitis, bronchospasm, cough, dyspnea, respiratory distress, upper respiratory tract infection
SKIN: Alopecia, dermatitis, diaphoresis, eczema, exfoliative dermatitis, flushing, pruritus, psoriasis, rash
Other: Angioedema, hyperkalemia, hyperuricemia, weight gain

Nursing Considerations

•Administer bisoprolol cautiously in patients with peripheral vascular disease because reduced cardiac output can cause or worsen arterial insufficiency. Assess patient's arms and legs for changes in color, temperature, and pulses; ask about numbness, tingling, and pain.
•Measure blood pressure with patient lying, sitting, and standing before initiating bisoprolol therapy and then every 4 to 8 hours, as appropriate, to evaluate effectiveness.
•If patient has diabetes, monitor closely for signs of hypoglycemia, which drug may mask.
•If patient has hyperthyroidism, watch for tachycardia and hypertension, which may be masked by bisoprolol.
•WARNING Keep in mind that abrupt withdrawal of bisoprolol may cause or worsen thyroid storm. During drug withdrawal, monitor patient closely.
•Expect to stop bisoprolol over 1 to 2 weeks to prevent MI, ventricular arrhythmias, and, possibly, death from catecholamine hypersensitivity caused by beta blocker therapy.
•If systolic blood pressure falls to less than 90 mm Hg, expect to discontinue drug. Prepare for hemodynamic monitoring, if needed.
•WARNING If patient is scheduled for surgery with general anesthesia, expect to discontinue bisoprolol about 48 hours beforehand to reduce risk of excessive myocardial depression during anesthesia.

PATIENT TEACHING
•Teach patient how to monitor her blood pressure, if appropriate, and to recognize signs of hypertension and hypotension.
•Instruct patient to avoid sudden position changes and to rise slowly from a sitting or lying position to minimize the effects of orthostatic hypotension.
•Advise patient to avoid driving and other activities that require mental alertness until bisoprolol's CNS effects are known.
•Instruct patient to contact prescriber before using any OTC product, such as a cold remedy or nasal decongestant.

bitolterol mesylate

Tornalate

Class and Category
Chemical class: Acid ester of colterol
Therapeutic class: Bronchodilator, sympathomimetic
Pregnancy category: C

Indications and Dosages
➤ *To prevent and treat asthma and other conditions associated with reversible bronchospasm, such as emphysema and chronic bronchitis*
INTERMITTENT AEROSOL SOLUTION
Adults and children age 12 and over. 1 mg of bitolterol diluted in 0.5 ml of normal saline solution and inhaled over 10 to 15 min t.i.d. *Maximum:* 8 mg daily.
CONTINUOUS AEROSOL SOLUTION
Adults and children age 12 and over. 2.5 mg of bitolterol diluted in 1.25 ml of normal saline solution and inhaled over 10 to 15 min t.i.d. *Maximum:* 14 mg daily.
METERED-DOSE INHALER
Adults and children age 12 and over. *To treat acute bronchospasm:* 2 inhalations over 1 to 3 min; then a third inhalation, if needed. *To prevent bronchospasm:* 2 inhalations every 8 hr not to exceed 3 inhalations every 6 hr or 2 inhalations every 4 hr.

Route	Onset	Peak	Duration
Aerosol, inhalation	In 2 to 3 min	30 to 60 min	6 to 8 hr
Metered-dose inhalation	3 to 5 min	30 min to 2 hr	4 to 8 hr

Mechanism of Action
Is hydrolyzed to active agent colterol (a long-acting agent that primarily affects beta$_2$-adrenergic receptors). Then it attaches to beta$_2$ receptors on bronchial cell membranes. This action stimulates the intracellular enzyme adenylate cyclase to convert adenosine triphosphate to cyclic adenosine monophosphate (cAMP). An increased intracellular level of cAMP relaxes bronchial smooth-muscle cells, stabilizes mast cells, and inhibits histamine release.

Incompatibilities
Don't mix bitolterol in inhalation solution with cromolyn sodium or acetylcysteine.

Contraindications
Hypersensitivity to bitolterol or its ingredients

Interactions
DRUGS
beta blockers: Possibly inhibition of bronchodilating effect of bitolterol
epinephrine, other sympathomimetic drugs: Possibly additive effects of either drug
MAO inhibitors, tricyclic antidepressants: Possibly potentiation of bitolterol's action on cardiovascular system

Adverse Reactions
CNS: Dizziness, fatigue, headache, hyperkinesia, insomnia, light-headedness, nervousness, paresthesia, somnolence, tremor, vertigo
CV: Chest pain, hypertension, irregular pulse, palpitations, tachycardia, transient ECG changes
EENT: Mouth and throat irritation, rhinitis
GI: Elevated liver function test results, nausea
HEME: Decreased hemoglobin level, hematocrit, and WBC count
RESP: Bronchospasm, cough

Nursing Considerations
•Assess respiratory rate, rhythm, and depth and breath sounds before, during, and after bitolterol therapy. Expect improved air movement and improvement in abnormal breath sounds.
•Because beta-adrenergic bronchodilators can significantly increase blood pressure and pulse rate, monitor them often.
•Expect therapy to begin with lowest effec-

tive dose because higher doses or more fre quent use may reduce drug effectiveness and cause paradoxical reactions or overdose.

PATIENT TEACHING
•Teach patient how to properly use and care for aerosol nebulizer or metered-dose inhaler. Before patient uses aerosol nebulizer, advise her to look for slight bubbling in solution-filled chamber and fine mist when nebulizer is turned on. Before patient uses inhaler for first time, instruct her to check that it's working properly by spraying it once in the air and looking for fine mist.
•Teach patient to mix nebulizer solution immediately before use. Afterward, he should clean nebulizer and solution chamber according to the manufacturer's recommendations.
•**WARNING** Advise patient not to use more than the recommended dosage of bitolterol; excessive use of sympathomimetic drugs may be fatal.
•Tell patient to wait 1 to 3 minutes between metered-dose inhalations.

bivalirudin

Angiomax

Class and Category
Chemical class: Hirudin analogue
Therapeutic class: Anticoagulant
Pregnancy category: B

Indications and Dosages
➤ *As adjunct to provide anticoagulation and prevent thrombosis in patients with unstable angina who are having percutaneous transluminal coronary angioplasty or percutaneous coronary intervention*

I.V. INFUSION
Adults. *Initial:* Immediately before angioplasty, 0.75-mg/kg bolus; then 1.75 mg/kg/hr as continuous infusion for duration of procedure. Five min after bolus dose and with continuous infusion running, another 0.3-mg/kg dose may be given if needed. After procedure, 1.75 mg/kg/hr may be given for 4 hr by continuous infusion, followed by 0.2 mg/kg/hr for up to 20 hr if needed.
DOSAGE ADJUSTMENT Infusion dosage possibly reduced to 1 mg/kg/hr for patients with severe renal impairment (glomerular filtra-

tion rate of 10 to 29 ml/min) and to 0.25 mg/kg/hr for patients undergoing dialysis.

Route	Onset	Peak	Duration
I.V.	Immediate	Unknown	1 hr after end of infusion

Mechanism of Action
Selectively binds to thrombin, including thrombin trapped in established clots. Without thrombin, fibrinogen can't convert to fibrin and clots can't form.

Incompatibilities
Don't mix other drugs in same I.V. line before or during bivalirudin administration. Mixing with alteplase, amiodarone, amphotericin B, chlorpromazine HCL, diazepam, prochlorperazine edisylate, reteplase, streptokinase, or vancomycin HCL can result in haze, particulate formation, or precipitation.

Contraindications
Active major bleeding, hypersensitivity to bivalirudin or its components

Interactions
DRUGS
alteplase, antineoplastics, antithymocyte globulin, heparin, NSAIDs, platelet inhibitors, reteplase, streptokinase, strontium chloride Sr 89, warfarin: Risk of bleeding
porfimer: Possibly decreased efficacy of porfimer photodynamic therapy
salicylates: Increased risk of hypoprothrombinemia and bleeding

Adverse Reactions
CNS: Headache, intracranial hemorrhage
CV: Hypotension, thrombosis (with gamma brachytherapy)
EENT: Epistaxis, gingival bleeding
GI: Abdominal cramps, diarrhea, GI or retroperitoneal bleeding, nausea, vomiting
GU: Hematuria, vaginal bleeding
MS: Back pain
RESP: Hemoptysis, hemothorax
SKIN: Ecchymosis
Other: Injection site bleeding, hematoma, or pain

Nursing Considerations
•To reconstitute bivalirudin, add 5 ml sterile

water for injection to 250-mg vial and swirl gently until dissolved. For initial infusion, dilute reconstituted vial in 50 ml of D_5W or normal saline solution to yield 5 mg/ml.
•For subsequent low-rate infusion, further dilute reconstituted drug in 500 ml of D_5W or normal saline solution to a final concentration of 0.5 mg/ml.
•Expect to give patient 300 to 325 mg of aspirin P.O. daily during bivalirudin therapy.
•WARNING Monitor blood coagulation tests before and regularly during therapy because bleeding is a major bivalirudin risk.
•WARNING Monitor patient often for bleeding because there's no antidote for bivalirudin. If life-threatening bleeding occurs, notify prescriber immediately, stop drug, and monitor APTT and other coagulation tests as ordered. Blood transfusions may be needed. Patients with increased bleeding risk include menstruating women; patients with vascular or organ abnormalities, such as severe uncontrolled hypertension, advanced renal disease, infective endocarditis, dissecting aortic aneurysm, diverticulitis, hemophilia, hepatic disease (especially from deficient vitamin K–dependent clotting factors), inflammatory bowel disease, or peptic ulcer disease; and those with recent stroke, major surgery (including eye, brain, or spinal cord), large vessel or lumbar puncture, organ biopsy, spinal anesthesia, or major bleeding (including intracranial, GI, intraocular, retroperitoneal, or pulmonary bleeding).
•If patient is receiving gamma brachytherapy, watch closely for evidence of thrombosis (weak or absent pulse, pallor, pain); use of bivalirudin may increase the risk in these patients.
•If possible, avoid I.M. injections of any kind to decrease the risk of bleeding.
•Discard any unused portion of drug.
PATIENT TEACHING
•Inform patient that bivalirudin is a blood thinner administered only in the hospital setting.
•Urge patient to check her skin for bruising or red spots and to immediately report back or stomach pain, trouble breathing, dizziness, fainting, and unusual bleeding (black, tarry stool; blood in urine; coughing blood; heavy menses; nosebleeds). Drug may be stopped.
•Encourage patient to reduce the risk of in-jury while receiving bivalirudin—as by brushing her teeth gently with a soft-bristled toothbrush.
•Caution patient not to take anti-inflammatories, such as ibuprofen, naproxen, ketoprofen, aspirin, and aspirin-like products, or other blood thinners, such as warfarin, while receiving bivalirudin unless directed.

bosentan

Tracleer

Class and Category
Chemical class: Endothelin receptor antagonist, pyrimidine derivative
Therapeutic class: Antihypertensive
Pregnancy category: X

Indications and Dosages
➤ *To treat pulmonary arterial hypertension in patients with World Health Organization class III or IV symptoms, to improve exercise ability, and to slow worsening of clinical condition*
TABLETS
Adults. *Initial:* 62.5 mg b.i.d. in the morning and evening for 4 wk. *Maintenance:* 125 mg b.i.d. in the morning and evening.
DOSAGE ADJUSTMENT For adults weighing less than 40 kg (88 lb), maintenance dosage is 62.5 mg b.i.d. morning and evening.

Contraindications
Hypersensitivity to bosentan or its components, concurrent use of cyclosporine or glyburide, pregnancy

Interactions
DRUGS
atorvastatin, lovastatin, simvastatin: Decreased blood level and efficacy of these drugs
cyclosporine: Markedly increased blood bosentan level
glyburide: Increased liver enzyme and possibly glucose levels; possibly decreased blood level of both drugs (and of other oral antidiabetics metabolized by CYP2C9 or CYP3A4)
hormonal contraceptives (oral, injected, implanted): Possibly decreased effects of these drugs
ketoconazole and other CYP3A4 inhibitors: Increased blood level and effects of bosentan

Mechanism of Action

Bosentan is an endothelin (ET) receptor antagonist that inhibits the effects of ET, a potent vasoconstrictor. ET, a neurohormone produced by endothelial cells that line blood vessels, normally increases during times of cardiovascular stress. Patients with pulmonary arterial hypertension have an abnormal increase in serum ET level.

ET binds with its receptors, ET_A and ET_B, which are located on endothelial and vascular smooth-muscle cells. When ET binds with these receptors, it causes vasoconstriction, as shown below left, and such long-term effects as fibrosis and hypertrophy. By binding to ET_A and ET_B receptors, as shown below right, bosentan blocks the vasoconstrictive effects of ET, causing pulmonary artery vasodilation and decreased pulmonary artery pressure. As a result, the patient experiences increased exercise tolerance and decreased breathlessness.

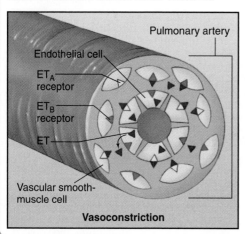

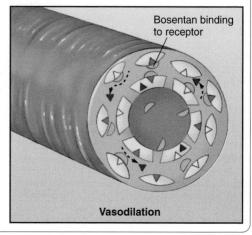

rifampicin: Possibly decreased blood bosentan level
tacrolimus: Possibly marked increase in blood bosentan level
warfarin: Increased elimination and decreased blood level of warfarin

Adverse Reactions

CNS: Fatigue, headache
CV: Edema, hypotension, palpitations
EENT: Nasopharyngitis
GI: Elevated liver function test results, hepatic injury, indigestion, liver failure
HEME: Decreased hemoglobin level and hematocrit, thrombocytopenia
SKIN: Flushing, pruritus, rash
Other: Hypersensitivity

Nursing Considerations

•Before giving bosentan, obtain baseline hemoglobin level and liver function test results, as ordered.

•WARNING Because bosentan use may cause major birth defects, make sure that female patient of childbearing age has had a negative pregnancy test before giving drug.
•WARNING Be aware that bosentan may put patient at risk for serious hepatic injury. Assess patient for signs and symptoms of hepatic dysfunction, including abdominal pain, fatigue, fever, jaundice, nausea, and vomiting. Monitor liver function test results every month, as ordered.
•Expect dosage to be adjusted or drug stopped if liver function test results become elevated. Expect treatment to be stopped if bilirubin level increases to twice the upper limit of normal (or higher) or if clinical symptoms occur in conjunction with liver function test elevations. Bosentan probably won't be prescribed for patients with moderate to severe hepatic dysfunction or for those with liver function test levels higher than three times the upper limit of normal.

B

•Monitor hemoglobin level 1 and 3 months after start of therapy and every 3 months thereafter, as ordered.

•Monitor patient's response to drug, and evaluate her activity tolerance.

PATIENT TEACHING

•**WARNING** Because major birth defects are associated with bosentan, caution female patient of childbearing age to have a urine or serum pregnancy test monthly during bosentan therapy to verify that she isn't pregnant. Advise her to notify prescriber immediately if she has a late or missed menstrual period. Instruct her to use a reliable nonhormonal method of contraception because bosentan may decrease effectiveness of hormonal contraceptives.

•Urge patient to immediately report signs or symptoms of hepatic dysfunction, including yellow skin or eyes, fever, nausea, vomiting, fatigue, and abdominal pain.

•Stress the importance of keeping appointments for follow-up testing so that drug's effects can be evaluated.

•Inform patient that bosentan is dispensed only by a special access program set up by the drug's manufacturer and isn't available from commercial pharmacies. Advise patient to allow for adequate delivery time when refilling prescription so that she doesn't run out of drug. Instruct her to review the medication guide that comes with each renewed prescription.

bretylium tosylate

Bretylate (CAN), Bretylol

Class and Category

Chemical class: Bromobenzyl quaternary ammonium compound
Therapeutic class: Class III antiarrhythmic
Pregnancy category: C

Indications and Dosages

➤ *To prevent and treat ventricular fibrillation and treat life-threatening ventricular arrhythmias that don't respond to first-line antiarrhythmics, such as lidocaine*

I.V. INFUSION, I.V. OR I.M. INJECTION

Adults with immediate life-threatening ventricular arrhythmias. *Initial:* 5 mg/kg, undiluted, by rapid I.V. injection; if ventricular fibrillation persists, 10 mg/kg repeated as often as needed. *Continuous suppression:* 1 to 2 mg/min or 5 to 10 mg/kg of diluted I.V. solution infused over at least 8 min every 6 hr.

Adults with other ventricular arrhythmias. *Initial:* 5 to 10 mg/kg of diluted I.V. solution infused over at least 8 min, repeated every 1 to 2 hr if arrhythmia continues; or 5 to 10 mg/kg undiluted I.M. injection, repeated every 1 to 2 hr if arrhythmia continues. *Maintenance:* 5 to 10 mg/kg diluted I.V. solution infused over at least 8 min every 6 hours, 1 to 2 mg/min infused continuously, or 5 to 10 mg/kg undiluted I.M. injection every 6 to 8 hr.

DOSAGE ADJUSTMENT Interval between dosages increased for patients with impaired renal function because bretylium is excreted primarily by kidneys.

Children with acute ventricular fibrillation. 5 mg/kg I.V. given over 8 to 10 min, followed by 10 mg/kg every 15 to 30 min up to total dose of 30 mg/kg. *Maintenance:* 5 to 10 mg/kg every 6 hr.

Children with other ventricular arrhythmias. 5 to 10 mg/kg every 6 hr.

Route	Onset	Peak	Duration
I.V.	5 to 10 min*	6 to 9 hr	6 to 24 hr
I.M.	20 to 60 min*	6 to 9 hr	6 to 24 hr

Contraindications

Digitalis toxicity, hypersensitivity to bretylium

Interactions

DRUGS

catecholamines (such as dopamine and norepinephrine): Increased vasopressor effects of catecholamines
digoxin: Possibly worsened digitalis toxicity

Adverse Reactions

CNS: Anxiety, confusion, dizziness, emotional lability, fever, lethargy, light-headedness, paranoia, psychosis, syncope, vertigo

CV: Angina, arrhythmias (including bradycardia and more frequent PVCs), hypotension, orthostatic hypotension, transient hypertension

---

* For suppression of ventricular fibrillation; 20 to 120 min for suppression of ventricular tachycardia.

Mechanism of Action
Bretylium prolongs the repolarization phase of the action potential and lengthens the effective refractory period, which helps terminate reentry arrhythmias. The drug also acts on adrenergic nerve terminals. Initially, it causes early release of norepinephrine, which increases the heart rate and blood pressure. Then it blocks the release of norepinephrine, as shown here. This reduces the heart rate and blood pressure. Bretylium also increases the ventricular threshold, making the ventricular myocardium less responsive to ectopic impulses and preventing ventricular fibrillation.

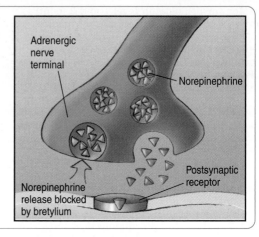

EENT: Mild conjunctivitis, nasal stuffiness
GI: Abdominal pain, diarrhea, hiccups, nausea, vomiting
GU: Renal impairment
RESP: Dyspnea
SKIN: Diaphoresis, erythematous macular rash, flushing
Other: Injection site pain

Nursing Considerations
•WARNING Use bretylium cautiously in patients with severe aortic stenosis or pulmonary hypertension because hypotension may occur.
•For I.V. infusion, dilute bretylium and administer at 1 to 2 mg/min.
•Dilute bretylium in compatible I.V. solution, such as D$_5$W, dextrose 5% in normal saline solution, dextrose 5% in lactated Ringer's solution, normal saline solution, 5% sodium bicarbonate, 20% mannitol, 1/6 molar sodium lactate, lactated Ringer's solution, calcium chloride in D$_5$W, and potassium chloride in D$_5$W.
•WARNING Be aware that patient may experience hypotension while supine. Have patient remain supine until tolerance develops. If her supine systolic blood pressure falls below 75 mm Hg, expect to give dopamine or norepinephrine and monitor her blood pressure closely because vasopressor effects are increased when these drugs are given together.
•Be alert for transient hypertension and increased frequency of arrhythmias because bretylium initially triggers release of norepi-

nephrine. Monitor patient's ECG tracings and blood pressure continuously, and notify prescriber of changes.
•Monitor blood bretylium level. Notify prescriber if level falls outside therapeutic range of 0.5 to 1.5 mcg/ml.
PATIENT TEACHING
•Advise patient to immediately report chest pain or pressure, pain at I.V. site, or rash.
•Warn patient that she may feel dizzy or light-headed even when lying down. Instruct her to remain supine and ask for help when attempting to move or sit up. Tell her that this sensation usually subsides in a few days.

bromocriptine mesylate

Alti-Bromocriptine (CAN), Apo-Bromocriptine (CAN), Parlodel, Parlodel SnapTabs

Class and Category
Chemical class: Ergot alkaloid derivative
Therapeutic class: Antidyskinetic, antihyperprolactinemic, dopamine-receptor agonist, growth hormone suppressant, infertility therapy adjunct
Pregnancy category: B

Indications and Dosages
➤ *To treat amenorrhea, galactorrhea, male hypogonadism, and infertility from hyperprolactinemia*
CAPSULES, TABLETS
Adults. *Initial:* 1.25 to 2.5 mg every at bedtime with snack. Increased by 2.5 mg every

3 to 7 days as needed to a total daily dose of 5 to 7.5 mg given in divided doses with snacks. *Maintenance:* 2.5 mg b.i.d. or t.i.d. with meals.

➤ *To treat prolactin-secreting adenoma*

CAPSULES, TABLETS

Adults and adolescents age 15 and over. *Initial:* 1.25 mg b.i.d. or t.i.d. with meals. Increased gradually over several weeks, if needed, to 10 to 20 mg daily in divided doses with meals. Some patients may need higher doses. *Maintenance:* 2.5 to 20 mg daily in divided doses with meals.

➤ *To treat Parkinson's disease*

CAPSULES, TABLETS

Adults. *Initial:* 1.25 mg every at bedtime with snack or b.i.d. with meals. Increased by 2.5 mg every 14 to 28 days, if needed. *Maintenance:* 2.5 to 40 mg daily in divided doses with meals.

➤ *To treat acromegaly*

CAPSULES, TABLETS

Adults and children age 15 and over. *Initial:* 1.25 to 2.5 mg every at bedtime with snack for 3 days. Then increased by 1.25 to 2.5 mg every 3 to 7 days, if needed, up to 30 mg daily. *Maintenance:* Usually 10 to 30 mg daily at bedtime with snack or in divided doses with meals.

Route	Onset	Peak	Duration
P.O.*	2 hr	8 hr	24 hr
P.O.†	30 to 90 min	2 hr	Unknown
P.O.‡	1 to 2 hr	4 to 8 wk	4 to 8 hr

Mechanism of Action

Inhibits release of prolactin and growth hormone from the anterior pituitary gland, thus restoring testicular or ovarian function and suppressing lactation. Bromocriptine decreases dopamine turnover in the CNS, depleting dopamine or blocking its receptors in the brain, alleviating dyskinesia.

---

* For amenorrhea, galactorrhea, male hypogonadism, infertility from hyperprolactinemia, and prolactin-secreting adenoma.
† For Parkinson's disease.
‡ For acromegaly.

Contraindications

Hypersensitivity to bromocriptine, other ergot alkaloids, or their components; severe ischemic heart disease or peripheral vascular disease

Interactions

DRUGS

antihypertensives: Increased hypotensive effects
clarithromycin, erythromycin, troleandomycin: Increased risk of bromocriptine toxicity
ergot alkaloids or derivatives: Increased risk of hypertension
haloperidol, loxapine, MAO inhibitors, methyldopa, metoclopramide, molindone, phenothiazines, pimozide, reserpine, risperidone, thioxanthenes: Increased serum prolactin level, decreased bromocriptine effectiveness
levodopa: Additive effects requiring reduced levodopa dose
ritonavir: Increased blood bromocriptine level

ACTIVITIES

alcohol use: Possibly disulfiram-like reaction

Adverse Reactions

CNS: Dizziness, drowsiness, fatigue, headache, light-headedness, syncope
CV: Hypertension, hypotension, orthostatic hypotension, Raynaud's phenomenon
EENT: Dry mouth, nasal congestion
GI: Abdominal cramps, anorexia, constipation, diarrhea, GI bleeding, indigestion, nausea, vomiting

Nursing Considerations

•Use bromocriptine cautiously if patient has a history of psychosis or cardiovascular disease, especially after MI with residual arrhythmia.
•Expect to perform a pregnancy test every 4 weeks during the amenorrheic period. Once menses resume, test whenever a period is missed, as ordered.
•Plan to withhold bromocriptine if patient becomes pregnant.
•If a rapidly expanding adenoma needs continued therapy, watch closely for hypertensive crisis.
•Be aware that bromocriptine shouldn't be given postpartum if patient has a history of coronary artery disease or other severe cardiovascular problem unless risk of withdrawing drug is greater than risk of use. If so, monitor closely for signs and symptoms of CV dysfunction, such as chest pain.
•Expect to give bromocriptine with levodopa

if patient is being treated for Parkinson's disease.
• Assess for hypotension when therapy starts and hypertension (typically during second week). Monitor blood pressure often if patient takes other antihypertensives.
• If patient has a history of peptic ulcer or GI bleeding, watch for new bleeding.
• Take safety precautions, such as keeping the bed in low position with side rails up, because bromocriptine can cause dizziness, drowsiness, light-headedness, and syncope.

PATIENT TEACHING
• Tell patient to take each dose with a meal, milk, or a snack to minimize nausea.
• Caution patient about possible dizziness, drowsiness, and light-headedness.
• Advise patient to avoid sudden position changes to minimize orthostatic hypotension.
• Warn patient to avoid alcohol while taking bromocriptine because it may cause disulfiram-like reactions, such as chest pain, confusion, a fast or pounding heartbeat, facial flushing, diaphoresis, nausea, vomiting, a throbbing headache, blurred vision, and severe weakness.
• Tell patient to take a missed dose as soon as she remembers it, unless it's almost time for the next dose. In that case, tell her to wait until the next scheduled dose. Warn her not to double the dose. Advise her to contact her prescriber if she misses more than one dose.
• Urge patient to report adverse reactions, such as an unremitting headache, nausea, vomiting, or other signs of CNS toxicity.
• Tell patient who takes large doses of bromocriptine to schedule regular dental check-ups because the drug can decrease salivary flow, which may encourage dental caries, periodontal disease, oral candidiasis, and discomfort.
• Tell patient with acromegaly to keep her fingers warm to prevent cold-sensitive digital vasospasm.

budesonide

Entocort EC, Pulmicort Flexhaler, Pulmicort Respules, Pulmicort Turbuhaler, Rhinocort, Rhinocort Aqua, Rhinocort Turbuhaler (CAN)

Class and Category
Chemical class: Glucocorticoid

Therapeutic class: Antiasthmatic, anti-inflammatory
Pregnancy category: B

Indications and Dosages
➤ *To manage symptoms of seasonal or perennial allergic rhinitis*
NASAL AEROSOL
Adults and children over age 6. 64 mcg in each nostril b.i.d. or 128 mcg in each nostril daily. *Maximum:* 256 mcg daily. *Maintenance:* Lowest dosage that controls symptoms.
NASAL POWDER
Adults and children over age 6. 200 mcg in each nostril daily. *Maximum:* 800 mcg daily (adults and adolescents); 400 mcg daily (children). *Maintenance:* Lowest dosage that controls symptoms.
NASAL SUSPENSION
Adults and children over age 6. 32 mcg in each nostril daily. *Maximum:* 256 mcg daily (adults and adolescents); 128 mcg daily (children). *Maintenance:* Lowest dosage that controls symptoms.

➤ *To manage symptoms of perennial non-allergic rhinitis*
NASAL AEROSOL
Adults and adolescents. 64 mcg in each nostril b.i.d. or 128 mcg in each nostril daily. *Maximum:* 256 mcg daily. *Maintenance:* Lowest dosage that controls symptoms.
NASAL POWDER
Adults and adolescents. 200 mcg in each nostril daily. *Maximum:* 800 mcg daily. *Maintenance:* Lowest dosage that controls symptoms.

➤ *To provide maintenance therapy in chronic bronchial asthma*
ORAL INHALATION
Adults previously on bronchodilators alone. 1 or 2 inhalations (200 to 400 mcg) b.i.d. *Maximum:* 800 mcg daily.
Adults previously on inhaled corticosteroids. 1 or 2 inhalations (200 to 400 mcg) b.i.d. *Maximum:* 800 mcg b.i.d. as needed and tolerated.
Adults previously on systemic corticosteroids. 2 to 4 inhalations (400 to 800 mcg) b.i.d. *Maximum:* 1,600 mcg daily.
Children age 6 and over. 1 inhalation (200 mcg) b.i.d. *Maximum:* 400 mcg b.i.d. as needed and tolerated.
ORAL INHALATION (PULMICORT FLEXHALER)

Adults and adolescents age 18 and over. *Initial:* 180 or 360 mcg b.i.d., increased as needed. *Maximum:* 720 mcg b.i.d.
Children ages 6 to 17. *Initial:* 180 or 360 mcg b.i.d. *Maximum:* 360 mcg b.i.d.

➤ *To prevent or provide maintenance therapy in chronic bronchial asthma*
NEBULIZED INHALATION (PULMICORT RESPULES)
Children ages 1 to 8 previously on bronchodilators alone. 0.25 mg b.i.d. or 0.5 mg daily by jet nebulizer. *Maximum:* 0.5 mg/day.
Children ages 1 to 8 previously on inhaled steroids. 0.25 mg b.i.d. or 0.5 mg daily inhaled by jet nebulizer. *Maximum:* 1 mg daily.
Children ages 1 to 8 previously on systemic corticosteroids. 0.5 mg b.i.d. or 1 mg daily inhaled by jet nebulizer. *Maximum:* 1 mg daily.

➤ *To treat mild to moderate active Crohn's disease involving the ileum, the ascending colon, or both*
CAPSULES
Adults. 9 mg daily in the morning for 8 weeks.

➤ *To maintain clinical remission of mild to moderate Crohn's disease involving the ileum, the ascending colon, or both*
CAPSULES
Adults. 6 mg daily in the morning for up to 3 months.
DOSAGE ADJUSTMENT Dosage reduced for patients with heptic insufficiency and those taking ketoconazole or other CYP3A4 inhibitor.

Route	Onset	Peak	Duration
Nasal aerosol	10 hr to 3 days	3 days to 3 wk	Unknown
Nasal powder or suspension, oral inhalation	In 4 wk	Unknown	Unknown
Nebulized inhalation	2 to 8 days	4 to 6 wk	Unknown
Oral capsules	Unknown	30 min to 10 hr	Unknown

Contraindications
Hypersensitivity to budesonide or its components, recent septal ulcers or nasal surgery or trauma (nasal spray); status asthmaticus or other acute asthma episodes (oral inhalation)

Mechanism of Action
Inhibits inflammatory cells and mediators, possibly by decreasing their influx into nasal passages or bronchial walls. As a result, nasal or airway inflammation decreases. Oral inhalation form also inhibits mucus secretion in airways, decreasing the amount and viscosity of sputum.

B

Interactions
DRUGS
clarithromycin, erythromycin, itraconazole, ketoconazole, other CYP3A4 inhibitors: Possibly increased blood budesonide level

Adverse Reactions
CNS: Amnesia, asthenia, dizziness, fatigue, fever, headache
EENT: Bad taste, cataracts, dry mouth, epistaxis, glaucoma, nasal irritation, oral or pharyngeal candidiasis, pharyngitis, rhinitis, sinusitis
ENDO: Growth suppression in children
GI: Abdominal pain, diarrhea, dyspepsia, flatulence, indigestion, nausea, vomiting
GU: UTI
MS: Arthralgia, back pain
RESP: Increased cough, respiratory tract infection
SKIN: Purpura, urticaria

Nursing Considerations
• Use budesonide cautiously if patient has tubercular infection; untreated fungal, bacterial, or systemic viral infection; or ocular herpes simplex.
• Closely monitor a child's growth pattern; budesonide may stunt growth.
• **WARNING** Assess patient who switches from a systemic corticosteroid to inhaled budesonide for adrenal insufficiency (fatigue, hypotension, lassitude, nausea, vomiting, weakness), which may be life-threatening. Hypothalamic-pituitary-adrenal axis function may take several months to recover after systemic corticosteroids stop. Stopping budesonide abruptly may cause adrenal insufficiency.
• Administer Respules by jet nebulizer connected to an air compressor.
• Patient exposed to chickenpox may receive varicella zoster immune globulin or pooled I.V. immunoglobulin. If chickenpox develops, give antiviral as ordered. A patient exposed

to measles may need pooled I.M. immuno-globulin.

•Assess patient for effectiveness of budesonide therapy, especially if patient is being weaned from a systemic corticosteroid. If patient has increased symptoms of asthma or an immunologic condition previously suppressed by the systemic corticosteroid—such as rhinitis, conjunctivitis, an eosinophilic condition, eczema, or arthritis—notify prescriber.

•Be aware that Pulmicort Flexhaler contains small amounts of lactose, which may trigger coughing, wheezing, or bronachospasm in a patient with a severe milk-protein allergy.

PATIENT TEACHING

•Urge patient taking oral capsules to swallow them whole and not to chew or break them.

•Instruct patient who uses nasal spray to shake container before each use. Instruct her to blow her nose, tilt her head slightly forward, and insert tube into a nostril, pointing toward inner corner of eye, away from nasal septum. Tell her to hold the other nostril closed and spray while inhaling gently. Then have her repeat in the other nostril.

•Instruct patient to prime oral inhaler before using it for first time by holding canister upright with mouthpiece on top and then twisting base of device fully to the right and then fully to the left until it clicks. Teach patient to load each subsequent dose just before use in the same manner. After loading a dose, caution patient not to shake device or blow into it. Instruct patient to turn her head away from device and exhale. Then have her hold device upright, place her lips around mouthpiece, and inhale deeply. The device will discharge a dose. Tell patient to remove her lips from mouthpiece to exhale.

•Caution patient not to use an oral inhaler with a spacer device.

•Advise patient to rinse her mouth with water after each dose and to spit the water out. Tell her to contact her prescriber if she develops a mouth or throat infection.

•Instruct patient not to use budesonide as a rescue inhaler.

•Instruct patient to contact prescriber if symptoms persist or have worsened after 3 weeks. Caution against increasing the dose on her own.

•Inform parents of small children using neb-ulized Respules that improvement may begin within 2 to 8 days but that full effect may not be evident for 4 to 6 weeks.

•Caution patient to avoid exposure to chickenpox and measles and, if exposed, to contact prescriber immediately.

•Caution against stopping budesonide abruptly.

•Instruct patient on long-term therapy to have regular eye examinations.

•Urge female patient to notify the prescriber if she is or could be pregnant.

bumetanide

Bumex

Class and Category

Chemical class: Sulfonamide derivative
Therapeutic class: Loop diuretic
Pregnancy category: C

Indications and Dosages

➤ *To treat edema caused by heart failure, hepatic disease, and renal disease, including nephrotic syndrome*

TABLETS

Adults. 0.5 to 2 mg daily, increased as needed, with a second or third dose every 4 to 5 hr or 0.5 to 2 mg every other day or daily for 3 or 4 days each week. *Maximum:* 10 mg daily.

I.V. INFUSION, I.V. OR I.M. INJECTION

Adults. 0.5 to 1 mg over 1 to 2 min daily, increased p.r.n. with a second or third dose every 2 to 3 hr. *Maximum:* 10 mg daily.

DOSAGE ADJUSTMENT Continuous infusion (12 mg over 12 hr) may be more effective and less toxic than intermittent infusion in patients with severe chronic renal insufficiency.

Route	Onset	Peak	Duration
P.O.	30 to 60 min	1 to 2 hr	4 to 6 hr
I.V.	In min	15 to 30 min	3.5 to 4 hr

Mechanism of Action

Inhibits the reabsorption of sodium, chloride, and water in the ascending limb of the loop of Henle, which promotes their excretion and reduces fluid volume.

Contraindications

Anuria, hepatic coma, hypersensitivity to bumetanide or its components, severe electrolyte depletion

Interactions

DRUGS

aminoglycosides: Increased risk of ototoxicity
antihypertensives: Increased antihypertensive effect
indomethacin: Slowed increase in urine and sodium excretion, inhibited plasma renin activity
lithium: Reduced lithium renal clearance, increased risk of lithium toxicity
probenecid: Reduced sodium excretion

Adverse Reactions

CNS: Dizziness, encephalopathy, headache
CV: Hypotension
EENT: Ototoxicity
ENDO: Hyperglycemia
GI: Nausea
GU: Azotemia, elevated serum creatinine level
MS: Muscle spasms
Other: Hyperuricemia, hypocalcemia, hypochloremia, hypokalemia, hyponatremia, hypovolemia

Nursing Considerations

•WARNING Know that a patient who is hypersensitive to sulfonamides may be hypersensitive to bumetanide. Monitor such a patient closely when starting therapy.
•Expect to use the parenteral route for patients with impaired GI absorption or in whom the oral route isn't practical. Switch to the oral route, as prescribed, as soon as possible.
•Discard unused parenteral solution 24 hours after preparation.
•Assess fluid and electrolyte balance closely because bumetanide is a potent diuretic (40 to 60 times more potent than furosemide). Monitor fluid intake and output once every 8 hours, evaluate serum electrolyte levels when ordered, and assess for imbalances.
•WARNING Be aware that high-dose or too-frequent administration can cause profound diuresis and water and electrolyte depletion, especially in elderly patients.
•Monitor serum potassium level regularly to check for hypokalemia, especially if patient takes a digitalis glycoside for heart failure or

has hepatic cirrhosis, ascites, aldosteronism, potassium-losing nephropathy, diarrhea, or a history of ventricular arrhythmias.
•Assess for signs of ototoxicity, such as tinnitus, daily. Rarely, bumetanide may cause ototoxicity, especially with I.V. administration, high doses, and increased frequency of dosing in a patient with renal impairment.
•Monitor results of renal function tests during therapy to detect adverse reactions.

PATIENT TEACHING

•Advise patient to avoid potentially hazardous activities until drug's CNS effects are known.
•Stress the importance of monitoring fluid intake and output and watching for signs and symptoms of electrolyte imbalances, such as dizziness, headache, and muscle spasms.
•Review adverse reactions, and tell patient to notify prescriber about severe or persistent reactions.
•Review potassium-rich foods, and encourage patient to include them in her daily diet.
•Encourage patient to return for appropriate follow-up care, especially if she's receiving bumetanide for a chronic condition.
•Tell diabetic patient to monitor blood glucose level regularly and to notify prescriber if hyperglycemia persistently occurs.

buprenorphine hydrochloride

Buprenex, Subutex

Class, Category, and Schedule

Chemical class: Opioid, thebaine derivative
Therapeutic class: Opioid analgesic
Pregnancy category: C
Controlled substance schedule: V

Indications and Dosages

➤ *To control moderate to severe pain*
I.V OR I.M. INJECTION
Adults and children age 12 and over. 0.3 mg every 6 hr or more, p.r.n. A second 0.3-mg dose given 30 to 60 min after first dose, if needed.
DOSAGE ADJUSTMENT In patients not at high risk for opioid toxicity, I.M. dose increased to 0.6 mg or frequency increased to every 4 hr, if needed, depending on pain severity and patient response. I.V. or I.M. dose re-

duced by half in elderly or debilitated patients and in those who have respiratory disease or also use another CNS depressant.
Children ages 2 to 12. 0.002 to 0.006 mg/kg every 4 to 6 hr, p.r.n.

➤ *To treat opioid dependence*
S.L. TABLETS
Adults. 12 to 16 mg daily.

Route	Onset	Peak	Duration
I.V.	Under 15 min	Under 1 hr	6 to 10 hr*
I.M.	15 min	1 hr	6 to 10 hr*

Mechanism of Action
May bind with CNS receptors to alter the perception of and emotional response to pain. Buprenorphine may act by displacing narcotic agonists from their binding sites and competitively inhibiting their actions.

Incompatibilities
Don't administer I.V. buprenorphine through the same I.V. line as diazepam or lorazepam.

Contraindications
Hypersensitivity to buprenorphine or its components

Interactions
DRUGS
CNS depressants, MAO inhibitors: Additive hypotensive and respiratory and CNS depressant effects of these drugs
opioid analgesics: Reduced therapeutic effects if buprenorphine is given before another narcotic analgesic

Adverse Reactions
CNS: Dizziness, headache, sedation, vertigo
CV: Bradycardia, hypertension, hypotension
EENT: Miosis
GI: Nausea, vomiting
RESP: Bronchospasm, hypoventilation
SKIN: Diaphoresis, pruritus, rash, urticaria
Other: Anaphylaxis; angioedema; injection site pain, redness, and swelling

Nursing Considerations
• Use buprenorphine cautiously in patients

---

* 4 to 5 hr in children ages 2 to 12.

with severe hepatic or renal impairment, myxedema, hypothyroidism, adrenal insufficiency, CNS depression, coma, toxic psychosis, prostatic hypertrophy, urethral stricture, acute alcoholism, alcohol withdrawal syndrome, kyphoscoliosis, or biliary tract dysfunction. Also use cautiously in patients who receive a drug that decreases hepatic clearance, are known drug abusers, or have been addicted to narcotics.
• Use drug cautiously in patients with head injury, intracranial lesions, or other conditions that could increase CSF pressure.
• To avoid causing withdrawal, buprenorphine shouldn't be given for opioid dependence until signs of withdrawal are evident.
• Administer I.V. form over at least 2 minutes.
• Inspect injection site for local reactions; don't use the same site twice.
• Monitor vital signs and response to drug often, especially after giving first dose.
PATIENT TEACHING
• Instruct patient taking S.L. form to place tablets under her tongue until they dissolve. If patient takes more than two tablets per dose, tell her to place all tablets under her tongue at the same time. If they won't fit, tell her to place two at a time under her tongue until full dose has dissolved. Caution her not to swallow the tablets.

bupropion hydrochloride
Wellbutrin, Wellbutrin SR, Wellbutrin XL, Zyban

bupropion hydrobromide
Aplenzin

Class and Category
Chemical class: Aminoketone derivative
Therapeutic class: Antidepressant, smoking cessation adjunct
Pregnancy category: C

Indications and Dosages
➤ *To treat depression*
E.R. TABLETS (WELLBUTRIN SR)
Adults. *Initial:* 150 mg daily in the morning for 3 days; then 150 mg b.i.d. and, after several weeks, 200 mg b.i.d., as needed and tolerated. *Maximum:* 400 mg daily or 200 mg/dose.
E.R. TABLETS (WELLBUTRIN XL)
Adults. *Initial:* 150 mg daily in the morning

for at least 3 days; then 300 mg daily and, after 4 wk, 450 mg daily, as needed and tolerated. *Maximum:* 450 mg daily.

E.R. TABLETS (APLENZIN)
Adults. *Initial:* 174 mg daily in the morning for 3 days. Then, if tolerated well, dosage increased to 348 mg daily in the morning. After 4 wk of therapy, dosage increased to 522 mg daily in the morning, if needed.

TABLETS
Adults. *Initial:* 100 mg b.i.d., increased after 3 or more days to 100 mg t.i.d., as needed. *Maximum:* 450 mg daily or 150 mg/dose.

➤ *To aid in smoking cessation*
E.R. TABLETS
Adults. *Initial:* 150 mg daily for 3 days and then 150 mg b.i.d. for 7 to 12 wk. *Maximum:* 300 mg daily or 150 mg/dose.

➤ *To prevent seasonal major depressive episodes in patient with seasonal affective disorder*
E.R. TABLETS
Adults. *Initial:* 150 mg once daily in morning starting in autumn, increased after 1 wk to 300 mg once daily in morning, if tolerated and needed. Decreased to 150 mg once daily 2 wk before stopping drug in early spring.
DOSAGE ADJUSTMENT For patients with severe hepatic cirrhosis, no more than 75 mg daily of Wellbutrin, 100 mg daily or 150 mg every other day of Wellbutrin SR, 150 mg every other day of Wellbutrin XL or Zyban, and 174 mg every other day of Aplenzin. In renal impairment, dosage or frequency decreased on an individual basis.

Route	Onset	Peak	Duration
P.O.	1 to 3 wk	Unknown	Unknown

Mechanism of Action
May inhibit norepinephrine, serotonin, and dopamine uptake by neurons, which significantly relieves evidence of depression.

Contraindications
Anorexia, bulimia, use of another form of bupropion, hypersensitivity to bupropion or its components, seizure disorder, treatment requiring abrupt discontinuation of alcohol or sedatives (including benzodiazepines), use within 14 days of an MAO inhibitor

Interactions
DRUGS
amantadine, levodopa: Increased adverse reactions to bupropion
carbamazepine, cimetidine, phenobarbital, phenytoin: Increased bupropion metabolism
clozapine, fluoxetine, haloperidol, lithium, loxapine, maprotiline, molindone, phenothiazines, thioxanthenes, trazodone, tricyclic antidepressants: Increased risk of major motor seizures
levodopa: Increased adverse bupropion effects
MAO inhibitors: Increased risk of acute bupropion toxicity
nicotine: Possibly increased blood pressure
warfarin: Possibly altered PT and INR; risk of hemorrhagic or thrombotic complications
ACTIVITIES
alcohol use, recreational drug abuse: Lowered seizure threshold

Adverse Reactions
CNS: Agitation, akathisia, anxiety, asthenia, CNS stimulation, coma, confusion, decreased concentration or memory, delusions, dizziness, euphoria, fever, general or migraine headache, hallucinations, hostility, insomnia, irritability, nervousness, paranoia, paresthesia, seizures, sleep disorder, somnolence, stroke, suicidal ideation, syncope, tremor, vertigo
CV: Arrhythmias, chest pain, complete AV block, hypertension, MI, orthostatic hypotension, palpitations, phlebitis, tachycardia, vasodilation
EENT: Altered taste, amblyopia, blurred vision, dry mouth, hearing loss, increased ocular pressure, pharyngitis, sinusitis, taste perversion, tinnitus
ENDO: Hyperglycemia, hypoglycemia, syndrome of inappropriate ADH secretion
GI: Abdominal pain, anorexia, constipation, diarrhea, dysphagia, flatulence, GI hemorrhage, GI ulceration, hepatitis, increased appetite, intestinal perforation, nausea, pancreatitis, vomiting
GU: Urinary frequency and urgency, UTI, vaginal hemorrhage
HEME: Anemia, leukocytosis, leukopenia, lym-phadenopathy, pancytopenia, thrombocytopenia
MS: Arthralgia, arthritis, muscle twitching, myalgia, rhabdomyolysis

RESP: Bronchospasm, cough, pulmonary embolism
SKIN: Diaphoresis, exfoliative dermatitis, flushing, pruritus, rash, urticaria
Other: Angioedema, generalized pain, hot flashes, infection, serum sicknesslike reaction, weight loss

Nursing Considerations

•Use cautiously in patients with renal impairment; drug is excreted by the kidneys.
•Monitor children, adolescents, and depressed patients closely for worsened depression and increased suicide risk, especially when therapy starts or dosage changes.
•To reduce the risk of seizures, allow at least 4 hours between doses of bupropion tablets and 8 hours between doses of E.R. tablets.
•Use seizure precautions, especially in patients who take OTC stimulants or anorectics; use excessive alcohol or sedatives; are addicted to opioids, cocaine, or stimulants; take drugs that lower the seizure threshold; have a history of seizures, head trauma, or CNS tumors; have severe hepatic cirrhosis; or take insulin or an oral antidiabetic.
•Using transdermal nicotine with bupropion may cause hypertension. Watch closely.

PATIENT TEACHING
•Advise patient to take bupropion for 7 or more days before stopping smoking.
•Tell patient to swallow E.R. tablets whole and not to cut, crush, or chew them.
•Tell patient to take bupropion with food.
•Urge patient to avoid or minimize consuming alcohol and sedatives during therapy and not to stop drug abruptly because seizures may occur.
•Urge caregivers to monitor depressed patient closely for worsened depression, especially when therapy starts or dosage changes.

buspirone hydrochloride

BuSpar, BuSpar DIVIDOSE, Bustab (CAN)

Class and Category

Chemical class: Azaspirodecanedione
Therapeutic class: Antianxiety
Pregnancy category: B

Indications and Dosages

➤ *To manage anxiety*
TABLETS
Adults. *Initial:* 5 mg t.i.d. or 7.5 mg b.i.d. in-

creased by 5 mg daily at 2- to 3-day intervals until desired response occurs. *Maintenance:* 20 to 30 mg daily (usual therapeutic range). *Maximum:* 60 mg daily.

DOSAGE ADJUSTMENT When used with nefazodone, dosage as little as 2.5 mg daily.

Route	Onset	Peak	Duration
P.O.	1 to 4 wk	3 to 6 wk	Unknown

Mechanism of Action

May act as a partial agonist at serotonin 5-hydroxytryptamine$_{1A}$ receptors in the brain, producing antianxiety effects.

Contraindications

Hypersensitivity to buspirone or its components, severe hepatic or renal impairment

Interactions

DRUGS
diltiazem, erythromycin, itraconazole, nefazodone, nordiazepam, verapamil: Increased blood level and adverse effects of buspirone
haloperidol: Increased blood haloperidol level
hepatic enzyme CYP3A4 inducers, such as dexamethasone and certain anticonvulsants (phenytoin, phenobarbital, carbamazepine): Possibly increased rate of buspirone metabolism
hepatic enzyme CYP3A4 inhibitors, such as ketoconazole and ritonavir: Possibly inhibited buspirone metabolism and increased blood level
MAO inhibitors: Increased risk of hypertension
rifampin: Decreased blood buspirone level and pharmacodynamic effects

FOODS
food: Possibly decreased clearance of buspirone
grapefruit juice: Increased blood buspirone level

Adverse Reactions

CNS: Akathisia, anger, ataxia, cogwheel rigidity, confusion, decreased concentration, depression, dizziness, dream disturbances, drowsiness, dyskinesias, dystonia, excitement, extrapyramidal symptoms, fatigue, headache, hostility, insomnia, lack of coordi-

nation, light-headedness, mood swings, nervousness, paresthesia, parkinsonism, restless leg syndrome, restlessness, serotonin syndrome, transient recall impairment, tremor, weakness
CV: Chest pain, palpitations, tachycardia
EENT: Blurred vision, dry mouth, nasal congestion, pharyngitis, tinnitus, tunnel vision
GI: Abdominal or gastric distress, constipation, diarrhea, nausea, vomiting
GU: Urine retention
MS: Myalgia
SKIN: Diaphoresis, ecchymosis, rash, urticaria
Other: Angioedema

Nursing Considerations
• Use buspirone cautiously in patients with hepatic or renal impairment.
• Institute safety precautions because of possible adverse CNS reactions.
• Follow closely if patient is being withdrawn from long-term therapy with benzodiazepines or other sedative-hypnotic drugs while starting buspirone therapy because buspirone won't prevent withdrawal symptoms.

PATIENT TEACHING
• Advise patient to take buspirone consistently, either always with or always without food.
• Caution patient to avoid drinking large amounts of grapefruit juice.
• Inform patient that 1 to 2 weeks of therapy may be needed before she notices drug's antianxiety effect.
• Stress the importance of not taking more buspirone than prescribed.
• Advise patient to avoid potentially hazardous activities until drug's CNS effects are known.

butabarbital sodium

Busodium, Butalan, Butisol, Sarisol No. 2

Class, Category, and Schedule
Chemical class: Barbiturate
Therapeutic class: Sedative-hypnotic
Pregnancy category: D
Controlled substance schedule: III

Indications and Dosages
➤ *To provide daytime sedation*
ELIXIR, TABLETS

Adults. 15 to 30 mg t.i.d. or q.i.d.
➤ *To treat insomnia*
ELIXIR, TABLETS
Adults. 50 to 100 mg every at bedtime.
➤ *To provide preoperative sedation*
ELIXIR, TABLETS
Adults. 50 to 100 mg 60 to 90 min before surgery.
Children. 2 to 6 mg/kg. *Maximum:* 100 mg/dose.
DOSAGE ADJUSTMENT Dosage reduced in patients with impaired renal or hepatic function and in elderly or debilitated patients because they may be more sensitive to drug.

Route	Onset	Peak	Duration
P.O.	45 to 60 min	Unknown	6 to 8 hr

Mechanism of Action
Inhibits the upward conduction of nerve impulses in the brain's reticular formation, which disrupts impulse transmission to the cortex. As a result, butabarbital depresses the CNS and produces drowsiness, sedation, and hypnosis.

Contraindications
History of addiction to sedative or hypnotic drug, hypersensitivity to butabarbital or its components, porphyria, severe hepatic or respiratory disease

Interactions
DRUGS
acetaminophen: Increased risk of hepatotoxicity (with large doses of or long-term therapy with butabarbital)
activated charcoal: Reduced butabarbital absorption
carbamazepine: Decreased blood carbamazepine level
chloramphenicol, corticosteroids, digitalis glycosides: Increased metabolism and decreased effects of these drugs
clonazepam: Increased clearance and reduced efficacy of clonazepam
CNS depressants, including OTC sedatives and hypnotics: Additive CNS depression
doxycycline: Shortened half-life and decreased effects of doxycycline
fenoprofen: Reduced bioavailability and ef-

fects of fenoprofen
griseofulvin: Reduced griseofulvin absorption
hydantoins, such as phenytoin: Unpredictable effects on barbiturate metabolism
MAO inhibitors: Prolonged barbiturate effects
meperidine: Prolonged CNS depressant effects of meperidine
methadone: Reduced methadone actions
methoxyflurane: Increased risk of nephrotoxicity
metronidazole: Decreased antimicrobial effect of metronidazole
oral anticoagulants: Decreased anticoagulant effect
oral contraceptives with estrogen: Decreased contraceptive effect
phenylbutazone: Reduced elimination half-life of phenylbutazone
rifampin: Decreased butabarbital effectiveness
sodium valproate, valproic acid: Decreased butabarbital metabolism and increased adverse CNS effects
theophylline: Decreased blood level and effects of theophylline
ACTIVITIES
alcohol use: Additive CNS depression

Adverse Reactions

CNS: Agitation, anxiety, ataxia, clumsiness, CNS depression, confusion, depression, dizziness, drowsiness, fever, hallucinations, headache, hyperkinesia, insomnia, irritability, nervousness, nightmares, psychiatric disturbance, sleep driving (see Patient Teaching section), somnolence, syncope
CV: Hypertension
EENT: Laryngospasm
GI: Constipation, hepatic dysfunction, nausea, vomiting
MS: Rickets
RESP: Apnea, bronchospasm, respiratory depression
SKIN: Exfoliative dermatitis, Stevens-Johnson syndrome
Other: Anaphylaxis, angioedema, drug tolerance, physical and psychological dependence

Nursing Considerations

• Use butabarbital cautiously, if at all, in patients with depression, suicidal tendency, history of drug abuse, or hepatic dysfunction. Don't administer drug to patients with pre-

monitory signs of hepatic coma.
• **WARNING** Monitor patient closely following butabarbital ingestion because anaphylaxis or angioedema, although rare, may occur with first dose or later doses. Notify prescriber immediately, and provide supportive emergency care.
• Expect to give drug for no more than 2 weeks to treat insomnia because, like all barbiturates, it loses effectiveness for sleep induction and sleep maintenance after 2 weeks.
• Monitor butabarbital intake closely during long-term use because tolerance and psychological and physical dependence may develop.
• Avoid abrupt withdrawal of butabarbital to prevent withdrawal symptoms.
• Monitor elderly and debilitated patients closely because drug may cause marked excitement, depression, and confusion in these patients.
• If patient experiencing pain receives butabarbital, monitor closely for paradoxical excitement.
• If pregnant woman took butabarbital during last trimester, monitor infant for withdrawal symptoms.
• Monitor patient for worsening of insomnia or emergence of abnormal thinking or behavior. If butabarbital unmasks them, patient will need further assessment.

PATIENT TEACHING
• Stress the importance of taking butabarbital exactly as prescribed because it can be addictive. Warn against increasing the dose or decreasing the dosage interval without consulting prescriber.
• Advise patient to notify prescriber if insomnia persists after 7 days of butabarbital therapy.
• Tell patient to avoid alcohol and OTC sedatives and hypnotics during butabarbital therapy because of additive CNS effects.
• Advise patient to avoid potentially hazardous activities until drug's CNS effects are known.
• Advise female patient not to rely on oral contraceptives during butabarbital therapy.
• Explain that butabarbital may cause sleep driving, in which the patient drives while not fully awake and typically cannot recall doing so. Tell family members to report any episodes of sleep driving.

butorphanol tartrate

Stadol, Stadol NS

Class, Category, and Schedule
Chemical class: Opioid
Therapeutic class: Anesthesia adjunct, opioid analgesic
Pregnancy category: C
Controlled substance schedule: II

Indications and Dosages
➤ *To manage pain*
I.V. INJECTION
Adults. 0.5 to 2 mg (usually 1 mg) every 3 to 4 hr, as needed.
I.M. INJECTION
Adults. 1 to 4 mg (usually 2 mg) every 3 to 4 hr, as needed. *Maximum:* 4 mg/single dose.
NASAL INHALATION
Adults. 1 spray (1 mg) in one nostril. Dose repeated after 60 to 90 min; two-dose sequence repeated every 3 to 4 hr, as needed. For severe pain, 2 sprays (1 in each nostril) every 3 to 4 hr, as needed.
DOSAGE ADJUSTMENT Dose reduced to 1 spray in one nostril for elderly patients and those with impaired hepatic or renal function. Dose repeated after 90 to 120 min; two-dose sequence repeated every 6 hr or more, as needed.
➤ *As adjunct to provide preoperative anesthesia*
I.V. OR I.M. INJECTION
Adults. Individualized. *Average:* 2 mg 60 to 90 min before surgery.
➤ *As adjunct to provide anesthesia*
I.V. INJECTION
Adults. Individualized. *Average:* 1 to 4 mg and then supplemental doses of 0.5 to 1 mg, p.r.n. Total usually required during surgery is 60 to 180 mcg/kg.
DOSAGE ADJUSTMENT Parenteral doses reduced by half for elderly patients and patients with impaired hepatic or renal function.

Route	Onset	Peak	Duration
I.V.	2 to 3 min	30 min	2 to 4 hr
I.M.	10 to 30 min	30 to 60 min	3 to 4 hr
Inhalation	In 15 min	1 to 2 hr	4 to 5 hr

Mechanism of Action
Binds with specific CNS receptors to alter the perception of and emotional response to pain.

Contraindications
Hypersensitivity to butorphanol or its components (including the preservative benzethonium chloride)

Interactions
DRUGS
CNS depressants: Additive CNS depression
nasal vasoconstrictors, such as oxymetazoline: Decreased absorption rate and delayed onset of butorphanol
ACTIVITIES
alcohol use: Additive CNS depression

Adverse Reactions
CNS: Anxiety, confusion, difficulty performing purposeful movements, difficulty speaking, dizziness, euphoria, floating feeling, headache, insomnia (with nasal form), lethargy, nervousness, paresthesia, sensation of heat, somnolence, syncope, tremor, vertigo
CV: Chest pain, hypotension, palpitations, tachycardia, vasodilation
EENT: Blurred vision, dry mouth, ear pain, epistaxis, nasal congestion or irritation (with nasal form), pharyngitis, rhinitis, sinus congestion, sinusitis, tinnitus, unpleasant taste
GI: Anorexia, constipation, epigastric pain, nausea, vomiting
RESP: Apnea, bronchitis, cough, dyspnea, respiratory depression, shallow breathing, upper respiratory tract infection
SKIN: Clammy skin, pruritus

Nursing Considerations
• Use butorphanol cautiously, if at all, in patients with depression, suicidal tendency, history of drug abuse, or hepatic or renal dysfunction.
• Because drug can raise CSF pressure, use it cautiously, if at all, in patients with head injury. Because it can increase cardiac workload, use with extreme caution in patients with acute MI, ventricular dysfunction, or coronary insufficiency.
• Be aware that butorphanol has a high potential for abuse.
• Monitor patient after first dose of nasal

form; hypotension and syncope may occur.
•Take safety precautions because butorphanol causes CNS depression.
•Assess respiratory status closely because drug causes respiratory depression.
•Frequently monitor blood pressure after giving drug. If severe hypertension develops (rare), stop drug at once and notify prescriber. If patient isn't narcotic-dependent, expect to administer naloxone to reverse butorphanol's effects.

PATIENT TEACHING
•Stress the importance of taking butorphanol exactly as prescribed because it can be addictive. Warn patient not to increase the dose or decrease the dosage interval without consulting prescriber.
•Advise patient to avoid hazardous activities until drug's CNS effects are known.
•Tell patient to avoid alcohol and other CNS depressants, including OTC drugs, while taking butorphanol because of additive adverse CNS reactions.
•Teach patient how to use nasal form properly. After blowing the nose to clear the nostrils, pull the clear cover from the pump unit and remove the protective clip from its neck. Prime the pump unit by placing the nozzle between the first and second fingers with the thumb on the bottom of the bottle. Then pump the sprayer unit firmly and quickly until a fine spray appears (7 or 8 strokes). Insert the spray tip about 1 cm (1/3") into one nostril, pointing the tip toward the back of the nose. Close the other nostril with one finger and tilt the head slightly forward. Then pump the sprayer firmly and quickly by pushing down on the pump unit's finger grips and against the thumb at the bottom of the bottle. Sniff gently with the mouth closed. After spraying, remove the pump from the nose, tilt the head back, and sniff gently for a few more seconds. Then replace the protective clip and clear cover.

C

cabergoline

Dostinex

Class and Category

Chemical class: Ergot alkaloid derivative
Therapeutic class: Antihyperprolactinemic
Pregnancy category: B

Indications and Dosages

➤ *To treat idiopathic or adenoma-induced hyperprolactinemic disorders*

TABLETS

Adults. 0.25 mg twice a week. Increased by 0.25 mg/wk at 4-wk intervals, if needed, up to 1 mg twice a week.

Route	Onset	Peak	Duration
P.O.	Unknown	48 hr	Up to 14 days

Mechanism of Action

Binds with dopamine D_2 receptors to block prolactin synthesis and secretion by the anterior pituitary gland, thereby reducing the serum prolactin level.

Contraindications

History of pulmonary, pericardial, cardiac valvular, or retroperitoneal fibrotic disorders; hypersensitivity to cabergoline, ergot derivatives, or their components; uncontrolled hypertension

Interactions

DRUGS

antihypertensives: Increased risk of hypotension
dopamine antagonists (butyrophenones, metoclopramide, phenothiazines, or thioxanthenes): Decreased cabergoline effectiveness

Adverse Reactions

CNS: Aggression, asthenia, depression, fatigue, headache, nervousness, paresthesia, pathological gambling behavior, somnolence, psychotic disorder, vertigo
CV: Orthostatic hypotension, valvulopathy
EENT: Dry mouth

ENDO: Breast pain
GI: Abdominal pain, constipation, diarrhea, flatulence, indigestion, nausea, vomiting
GU: Dysmenorrhea, increased libido
RESP: Pulmonary effusion or fibrosis
SKIN: Alopecia

Nursing Considerations

•Before each dose increase, check serum prolactin level to assess cabergoline's effectiveness.

•If patient has moderate to severe hepatic impairment, monitor closely for adverse reactions because of decreased cabergoline metabolism.

•Expect patient who takes cabergoline long-term to undergo periodic reassessment of cardiac status, including echocardiography, because valvulopathy can occur with prolonged cabergoline use.

•Be aware that erythrocyte sedimentation rate may increase in a patient with pleural effusion or pleural fibrosis.

•**WARNING** If you detect evidence of overdose, such as syncope, hallucinations, light-headedness, tachycardia, and nasal congestion, notify prescriber and treat as ordered.

PATIENT TEACHING

•Urge patient to read and follow printed information that explains how to use cabergoline for maximum therapeutic results.

•Advise patient to take drug with meals to help decrease GI distress.

•Tell patient to take a missed dose as soon as possible within 1 to 2 days. If the missed dose isn't remembered until it's time for the next dose, instruct him to double the dose if the drug is generally well tolerated and doesn't cause nausea. If the drug isn't well tolerated, instruct him to consult prescriber before taking the missed dose.

•Instruct patient to change positions slowly to avoid the effects of orthostatic hypotension. Tell him to notify prescriber if such effects occur.

•Encourage patient to keep regular appointments to monitor drug effectiveness.

•Advise patient that drug therapy will end when serum prolactin level is normal for 6 months. Explain that he'll need periodic monitoring of the level to determine whether therapy should resume.

•Tell female patient to notify prescriber if she

is, could be, or plans to become pregnant during therapy; drug may need to be discontinued.

• Caution patient to avoid gambling during cabergoline therapy because drug may increase the risk of pathological gambling behaviors.

calcifediol

Calderol

Class and Category

Chemical class: Sterol derivative, vitamin D analogue
Therapeutic class: Antihypocalcemic
Pregnancy category: C

Indications and Dosages

➤ *To treat metabolic bone disease or hypocalcemia in patients receiving renal dialysis*

CAPSULES

Adults and children age 10 and over. 300 to 350 mcg/wk given in divided doses daily or every other day. Increased at 4-wk intervals, p.r.n. Most patients respond to 50 to 100 mcg daily or 100 to 200 mcg every other day.
Children ages 2 to 10. 0.05 mg daily.
Children up to age 2. 0.02 to 0.05 mg daily.
DOSAGE ADJUSTMENT Dosage decreased as low as 20 mcg every other day in patients with normal serum calcium level.

Route	Onset	Peak	Duration
P.O.	Unknown	Unknown	15 to 20 days

Mechanism of Action

Is converted to calcitriol in the kidneys and then binds to specific receptors in the intestinal mucosa to increase calcium absorption from the intestines. Calcifediol may also regulate calcium ion transfer from bone to blood and stimulate calcium reabsorption in the distal renal tubules, making more calcium available in the body.

Contraindications

Abnormal sensitivity to vitamin D's effects, decreased renal function, hypercalcemia, hyperphosphatemia, hypervitaminosis, malabsorption syndrome, vitamin D toxicity

Interactions
DRUGS

aluminum-containing antacids: Increased blood aluminum level, especially in patients with chronic renal failure
barbiturates, corticosteroids, hydantoin anticonvulsants, primidone: Decreased effects of vitamin D
calcitonin, etidronate, gallium nitrate, pamidronate, plicamycin: Decreased effects of these drugs
calcium (high doses), thiazide diuretics: Increased risk of hypercalcemia
cholestyramine, colestipol, mineral oil: Decreased vitamin D absorption
digitalis glycosides: Increased risk of arrhythmias from hypercalcemia
magnesium-containing antacids: Hypermagnesemia, especially in chronic renal failure
phosphorous-containing drugs: Increased risk of hyperphosphatemia
verapamil: Increased risk of atrial fibrillation
vitamin D derivatives, such as calcitriol, dihydrotachysterol, ergocalciferol: Increased risk of vitamin D toxicity

Adverse Reactions

None with usual dosages

Nursing Considerations

• Use calcifediol cautiously in patients with sarcoidosis or other granulomatous disease because of increased sensitivity to effects of vitamin D.
• If hypercalcemia develops, expect to discontinue therapy. Calcium level usually returns to normal in 2 to 4 weeks. To manage acute hypercalcemia, administer I.V. normal saline solution and, possibly, a loop diuretic as prescribed to enhance diuresis or prepare for dialysis with a calcium-free dialysate if needed. Be aware that chronic hypercalcemia may lead to diffuse vascular calcification, nephrocalcinosis, and other soft-tissue calcification.
• If patient receives high-dose or long-term calcifediol therapy, be alert for vitamin D toxicity. Early signs and symptoms include bone pain, constipation, dry mouth, headache, metallic taste, myalgia, nausea, somnolence, vomiting, and weakness. Late signs and symptoms include albuminuria, anorexia, arrhythmias, azotemia, conjunctivitis (calcific), decreased libido, elevated AST and

ALT levels, elevated BUN level, generalized vascular calcification, hypercholesterolemia, hypertension, hyperthermia, irritability, mild acidosis, nephrocalcinosis, nocturia, pancreatitis, photophobia, polydipsia, polyuria, pruritus, rhinorrhea, and weight loss.

PATIENT TEACHING
• Instruct patient to swallow capsule whole and not to crush or chew it.
• Advise patient to consult prescriber before taking OTC drugs.
• Instruct patient to store drug tightly capped in a cool, dry place away from direct light.
• Encourage patient to eat a balanced diet that includes foods high in vitamin D and calcium. Calcifediol is most effective when patient follows a high-calcium diet.
• If patient takes vitamin supplements, warn him not to exceed recommended amounts.
• Tell patient to avoid calcium-, magnesium-, and phosphate-containing laxatives and antacids; mineral oil; and vitamin D preparations because they may increase the risk of calcifediol's toxic effects.
• Advise patient to notify prescriber immediately if signs of toxicity, such as headache, irritability, nausea, photophobia, vomiting, weakness, and weight loss, develop.
• Stress the importance of follow-up care, including laboratory tests to evaluate progress and identify signs of toxicity early.

calcitonin, human

Cibacalcin

calcitonin, salmon

Calcimar, Miacalcin

Class and Category
Chemical class: Polypeptide hormone
Therapeutic class: Antihypercalcemic, bone resorption inhibitor, osteoporosis therapy adjunct
Pregnancy category: C

Indications and Dosages
➤ *To treat hypercalcemic emergency*
I.M. OR SUBCUTANEOUS INJECTION
Adults. *Initial:* 4 international units/kg every 12 hr. Increased after 1 or 2 days, if needed, to 8 international units/kg every 12 hr. *Maximum:* 8 international units/kg every 6 hr.

➤ *To treat postmenopausal osteoporosis*
I.M. OR SUBCUTANEOUS INJECTION (CALCITONIN, SALMON)
Adults. *Initial:* 100 international units daily, every other day, or 3 times weekly. *Maximum:* 100 international units daily.
NASAL SPRAY
Adults. 200 international units (1 spray) daily, alternating nostrils.

➤ *To treat Paget's disease of the bone*
I.M. OR SUBCUTANEOUS INJECTION (CALCITONIN, SALMON)
Adults. *Initial:* 100 international units daily. *Maintenance:* 50 to 100 international units daily or every other day. *Maximum:* 100 international units daily.
SUBCUTANEOUS INJECTION (CALCITONIN, HUMAN)
Adults. 0.5 mg daily, 0.5 mg 2 or 3 times/wk, or 0.25 mg daily.

Route	Onset	Peak	Duration
I.M., SubQ	In 15 min*	2 hr†	6 to 8 hr†

> **Mechanism of Action**
> Directly inhibits bone resorption. Besides reducing the serum calcium level, this action slows bone metabolism (a major factor in the development of Paget's disease) and calcium loss from the bone (a major factor in the development of osteoporosis).

Contraindications
Hypersensitivity to calcitonin, human; calcitonin, salmon; or their components

Adverse Reactions
CNS: Agitation, anxiety, dizziness, headache, insomnia, neuralgia, paresthesia, stroke, vertigo
CV: Bundle-branch block, hypertension, MI, palpitations, peripheral edema, tachycardia, thrombophlebitis
EENT: Blurred vision; dry mouth; earache; epistaxis; eye pain; hearing loss; nasal irritation, lesions, or redness; pharyngitis; rhinitis; salty taste; sinusitis; taste perversion; tinnitus; vitreous floaters

---

* For hypercalcemia; 6 to 24 mo for Paget's disease.
† For hypercalcemia; unknown for other indications.

ENDO: Goiter, hyperthyroidism
GI: Anorexia, cholelithiasis, epigastric discomfort, flatulence, gastritis, hepatitis, increased appetite, nausea, thirst, vomiting
GU: Hematuria, nocturia, pyelonephritis, renal calculi
HEME: Anemia
MS: Arthritis, arthrosis, back pain, joint stiffness, polymyalgia rheumatica
RESP: Bronchitis, cough, dyspnea, pneumonia, upper respiratory tract infection
SKIN: Alopecia, diaphoresis, eczema, flushing of face or hands, pruritus of earlobes, rash, ulceration
Other: Antibody formation, feverish sensation, injection site inflammation, lymphadenopathy, mild tetanic symptoms

Nursing Considerations

•If sensitivity to calcitonin, human; calcitonin, salmon; or their components is suspected, expect to perform a skin test before administering drug. Prepare a mixture of 10 international units/ml by withdrawing 0.05 ml from a 200–international units solution in a tuberculin syringe and filling the syringe to 1 ml with sodium chloride for injection. Mix well, discard 0.9 ml, and inject 0.1 ml intradermally on the inner forearm. Observe the site for 15 minutes after injection. If you detect evidence of sensitivity, such as more than mild erythema or a wheal, notify prescriber.
•If patient receives calcitonin for hypercalcemia, monitor serum calcium level. During first several doses, keep parenteral calcium available in case the calcium level is inadvertently overcorrected.
•If prescribed calcitonin dose exceeds 2 ml, expect to use I.M. route and multiple injection sites.
•For patient receiving calcitonin for postmenopausal osteoporosis, also expect to give 1.5 g of supplemental calcium carbonate and at least 400 units of vitamin D daily. Plan to provide a balanced diet that includes foods high in calcium and vitamin D.
•Assess for nausea, especially with the first dose. Nausea tends to decrease or disappear with continued use.
•If patient with Paget's disease relapses after treatment, check for antibody formation, as ordered.

PATIENT TEACHING

•Tell patient to refrigerate injection or unopened nasal spray container.
•Teach patient how to self-administer injections.
•If patient has postmenopausal osteoporosis, teach her about dietary needs, including foods rich in calcium and vitamin D.
•For a nasal spray user, explain how to activate the nasal pump by holding the bottle upright and depressing two white side arms toward the bottle six times. When the bottle emits a faint spray, the pump is activated. Tell patient to store the activated nasal pump upright at room temperature and to discard it after 30 days.
•Instruct patient to place the nozzle firmly into one nostril while holding the head upright. Tell him to then depress the pump toward the bottle.
•Remind patient that he doesn't need to reactivate the pump before each daily dose.
•Instruct patient to report nasal symptoms, such as redness, lesions, sinusitis, and rhinitis, to prescriber.

calcitriol
(1,25-dihydroxycholecalciferol)

Calcijex, Rocaltrol

Class and Category

Chemical class: Sterol derivative, vitamin D analogue
Therapeutic class: Antihypocalcemic, antihypoparathyroid
Pregnancy category: C

Indications and Dosages

➤ *To treat hypocalcemia in dialysis patients*

CAPSULES, ORAL SOLUTION

Adults. *Initial:* 0.25 mcg daily. Increased by 0.25 mcg daily every 4 to 8 wk, if needed to achieve normal serum calcium level. *Maintenance:* 0.5 to 3 mcg daily.

➤ *To treat hypocalcemia in predialysis patients*

CAPSULES, ORAL SOLUTION

Adults and children age 3 and over. *Initial:* 0.25 mcg daily. Increased after 4 to 8 wk, if needed, to 0.5 mcg daily.

ORAL SOLUTION

Children up to age 3. 10 to 15 ng/kg daily.

➤ *To treat hypoparathyroidism*

TABLETS

Adults and children age 6 and over. *Initial:* 0.25 mcg daily in the morning. Increased every 2 to 4 wk, if needed to achieve normal serum calcium level. *Usual:* 0.5 to 2 mcg daily.

Children ages 1 to 5. 0.25 to 0.75 mcg daily in the morning.

I.V. INJECTION

Adults. *Initial:* 1 to 2 mcg 3 times/wk given every other day. Each dose increased 0.5 to 1 mcg at 2- to 4-wk intervals, if needed.

Route	Onset	Peak	Duration
P.O.	2 to 6 hr	10 hr	3 to 5 days

Mechanism of Action

Binds to specific receptors of the intestinal mucosa to increase calcium absorption from the intestines. It also may regulate calcium ion transfer from bone to blood and stimulate calcium reabsorption in the distal renal tubules, making more calcium available in the body.

Contraindications

Hypercalcemia, vitamin D toxicity

Interactions

DRUGS

cholestyramine: Decreased calcitriol absorption

digitalis glycosides: Possibly arrhythmias

ketoconazole: Decreased blood calcitriol level

magnesium-containing antacids (I.V. form): Hypermagnesemia

mineral oil: Decreased blood calcitriol level (with prolonged use of mineral oil)

phenobarbital, phenytoin: Decreased synthesis and blood level of calcitriol

thiazide diuretics: Hypercalcemia

Adverse Reactions

SKIN: Erythema multiforme, lip swelling, pruritus, rash, urticaria

Other: Anaphylaxis

Nursing Considerations

•Make sure patient receives enough calcium.

•Store drug at room temperature and protect from heat and direct light.

•In high-dose or long-term calcitriol therapy, be alert for vitamin D toxicity. Early evidence includes abdominal or bone pain, constipation, dry mouth, headache, metallic taste, myalgia, nausea, somnolence, vomiting, and weakness. Late evidence includes albuminuria, anorexia, arrhythmias, azotemia, conjunctivitis (calcific), decreased libido, elevated AST and ALT levels, elevated BUN level, vascular calcification, hypercholesterolemia, hypertension, hyperthermia, irritability, mild acidosis, nephrocalcinosis, nocturia, pancreatitis, photophobia, polydipsia, polyuria, pruritus, rhinorrhea, and weight loss.

PATIENT TEACHING

•Warn patient not to take other forms of vitamin D while taking calcitriol.

•Instruct patient to take a missed dose as soon as possible.

•Advise patient to notify prescriber immediately if signs of toxicity, such as headache, irritability, nausea, photophobia, vomiting, weakness, and weight loss, develop.

calcium acetate

PhosLo

calcium carbonate

Apo-Cal (CAN), Calci-Mix, Calsan (CAN), Liqui-Cal, Liquid Cal-600, Titralac

calcium chloride

Calciject (CAN)

calcium citrate

Citracal, Citracal Liquitabs

calcium glubionate

Calcionate, Calcium-Sandoz (CAN), Neo-Calglucon

calcium gluceptate

Calcium Stanley (CAN)

calcium gluconate

calcium lactate

Class and Category

Chemical class: Elemental cation

Therapeutic class: Antacid, antihypermagnesemic, antihyperphosphatemic, antihypocalcemic, calcium replacement, cardiotonic

Pregnancy category: C (Not rated for calcium carbonate, citrate, and lactate)

Indications and Dosages

➤ *To treat hyperphosphatemia*
TABLETS (CALCIUM ACETATE)
Adults. *Initial:* 2 tablets (338 mg elemental calcium, 1,334 mg calcium acetate) t.i.d. with meals. Dosage increased to reduce serum phosphorous level below 6 mg/dl as long as hypercalcemia doesn't develop. *Maintenance:* 3 or 4 tablets t.i.d. with each meal.

➤ *To prevent hypocalcemia*
CAPSULES, ORAL SUSPENSION, TABLETS (CALCIUM CARBONATE); EFFERVESCENT TABLETS, TABLETS (CALCIUM CITRATE); SYRUP (CALCIUM GLUBIONATE); TABLETS (CALCIUM GLUCONATE OR LACTATE)
Adults and children over age 10. 800 to 1,200 mg daily.
Pregnant and breastfeeding women. 1,200 mg daily.
Children ages 4 to 10. 800 mg daily.
Children up to age 4. 400 to 800 mg daily.

➤ *To provide antacid effects*
CHEWABLE TABLETS, ORAL SUSPENSION, TABLETS (CALCIUM CARBONATE)
Adults and children age 12 and over. 350 to 1,500 mg 1 hr after meals and at bedtime, p.r.n.

➤ *To replace calcium in hypocalcemia*
I.V. INFUSION (CALCIUM CHLORIDE)
Adults. 0.5 to 1 g every 1 to 3 days, infused at less than 1 ml/min.
Children. 25 mg/kg given over several minutes.
I.V. OR I.M. INJECTION (CALCIUM GLUCEPTATE)
Adults and children. 0.44 to 1.1 g I.M. or 1.1 to 4.4 g I.V. at a rate not to exceed 2 ml (36 mg)/min.
I.V. INJECTION (CALCIUM GLUCONATE)
Adults. 970 mg given slowly, repeated if needed until tetany is controlled.
Children. 200 to 500 mg as a single dose given slowly, repeated if needed until tetany is controlled.

➤ *As adjunct to treat magnesium intoxication*
I.V. INJECTION (CALCIUM CHLORIDE)
Adults. 500 mg promptly and repeated p.r.n., based on response.

➤ *As adjunct in cardiac resuscitation*
I.V. INJECTION (CALCIUM CHLORIDE)
Adults. 0.5 to 1 g.

Children. 0.2 ml/kg.

➤ *As adjunct in exchange transfusion*
I.V. INJECTION (CALCIUM GLUCONATE)
Adults. 1.35 mEq with each 100 ml of citrated blood exchanged.
Neonates. 0.45 mEq after each 100 ml of citrated blood exchanged.
I.V. INJECTION (CALCIUM GLUCEPTATE)
Neonates. 110 mg after each 100 ml of citrated blood exchanged.

Mechanism of Action

Increases levels of intracellular and extracellular calcium, which is needed to maintain homeostasis, especially in the nervous and musculoskeletal systems. Also plays a role in normal cardiac and renal function, respiration, coagulation, and cell membrane and capillary permeability. Helps regulate the release and storage of neurotransmitters and hormones. Oral forms also neutralize or buffer stomach acid to relieve discomfort caused by hyperacidity.

Contraindications

Hypercalcemia, hypersensitivity to calcium salts or their components, hypophosphatemia, renal calculi

Incompatibilities

To avoid precipitation, don't give I.V. calcium chloride, gluceptate, or gluconate through same I.V. line as bicarbonates, carbonates, phosphates, sulfates, or tartrates.

Interactions
DRUGS
aluminum-containing antacids: Enhanced aluminum absorption with use of calcium citrate
atenolol: Decreased blood atenolol level and beta blockade
calcitonin: Possibly antagonized effects of calcitonin in hypercalcemia treatment
calcium supplements, magnesium-containing preparations: Increased serum calcium or magnesium level, especially in patients with impaired renal function
cellulose sodium phosphate: Decreased effectiveness of cellulose sodium phosphate in preventing hypercalciuria

digitalis glycosides: Increased risk of arrhythmias
estrogens, oral contraceptives (estrogen-containing): Increased calcium absorption
etidronate: Decreased etidronate absorption
fluoroquinolones: Reduced fluoroquinolone absorption by calcium carbonate
gallium nitrate: Antagonized effects of gallium nitrate
iron salts: Decreased gastric absorption of iron
magnesium sulfate (parenteral): Neutralized effects of magnesium by parenteral calcium salts
neuromuscular blockers (except succinylcholine): Possibly reversal of neuromuscular blockade by parenteral calcium salts; enhanced or prolonged neuromuscular blockade induced by tubocurarine
norfloxacin: Decreased norfloxacin bioavailability
phenytoin: Decreased bioavailability of phenytoin and calcium
potassium phosphates, potassium and sodium phosphates: Increased risk of calcium deposition in soft tissue
sodium bicarbonate: Possibly milk-alkali syndrome
sodium fluoride: Reduced fluoride and calcium absorption
sodium polystyrene sulfonate: Possibly metabolic alkalosis if patient has renal impairment
tetracyclines: Decreased tetracycline absorption and blood level, leading to decreased anti-infective response
thiazide diuretics: Possibly hypercalcemia
verapamil: Reversed verapamil effects
vitamin A (more than 25,000 units daily): Possibly stimulation of bone loss, decreased effects of calcium supplementation, and hypercalcemia
vitamin D (high doses): Excessively increased calcium absorption

FOODS
caffeine, high-fiber food: Possibly decreased calcium absorption

ACTIVITIES
alcohol use (excessive), smoking: Possibly decreased calcium absorption

Adverse Reactions
CNS: Paresthesia (parenteral form)
CV: Hypotension, irregular heartbeat (parenteral form)

GI: Nausea or vomiting (parenteral form)
SKIN: Diaphoresis, flushing, or sensation of warmth (parenteral form)
Other: Hypercalcemia; injection site burning, pain, rash, or redness (parenteral form)

Nursing Considerations
• Store at room temperature and protect from heat, moisture, and direct light. Don't freeze.
• Warm solution to room temperature before parenteral administration.
• Maintain patient in a recumbent position for 30 minutes after parenteral administration to prevent dizziness from hypotension.
• Administer I.V. calcium through an infusing I.V. solution, using a small-bore needle inserted into a large vein to minimize irritation. Give calcium slowly to prevent excess calcium from reaching the heart and causing adverse cardiovascular reactions. Adverse reactions often result from too-rapid administration. If ECG tracings are abnormal or patient reports injection site discomfort, expect to temporarily discontinue administration.
• Check regularly for infiltration because calcium causes necrosis. If infiltration occurs, stop infusion and tell prescriber immediately.
• Divide I.M. calcium gluceptate dose of 5 ml or more in half and inject in gluteal region.
• Regularly monitor serum calcium level and evaluate therapeutic response by assessing for Chvostek's and Trousseau's signs, which shouldn't appear.
• Be aware that calcium chloride injection contains three times as much calcium per milliliter as calcium gluconate injection.

PATIENT TEACHING
• For chewable tablets, urge patient to chew thoroughly before swallowing and to drink a glass of water afterward.
• If suspension is prescribed, tell patient to shake bottle well before each use.
• If calcium citrate effervescent tablets are prescribed, tell patient to dissolve them in water and drink immediately.
• Instruct patient to take calcium carbonate tablets 1 to 2 hours after meals, calcium glubionate syrup before meals (diluted in water or fruit juice, if desired, for an infant or a child), and other calcium forms with meals.
• Advise storing calcium at room temperature away from heat, moisture, and direct light. Warn against freezing suspension or syrup.
• Instruct patient to avoid taking calcium within 2 hours of taking another oral drug

because of risk of interactions.
•Urge patient to see prescriber before taking OTC drugs because of risk of interactions.
•Tell patient to avoid excessive use of tobacco and excessive consumption of alcoholic beverages, caffeine-containing products, and high-fiber foods because these substances may decrease calcium absorption.

candesartan cilexetil

Atacand

Class and Category
Chemical class: Angiotensin II receptor antagonist
Therapeutic class: Antihypertensive
Pregnancy category: C (first trimester), D (later trimesters)

Indications and Dosages
➤ *To manage, or as adjunct in managing, hypertension*
TABLETS
Adults. *Initial:* 16 mg daily. *Maintenance:* 8 to 32 mg daily or 4 to 16 mg every 12 hr. *Maximum:* 32 mg daily.
DOSAGE ADJUSTMENT Initial dosage decreased to 2 mg for patients with moderate to severe hepatic impairment and to 4 mg for those with renal impairment, need for hemodialysis, or possibly a risk of hypotension.
➤ *To treat heart failure in patients with an ejection fraction of 40% or less and NYHA class II–IV to reduce the risk of death from cardiovascular causes and reduce hospitalizations for heart failure*
TABLETS
Adults. *Initial:* 4 mg daily for 2 wk; then doubled every 2 wk as tolerated until reaching target dose of 32 mg daily.

Route	Onset	Peak	Duration
P.O.	In 2 wk	In 4 to 5 wk	Unknown

Mechanism of Action
Selectively blocks binding of angiotensin (AT) II to AT$_1$ receptor sites in many tissues, including vascular smooth muscle and adrenal glands. This inhibits vasoconstrictive and aldosterone-secreting effects of AT II, which reduces blood pressure.

Contraindications
Hypersensitivity to candesartan or its components

Interactions
DRUGS
diuretics, other antihypertensives: Possibly increased risk of hypotension
heparin, potassium-sparing diuretics, potassium supplements, potassium-containing salt substitutes: Possibly increased risk of hyperkalemia
lithium: Increased blood lithium level

Adverse Reactions
CNS: Dizziness, headache
CV: Hypotension
EENT: Pharyngitis, rhinitis
GI: Elevated liver function test results, hepatitis
GU: Elevated BUN and serum creatinine levels
HEME: Agranulocytosis, leukopenia, neutropenia
MS: Back pain, rhabdomyolysis
RESP: Upper respiratory tract infection
Other: Hyperkalemia, hyponatremia

Nursing Considerations
•If patient has known or suspected hypovolemia, expect to provide treatment, such as I.V. normal saline solution, as prescribed, to correct it before starting candesartan.
•Monitor patient closely during major surgery and anesthesia because candesartan increases the risk of hypotension by blocking the renin-angiotensin system.
•Watch for elevated BUN and serum creatinine levels, especially if patient has heart failure or impaired renal function; drug may cause acute renal failure. Report significant or persistent increases immediately.
•If blood pressure isn't controlled with candesartan alone, expect to give a diuretic, such as hydrochlorothiazide, as prescribed.
•**WARNING** If patient receives a diuretic or antihypertensive with candesartan, has heart failure, or is elderly, assess blood pressure often because of added risk of hypotension.
•If patient develops hypotension, expect to stop drug temporarily. Immediately place patient in supine position and prepare to give I.V. normal saline solution, as prescribed. Expect to resume therapy after blood pressure stabilizes.

•If patient receives a diuretic, provide hydration, as ordered, to help prevent hypovolemia and watch for evidence, such as hypotension with dizziness and fainting. If patient has heart failure and develops hypotension, dosage of diuretic, candesartan, or both may be reduced when blood pressure stablizes and therapy resumes.

•Check patient's CBC for decreases in hemoglobin and hematocrit. If they're significant or persistent, notify prescriber immediately.

PATIENT TEACHING

•Advise patient that full effects of candesartan may not occur for 4 to 5 weeks.

•Explain the importance of lifestyle choices in controlling hypertension.

•Advise female patient to immediately report known or suspected pregnancy. Explain that if she becomes pregnant, prescriber may replace candesartan with another antihypertensive that is safe to use during pregnancy.

capreomycin sulfate

Capastat

Class and Category

Chemical class: Polypeptide antibiotic isolated from *Streptomyces capreolus*
Therapeutic class: Antitubercular
Pregnancy category: C

Indications and Dosages

➤ *As adjunct to treat pulmonary tuberculosis caused by* Mycobacterium tuberculosis *in which primary drugs are ineffective or can't be used because of toxicity*

I.V. INFUSION, I.M. INJECTION

Adults. 1 g daily for 60 to 120 days followed by 1 g 2 or 3 times/wk for 12 to 24 mo. *Maximum:* 20 mg/kg daily.

DOSAGE ADJUSTMENT For patient with renal impairment, dosage reduced according to patient's creatinine clearance.

Mechanism of Action

May interfere with lipid and nucleic acid biosynthesis in actively growing tubercle bacilli.

Contraindications

Hypersensitivity to capreomycin or its components

Interactions

DRUGS

aminoglycosides (parenteral): Increased risk of ototoxicity, nephrotoxicity, and neuromuscular blockade
nephrotoxic drugs, such as amphotericin B: Increased risk of nephrotoxicity
nondepolarizing neuromuscular blockers: Enhanced neuromuscular blockade
ototoxic drugs, such as quinidine: Increased risk of ototoxicity
polymyxins (parenteral): Increased risk of nephrotoxicity and neuromuscular blockade

Adverse Reactions

CNS: Dizziness, vertigo
EENT: Ototoxicity
GI: Elevated liver function test results
GU: Nephrotoxicity
HEME: Leukocytosis, leukopenia
SKIN: Maculopapular rash, sterile abscess, urticaria
Other: Hypocalcemia, hypokalemia, hypomagnesemia, injection site pain, induration, and bleeding

Nursing Considerations

•Use capreomycin cautiously in patients with renal insufficiency, impaired hearing, or a history of hypersensitivity, especially to other drugs.

•Expect to obtain baseline renal function studies, as ordered, before starting capreomycin therapy and weekly throughout therapy because drug may alter renal function.

•To reconstitute drug for I.V. injection, add 100 ml of normal saline solution. Administer over 60 minutes.

•To reconstitute drug for I.M. injection, add 2 ml of sodium chloride for injection or sterile water for injection to each 1-g vial. Allow 2 to 3 minutes for complete dissolution.

•Give I.M. injection deep into a large muscle mass, such as the gluteus maximus.

•Observe injection site for excessive bleeding or sterile abscess.

•Make sure patient receives audiometric tests and vestibular function assessment regularly.

•Closely monitor patient for urticaria and maculopapular rash.

•Check serum electrolyte levels periodically, as ordered, because capreomycin may cause imbalances such as hypocalcemia, hypokalemia, and hypomagnesemia.

- Advise patient to alert nurse or prescriber if injection site bleeds excessively.
- Warn patient to contact prescriber immediately about hearing loss or tinnitus.
- Explain the need for frequent laboratory tests to monitor renal function.
- Tell patient that tuberculosis therapy lasts for 12 to 24 months.
- Explain that noncompliance may decrease effectiveness and lengthen treatment.

captopril

Capoten

Class and Category

Chemical class: ACE inhibitor
Therapeutic class: Antihypertensive
Pregnancy category: C (first trimester), D (later trimesters)

Indications and Dosages

➤ *To control hypertension*
TABLETS
Adults and adolescents. *Initial:* 25 mg b.i.d. or t.i.d. Increased to 50 mg b.i.d. or t.i.d. after 1 to 2 wk, if needed. If blood pressure isn't well controlled at this dosage and with the addition of a diuretic, dosage increased to 100 mg b.i.d. or t.i.d. and then, if needed, to 150 mg b.i.d. or t.i.d. while continuing diuretic. *Maximum:* 450 mg daily.

➤ *To control accelerated or malignant hypertension when temporary discontinuation of current antihypertensive therapy isn't practical or when prompt titration of blood pressure is needed*
TABLETS
Adults and adolescents. *Initial:* 25 mg b.i.d. or t.i.d while continuing diuretic but discontinuing current antihypertensive drug. Increased every 24 hr as needed until satisfactory response is obtained or maximum dosage is reached. *Maximum:* 450 mg daily.

➤ *To treat heart failure that's unresponsive to conventional therapy*
TABLETS
Adults and adolescents. *Initial:* 25 mg b.i.d. or t.i.d. Increased to 50 mg b.i.d. or t.i.d., as needed. After 14 days, increased to 100 mg t.i.d. and then to 150 mg t.i.d, if needed. *Maximum:* 450 mg daily.

➤ *To treat left-sided heart failure after MI*
TABLETS
Adults and adolescents. *Initial:* 6.25 mg as a single dose starting 3 days after MI and then 12.5 mg t.i.d. Increased to 25 mg t.i.d. for several days and then increased again to maintenance dosage. *Maintenance:* 50 mg t.i.d.

➤ *To treat diabetic nephropathy*
TABLETS
Adults and adolescents. 25 mg t.i.d.
DOSAGE ADJUSTMENT Starting dosage reduced to 6.25 mg b.i.d. or t.i.d. if patient with hypertension also has heart failure, is undergoing dialysis, or is being vigorously treated with diuretics that result in hyponatremia or hypovolemia.

Route	Onset	Peak	Duration
P.O.	15 to 60 min	60 to 90 min	6 to 12 hr

Mechanism of Action

May reduce blood pressure by affecting the renin-angiotensin-aldosterone system. By inhibiting angiotensin-converting enzyme, captopril:
- prevents conversion of angiotensin I to angiotensin II, a potent vasoconstrictor that also stimulates the adrenal cortex to secrete aldosterone. Inhibiting aldosterone increases sodium and water excretion, reducing blood pressure.
- may inhibit renal and vascular production of angiotensin II.
- decreases serum angiotensin II level and increases renin activity. This decreases aldosterone secretion, slightly increasing serum potassium level and fluid loss.
- decreases vascular tone and blood pressure.

Contraindications

Hypersensitivity to captopril, other ACE inhibitors, or their components

Interactions
DRUGS
allopurinol: Increased risk of hypersensitivity reactions, including Stevens-Johnson syndrome, skin eruptions, fever, arthralgia
antacids: Possibly impaired captopril absorption

capsaicin: Possibly initiation or worsening of cough caused by ACE inhibitor
cyclosporine, potassium-containing drugs, potassium-sparing diuretics, potassium supplements: Increased risk of hyperkalemia
digoxin: Increased blood digoxin level
diuretics; hypotension-producing drugs, such as hydralazine: Additive hypotensive effects
gold: Increased risk of nitritoid reaction, including facial flushing, nausea, vomiting, and hypotension
lithium: Increased risk of lithium toxicity
NSAIDs: Decreased antihypertensive response to ACE inhibition
probenecid: Increased blood level and decreased total clearance of captopril

ACTIVITIES
alcohol use: Additive hypotensive effects

Adverse Reactions
CNS: Fever
CV: Chest pain, hypotension, orthostatic hypotension, palpitations, tachycardia
EENT: Loss of taste
GU: Dysuria, impotence, nephrotic syndrome, nocturia, oliguria, polyuria, proteinuria, urinary frequency
HEME: Eosinophilia
MS: Arthralgia
RESP: Cough
SKIN: Photosensitivity, pruritus, rash
Other: Angioedema, hyperkalemia, hyponatremia, positive ANA titer

Nursing Considerations
• Closely monitor patient's blood pressure, especially when therapy starts and dosage increases. Keep patient supine if hypotension occurs.
• Monitor renal function tests for signs of nephrotic syndrome, such as proteinuria and increased BUN and serum creatinine levels. Also watch for renal symptoms, such as oliguria, polyuria, and urinary frequency.
• Monitor WBC regularly, as ordered, especially if patient has collagen vascular disease or renal disease.

PATIENT TEACHING
• Instruct patient to take captopril 1 hour before meals.
• Tell patient to rise slowly from sitting or lying down to minimize orthostatic hypotension.
• Tell patient to avoid sunlight or to wear sunscreen in direct sunlight because photo-

sensitivity may occur.
• Warn patient not to stop drug abruptly.
• Advise patient not to use salt substitutes that contain potassium and to consult prescriber before increasing potassium intake to avoid increasing the risk of hyperkalemia.
• Urge patient to tell prescriber about signs and symptoms of infection, such as sore throat or fever.

carbamazepine

Apo-Carbamazepine (CAN), Atretol, Carbatrol, Epitol, Equetro, Novo-Carbamaz (CAN), Tegretol, Tegretol-XR

Class and Category
Chemical class: Tricyclic iminostilbene derivative
Therapeutic class: Analgesic, anticonvulsant
Pregnancy category: C

Indications and Dosages
➤ *To treat epilepsy*
E.R. CAPSULES (CARBATROL), E.R. TABLETS (TEGRETOL-XR)
Adults and children age 12 and over. *Initial:* 200 mg b.i.d. Increased weekly by 200 mg daily, if needed. *Maximum:* 1,600 mg daily in adults, 1,200 mg daily in children age 16 and over, and 1,000 mg daily in children ages 12 to 16.
Children ages 6 to 12. *Initial:* 100 mg b.i.d. Increased weekly by 100 mg daily, if needed. *Maximum:* 1,000 mg daily.
ORAL SUSPENSION
Adults and children age 12 and over. *Initial:* 100 mg q.i.d. Increased weekly by 200 mg daily, if needed, given in divided doses t.i.d or q.i.d. *Maximum:* 1,600 mg daily in adults, 1,200 mg daily in children age 16 and over, and 1,000 mg daily in children ages 12 to 16.
Children ages 6 to 12. *Initial:* 50 mg q.i.d. Increased weekly by 100 mg daily, if needed, given in divided doses t.i.d or q.i.d. *Maximum:* 1,000 mg daily.
Children up to age 6. *Initial:* 10 to 20 mg/kg/day in divided doses q.i.d. *Maximum:* 35 mg/kg daily.
TABLETS
Adults and children age 12 and over. *Initial:* 200 mg b.i.d. Increased weekly by 200 mg/day, if needed, given in divided doses t.i.d. or q.i.d. *Maximum:* 1,600 mg daily in adults,

1,200 mg daily in children age 16 and over, and 1,000 mg daily in children ages 12 to 16. **Children ages 6 to 12.** *Initial:* 100 mg b.i.d. Increased weekly by 100 mg daily, if needed, given in divided doses t.i.d. or q.i.d. *Maximum:* 1,000 mg daily.

Children up to age 6. *Initial:* 10 to 20 mg/kg daily in divided doses b.i.d. or t.i.d. Increased weekly, if needed, divided and given t.i.d. or q.i.d. *Maximum:* 35/kg daily.

➤ *To relieve pain in trigeminal neuralgia*
E.R. CAPSULES (CARBATROL), E.R. TABLETS (TEGRETOL-XR), TABLETS
Adults. *Initial:* 100 mg b.i.d. Increased by up to 200 mg daily, if needed, in increments of 100 mg every 12 hr. *Maintenance:* 400 to 800 mg/day. *Maximum:* 1,200 mg daily.

ORAL SUSPENSION (100 MG/5 ML)
Adults. 50 mg q.i.d. Increased by up to 200 mg daily, if needed, in increments of 50 mg q.i.d. *Maintenance:* 400 to 800 mg daily. *Maximum:* 1,200 mg daily.

➤ *To treat acute manic and mixed episodes in bipolar disorder*
E.R. CAPSULES (EQUETRO)
Adults. *Initial:* 200 mg b.i.d., increased as needed in 200-mg increments. *Maximum:* 1,600 mg daily.

Route	Onset	Peak	Duration
P.O. (all forms)	In 1 mo*	Unknown	Unknown

Contraindications

History of bone marrow depression; hypersensitivity to carbamazepine, tricyclic compounds, or their components; MAO inhibitor or nefazodone therapy

Interactions

DRUGS
acetaminophen (long-term use): Increased metabolism, leading to acetaminophen-induced hepatotoxicity or decreased acetaminophen effectiveness
acetazolamide, cimetidine, clarithromycin, danazol, diltiazem, erythromycin, fluconazole, fluoxetine, fluvoxamine, isoniazid, itraconazole, ketoconazole, loratadine, niacinamide, nicotinamide, propoxyphene, protease inhibitors, terfenadine, troleandomycin,

---

* For anticonvulsant use; 8 to 72 hr for use in trigeminal neuralgia.

valproate, verapamil: Increased blood carbamazepine level
alprazolam, amitriptyline, bupropion, buspirone, citalopram, clobazam, clonazepam, clozapine, cyclosporine, delavirdine, desipramine, diazepam, dicumarol, doxycycline, ethosuximide, felodipine, glucocorticoids, haloperidol, itraconazole, lamotrigine, levothyroxine, lorazepam, methadone, methsuximide, midazolam, mirtazapine, nortriptyline, olanzapine, oral contraceptives, oxcarbazepine, phenytoin, praziquantel, protease inhibitors, quetiapine, risperidone, theophylline, tiagabine, topiramate, tramadol, triazolam, trazodone, valproate, warfarin, ziprasidone, zonisamide: Decreased blood levels of these drugs
cisplatin, doxorubicin, felbamate, methsuximide, phenytoin, rifampin, theophylline: Decreased blood carbamazepine level
clomipramine, phenytoin, primidone: Increased blood levels of these drugs
felbamate: Decreased blood level of felbamate or carbamazepine
isoniazid: Increased risk of carbamazepine toxicity and isoniazid hepatotoxicity
lamotrigine, phenobarbital, primidone, tricyclic antidepressants, valproic acid: Decreased blood levels of these drugs, increased blood level of carbamazepine
lithium: Increased risk of CNS toxicity
nefazodone: Decreased nefazodone effectiveness and increased blood carbamazepine level
nondepolarizing neuromuscular blockers: Possibly reduced duration or decreased effectiveness of neuromuscular blocker
oral anticoagulants: Increased metabolism and decreased effectiveness of anticoagulant

FOODS
grapefruit juice: Increased blood carbamazepine level

ACTIVITIES
alcohol use: Increased sedative effect

Adverse Reactions

CNS: Chills, confusion, dizziness, drowsiness, fatigue, fever, headache, syncope, talkativeness, unsteadiness, visual hallucinations
CV: Arrhythmias, including AV block; edema; heart failure; hypertension; hypotension; thromboembolism; thrombophlebitis; worsened coronary artery disease
EENT: Blurred vision, conjunctivitis, dry

Mechanism of Action

Normally, sodium moves into a neuronal cell by passing through a gated sodium channel in the cell membrane. Carbamazepine may prevent or halt seizures by closing or blocking sodium channels, as shown, thus preventing sodium from entering the cell. Keeping sodium out of the cell may slow nerve impulse transmission, thus slowing the rate at which neurons fire.

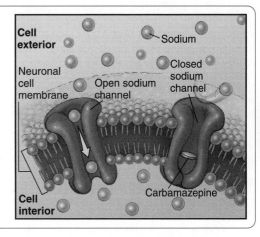

mouth, glossitis, nystagmus, oculomotor disturbances, stomatitis, tinnitus, transient diplopia

ENDO: Syndrome of inappropriate ADH secretion, water intoxication

GI: Abdominal pain, anorexia, constipation, diarrhea, dyspepsia, elevated liver function test results, hepatitis, nausea, pancreatitis, vomiting

GU: Acute urine retention, albuminuria, azotemia, glycosuria, impotence, oliguria, renal failure, urinary frequency

HEME: Acute intermittent porphyria, agranulocytosis, aplastic anemia, bone marrow depression, eosinophilia, leukocytosis, leukopenia, pancytopenia, thrombocytopenia

MS: Arthralgia, leg cramps, myalgia

RESP: Pulmonary hypersensitivity (dyspnea, fever, pneumonia, or pneumonitis)

SKIN: Aggravation of disseminated lupus erythematosus, alopecia, altered skin pigmentation, diaphoresis, erythema multiforme, erythema nodosum, exfoliative dermatitis, jaundice, Lyell's syndrome, photosensitivity reactions, pruritic and erythematous rash, purpura, Stevens-Johnson syndrome, urticaria

Other: Adenopathy, lymphadenopathy

Nursing Considerations

•Avoid using carbamazepine in patients with a history of hepatic porphyria because it may prompt an acute attack.

•**WARNING** If patient has Asian ancestry, make sure he has been evaluated for the genetic allelic variant HLA-B 1502 before starting carbamazepine therapy. Patients positive for HLA-B 1502 shouldn't take carbamazepine because the risk of serious, sometimes fatal, dermatologic reactions is ten times higher than in patients without this variant.

•Use carbamazepine cautiously in patients with impaired hepatic function because it's mainly metabolized in the liver. Monitor results of liver function tests, as directed.

•Monitor patient closely for adverse reactions because many are serious.

•Periodically monitor blood carbamazepine level to assess for therapeutic and toxic levels; a blood level of 6 to 12 mcg/ml is optimal for anticonvulsant effects.

•**WARNING** Monitor WBC and platelet counts monthly for first 2 months. Decreased counts may indicate bone marrow depression.

•Withdraw carbamazepine therapy gradually to minimize the risk of seizures.

PATIENT TEACHING

•Tell patient to take carbamazepine with food (except the oral suspension form, which shouldn't be taken with other liquid drugs or diluents).

•Warn patient about possible dizziness, blurred vision, and unsteadiness.

•Inform patient that the coating of E.R. tablets isn't absorbed and may appear in stool.

•Advise patient not to crush or chew E.R. capsules or tablets. If he can't swallow capsules whole, have him open them and sprinkle contents on food.

•Urge patient to wear sunscreen and protective clothing to prevent photosensitivity.
•Tell patient to report unusual bleeding or bruising, fever, rash, or mouth ulcers.
•Warn female patients that drug decreases oral contraceptive effectiveness, and urge her to use another form of contraception. Because drug may cause fetal harm, urge her to notify prescriber if pregnancy is suspected or occurs.

carisoprodol

Soma, Vanadom

Class and Category
Chemical class: Dicarbamate
Therapeutic class: Skeletal muscle relaxant
Pregnancy category: C

Indications and Dosages
➤ *As adjunct to relieve acute musculo-skeletal pain and stiffness*
TABLETS (SOMA)
Adults and children over age 16. 250 to 350 mg t.i.d. and at bedtime.
TABLETS (VANADOM)
Children ages 5 to 12. 6.25 mg/kg t.i.d. and at bedtime.

Route	Onset	Peak	Duration
P.O.	30 min	Unknown	4 to 6 hr

Mechanism of Action
Blocks interneuronal activity in the descending reticular formation and spinal cord, producing muscle relaxation and sedation.

Contraindications
Hypersensitivity or idiosyncratic reactions to carisoprodol, to its components, or to meprobamate-related compounds; intermittent porphyria

Interactions
DRUGS
CNS depressants, psychotropic drugs: Additive CNS depression
fluvoxamine, omeprazole: Increased blood carisoprodol level
rifampin, St. John's wort: Decreased blood carisoprodol level

ACTIVITIES
alcohol use: Additive CNS depression

Adverse Reactions
CNS: Agitation, ataxia, depression, dizziness, drowsiness, fever, headache, insomnia, irritability, seizures, somnolence, syncope, tremor, vertigo
CV: Orthostatic hypotension, tachycardia
EENT: Diplopia, transient vision loss
GI: Epigastric discomfort, hiccups, nausea, vomiting
HEME: Eosinophilia
SKIN: Erythema multiforme, facial flushing, pruritus, rash
Other: Drug dependence or withdrawal

Nursing Considerations
•Use carisoprodol cautiously in patients with history of drug addiction.
•Carisoprodol therapy should last no longer than 3 weeks.
•Monitor patient closely for hypersensitivity or idiosyncratic reactions. They typically occur before the fourth dose in patients with no previous exposure to carisoprodol.
•Provide rest and other pain-relief measures.
•To avoid mild withdrawal symptoms, expect to taper therapy as prescribed, rather than stopping it abruptly.
PATIENT TEACHING
•Tell patient to take carisoprodol with meals if GI distress occurs.
•Caution patient that drug dependence and withdrawal may occur, especially if patient takes carisoprodol for a long time or changes dosage without consulting prescriber.
•Warn patient about possible dizziness, drowsiness, syncope, and vertigo; discourage hazardous activities, such as driving, until the effects of the drug are known.
•Inform patient that abruptly stopping drug can cause headache, insomnia, nausea, and other adverse reactions.
•Instruct patient to avoid alcohol and other CNS depressants while taking drug.
•Inform patient that saliva, urine, and sweat may appear darker (red, brown, or black). Reassure him that this discoloration is harmless but may stain garments.
•Tell patient to store drug in a tightly capped container at room temperature.
•Tell patient not to store drug in bathroom, near kitchen sink, or in other damp places to protect it from heat and moisture.

carteolol hydrochloride

Cartrol

Class and Category

Chemical: Beta-adrenergic blocker
Therapeutic: Antihypertensive
Pregnancy category: C

Indications and Dosages

➤ *To control hypertension*

TABLETS

Adults. *Initial:* 2.5 mg daily. If response is inadequate, dosage increased to 5 mg and then 10 mg daily, p.r.n. *Maintenance:* 2.5 or 5 mg daily.

DOSAGE ADJUSTMENT Interval increased to every 48 hr for patients with creatinine clearance of 20 to 60 ml/min/1.73 m^2 or to every 72 hr for clearance of less than 20 ml/min/1.73 m^2.

Route	Onset	Peak	Duration
P.O.	Unknown	1 to 3 hr	Unknown

Mechanism of Action

May reduce blood pressure by competing with beta-adrenergic receptor agonists, which helps reduce cardiac output, decrease sympathetic outflow to peripheral blood vessels, and inhibit renin.

Contraindications

Asthma, bradycardia (less than 45 beats/min), cardiogenic shock, hypersensitivity to carteolol or its components, second- or third-degree heart block

Interactions

DRUGS

allergen immunotherapy, allergenic extracts for skin testing: Increased risk of serious systemic reaction or anaphylaxis
catecholamine-depleting drugs, such as reserpine: Additive effects, increased risk of hypotension and bradycardia
clonidine: Increased risk of tachycardia and hypertension after clonidine discontinuation
diltiazem, nifedipine, verapamil: Potentiated effects of carteolol
general anesthetics: Exaggeration of hypotension
NSAIDs: Reduced antihypertensive effect of carteolol
oral antidiabetic drugs: Reduced symptomatic responses to hypoglycemia
sympathomimetics with alpha- and beta-adrenergic effects, such as pseudoephedrine: Possibly hypertension and excessive bradycardia or heart block

Adverse Reactions

CNS: Fatigue, insomnia, lassitude, paresthesia, tiredness, weakness
CV: Chest pain, heart failure, peripheral edema
EENT: Dry mouth, nasal congestion, pharyngitis
GI: Abdominal pain, diarrhea, flatulence, nausea
MS: Arthralgia, back pain, leg pain, muscle spasms
SKIN: Rash

Nursing Considerations

•**WARNING** Be aware that stopping carteolol abruptly in patients with angina may cause worsening of angina or MI; abrupt cessation in patients with hyperthyroidism may cause thyroid storm.
•Carefully monitor blood glucose level in diabetic patient because carteolol can mask hypoglycemic symptoms. It also can interfere with endogenous insulin release in response to hyperglycemia, requiring dosage adjustment of oral antidiabetic drug.

PATIENT TEACHING

•Advise patient to follow dosing schedule even if he feels better and not to discontinue therapy abruptly.
•Instruct patient to report signs of heart failure, such as fatigue, difficulty breathing, cough, and unusually fast heartbeat.
•Tell diabetic patient to frequently monitor his blood glucose level.
•Advise patient to consult prescriber before taking OTC preparations, such as nasal decongestants and cold preparations that contain sympathomimetics, because of the risk of serious drug interactions.

carvedilol

Coreg, Coreg CR

Class and Category

Chemical class: Nonselective beta-adrenergic blocker with alpha$_1$-adrenergic blocking activity

C

Therapeutic class: Antihypertensive, heart failure treatment adjunct
Pregnancy category: C

Indications and Dosages

➤ *To control hypertension*

TABLETS

Adults. 6.25 mg b.i.d. for 7 to 14 days, if tolerated. Then dosage increased to 12.5 mg b.i.d. for 7 to 14 days, and up to 25 mg, if tolerated and needed. *Maximum:* 50 mg daily.

E.R. CAPSULES

Adults. *Initial:* 20 mg once daily with food. After 7 to 14 days, increased to 40 mg once daily. After another 7 to 14 days, increased to 80 mg once daily. *Maximum:* 80 mg once daily.

➤ *As adjunct to treat mild to severe heart failure of ischemic or cardiomyopathic origin*

TABLETS

Adults. 3.125 mg b.i.d. for 2 wk, then increased to 6.25, 12.5, and 25 mg b.i.d. at successive 2-wk intervals, as tolerated. *Maximum (for patients with mild to moderate heart failure):* 50 mg b.i.d. if patient weighs more than 85 kg (187 lb).

E.R. CAPSULES

Adults. *Initial:* 10 mg once daily with food for 2 wk. Then increased to 20 mg once daily, as needed. Subsequent dosage increased by 20 mg every 2 wk, as needed. *Maximum:* 80 mg once daily.

➤ *To reduce CV mortality after acute phase of MI in patients with left ventricular ejection fraction of 40% or less*

TABLETS

Adults. 6.25 mg b.i.d. for 3 to 10 days, if tolerated. Then dosage increased to 12.5 mg b.i.d. for 3 to 10 days and up to 25 mg b.i.d., if needed and tolerated.

E.R. CAPSULES

Adults. *Initial:* 10 to 20 mg once daily. After 3 to 10 days, increased to 20 to 40 mg once daily. Increased again as needed every 3 to 10 days until reaching tolerance or target dose of 80 mg once daily. *Maximum:* 80 mg once daily.

DOSAGE ADJUSTMENT For patient with fluid retention or low blood pressure or heart rate, starting dosage may be decreased to 3.125 mg b.i.d., increase may be slowed, or both for tablet form. For patient with heart rate below 55 beats/min, extended release dosage decreased as clinical condition indicates.

Route	Onset	Peak	Duration
P.O.	In 30 min	1.5 to 7 hr	Unknown

Mechanism of Action

Reduces cardiac output and tachycardia, causes vasodilation, and decreases peripheral vascular resistance, which reduces blood pressure and cardiac workload. When administered for at least 4 weeks, carvedilol reduces plasma renin activity.

Contraindications

Asthma or related bronchospastic conditions; cardiogenic shock; decompensated heart failure that requires I.V. inotropics; hypersensitivity to carvedilol or its components; and second- or third-degree AV block, severe bradycardia or hepatic impairment, or sick sinus syndrome unless pacemaker is in place

Interactions

DRUGS

beta blockers, digoxin: Increased risk of bradycardia
calcium channel blockers (especially diltiazem and verapamil): Abnormal cardiac conduction and, possibly, increased adverse effects of calcium channel blockers
catecholamine-depleting drugs (such as reserpine and MAO inhibitors): Additive effects, increased risk of hypotension and bradycardia
cimetidine: Increased blood carvedilol level
clonidine: Risk of tachycardia and hypertension when clonidine is discontinued
cyclosporine, digoxin: Increased blood levels of these drugs
digoxin: Possibly increased blood digoxin level
oral antidiabetic drugs: Increased risk of hypoglycemia
rifampin: Decreased blood carvedilol level

Adverse Reactions

CNS: Asthenia, depression, dizziness, fatigue, fever, headache, hypesthesia, hypo-tonia, insomnia, light-headedness, malaise, paresthesia, somnolence, stroke, syncope, vertigo
CV: Angina, AV block, bradycardia, edema, heart failure, hypertension, hypertriglyceridemia, orthostatic hypotension, palpita-

tions, peripheral vascular disorder
EENT: Blurred vision, dry eyes, periodontitis, pharyngitis, rhinitis
ENDO: Hyperglycemia, hypoglycemia
GI: Abdominal pain, diarrhea, elevated liver function test results, melena, nausea, vomiting
GU: Albuminuria, hematuria, elevated BUN and creatinine levels, impotence, renal insufficiency, UTI
HEME: Aplastic anemia, decreased PT, thrombocytopenia, unusual bleeding or bruising
MS: Arthralgia, arthritis, back pain, muscle cramps
RESP: Dyspnea, increased cough
SKIN: Jaundice, pruritus, purpura
Other: Anaphylaxis, fluid overload, gout, hyperkalemia, hyperuricemia, hyponatremia, hypovolemia, viral infection, weight gain or loss

Nursing Considerations
• Use carvedilol cautiously in patients with peripheral vascular disease because it may aggravate symptoms of arterial insufficiency; in patients with diabetes mellitus it may mask signs of hypoglycemia, such as tachycardia, and may delay recovery.
• Monitor patient's blood glucose level, as ordered, throughout carvedilol therapy because drug may alter blood glucose level.
• WARNING Avoid stopping drug abruptly in patients with hyperthyroidism because thyroid storm may occur and in patients with angina because it may worsen or MI may occur.
• If patient has heart failure, expect to also give digoxin, a diuretic, and an ACE inhibitor.

PATIENT TEACHING
• Instruct patient prescribed extended-release capsules to swallow them whole. If swallowing capsules is difficult, tell patient he may open capsule and sprinkle beads on a spoonful of cold applesauce and then eat the applesauce immediately without chewing.
• Warn patient that drug may cause orthostatic hypotension, light-headedness, and dizziness; advise him to take safety precautions.
• Tell patient with heart failure to notify prescriber if he gains 5 lb or more in 2 days or if shortness of breath increases. These changes may signal worsening heart failure.

• Alert patient with diabetes to monitor his glycemic control closely because drug may increase blood glucose level or mask symptoms of hypoglycemia.

caspofungin acetate
Cancidas

Class and Category
Chemical class: Echinocandins
Therapeutic class: Antifungal
Pregnancy category: C

Indications and Dosages
➤ *To treat invasive aspergillosis in patients refractory to or intolerant of other therapies; to treat candidemia and candidal infections in intra-abdominal abscesses, peritonitis, and pleural space infections*

I.V. INFUSION
Adults. *Initial:* 70 mg on day 1, followed by 50 mg daily. *Maximum:* 70 mg daily.
Children ages 3 months to 17 years. *Initial:* 70 mg/m^2 on day 1, followed by 50 mg/m^2 daily. *Maximum:* 70 mg daily regardless of dose calculated based on patient's body surface area.

➤ *To treat presumed fungal infections in febrile, neutropenic patients*

I.V. INFUSION
Adults. *Initial:* 70 mg on day 1, followed by 50 mg daily for at least 14 days, including at least 7 days after neutropenia and symptoms have resolved. Increased to 70 mg daily as needed. *Maximum:* 70 mg daily.
Children ages 3 months to 17 years. *Initial:* 70 mg/m^2 on day 1, followed by 50 mg/m^2 daily for at least 14 days, including at least 7 days after neutropenia and symptoms have resolved. *Maximum:* 70 mg daily regardless of dose calculated based on patient's body surface area.

DOSAGE ADJUSTMENT Dosage reduced to 35 mg daily after initial 70-mg loading dose in moderate hepatic insufficiency.

➤ *To treat esophageal candidiasis*

I.V. INFUSION
Adults. 50 mg daily.
Children ages 3 months to 17 years. *Initial:* 70 mg/m^2 on day 1, followed by 50 mg/m^2

daily. *Maximum:* 70 mg daily regardless of dose calculated based on patient's body surface area.

DOSAGE ADJUSTMENT Dosage reduced to 35 mg daily in moderate hepatic insufficiency.

Mechanism of Action

Caspofungin acetate interferes with fungal cell membrane synthesis by inhibiting the synthesis of β (1,3)-D-glucan. A polypeptide, β (1,3)-D-glucan is the essential component of the fungal cell membrane that makes it rigid and protective. Without it, fungal cells rupture and die. This mechanism of action is most effective against susceptible filamentous fungi, such as *Aspergillus*.

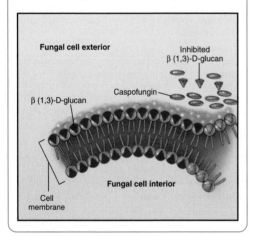

Incompatibilities

Don't mix or infuse with other drugs. Don't admix with diluents that contain dextrose.

Contraindications

Hypersensitivity to caspofungin acetate or its components

Interactions

DRUGS

carbamazepine, dexamethasone, efavirenz, nelfinavir, nevirapine, phenytoin, rifampin: Possibly decreased blood caspofungin level
cyclosporine: Transient increases in ALT and AST levels
tacrolimus: Possibly decreased blood tacrolimus level

Adverse Reactions

CNS: Chills, dizziness, fever, headache, insomnia, paresthesia, tremor
CV: Edema, hypertension, hypotension, phlebitis, tachycardia, thrombophlebitis
GI: Abdominal pain, diarrhea, elevated liver function test results, hepatic dysfunction, jaundice, nausea, vomiting
GU: Elevated BUN or serum creatinine level, proteinuria, renal insufficiency
HEME: Decreased hemoglobin and hematocrit
MS: Back pain, myalgia
RESP: Bronchospasm, dyspnea, stridor, tachypnea
SKIN: Diaphoresis, erythema, flushing, pruritus, rash, sensation of warmth
Other: Decreased serum bicarbonate level, facial edema, hypercalcemia, hyperkalemia, hyperphosphatemia, hypokalemia, hypomagnesemia, infusion site reaction

Nursing Considerations

• To prepare 70-mg loading dose, let vial reach room temperature. Reconstitute by adding 10.5 ml normal saline solution to vial. Dilute for administration by transferring 10 ml of reconstituted drug to 250 ml normal saline solution.
• To prepare 70-mg loading dose from two 50-mg vials, add 10.5 ml normal saline solution to each vial; then transfer 14 ml prepared solution to 250 ml normal saline solution.
• To prepare daily 50-mg infusion, let vial reach room temperature. Reconstitute by adding 10.5 ml normal saline solution to vial. Dilute for administration by transferring only 10 ml reconstituted drug to 250 ml normal saline solution.
• To prepare daily 50-mg infusion at reduced volume, add 10 ml reconstituted drug to 100 ml normal saline solution.
• To prepare 35-mg daily dose for patient with moderate hepatic insufficiency, reconstitute 50-mg vial with 10.5 ml normal saline solution. To dilute, transfer only 7 ml reconstituted drug to 250 ml normal saline solution or, if needed, to 100 ml normal saline solution.
• When preparing powder for reconstitution, mix gently to obtain clear solution. Don't use if solution is cloudy or contains precipitate. Discard unused solution after 24 hours.

•Infuse drug slowly over about 1 hour.
•Expect to increase daily dose to 70 mg for adults and 70 mg/m² for children (not to exceed the adult dose of 70 mg regardless of calculated dose), as prescribed, for patients also receiving carbamazepine, dexamethasone, efavirenz, nelfinavir, nevirapine, phenytoin, or rifampin.
•Watch for flushed skin, and assess patient often for unexplained temperature elevation.
•Assess for airway patency if patient develops excessive facial edema or respiratory stridor. Provide emergency airway management if complete obstruction occurs.
•Monitor patient's liver function test results, as ordered, and report abnormalities.

PATIENT TEACHING
•Urge patient to notify prescriber immediately if he has difficulty talking, swallowing, or breathing during drug administration.

cefaclor

Apo-Cefaclor (CAN), Ceclor, Ceclor CD, Raniclor

Class and Category
Chemical class: Second-generation cephalosporin, 7-aminocephalosporanic acid
Therapeutic class: Antibiotic
Pregnancy category: B

Indications and Dosages
➤ *To treat otitis media caused by* Haemophilus influenzae, *staphylococci,* Streptococcus pneumoniae, *and* Streptococcus pyogenes; *lower respiratory tract infections, including pneumonia caused by* H. influenzae, S. pneumoniae, *and* S. pyogenes; *pharyngitis and tonsillitis caused by* S. pyogenes; *UTI, including cystitis and pyelonephritis, caused by* Escherichia coli, Klebsiella *species,* Proteus mirabilis, *and coagulase-negative staphylococci; and skin and soft-tissue infections caused by* S. pyogenes *and* Staphylococcus aureus

CAPSULES
Adults and adolescents. 250 mg every 8 hr. For severe infections, such as pneumonia, or those caused by less susceptible organisms, 500 mg every 8 hr. *Maximum:* 4 g daily.
CHEWABLE TABLETS, ORAL SUSPENSION
Adults and adolescents. 250 mg every 8 hr.

For severe infections, such as pneumonia, or those caused by less susceptible organisms, 500 mg every 8 hr. *Maximum:* 4 g daily.
Children. 20 mg/kg daily in divided doses every 8 hr. For serious infections, such as otitis media, and infections caused by less susceptible organisms, 40 mg/kg daily in divided doses every 8 hr. For otitis media and pharyngitis, total daily dosage divided and given every 12 hr, if needed. *Maximum:* 1 g daily.
➤ *To treat acute bacterial infection in chronic bronchitis or secondary bacterial infection in acute bronchitis (not caused by* H. influenzae)
E.R. TABLETS
Adults and adolescents age 16 and over. 500 mg every 12 hr for 7 days.
➤ *To treat pharyngitis and tonsillitis (not caused by* H. influenzae)
E.R. TABLETS
Adults and adolescents age 16 and over. 375 mg every 12 hr for 10 days.
➤ *To treat uncomplicated skin and soft-tissue infections caused by* S. aureus
E.R. TABLETS
Adults and adolescents age 16 and over. 375 mg every 12 hr for 7 to 10 days.

Mechanism of Action
Interferes with bacterial cell wall synthesis by inhibiting cross-linking of peptidoglycan strands, which stiffen cell membranes. As a result, bacterial cells rupture.

Contraindications
Hypersensitivity to cephalosporins or their components

Interactions
DRUGS
aminoglycosides, loop diuretics: Increased risk of nephrotoxicity
antacids: Decreased blood cefaclor level (E.R. tablets)
oral anticoagulants: Increased anticoagulation

Adverse Reactions
CNS: Chills, fever, headache, seizures
CV: Edema
EENT: Hearing loss
GI: Abdominal cramps, diarrhea, elevated

liver function test results, hepatic failure, hepatomegaly, nausea, oral candidiasis, pseudomembranous colitis, vomiting
GU: Elevated BUN level, nephrotoxicity, renal failure, vaginal candidiasis
HEME: Eosinophilia, hemolytic anemia, hypoprothrombinemia, neutropenia, thrombocytopenia, unusual bleeding
MS: Arthralgia
RESP: Dyspnea
SKIN: Ecchymosis, erythema, erythema multiforme, pruritus, rash, Stevens-Johnson syndrome
Other: Anaphylaxis, superinfection

Nursing Considerations
• Use cefaclor cautiously in patients with impaired renal function or a history of GI disease, particularly colitis, and in patients who are hypersensitive to penicillin; about 10% of such patients have cross-sensitivity.
• If possible, obtain culture and sensitivity test results, as ordered, before giving drug.
• Monitor BUN and serum creatinine levels for early signs of nephrotoxicity. Also monitor fluid intake and output; decreasing urine output may indicate nephrotoxicity.
• Be aware that an allergic reaction may occur a few days after therapy starts.
• Assess bowel pattern daily; severe diarrhea may indicate pseudomembranous colitis.
• Assess patient for superinfection: perineal itching, fever, malaise, redness, pain, swelling, rash, drainage, diarrhea, cough, sputum changes.

PATIENT TEACHING
• Instruct patient to complete the prescribed course of therapy, even if he feels better.
• Tell patient to swallow E.R. tablets whole and not to crush, break, or chew them.
• Advise patient to take E.R. tablets with food to enhance absorption.
• Instruct patient to take capsules or E.R. tablets with a full glass of water.
• Tell patient to shake oral suspension well before measuring and to use a calibrated measuring device to ensure accurate dose.
• Tell patient to refrigerate oral suspension and to discard unused portion after 14 days.
• Instruct patient to immediately report severe diarrhea to prescriber.
• Explain that yogurt and buttermilk protect intestinal flora and decrease diarrhea.
• Urge patient to report evidence of superinfection.

cefadroxil
Duricef

Class and Category
Chemical class: First-generation cephalosporin, 7-aminocephalosporanic acid
Therapeutic class: Antibiotic
Pregnancy category: B

Indications and Dosages
➤ *To treat UTI caused by* Escherichia coli, Klebsiella *species, or* Proteus mirabilis
CAPSULES, TABLETS
Adults. For uncomplicated lower UTI, 1 to 2 g daily or in divided doses every 12 hr. For all other UTIs, 2 g every 12 hr.
ORAL SUSPENSION
Adults. For uncomplicated lower UTI, 1 to 2 g daily or in divided doses every 12 hr. For all other UTIs, 2 g every 12 hr.
Children. 30 mg/kg daily in divided doses every 12 hr. *Maximum:* Adult dosage.
➤ *To treat skin and soft-tissue infections caused by staphylococci or streptococci*
CAPSULES, TABLETS
Adults. 1 g daily or 500 mg every 12 hr.
ORAL SUSPENSION
Adults. 1 g daily or 500 mg every 12 hr.
Children. 30 mg/kg daily in divided doses every 12 hr. *Maximum:* Adult dosage.
➤ *To treat pharyngitis and tonsillitis caused by group A beta-hemolytic streptococci*
CAPSULES, TABLETS
Adults. 1 g daily or 500 mg b.i.d for 10 days.
ORAL SUSPENSION
Adults. 1 g daily or 500 mg b.i.d. for 10 days.
Children. 30 mg/kg daily in divided doses every 12 hr for 10 days. *Maximum:* 1 g daily or 500 mg b.i.d. for 10 days.
DOSAGE ADJUSTMENT Initial dose of 1 g; then maintenance of 0.5 g every 12 hr if creatinine clearance is 25 to 50 ml/min/1.73 m^2; 0.5 g every 24 hr if creatinine clearance is 10 to 25 ml/min/1.73 m^2; and 0.5 g every 36 hr if creatinine clearance is 0 to 10 ml/min/1.73 m^2.

Contraindications
Hypersensitivity to cephalosporins or their components

Interactions
DRUGS
aminoglycosides, loop diuretics: Increased toxicity of these drugs

Mechanism of Action
Interferes with bacterial cell wall synthesis by inhibiting the final step in the cross-linking of peptidoglycan strands. Peptidoglycan makes cell membranes rigid and protective. Without it, bacterial cells rupture and die.

Adverse Reactions
CNS: Chills, fever, headache, seizures
CV: Edema
EENT: Hearing loss
GI: Abdominal cramps, diarrhea, elevated liver function test results, hepatic failure, hepatomegaly, nausea, oral candidiasis, pseudomembranous colitis, vomiting
GU: Elevated BUN level, nephrotoxicity, renal failure, vaginal candidiasis
HEME: Eosinophilia, hemolytic anemia, hypoprothrombinemia, neutropenia, thrombocytopenia, unusual bleeding
MS: Arthralgia
RESP: Dyspnea
SKIN: Ecchymosis, erythema, erythema multiforme, pruritus, rash, Stevens-Johnson syndrome
Other: Anaphylaxis, superinfection

Nursing Considerations
• Use cefadroxil cautiously in patients with impaired renal function or a history of GI disease, particularly colitis. Also use drug cautiously in patients who are hypersensitive to penicillin because cross-sensitivity has occurred in about 10% of such patients.
• If possible, obtain culture and sensitivity test results, as ordered, before giving drug.
• Be aware that an allergic reaction may occur a few days after therapy starts.
• Monitor BUN and serum creatinine levels for early signs of nephrotoxicity. Also monitor fluid intake and output; decreasing urine output may indicate nephrotoxicity.
• Assess bowel pattern daily; severe diarrhea may indicate pseudomembranous colitis.
• Assess for signs of superinfection, such as perineal itching, fever, malaise, redness, pain, swelling, drainage, rash, diarrhea, and cough or sputum changes.
PATIENT TEACHING
• Instruct patient to complete the prescribed course of therapy.
• Tell patient to shake oral suspension before measuring and to use a liquid-measuring device to ensure accurate doses.
• Tell patient to refrigerate oral suspension and to discard the unused portion after 14 days.
• Urge patient to report watery, bloody stools to prescriber immediately, even up to 2 months after drug therapy has ended.
• Inform patient that yogurt and buttermilk can help maintain intestinal flora and decrease diarrhea.
• Teach patient to recognize and report evidence of superinfection, such as furry tongue, perineal itching, and loose, foul-smelling stools.

cefazolin sodium
Ancef

Class and Category
Chemical class: First-generation cephalosporin, 7-aminocephalosporanic acid
Therapeutic class: Antibiotic
Pregnancy category: B

Indications and Dosages
➤ *To treat respiratory tract infections caused by group A beta-hemolytic streptococci,* Haemophilus influenzae, Klebsiella *species,* Staphylococcus aureus, *and* Streptococcus pneumoniae; *skin and soft-tissue infections caused by* S. aureus, *group A beta-hemolytic and other strains of streptococci; biliary tract infections caused by* Escherichia coli, Klebsiella *species,* Proteus mirabilis, S. aureus, *and various strains of streptococci; bone and joint infections caused by* S. aureus; *genital infections, such as epididymitis and prostatitis, caused by* E. coli, Klebsiella *species,* P. mirabilis, *and some strains of enterococci; septicemia caused by* E. coli, Klebsiella *species,* P. mirabilis, S. aureus, *and* S. pneumoniae; *and endocarditis caused by group A beta-hemolytic streptococci and* S. aureus
I.V. INFUSION, I.V. OR I.M. INJECTION
Adults. For mild infections, 250 to 500 mg every 8 hr; for moderate to severe infections, 500 to 1,000 mg every 6 to 8 hr; and for severe life-threatening infections, 1,000 to 1,500 mg every 6 hr. *Maximum:* 6 g daily.

Children: For mild to moderate infections, 25 to 50 mg/kg daily divided equally and given t.i.d. or q.i.d.; for severe infections, 100 mg/kg daily divided equally and given t.i.d. or q.i.d.

➤ *To treat pneumococcal pneumonia*
I.V. INFUSION, I.V. OR I.M. INJECTION
Adults. 500 mg every 12 hr.

➤ *To treat acute uncomplicated UTI caused by* E. coli, Klebsiella *species,* P. mirabilis, *and some strains of* Enterobacter *and* Enterococcus
I.V. INFUSION, I.V. OR I.M. INJECTION
Adults. 1 g every 12 hr.

➤ *To provide surgical prophylaxis*
I.V. INFUSION, I.V. OR I.M. INJECTION
Adults. 1 g 30 to 60 min before surgery; 0.5 to 1 g during surgery if it lasts 2 hr or longer; 0.5 to 1 g every 6 to 8 hr for 24 hr after surgery.

DOSAGE ADJUSTMENT After initial loading dose appropriate to infection's severity, dosage interval restricted to at least 8 hr for adults with creatinine clearance of 35 to 54 ml/min/1.73 m^2; dosage reduced by 50% and given every 12 hr for adults with creatinine clearance of 11 to 34 ml/min/1.73 m^2; and dosage reduced by 50% and given every 18 to 24 hr for adults with creatinine clearance of 10 ml/min/1.73 m^2 or less. Dosage reduced to 60% and given every 12 hr for children with creatinine clearance of 40 to 70 ml/min/1.73 m^2; dosage reduced to 25% and given every 12 hr for children with creatinine clearance of 20 to 40 ml/min/1.73 m^2; and dosage reduced to 10% and given every 24 hr for children with creatinine clearance of 5 to 20 ml/min/1.73 m^2.

Mechanism of Action
Interferes with bacterial cell wall synthesis by inhibiting the final step in the cross-linking of peptidoglycan strands. Peptidoglycan makes cell membranes rigid and protective. Without it, bacterial cells rupture and die.

Incompatibilities
To prevent mutual inactivation, don't mix cefazolin with aminoglycosides. Also avoid mixing cefazolin with other drugs, including pentamidine isethionate.

Contraindications
Hypersensitivity to cephalosporins or their components

Interactions
DRUGS
aminoglycosides, loop diuretics: Additive nephrotoxicity
probenecid: Increased and prolonged blood cefazolin level

Adverse Reactions
CNS: Chills, fever, headache, seizures
CV: Edema
EENT: Hearing loss
GI: Abdominal cramps, diarrhea, elevated liver function test results, hepatic failure, hepatitis, hepatomegaly, nausea, oral candidiasis, pseudomembranous colitis, vomiting
GU: Elevated BUN and serum creatinine levels, nephrotoxicity, renal failure, vaginal candidiasis
HEME: Eosinophilia, hemolytic anemia, hypoprothrombinemia, neutropenia, thrombocytopenia, unusual bleeding
MS: Arthralgia
RESP: Dyspnea
SKIN: Ecchymosis, erythema, erythema multiforme, pruritus, rash, Stevens-Johnson syndrome
Other: Anaphylaxis; injection site pain, redness, and swelling; superinfection

Nursing Considerations
•Use cefazolin cautiously in patients with impaired renal function or a history of GI disease, particularly colitis. Also use drug cautiously in patients who are hypersensitive to penicillin because cross-sensitivity has occurred in about 10% of such patients.

•If possible, obtain culture and sensitivity test results, as ordered, before giving drug.

•WARNING To prevent unintentional overdose, cefazolin for injection USP and dextrose injection USP shouldn't be used in children who require less than the full adult dose.

•Reconstitute 500-mg vial of drug with 2 ml of sterile water for injection (or 1-g vial with 2.5 ml). Shake well until dissolved.

•For direct I.V. injection, further dilute reconstituted solution with at least 5 ml of sterile water for injection. Inject slowly over 3 to 5 minutes through tubing of a flowing compatible I.V. solution.

•For intermittent I.V. infusion, reconstitute

500 to 1,000 mg in 50 to 100 ml of normal saline solution, D_5W, $D_{10}W$, dextrose 5% in lactated Ringer's solutoin, dextrose 5% in quarter-normal (0.2) saline solution, dextrose 5% in half-normal (0.45) saline solution, dextrose 5% in normal saline solution, lactated Ringer's injection, 5% or 10% invert sugar in sterile water for injection, 5% sodium bicarbonate (Ancef), or Ringer's injection.

• Administer I.M injection deep into large muscle mass, such as the gluteus maximus.
• Store reconstituted drug up to 24 hours at room temperature or 10 days refrigerated.
• Monitor I.V. site for irritation, phlebitis, and extravasation.
• Monitor BUN and serum creatinine levels for early signs of nephrotoxicity. Also monitor fluid intake and output; decreasing urine output may indicate nephrotoxicity.
• Be aware that an allergic reaction may occur a few days after therapy starts.
• Assess bowel pattern daily; severe diarrhea may indicate pseudomembranous colitis.
• Watch for evidence of superinfection: cough, diarrhea, drainage, fever, malaise, pain, perineal itching, rash, redness, swelling.
• Assess for pharyngitis, ecchymosis, bleeding, and arthralgia; they may indicate a blood dyscrasia.

PATIENT TEACHING
• Instruct patient to complete the prescribed course of therapy.
• Reassure patient that I.M. injection doesn't typically cause pain.
• Tell patient to report watery, bloody stools to prescriber immediately, even up to 2 months after drug therapy has ended.

cefdinir

Omnicef

Class and Category
Chemical class: Cephalosporin
Therapeutic class: Antibiotic
Pregnancy category: B

Indications and Dosages
➤ *To treat community-acquired pneumonia caused by* Haemophilus influenzae *(including beta-lactamase–producing strains),* Haemophilus parainfluenzae *(including beta-lactamase–producing strains),* Streptococcus pneumoniae *(penicillin-susceptible strains only), and* Moraxella catarrhalis *(including beta-lactamase–producing strains)*

CAPSULES
Adults and adolescents. 300 mg every 12 hr for 10 days. *Maximum:* 600 mg daily.
➤ *To treat pharyngitis or tonsillitis caused by* Streptococcus pyogenes *and acute exacerbations of chronic bronchitis caused by* H. influenzae *(including beta-lactamase–producing strains),* H. parainfluenzae *(including beta-lactamase–producing strains),* S. pneumoniae *(penicillin-susceptible strains only), and* M. catarrhalis *(including beta-lactamase–producing strains)*

CAPSULES
Adults and adolescents. 300 mg every 12 hr for 5 to 10 days or 600 mg every 24 hr for 10 days. *Maximum:* 600 mg daily.
ORAL SUSPENSION
Children ages 6 months to 12 years. 7 mg/kg every 12 hr for 5 to 10 days or 14 mg/kg every 24 hr for 10 days (for pharyngitis or tonsillitis).
➤ *To treat acute maxillary sinusitis caused by* H. influenzae *(including beta-lactamase–producing strains),* S. pneumoniae *(penicillin-susceptible strains only), and* M. catarrhalis *(including beta-lactamase–producing strains)*

CAPSULES
Adults and adolescents. 300 mg every 12 hr or 600 mg every 24 hr for 10 days. *Maximum:* 600 mg daily.
ORAL SUSPENSION
Children ages 6 months to 12 years. 7 mg/kg every 12 hr or 14 mg/kg every 24 hr for 10 days.
➤ *To treat uncomplicated skin and soft-tissue infections caused by* Staphylococcus aureus *(including beta-lactamase–producing strains) and* Streptococcus pyogenes

CAPSULES
Adults and adolescents. 300 mg every 12 hr for 10 days. *Maximum:* 600 mg daily.
ORAL SUSPENSION
Children ages 6 months to 12 years. 7 mg/kg every 12 hr for 10 days.
➤ *To treat acute bacterial otitis media*

caused by H. influenzae *(including beta-lactamase–producing strains),* S. pneumoniae *(penicillin-susceptible strains only), and* M. catarrhalis *(including beta-lactamase–producing strains)*

ORAL SUSPENSION

Children ages 6 months to 12 years. 7 mg/kg every 12 hr for 5 to 10 days or 14 mg/kg every 24 hr for 10 days.

DOSAGE ADJUSTMENT For adults with creatinine clearance of less than 30 ml/min/1.73 m², expect to reduce cefdinir dosage to 300 mg daily; for children with creatinine clearance of less than 30 ml/min/1.73 m², dosage is 7 mg/kg (up to 300 mg) daily. For patients undergoing intermittent hemodialysis, dosage is 300 mg or 7 mg/kg every other day, beginning at the end of each hemodialysis session, as prescribed.

Mechanism of Action

Interferes with bacterial cell wall synthesis by inhibiting the final step in the cross-linking of peptidoglycan strands. Peptidoglycan makes cell membranes rigid and protective. Without it, bacterial cells rupture and die. Because cefdinir is not degraded by some bacterial beta-lactamase enzymes, it's effective against many organisms that are resistant to both penicillins and some cephalosporins.

Contraindications

Hypersensitivity to cefdinir, other cephalosporins, or their components

Interactions

DRUGS

antacids that contain aluminum or magnesium: Decreased cefdinir absorption if given within 2 hours of antacid
iron salts: Reduced cefdinir absorption if given within 2 hours of iron
probenecid: Increased blood level and prolonged half-life of cefdinir

Adverse Reactions

CNS: Asthenia, dizziness, drowsiness, headache, insomnia, somnolence
EENT: Dry mouth, pharyngitis, rhinitis
GI: Abdominal pain, anorexia, constipation, diarrhea, flatulence, indigestion, nausea, pseudomembranous colitis, stool discoloration, vomiting
GU: Leukorrhea, vaginal candidiasis, vaginitis
HEME: Leukopenia
SKIN: Pruritus, rash
Other: Anaphylaxis, serum sicknesslike reaction

Nursing Considerations

• To reconstitute cefdinir powder for oral suspension, tap bottle to loosen powder, and then dilute with water to 125 mg/5 ml. Shake well before each use. Discard any unused portion after 10 days. Keep suspension bottle tightly closed, and store it at room temperature.
• Administer antacids that contain aluminum or magnesium and iron salts at least 2 hours before or after cefdinir because they may interfere with cefdinir absorption.
• Monitor patient who is allergic to penicillin for evidence of hypersensitivity reaction, ranging from a mild rash to fatal anaphylaxis, because cross-sensitivity can occur.
• Monitor patient with a chronic GI condition, such as colitis, for signs and symptoms of a drug-related exacerbation.
• Because all cephalosporins have the potential to cause bleeding, monitor elderly patients and patients with a preexisting coagulopathy, including vitamin K deficiency, for elevated PT or APTT.
• Assess patient's bowel pattern daily; severe diarrhea may indicate pseudomembranous colitis. Notify prescriber immediately if you detect signs or symptoms of this adverse reaction.
• Assess for other evidence of superinfection, including perineal itching; loose, foul-smelling stools; and vaginal drainage.

PATIENT TEACHING

• Advise patient taking cefdinir oral suspension to shake bottle well before use and to use a liquid-measuring device to ensure accurate dose.
• Inform patient that tablet coating may cause stools to become a reddish color.
• Instruct patient to complete entire course of therapy, even if he feels better.
• Advise patient to take iron salts and aluminum- or magnesium-containing antacids at least 2 hours before or after taking cefdinir.
• Inform patient with history of colitis that

cefdinir may worsen it; urge him to notify prescriber immediately if symptoms develop.
•Inform patient with diabetes mellitus that oral suspension contains 2.86 g of sucrose per teaspoon; advise him to monitor his blood glucose levels as appropriate.
•Teach patient to recognize and report evidence of superinfection, such as perineal itching; loose, foul-smelling stools; and vaginal drainage.
•Inform patient that yogurt and buttermilk can help prevent superinfection and may decrease diarrhea.

cefditoren pivoxil

Spectracef

Class and Category
Chemical class: Cephalosporin
Therapeutic class: Antibiotic
Pregnancy category: B

Indications and Dosages
➤ *To treat mild to moderate acute bacterial exacerbation of chronic bronchitis or community-acquired pneumonia caused by* Haemophilus influenzae *(including beta-lactamase–producing strains),* H. parainfluenzae *(including beta-lactamase–producing strains),* Streptococcus pneumoniae *(penicillin-susceptible strains), or* Moraxella catarrhalis *(including beta-lactamase–producing strains)*

TABLETS
Adults and children age 12 and over. 400 mg b.i.d. for 10 days or for 14 days for community-acquired pneumonia.

➤ *To treat mild to moderate pharyngitis and tonsillitis caused by* Streptococcus pyogenes

TABLETS
Adults and children age 12 and over. 200 mg b.i.d. for 10 days.

➤ *To treat mild to moderate uncomplicated skin and soft-tissue infections caused by* Staphylococcus aureus *(including beta-lactamase–producing strains) or* S. pyogenes

TABLETS
Adults and children age 12 and over. 200 mg b.i.d. for 10 days.

DOSAGE ADJUSTMENT For patients with moderate renal impairment (creatinine clearance of 30 to 49 ml/min/1.73 m^2), maximum dosage reduced to 200 mg b.i.d. For patients with severe renal impairment (creatinine clearance less than 30 ml/min/1.73 m^2), maximum dosage reduced to 200 mg daily.

Mechanism of Action
Interferes with bacterial cell wall synthesis by inhibiting the final step in the cross-linking of peptidoglycan strands. Peptidoglycan makes the cell membrane rigid and protective. Without it, bacterial cells rupture and die. This mechanism of action is most effective against bacteria that divide rapidly, including many gram-positive and gram-negative bacteria. Cefditoren isn't inactivated by beta lactamase produced by some bacteria.

Contraindications
Carnitine deficiency or inborn metabolic disorder that causes it; hypersensitivity to cephalosporins or their components

Interactions
DRUGS
aluminum- and magnesium-containing antacids, H$_2$-receptor antagonists: Reduced cefditoren absorption
probenecid: Increased and prolonged blood cefditoren level
FOODS
food: Increased cefditoren absorption

Adverse Reactions
CNS: Headache, hyperactivity, hypertonia, seizures
GI: Abdominal pain, diarrhea, dyspepsia, hepatic dysfunction, nausea, pseudomembranous colitis, vomiting
GU: Acute renal failure, renal dysfunction, toxic nephropathy
HEME: Aplastic anemia, hemolytic anemia, hemorrhage, thrombocytopenia
MS: Arthralgia
RESP: Pneumonia
SKIN: Erythema multiforme, Stevens-Johnson syndrome, toxic epidermal necrolysis
Other: Allergic reaction, anaphylaxis, carnitine deficiency, drug fever, serum sicknesslike reaction, superinfection

Nursing Considerations

•**WARNING** Before instituting cefditoren therapy, determine if patient is hypersensitive to milk protein because cefditoren contains sodium caseinate, a milk protein. Be aware that drug should not be given to patient with this hypersensitivity. Also determine if patient has had a hypersensitivity reaction to cefditoren or other cephalosporins (because drug is contraindicated in these patients) or to penicillin (because cross-sensitivity has occurred in about 10% of patients).

•Cefditoren shouldn't be used for prolonged treatment because of the risk of carnitine deficiency.

•If possible, obtain culture and sensitivity test results before giving cefditoren.

•Assess patient for evidence of *Clostridium difficile* infection and pseudomembranous colitis, such as profuse, watery diarrhea. For mild cases, expect to discontinue cefditoren. For moderate to severe cases, expect to also administer fluids and electrolytes, protein supplementation, and an antibacterial drug effective against *C. difficile* colitis, as prescribed.

•If an allergic reaction occurs, expect to discontinue drug, as prescribed. For serious acute hypersensitivity reactions, expect to also administer epinephrine, oxygen, I.V. fluids, I.V. antihistamines, I.V. corticosteroids, and I.V. vasopressors, as prescribed.

•Monitor BUN and serum creatinine levels to detect early signs of renal dysfunction. Also monitor fluid intake and output.

•Watch for a decreased PT, as ordered, in at-risk patients, such as those with renal or hepatic impairment, those with a poor nutritional state, and those receiving anticoagulant or prolonged antibiotic therapy. Notify prescriber if a decrease occurs, and give vitamin K as ordered.

PATIENT TEACHING

•Urge patient to complete prescribed course of therapy.

•Instruct patient to take cefditoren with meals to enhance drug absorption.

•Advise patient not to take cefditoren with aluminum- or magnesium-containing antacids or other drugs used to reduce stomach acids because these drugs may interfere with cefditoren absorption.

•Explain that yogurt and buttermilk help maintain normal intestinal flora and can decrease diarrhea during therapy.

•Instruct patient to immediately report severe diarrhea to prescriber.

cefepime hydrochloride

Maxipime

Class and Category

Chemical class: Fourth-generation cephalosporin, 7-aminocephalosporanic acid
Therapeutic class: Antibiotic
Pregnancy category: B

Indications and Dosages

➤ *To treat mild to moderate UTI caused by* Escherichia coli, Klebsiella pneumoniae, *and* Proteus mirabilis

I.V. INFUSION, I.M. INJECTION (ONLY FOR UTI CAUSED BY *E. COLI*)

Adults and children age 12 and over. 500 to 1,000 mg every 12 hr for 7 to 10 days.

➤ *To treat severe UTI caused by* E. coli *or* K. pneumoniae, *moderate to severe skin and soft-tissue infections caused by* Staphylococcus aureus *or* Streptococcus pyogenes

I.V. INFUSION

Adults and children age 12 and over. 2 g every 12 hr for 10 days.

➤ *To treat moderate to severe pneumonia caused by* Enterobacter *species,* K. pneumoniae, Pseudomonas aeruginosa, *or* Streptococcus pneumoniae

I.V. INFUSION

Adults and children age 12 and over. 1 to 2 g every 12 hr for 10 days.

➤ *To treat febrile neutropenia*

I.V. INFUSION

Adults and children age 12 and over. 2 g every 8 hr for 7 days or until neutropenia resolves.

➤ *To treat complicated intra-abdominal infections (together with metronidazole) caused by alpha-hemolytic streptococci,* Bacteroides fragilis, E. coli, Enterobacter *species,* K. pneumoniae, *or* P. aeruginosa

I.V. INFUSION

Adults and children age 12 and over. 2 g every 12 hr for 7 to 10 days.

DOSAGE ADJUSTMENT Dosing interval increased from 12 to 24 hr and from 8 to 12 hr for patients with creatinine clearance of 30 to 60 ml/min/1.73 m²; dosing interval increased from 8 or 12 hr to 24 hr and dose decreased from 2 g every 12 hr to 1 g every 24 hr (all other doses remain unchanged) for patients with creatinine clearance of 11 to 29 ml/min/1.73 m²; dosage decreased from 500 mg every 12 hr to 250 mg every 24 hr, from 1,000 mg every 12 hr to 250 mg every 24 hr, from 2,000 mg every 12 hr to 500 mg every 24 hr, and from 2 g every 8 hr to 1 g every 24 hr if creatinine clearance is less than 11 ml/min/1.73 m².

Mechanism of Action

Interferes with bacterial cell wall synthesis by inhibiting the final step in the cross-linking of peptidoglycan strands. Peptidoglycan makes cell membranes rigid and protective. Without it, bacterial cells rupture and die.

Incompatibilities

Don't add cefepime to solutions that contain ampicillin in a concentration of more than 40 mg/ml. Don't add drug to solutions that contain aminophylline, gentamycin, metronidazole, netilmicin sulfate, tobramycin, or vancomycin.

Contraindications

Hypersensitivity to cephalosporins or their components

Interactions
DRUGS
aminoglycosides, loop diuretics: Increased risk of renal failure in renal disease

Adverse Reactions
CNS: Chills, fever, headache, seizures
CV: Edema
EENT: Hearing loss
GI: Abdominal cramps, diarrhea, elevated liver function test results, hepatic failure, hepatomegaly, nausea, oral candidiasis, pseudomembranous colitis, vomiting
GU: Elevated BUN level, nephrotoxicity, renal failure, vaginal candidiasis
HEME: Eosinophilia, hemolytic anemia, hypoprothrombinemia, neutropenia, thrombocytopenia, unusual bleeding

MS: Arthralgia
RESP: Dyspnea
SKIN: Ecchymosis, erythema, erythema multiforme, pruritus, rash, Stevens-Johnson syndrome
Other: Anaphylaxis; injection site pain, redness, and swelling; superinfection

Nursing Considerations
• Use cefepime cautiously in patients with impaired renal function or a history of GI disease, particularly colitis. Also use drug cautiously in patients who are hypersensitive to penicillin because cross-sensitivity has occurred in about 10% of such patients.
• If possible, obtain culture and sensitivity test results, as ordered, before giving drug.
• For I.V. infusion, reconstitute using manufacturer's guidelines. Give over 30 minutes.
• For I.M. injection, reconstitute 500-mg vial of drug with 1.3 ml of diluent, such as sterile water for injection (or 1-g vial with 2.4 ml of diluent). See manufacturer's guidelines for complete list of appropriate diluents.
• Be aware that an allergic reaction may occur a few days after therapy starts.
• Monitor BUN and serum creatinine levels for early signs of nephrotoxicity. Also monitor fluid intake and output; decreasing urine output may indicate nephrotoxicity. Be aware that unadjusted dosages of cefepime in renally impaired patients may cause myoclonus and seizures.
• Assess bowel pattern daily; severe diarrhea may indicate pseudomembranous colitis.
• Assess for signs of superinfection, such as perineal itching, fever, malaise, redness, pain, swelling, drainage, rash, diarrhea, and cough or sputum changes.
• Assess for pharyngitis, ecchymosis, bleeding, and arthralgia; they may indicate a blood dyscrasia.
PATIENT TEACHING
• Tell patient to immediately report severe diarrhea to prescriber.

cefixime

Suprax

Class and Category
Chemical class: Third-generation cephalosporin, 7-aminocephalosporanic acid

Therapeutic class: Antibiotic
Pregnancy category: B

Indications and Dosages

➤ *To treat uncomplicated UTI caused by* Escherichia coli *and* Proteus mirabilis; *otitis media caused by* Haemophilus influenzae, Moraxella catarrhalis, *and* Streptococcus pyogenes; *pharyngitis and tonsillitis caused by* S. pyogenes; *acute bronchitis and acute exacerbations of chronic bronchitis caused by* H. influenzae *and* Streptococcus pneumoniae

ORAL SUSPENSION

Children. 8 mg/kg daily or 4 mg/kg every 12 hr.

TABLETS

Adults and children over 50 kg (110 lb) or age 12. 400 mg daily or 200 mg every 12 hr.

➤ *To treat uncomplicated gonorrhea caused by* Neisseria gonorrhoeae

TABLETS

Adults and children over 50 kg or age 12. 400 mg daily.

DOSAGE ADJUSTMENT Dosage reduced to 75% for patients who have creatinine clearance of 21 to 60 ml/min/1.73 m^2 or receive hemodialysis. Dosage reduced to 50% for patients who have creatinine clearance of 20 ml/min/1.73 m^2 or less.

Mechanism of Action

Interferes with bacterial cell wall synthesis by inhibiting the final step in the cross-linking of peptidoglycan strands. Peptidoglycan makes cell membranes rigid and protective. Without it, bacterial cells rupture and die.

Contraindications

Hypersensitivity to cephalosporins or their components

Interactions

DRUGS

aminoglycosides, loop diuretics: Increased risk of nephrotoxicity
carbamazepine: Increased blood carbamazepine level

Adverse Reactions

CNS: Chills, fever, headache, seizures

CV: Edema
EENT: Hearing loss
GI: Abdominal cramps, diarrhea, elevated liver function test results, hepatic failure, hepatitis, hepatomegaly, jaundice, nausea, oral candidiasis, pseudomembranous colitis, vomiting
GU: Elevated BUN level, nephrotoxicity, renal failure, vaginal candidiasis
HEME: Eosinophilia, hemolytic anemia, hypoprothrombinemia, neutropenia, thrombocytopenia, unusual bleeding
MS: Arthralgia
RESP: Dyspnea
SKIN: Ecchymosis, erythema, erythema multiforme, pruritus, rash, Stevens-Johnson syndrome, toxic epidermal necrolysis
Other: Anaphylaxis, angioedema, facial edema, superinfection

Nursing Considerations

•Use cefixime cautiously in patients with impaired renal function or a history of GI disease, especially colitis. Also use drug cautiously in patients who are hypersensitive to penicillin because cross-sensitivity has occurred in about 10% of such patients.
•If possible, obtain culture and sensitivity test results, as ordered, before giving drug.
•Be aware that tablets shouldn't be substituted for oral suspension to treat otitis media because cefixime suspension produces a higher peak blood level than do tablets when administered at the same dose.
•Monitor BUN and serum creatinine levels to detect early signs of nephrotoxicity. Also monitor fluid intake and output; decreasing urine output may indicate nephrotoxicity.
•Be aware that an allergic reaction may occur a few days after therapy starts.
•Assess bowel pattern daily; severe diarrhea may indicate pseudomembranous colitis.
•Assess for signs of superinfection, such as perineal itching, fever, malaise, redness, pain, swelling, drainage, rash, diarrhea, and cough or sputum changes.
•Assess for pharyngitis, ecchymosis, bleeding, and arthralgia; they may indicate a blood dyscrasia.

PATIENT TEACHING

•Instruct patient to complete the prescribed course of therapy.
•Advise patient to shake oral suspension well before pouring dose and to use a liquid-measuring device to obtain an accurate dose.

•Instruct patient to store oral suspension at room temperature and to discard unused portion after 14 days.
•Tell patient to immediately report severe diarrhea to prescriber.
•Inform patient that yogurt and buttermilk can help maintain intestinal flora and decrease diarrhea.
•Teach patient to recognize and report signs of superinfection, such as furry tongue, perineal itching, and loose, foul-smelling stools.

cefmetazole sodium

Zefazone

Class and Category

Chemical class: Second-generation cephalosporin, 7-aminocephalosporanic acid
Therapeutic class: Antibiotic
Pregnancy category: B

Indications and Dosages

➤ *To treat UTI caused by* Escherichia coli; *lower respiratory tract infections, such as bronchitis and pneumonia, caused by* E. coli, Haemophilus influenzae, Staphylococcus aureus, *and* Streptococcus pneumoniae; *skin and soft-tissue infections caused by* Bacteroides fragilis, Bacteroides melaninogenicus, E. coli, Klebsiella oxytoca, Klebsiella pneumoniae, Morganella morganii, Proteus mirabilis, Proteus vulgaris, S. aureus, Staphylococcus epidermidis, Streptococcus agalactiae, *and* Streptococcus pyogenes; *intra-abdominal infections caused by* B. fragilis, Clostridium perfringens, E. coli, K. oxytoca, *and* K. pneumoniae

I.V. INFUSION
Adults. 2 g every 6 to 12 hr for 5 to 14 days.
DOSAGE ADJUSTMENT Dosage reduced to 1 to 2 g every 12 hr if creatinine clearance is 50 to 90 ml/min/1.73 m²; 1 to 2 g every 16 hr if creatinine clearance is 30 to 49 ml/min/1.73 m²; 1 to 2 g every 24 hr if creatinine clearance is 10 to 29 ml/min/1.73 m²; and 1 to 2 g every 48 hr if creatinine clearance is less than 10 ml/min/1.73 m².

➤ *To provide surgical prophylaxis for vaginal hysterectomy*
I.V. INFUSION
Adults. 2 g as a single dose 30 to 90 min before surgery or 1 g 30 to 90 min before surgery and repeated 8 and 16 hr later.

➤ *To provide surgical prophylaxis for abdominal hysterectomy and for high-risk cholecystectomy*
I.V. INFUSION
Adults. 1 g 30 to 90 min before surgery and repeated 8 and 16 hr later.

➤ *To provide surgical prophylaxis for cesarean section*
I.V. INFUSION
Adults. 2 g as a single dose after cord is clamped or 1 g after cord is clamped and then repeated 8 and 16 hr later.

➤ *To provide surgical prophylaxis for colorectal surgery*
I.V. INFUSION
Adults. 2 g as a single dose 30 to 90 min before surgery or 2 g 30 to 90 min before surgery and repeated 8 and 16 hr later.

Mechanism of Action
Interferes with bacterial cell wall synthesis by inhibiting the final step in the cross-linking of peptidoglycan strands. Peptidoglycan makes cell membranes rigid and protective. Without it, bacterial cells rupture and die.

Contraindications
Hypersensitivity to cephalosporins or their components

Interactions
DRUGS
aminoglycosides, loop diuretics: Increased risk of nephrotoxicity
anticoagulants: Possibly increased anticoagulant effect
probenecid: Increased and prolonged blood cefmetazole level
ACTIVITIES
alcohol use: Possibly disulfiram-like reaction

Adverse Reactions
CNS: Chills, fever, headache, seizures
CV: Edema
EENT: Hearing loss
GI: Abdominal cramps, diarrhea, elevated liver function test results, hepatic failure, hepatomegaly, nausea, oral candidiasis, pseudomembranous colitis, vomiting

GU: Elevated BUN level, nephrotoxicity, renal failure, vaginal candidiasis
HEME: Eosinophilia, hemolytic anemia, hypoprothrombinemia, neutropenia, thrombocytopenia, unusual bleeding
MS: Arthralgia
RESP: Dyspnea
SKIN: Ecchymosis, erythema, erythema multiforme, pruritus, rash, Stevens-Johnson syndrome
Other: Anaphylaxis; injection site pain, redness, and swelling; superinfection

Nursing Considerations
•Use cefmetazole cautiously in patients hypersensitive to penicillin; cross-sensitivity has occurred in about 10% of such patients.
•If possible, obtain culture and sensitivity test results, as ordered, before giving drug.
•Reconstitute drug with sterile or bacteriostatic water for injection or sodium chloride for injection.
•Dilute primary solution as needed to 1 to 20 mg/ml in D$_5$W, normal saline solution, lactated Ringer's solution, or 1% lidocaine solution without epinephrine.
•Store reconstituted solution for up to 24 hours at room temperature or 7 days refrigerated.
•Monitor BUN and serum creatinine levels and fluid intake and output to detect early signs of nephrotoxicity.
•Assess bowel pattern daily; severe diarrhea may indicate pseudomembranous colitis.
•Assess for signs of superinfection, such as perineal itching, fever, malaise, redness, rash, diarrhea, and cough or sputum changes.
•Assess for pharyngitis, bleeding, and arthralgia, which may indicate blood dyscrasia. Monitor PT and bleeding time, as ordered.

PATIENT TEACHING
•Advise patient to immediately report severe diarrhea to prescriber.
•Instruct patient to avoid alcohol during therapy and for at least 3 days after last dose.

cefonicid sodium

Monocid

Class and Category
Chemical class: Second-generation cephalosporin, 7-aminocephalosporanic acid

Therapeutic class: Antibiotic
Pregnancy category: B

Indications and Dosages
➤ *To treat lower respiratory tract infections caused by* Escherichia coli, Haemophilus influenzae, Klebsiella pneumoniae, *and* Streptococcus pneumoniae; *UTI caused by* E. coli, K. pneumoniae, Morganella morganii, Proteus mirabilis, Proteus vulgaris, *and* Providencia rettgeri; *skin and soft-tissue infections caused by* Staphylococcus aureus, Staphylococcus epidermidis, Streptococcus agalactiae, *and* Streptococcus pyogenes; *septicemia caused by* E. coli *and* S. pneumoniae; *and bone and joint infections caused by* S. aureus
I.V. INFUSION, I.V. OR I.M. INJECTION
Adults. For mild to moderate infections, 1 g every 24 hr. For severe or life-threatening infections, 2 g every 24 hr.

➤ *To treat uncomplicated UTI*
I.V. INFUSION, I.V. OR I.M. INJECTION
Adults. 500 mg every 24 hr.
DOSAGE ADJUSTMENT Initial dose reduced to 75 mg/kg I.V. or I.M. in patients with impaired renal function. Then dosage reduced to 10 to 25 mg/kg every 24 hr if creatinine clearance is 60 to 79 ml/min/1.73 m^2; 8 to 20 mg/kg every 24 hr if creatinine clearance is 40 to 59 ml/min/1.73 m^2; 4 to 15 mg/kg every 24 hr if creatinine clearance is 20 to 39 ml/min/1.73 m^2; 4 to 15 mg/kg every 48 hr if creatinine clearance is 10 to 19 ml/min/1.73 m^2; 4 to 15 mg/kg every 3 to 5 days if creatinine clearance is 5 to 9 ml/min/1.73 m^2; and 3 to 4 mg/kg every 3 to 5 days if creatinine clearance is less than 5 ml/min/1.73 m^2.

➤ *To provide surgical prophylaxis*
I.V. INFUSION, I.V. OR I.M. INJECTION
Adults. 1 g 60 min before surgery. Dose repeated once daily, if needed, for 2 days after prosthetic arthroplasty or open-heart surgery.

Incompatibilities
To prevent mutual inactivation, don't mix cefonicid with aminoglycosides.

Contraindications
Hypersensitivity to cephalosporins or their components

Mechanism of Action
Interferes with bacterial cell wall synthesis by inhibiting the final step in the cross-linking of peptidoglycan strands. Peptidoglycan makes cell membranes rigid and protective. Without it, bacterial cells rupture and die.

Interactions
DRUGS
aminoglycosides, loop diuretics: Increased risk of nephrotoxicity

Adverse Reactions
CNS: Chills, fever, headache, seizures
CV: Edema
EENT: Hearing loss
GI: Abdominal cramps, diarrhea, elevated liver function test results, hepatic failure, hepatomegaly, nausea, oral candidiasis, pseudomembranous colitis, vomiting
GU: Elevated BUN level, nephrotoxicity, renal failure, vaginal candidiasis
HEME: Eosinophilia, hemolytic anemia, hypoprothrombinemia, neutropenia, thrombocytopenia, unusual bleeding
MS: Arthralgia
RESP: Dyspnea
SKIN: Ecchymosis, erythema, erythema multiforme, pruritus, rash, Stevens-Johnson syndrome
Other: Anaphylaxis; injection site pain, redness, and swelling; superinfection

Nursing Considerations
• Use cefonicid cautiously in patients with impaired renal function. Also use drug cautiously in patients hypersensitive to penicillin because cross-sensitivity has occurred in about 10% of such patients.
• If possible, obtain culture and sensitivity test results, as ordered, before giving drug.
• Reconstitute each 500-mg vial of drug with 2 ml of sterile water for injection (or each 1-g vial with 2.5 ml).
• For I.V. infusion, dilute further in 50 to 100 ml compatible solution, such as D_5W, $D_{10}W$, dextrose 5% in quarter-normal (0.2) saline solution, dextrose 5% in half-normal (0.45) saline solution, or dextrose 5% in normal saline solution.
• Give I.V. injection slowly over 3 to 5 minutes through tubing of a flowing compatible I.V. solution.
• For I.M. dose larger than 1 g, divide dose in half and give into large muscle mass, such as the gluteus maximus, at two different sites.
• Store reconstituted solution for 24 hours at room temperature, 72 hours refrigerated.
• Monitor patient's BUN and serum creatinine levels to detect early signs of nephrotoxicity. Also monitor fluid intake and output; decreasing urine output may indicate nephrotoxicity.
• Assess patient's bowel pattern daily; severe diarrhea may indicate pseudomembranous colitis.
• Watch for signs of superinfection, such as perineal itching, fever, malaise, redness, pain, swelling, drainage, rash, diarrhea, and cough or sputum changes.
• Assess patient for pharyngitis, ecchymosis, bleeding, and arthralgia; they may indicate a blood dyscrasia.

PATIENT TEACHING
• Warn patient that I.M. injection may be painful.
• Tell patient to immediately report severe diarrhea to prescriber.

cefoperazone sodium
Cefobid

Class and Category
Chemical class: Third-generation cephalosporin, 7-aminocephalosporanic acid
Therapeutic class: Antibiotic
Pregnancy category: B

Indications and Dosages
➤ *To treat respiratory tract infections caused by* Enterobacter *species,* Escherichia coli, Haemophilus influenzae, Klebsiella pneumoniae, Proteus mirabilis, Pseudomonas aeruginosa, Staphylococcus aureus, Streptococcus pneumoniae, Streptococcus pyogenes, *and other streptococci (excluding enterococci); UTI caused by* E. coli *and* P. aeruginosa; *uncomplicated gonorrhea caused by* Neisseria gonorrhoeae; *gynecologic infections caused by anaerobic gram-positive cocci,* Bacteroides *species,* Clostridium *species,* E. coli, *Staphylococcus epidermidis, and* Streptococcus

agalactiae; *bacterial septicemia caused by* E. coli, Klebsiella *species,* S. aureus, Serratia marcescens, *and streptococci; skin and soft-tissue infections caused by* P. aeruginosa, S. aureus, *and* S. pyogenes; *and intra-abdominal infections caused by anaerobic gram-negative bacilli,* E. coli, *and* P. aeruginosa

I.V. INFUSION, I.M. INJECTION

Adults. 1 to 2 g every 12 hr. For severe infections or those caused by less sensitive organisms, 6 to 12 g daily divided into equal doses and given b.i.d., t.i.d., or q.i.d. *Maximum:* 12 g daily.

Mechanism of Action

Interferes with bacterial cell wall synthesis by inhibiting the final step in the cross-linking of peptidoglycan strands. Peptidoglycan makes cell membranes rigid and protective. Without it, bacterial cells rupture and die.

Incompatibilities

To prevent mutual inactivation, don't mix cefoperazone with aminoglycosides. Also avoid mixing cefoperazone with other drugs, including pentamidine isethionate.

Contraindications

Hypersensitivity to cephalosporins or their components

Interactions

DRUGS

aminoglycosides, loop diuretics: Increased risk of nephrotoxicity
oral anticoagulants, other drugs that affect blood clotting: Increased anticoagulant effect

ACTIVITIES

alcohol use: Disulfiram-like reaction

Adverse Reactions

CNS: Chills, fever, headache, seizures
CV: Edema
EENT: Hearing loss
GI: Abdominal cramps, diarrhea, elevated liver function test results, hepatic failure, hepatomegaly, nausea, oral candidiasis, pseudomembranous colitis, vomiting
GU: Elevated BUN level, nephrotoxicity, renal failure, vaginal candidiasis
HEME: Eosinophilia, hemolytic anemia, hypoprothrombinemia, neutropenia, thrombocytopenia, unusual bleeding
MS: Arthralgia
RESP: Dyspnea
SKIN: Ecchymosis, erythema, erythema multiforme, pruritus, rash, Stevens-Johnson syndrome
Other: Anaphylaxis; injection site pain, redness, and swelling; superinfection

Nursing Considerations

• Use cefoperazone cautiously in patients with a history of bleeding problems, GI disease (especially colitis), or severely impaired hepatic or renal function. Also use drug cautiously in patients who are hypersensitive to penicillin because cross-sensitivity has occurred in about 10% of such patients.
• If possible, obtain culture and sensitivity test results, as ordered, before giving drug.
• For I.V. use, reconstitute drug with required amount of diluent. Then further dilute in compatible solution, such as D_5W, $D_{10}W$, dextrose 5% in lactated Ringer's solution, dextrose 5% in quarter-normal (0.2) saline solution, dextrose 5% in normal saline solution, lactated Ringer's injection, normal saline solution, Normosol M and D_5W, or Normosol R. (See manufacturer's guidelines for details.)
• Administer I.V. drug as intermittent infusion over 15 to 30 minutes or as continuous infusion. Direct bolus injection isn't recommended.
• For I.M. injection, reconstitute drug with bacteriostatic water for injection (that contains benzyl alcohol or parabens) or sterile water for injection.
• After reconstitution, let foam dissipate and inspect the solution to ensure complete dissolution.
• Store reconstituted solution at room temperature for 24 hours.
• Monitor BUN and serum creatinine levels to detect early signs of nephrotoxicity. Also monitor fluid intake and output; decreasing urine output may indicate nephrotoxicity.
• Assess bowel pattern daily; severe diarrhea may indicate pseudomembranous colitis.
• Assess for pharyngitis, ecchymosis, bleeding, and arthralgia; they may indicate a blood dyscrasia.
• Assess for signs of superinfection, such as perineal itching, fever, malaise, redness, pain,

swelling, drainage, rash, diarrhea, and cough or sputum changes.

PATIENT TEACHING
• Advise patient to avoid alcohol during therapy and for at least 3 days after last dose.
• Explain that I.M. injection may cause pain.
• Tell patient to immediately report severe diarrhea to prescriber.

cefotaxime sodium

Claforan

Class and Category

Chemical class: Third-generation cephalosporin, 7-aminocephalosporanic acid
Therapeutic class: Antibiotic
Pregnancy category: B

Indications and Dosages

➤ *To provide perioperative prophylaxis*
I.V. INFUSION, I.V. OR I.M. INJECTION
Adults and children weighing more than 50 kg (110 lb). 1 g 30 to 90 min before surgery.

➤ *To provide perioperative prophylaxis related to cesarean section*
I.V. INFUSION, I.V. OR I.M. INJECTION
Adults. 1 g as soon as cord is clamped, then 1 g every 6 hr for up to two doses.

➤ *To treat gonococcal urethritis and cervicitis in men and women*
I.M. INJECTION
Adults weighing more than 50 kg. 500 mg as a single dose.

➤ *To treat rectal gonorrhea in women*
I.M. INJECTION
Adults weighing more than 50 kg. 500 mg as a single dose.

➤ *To treat rectal gonorrhea in men*
I.M. INJECTION
Adults weighing more than 50 kg. 1 g as a single dose.

➤ *To treat disseminated gonorrhea*
I.V. INFUSION OR INJECTION
Adults and children weighing more than 50 kg. 1 g every 8 hr.

➤ *To treat uncomplicated infections caused by susceptible organisms*
I.V. INFUSION, I.V. OR I.M. INJECTION
Adults and children weighing more than 50 kg. 1 g every 12 hr.

Children ages 1 month to 12 years weighing less than 50 kg. 50 to 180 mg/kg daily in four to six divided doses.
Children ages 1 to 4 weeks. 50 mg/kg I.V. every 8 hr.
Children age 1 week and under. 50 mg/kg I.V. every 12 hr.

➤ *To treat moderate to severe infections caused by susceptible organisms*
I.V. INFUSION, I.V. OR I.M. INJECTION
Adults and children weighing more than 50 kg. 1 to 2 g every 8 hr.
Children ages 1 month to 12 years weighing less than 50 kg. 50 to 180 mg/kg daily in four to six divided doses. For more serious infections, including meningitis, higher dosages are used.
Children ages 1 to 4 weeks. 50 mg/kg I.V. every 8 hr.
Children age 1 week and younger. 50 mg/kg I.V. every 12 hr.

➤ *To treat septicemia and other infections that commonly require antibiotics in higher doses than those used to treat moderate to severe infections*
I.V. INFUSION OR INJECTION
Adults and children weighing more than 50 kg. 2 g every 6 to 8 hr.

➤ *To treat life-threatening infections caused by susceptible organisms*
I.V. INFUSION OR INJECTION
Adults and children weighing more than 50 kg. 2 g every 4 hr. *Maximum:* 12 g daily.
Children ages 1 month to 12 years weighing less than 50 kg. 50 to 180 mg/kg daily in four to six divided doses.
Children ages 1 to 4 weeks. 50 mg/kg every 8 hr.
Children age 1 week and younger. 50 mg/kg every 12 hr.
DOSAGE ADJUSTMENT Dosage reduced by 50% for patients with estimated creatinine clearance below 20 ml/min/1.73 m^2.

Mechanism of Action

Interferes with bacterial cell wall synthesis by inhibiting the cross-linking of peptidoglycan strands. Peptidoglycan makes cell membranes rigid and protective. Without it, bacterial cells rupture and die.

Incompatibilities

To prevent mutual inactivation, don't mix cefotaxime with aminoglycosides. Also avoid mixing cefotaxime with other drugs, including pentamidine isethionate.

Contraindications

Hypersensitivity to cephalosporins or their components

Interactions

DRUGS

aminoglycosides, loop diuretics: Increased risk of nephrotoxicity
probenecid: Increased and prolonged blood cefotaxime level

Adverse Reactions

CNS: Chills, fever, headache, seizures
CV: Edema
EENT: Hearing loss
GI: Abdominal cramps, diarrhea, elevated liver function test results, hepatic failure, hepatomegaly, nausea, oral candidiasis, pseudomembranous colitis, vomiting
GU: Elevated BUN level, nephrotoxicity, renal failure, vaginal candidiasis
HEME: Eosinophilia, hemolytic anemia, hypoprothrombinemia, neutropenia, thrombocytopenia, unusual bleeding
MS: Arthralgia
RESP: Dyspnea
SKIN: Ecchymosis, erythema, erythema multiforme, pruritus, rash, Stevens-Johnson syndrome, toxic epidermal necrolysis
Other: Anaphylaxis; injection site pain, redness, and swelling; superinfection

Nursing Considerations

• Use cefotaxime cautiously in patients with impaired renal function, a history of GI disease (especially colitis), or hypersensitivity to penicillin because cross-sensitivity has occurred in about 10% of such patients.
• If possible, obtain culture and sensitivity test results, as ordered, before giving drug.
• For I.V. use, reconstitute each 0.5-, 1-, or 2-g vial with 10 ml of sterile water for injection. Shake to dissolve.
• For intermittent I.V. infusion, further dilute in 50 to 100 ml of D₅W or normal saline solution.
• For I.M. use, reconstitute each 500-mg vial with 2 ml of sterile water for injection or bacteriostatic water for injection; each 1-g

vial with 3 ml of diluent; and each 2-g vial with 5 ml of diluent. Shake to dissolve.
• **WARNING** When preparing drug for a neonate, don't use diluent that contains benzyl alcohol; it could cause a fatal toxic syndrome.
• Give cefotaxime by I.V. injection over 3 to 5 minutes through tubing of a free-flowing compatible I.V. solution. Temporarily stop other solutions being given through same I.V. site.
• Discard unused drug after 24 hours if stored at room temperature, 5 days if refrigerated.
• Protect cefotaxime powder and solution from light and heat.
• Monitor I.V. sites for signs of phlebitis or extravasation. Rotate I.V. sites every 72 hours.
• Monitor BUN and serum creatinine levels and fluid intake and output for signs of nephrotoxicity.
• Be aware that an allergic reaction may occur a few days after cefotaxime therapy starts.
• Assess bowel pattern daily; severe diarrhea may indicate pseudomembranous coliti caused by *Clostridium difficile*. If diarrhea occurs, notify prescriber and expect to withhold cefotaxime and treat with fluids, electrolytes, protein, and an antibiotic effective against *C. difficile*.
• Assess patient for pharyngitis, ecchymosis, bleeding, and arthralgia, which may indicate a blood dyscrasia. Monitor CBC, PT, and bleeding time, as ordered.
• Monitor patient closely for superinfection. If signs appear, notify prescriber and expect to stop drug and give appropriate care.

PATIENT TEACHING

• Explain that I.M. injection may be painful.
• Instruct patient to report watery, bloody stools to prescriber immediately, even up to 2 months after drug therapy has ended.

cefotetan disodium

Cefotan

Class and Category

Chemical class: Second-generation cephalosporin, 7-aminocephalosporanic acid
Therapeutic class: Antibiotic
Pregnancy category: B

Indications and Dosages

➤ *To provide surgical prophylaxis*
I.V. INJECTION
Adults. 1 to 2 g 30 to 60 min before surgery or, in cesarean section, as soon as cord is clamped.

➤ *To treat lower respiratory tract infections caused by* Escherichia coli, Haemophilus influenzae, Klebsiella *species,* Proteus mirabilis, Serratia marcescens, Staphylococcus aureus, *and* Streptococcus pneumoniae; *gynecologic infections caused by* Bacteroides *species (excluding* B. distasonis, B. ovatus, *and* B. thetaiotaomicron), E. coli, Fusobacterium *species, gram-positive anaerobic cocci,* Neisseria gonorrhoeae, P. mirabilis, S. aureus, Staphylococcus epidermidis, *and* Streptococcus *species (excluding enterococci); intra-abdominal infections caused by* Bacteroides *species (excluding* B. distasonis, B. ovatus, *and* B. thetaiotaomicron), Clostridium *species,* E. coli, Klebsiella *species, and* Streptococcus *species (excluding enterococci); and bone and joint infections caused by* S. aureus
I.V. INFUSION, I.V. OR I.M. INJECTION
Adults. For mild to moderate infections, 1 to 2 g every 12 hr.
I.V. INFUSION OR INJECTION
Adults. For severe infections, 2 g every 12 hr; for life-threatening infections, 3 g every 12 hr.

➤ *To treat UTI caused by* E. coli, Klebsiella *species, or* Proteus *species*
I.V. INFUSION, I.V. OR I.M. INJECTION
Adults. 0.5 to 2 g every 12 hr or 1 to 2 g every 24 hr.

➤ *To treat skin and soft-tissue infections caused by* E. coli, Klebsiella pneumoniae, Peptostreptococcus *species,* S. aureus, S. epidermidis, Streptococcus pyogenes, *and* Streptococcus *species (excluding enterococci)*
I.V. INFUSION, I.V. OR I.M. INJECTION
Adults. For mild to moderate infections due to *K. pneumoniae,* 1 or 2 g every 12 hr. For mild to moderate infections caused by other organisms, 1 g I.M. or I.V. every 12 hr or 2 g I.V. every 24 hr; for severe infections, 2 g I.V. every 12 hr.

DOSAGE ADJUSTMENT Dosing interval reduced to 24 hr in patients with creatinine clearance of 10 to 30 ml/min/1.73 m^2 and to 48 hr in patients with creatinine clearance less than 10 ml/min/1.73 m^2.

Mechanism of Action
Interferes with bacterial cell wall synthesis by inhibiting the final step in the cross-linking of peptidoglycan strands. Peptidoglycan makes cell membranes rigid and protective. Without it, bacterial cells rupture and die.

Incompatibilities
To prevent mutual inactivation, don't mix cefotetan with aminoglycosides.

Contraindications
Hypersensitivity to cephalosporins or their components

Interactions
DRUGS
aminoglycosides, loop diuretics: Increased risk of nephrotoxicity
oral anticoagulants, other drugs that affect blood clotting: Enhanced anticoagulant effect
probenecid: Increased and prolonged blood cefotetan level
ACTIVITIES
alcohol use: Disulfiram-like reaction

Adverse Reactions
CNS: Chills, fever, headache, seizures
CV: Edema
EENT: Hearing loss
GI: Abdominal cramps, diarrhea, elevated liver function test results, hepatic failure, hepatomegaly, nausea, oral candidiasis, pseudomembranous colitis, vomiting
GU: Elevated BUN level, nephrotoxicity, renal failure, vaginal candidiasis
HEME: Eosinophilia, hemolytic anemia, hypoprothrombinemia, neutropenia, thrombocytopenia, unusual bleeding
MS: Arthralgia
RESP: Dyspnea
SKIN: Ecchymosis, erythema, erythema multiforme, pruritus, rash, Stevens-Johnson syndrome
Other: Anaphylaxis; injection site pain, redness, and swelling; superinfection

C

Nursing Considerations
•Use cefotetan cautiously in patients with impaired renal function or a history of GI disease, especially colitis. Also use drug cautiously in patients who are hypersensitive to penicillin because cross-sensitivity has occurred in about 10% of such patients.
•If possible, obtain culture and sensitivity test results, as ordered, before giving drug.
•For I.V. use, reconstitute each 1-g vial of drug with 10 ml of sterile water for injection. For each 2-g vial, use 10 to 20 ml of diluent. For I.V. infusion, further dilute solution in 50 to 100 ml of D_5W or normal saline solution.
•For direct I.V. injection, administer drug slowly over 3 to 5 minutes through tubing of a flowing compatible I.V. solution.
•For I.M. use, reconstitute each 1-g vial of drug with 2 ml of sterile or bacteriostatic water for injection, or sodium chloride for injection. For a 2-g vial, use 3 ml of diluent.
•Monitor I.V. site for signs and symptoms of phlebitis and extravasation; rotate sites every 72 hours.
•Protect reconstituted solution from light and store for up to 24 hours at room temperature or 96 hours under refrigeration.
•Be aware than an allergic reaction may occur a few days after therapy starts.
•Monitor BUN and serum creatinine levels and fluid intake and output for signs of nephrotoxicity.
•Monitor patient receiving even short-term cefotetan therapy for signs and symptoms of hemolytic anemia, such as marked pallor and fatigue.
•If patient receives long-term therapy, monitor CBC and serum AST, ALT, bilirubin, LD, and alkaline phosphatase levels.
•Assess patient's bowel pattern daily; severe diarrhea may indicate pseudomembranous colitis.
•Watch for pharyngitis, ecchymosis, bleeding, and arthralgia, which may indicate a blood dyscrasia. Monitor PT and bleeding time, as ordered. Be prepared to give vitamin K, if ordered, to treat hypoprothrombinemia.

PATIENT TEACHING
•Explain that I.M. injection may be painful.
•Tell patient to immediately report severe diarrhea to prescriber.
•Urge patient to avoid alcohol during and for at least 3 days after cefotetan therapy.

cefoxitin sodium

Mefoxin

Class and Category
Chemical class: Second-generation cephalosporin, 7-aminocephalosporanic acid
Therapeutic class: Antibiotic
Pregnancy category: B

Indications and Dosages
➤ *To provide surgical prophylaxis*
I.V. INFUSION OR INJECTION
Adults. 2 g 30 to 60 min before surgery and then 2 g every 6 hr after first dose for up to 24 hr.
Children age 3 months or over. 30 to 40 mg/kg 30 to 60 min before surgery and then every 6 hr after first dose for up to 24 hr.

➤ *To provide surgical prophylaxis for cesarean section*
I.V. INFUSION OR INJECTION
Adults. 2 g as a single dose as soon as cord is clamped or 2 g as soon as cord is clamped followed by 2 g 4 and 8 hr after initial dose.

➤ *To provide surgical prophylaxis for transurethral prostatectomy*
I.V. INFUSION OR INJECTION
Adults. 1 g 30 to 60 min before surgery and then 1 g every 8 hr for up to 5 days.

➤ *To treat infections, including septicemia, gynecologic infections, intra-abdominal infections, UTI, and infections of the lower respiratory tract, skin, soft tissue, bones, and joints caused by anaerobes (including* Bacteroides *species,* Clostridium *species,* Fusobacterium *species,* Peptococcus niger, *and* Peptostreptococcus *species), gram-negative organisms (including* Escherichia coli, Haemophilus influenzae *[also ampicillin-resistant strains],* Klebsiella, *and* Proteus *species), and gram-positive organisms (including* Staphylococcus aureus *[penicillinase- and non–penicillinase-producing strains],* Staphylococcus epidermidis, Streptococcus agalactiae, Streptococcus pneumoniae, *and* Streptococcus pyogenes)*
I.V. INFUSION OR INJECTION
Adults. For uncomplicated infections, 1 g every 6 to 8 hr; for moderate to severe infections, 1 g every 4 hr or 2 g every 6 to 8 hr;

for infections that commonly require high-dose antibiotics (such as gas gangrene), 2 g every 4 hr or 3 g every 6 hr.

Children age 3 months or over. 80 to 160 mg/kg daily in equal doses and given every 4 to 6 hr (with higher dosages used for more severe infections). *Maximum:* 12 g daily.

➤ *To treat uncomplicated gonorrhea*

I.M. INJECTION

Adults. 2 g as a single dose along with 1 g oral probenecid concurrently or within 30 min of cefoxitin.

DOSAGE ADJUSTMENT Dosage reduced to 1 to 2 g every 8 to 12 hr if creatinine clearance is 30 to 50 ml/min/1.73 m^2; 1 to 2 g every 12 to 24 hr if clearance is 10 to 29 ml/min/1.73 m^2; 0.5 to 1 g every 12 to 24 hr if clearance is 5 to 9 ml/min/1.73 m^2; and 0.5 to 1 g every 24 to 48 hr if clearance is less than 5 ml/min/1.73 m^2.

Mechanism of Action

Interferes with bacterial cell wall synthesis by inhibiting the final step in the cross-linking of peptidoglycan strands. Peptidoglycan makes cell membranes rigid and protective. Without it, bacterial cells rupture and die.

Incompatibilities

To prevent mutual inactivation, don't mix cefoxitin with aminoglycosides. Also avoid mixing cefoxitin with other drugs, including pentamidine isethionate.

Contraindications

Hypersensitivity to cephalosporins or their components

Interactions

DRUGS

aminoglycosides, loop diuretics: Increased risk of nephrotoxicity

Adverse Reactions

CNS: Chills, fever, headache, seizures
CV: Edema
EENT: Hearing loss
GI: Abdominal cramps, diarrhea, elevated liver function test results, hepatic failure, hepatomegaly, nausea, oral candidiasis, pseudomembranous colitis, vomiting
GU: Elevated BUN level, nephrotoxicity,

renal failure, vaginal candidiasis
HEME: Eosinophilia, hemolytic anemia, hypoprothrombinemia, neutropenia, thrombocytopenia, unusual bleeding
MS: Arthralgia
RESP: Dyspnea
SKIN: Ecchymosis, erythema, erythema multiforme, flushing, pruritus, rash, Stevens-Johnson syndrome, urticaria
Other: Anaphylaxis; injection site pain, redness, and swelling; superinfection

Nursing Considerations

• Use cefoxitin cautiously in patients hypersensitive to penicillin; cross-sensitivity has occurred in about 10% of such patients. Also use cautiously in patients with a history of GI disease, particularly colitis, because of an increased risk of pseudomembranous colitis.
• If possible, obtain culture and sensitivity test results, as ordered, before giving drug.
• For I.V. use, reconstitute 1 g with 10 ml of sterile water for injection or 2 g with 10 to 20 ml of diluent.
• For I.V. injection, administer slowly over 3 to 5 minutes through tubing of a flowing compatible I.V. solution.
• For intermittent infusion, further dilute with 50 to 100 ml of D$_5$W or normal saline solution.
• For continuous high-dose infusion, add cefoxitin to I.V. solutions of D$_5$W, normal saline solution, or dextrose 5% in normal saline solution.
• For I.M. use, reconstitute each 1 g with 2 ml of sterile water for injection.
• Discard unused drug after 24 hours if stored at room temperature or after 1 week if refrigerated.
• Be aware that powder or solution may darken during storage, a change that doesn't reflect altered potency.
• Be aware that an allergic reaction may occur a few days after therapy starts.
• Monitor BUN and serum creatinine levels for early signs of nephrotoxicity. Also monitor fluid intake and output; decreasing urine output may indicate nephrotoxicity.
• Assess patient's bowel pattern daily; severe diarrhea may indicate pseudomembranous colitis.
• Assess for pharyngitis, ecchymosis, bleeding, and arthralgia; they may indicate a blood dyscrasia.

PATIENT TEACHING
•Tell patient to immediately report severe diarrhea to prescriber.
•Instruct patient to complete the course of therapy as prescribed.

cefpodoxime proxetil

Vantin

Class and Category

Chemical class: Third-generation cephalosporin, 7-aminocephalosporanic acid
Therapeutic class: Antibiotic
Pregnancy category: B

Indications and Dosages

➤ *To treat acute community-acquired pneumonia caused by* Haemophilus influenzae *or* Streptococcus pneumoniae
ORAL SUSPENSION, TABLETS
Adults and adolescents over age 13. 200 mg every 12 hr for 14 days.

➤ *To treat acute bacterial exacerbation of chronic bronchitis caused by* H. influenzae, Moraxella catarrhalis, *or* S. pneumoniae
TABLETS
Adults and adolescents over age 13. 200 mg every 12 hr for 10 days.

➤ *To treat uncomplicated gonorrhea in men and women and rectal gonococcal infections in women caused by* Neisseria gonorrhoeae
ORAL SUSPENSION, TABLETS
Adults. 200 mg as a single dose.

➤ *To treat uncomplicated UTI caused by* Escherichia coli, Klebsiella pneumoniae, Proteus mirabilis, *or* Staphylococcus saprophyticus
ORAL SUSPENSION, TABLETS
Adults. 100 mg every 12 hr for 7 days.

➤ *To treat skin and soft-tissue infections caused by* Staphylococcus aureus *or* Staphylococcus pyogenes
ORAL SUSPENSION, TABLETS
Adults and adolescents over age 13. 400 mg every 12 hr for 7 to 14 days.

➤ *To treat acute otitis media caused by* H. influenzae, M. catarrhalis, *or* S. pneumoniae
ORAL SUSPENSION, TABLETS

Children ages 5 months through 12 years. 5 mg/kg every 12 hr (*maximum:* 200 mg/dose) or 10 mg/kg every 24 hr (*maximum:* 400 mg/dose) for 10 days.

➤ *To treat pharyngitis and tonsillitis caused by* S. pyogenes
ORAL SUSPENSION, TABLETS
Adults and adolescents over age 13. 100 mg every 12 hr for 5 to 10 days.
Children ages 2 months through 12 years. 5 mg/kg every 12 hr for 5 to 10 days. *Maximum:* 100 mg/dose.
DOSAGE ADJUSTMENT Dosing interval increased to 24 hr in patients with creatinine clearance of less than 30 ml/min/1.73 m^2.

Mechanism of Action
Interferes with bacterial cell wall synthesis by inhibiting the final step in the cross-linking of peptidoglycan strands. Peptidoglycan makes cell membranes rigid and protective. Without it, bacterial cells rupture and die.

Contraindications
Hypersensitivity to cephalosporins or their components

Interactions
DRUGS
aminoglycosides, loop diuretics: Increased risk of nephrotoxicity
antacids, H$_2$-receptor antagonists: Reduced bioavailability and blood level of cefpodoxime
oral anticholinergics: Delayed peak blood level of cefpodoxime
probenecid: Possibly increased and prolonged blood cefpodoxime level

Adverse Reactions
CNS: Chills, fever, headache, seizures
CV: Edema
EENT: Hearing loss
GI: Abdominal cramps, diarrhea, elevated liver function test results, hepatic failure, hepatomegaly, nausea, oral candidiasis, pseudomembranous colitis, vomiting
GU: Elevated BUN level, nephrotoxicity, renal failure, vaginal candidiasis
HEME: Eosinophilia, hemolytic anemia, hypoprothrombinemia, neutropenia, thrombocytopenia, unusual bleeding
MS: Arthralgia

RESP: Dyspnea
SKIN: Ecchymosis, erythema, erythema multiforme, pruritus, rash, Stevens-Johnson syndrome
Other: Anaphylaxis, superinfection

Nursing Considerations

•Use cefpodoxime cautiously in patients who have impaired renal function or are receiving potent diuretics. Also use drug cautiously in patients who are hypersensitive to penicillin because cross-sensitivity has occurred in about 10% of such patients.
•If possible, obtain culture and sensitivity test results, as ordered, before giving cefpodoxime.
•Assess patient's bowel pattern daily; severe diarrhea may indicate pseudomembranous colitis.
•Be aware that an allergic reaction may occur a few days after therapy starts.

PATIENT TEACHING
•Urge patient to complete the prescribed course of therapy.
•Tell patient to take tablets with food to enhance absorption.
•Advise patient to refrigerate oral suspension and discard after 14 days.
•Instruct patient to shake oral suspension bottle well before pouring dose and to use a liquid-measuring device to ensure accurate doses.
•Inform patient that yogurt and buttermilk can help maintain intestinal flora and decrease diarrhea.
•Warn patient not to take an antacid within 2 hours before or after taking cefpodoxime.
•Tell patient to report watery, bloody stools to prescriber immediately, even up to 2 months after drug therapy has ended.

cefprozil

Cefzil

Class and Category

Chemical class: Second-generation cephalosporin, 7-aminocephalosporanic acid
Therapeutic class: Antibiotic
Pregnancy category: B

Indications and Dosages

➤ *To treat secondary bacterial infections in patients with acute bronchitis and acute bacterial exacerbations of acute* bronchitis caused by Haemophilus influenzae, Moraxella catarrhalis, *and* Streptococcus pneumoniae

ORAL SUSPENSION, TABLETS
Adults and adolescents. 500 mg every 12 hr for 10 days.

➤ *To treat uncomplicated skin and soft-tissue infections caused by* Staphylococcus aureus *and* Streptococcus pyogenes

ORAL SUSPENSION, TABLETS
Adults and adolescents. 250 mg every 12 hr or 500 mg every 12 to 24 hr for 10 days.
Children ages 2 to 12. 20 mg/kg every 24 hr for 10 days.

➤ *To treat pharyngitis and tonsillitis caused by* S. pyogenes

ORAL SUSPENSION, TABLETS
Adults and adolescents. 500 mg every 24 hr for 10 days.
Children ages 2 to 12. 7.5 mg/kg every 12 hr for 10 days.

➤ *To treat otitis media caused by* H. influenzae, M. catarrhalis, *and* S. pneumoniae

ORAL SUSPENSION, TABLETS
Children ages 6 months to 12 years. 15 mg/kg every 12 hr for 10 days.

➤ *To treat acute sinusitis caused by* H. influenzae, M. catarrhalis, *and* S. pneumoniae

ORAL SUSPENSION, TABLETS
Adults and adolescents. 250 to 500 mg every 12 hr for 10 days.
Children ages 6 months to 12 years. 7.5 or 15 mg/kg every 12 hr for 10 days.
DOSAGE ADJUSTMENT Dosage reduced by half and given at usual intervals in patients with creatinine clearance of less than 30 ml/min/ 1.73 m^2.

> ### Mechanism of Action
> Interferes with bacterial cell wall synthesis by inhibiting the final step in the cross-linking of peptidoglycan strands. Peptidoglycan makes the cell membrane rigid and protective. Without it, bacterial cells rupture and die.

Contraindications

Hypersensitivity to cephalosporins or their components

Interactions

DRUGS

aminoglycosides, loop diuretics: Increased risk of nephrotoxicity
probenecid: Increased blood cefprozil level

Adverse Reactions

CNS: Chills, fever, headache, seizures
CV: Edema
EENT: Hearing loss
GI: Abdominal cramps, diarrhea, elevated liver function test results, hepatic failure, hepatomegaly, nausea, oral candidiasis, pseudomembranous colitis, vomiting
GU: Elevated BUN level, nephrotoxicity, renal failure, vaginal candidiasis
HEME: Eosinophilia, hemolytic anemia, hypoprothrombinemia, neutropenia, thrombocytopenia, unusual bleeding
MS: Arthralgia
RESP: Dyspnea
SKIN: Ecchymosis, erythema, erythema multiforme, pruritus, rash, Stevens-Johnson syndrome
Other: Anaphylaxis, superinfection

Nursing Considerations

• Use cefprozil cautiously in patients with impaired renal function or a history of GI disease, especially colitis. Also use drug cautiously in patients who are hypersensitive to penicillin because cross-sensitivity has occurred in about 10% of such patients.
• If possible, obtain culture and sensitivity test results, as ordered, before giving drug.
•**WARNING** Don't administer oral suspension to patients with phenylketonuria because it contains phenylalanine 28 mg/5 ml.
• Monitor BUN and serum creatinine levels to detect early signs of nephrotoxicity. Also monitor fluid intake and output; decreasing urine output may indicate nephrotoxicity.
• Be aware that an allergic reaction may occur a few days after therapy starts.
• Assess patient's bowel pattern daily; severe diarrhea may indicate pseudomembranous colitis.

PATIENT TEACHING

• Urge patient to complete the prescribed course of therapy.
• Tell patient to refrigerate oral suspension and discard after 14 days.
• Instruct patient to shake oral suspension well before pouring and to use a calibrated measuring device to ensure accurate doses.
• Inform patient that yogurt and buttermilk can help maintain intestinal flora and decrease diarrhea.
• Tell patient to report watery, bloody stools to prescriber immediately, even up to 2 months after drug therapy has ended.

ceftazidime

Ceptaz, Fortaz, Tazicef, Tazidime

Class and Category

Chemical class: Third-generation cephalosporin, 7-aminocephalosporanic acid
Therapeutic class: Antibiotic
Pregnancy category: B

Indications and Dosages

➤ *To treat infections caused by gram-negative organisms (including* Acinetobacter, Citrobacter, Enterobacter, Escherichia coli, Haemophilus influenzae, Klebsiella, Neisseria, Proteus mirabilis, Proteus vulgaris, Pseudomonas aeruginosa, Salmonella, Serratia, *and* Shigella*), gram-positive organisms (including* Streptococcus agalactiae, Streptococcus pneumoniae, *and* Streptococcus pyogenes *[group B streptococci]), as well as* Staphylococcus aureus *(penicillinase- and non–penicillinase-producing strains)*

I.V. INFUSION, I.M. INJECTION

Adults and children age 12 and over. 1 g every 8 to 12 hr.

I.V. INFUSION

Children ages 1 month to 12 years. 30 to 50 mg/kg every 8 hr.
Neonates up to age 1 month. 30 mg/kg every 12 hr. *Maximum:* 6 g daily.

➤ *To treat uncomplicated UTI*

I.V. INFUSION, I.M. INJECTION

Adults and children age 12 and over. 250 mg every 12 hr.

➤ *To treat complicated UTI*

I.V. INFUSION, I.M. INJECTION

Adults and children age 12 and over. 500 mg every 8 to 12 hr.

➤ *To treat uncomplicated pneumonia and mild skin and soft-tissue infections*

I.V. INFUSION, I.M. INJECTION

Adults and children age 12 and over. 0.5 to 1 g every 8 hr.

➤ *To treat bone and joint infections*
I.V. INFUSION
Adults and children age 12 and over. 2 g every 12 hr.

➤ *To treat serious gynecologic and intra-abdominal infections, meningitis, and life-threatening infections, especially in immunocompromised patients*
I.V. INFUSION
Adults and children age 12 and over. 2 g every 8 hr.

➤ *To treat pseudomonal lung infection in patients with cystic fibrosis and normal renal function*
I.V. INFUSION
Adults and children age 1 month and over. 30 to 50 mg/kg every 8 hr. *Maximum:* 6 g daily.
Neonates up to age 1 month. 30 mg/kg every 12 hr.
DOSAGE ADJUSTMENT Dosage reduced to 1 g every 12 hr if creatinine clearance is 31 to 50 ml/min/1.73 m^2; to 1 g every 24 hr if 16 to 30 ml/min/1.73 m^2; to 0.5 g every 24 hr if 6 to 15 ml/min/1.73 m^2; and to 0.5 g every 48 hr if less than 6 ml/min/1.73 m^2.

Mechanism of Action
Interferes with bacterial cell wall synthesis by inhibiting the cross-linking of peptidoglycan strands. Peptidoglycan makes the cell membrane rigid and protective. Without it, bacterial cells rupture and die.

Incompatibilities
Don't mix ceftazidime with aminoglycosides to prevent mutual inactivation. Vancomycin is physically incompatible with ceftazidime (precipitate may form); flush I.V. line between these drugs if given through same tubing. Avoid mixing ceftazidime with other drugs, including pentamidine isethionate.

Contraindications
Hypersensitivity to cephalosporins or their components

Interactions
DRUGS
aminoglycosides, loop diuretics: Increased risk of nephrotoxicity
oral combined estrogen-progesterone contra-ceptives: Decreased effectiveness of oral contraceptive

Adverse Reactions
CNS: Chills, fever, headache, seizures
CV: Edema
EENT: Hearing loss
GI: Abdominal cramps, diarrhea, elevated liver function test results, hepatic failure, hepatomegaly, nausea, oral candidiasis, pseudomembranous colitis, vomiting
GU: Elevated BUN level, nephrotoxicity, renal failure, vaginal candidiasis
HEME: Eosinophilia, hemolytic anemia, hypoprothrombinemia, neutropenia, thrombocytopenia, unusual bleeding
MS: Arthralgia
RESP: Dyspnea
SKIN: Ecchymosis, erythema, erythema multiforme, pruritus, rash, Stevens-Johnson syndrome
Other: Anaphylaxis; injection site pain, redness, and swelling; superinfection

Nursing Considerations
• Use ceftazidime cautiously in patients hypersensitive to penicillin because cross-sensitivity occurs in about 10% of them. Watch for allergic reactions a few days after therapy starts.
• Use cautiously in patients with a history of GI disease, particularly colitis, because risk of pseudomembranous colitis is increased.
• Ceftazidime L-arginine (Ceptaz) is not recommended for children under age 12.
• If possible, obtain culture and sensitivity test results, as ordered, before giving drug.
• Protect ceftazidime powder and reconstituted drug from heat and light; both tend to darken during storage.
• If pharmacy delivers frozen solution, thaw it at room temperature, not in water bath or microwave. Store thawed solution for up to 12 hours at room temperature or 7 days in refrigerator; don't refreeze.
• **WARNING** When preparing drug for neonates or immature infants, don't use diluents containing benzyl alcohol because they are linked to a fatal toxic syndrome.
• For I.V. bolus, reconstitute 1 to 2 g with 10 ml sterile water for injection, D$_5$W, or sodium chloride for injection. Shake to dissolve. Administer I.V. injection slowly over 3 to 5 minutes through tubing of a flowing compatible I.V. fluid.

C

•For intermittent infusion, further dilute in 50 to 100 ml of D_5W or normal saline solution. Avoid using sodium bicarbonate injection as a diluent because drug is least stable in it. During ceftazidime administration, temporarily stop other solutions being given at the same I.V. site.

•For I.M. use, reconstitute each gram with 3 ml sterile water for injection or bacteriostatic water for injection.

•Give I.M. injection deep into large muscle mass, such as gluteus maximus.

•Rotate I.V. sites every 72 hours. Assess for phlebitis and extravasation.

•Assess bowel pattern daily; severe diarrhea may indicate pseudomembranous colitis.

•Monitor CBC, hematocrit, and serum AST, ALT, bilirubin, LD, and alkaline phosphatase levels during long-term therapy.

•Monitor PT, as ordered, in at-risk patients, such as those with renal or hepatic impairment or poor nutritional state and those receiving anticoagulant or prolonged antibiotic therapy. Notify prescriber if PT decreases, and expect to give vitamin K.

•Assess patient for perineal itching, fever, malaise, redness, swelling, rash, and change in cough or sputum; they may indicate a superinfection.

•Watch for pharyngitis, ecchymosis, bleeding, and arthralgia (possible blood dyscrasia). Monitor PT and bleeding time.

PATIENT TEACHING

•Tell patient to take ceftazidine exactly as prescribed.

•Tell patient to immediately report evidence of blood dyscrasia or superinfection to prescriber.

•Urge patient to report watery, bloody stools to prescriber immediately, even up to 2 months after drug therapy has ended.

ceftibuten

Cedax

Class and Category

Chemical class: Third-generation cephalosporin, 7-aminocephalosporanic acid
Therapeutic class: Antibiotic
Pregnancy category: B

Indications and Dosages

➤ *To treat acute bacterial exacerbations of chronic bronchitis caused by* Haemophilus influenzae, Moraxella catarrhalis, *or* Streptococcus pneumoniae; *pharyngitis and tonsillitis caused by* Streptococcus pyogenes; *and acute bacterial otitis media caused* by H. influenzae, M. catarrhalis, *or* S. pneumoniae

CAPSULES, ORAL SUSPENSION

Adults and children age 12 and over. 400 mg daily for 10 days.

➤ *To treat pharyngitis and tonsillitis caused by* S. pyogenes *and acute bacterial otitis media caused* by H. influenzae, M. catarrhalis, *or* S. pneumoniae

ORAL SUSPENSION

Children under age 12. 9 mg/kg daily for 10 days. *Maximum:* 400 mg daily.

DOSAGE ADJUSTMENT Dosage reduced to 4.5 mg/kg or 200 mg every 24 hr if creatinine clearance is 30 to 49 ml/min/1.73 m^2; to 2.25 mg/kg or 100 mg every 24 hr if it's 5 to 29 ml/min/1.73 m^2.

Mechanism of Action

Interferes with bacterial cell wall synthesis by inhibiting the cross-linking of peptidoglycan strands. Peptidoglycan makes the cell membrane rigid and protective. Without it, bacterial cells rupture and die.

Contraindications

Hypersensitivity to cephalosporins or their components

Interactions

DRUGS

aminoglycosides, loop diuretics: Increased risk of nephrotoxicity

Adverse Reactions

CNS: Chills, fever, headache, seizures
CV: Edema
EENT: Hearing loss
GI: Abdominal cramps, diarrhea, elevated liver function test results, hepatic failure, hepatomegaly, nausea, oral candidiasis, pseudomembranous colitis, vomiting
GU: Elevated BUN level, nephrotoxicity, renal failure, vaginal candidiasis
HEME: Eosinophilia, hemolytic anemia, hypoprothrombinemia, neutropenia, thrombocytopenia, unusual bleeding

MS: Arthralgia
RESP: Dyspnea
SKIN: Ecchymosis, erythema, erythema multiforme, pruritus, rash, Stevens-Johnson syndrome
Other: Anaphylaxis, superinfection

Nursing Considerations
•Use ceftibuten cautiously in patients hypersensitive to penicillins because cross-sensitivity occurs in up to 10% of such patients.
•If possible, obtain culture and sensitivity test results, as ordered, before giving drug.
•Refrigerate oral suspension; shake well before using. Discard after 14 days.
•Monitor BUN and serum creatinine levels to detect early signs of nephrotoxicity. Also, monitor fluid intake and output; decreasing urine output may indicate nephrotoxicity.
•Be aware that an allergic reaction may occur a few days after therapy starts.
•Assess bowel pattern daily; severe diarrhea may indicate pseudomembranous colitis.
•Assess patient for perineal itching, fever, malaise, redness, swelling, rash, and change in cough or sputum; they may indicate a superinfection.
•Assess for pharyngitis, ecchymosis, bleeding, and arthralgia; they may indicate a blood dyscrasia.

PATIENT TEACHING
•Urge patient to complete the drug therapy as prescribed.
•Instruct patient to take drug on an empty stomach at least 2 hours before or 1 hour after meals.
•Inform patient that unflavored oral suspension has a bitter taste. Suggest that he have a flavor added when prescription is filled.
•Advise patient that yogurt and buttermilk can help maintain intestinal flora and decrease diarrhea during therapy.
•Tell patient to immediately report hypersensitivity reactions, severe diarrhea, and evidence of blood dyscrasia or superinfection.

ceftizoxime sodium

Cefizox

Class and Category
Chemical class: Third-generation cephalosporin, 7-aminocephalosporanic acid
Therapeutic class: Antibiotic
Pregnancy category: B

Indications and Dosages
➤ *To treat mild to moderate infections of the lower respiratory tract, skin, soft tissue, bones, and joints; septicemia; meningitis; and intra-abdominal infections caused by anaerobes (such as* Bacteroides *species,* Peptococcus, *and* Peptostreptococcus), *gram-negative organisms (including* Escherichia coli, Haemophilus influenzae, Klebsiella, *and* Proteus mirabilis), *and gram-positive organisms (including* Enterobacter *species,* Serratia *species,* Staphylococcus aureus, Staphylococcus epidermidis, Streptococcus agalactiae, Streptococcus pneumoniae, *and* Streptococcus pyogenes)

I.V. INFUSION, I.V. OR I.M. INJECTION
Adults and children age 12 and over. 1 to 2 g every 8 to 12 hr.
➤ *To treat severe or refractory infections of the type listed above*

I.V. INFUSION OR INJECTION
Adults and children age 12 and over. 1 g every 8 hr or 2 g every 8 to 12 hr.
➤ *To treat life-threatening infections of the type listed above*

I.V. INFUSION OR INJECTION
Adults and children age 12 and over. 3 to 4 g every 8 hr or, if required, up to 2 g every 4 hr.
➤ *To treat bacterial infections in children*

I.V. INFUSION, I.V. OR I.M. INJECTION
Children age 6 months and over. 50 mg/kg every 6 to 8 hr.
➤ *To treat uncomplicated UTI*

I.V. INFUSION, I.V. OR I.M. INJECTION
Adults. 500 mg every 12 hr.
➤ *To treat pelvic inflammatory disease*

I.V. INFUSION OR INJECTION
Adults. 2 g every 8 hr.
➤ *To treat uncomplicated gonococcal infections*

I.M. INJECTION
Adults. 1 g as a single dose.
DOSAGE ADJUSTMENT Dosage reduced to 0.5 g every 8 hr for less severe infections and 0.75 to 1.5 g every 8 hr for life-threatening infections if creatinine clearance is 50 to 79 ml/min/1.73 m^2; to 0.25 to 0.5 g every 12 hr for less severe infections and 0.5 to 1 g every 12 hr for life-threatening infections if creati-

nine clearance is 5 to 49 ml/min/1.73 m^2; and to 0.5 g every 48 hr or 0.25 g every 24 hr for less severe infections and 0.5 to 1 g every 48 hr or 0.5 g every 24 hr for life-threatening infections if creatinine clearance is 4 ml/min/1.73 m^2 or less.

> ## Mechanism of Action
> Interferes with bacterial cell wall synthesis by inhibiting the final step in the cross-linking of peptidoglycan strands. Peptidoglycan makes the cell membrane rigid and protective. Without it, bacterial cells rupture and die.

Contraindications
Hypersensitivity to cephalosporins or their components

Interactions
DRUGS
aminoglycosides, loop diuretics: Increased risk of nephrotoxicity

Adverse Reactions
CNS: Chills, fever, headache, seizures
CV: Edema
EENT: Hearing loss
GI: Abdominal cramps, diarrhea, elevated liver function test results, hepatic failure, hepatomegaly, nausea, oral candidiasis, pseudomembranous colitis, vomiting
GU: Elevated BUN level, nephrotoxicity, renal failure, vaginal candidiasis
HEME: Eosinophilia, hemolytic anemia, hypoprothrombinemia, neutropenia, thrombocytopenia, unusual bleeding
MS: Arthralgia
RESP: Dyspnea
SKIN: Ecchymosis, erythema, erythema multiforme, pruritus, rash, Stevens-Johnson syndrome
Other: Anaphylaxis; injection site pain, redness, and swelling; superinfection

Nursing Considerations
• Use ceftizoxime cautiously in patients who are hypersensitive to penicillin because cross-sensitivity has occurred in about 10% of such patients.
• If possible, obtain culture and sensitivity test results, as ordered, before giving drug.
• For I.V. administration, reconstitute with sterile water for injection as follows: for 500-mg vial, add 5 ml; for 1-g vial, add 10 ml; and for 2-g vial, add 20 ml. Shake well. Dilute reconstituted solution further with 50 to 100 ml of a compatible solution, such as normal saline solution or D$_5$W, before administration. Administer I.V. injection slowly over 3 to 5 minutes through tubing of a flowing compatible I.V. fluid.
• For I.M. administration, reconstitute with sterile water for injection as follows: for 500-mg vial, add 1.5 ml; for 1-g vial, add 3 ml; and for 2-g vial, add 6 ml. Shake well. Divide 2-g doses and administer in different sites. Inject deeply in large muscle mass, such as the gluteus maximus.
• Reconstituted drug may be stored for 24 hours at room temperature or 96 hours if refrigerated.
• Assess I.V. site for extravasation and phlebitis.
• Monitor BUN and serum creatinine levels to detect early signs of nephrotoxicity. Also, monitor fluid intake and output; decreasing urine output may indicate nephrotoxicity.
• Assess bowel pattern daily; severe diarrhea may indicate pseudomembranous colitis.
• Monitor for allergic reactions a few days after therapy starts.
• Assess CBC, hematocrit, and serum AST, ALT, bilirubin, LD, and alkaline phosphatase levels during long-term therapy.
• Assess for pharyngitis, ecchymosis, bleeding, and arthralgia; they may indicate a blood dyscrasia.
PATIENT TEACHING
• Advise patient to immediately report severe or persistent diarrhea or evidence of blood dyscrasia to prescriber.

ceftriaxone sodium
Rocephin

Class and Category
Chemical class: Third-generation cephalosporin, 7-aminocephalosporanic acid
Therapeutic class: Antibiotic
Pregnancy category: B

Indications and Dosages
➤ *To treat infections of the lower respiratory tract, skin, soft tissue, urinary tract, bones, and joints; sinusitis; intra-*

abdominal infections; and septicemia caused by anaerobes (including Bacteroides bivius, Bacteroides fragilis, Bacteroides melaninogenicus, and Peptostreptococcus species), gram-negative organisms (including Citrobacter species, Enterobacter aerogenes, Escherichia coli, Haemophilus influenzae, Klebsiella species, Neisseria species, Proteus mirabilis, Proteus vulgaris, Providencia species, Salmonella species, Serratia marcescens, Shigella, and some strains of Pseudomonas aeruginosa), and gram-positive organisms (including Staphylococcus aureus, Streptococcus pneumoniae, and Streptococcus pyogenes)

I.V. INFUSION, I.M. INJECTION
Adults. 1 to 2 g daily or in equally divided doses b.i.d. *Maximum:* 4 g daily.
Children. 50 to 75 mg/kg daily in divided doses every 12 hr. *Maximum:* 2 g daily.

➤ *To treat meningitis*
I.V. INFUSION
Children. *Initial:* 100 mg/kg on first day, then 100 mg/kg daily or in divided doses every 12 hr for 7 to 14 days. *Maximum:* 4 g daily.

➤ *To treat acute bacterial otitis media*
I.M. INJECTION
Children. 50 mg/kg as a single dose. *Maximum:* 1 g.

➤ *To treat chancroid (*Haemophilus ducreyi *infection) and uncomplicated gonorrhea*
I.M. INJECTION
Adults. 250 mg as a single dose.

➤ *To treat gonococcal conjunctivitis*
I.M. INJECTION
Adults. 1 g as a single dose.

➤ *To treat disseminated gonoccocal infection and pelvic inflammatory disease*
I.V. INFUSION, I.M. INJECTION
Adults: 1 g every 24 hr.

➤ *To treat gonococcal meningitis and endocarditis*
I.V. INFUSION
Adults. 1 to 2 g every 12 hr for 10 to 14 days (meningitis) or for 4 wk or longer (endocarditis).

➤ *To provide surgical prophylaxis*

I.V. INFUSION
Adults. 1 g 30 min to 2 hr before surgery.

Incompatibilities
Don't admix ceftriaxone with pentamidine isethionate, labetalol, or other antibiotics, such as aminoglycosides, because of potential for incompatibility, such as substantial mutual inactivation. Also don't mix with calcium-containing solutions or products because a ceftriaxone-calcium salt may precipitate in the lungs and kidneys and may be fatal, especially in newborns.

Mechanism of Action
Interferes with bacterial cell wall synthesis by inhibiting cross-linking of peptidoglycan strands. Peptidoglycan makes the cell membrane rigid and protective. Without it, bacterial cells rupture and die.

Contraindications
Calcium-containing I.V. solutions; hyperbilirubinemic neonates 28 days old or less; hypersensitivity to ceftriaxone, other cephalosporins, or their components

Interactions
DRUGS
aminoglycosides, loop diuretics: Increased risk of nephrotoxicity

Adverse Reactions
CNS: Chills, fever, headache, hypertonia, reversible hyperactivity, seizures
CV: Edema
EENT: Glossitis, hearing loss, stomatitis
GI: Abdominal cramps, cholestasis, diarrhea, elevated liver function test results, gallbladder dysfunction, hepatic failure, hepatomegaly, nausea, oral candidiasis, pancreatitis, pseudolithiasis, pseudomembranous colitis, vomiting
GU: Elevated BUN level, nephrotoxicity, oliguria, renal failure, vaginal candidiasis
HEME: Aplastic anemia, eosinophilia, hemolytic anemia, hemorrhage, hypoprothrombinemia, neutropenia, thrombocytopenia, unusual bleeding
MS: Arthralgia
RESP: Allergic pneumonitis, dyspnea
SKIN: Allergic dermatitis, ecchymosis, erythema, erythema multiforme, exanthema,

C

pruritus, rash, Stevens-Johnson syndrome, toxic epidermal necrolysis, urticaria
Other: Anaphylaxis; drug fever; injection site pain, redness, and swelling; serum sickness; superinfection

Nursing Considerations

•**WARNING** Calcium-containing products must not be given I.V. within 48 hours of ceftriaxone, including solutions given through a different I.V. line and at a different site, because a ceftriaxone-calcium salt may precipitate in the lungs and kidneys and could be fatal.

•Use ceftriaxone cautiously in patients who are hypersensitive to penicillins because cross-sensitivity has occurred in about 10% of such patients.

•If possible, obtain culture and sensitivity results, as ordered, before giving drug.

•Protect powder from light.

•For I.V. use, reconstitute with an appropriate diluent, such as sterile water for injection or sodium chloride for injection, as follows: for 250-mg vial, add 2.4 ml; for 500-mg vial, add 4.8 ml; for 1-g vial, add 9.6 ml; and for 2-g vial, add 19.2 ml to yield 100 mg/ml. For piggyback bottles, reconstitute with 10 ml of diluent indicated above for 1-g bottle and 20 ml for 2-g bottle. After reconstitution, further dilute to 50 to 100 ml with diluent indicated above and infuse over 30 minutes.

•For I.M. administration, reconstitute with an appropriate diluent, such as sterile water for injection or sodium chloride for injection, as follows: for 250-mg vial, add 0.9 ml; for 500-mg vial, add 1.8 ml; for 1-g vial, add 3.6 ml; and for 2-g vial, add 7.2 ml to make a 250-mg/ml concentration. Shake well. Inject deep into large muscle mass, such as the gluteus maximus.

•Monitor BUN and serum creatinine levels to detect early signs of nephrotoxicity. Also, monitor fluid intake and output; decreasing urine output may indicate nephrotoxicity.

•Monitor patient for allergic reactions a few days after therapy starts.

•Assess CBC, hematocrit, and serum AST, ALT, bilirubin, LD, and alkaline phosphatase levels during long-term therapy.

•Assess bowel pattern daily; severe diarrhea may indicate pseudomembranous colitis caused by *Clostridium difficile.* If diarrhea

occurs, notify prescriber and expect to withhold cefotaxime and treat with fluids, electrolytes, protein, and an antibiotic effective against *C. difficile.*

•Monitor patient for evidence of gallbladder disease (abdominal pain, nausea, vomiting) because drug may cause a ceftriaxone-calcium salt to deposit in the gallbladder, which may mimic gallstones. Expect drug to be discontinued if gallbladder disorders arise.

•Assess for perineal itching, fever, malaise, redness, swelling, rash, and change in cough or sputum; they may indicate a superinfection.

•Assess for pharyngitis, ecchymosis, bleeding, and arthralgia; they may indicate a blood dyscrasia.

PATIENT TEACHING

•Tell patient to immediately report evidence of blood dyscrasia or superinfection to prescriber.

•Urge patient to report watery, bloody stools to prescriber immediately, even up to 2 months after drug therapy has ended.

cefuroxime axetil

Ceftin

cefuroxime sodium

Zinacef

Class and Category

Chemical class: Second-generation cephalosporin, 7-aminocephalosporanic acid
Therapeutic class: Antibiotic
Pregnancy category: B

Indications and Dosages

➤ *To treat pharyngitis and tonsillitis*
ORAL SUSPENSION
Children ages 3 months to 12 years. 10 mg/kg daily in equally divided doses b.i.d. for 10 days. *Maximum:* 500 mg daily.
TABLETS
Adults and children age 13 and over. 250 mg b.i.d. for 10 days.
Children under age 13 who can swallow tablets. 125 mg b.i.d. for 10 days.

➤ *To treat acute otitis media*
ORAL SUSPENSION
Children ages 3 months to 12 years. 30 mg/kg daily in equally divided doses b.i.d. for

10 days. *Maximum:* 1,000 mg daily.

TABLETS

Children under age 13 who can swallow tablets. 250 mg b.i.d. for 10 days.

➤ *To treat impetigo*

ORAL SUSPENSION

Children ages 3 months to 12 years. 30 mg/kg daily in equally divided doses b.i.d. for 10 days. *Maximum:* 1,000 mg daily.

➤ *To treat acute bacterial maxillary sinusitis*

ORAL SUSPENSION

Children ages 3 months to 12 years. 30 mg/kg/day in equally divided doses b.i.d. for 10 days. *Maximum:* 1,000 mg daily.

TABLETS

Adults and children age 13 and over and children under age 13 who can swallow tablets. 250 mg b.i.d. for 10 days.

➤ *To treat acute bacterial exacerbations of chronic bronchitis and uncomplicated skin and soft-tissue infections*

TABLETS

Adults and children age 13 and over. 250 to 500 mg b.i.d. for 10 days.

I.V. INFUSION, I.V. OR I.M. INJECTION

Adults. 750 mg every 8 hr.

➤ *To treat secondary bacterial infection in patients with acute bronchitis*

Adults and children age 13 and over. 250 to 500 mg b.i.d. for 5 to 10 days.

➤ *To treat early Lyme disease*

TABLETS

Adults and children age 13 and over. 500 mg b.i.d. for 20 days.

➤ *To treat uncomplicated UTI*

TABLETS

Adults. 125 to 250 mg b.i.d. for 7 to 10 days.

I.V. INFUSION, I.V. OR I.M. INJECTION

Adults. 750 mg every 8 hr.

➤ *To treat uncomplicated gonorrhea*

TABLETS

Adults. 1 g as a single dose.

I.M. INJECTION

Adults. 1.5 g as a single dose divided equally and injected into two different sites; given with oral probenecid 1 g.

➤ *To treat disseminated gonococcal infection and uncomplicated pneumonia*

I.V. INFUSION, I.V. OR I.M. INJECTION

Adults. 750 mg every 8 hr.

➤ *To treat bone and joint infections*

I.V. INFUSION, I.V. OR I.M. INJECTION

Adults. 1.5 g every 8 hr.

Children over age 3 months. 50 to 150 mg/kg daily in divided doses every 8 hr. *Maximum:* Adult dose.

➤ *To treat bacterial meningitis*

I.V. INFUSION

Adults. 1.5 to 3 g every 8 hr..

Children over age 1 month. 50 to 80 mg/kg every 6 to 8 hr.

Neonates up to age 1 month. 33.3 to 50 mg/kg every 8 to 12 hr.

➤ *To treat moderate infections other than those listed above*

I.V. INFUSION, I.V. OR I.M. INJECTION

Adults. 750 mg every 8 hr for 5 to 10 days.

I.V. INFUSION OR INJECTION

Children over age 3 months. 50 mg/kg daily in equally divided doses every 6 to 8 hr.

➤ *To treat severe or complicated infections other than those listed above*

I.V. INFUSION OR INJECTION

Adults. 1.5 g every 8 hr.

Children over age 3 months. 100 mg/kg daily in equally divided doses every 6 to 8 hr.

➤ *To treat life-threatening infections other than those listed above*

I.V. INFUSION OR INJECTION

Adults. 1.5 g every 6 hr.

➤ *To provide perioperative prophylaxis*

I.V. INFUSION OR INJECTION

Adults. 1.5 g 30 to 60 min before surgery (at induction of anesthesia for open-heart surgery), and then 0.75 g every 8 hr thereafter (1.5 g every 12 hr for total of 6 g with open-heart surgery).

DOSAGE ADJUSTMENT Parenteral dosage reduced to 0.75 g every 12 hr if creatinine clearance is 10 to 20 ml/min/1.73 m^2 or to 0.75 g every 24 hr if creatinine clearance less than 10 ml/min/1.73 m^2.

Mechanism of Action

Interferes with bacterial cell wall synthesis by inhibiting the final step in the cross-linking of peptidoglycan strands. Peptidoglycan makes the cell membrane rigid and protective. Without it, bacterial cells rupture and die.

Incompatibilities

Don't admix parenteral cefuroxime with other antibiotics, such as aminoglycosides, because of potential for incompatibility, such as substantial mutual inactivation. If they're administered concurrently, don't mix them in the same I.V. bag or bottle.

Contraindications

Hypersensitivity to cephalosporins or their components

Interactions

DRUGS

aminoglycosides, loop diuretics: Increased risk of nephrotoxicity
antacids, H₂-receptor antagonists, omeprazole: Decreased cefuroxime axetil absorption
probenecid: Increased and prolonged blood cefuroxime level

Adverse Reactions

CNS: Chills, fever, headache, seizures
CV: Edema
EENT: Hearing loss, oral candidiasis
GI: Abdominal cramps, diarrhea, elevated liver function test results, hepatic failure, hepatomegaly, nausea, pseudomembranous colitis, vomiting
GU: Elevated BUN level, nephrotoxicity, renal failure, vaginal candidiasis
HEME: Eosinophilia, hemolytic anemia, hypoprothrombinemia, neutropenia, thrombocytopenia, unusual bleeding
MS: Arthralgia
RESP: Dyspnea
SKIN: Ecchymosis, erythema, erythema multiforme, pruritus, rash, Stevens-Johnson syndrome
Other: Anaphylaxis; injection site edema, pain, and redness; superinfection

Nursing Considerations

•Use cefuroxime cautiously in patients hypersensitive to penicillin because cross-sensitivity has occurred in about 10% of such patients.
•If possible, obtain culture and sensitivity results, as ordered, before giving drug.
•Give oral form with food to decrease GI distress, as needed.
•Remember that oral forms—tablets and suspension—aren't bioequivalent.
•For I.V. use, reconstitute following manufacturer's instructions according to type of preparation available. Solution ranges in color from light yellow to amber.
•For I.M. use, add 3 or 3.6 ml of sterile water for injection to each 750-mg vial to yield 220 mg/ml.
•If using a container of frozen parenteral solution, thaw at room temperature or under refrigeration before administration; make sure all ice crystals have melted. Don't force thawing by microwave irradiation.
•Store reconstituted parenteral drug for up to 24 hours at room temperature or 96 hours in refrigerator. (Thawed solutions may be stable for 24 hours at room temperature or 28 days if refrigerated.) Store reconstituted oral suspension in refrigerator or at room temperature for up to 10 days.
•Administer I.V. injection over 3 to 5 minutes through tubing of a flowing compatible I.V. fluid.
•Monitor I.V. site for extravasation and phlebitis.
•Monitor BUN and serum creatinine levels and fluid intake and output to detect signs of nephrotoxicity. Monitor patients with renal impairment closely because they may have greater toxic reactions to cefuroxime.
•Monitor patient for allergic reactions continuing up to a few days after therapy starts. Patients with a history of some form of allergy, especially to drugs, are at increased risk for an allergic reaction.
•Assess bowel pattern daily; severe diarrhea may indicate pseudomembranous colitis. If it's suspected, stop drug, as ordered, and provide treatment as prescribed.
•Assess patient for pharyngitis, ecchymosis, bleeding, and arthralgia, which may indicate a blood dyscrasia.
•Monitor PT and bleeding time, as ordered. Be prepared to administer vitamin K, if ordered, to treat hypothrombinemia.

PATIENT TEACHING

•Instruct patient to shake oral suspension well before measuring each dose and to use an accurate liquid-measuring device.
•Advise patient using single-dose packets of oral suspension to empty the contents of one packet into a glass and add at least 10 ml (2 tsp) of cold water; apple, grape, or orange juice; or lemonade. Tell him to stir well and consume entire mixture at once.
•Inform patient that yogurt and buttermilk help maintain intestinal flora and can de-

crease diarrhea during therapy.
•Instruct patient to report evidence of blood dyscrasia to prescriber immediately.
•Urge patient to report watery, bloody stools to prescriber immediately, even up to 2 months after drug therapy has ended.

celecoxib

Celebrex

Class and Category
Chemical class: Diaryl-substituted pyrazole derivative
Therapeutic class: Anti-inflammatory, antirheumatic
Pregnancy category: C

Indications and Dosages
➤ *To relieve signs and symptoms of osteoarthritis*
CAPSULES
Adults. 200 mg daily or 100 mg b.i.d.
➤ *To relieve signs and symptoms of rheumatoid arthritis*
CAPSULES
Adults. 100 to 200 mg b.i.d.
➤ *To relieve signs and symptoms of juvenile rheumatoid arthritis*
CAPSULES
Children age 2 and older weighing between 10 and 25 kg (22 and 55 lb). 50 mg b.i.d.
Children age 2 and older weighing more than 25 kg. 100 mg b.i.d.
➤ *To relieve pain from ankylosing spondylitis*
CAPSULES
Adults. 200 mg daily or 100 mg b.i.d. Dosage increased to 400 mg daily or 200 mg b.i.d. after 6 weeks if needed.
➤ *As adjunct to reduce adenomatous colorectal polyps in patients with familial adenomatous polyposis*
CAPSULES
Adults. 400 mg b.i.d.
➤ *To manage acute pain, to treat primary dysmenorrhea*
CAPSULES
Adults. 400 mg, followed by 200 mg if needed, on 1st day. On subsequent days, 200 mg b.i.d. as needed.
DOSAGE ADJUSTMENT Daily dosage reduced

for patients with hepatic impairment. For those weighing less than 50 kg (110 lb), expect to start with lowest recommended dose.

Mechanism of Action
Selectively inhibits the enzymatic activity of cyclooxygenase-2 (COX-2), the enzyme needed to convert arachidonic acid to prostaglandin. Prostaglandins are responsible for mediating the inflammatory response and causing local vasodilation, swelling, and pain. Prostaglandins also play a role in peripheral pain transmission to the spinal cord. By inhibiting COX-2 activity and prostaglandin production, this NSAID reduces inflammatory symptoms and relieves pain. Celecoxib's mechanism of action in reducing the number of colorectal polyps is unknown.

Contraindications
Allergic reaction (such as anaphylaxis or angioedema) to aspirin, other NSAIDs, or sulfonamide derivatives or history of aspirin-induced nasal polyps with bronchospasm; hypersensitivity to celecoxib or its components; treatment of perioperative pain after coronary artery bypass graft surgery

Interactions
DRUGS
ACE inhibitors, angiotensin II receptor antagonists: Decreased antihypertensive effect of ACE inhibitors and angiotensin II receptor antagonists, increased risk of renal failure
aspirin: Increased risk of GI ulceration and other GI complications
fluconazole: Increased blood celecoxib level
furosemide, thiazide diuretics: Reduced diuretic effects of these drugs, increased risk of renal failure
lithium: Possibly elevated blood lithium level
warfarin: Possibly increased PT and risk of bleeding

Adverse Reactions
CNS: Asceptic meningitis, cerebral hemorrhage, depression, dizziness, fever, headache, insomnia, ischemic stroke, suicidal ideation, syncope, transient ischemic attacks, vertigo
CV: Aortic valve incompetence, chest pain,

congestive heart failure, deep vein thrombosis, fluid retention, hypertension, MI, palpitations, peripheral edema or gangrene, sinus bradycardia, tachycardia, unstable angina, vasculitis, ventricular fibrillation, ventricular hypertrophy
EENT: Conjunctival hemorrhage, deafness, labyrinthitis, nasopharyngitis, pharyngitis, rhinitis, sinusitis, vitreous floaters
ENDO: Hyperglycemia, hypoglycemia
GI: Abdominal pain, diarrhea, elevated liver function test results, esophageal perforation, flatulence, GI bleeding or ulceration, hepatic failure, ileus, indigestion, jaundice, nausea, pancreatitis, perforation of stomach or intestine, vomiting
GU: Acute renal failure, interstitial nephritis, ovarian cyst, proteinuria, UTI, urinary incontinence
HEME: Agranulocytosis, aplastic anemia, decreased hematocrit and hemoglobin, leukopenia, pancytopenia, prolonged APTT, thrombocytopenia
MS: Arthralgia, back pain, elevated serum CK level, epicondylitis, tendon rupture
RESP: Bronchospasm, cough, dyspnea, pneumonia, pulmonary embolism, upper respiratory tract infection
SKIN: Erythema multiforme, exfoliative dermatitis, phototoxicity, rash, Stevens-Johnson syndrome, toxic epidermal necrolysis, urticaria
Other: Anaphylaxis, angioedema, hyperkalemia, hypernatremia, hyponatremia, sepsis

Nursing Considerations
•Use celecoxib with extreme caution in patients who have a history of ulcer disease or GI bleeding because NSAIDs, such as celecoxib, increase the risk of GI bleeding and ulceration. In these patients, drug should be used for the shortest time possible.
•Be aware that serious GI tract ulceration and bleeding as well as perforation of the stomach or intestine can occur without warning or symptoms. Elderly patients are at greatest risk. To minimize this risk, give celecoxib with food. If patient develops GI distress, withhold celecoxib and notify prescriber immediately.
•Use celecoxib cautiously in patients with hypertension, and monitor blood pressure closely throughout therapy because drug can

start or worsen hypertension.
•Use celecoxib cautiously in children with systemic onset juvenile rheumatoid arthritis because serious adverse reactions can occur, including disseminated intravascular coagulation.
•**WARNING** Monitor patient closely for thrombotic events, including MI and stroke, because use of NSAIDs, such as celecoxib, increases the risk.
•**WARNING** In patient who has bone marrow suppression or is receiving antineoplastic drug therapy, monitor laboratory results (including WBC) and assess for evidence of infection because celecoxib has anti-inflammatory and antipyretic actions that may mask signs and symptoms, such as fever and pain.
•Monitor patient—especially if he's elderly or receiving long-term celecoxib therapy—for less common but serious adverse GI reactions, including anorexia, constipation, diverticulitis, dysphagia, esophagitis, gastritis, gastroenteritis, gastroesophageal reflux disease, hemorrhoids, hiatal hernia, melena, stomatitis, and vomiting.
•Monitor liver function test results because, in rare cases, elevations may progress to severe hepatic reactions, including fatal hepatitis, hepatic necrosis, and hepatic failure.
•Monitor BUN and serum creatinine levels in elderly patients; patients taking diuretics, ACE inhibitors, or angiotensin II receptor antagonists; and patients with heart failure, impaired renal function, or hepatic dysfunction because drug may cause renal failure.
•Monitor CBC for decreased hemoglobin level and hematocrit because drug may worsen anemia.
•Assess patient's skin regularly for signs of rash or other hypersensitivity reaction because celecoxib is a sulfur drug and may cause serious skin reactions without warning, even in patients with no history of sensitivity to sulfur. At first sign of reaction, stop drug and notify prescriber.
•Avoid using celecoxib with a non-aspirin NSAID, regardless of the dose, because celecoxib reduces inflammation and fever, which may mask signs of infection.
PATIENT TEACHING
•Instruct patient to swallow celecoxib capsules whole with a full glass of water and with food or milk to prevent stomach upset.
•Advise patient to notify prescriber if pain

continues or is poorly controlled.

•Explain that celecoxib may increase the risk of serious adverse CV events; urge patient to seek immediate medical attention if signs or symptoms arise, such as chest pain, shortness of breath, slurred speech, and weakness.

•Tell patient that celecoxib may increase the risk of serious adverse GI reactions. Stress the need to seek immediate medical attention if signs or symptoms develop, such as epigastric or abdominal pain, indigestion, black or tarry stools, and vomiting blood or material that resembles coffee grounds.

•Alert patient that celecoxib may cause serious skin reactions. Advise seeking immediate medical attention if signs or symptoms develop, such as rash, blisters, fever, itching, or other evidence of hypersensitivity.

•Urge patient to avoid smoking and alcohol consumption during celecoxib therapy because they may increase the risk of adverse GI reactions.

cephalexin hydrochloride

Keftab

cephalexin monohydrate

Apo-Cephalex (CAN), Keflex, Novo-Lexin (CAN), Nu-Cephalex (CAN), PMS-Cephalexin (CAN)

Class and Category

Chemical class: First-generation cephalosporin, 7-aminocephalosporanic acid
Therapeutic class: Antibiotic
Pregnancy category: B

Indications and Dosages

➤ *To treat streptococcal tonsillitis, pharyngitis, and skin and soft-tissue infections*

CAPSULES, ORAL SUSPENSION, TABLETS

Adults and adolescents age 15 and over. 500 mg every 12 hr. *Maximum:* 4 g daily.
Children and adolescents ages 2 to 15. 25 to 50 mg/kg daily divided into two equal doses and given every 12 hr. If infection is severe, dose may be doubled.

➤ *To treat mild to moderate respiratory tract, skin, soft-tissue, bone, and GU infections caused by susceptible organisms other than streptococci*

CAPSULES, ORAL SUSPENSION, TABLETS

Adults. 250 mg every 6 hr.

ORAL SUSPENSION

Children. 25 to 50 mg/kg daily in equally divided doses b.i.d. or q.i.d.

➤ *To treat severe respiratory tract, skin, soft-tissue, bone, and GU infections*

CAPSULES, ORAL SUSPENSION, TABLETS

Adults. 0.5 to 1 g every 6 hr. *Maximum:* 4 g daily.
Children. 50 to 100 mg/kg daily in equally divided doses q.i.d.

➤ *To treat otitis media*

ORAL SUSPENSION

Children. 75 to 100 mg/kg daily in equally divided doses q.i.d.

➤ *To treat uncomplicated cystitis*

CAPSULES, ORAL SUSPENSION, TABLETS

Adults and adolescents age 15 and over. 500 mg every 12 hr.

Contraindications

Hypersensitivity to cephalosporins or their components

Interactions

DRUGS

aminoglycosides, loop diuretics: Increased risk of nephrotoxicity
probenecid: Increased and prolonged blood cephalexin level

Adverse Reactions

CNS: Chills, fever, headache, seizures
CV: Edema
EENT: Hearing loss
GI: Abdominal cramps, diarrhea, elevated liver function test results, hepatic failure, hepatomegaly, nausea, oral candidiasis, pseudomembranous colitis, vomiting
GU: Elevated BUN level, nephrotoxicity, renal failure, vaginal candidiasis
HEME: Eosinophilia, hemolytic anemia, hypoprothrombinemia, neutropenia, thrombocytopenia, unusual bleeding
MS: Arthralgia
RESP: Dyspnea
SKIN: Ecchymosis, erythema, erythema multiforme, pruritus, rash, Stevens-Johnson syndrome
Other: Anaphylaxis, superinfection

Nursing Considerations

•Use cephalexin cautiously in patients who are hypersensitive to penicillin because

Mechanism of Action

Like all cephalosporins, cephalexin interferes with bacterial cell wall synthesis by inhibiting the final step in the cross-linking of peptidoglycan strands. Peptidoglycan makes the cell membrane rigid and protective. Without it, bacterial cells rupture and die. This mechanism of action is most effective against bacteria that divide rapidly, including many gram-positive and gram-negative bacteria.

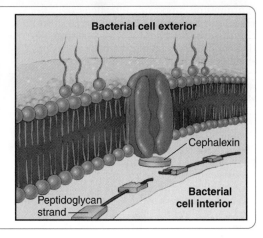

cross-sensitivity occurs in about 10% of them.
•If possible, obtain culture and sensitivity test results, as ordered, before giving drug.
•Monitor patient's BUN and serum creatinine levels to detect early signs of nephrotoxicity. Also, monitor fluid intake and output; decreasing urine output may indicate nephrotoxicity.
•Monitor for allergic reactions a few days after therapy starts.
•Assess CBC, hematocrit, and serum AST, ALT, bilirubin, LD, and alkaline phosphatase levels during long-term therapy.
•Assess patient's bowel pattern daily; severe diarrhea may indicate pseudomembranous colitis caused by *Clostridium difficile*. If diarrhea occurs, notify prescriber and expect to withhold cefotaxime and treat with fluids, electrolytes, protein, and an antibiotic effective against *C. difficile*.
•Assess patient for pharyngitis, ecchymosis, bleeding, and arthralgia; they may indicate a blood dyscrasia.

PATIENT TEACHING
•Advise patient to complete prescribed course of therapy.
•Instruct patient to shake oral suspension well before measuring each dose and to use a calibrated liquid-measuring device to ensure an accurate dose.
•Tell patient that yogurt and buttermilk can help maintain intestinal flora and decrease diarrhea during therapy.
•Urge patient to immediately report watery,

bloody stools to prescriber, even if they occur up to 2 months after cephalexin therapy has ended.

cephapirin sodium

Cefadyl

Class and Category

Chemical class: First-generation cephalosporin, 7-aminocephalosporanic acid
Therapeutic class: Antibiotic
Pregnancy category: B

Indications and Dosages

➤ *To treat respiratory tract infection, skin and soft-tissue infections, UTI, septicemia, endocarditis, and osteomyelitis caused by gram-negative organisms (including* Escherichia coli, Haemophilus influenzae, Klebsiella *species, and* Proteus mirabilis*) and gram-positive organisms (including group A beta-hemolytic streptococci,* Streptococcus pneumoniae, *and staphylococci, including coagulase-positive, coagulase-negative, and penicillinase-producing strains but not methicillin-resistant* Staphylococcus aureus*)*

I.V. INFUSION, I.V. OR I.M. INJECTION
Adults. 0.5 to 1 g every 4 to 6 hr. *Maximum:* 12 g daily. For serious infections, higher doses are given by I.V. route.
Children over age 3 months. 40 to 80 mg/kg daily divided into four equal doses and given every 6 hr. *Maximum:* 12 g daily.

➤ *To provide surgical prophylaxis*
I.V. INFUSION, I.V. OR I.M. INJECTION
Adults. 1 to 2 g 30 to 60 min before surgery, 1 to 2 g during long procedure, and 1 to 2 g every 6 hr after surgery for 24 hr.
DOSAGE ADJUSTMENT For open-heart surgery or prosthetic arthroplasty, prophylaxis continued 3 to 5 days after procedure, if needed.

Mechanism of Action
Interferes with bacterial cell wall synthesis by inhibiting the final step in the cross-linking of peptidoglycan strands. Peptidoglycan makes the cell membrane rigid and protective. Without it, bacterial cells rupture and die.

Contraindications
Hypersensitivity to cephalosporins or their components

Interactions
DRUGS
aminoglycosides, loop diuretics: Increased risk of nephrotoxicity
probenecid: Increased and prolonged blood cephapirin level

Adverse Reactions
CNS: Chills, fever, headache, seizures
CV: Edema
EENT: Hearing loss
GI: Abdominal cramps, diarrhea, elevated liver function test results, hepatic failure, hepatomegaly, nausea, oral candidiasis, pseudomembranous colitis, vomiting
GU: Elevated BUN level, nephrotoxicity, renal failure, vaginal candidiasis
HEME: Eosinophilia, hemolytic anemia, hypoprothrombinemia, neutropenia, thrombocytopenia, unusual bleeding
MS: Arthralgia
RESP: Dyspnea
SKIN: Ecchymosis, erythema, erythema multiforme, pruritus, rash, Stevens-Johnson syndrome
Other: Anaphylaxis; injection site pain, redness, and swelling; superinfection

Nursing Considerations
•Use cephapirin cautiously in patients who are hypersensitive to penicillins because cross-sensitivity has occurred in about 10%

of such patients.
•If possible, obtain culture and sensitivity test results, as ordered, before giving drug.
•For I.V. injection, reconstitute 1 g with 10 ml or more of appropriate diluent, such as sterile water for injection. Administer I.V. injection slowly over 3 to 5 minutes through tubing of a flowing compatible I.V. fluid.
•For I.V. infusion, dilute further in 50 ml of D_5W or normal saline solution and infuse over 15 to 30 minutes. Stop primary I.V. solution during cephapirin administration.
•For I.M. injection, reconstitute 1-g vial with 2 ml of sterile water for injection or bacteriostatic water for injection. Inject deep into large muscle mass, such as the gluteus maximus.
•Store reconstituted drug for up to 24 hours at room temperature or 10 days refrigerated.
•Don't give a cloudy solution.
•Assess I.V. site for extravasation and phlebitis.
•Monitor BUN and serum creatinine levels to detect early signs of nephrotoxicity. Also, monitor fluid intake and output; decreasing urine output may indicate nephrotoxicity.
•Monitor for allergic reactions a few days after therapy starts.
•Assess CBC, hematocrit, and serum AST, ALT, bilirubin, LD, and alkaline phosphatase levels during long-term therapy.
•Assess patient's bowel pattern daily; severe diarrhea may indicate pseudomembranous colitis.
•Assess for pharyngitis, ecchymosis, bleeding, and arthralgia; they may indicate a blood dyscrasia.
•Assess for furry tongue, perineal itching, and loose, foul-smelling stool; they may indicate superinfection.
PATIENT TEACHING
•Instruct patient to immediately report severe diarrhea or evidence of blood dyscrasia or superinfection to prescriber.

cephradine
Velosef

Class and Category
Chemical class: First-generation cephalosporin, 7-aminocephalosporanic acid
Therapeutic class: Antibiotic
Pregnancy category: B

Indications and Dosages

➤ *To treat respiratory tract infections (other than lobar pneumonia) and skin and soft-tissue infections*

CAPSULES, ORAL SUSPENSION

Adults. 250 mg every 6 hr or 500 mg every 12 hr. *Maximum:* 4 g daily.

ORAL SUSPENSION

Children age 9 months and over. 25 to 50 mg/kg daily in equally divided doses every 6 or 12 hr. *Maximum:* 4 g daily.

➤ *To treat lobar pneumonia*

CAPSULES, ORAL SUSPENSION

Adults. 0.5 g every 6 hr or 1 g every 12 hr. *Maximum:* 4 g daily.

ORAL SUSPENSION

Children age 9 months and over. 25 to 50 mg/kg daily in equally divided doses every 6 or 12 hr. *Maximum:* 4 g daily.

➤ *To treat uncomplicated UTI*

CAPSULES, ORAL SUSPENSION

Adults. 500 mg every 12 hr. For more serious infections, 500 mg every 6 hr or 1,000 mg every 12 hr. *Maximum:* 4 g daily.

➤ *To treat otitis media caused by* Haemophilus influenzae

ORAL SUSPENSION

Children. 75 to 100 mg/kg daily in equally divided doses every 6 to 12 hr. *Maximum:* 4 g daily.

DOSAGE ADJUSTMENT Dosage reduced to 500 mg every 6 hr if creatinine clearance exceeds 20 ml/min/1.73 m^2; 250 mg every 6 hr if creatinine clearance is 5 to 20 ml/min/1.73 m^2; and 250 mg every 12 hr if creatinine clearance is less than 5 ml/min/1.73 m^2.

Mechanism of Action

Interferes with bacterial cell wall synthesis by inhibiting the final step in the cross-linking of peptidoglycan strands. Peptidoglycan makes the cell membrane rigid and protective. Without it, bacterial cells rupture and die.

Contraindications

Hypersensitivity to cephalosporins or their components

Interactions

DRUGS

aminoglycosides, loop diuretics: Increased risk of nephrotoxicity

probenecid: Increased and prolonged blood cephradine level

Adverse Reactions

CNS: Chills, fever, headache, seizures

CV: Edema

EENT: Hearing loss, oral candidiasis

GI: Abdominal cramps, diarrhea, elevated liver function test results, hepatic failure, hepatomegaly, nausea, pseudomembranous colitis, vomiting

GU: Elevated BUN level, nephrotoxicity, renal failure, vaginal candidiasis

HEME: Eosinophilia, hemolytic anemia, hypoprothrombinemia, neutropenia, thrombocytopenia, unusual bleeding

MS: Arthralgia

RESP: Dyspnea

SKIN: Ecchymosis, erythema, erythema multiforme, pruritus, rash, Stevens-Johnson syndrome

Other: Anaphylaxis, superinfection

Nursing Considerations

• If possible, obtain culture and sensitivity test results, as ordered, before giving drug.

• Monitor patients who are hypersensitive to penicillin for evidence of a hypersensitivity reaction because cross-sensitivity has occurred in about 10% of such patients.

• Store oral suspension for 7 days at room temperature or for 14 days if refrigerated.

• Monitor BUN and serum creatinine levels to detect early signs of nephrotoxicity. Also monitor fluid intake and output; decreasing urine output may indicate nephrotoxicity.

• Monitor patient for allergic reactions a few days after therapy starts. If patient develops hypersensitivity, be prepared to discontinue the drug and administer antihistamines, corticosteroids, and vasopressors, as ordered. Also prepare to administer oxygen, maintain an open airway, and assist with endotracheal intubation, as appropriate.

• Assess CBC, hematocrit, and serum AST, ALT, bilirubin, LD, and alkaline phosphatase levels during long-term therapy.

• Assess bowel pattern daily; severe diarrhea may indicate pseudomembranous colitis. Obtain a stool specimen to test for *Clostridium difficile.* Keep in mind that this serious adverse reaction can occur during therapy or up to several weeks after therapy is discontinued. Also avoid giving antiperistaltic antidiarrheals, such as atropine and diphenoxylate or loperamide, because they may delay elimination of toxins from the bowel and cause damage to the colon from toxin retention. Mild cases may respond after cephradine is discontinued. For moderate or severe cases, be prepared to administer fluids, electrolytes, and protein replacement as ordered.

•If patient has a history of GI disease, especially ulcerative colitis, regional enteritis, or antibiotic-associated colitis, assess him frequently for diarrhea because he is at risk for pseudomembranous colitis.

•Assess for pharyngitis, ecchymosis, bleeding, and arthralgia; these may indicate a blood dyscrasia.

•If patient has a seizure, notify prescriber immediately and expect to discontinue drug. Institute seizure precautions according to facility policy.

PATIENT TEACHING

•If patient develops GI distress, advise him to take cephradine with food.

•Advise patient to complete prescribed course of therapy.

•Explain that patient should avoid missing doses and that he should take the drug at evenly spaced intervals. If patient misses a dose, instruct him to take the dose as soon as possible unless it's almost time for the next dose. Emphasize that he shouldn't double the dose.

•Tell patient that yogurt and buttermilk help maintain intestinal flora and can decrease diarrhea during therapy.

•Instruct patient to immediately report to prescriber severe diarrhea or evidence of blood dyscrasia or superinfection. Warn patient not to take any OTC antidiarrheals before consulting prescriber.

•Advise patient to notify prescriber if symptoms don't improve within a few days.

certolizumab pegol

Cimzia

Class and Category

Chemical class: Recombinant, humanized antibody Fab fragment
Therapeutic class: Disease modifying anti-inflammatory
Pregnancy category: B

Indications and Dosages

➤ *To reduce signs and symptoms of Crohn's disease and maintain clinical response in patients with moderately to severely active disease who have had an inadequate response to conventional therapy*

SUBCUTANEOUS INJECTION

Adults. *Initial:* 400 mg (given as two 200-mg injections) and repeated at wk 2 and 4. *Maintenance:* 400 mg (given as two 200-mg injections) every 4 wk if clinical response occurs.

Route	Onset	Peak	Duration
SubQ	Unknown	54 to 171 hr	Unknown

Mechanism of Action

Binds to human tumor necrosis factor (TNF) alpha, inhibiting it. TNF alpha stimulates production of inflammatory mediators, including interleukin-1, prostaglandins, platelet activating factor, and nitric oxide. TNF alpha level is increased in patients with Crohn's disease. Inhibition of TNF alpha causes C-reactive protein level to decline in patients with Crohn's disease, and the disease improves.

Contraindications

Active infection, hypersensitivity to cetolizumab or its components, I.V. administration

Interactions

DRUGS

anakinra: Possibly increased risk of serious infection and neutropenia
immunosuppressants: Possibly increased risk of infection
live-virus vaccines: Increased risk of adverse vaccine effects

Adverse Reactions

CNS: Anxiety, bipolar disorder, dizziness, fever, malaise, suicidal ideation, syncope
CV: Angina, arrhythmias, heart failure, hypertension, hypotension, MI, pericardial effusion, pericarditis, peripheral edema, vasculitis
EENT: Optic neuritis, retinal hemorrhage, uveitis
ENDO: Hot flashes

GI: Abdominal pain, diarrhea, elevated liver enzymes, hepatitis, intestinal obstruction
GU: Menstrual dysfunction, nephrotic syndrome, pyelonephritis, renal failure, UTI
HEME: Anemia, leukopenia, lymphadenopathy, pancytopenia, thrombophilia
MS: Arthralgia, extremity pain
RESP: Dyspnea, pneumonia, upper respiratory infection
SKIN: Allergic dermatitis, alopecia, erythema multiforme, erythema nodosum, rash, Stevens-Johnson sydrome, toxic epidermal necrolysis
Other: Angioedema, bacterial and viral infections, injection site reactions (redness, pain), lupus-like syndrome, malignancies, serum sickness, tuberculosis

Nursing Considerations

•Use certolizumab cautiously in patients with recurrent or increased risk of infection, patients who live in regions where tuberculosis and histoplasmosis are endemic, and patients with a history of CNS demyelinating disorders because any of these disorders can occur, rarely, during certolizumab therapy.

•Use cautiously in patients who are chronic carriers of hepatitis B virus because drug may reactivate the virus. Assess patient for evidence of hepatitis B viral infection before starting and periodically throughout certolizumab therapy. If HBV reactivation occurs, notify prescriber, discontinue drug, and start appropriate therapy, as ordered.

•**WARNING** If patient has evidence of an active infection when drug is prescribed, therapy shouldn't begin until infection has been treated. Monitor all patients for infection during therapy, especially those receiving immunosuppressants. If serious infection develops, expect prescriber to stop drug.

•Make sure patient has a tuberculin skin test before therapy starts. If skin test is positive, treatment of latent tuberculosis must start before certolizumab is given, as prescribed.

•Reconstitute two 200-mg certolizumab vials for each dose after drug has reached room temperature. Inject 1 ml sterile water for injection using a 20G needle into each vial. Gently swirl each vial without shaking. Then leave vials undisturbed for up to 30 minutes to allow time for powder to completely dissolve. Do not leave at room temperature, once reconstituted, for more than 2 hours before administration. If administration will be delayed, reconstituted drug can be refrigerated up to 24 hours. Do not let drug freeze.

•Administer drug only when solution has reached room temperature. Using a 20G needle, withdraw drug from vial using a separate syringe and needle for each vial. Switch needle to a 23G needle and administer subcutaneously into two separate areas on patient's abdomen or thigh.

•**WARNING** Stop drug immediately and notify prescriber if patient has an allergic reaction. Expect to provide supportive care.

•Monitor patient closely for evidence of congestive heart failure (sudden, unexplained weight gain; dyspnea; crackles; anxiety), and notify prescriber if they occur.

•Monitor patient's CBC, as ordered, because certolizumab may have adverse hematologic effects. Notify prescriber about persistent fever, bruising, bleeding, or pallor.

PATIENT TEACHING

•Review signs and symptoms of an allergic reaction (rash, swollen face, trouble breathing), and tell patient to seek emergency care immediately if these occur.

•Inform patient that injection site reactions such as redness or pain may occur and usually are mild and transient. Instruct him to apply a towel soaked in cold water to the site if it hurts. If reaction persists or seems to worsen, tell patient to call prescriber.

•Inform patient that tuberculosis may occur during certolizumab theray. Instruct him to report persistent cough, wasting or weight loss, and low-grade fever to prescriber.

•Tell patient to report evidence of infections and bleeding disorders to prescriber; drug may need to be stopped. Advise patient to avoid people with infections and to comply with all prescribed laboratory tests.

•Inform patient that certain kinds of cancer, especially lymphomas, are more likely in patients taking certolizumab but still rare. Stress needto keep follow-up visits and report unusual or sudden signs or symptoms.

•Caution patient against receiving live-virus vaccines while taking certolizumab; doing so may adversely effect the immune system.

•Instruct patient to report lupus-like signs and symptoms that, although rare, may occur during therapy, such as chest pain that doesn't go away, shortness of breath, joint pain, or a rash on the cheeks or arms that's sensitive to the sun. Explain that drug may need to be discontinued if these occur.

•Advise patient to inform all health care providers about certolizumab use and to inform prescriber about any OTC medications, herbal remedies, and vitamin and mineral supplements being taken.

cevimeline hydrochloride

Evoxac

Class and Category

Chemical class: Quinuclidine derivative of acetylcholine
Therapeutic class: Cholinergic enhancer, dry mouth reliever
Pregnancy category: C

Indications and Dosages

➤ *To treat dry mouth associated with Sjögren's syndrome*

CAPSULES

Adults. 30 mg t.i.d. *Maximum:* 90 mg daily.

Mechanism of Action

As a cholinergic agonist, binds to and activates muscarinic receptors of the parasympathetic nervous system and increases secretions of the exocrine glands, such as salivary glands.

Contraindications

Acute iritis, angle-closure glaucoma, hypersensitivity to cevimeline or its components, uncontrolled asthma

Interactions

DRUGS

amiodarone, cimetidine, clarithromycin, diltiazem, erythromycin, fluconazole, haloperidol, itraconazole, ketoconazole, metoclopramide, mibefradil, nefazodone, propafenone, quinidine, ritonavir, selective serotonin reuptake inhibitors, thioridazine, tricyclic antidepressants, troleandomycin, verapamil: Possibly inhibited metabolism and increased blood level of cevimeline
anticholinergics: Decreased effectiveness of anticholinergics
antimuscarinics: Altered effects of antimuscarinics and decreased therapeutic action of cevimeline

beta blockers: Possibly cardiac conduction disturbances
parasympathomimetics: Additive effects of either drug

Adverse Reactions

CNS: Depression, fatigue, fever, hypoesthesia, insomnia, migraine headache, tremor
CV: Edema, palpitations
EENT: Abnormal vision, conjunctivitis, dry mouth, earache, epistaxis, excessive salivation, eye pain, rhinitis, salivary gland pain
GI: Abdominal pain, anorexia, cholecystitis, constipation, eructation, heartburn, hiccups, nausea, vomiting
HEME: Anemia
MS: Arthralgia, leg cramps, myalgia
RESP: Cough, dyspnea
SKIN: Diaphoresis, pruritus
Other: Flulike symptoms, hot flashes

Nursing Considerations

•Give cevimeline on an empty stomach because food may decrease rate and extent of absorption, delaying peak concentration.
•Assess patient with a pulmonary disorder for wheezing and increased respiratory secretions because drug may cause increased bronchiolar smooth-muscle contractions, airway resistance, and respiratory secretions.
•Monitor patient with known or suspected gallbladder disease for abdominal pain and other warnings of biliary obstruction, cholecystitis, or cholangitis; each of these conditions may be precipitated by cevimeline.

PATIENT TEACHING

•Instruct patient to take cevimeline on an empty stomach.
•Inform patient that drug may cause vision changes; advise him to avoid driving at night or performing potentially hazardous activities until drug's adverse effects are known.
•Urge patient to drink plenty of fluids during hot weather and while exercising because drug may cause excessive sweating and dehydration.

chloral hydrate

Aquachloral Supprettes, Novo-Chlorhydrate (CAN), PMS-Chloral Hydrate (CAN)

Class, Category, and Schedule

Chemical class: Chloral derivative
Therapeutic class: Sedative-hypnotic

Pregnancy category: C
Controlled substance schedule: IV

Indications and Dosages

➤ *To prevent or suppress alcohol with-drawal symptoms, act as an adjunct to opioids and analgesics to control post-operative pain*

CAPSULES, SYRUP, SUPPOSITORIES

Adults. 250 mg t.i.d. after meals. *Maximum:* 2,000 mg.

➤ *To produce nocturnal sedation*

CAPSULES, SYRUP, SUPPOSITORIES

Adults. 0.5 to 1 g 30 min before bedtime. *Maximum:* 2 g.

➤ *To produce preoperative sedation*

CAPSULES, SYRUP, SUPPOSITORIES

Adults. 0.5 to 1 g 30 min before surgery.

➤ *To provide sedation before dental or medical procedure*

SYRUP, SUPPOSITORIES

Children. 25 mg/kg up to 500 mg/single dose; up to 75 mg/kg for dental procedure supplemented by nitrous oxide.

Route	Onset	Peak	Duration
P.O.	30 min to 1 hr	Unknown	4 to 8 hr
P.R.	Unknown	Unknown	4 to 8 hr

Mechanism of Action

Produces CNS depression by an unknown mechanism involving trichloroethanol, the drug's active metabolite.

Contraindications

Gastritis; hypersensitivity or idiosyncrasy to chloral hydrate or its components; severe cardiac, hepatic, or renal disease

Interactions

DRUGS

CNS depressants: Increased CNS effects of chloral hydrate

furosemide (I.V.): Increased incidence of adverse effects when administered after chloral hydrate

phenytoin: Increased excretion and subsequent decreased effectiveness of phenytoin

warfarin: Transient increase in anticoagulant effect

ACTIVITIES

alcohol use: Increased CNS effects of chloral hydrate

Adverse Reactions

CNS: Ataxia, disorientation, hangover, incoherence, paranoia, somnolence

GI: Gastric irritation, nausea, vomiting

SKIN: Rash, urticaria

Other: Drug dependence

Nursing Considerations

• Administer with full glass of water or juice to minimize GI distress from chloral hydrate capsules. Dilute syrup in a half-glass of water, ginger ale, or fruit juice.

• **WARNING** Monitor carefully for hypersensitivity reaction in patients with a history of tartrazine sensitivity.

• Suspect physical or psychological dependence if withdrawal of chloral hydrate produces confusion, hallucinations, nausea, nervousness, restlessness, stomach pain, tremor, unusual excitement, or vomiting.

PATIENT TEACHING

• Advise patient to take capsules with a full glass of water or juice or to mix syrup in a half-glass of water, ginger ale, or fruit juice.

• Advise patient to avoid hazardous activities until drug's CNS effects are known.

• Caution patient that drug may be habit-forming. Advise taking it exactly as prescribed and not to stop taking it abruptly because withdrawal symptoms could occur.

• Instruct patient to notify prescriber right away about stomach pains or tarry stools.

chloramphenicol

Chloromycetin, Novochlorocap (CAN)

chloramphenicol palmitate

Chloromycetin

chloramphenicol sodium succinate

Chloromycetin

Class and Category

Chemical class: Dichloroacetic acid derivative

Therapeutic class: Antibiotic

Pregnancy category: Not rated

Indications and Dosages

➤ *To treat serious infections for which less potentially dangerous drugs are ineffective or contraindicated*

I.V. INFUSION

Adults. 12.5 mg/kg every 6 hr. *Maximum:* 4 g daily.

Children. 50 to 75 mg/kg daily in divided doses every 6 hr.

Full-term infants age 2 weeks and over. 12.5 mg/kg every 6 hr or 25 mg/kg every 12 hr.

Preterm and full-term infants up to age 2 weeks. 6.25 mg/kg every 6 hr.

➤ *To treat bacteremia or meningitis*

I.V. INFUSION

Children. 50 to 100 mg/kg daily in divided doses every 6 hr.

DOSAGE ADJUSTMENT Dosage limited to 25 mg/kg daily for infants and children with immature metabolic processes.

Mechanism of Action

Produces a bacteriostatic effect on susceptible organisms by inhibiting protein synthesis, thereby preventing amino acids from being transferred to growing polypetide chains.

Contraindications

Hypersensitivity to chloramphenicol or its components

Interactions

DRUGS

alfentanil: Prolonged alfentanil effect

barbiturates: Increased blood barbiturate level; decreased blood chloramphenicol level

blood-dyscrasia–causing drugs (such as captopril and cephalosporins), bone marrow depressants (including colchicine and methotrexate): Increased bone marrow depression

chlorpropamide, tolbutamide: Increased hypoglycemic effects

clindamycin, erythromycin, lincomycin: Decreased antibacterial effects of these drugs

cyclophosphamide: Decreased or delayed activation of cyclophosphamide, increased bone marrow depression

hepatic enzyme inducers (including rifampin): Decreased blood chloramphenicol level

hydantoins: Increased blood hydantoin level, possibly resulting in toxicity; increased or decreased blood chloramphenicol level

iron salts: Increased serum iron level

oral anticoagulants: Enhanced anticoagulant action

oral contraceptives containing estrogen: Decreased contraceptive effect with prolonged chloramphenicol use

penicillins: Decreased penicillin activity; synergistic effects with treatment of certain microorganisms

vitamin B$_{12}$: Antagonized hematopoietic response to vitamin B$_{12}$

Adverse Reactions

CNS: Confusion, delirium, depression, fever, headache, peripheral neuropathy

CV: Gray syndrome in neonates

EENT: Optic neuritis

GI: Diarrhea, nausea, vomiting

HEME: Aplastic anemia, bone marrow depression, granulocytopenia, hypoplastic anemia, leukopenia, reticulocytopenia, thrombocytopenia

SKIN: Rash

Other: Anaphylaxis, angioedema

Nursing Considerations

•As appropriate and ordered, obtain specimen for culture and sensitivity testing before beginning chloramphenicol therapy.

•Keep in mind that chloramphenicol should never be used to treat minor infections or for prophylaxis because of the many serious toxicities associated with its use.

•Be aware that repeated courses of therapy should be avoided because of the risk of serious adverse reactions.

•For I.V. use, prepare a 10% solution by adding 10 ml of sterile water for injection or D$_5$W to each 1-g vial. Administer over at least 1 minute.

•Know that diluted I.V. solution is stable for 24 to 48 hours when stored at room temperature or refrigerated. Don't use if cloudy.

•Assess patient for fever, sore throat, tiredness, unusual bleeding, or ecchymosis; these may indicate a blood dyscrasia.

•Perform neurologic assessments regularly, looking for signs of peripheral neuropathy.

•**WARNING** If early signs of gray syndrome appear (failure to eat, pallor, cyanosis, abdominal distention, irregular respirations, and vasomotor collapse), notify prescriber and be prepared to stop drug immediately.

•Monitor blood chloramphenicol level as ap-

propriate. Keep in mind that therapeutic peak levels are 10 to 20 mcg/ml and trough levels are 5 to 10 mcg/ml.
•Monitor CBC and platelet and reticulocyte counts as ordered to detect signs of blood dyscrasia. Notify prescriber immediately about abnormal results.

PATIENT TEACHING
•Instruct patient to immediately report to prescriber signs of blood dyscrasia.
•**WARNING** Tell patient to stay alert for signs of potentially fatal, irreversible bone marrow depression that leads to aplastic anemia and is characterized by fever, pallor, pharyngitis, severe fatigue and weakness, and unusual bleeding or bruising. Bone marrow depression may occur weeks to months after therapy stops. Stress the need for follow-up care.

chlordiazepoxide hydrochloride

Apo-Chlordiazepoxide (CAN), Librium, Novo-Poxide (CAN)

Class, Category, and Schedule
Chemical class: Benzodiazepine
Therapeutic class: Antianxiety
Pregnancy category: Not rated
Controlled substance schedule: IV

Indications and Dosages
➤ *To provide short-term management of mild anxiety*
CAPSULES, TABLETS
Adults. 5 to 10 mg t.i.d. or q.i.d.
Children over age 6. 5 mg b.i.d. to q.i.d. increased as needed to 10 mg b.i.d. or t.i.d., or 0.5 mg/kg daily in equally divided doses every 6 to 8 hr.
➤ *To provide short-term management of severe anxiety*
CAPSULES, TABLETS
Adults. 20 to 25 mg t.i.d. or q.i.d.
I.V. OR I.M. INJECTION
Adults. *Initial:* 50 to 100 mg. Then, 25 to 50 mg t.i.d. or q.i.d., p.r.n. *Maximum:* 300 mg daily.
I.M. INJECTION
Children age 12 and over. 0.5 mg/kg daily in equally divided doses every 6 to 8 hr.
➤ *To provide short-term treatment of acute alcohol withdrawal*

CAPSULES, TABLETS, I.V. OR I.M. INJECTION
Adults. *Initial:* 50 to 100 mg, usually given I.V. or I.M. Repeated in 2 to 4 hr followed by individualized oral dosage if needed to control symptoms. *Maximum:* 300 mg daily.
➤ *To provide perioperative relaxation and reduce apprehension and anxiety*
CAPSULES, TABLETS, I.M. INJECTION
Adults. 5 to 10 mg P.O. t.i.d. or q.i.d. several days before surgery; 50 to 100 mg I.M. 1 hr before surgery.
DOSAGE ADJUSTMENT Dosage reduced to 5 mg P.O. b.i.d. to q.i.d., p.r.n., for elderly or debilitated patients.

Mechanism of Action
May potentiate the effects of gamma-aminobutyric acid (GABA) and other inhibitory neurotransmitters by binding to specific benzodiazepine receptors in the limbic and cortical areas of the CNS. By binding to these receptors, chlordiazepoxide increases GABA's inhibitory effects and blocks cortical and limbic arousal, which helps control emotional behavior. It also helps relieve symptoms of alcohol withdrawal by causing CNS depression.

Contraindications
Hypersensitivity to chlordiazepoxide or its components

Interactions
DRUGS
antacids: Altered rate of chlordiazepoxide absorption
cimetidine, disulfiram, fluoxetine, isoniazid, ketoconazole, metoprolol, oral contraceptives, propoxyphene, propranolol, valproic acid: Increased blood chlordiazepoxide level
CNS depressants: Increased CNS effects
digoxin: Increased blood digoxin level and risk of digitalis toxicity
levodopa: Decreased efficacy of levodopa's antiparkinsonian effects
neuromuscular blockers: Potentiated, counteracted, or diminished effects of neuromuscular blockers
phenytoin: Possibly increased phenytoin toxicity
probenecid: Shortened onset of action or prolonged effect of chlordiazepoxide

rifampin: Decreased chlordiazepoxide effect
theophyllines: Antagonized sedative effects
of chlordiazepoxide
ACTIVITIES
alcohol use: Increased CNS effects

Adverse Reactions

CNS: Ataxia, confusion, depression, drowsiness, suicidal ideation
CV: ECG changes, hypotension, tachycardia
GI: Hepatic dysfunction
HEME: Agranulocytosis
SKIN: Jaundice
Other: Injection site pain, redness, and swelling

Nursing Considerations

• Use chlordiazepoxide cautiously in patients with renal or hepatic impairment or porphyria.
• **WARNING** Be aware that prolonged use of chlordiazepoxide at therapeutic doses can lead to dependence.
• For I.V. use, reconstitute ampule contents with 5 ml sterile water for injection or sodium chloride for injection. Agitate gently until completely dissolved. Give slowly over 1 minute.
• For I.M. use, reconstitute only with diluent provided by manufacturer.
• **WARNING** Don't use supplied diluent to prepare drug for I.V. use because air bubbles form on the surface.
• Don't give opalescent or hazy solution.
• Monitor patient for evidence of phlebitis or thrombophlebitis after I.V. chlordiazepoxide administration.
• Monitor liver function test results during therapy.
• If patient is a hyperactive, aggressive child or has a history of psychiatric disorders, watch for paradoxical reactions, such as excitement, stimulation, and acute rage, during first 2 weeks of therapy.
• Watch patients closely (especially children, adolescents, and young adults) for suicidal tendencies, particularly when chlordiazepoxide therapy starts and dosage changes.
PATIENT TEACHING
• Warn that drug may cause drowsiness.
• Advise patient to avoid other CNS depressants during therapy.
• Warn patient not to take antacids with chlordiazepoxide.
• Urge family or caregiver to watch patient closely for suicidal tendencies, especially when therapy starts or dosage changes and particularly if patient is a child, teenager, or young adult.

chlorothiazide
Diuril
chlorothiazide sodium
Diuril

Class and Category
Chemical class: Sulfonamide derivative
Therapeutic class: Antihypertensive, diuretic
Pregnancy category: B

Indications and Dosages
➤ *To treat hypertension*
ORAL SUSPENSION, TABLETS
Adults. 250 to 1,000 mg daily in a single dose or divided doses b.i.d. *Maximum:* 2,000 mg daily in divided doses.
Children age 6 months and over. 10 to 20 mg/kg daily in a single dose or divided doses b.i.d. *Maximum:* 1,000 mg daily for ages 2 to 12; 375 mg daily for ages 6 months to 2 years.
Children under age 6 months. Up to 30 mg/kg daily in divided doses given b.i.d.
➤ *To produce diuresis*
ORAL SUSPENSION, TABLETS
Adults. 250 mg every 6 to 12 hr. Administered on an intermittent schedule, if needed, such as alternate days or 3 to 5 days/wk.
Children age 6 months and over. 10 to 20 mg/kg daily in a single dose or divided doses b.i.d. *Maximum:* 1,000 mg daily for children ages 2 to 12; 375 mg daily for children ages 6 months to 2 years.
Children under age 6 months. Up to 33 mg/kg daily in divided doses b.i.d.
I.V. INFUSION OR INJECTION
Adults. 250 mg every 6 to 12 hr.

Route	Onset	Peak	Duration
P.O.	2 hr	4 hr	6 to 12 hr
I.V.	15 min	4 hr	6 to 12 hr

Contraindications
Anuria; hepatic coma; hypersensitivity to chlorothiazide or its components, sulfonamides, or related thiazide diuretics; renal failure

Mechanism of Action

May promote sodium, chloride, and water excretion by inhibiting sodium reabsorption in the kidneys' distal tubules. Initially, chlorothiazide may reduce blood pressure by decreasing extracellular fluid volume, plasma volume, and cardiac output. It also may dilate arteries directly, reducing peripheral vascular resistance. After several weeks, extracellular fluid and plasma volume and cardiac output return to normal, but peripheral vascular resistance remains decreased.

Interactions

DRUGS

allopurinol: Increased risk of allopurinol hypersensitivity

amiodarone: Increased risk of arrhythmias from hypokalemia

amphotericin B, glucocorticoids: Intensified electrolyte depletion

anesthetics: Potentiated effects of anesthetics

anticholinergics: Increased chlorothiazide absorption

anticoagulants, methenamines, sulfonylureas: Decreased effects of these drugs

antihypertensives: Increased antihypertensive effect

antineoplastics: Prolonged antineoplastic-induced leukopenia

calcium: Possibly increased blood calcium level

cholestyramine, colestipol: Decreased chlorothiazide absorption

diazoxide: Hyperglycemia, hypotension

digitalis glycosides: Increased risk of digitalis-induced arrhythmias

dopamine: Increased diuretic effect

lithium: Increased risk of lithium toxicity

loop diuretics: Synergistic effects, resulting in profound diuresis and serious electrolyte imbalances

methyldopa: Potential development of hemolytic anemia

neuromuscular blockers: Increased neuromuscular blockade

NSAIDs: Possibly reduced diuretic effect of chlorothiazide; increased risk of renal failure if patient has compromised renal function

sympathomimetics: Possibly inhibited antihypertensive effect of chlorothiazide

vitamin D: Enhanced vitamin D action

Adverse Reactions

CNS: Dizziness, headache, paresthesia, restlessness, vertigo, weakness

CV: Orthostatic hypotension

ENDO: Hyperglycemia

GI: Abdominal cramps, anorexia, constipation, diarrhea, gastric irritation, nausea, pancreatitis, vomiting

GU: Glycosuria, hematuria (I.V. form), impotence, interstitial nephritis, renal dysfunction or failure

HEME: Agranulocytosis, aplastic anemia, hemolytic anemia, leukopenia, thrombocytopenia

MS: Muscle spasms

SKIN: Jaundice, photosensitivity, purpura, rash, urticaria

Other: Anaphylactic reactions, hypercalcemia, hyperuricemia, hypochloremic alkalosis, hypokalemia, hypomagnesemia, hyponatremia, hypovolemia

Nursing Considerations

• Don't give parenteral form of chlorothiazide by I.M. or subcutaneous route.

• For I.V. use, reconstitute with at least 18 ml of sterile water for injection. Discard unused solution after 24 hours. Reconstituted solution is compatible with dextrose solution or normal saline solution for infusion.

• Watch I.V. site closely. If extravasation occurs, stop infusion and tell prescriber at once.

• Weigh patient daily to assess fluid loss and drug effectiveness. Also, check blood pressure often if used to treat hypertension; antihypertensive effect may not appear for days.

• Assess patient for electrolyte imbalances.

• Monitor renal function closely, especially in elderly patients, because the risk of toxicity increases with renal impairment.

PATIENT TEACHING

• Tell patient to take chlorothiazide early in the day to avoid nocturia and to take it with food or milk if GI distress occurs.

• Encourage patient to eat a high-potassium diet.

• Instruct patient to rise slowly to minimize effects of orthostatic hypotension.

• Urge patient to weigh himself at least weekly and to notify prescriber if weight rises or falls by 5 lb (2.25 kg) or more in 2 days.

• Tell patient to immediately notify pre-

scriber about weakness, cramps, nausea, vomiting, restlessness, excessive thirst, drowsiness, tiredness, increased heart rate, diarrhea, sudden joint pain, or dizziness.
•If patient has diabetes mellitus, tell him to monitor his blood glucose level often. Oral antidiabetic dosage may need to be increased.
•Tell patient to avoid prolonged exposure to sun, use sunscreen, and wear protective clothing.
•Advise patient to consult prescriber or pharmacist before using alcohol and such OTC drugs as those used for appetite control, colds, cough, hay fever, and sinus problems.

chlorphenesin carbamate

Maolate

Class and Category

Chemical class: Chemically related to mephenesin
Therapeutic class: Skeletal muscle relaxant
Pregnancy category: Not rated

Indications and Dosages

➤ *As adjunct to relieve pain in acute musculoskeletal conditions*
TABLETS
Adults: 800 mg t.i.d. until desired effect occurs. *Maintenance:* 400 mg q.i.d or less, p.r.n.

Mechanism of Action
May act on the CNS, rather than directly on skeletal muscle, producing a sedative effect that aids in muscle relaxation.

Contraindications
Hypersensitivity to chlorphenesin or its components

Interactions
DRUGS
CNS depressants: Increased adverse CNS effects
ACTIVITIES
alcohol use: Increased adverse CNS effects

Adverse Reactions
CNS: Confusion, dizziness, drowsiness, headache, insomnia, nervousness, paradoxical stimulation
EENT: Diplopia, transient vision loss

GI: Epigastric discomfort, nausea
Other: Anaphylaxis, drug-induced fever

Nursing Considerations
•**WARNING** Use chlorphenesin cautiously in patients hypersensitive to aspirin; it contains tartrazine, which may cause hypersensitivity.
•Expect drug therapy to last for no more than 8 weeks because safety beyond this point is unknown.
•Provide rest and other pain-relief measures.
PATIENT TEACHING
•Because of possible reduced alertness, advise patient to avoid potentially hazardous activities until drug's CNS effects are known.
•Instruct patient to notify prescriber if these symptoms occur: confusion, dizziness, drowsiness, insomnia, nervousness, or paradoxical stimulation.
•Tell patient to immediately notify prescriber if he develops a fever or any signs or symptoms of an allergic reaction, such as rash, hives, itching, facial swelling, or difficulty breathing.

chlorpromazine

Largactil (CAN), Thorazine

chlorpromazine hydrochloride

Chlorpromanyl (CAN), Novo-Chlorpromazine (CAN), Thorazine, Thorazine Spansule

Class and Category

Chemical class: Propylamine derivative of phenothiazine
Therapeutic class: Antiemetic, antipsychotic, tranquilizer
Pregnancy category: Not rated

Indications and Dosages

➤ *To manage symptoms of psychotic disorders or control manic manifestations of manic-depression in outpatients*
E.R. CAPSULES
Adults. 30 to 300 mg 1 to 3 times daily, with dosage adjusted as needed. *Maximum:* 1 g daily.
ORAL CONCENTRATE, SYRUP, TABLETS
Adults. 10 mg t.i.d. or q.i.d., or 25 mg b.i.d. or t.i.d. After 1 or 2 days, dose increased by 20 to 50 mg semiweekly until patient is calm. After 2 wk of calmness, dosage gradu-

ally reduced to maintenance level of 200 to 800 mg daily in equally divided doses.

➤ *To control acutely disturbed or manic hospitalized patients*

I.M. INJECTION

Adults. 25 mg. Repeated 25 to 50 mg in 1 hr, if needed. Increased gradually over several days up to 400 mg every 4 to 6 hr for severe cases until behavior is controlled. Then, regimen switched to oral form and outpatient dosage.

➤ *To treat severe behavioral problems in children*

ORAL CONCENTRATE, SYRUP, TABLETS

Children ages 6 months to 12 years. 0.55 mg/kg every 4 to 6 hr, p.r.n.

SUPPOSITORIES

Children ages 6 months to 12 years. 1 mg/kg every 6 to 8 hr, p.r.n.

I.M. INJECTION

Children ages 6 months to 12 years. 0.55 mg/kg every 6 to 8 hr. *Maximum:* 75 mg daily for children ages 5 to 12 years or weighing 50 to 100 lb (23 to 45 kg), except in unmanageable cases; 40 mg daily for children up to age 5 or weighing up to 50 lb.

➤ *To treat nausea and vomiting*

ORAL CONCENTRATE, SYRUP, TABLETS

Adults and adolescents. 10 to 25 mg every 4 to 6 hr, p.r.n.

Children ages 6 months to 12 years. 0.55 mg/kg every 4 to 6 hr, p.r.n.

I.M. INJECTION

Adults. 25 mg. If no hypotension occurs, 25 to 50 mg every 3 to 4 hr, p.r.n., until vomiting stops; then drug switched to oral form.

Children age 6 months and over. 0.55 mg/kg every 6 to 8 hr, p.r.n. *Maximum:* 75 mg daily for children ages 5 to 12 or weighing 50 to 100 lb; 40 mg daily for children up to age 5 or weighing up to 50 lb.

SUPPOSITORIES

Adults and adolescents. 50 to 100 mg every 6 to 8 hr, p.r.n.

Children ages 6 months to 12 years. 1 mg/kg every 6 to 8 hr, p.r.n.

➤ *To provide intraoperative control of nausea and vomiting*

I.V. INJECTION

Adults. 25 mg diluted to 1 mg/ml with sodium chloride for injection and given at no more than 2 mg every 2 min. *Maximum:* 25 mg.

Children age 6 months and over. 0.275 mg/kg diluted to at least 1 mg/ml with sodium chloride for injection and given at no more than 1 mg every 2 min. *Maximum:* 75 mg/day for children ages 5 to 12 years or weighing 50 to 100 lb; 40 mg daily for children up to age 5 years or weighing up to 50 lb.

I.M. INJECTION

Adults. 12.5 mg. Repeated in 30 min if needed and no hypotension occurs.

Children age 6 months and over. 0.275 mg/kg. Repeated in 30 min if needed and tolerated.

➤ *To treat intractable hiccups*

TABLETS

Adults. 25 to 50 mg t.i.d. or q.i.d. If hiccups last longer than 2 days, route switched to I.M., as prescribed.

I.V. INFUSION

Adults. 25 to 50 mg diluted in 500 to 1,000 ml of normal saline solution and given at 1 mg/min with patient in supine position.

I.M. INJECTION

Adults. 25 to 50 mg given only if oral route is ineffective. If symptoms persist, route switched to I.V., as prescribed.

➤ *To provide preoperative relaxation*

ORAL CONCENTRATE, SYRUP, TABLETS

Adults and adolescents. 25 to 50 mg 2 to 3 hr before surgery.

Children ages 6 months to 12 years. 0.55 mg/kg 2 to 3 hr before surgery.

I.M. INJECTION

Adults. 12.5 to 25 mg 1 to 2 hr before surgery.

Children age 6 months and over. 0.55 mg/kg 1 to 2 hr before surgery.

➤ *To treat acute intermittent porphyria*

ORAL CONCENTRATE, SYRUP, TABLETS

Adults and adolescents. 25 to 50 mg t.i.d. or q.i.d.

I.M. INJECTION

Adults. 25 mg t.i.d. or q.i.d. until oral route is possible.

➤ *To treat tetanus (usually as adjunct with barbiturates)*

I.V. INFUSION

Adults. 25 to 50 mg diluted to at least 1 mg/ml and given at no more than 1 mg/min.

Children age 6 months and over. 0.55 mg/kg every 6 to 8 hr, diluted to at least 1 mg/ml and given at no more than 1 mg/2 min. *Maximum:* 75 mg daily for children ages 5 to 12 years or weighing 50 to 100 lb; 40 mg daily for children up to age 5 years or weighing up to 50 lb.

I.M. INJECTION
Adults. 25 to 50 mg t.i.d. or q.i.d.
Children age 6 months and over. 0.55 mg/kg every 6 to 8 hr. *Maximum:* 75 mg daily for children ages 5 to 12 years or weighing 50 to 100 lb; 40 mg daily for children up to age 5 years or weighing up to 50 lb.
DOSAGE ADJUSTMENT Dosage possibly reduced for patients with hepatic dysfunction. Dosage reduced to one-third to one-half the normal adult dosage for elderly or debilitated patients.

Mechanism of Action
Depresses brain areas that control activity and aggression, including the cerebral cortex, hypothalamus, and limbic system, by an unknown mechanism. Prevents nausea and vomiting by inhibiting or blocking dopamine receptors in the medullary chemoreceptor trigger zone and peripherally by blocking the vagus nerve in the GI tract. May relieve anxiety by indirect reduction in arousal and increased filtering of internal stimuli to the reticular activating system in the brain stem.

Incompatibilities
Don't mix chlorpromazine with thiopental, atropine, or solutions that don't have a pH of 4 to 5 because a precipitate will form. Don't mix chlorpromazine injection with other drugs in a syringe.

Contraindications
Comatose states; hypersensitivity to chlorpromazine, phenothiazines, or their components; use of large amounts of CNS depressants

Interactions
DRUGS
amphetamines: Decreased amphetamine effectiveness, decreased antipsychotic effectiveness of chlorpromazine
antacids (aluminum hydroxide or magnesium trisilicate gel): Decreased chlorpromazine absorption and effectiveness
barbiturates: Decreased plasma level and, possibly, effectiveness of chlorpromazine
CNS depressants: Prolonged and intensified CNS depression
metrizamide: Possibly lowered seizure threshold

oral anticoagulants: Decreased anticoagulation
phenytoin: Interference with phenytoin metabolism, increased risk of phenytoin toxicity
propranolol: Increased plasma levels of both drugs
thiazide diuretics: Possibly increased orthostatic hypotension
ACTIVITIES
alcohol use: Prolonged and intensified CNS depression

Adverse Reactions
CNS: Drowsiness, extrapyramidal reactions (such as dystonia, fever, motor restlessness, pseudoparkinsonism, and tardive dyskinesia), neuroleptic malignant syndrome, seizures
CV: ECG changes, such as nonspecific, usually reversible Q- and T-wave changes; orthostatic hypotension; tachycardia
EENT: Blurred vision, dry mouth, nasal congestion, ocular changes (fine particle deposits in lens and cornea) with long-term therapy
ENDO: Gynecomastia, hyperglycemia, hypoglycemia, lactation, moderate breast engorgement
GI: Constipation, ileus, nausea
GU: Amenorrhea, ejaculation disorders, impotence, priapism, urine retention
HEME: Agranulocytosis, aplastic anemia, eosinophilia, hemolytic anemia, leukopenia, pancytopenia, thrombocytopenic purpura
SKIN: Exfoliative dermatitis, jaundice, photosensitivity, tissue necrosis, urticaria

Nursing Considerations
• Don't open or crush E.R. capsules.
• Chlorpromazine shouldn't be used to treat dementia-related psychosis in the elderly because of an increased risk of death.
• Use chlorpromazine cautiously in patients (especially children) with chronic respiratory disorders (such as severe asthma or emphysema) or acute respiratory tract infections because drug has CNS depressant effect. Also use cautiously in patients with cardiovascular, hepatic, or renal disease because of increased risk of developing hypotension, heart failure, and arrhythmias.
• Because of chlorpromazine's anticholinergic effects, use it cautiously in patients with glaucoma. Also use it cautiously in those who are exposed to extreme heat or organophosphorus insecticides and those receiving atropine or related drugs.

C

•Protect concentrate from light. Refrigeration isn't required.

•Dilute concentrate in at least 60 ml of diluent just before administering it. Use tomato or fruit juice, milk, simple syrup, orange syrup, a carbonated beverage, coffee, tea, water, or semisolid food, such as pudding and soup.

•Protect parenteral solution from light. Solution should be clear and colorless to pale yellow. Discard markedly discolored solution.

•Don't inject drug by subcutaneous route because it can cause severe tissue necrosis.

•Wear gloves when working with liquid or injectable form because parenteral solution may cause contact dermatitis.

•For I.V. injection, dilute chlorpromazine with sodium chloride to a concentration of 1 mg/ml.

•Give I.M. injection slowly and deep into upper outer quadrant of buttocks, such as in the gluteus maximus. To minimize hypotensive effects, keep patient lying flat and monitor blood pressure for 30 minutes after injection.

•**WARNING** Stay alert for possible suppressed cough reflex, which increases the risk of the patient's aspirating vomitus.

•Monitor patient for increased sensitivity to drug's CNS effects if patient has a history of hepatic encephalopathy from cirrhosis.

•**WARNING** If neuroleptic malignant syndrome (hyperpyrexia, muscle rigidity, altered mental status, autonomic instability) develops, notify prescriber immediately and expect to stop drug and start intensive treatment. Watch for recurrence if patient resumes antipsychotic therapy.

PATIENT TEACHING

•Instruct patient to swallow E.R. capsules whole and not to crush, break, or chew them.

•Tell patient not to take drug within 2 hours of taking an antacid. Allow him to take drug with food or a full glass of milk or water.

•If patient uses suppository form of chlorpromazine, tell him to chill the suppository, moisten it with cold water, and insert it well inside the rectum.

•Tell patient to store oral concentrate at room temperature, away from light ,and to measure it with the dropper provided and to dilute it in 4 oz of fluid just before use.

•Because of possible drowsiness, dizziness, and blurred vision (especially during the first few days of therapy), advise the patient to avoid potentially hazardous activities until drug's CNS effects are known.

•Tell patient to avoid alcohol because of possible additive effects and hypotension.

•Advise patient, especially if elderly, to rise slowly from a supine or seated position to avoid dizziness, light-headedness, and fainting.

•Tell patient to inform doctors and dentists that he's taking chlorpromazine before he undergoes surgery, medical tests, or dental work.

•Explain that drug may reduce the body's response to heat and cold; tell patient to avoid temperature extremes, as in a sauna, hot tub, or very cold or hot shower. Remind patient to dress warmly in cold weather.

•Warn patient not to take OTC drugs for a cold or an allergy because they can increase the risk of heatstroke and other unwanted effects.

•Inform patient that drug increases sensitivity to sunlight; tell him to stay out of the sun as much as possible and to protect his skin.

•If patient reports dry mouth, suggest sugarless chewing gum, hard candy, and fluids.

•Urge patient to report sudden sore throat or other signs of infection.

chlorpropamide

Apo-Chlorpropamide (CAN), Diabinese, Novo-Propamide (CAN)

Class and Category

Chemical class: Sulfonylurea
Therapeutic class: Antidiabetic
Pregnancy category: C

Indications and Dosages

➤ *As adjunct to manage non–insulin-dependent diabetes when diet alone fails to lower blood glucose level*

TABLETS

Adults. *Initial:* 250 mg daily for 5 to 7 days. After therapy begins, dosage may be adjusted up or down by increments of 50 to 125 mg at intervals of 3 to 5 days to obtain optimal control. *Maintenance:* 100 to 500 mg daily. *Maximum:* 750 mg daily.

DOSAGE ADJUSTMENT If patient takes more than 40 units of insulin daily, dosage reduced to half usual insulin dose for first few days of chlorpropamide therapy. Insulin dose can be reduced, depending on response. If patient takes oral antidiabetic drug or less than 40 units of insulin daily, it may be stopped abruptly when chlorpropamide starts.

Dosage reduced to half usual dose if patient has mild renal failure because metabolites and unchanged drug are excreted in urine. To avoid hypoglycemic reactions, initial dosage reduced to 100 to 125 mg daily for elderly, debilitated, or malnourished patients and patients with impaired hepatic function.

Route	Onset	Peak	Duration
P.O.	1 hr	3 to 6 hr	24 to 72 hr

Mechanism of Action
Lowers blood glucose level by stimulating release of insulin from the pancreas in patients who have functioning beta cells. It also may increase insulin sensitivity in target tissues, which may result in a decrease in liver breakdown of glycogen to glucose or the liver's production of new glucose.

Contraindications
Diabetic ketoacidosis (with or without coma), hypersensitivity to chlorpropamide or its components, type I diabetes mellitus

Interactions
DRUGS
androgens, anticoagulants, azole antifungals, chloramphenicol, clofibrate, fenfluramine, fluconazole, gemfibrozil, H₂-receptor antagonists, magnesium salts, MAO inhibitors, methyldopa, probenecid, salicylates, sulfinpyrazone, sulfonamides, tricyclic antidepressants, urinary acidifiers: Increased hypoglycemic effect
barbiturates: Prolonged barbiturate action
beta blockers, calcium channel blockers, cholestyramine, corticosteroids, diazoxide, estrogens, hydantoins, isoniazid, nicotinic acid, oral contraceptives, phenothiazines, rifampin, sympathomimetics, thiazide diuretics, thyroid drugs, urinary alkalinizers: Decreased hypoglycemic effect
digitalis glycosides: Increased blood digitalis level
oral miconazole: Risk of severe hypoglycemia

ACTIVITIES
alcohol use: Disulfiram-like reaction

Adverse Reactions
ENDO: Hypoglycemia
GI: Anorexia, diarrhea, hunger, nausea, vomiting
SKIN: Maculopapular eruptions, photosensitivity, pruritus, urticaria
Other: Disulfiram-like reaction

Nursing Considerations
• Use chlorpropamide cautiously in patients with renal or hepatic dysfunction; in elderly, debilitated, or malnourished patients; and in those with adrenal or pituitary insufficiency because of increased susceptibility to drug's hypoglycemic action.
• Monitor patient's blood glucose level frequently at start of therapy and during dosage adjustments or changes in patient's life, such as during stress and illness. Hypoglycemia may be difficult to recognize in elderly patients and those who take beta-adrenergic blockers.
• Assess patient for hypoglycemia—the most common adverse reaction to chlorpropamide—especially in patients whose caloric intake is deficient, who have just engaged in strenuous or prolonged exercise, who have ingested alcohol, or who receive more than one glucose-lowering drug.
• Treat hypoglycemia promptly by giving 15 g of simple carbohydrate, such as 4 oz of orange juice or soda or 8 oz of milk. Repeat in 15 minutes, if needed. Because of drug's long half-life, careful monitoring and frequent feedings are required for 3 to 5 days after a hypoglycemic episode. Hospitalization and I.V. glucose may be needed.
• Monitor patients receiving long-term chlorpropamide therapy for secondary failure, which causes loss of blood glucose control despite adherence to prescribed drug therapy and diet and exercise guidelines. If secondary failure occurs, therapy should be discontinued and a different antidiabetic drug substituted.

PATIENT TEACHING
• Instruct patient to store chlorpropamide in a sealed container, protected from heat and light.
• Tell patient to take chlorpropamide with breakfast.
• Stress that drug works with diet and exer-

cise to help control blood glucose level and isn't a substitute for them.
•Tell patient to monitor blood glucose level as instructed.
•Instruct patient not to skip meals or exercise excessively.
•Teach patient how to recognize and treat hypoglycemia. Tell him to report frequent or severe hypoglycemia to prescriber.
•Caution patient with confirmed or suspected hypoglycemia not to drive or operate machinery until blood glucose levels return to normal.
•Tell patient to take a missed dose as soon as he remembers it unless it's almost time for the next scheduled dose.
•Urge patient to wear or carry medical identification showing that he has diabetes and listing his drugs.
•Advise the patient to protect his skin from the sun.
•Instruct patient to notify prescriber about fever, sore throat, dark yellow or brown urine, yellow skin and eyes, bleeding, and bruising.

chlorthalidone

Apo-Chlorthalidone (CAN), Hygroton, Novo-Thalidone (CAN), Thalitone, Uridon (CAN)

Class and Category

Chemical class: Phthalimidine derivative of benzenesulfonamide (thiazide-like diuretic)
Therapeutic class: Antihypertensive, diuretic
Pregnancy category: B

Indications and Dosages

➤ *To reduce edema caused by heart failure, hepatic cirrhosis, corticosteroid or estrogen therapy, or renal dysfunction*

TABLETS

Adults. *Initial:* 50 to 100 mg (Thalitone, 30 to 60 mg) daily, 100 mg (Thalitone, 60 mg) every other day, or 150 to 200 mg (Thalitone, 90 to 120 mg) daily or every other day. *Maintenance:* Individualized; may be lower than initial dosage.

➤ *To treat hypertension*

TABLETS

Adults. *Initial:* 25 mg daily (Thalitone, 15 mg daily). If response is insufficient, dosage increased to 50 mg daily (Thalitone, 30 to 50 mg daily). If additional control is re-

quired, dosage increased to 100 mg daily (except Thalitone) or a second antihypertensive added. *Maintenance:* Individualized; may be lower than initial dosage.

Route	Onset	Peak	Duration
P.O.	2 to 3 hr	2 to 6 hr	24 to 72 hr

Mechanism of Action

May promote sodium, chloride, and water excretion by inhibiting sodium reabsorption in the distal tubules of the kidneys. Initially, chlorthalidone may decrease extracellular fluid volume, plasma volume, and cardiac output, which helps explain how it reduces blood pressure. It also may dilate arteries directly, which helps reduce peripheral vascular resistance and blood pressure. After several weeks, extracellular fluid and plasma volume and cardiac output return to normal, but peripheral vascular resistance remains decreased.

Contraindications

Anuria; hypersensitivity to chlorthalidone, other sulfonamides, or their components; renal decompensation

Interactions

DRUGS

allopurinol: Increased risk of allopurinol hypersensitivity
amphotericin B, glucocorticoids: Intensified electrolyte depletion
anesthetics: Potentiated effects of anesthetics
anticholinergics: Increased chlorthalidone absorption
antidiabetics, methenamines, oral anticoagulants, sulfonylureas: Decreased effects of these drugs
antihypertensives: Potentiated action of antihypertensives and chlorthalidone
antineoplastics: Prolonged antineoplastic-induced leukopenia
cholestyramine, colestipol: Decreased chlorthalidone absorption
diazoxide: Increased risk of hyperglycemia and hypotension
digitalis glycosides: Increased risk of digitalis-induced arrhythmias
lithium: Decreased renal lithium clearance and increased risk of lithium toxicity

loop diuretics: Increased synergistic effects, resulting in profound diuresis and serious electrolyte imbalances
methyldopa: Potential development of hemolytic anemia
neuromuscular blockers: Increased neuromuscular blockade
NSAIDs: Possibly reduced diuretic effect of chlorthalidone
vitamin D: Enhanced vitamin D action

Adverse Reactions

CNS: Dizziness, headache, insomnia, lightheadedness, paresthesia, restlessness, vertigo, weakness
CV: Orthostatic hypotension, vasculitis
EENT: Yellow vision
ENDO: Hyperglycemia
GI: Abdominal cramps or pain, anorexia, bloating, constipation, diarrhea, gastric irritation, nausea, pancreatitis, vomiting
GU: Decreased libido, impotence
HEME: Agranulocytosis, aplastic anemia, hypoplastic anemia, leukopenia, thrombocytopenia
MS: Gout attacks, muscle spasms
SKIN: Cutaneous vasculitis, exfoliative dermatitis, jaundice, necrotizing vasculitis, photosensitivity, purpura, rash, urticaria
Other: Hyperuricemia

Nursing Considerations

• Use chlorthalidone cautiously in patients with impaired hepatic function or progressive hepatic disease because minor changes in fluid and electrolyte balance may cause hepatic coma.
• Assess BUN, serum electrolyte, uric acid, and blood glucose levels before therapy and periodically throughout therapy. Monitor patient for signs of fluid and electrolyte imbalance.
• **WARNING** Monitor renal function periodically to detect cumulative drug effects, which may cause azotemia in patients with impaired renal function.

PATIENT TEACHING
• Stress the importance of taking chlorthalidone even when feeling well.
• Tell patient to store drug at room temperature in tightly closed container.
• Tell patient to take drug in the morning with food or milk.
• To minimize effects of orthostatic hypotension, instruct patient to rise slowly from a seated or lying position.
• Advise patient to check blood pressure regularly.
• Instruct patient to report signs of low potassium level, such as muscle weakness and fatigue.
• Advise patient to protect his skin from the sun.
• Urge patient to immediately report sudden joint pain to prescriber because drug can cause sudden gout attacks.
• Instruct patient to take a missed dose as soon as he remembers it. If he misses one day in an every-other-day schedule, tell him to take the dose on the off day and then resume usual dosing schedule. Warn against taking double or extra doses.

chlorzoxazone

EZE-DS, Paraflex, Parafon Forte DSC, Relaxazone, Remular, Remular-S, Strifon Forte DSC

Class and Category

Chemical class: Benzoxazole derivative
Therapeutic class: Skeletal muscle relaxant
Pregnancy category: C (Parafon Forte DSC, not rated)

Indications and Dosages

➤ *As adjunct to relieve acute musculoskeletal pain and stiffness*

TABLETS
Adults. 250 to 750 mg t.i.d. or q.i.d., usually 500 mg t.i.d. or q.i.d., increased or decreased according to patient response.

Route	Onset	Peak	Duration
P.O.	In 1 hr	Unknown	3 to 4 hr

Mechanism of Action

Reduces muscle spasm by inhibiting multisynaptic reflex arcs at the level of the spinal cord and subcortical areas of the brain that are active in producing and maintaining skeletal muscle spasm.

Contraindications

Hypersensitivity or known intolerance to chlorzoxazone or any of its components

Interactions
DRUGS
CNS depressants: Additive CNS depression
ACTIVITIES
alcohol use: Additive CNS depression

Adverse Reactions
CNS: Dizziness, drowsiness, headache, light-headedness, malaise, paradoxical stimulation
GI: Abdominal cramps or pain, constipation, diarrhea, GI bleeding, heartburn, hepatotoxicity, nausea, vomiting
GU: Urine discoloration
HEME: Agranulocytosis, anemia
SKIN: Allergic dermatitis, ecchymosis, petechiae
Other: Anaphylaxis, angioedema

Nursing Considerations
•If needed, crush chlorzoxazone tablets and mix with food or liquid for easier swallowing.
•Assess patients, especially those with a history of allergies, for signs and symptoms of hypersensitivity, such as rash, hives, and itching.
•**WARNING** Monitor patient for signs of hepatotoxicity, including fever, rash, jaundice, and darkened urine. Notify prescriber immediately and expect to discontinue drug if any of these signs or symptoms occur. Monitor patient for abnormal liver function test results, such as elevated AST, ALT, alkaline phosphatase, and bilirubin levels, and expect to discontinue drug, as ordered, if any of these occurs.
•Ensure adequate rest, and provide other pain-relief measures as needed.
•Institute safety measures to prevent falls or injury (such as raising bed rails and assisting with ambulation) until drug's full CNS effects are known.
PATIENT TEACHING
•Advise patient to take a missed dose of chlorzoxazone as soon as possible unless it's almost time for the next dose.
•Advise patient to avoid hazardous activities until drug's CNS effects are known.
•Instruct patient to avoid alcohol and other CNS depressants during therapy.
•Inform patient that, in rare instances, urine may turn orange or reddish purple during therapy.
•Advise patient to store drug in a tightly capped container at room temperature.

cholestyramine
Questran, Questran Light

Class and Category
Chemical class: Quaternary ammonium anion exchange resin
Therapeutic class: Antihyperlipidemic, antipruritic (cholestasis)
Pregnancy category: Not rated

Indications and Dosages
➤ *As adjunct to reduce serum cholesterol level in patients with primary hypercholesterolemia, to relieve pruritus associated with partial biliary obstruction*
ORAL SUSPENSION
Adults. *Initial:* 4 g once or twice daily before meals. *Maintenance:* 8 to 24 g equally divided and given 2 to 6 times a day. *Maximum:* 24 g daily when used as antihyperlipidemic drug and 16 g daily when used as antipruritic drug.

Route	Onset	Peak	Duration
P.O.	In 1 to 2 wk*	Unknown	2 to 4 wk†

Mechanism of Action
Increases bile acid excretion in the feces. The resulting decreased bile acid level increases the activity of the enzyme that regulates cholesterol synthesis in the liver. As a result, the liver increases its cholesterol synthesis to produce more bile acids. However, the liver's synthesis of cholesterol typically can't match the amount needed to synthesize bile acids, which reduces the cholesterol level. Also, a decreased cholesterol level causes liver cells to increase their uptake of LDLs, which further reduces the cholesterol level. Cholestyramine may relieve pruritus by decreasing the body's bile acid level. This reduces the amount of excess bile acids that are deposited in the dermis and that typically cause pruritus in patients with cholestasis.

---

* For hypercholesterolemia; in 1 to 3 wk for pruritus.
† For hypercholesterolemia; 1 to 2 wk for pruritus.

Contraindications

Complete biliary obstruction (when bile isn't excreted into intestine), hypersensitivity to cholestyramine or its components

Interactions

DRUGS

chenodiol, digitalis glycosides, fat-soluble vitamins, folic acid, gemfibrozil, penicillin G (oral), phenylbutazone, propranolol (oral), tetracyclines (oral), thiazide diuretics (oral), thyroid hormones, ursodiol, vancomycin (oral): Decreased absorption and effects of these drugs
oral anticoagulants: Decreased or increased anticoagulant effect

Adverse Reactions

CNS: Headache, dizziness
GI: Bloating, constipation, diarrhea, epigastric pain, eructation, fecal impaction, flatulence, indigestion, nausea, vomiting

Nursing Considerations

• Store cholestyramine at room temperature.
• Don't give dry powder because it may cause esophageal distress; mix it in a beverage .
• **WARNING** Be aware that long-term use may increase bleeding tendency from hyperprothrombinemia caused by vitamin K deficiency. If this occurs, patient will require treatment with vitamin K_1.
• Monitor for deficiencies of fat-soluble vitamins, such as A and D. If long-term therapy prevents absorption of these vitamins, expect to provide supplementation.

PATIENT TEACHING

• Urge patient to follow a low-fat, low-cholesterol diet and regular exercise program.
• Tell patient to take drug before meals.
• Instruct patient to mix dry powder as follows: Place the amount of powder needed for dose in any beverage and stir vigorously. Then, vigorously stir in another 2 to 4 oz of beverage. After drinking mixture, rinse glass with more liquid, and swallow it to make sure full dose is taken. Patient also may mix drug in thin soups or moist, pulpy fruits, such as applesauce and crushed pineapple.
• Tell patient to drink plenty of fluids and increase bulk in his diet to minimize constipation; remind him to notify prescriber if constipation, nausea, or other adverse GI reactions develop.
• Explain that the serum cholesterol level will need to be measured often for first few months of therapy and periodically thereafter.
• Advise patient to take other drugs at least 1 hour before or 4 to 6 hours after cholestyramine to avoid interference with their absorption.
• Tell patient to take a missed dose as soon as he remembers but not to take double or extra doses.

choline salicylate

Arthropan

Class and Category

Chemical class: Salicylate
Therapeutic class: Analgesic, anti-inflammatory, antipyretic
Pregnancy category: C (first trimester), Not rated (later trimesters)

Indications and Dosages

➤ *To treat mild to moderate pain, reduce fever*

LIQUID

Adults and adolescents. 435 to 870 mg every 4 hr, p.r.n. *Maximum:* 5,325 mg daily.
Children ages 11 to 12. 435 to 652.5 mg every 4 hr, p.r.n. *Maximum:* Five doses daily.
Children ages 9 to 11. 435 to 543.8 mg every 4 hr, p.r.n. *Maximum:* Five doses daily.
Children ages 6 to 9. 435 mg every 4 hr, p.r.n. *Maximum:* Five doses daily.
Children ages 4 to 6. 326.5 mg every 4 hr, p.r.n. *Maximum:* Five doses daily.
Children ages 2 to 4. 217.5 mg every 4 hr, p.r.n. *Maximum:* Five doses daily.
Children up to age 2. Individualized dosage. *Maximum:* Five doses daily.

➤ *To treat rheumatoid arthritis*

LIQUID

Adults and adolescents. 870 to 1,740 mg up to four times daily.
Children age 12 and younger. 107 to 133 mg/ kg daily in divided doses.

Route	Onset	Peak	Duration
P.O.	Unknown	Several wk*	Unknown

Contraindications

Hypersensitivity to nonacetylated salicylates

---

* For rheumatoid arthritis.

Mechanism of Action

Blocks cyclooxygenase, an enzyme needed for prostaglandin synthesis. As mediators in the inflammatory process, prostaglandins cause local vasodilation, swelling, and pain. They also influence pain transmission from the periphery to the spinal cord. By blocking cyclooxygenase and inhibiting prostaglandins, this NSAID decreases inflammatory symptoms and relieves pain. It also acts on the heat-regulating center in the hypothalamus and causes peripheral vasodilation, sweating, and heat loss.

Interactions
DRUGS

antacids: Increased clearance and decreased blood level of salicylate

carbonic anhydrase inhibitors, phenytoin, valproic acid: Decreased blood levels and therapeutic effects of these drugs

corticosteroids: Decreased blood salicylate level, increased salicylate dosage requirements

insulin, sulfonylureas: Increased hypoglycemic response

methotrexate: Increased therapeutic and toxic effects of methotrexate, especially when given in chemotherapeutic doses

oral anticoagulants: Increased blood level of unbound anticoagulant and risk of bleeding

salicylate-containing products: Increased plasma salicylate level, possibly to toxic level

uricosuric drugs: Decreased uricosuric drug efficacy

Adverse Reactions

CNS: Confusion, dizziness, drowsiness, hallucinations, headache, light-headedness
CV: Tachycardia
EENT: Hearing loss, tinnitus
GI: Constipation, diarrhea, epigastric pain, heartburn, indigestion, nausea, vomiting
HEME: Easy bruising, unusual bleeding

Nursing Considerations

•Use choline salicylate cautiously in patients with renal impairment.
•Don't give salicylates to children and adolescents with chickenpox or influenza symptoms because of the risk of Reye's syndrome.
•WARNING During high-dose or long-term

therapy, watch for salicylate intoxication, (headache, dizziness, tinnitus, hearing loss, confusion, drowsiness, diaphoresis, vomiting, diarrhea, hyperventilation, and possibly CNS disturbance, electrolyte imbalance, respiratory acidosis, hyperthermia, and dehydration). Prepare for induced vomiting, gastric lavage, activated charcoal, and peritoneal dialysis or hemodialysis, as ordered.

PATIENT TEACHING

•Tell patient to store drug at room temperature, away from heat, light, and moisture.
•Instruct patient to take drug with full glass of water or with food.
•Tell patient to take a missed dose as soon as he remembers but to avoid doubling the dose.
•If patient has arthritis, explain that optimal drug effects may not occur for 2 to 3 weeks.
•Teach patient to recognize and immediately report signs of salicylate toxicity.
•Because drug is closely related to aspirin, advise against taking aspirin-containing OTC products during therapy.

ciclesonide

Alvesco

Class and Category

Chemical class: Non-halogenated glucocorticoid
Therapeutic class: Antiasthmatic, anti-inflammatory
Pregnancy category: C

Indications and Dosages

➤ *To prevent asthma attacks as part of maintenance therapy*

INHALATION AEROSOL

Adults and children age 12 and over using bronchodilator therapy. *Initial:* 80 mcg b.i.d. *Maximum:* 160 mcg b.i.d.

Adults and children age 12 and over switching from another inhaled corticosteroid. *Initial:* 80 mcg b.i.d., adjusted to lowest effective dose when stabilized. *Maximum:* 320 mg b.i.d.

Adults and children age 12 and older using oral corticosteroid therapy. *Initial and maximum:* 320 mcg b.i.d., adjusted to lowest effective dose when stabilized.

➤ *To treat nasal congestion in seasonal or allergic rhinitis*

INHALATION AEROSOL
Adults and children age 6 and over. 200 mcg
daily as 2 sprays in each nostril.

Route	Onset	Peak	Duration
Inhala-tion	Unknown	4 wk or longer	Several days

Mechanism of Action
Inhibits cells involved in the asthma inflammatory response, such as mast cells,
eosinophils, basophils, lymphocytes, macrophages, and neutrophils. Ciclesonide
also inhibits production or secretion of
chemical mediators, such as histamine,
eicosanoids, leukotrienes, and cytokines.

Contraindications
Hypersensitivity to ciclesonide or its components, primary treatment of status asthmaticus or other acute asthma episodes that require intensive measures

Interactions
DRUGS
ketoconazole: Increased exposure time of ciclesonide

Adverse Reactions
CNS: Dizziness, fatigue, headache
EENT: Cataracts, conjunctivitis, dry mouth
or throat, dysphonia, glaucoma, hoarseness,
nasal congestion, nasopharyngitis, oral can-
didiasis, pharyngolaryngeal pain, sinusitis
ENDO: Adrenal insufficiency, cushingoid
symptoms, decreased bone mineral density,
hyperglycemia, slower growth in children
GI: Nausea
MS: Arthralgia, back or limb pain, muscu-
loskeletal chest pain
RESP: Bronchospasm, cough, pneumonia,
upper respiratory tract infection
SKIN: Facial edema, urticaria
Other: Angioedema, influenza

Nursing Considerations
•Use cautiously in patients with tuberculosis; fungal, bacterial, viral, or parasitic infection; ocular herpes simplex; or measles or
chickenpox because these conditions may
worsen with ciclesonide therapy.
•Also use cautiously in patients with a history of increased intraocular pressure, glau-

coma, or cataracts because ciclesonide may
increase intraocular pressure or cause cataract formation and in patients with major
risk factors for decreased bone mineral content, such as prolonged immobilization, family history of osteoporosis, or long-term use
of drugs that can reduce bone mass, such as
anticonvulsants and oral corticoseroids.
•Inspect patient's oral cavity regularly for
abnormalities. Have patient rinse mouth following inhalation of ciclesonide to reduce
risk of oral candidiasis. If oral candidiasis
occurs, expect to continue ciclesonide therapy, unless severe.
•If patient takes a systemic corticosteroid,
expect to taper dosage by no more than
2.5 mg/day at weekly intervals, starting
1 week after ciclesonide therapy begins.
•**WARNING** If patient is switched from systemic corticosteroid to ciclesonide, assess for
adrenal insufficiency (fatigue, hypotension,
lassitude, nausea, vomiting, weakness) early
in therapy and whenever patient has infection, stress, trauma, surgery, or other steroid-
depleting conditions or procedures. Notify
prescriber immediately if signs or symptoms
develop.
•As prescribed, administer a fast-acting inhaled bronchodilator if an acute asthma attack occurs. Ciclesonide is not a bronchodilator and its action takes longer than
needed to abort acute asthma symptoms. If
bronchospasm occurs immediately after ciclesonide use, expect to stop drug and start
another drug regimen.
•Monitor growth in children because ciclesonide may suppress growth
PATIENT TEACHING
•Urge patient to use ciclesonide regularly, as
prescribed, but not for acute bronchospasm.
Also tell her never to increase or decrease
the dosage without consulting prescriber.
•Tell patient to use ciclesonide only with the
actuator supplied with the product. Explain
that when the dose indicator shows a red
zone in the window, about 20 inhalations are
left, indicating a need for a refill. When the
indicator shows zero, she should discard the
inhaler. Advise against relying solely on the
dose indicator, especially if inhaler has been
dropped, but to keep track of number of inhalations used separately.
•Instruct patient to use inhaler according to
package instructions. Stress need to make

sure canister is firmly seated in the plastic mouthpiece adapter before each use and to press inhaler slowly but firmly until it can go no further in the adapter for each spray. Inform patient that she doesn't need to shake inhaler before use.

•On first use, advise her to spray three times into the air (away from her eyes) looking for a fine mist. If inhaler hasn't been used for more than 10 days, it should be primed again.

•Instruct patient to gargle and rinse her mouth after each dose to help prevent dry mouth and throat, relieve throat irritation, and prevent oral yeast infection.

•Tell patient to always replace cap after use, to keep mouthpiece clean, and to clean mouthpiece once a week with a clean, dry tissue or cloth.

•Explain that the full effect of drug may not occur for 4 weeks or more.

•Stress importance of notifying prescriber if symptoms continue or worsen.

•Instruct patient to notify prescriber immediately if asthma attacks don't respond to bronchodilators during ciclesonide use.

•If patient is switching from an oral corticosteroid to ciclesonide, urge her to carry medical identification indicating the need for supplemental systemic corticosteroids during stress or severe asthma attack.

•Caution patient to avoid contact with people who have infections because ciclesonide suppresses the immune system, increasing the risk of infection. Instruct patient to notify prescriber about exposure to chickenpox, measles, or other infections because additional treatment may be needed.

cilostazol

Pletal

Class and Category

Chemical class: Quinolinone derivative
Therapeutic class: Phosphodiesterase III inhibitor, platelet aggregation inhibitor
Pregnancy category: C

Indications and Dosages

➤ *To reduce symptoms of intermittent claudication*

TABLETS

Adults. 100 mg b.i.d. taken at least 30 min before or 2 hr after breakfast and dinner.

Mechanism of Action

May inhibit phosphodiesterase, decreasing phosphodiesterase activity and suppressing cyclic adenosine monophosphate (cAMP) degradation. This action increases cAMP in platelets and blood vessels, which inhibits platelet aggregation and causes vasodilation. This in turn relieves symptoms of claudication.

Contraindications

Heart failure, hypersensitivity to cilostazol or its components

Interactions

DRUGS

diltiazem, erythromycin, itraconazole, ketoconazole, omeprazole: Increased plasma cilostazol level

FOODS

grapefruit: Increased risk of adverse reactions
high-fat foods: Faster cilostazol absorption and increased risk of adverse reactions

ACTIVITIES

smoking: Decreased cilostazol effects by about 20%

Adverse Reactions

CNS: Cerebral hemorrhage, dizziness, headache, paresthesia
CV: Angina, chest pain, hypertension, hypotension, palpitations, peripheral edema, prolonged QT interval, subacute thrombosis, tachycardia, torsades de pointes
EENT: Pharyngitis, rhinitis
ENDO: Diabetes mellitus, hot flashes, hyperglycemia
GI: Abdominal pain, abnormal stool, diarrhea, elevated liver function test results, flatulence, GI hemorrhage, hepatic dysfunction, indigestion, jaundice, vomiting
GU: Elevated BUN level, hematuria
HEME: Agranulocytosis, aplastic anemia, bleeding tendency, decreased platelet count, granulocytopenia, leukopenia, thrombocytopenia
MS: Back pain, myalgia
RESP: Cough, interstitial pneumonia, pulmonary hemorrhage
SKIN: Eruptions, pruritus, rash, Stevens-Johnson syndrome
Other: Infection, increased blood uric acid level

Nursing Considerations
• Monitor patient's vital signs and cardiovascular status closely because cilostazol may cause cardiovascular lesions, which could lead to problems, such as endocardial hemorrhage.
• Monitor blood glucose level to detect hyperglycemia. Also assess for signs of type 2 diabetes mellitus, such as polyuria, polydipsia, polyphagia, and fatigue.

PATIENT TEACHING
• Instruct patient to take cilostazol on an empty stomach because high-fat foods can increase the risk of adverse reactions.
• Warn patent to avoid grapefruit juice during therapy because it can increase the risk of adverse reactions.
• Urge patient not to smoke because it decreases drug's effects.
• Explain that assessment of drug effectiveness is based on ability to walk increased distances. Stress that drug effects won't appear until 2 to 4 weeks after therapy starts and that full effects may take up to 12 weeks.

cimetidine

Apo-Cimetidine (CAN), Gen-Cimetidine (CAN), Novo-Cimetine (CAN), Nu-Cimet (CAN), PMS-Cimetidine (CAN), Tagamet, Tagamet HB

cimetidine hydrochloride

Novo-Cimetine (CAN), Tagamet

Class and Category
Chemical class: Imidazole derivative
Therapeutic class: Antiulcer agent, gastric acid secretion inhibitor, H_2-receptor antagonist
Pregnancy category: B

Indications and Dosages
➤ *To treat and prevent recurrence of duodenal ulcer*

ORAL SOLUTION, TABLETS
Adults and adolescents. *Initial:* 800 mg at bedtime, 300 mg q.i.d. with meals and at bedtime, or 400 to 600 mg in morning and at bedtime for 4 to 6 wk. *Maintenance:* 400 mg at bedtime.
Children. 20 to 40 mg/kg daily in divided doses q.i.d. with meals and at bedtime.

I.V. OR I.M. INJECTION
Adults. *Initial:* 300 mg every 6 to 8 hr. Dosage increased, if needed, by increasing frequency. *Maximum:* 2,400 mg daily.

➤ *To treat active, benign gastric ulcer*

ORAL SOLUTION, TABLETS
Adults and adolescents. 800 mg at bedtime, 300 mg q.i.d. with meals and at bedtime, or 600 mg b.i.d. in morning and at bedtime, or 800 mg at bedtime for up to 8 wk.
Children. 20 to 40 mg/kg daily in divided doses q.i.d. with meals and at bedtime.

I.V. OR I.M. INJECTION
Adults and adolescents. *Initial:* 300 mg every 6 to 8 hr. Dosage increased, if needed, by increasing frequency. *Maximum:* 2,400 mg daily.

➤ *To manage gastroesophageal reflux disease*

ORAL SOLUTION, TABLETS
Adults and adolescents. 1,600 mg daily in divided doses (800 mg b.i.d or 400 mg q.i.d.) for up to 12 wk.
Children. 40 to 80 mg/kg daily in divided doses q.i.d.

➤ *To treat pathological hypersecretory conditions, such as Zollinger-Ellison syndrome*

ORAL SOLUTION, TABLETS
Adults and adolescents. 300 mg q.i.d. with meals and at bedtime. Given more often, if needed. *Maximum:* 2,400 mg daily.

I.V. OR I.M. INJECTION
Adults and adolescents. *Initial:* 300 mg every 6 to 8 hr. Dosage increased, if needed, by increasing frequency. *Maximum:* 2,400 mg daily.

➤ *To treat heartburn and acid indigestion*

ORAL SOLUTION, TABLETS
Adults and adolescents. *Initial:* 200 mg with water at onset of symptoms. *Maximum:* 400 mg every 24 hr for no more than 2 wk unless prescribed.

DOSAGE ADJUSTMENT Oral dosage for all indications reduced to 300 mg every 12 hr (and increased to every 8 hr with caution, if needed) for patients with renal impairment.

➤ *To prevent stress-related upper GI bleeding during hospitalization*

I.V. INFUSION
Adults. 50 mg/hr by continuous infusion for 7 days.

Route	Onset	Peak	Duration
P.O.	Unknown	1 to 2 hr	4 to 5 hr
I.V., I.M.	Unknown	Unknown	4 to 5 hr

Mechanism of Action

Blocks histamine's action at H_2-receptor sites on the stomach's parietal cells. This action reduces gastric fluid volume and acidity. Cimetidine also decreases the amount of gastric acid that's secreted in response to food, caffeine, insulin, betazole, or pentagastrin.

Incompatibilities

Don't mix cimetidine with aminophylline or barbiturates in I.V. solution. Don't mix drug with pentobarbital sodium in the same syringe.

Contraindications

Hypersensitivity to cimetidine or its components

Interactions

DRUGS

antacids, anticholinergics, metoclopramide: Decreased cimetidine absorption

benzodiazepines, calcium channel blockers, carbamazepine, chloroquine, labetalol, lidocaine, metoprolol, metronidazole, moricizine, pentoxifylline, phenytoin, propafenone, propranolol, quinidine, quinine, sulfonylureas, tacrine, theophyllines, triamterene, tricyclic antidepressants, valproic acid, warfarin: Reduced metabolism and increased blood levels and effects of these drugs, possibly toxicity from these drugs

carmustine: Increased carmustine myelotoxicity

digoxin, fluconazole: Possibly decreased blood levels of these drugs

ferrous salts, indomethacin, ketoconazole, tetracyclines: Decreased effects of these drugs

flecainide: Increased flecainide effects

fluorouracil: Increased blood fluorouracil level after long-term cimetidine use

ketoconazole: Decreased blood ketoconazole level

narcotic analgesics: Increased toxic effects of narcotic analgesics

oral anticoagulants: Increased anticoagulant effect

procainamide: Increased blood procainamide level

succinylcholine: Increased neuromuscular blockade

tocainide: Decreased tocainide effects

FOODS

caffeine: Reduced metabolism and increased blood level and effects of caffeine

ACTIVITIES

alcohol use: Possibly increased blood alcohol level

Adverse Reactions

CNS: Confusion, dizziness, hallucinations, headache, peripheral neuropathy, somnolence

ENDO: Mild gynecomastia if used longer than 1 month

GI: Mild and transient diarrhea

GU: Impotence, transiently elevated serum creatinine level

SKIN: Rash

Other: Pain at I.M. injection site

Nursing Considerations

•**WARNING** Be aware that rapid administration of cimetidine can increase the patient's risk of developing arrhythmias and hypotension.

•For I.V. injection, dilute cimetidine in normal saline solution to a total volume of 20 ml. Inject cimetidine over 5 minutes or more.

•For intermittent I.V. infusion, dilute cimetidine in at least 50 ml of D_5W or other compatible I.V. solution. Infuse over 15 to 20 minutes.

•For I.M. injection, don't dilute cimetidine before administering it.

•Be especially alert for confusion in elderly or debilitated patients who receive cimetidine.

PATIENT TEACHING

•Tell patient to use a liquid-measuring device to ensure accurate measurement of oral solution.

•Advise patient to avoid alcohol while taking cimetidine to prevent interactions.

•Instruct patient to avoid taking antacids within 1 hour of taking cimetidine.

•Warn patient that cigarette smoking increases gastric acid secretion and can worsen gastric disease.

•Caution patient not to take drug for more than 14 days, unless prescribed.

cinacalcet hydrochloride

Sensipar

Class and Category

Chemical class: Calcimimetic
Therapeutic class: Calcium reducer
Pregnancy category: C

Indications and Dosages

➤ *To treat secondary hyperparathyroidism in patients with chronic renal disease who are on dialysis*

TABLETS

Adults. Initial: 30 mg daily P.O., increased every 2 to 4 wk in sequential doses of 60, 90, 120, and 180 mg daily, as needed.

➤ *To treat hypercalcemia in patients with parathyroid carcinoma*

TABLETS

Adults. Initial: 30 mg daily P.O., increased every 2 to 4 wk in sequential doses of 30 mg b.i.d., 60 mg b.i.d., 90 mg b.i.d., and then 90 mg t.i.d. or q.i.d., as needed to normalize serum calcium level.

Route	Onset	Peak	Duration
P.O.	Unknown	2 to 6 hr	Unknown

Mechanism of Action

Increases sensitivity of calcium-sensing receptors on the surface of parathyroid cells to extracellular calcium. This sensitivity directly reduces parathyroid hormone (PTH) level, which in turn decreases serum calcium level.

Contraindications

Hypersensitivity to cinacalcet or its components

Interactions

DRUGS

amitriptyline, flecainide, thioridazine, tricyclic antidepressants (most), vinblastine: Possibly increased blood level of these drugs
erythromycin, itraconazole, ketoconazole: Possibly increased blood cinacalcet level

Adverse Reactions

CNS: Asthenia, dizziness
CV: Hypertension, hypotension, worsening heart failure
ENDO: Hypocalcemia
GI: Anorexia, diarrhea, nausea, vomiting
MS: Myalgia
SKIN: Rash
Other: Allergic reaction, noncardiac chest pain

Nursing Considerations

- Use cinacalcet cautiously in patients with a history of seizures because reduced blood calcium level may lower seizure threshold. Also use cautiously in patients with hepatic insufficiency because cinacalcet metabolism may be reduced.
- Monitor patient for hypocalcemia exhibited by cramping, myalgia, paresthesia, seizures, and tetany. Also monitor patient's blood calcium and phosphorus levels within 1 week after starting therapy or adjusting dosage, and every month or two once the maintenance dose is established, as ordered. If hypocalcemia develops, notify prescriber immediately because treatment to raise calcium level will be needed. Treatment may include giving supplemental calcium, initiating or increasing dosage of calcium-based phosphate binder or vitamin D sterols, or temporarily withholding cinacalcet.
- Be aware that if patient starts or stops therapy with a strong CYP3A4 inhibitor, such as erythromycin, itraconazole, or ketoconazole, cinacalcet dosage may need to be adjusted.
- Monitor dialysis patient's intact PTH levels 1 to 4 weeks after therapy starts or dose is adjusted and then every 1 to 3 months thereafter, as ordered. Expect to reduce dosage or discontinue cinacalcet therapy, as ordered, in a patient whose intact PTH level falls below the target range of 150 to 300 pg/ml.

PATIENT TEACHING

- Instruct patient to take cinacalcet with food or shortly after a meal.
- Caution patient to take tablet whole and not divide it or crush it.
- Review signs and symptoms of hypocalcemia with patient and urge him to notify prescriber of changes.

cinoxacin

Cinobac

Class and Category

Chemical class: Quinolone derivative
Therapeutic class: Antibiotic

C

Pregnancy category: B

Indications and Dosages

➤ *To treat UTI caused by* Enterobacter *species,* Escherichia coli, Klebsiella *species,* Proteus mirabilis, *or* Proteus vulgaris

CAPSULES

Adults. 1 g daily in divided doses b.i.d. to q.i.d. for 7 to 14 days.

DOSAGE ADJUSTMENT After initial 500-mg dose, dosage reduced to 250 mg t.i.d. if creatinine clearance is 50 to 80 ml/min/1.73 m^2, 250 mg b.i.d. if clearance is 20 to 50 ml/min/1.73 m^2, and 250 mg daily if clearance is less than 20 ml/min/1.73 m^2.

➤ *To prevent UTI in women with a history of chronic UTI*

CAPSULES

Adults. 250 mg at bedtime for up to 5 mo.

Mechanism of Action

Inhibits the enzyme DNA gyrase, which is responsible for the unwinding and supercoiling of bacterial DNA before it replicates. By inhibiting this enzyme, cinoxacin causes bacterial cells to die.

Contraindications

Hypersensitivity to cinoxacin, other quinolones, or their components

Interactions

DRUGS

antacids that contain aluminum or magnesium, didanosine (chewable tablets, buffered tablets, pediatric powder for oral solution), metal cations (such as iron), multivitamins that contain zinc, sucralfate: Possibly interference with cinoxacin absorption
probenecid: Increased blood cinoxacin level
theophylline: Possibly increased blood theophylline level

FOODS

caffeine: Decreased metabolism of caffeine, resulting in increased blood caffeine level

Adverse Reactions

CNS: Dizziness, headache
CV: Edema
EENT: Altered taste
GI: Abdominal cramps, anorexia, diarrhea, elevated liver function test results, nausea, vomiting
GU: Perineal burning
HEME: Eosinophilia
SKIN: Angioedema, photosensitivity, pruritus, rash, urticaria

Nursing Considerations

• Obtain results of urine culture and sensitivity test before administering first dose of cinoxacin.

• Review results of liver function tests, as indicated, during treatment.

• Administer drug with food, if needed; food decreases peak blood level but doesn't change total absorption.

PATIENT TEACHING

• Tell patient to take cinoxacin with food, if needed, to avoid GI distress.

• Instruct patient to drink 2 to 3 L of fluid daily unless contraindicated.

• Inform patient not to take antacids that contain aluminum or magnesium; didanosine chewable tablets, buffered tablets, or pediatric powder for oral solution; sucralfate; metal cations such as iron; or multivitamins that contain zinc for at least 2 hours before or after taking cinoxacin because they can interfere with absorption of the drug.

• Advise patient to limit caffeine intake while taking cinoxacin because the drug may cause caffeine to accumulate in the body.

• Advise patient to immediately report edema, rash, or severe adverse GI reactions.

• Tell patient to immediately report tendon inflammation, pain, or rupture to prescriber because other drugs in the same class as cinoxacin have caused tendon rupture, requiring drug therapy to be discontinued.

• Warn patient about the potential for seizures, which have occurred with other drugs in the same class as cinoxacin.

ciprofloxacin

Cipro, Cipro I.V., Cipro XR, Proquin XR

Class and Category

Chemical class: Fluoroquinolone derivative
Therapeutic class: Antibiotic
Pregnancy category: C

Indications and Dosages

➤ *To prevent inhalation anthrax after exposure or to treat inhalation anthrax*

ORAL SUSPENSION, TABLETS
Adults and adolescents. 500 mg every 12 hr for 60 days.
Children. 15 mg/kg every 12 hr for 60 days. *Maximum:* 500 mg/dose.
I.V. INFUSION
Adults and adolescents. 400 mg every 12 hr for 60 days.
Children. 10 mg/kg every 12 hr for 60 days. *Maximum:* 400 mg/dose or 800 mg daily.

➤ *To treat acute sinusitis caused by gram-negative organisms (including* Campylobacter jejuni, Citrobacter diversus, Citrobacter freundii, Enterobacter cloacae, Escherichia coli, Haemophilus influenzae, Haemophilus parainfluenzae, Klebsiella pneumoniae, Morganella morganii, Neisseria gonorrhoeae, Proteus mirabilis, Proteus vulgaris, Providencia rettgeri, Providencia stuartii, Pseudomonas aeruginosa, Serratia marcescens, Shigella flexneri, *and* Shigella sonnei*) and gram-positive organisms (including* Enterococcus faecalis, Staphylococcus aureus, Staphylococcus epidermidis, *and* Streptococcus pneumoniae*)*

ORAL SUSPENSION, TABLETS
Adults. 500 mg every 12 hr for 10 days.
I.V. INFUSION
Adults. For mild to moderate infections, 400 mg every 12 hr.

➤ *To treat bone and joint infections caused by susceptible organisms listed above*
ORAL SUSPENSION, TABLETS
Adults. For mild to moderate infections, 500 mg every 12 hr for 4 to 6 wk. For severe or complicated infections, 750 mg every 12 hr for 4 to 6 wk.
I.V. INFUSION
Adults. For mild to moderate infections, 400 mg every 12 hr for 4 to 6 wk. For severe or complicated infections, 400 mg every 8 hr.

➤ *To treat skin and soft-tissue infections caused by susceptible organisms listed above*
ORAL SUSPENSION, TABLETS
Adults. For mild to moderate infections, 500 mg every 12 hr for 7 to 14 days. For severe or complicated infections, 750 mg every 12 hr for 7 to 14 days.
I.V. INFUSION
Adults. For mild to moderate infections,

400 mg every 12 hr. For severe or complicated infections, 400 mg every 8 hr.

➤ *To treat chronic bacterial prostatitis caused by susceptible organisms listed above*
ORAL SUSPENSION, TABLETS
Adults. 500 mg every 12 hr for 28 days.
I.V. INFUSION
Adults. 400 mg every 12 hr.

➤ *To treat infectious diarrhea caused by susceptible organisms listed above*
ORAL SUSPENSION, TABLETS
Adults. 500 mg every 12 hr for 5 to 7 days.

➤ *To treat UTI caused by susceptible organisms listed above*
ORAL SUSPENSION, TABLETS
Adults. For acute uncomplicated infections, 100 mg every 12 hr for 3 days. For mild to moderate infections, 250 mg every 12 hr for 7 to 14 days. For severe or complicated infections, 500 mg every 12 hr for 7 to 14 days.
I.V. INFUSION
Adults. For mild to moderate infections, 200 mg every 12 hr. For severe or complicated infections, 400 mg every 12 hr.

➤ *To treat complicated UTI caused by* E. coli, K. pneumoniae, Enterococcus faecalis, P. mirabilis, *or* P. aeruginosa *or acute uncomplicated pyelonephritis caused by* E. coli
E.R. TABLETS
Adults. 1,000 mg daily for 7 to 14 days.

➤ *To treat acute cystitis caused by* E. coli, P. mirabilis, E. faecalis, *or* Staphylococcus saprophyticus
E.R. TABLETS
Adults. 500 mg daily for 3 days.

➤ *To treat lower respiratory tract infections caused by susceptible organisms listed above*
ORAL SUSPENSION, TABLETS
Adults. For mild to moderate infections, 500 mg every 12 hr for 7 to 14 days. For severe or complicated infections, 750 mg every 12 hr for 7 to 14 days.
I.V. INFUSION
Adults. For mild to moderate infections, 400 mg every 12 hr. For severe or complicated infections, 400 mg every 8 hr.

➤ *To treat intra-abdominal infections caused by susceptible organisms listed above*
I.V. INFUSION

C

Adults. 400 mg every 8 hr along with parenteral metronidazole.

➤ *To treat mild to severe nosocomial pneumonia caused by susceptible organisms listed above*

I.V. INFUSION

Adults. 400 mg every 8 hr.

➤ *To treat typhoid fever caused by* Salmonella typhi *or infectious diarrhea caused by* C. jejuni, E. coli, S. flexneri, *or* S. sonnei

ORAL SUSPENSION, TABLETS

Adults. 500 mg every 12 hr for 10 days.

➤ *To treat uncomplicated urethral or cervical gonococcal infections caused by* N. gonorrhoeae

ORAL SUSPENSION, TABLETS

Adults. 250 mg as a single dose.

DOSAGE ADJUSTMENT Dosage reduced to 250 to 500 mg every 12 hr in patients with creatinine clearance of 30 to 50 ml/min/1.73 m^2; and to 250 to 500 mg P.O. or 200 to 400 mg I.V. every 18 hr in patients with creatinine clearance of 5 to 29 ml/min/1.73 m^2.

➤ *To treat acute cystitis caused by* E. coli *or* K. pneumoniae

E.R. TABLETS (PROQUIN XR)

Adults. 500 mg daily for 3 days with evening meal.

Mechanism of Action

Inhibits the enzyme DNA gyrase, which is responsible for the unwinding and supercoiling of bacterial DNA before it replicates. By inhibiting this enzyme, ciprofloxacin causes bacterial cells to die.

Incompatibilities

Don't administer parenteral ciprofloxacin with aminophylline, amoxicillin, cefepime, clindamycin, dexamethasone, floxacillin, furosemide, heparin, or phenytoin.

Contraindications

Hypersensitivity to ciprofloxacin, quinolones, or their components

Interactions

DRUGS

antacids, didanosine, iron supplements, sucralfate, multivitamins that contain iron or zinc: Decreased ciprofloxacin absorption
cyclosporine: Elevated serum creatinine and blood cyclosporine levels
glyburide: Severe hypoglycemia
methotrexate: Increased blood methotrexate level and increased risk of toxicity
NSAIDs (except acetylsalicylic acid): Increased risk of seizures with high doses of ciprofloxacin
oral anticoagulants: Enhanced anticoagulant effects
phenytoin: Increased or decreased blood phenytoin level
probenecid: Increased blood ciprofloxacin level and, possibly, toxicity
theophylline: Increased blood level, half-life, and risk of adverse effects of theophylline
tizanidine: Increased tizanidine effects

FOODS

caffeine: Increased caffeine effects
dairy products: Delayed drug absorption

Adverse Reactions

CNS: Agitation, anxiety, cerebral thrombosis, confusion, dizziness, headache, insomnia, light-headedness, migraine, nightmares, paranoia, peripheral neuropathy, restlessness, seizures, syncope, toxic psychosis

CV: Angina, atrial flutter, cardiopulmonary arrest, cardiovascular collapse, hypertension, MI, orthostatic hypotension, palpitations, phlebitis, tachycardia, torsades de pointes, vasculitis, ventricular ectopy

EENT: Oral candidiasis

GI: Abdominal pain, constipation, diarrhea, elevated liver function test results, flatulence, GI bleeding, hepatic failure or necrosis, hepatitis, indigestion, intestinal perforation, jaundice, nausea, pancreatitis, pseudomembranous colitis, vomiting

GU: Crystalluria, hematuria, increased serum creatinine level, interstitial nephritis, nephrotoxicity, renal calculi, renal failure, urine retention, vaginal candidiasis

HEME: Agranulocytosis, bone marrow depression, hemolytic anemia, lymphadenopathy, pancytopenia

MS: Tendinitis, tendon rupture

SKIN: Erythema multiforme, exfoliative dermatitis, photosensitivity, rash, Stevens-Johnson syndrome, toxic epidermal necrolysis, urticaria

RESP: Bronchospasm, pulmonary embolism, respiratory arrest

Other: Acidosis, anaphylaxis, angioedema, serum sicknesslike reaction

Nursing Considerations
• Obtain culture and sensitivity test results, as ordered, before giving ciprofloxacin.
• Use drug cautiously in patients with CNS disorders and patients who may be more susceptible to drug's effect on QT interval, such as those taking Class IA or III antiarrhythmics or those with uncorrected hypokalemia or a history of QT-interval prolongation.
• Dilute I.V. ciprofloxacin concentrate to 1 to 2 mg/ml using D_5W or sodium chloride for injection. Don't dilute solutions that come from the manufacturer in D_5W before I.V. infusion. Infuse slowly over 1 hour.
• Store reconstituted solution for up to 14 days at room temperature or refrigerated.
• Don't give oral suspension by feeding tube.
• Be aware that E.R. and immediate-release tablets aren't interchangeable and that Proquin XR and Cipro XR aren't interchangeable.
• Be aware that patient should be well hydrated during therapy to help prevent alkaline urine, which may lead to crystalluria and nephrotoxicity.
• Assess patient's hepatic, renal, and hematologic functions periodically, as ordered, if he's receiving prolonged therapy.
• Monitor patient closely for diarrhea, which may reflect pseudomembranous colitis. If it occurs, notify prescriber and expect to withhold ciprofloxacin and treat diarrhea.
• Assess patient for evidence of peripheral neuropathy. Notify prescriber and expect to stop drug if patient complains of burning, numbness, pain, tingling, or weakness in extremities or if physical examination reveals deficits in light touch, pain, temperature, position sense, vibratory sensation, or motor strength.
• Monitor patients (especially children, elderly patients, patients receiving corticosteroids, and patients who have renal failure or who have had a kidney, heart, or lung transplant) for evidence of tendon rupture, such as inflammation, pain, and swelling at the site. Be aware that tendon rupture may occur during or after ciprofloxacin therapy. Notify prescriber about suspected tendon rupture, and have patient rest and refrain from exercise until tendon rupture has been ruled out. If present, expect to provide supportive care as ordered.

• Assess patient routinely for signs of rash or other hypersensitivity reactions, even after patient has received multiple doses. Stop drug at first sign of rash, jaundice, or other sign of hypersensivitity, and notify prescriber immediately. Be prepared to provide supportive emergency care.

PATIENT TEACHING
• Urge patient to complete the prescribed course of therapy, even if he feels better before it's finished.
• Tell patient not to take drug with dairy products or calcium-fortified juices alone.
• Advise patient to take ciprofloxacin 2 hours before or 6 hours after antacids, iron supplements, or multivitamins that contain iron or zinc. Tell him to shake oral suspension for 15 seconds, not to chew microcapsules, and not to split, crush, or chew E.R. tablets.
• Encourage patient to drink plenty of fluids during therapy to help prevent crystalluria.
• Urge patient to avoid caffeinated products because caffeine may accumulate in the body during ciprofloxacin therapy and cause excessive stimulation.
• Caution patient to avoid excessive exposure to sunlight or artificial ultraviolet light because severe sunburn may result. Tell patient to notify prescriber if sunburn develops because ciprofloxacin will need to be stopped.
• Urge patient to avoid hazardous activities until CNS effects of drug are known.
• Advise patient to notify prescriber about changes in limb sensation or movement and about inflammation, pain, or swelling over a joint. Urge patient to rest the affected limb at the first sign of discomfort.
• Tell patient to stop taking drug and to notify prescriber at first sign of rash or other hypersensitivity reaction.
• Urge patient to report watery, bloody stools to prescriber immediately, even up to 2 months after drug therapy has ended.

citalopram hydrobromide

Celexa

Class and Category
Chemical class: Racemic, bicyclic phthalate derivative
Therapeutic class: Antidepressant

Pregnancy category: C

Indications and Dosages

➤ *To treat depression*

ORAL SOLUTION, TABLETS

Adults. *Initial:* 20 mg daily. Increased by 20 mg at weekly intervals, as prescribed. *Usual:* 40 mg daily. *Maximum:* 60 mg daily. **DOSAGE ADJUSTMENT** For elderly patients, maximum dosage is 40 mg daily.

Route	Onset	Peak	Duration
P.O.	1 to 4 wk	Unknown	Unknown

Mechanism of Action

Blocks serotonin reuptake by adrenergic nerves, which normally release this neurotransmitter from their storage sites when activated by a nerve impulse. This blocked reuptake increases serotonin levels at nerve synapses, which may elevate mood and reduce depression.

Contraindications

Hypersensitivity to citalopram or its components, use within 14 days of MAO inhibitor therapy

Interactions

DRUGS

amitriptyline, bromocriptine, buspirone, clomipramine, dextromethorphan, fluoxetine, fluvoxamine, furazolidone, imipramine, levodopa, lithium, meperidine, naratriptan, nefazodone, paroxetine, pentazocine, phenelzine, procarbazine, selegiline, sertraline, sibutramine, sumatriptan, tramadol, tranylcypromine, trazodone, venlafaxine, zolmitriptan: Possibly enhanced serotonergic effects of citalopram, resulting in agitation, chills, confusion, diaphoresis, diarrhea, fever, hyperreflexia, hypomania, incoordination, myoclonus, or tremor

aspirin, NSAIDs, warfarin: Increased risk of bleeding ranging from ecchymoses to life-threatening hemorrhage

carbamazepine: Possibly increased clearance of citalopram

cimetidine: Possibly increased blood citalopram level

desipramine, metoprolol: Increased blood levels of these drugs

furazolidone, procarbazine, selegiline: Possi-

bly hyperthermia, rigidity, myoclonus, and extreme agitation progressing to delirium and coma

itraconazole, ketoconazole, macrolide antibiotics, omeprazole: Possibly decreased clearance of citalopram

MAO inhibitors: Increased risk of life-threatening serotonin syndrome or neuroleptic malignant syndrome

warfarin: Possibly increased PT

Adverse Reactions

CNS: Agitation, akathisia, anxiety, asthenia, delirium, dizziness, drowsiness, dyskinesia, fatigue, fever, insomnia, myoclonus, neuroleptic malignant syndrome, seizures, serotonin syndrome, suicidal ideation, tremor

CV: Chest pain, prolonged QT interval, thrombosis, ventricular arrhythmias

EENT: Blurred vision, dry mouth, rhinitis, sinusitis

GI: Abdominal pain, anorexia, diarrhea, GI bleeding, hepatic necrosis, indigestion, nausea, pancreatitis, vomiting

GU: Acute renal failure, anorgasmia, decreased libido, dysmenorrhea, ejaculation disorders, impotence, priapism

HEME: Abnormal bleeding, decreased PT, hemolytic anemia, thrombocytopenia

MS: Arthralgia, myalgia, rhabdomyolysis

RESP: Upper respiratory tract infection

SKIN: Diaphoresis, ecchymosis, erythema multiforme

Other: Anaphylaxis, angioedema, hyponatremia, weight gain or loss

Nursing Considerations

•**WARNING** Whenever citalopram dosage is increased, monitor patient for possible serotonin syndrome, characterized by agitation, chills, confusion, diaphoresis, diarrhea, fever, hyperactive reflexes, poor coordination, restlessness, shaking, talking or acting with uncontrolled excitement, tremor, and twitching.

•Be aware that effective antidepressant therapy may convert depression into mania in predisposed people. If patient develops symptoms of mania, notify prescriber immediately and expect to discontinue citalopram.

•Monitor patient with hepatic disease for increased adverse reactions because drug is extensively metabolized in the liver.

•Assess elderly patients and those taking diuretics for signs suggesting syndrome of inappropriate secretion of antidiuretic hormone, including hyponatremia and increased serum and urine osmolarity.

•If patient (especially a child or adolescent) takes citalopram for depression, monitor him closely for suicidal tendencies, especially when therapy starts or dosage changes, because depression may worsen at these times.

•To stop therapy, expect to reduce dosage gradually to avoid serious adverse reactions.

PATIENT TEACHING

•Inform patient that citalopram's full effects may take up to 4 weeks to occur.

•Advise patient not to self-medicate for coughs, colds, or allergies without consulting prescriber because these preparations can increase the risk of adverse reactions.

•Caution patient not to stop citalopram abruptly because doing so may lead to serious adverse reactions.

•If patient (especially a child or adolescent) takes citalopram for depression, urge caregivers to monitor him closely for suicidal tendencies, especially when therapy starts or dosage changes.

•Caution against taking OTC NSAIDs, aspirin, or other remedies (including herbal products, such as St. John's wort) while taking citalopram because they may increase the risk of bleeding.

clarithromycin

Biaxin, Biaxin XL, Biaxin XL-PAK

Class and Category

Chemical class: Macrolide derivative
Therapeutic class: Antibiotic
Pregnancy category: C

Indications and Dosages

➤ *To treat pharyngitis and tonsillitis caused by* Streptococcus pyogenes

ORAL SUSPENSION, TABLETS

Adults and adolescents. 250 mg every 12 hr for 10 days.

Children. 15 mg/kg daily in divided doses every 12 hr for 10 days.

➤ *To treat acute maxillary sinusitis caused by* Haemophilus influenzae, Moraxella catarrhalis, *or* Streptococcus pneumoniae

ORAL SUSPENSION, TABLETS

Adults and adolescents. 500 mg every 12 hr for 14 days.

Children. 15 mg/kg daily in divided doses every 12 hr for 10 days.

EXTENDED-RELEASE TABLETS

Adults and adolescents. 1,000 mg every 24 hr for 14 days.

➤ *To treat acute exacerbations of chronic bronchitis caused by* H. influenzae, M. catarrhalis, *or* S. pneumoniae

ORAL SUSPENSION, TABLETS

Adults and adolescents. 250 to 500 mg every 12 hr for 7 to 14 days.

Children. 15 mg/kg daily in divided doses every 12 hr for 10 days.

EXTENDED-RELEASE TABLETS

Adults and adolescents. 1,000 mg every 24 hr for 7 days.

➤ *To treat uncomplicated skin and soft-tissue infections caused by* Staphylococcus aureus *or* S. pyogenes

ORAL SUSPENSION, TABLETS

Adults and adolescents. 250 mg every 12 hr for 7 to 14 days.

Children. 15 mg/kg daily in divided doses every 12 hr for 10 days.

➤ *To treat pneumonia caused by* Chlamydia pneumoniae, Mycoplasma pneumoniae, *or* S. pneumoniae

ORAL SUSPENSION, TABLETS

Adults and adolescents. 250 mg every 12 hr for 7 to 14 days.

Children. 15 mg/kg daily in divided doses every 12 hr for 10 days.

➤ *To treat pneumonia caused by* H. influenzae

ORAL SUSPENSION, TABLETS

Adults and adolescents. 250 mg every 12 hr for 7 days.

Children. 15 mg/kg daily in divided doses every 12 hr for 10 days.

➤ *To treat acute otitis media caused by* H. influenzae, M. catarrhalis, *or* S. pneumoniae

ORAL SUSPENSION, TABLETS

Children. 15 mg/kg daily in divided doses every 12 hr for 10 days.

➤ *To treat active duodenal ulcer caused by* Helicobacter pylori

ORAL SUSPENSION, TABLETS

Adults and adolescents. 500 mg every 8 hr for 14 days with omeprazole 40 mg daily in the morning. Then, omeprazole continued at 20 mg daily in the morning days 15 through 28. Or, 500 mg every 12 hr for 14 days with lansoprazole 30 mg and amoxicillin 1 g every 12 hr for 14 days.

➤ *To prevent or treat* Mycobacterium avium *complex in patients with HIV infection*

ORAL SUSPENSION, TABLETS

Adults and adolescents. 500 mg every 12 hr for 7 to 14 days.

Children. 7.5 mg/kg every 12 hr. *Maximum:* 500 mg b.i.d.

Mechanism of Action

Inhibits RNA-dependent protein synthesis in many types of aerobic, anaerobic, gram-positive, and gram-negative bacteria. By binding with the 50S ribosomal subunit of the bacterial 70S ribosome, clarithromycin causes bacterial cells to die.

Contraindications

Concurrent therapy with astemizole, cisapride, pimozide, or terfenadine; hypersensitivity to clarithromycin, erythromycin, or any macrolide antibiotic

Interactions

DRUGS

astemizole, disopyramide, quinidine: Possibly prolonged QT interval or torsades de pointes
carbamazepine, other drugs metabolized by cytochrome P450 enzyme system: Increased blood levels of these drugs
cisapride, disopyramide, pimozide, quinidine, terfenadine: Increased risk of arrhythmias
colchicine: Increased risk of colchicine toxicity
digoxin: Increased serum digoxin level
dihydroergotamine, ergotamine: Risk of acute ergot toxicity
lovastatin, simvastatin: Risk of rhabdomyolysis
oral anticoagulants: Potentiated anticoagulant effects
rifabutin, rifampin: Decreased blood clarithromycin level by more than 50%
sildenafil: Possibly prolonged blood sildenafil level
theophylline: Increased blood theophylline level
triazolam: Possibly increased CNS effects
zidovudine: Decreased blood zidovudine level

Adverse Reactions

CNS: Anxiety, confusion, dizziness, fatigue, hallucinations, headache, insomnia, mania, nightmares, seizures, somnolence, tremor, vertigo
CV: Prolonged QT interval, ventricular arrhythmias
EENT: Altered smell, altered taste, glossitis, hearing loss, oral moniliasis, stomatitis, tinnitus, tongue or tooth discoloration
ENDO: Hypoglycemia
GI: Abdominal pain, diarrhea, indigestion, nausea, pancreatitis, pseudomembranous colitis
GU: Anorexia, elevated BUN level, hepatic dysfunction, vomiting
HEME: Leukopenia, neutropenia, increased prothrombin time, thrombocytopenia
SKIN: Pruritus, rash, Stevens-Johnson syndrome, toxic epidermal necrolysis, urticaria
Other: Anaphylaxis, new or worsening myasthenia gravis symptoms, superinfection

Nursing Considerations

•Expect to obtain a specimen for culture and sensitivity tests before giving first dose.
•Use clarithromycin cautiously in patients with renal impairment. Be aware that patients with severe renal impairment may need decreased dosage or prolonged dosage interval and that clarithromycin is not recommended in combination with ranitidine bismuth citrate therapy if patient has a creatinine clearance less than 2.5 ml/min/1.73 m^2 or a history of acute porphyria.
•Assess patient's bowel pattern daily; severe diarrhea may indicate pseudomembranous colitis caused by *Clostridium difficile*. If diarrhea occurs, notify prescriber and expect to withhold clarithromycin and treat with fluids, electrolytes, protein, and an antibiotic effective against *C. difficile*.

PATIENT TEACHING

•Stress the importance of taking the full course of clarithromycin exactly as prescribed, even after feeling better.
•Caution patient not to crush or chew E.R. tablets.
•Advise patient to take drug with food if he takes E.R. tablets or experiences GI distress.
•If patient takes suspension form, instruct him not to refrigerate it.
•Tell patient to report severe nausea, rash, or itching.
•Instruct patient not to take OTC or pre-

scription drugs without consulting prescriber of clarithromycin.
•Urge patient to immediately report watery, bloody stools to prescriber, even if they occur up to 2 months after therapy has ended.

clidinium bromide

Quarzan

Class and Category
Chemical class: Synthetic quaternary ammonium derivative
Therapeutic class: Anticholinergic
Pregnancy category: Not rated

Indications and Dosages
➤ *As adjunct to treat peptic ulcer*
CAPSULES
Adults. 2.5 to 5 mg t.i.d. or q.i.d. 30 to 60 min before meals and at bedtime.
DOSAGE ADJUSTMENT Dosage limited to 2.5 mg t.i.d. before meals for elderly or debilitated patients.

Route	Onset	Peak	Duration
P.O.	1 hr	Unknown	Up to 3 hr

Mechanism of Action
Inhibits acetylcholine's muscarinic actions at postganglionic parasympathetic receptor sites, including smooth muscles, secretory glands, and the CNS. These actions relax smooth muscles and diminish GI, GU, and biliary tract secretions.

Contraindications
Angle-closure glaucoma, benign bladder neck obstruction, hypersensitivity to clidinium bromide or its components, ileus, intestinal atony (elderly or debilitated patients), intestinal obstruction, myasthenia gravis, myocardial ischemia, ocular adhesions between lens and iris, prostatic hypertrophy, renal disease, severe ulcerative colitis, tachycardia, toxic megacolon, unstable cardiovascular status in acute hemorrhage

Interactions
DRUGS
amantadine: Increased risk of clidinium adverse effects
atenolol: Increased atenolol effects

CNS depressants: Increased clidinium effects
phenothiazines: Decreased antipsychotic effectiveness
tricyclic antidepressants: Increased clidinium adverse effects
ACTIVITIES
alcohol use: Increased clidinium effects

Adverse Reactions
CNS: Confusion, dizziness, drowsiness, excitement, fever, headache, insomnia, memory loss, nervousness, weakness
CV: Palpitations, tachycardia
EENT: Blurred vision, cycloplegia, dry mouth, increased intraocular pressure, loss of taste, mydriasis, nasal congestion, pharyngitis, photophobia
GI: Bloating, constipation, dysphagia, heartburn, ileus, nausea, vomiting
GU: Impotence, urinary hesitancy, urine retention
SKIN: Decreased sweating, flushing, rash, urticaria

Nursing Considerations
•Avoid high doses in patients with ulcerative colitis because clidinium may inhibit intestinal motility and cause or worsen toxic megacolon. Also avoid high doses in patients with hiatal hernia or reflux esophagitis because drug may aggravate esophagitis.
•Use drug cautiously in patients with heart failure, arrhythmias, hypertension, autonomic neuropathy, hyperthyroidism, allergies, asthma, or debilitating chronic lung disease.
•**WARNING** Monitor patient for excitement, agitation, drowsiness, and confusion in elderly patients, even with small doses, because they're more sensitive to clidinium's effects. If these reactions occur, notify prescriber and expect to decrease dosage.
•Take safety precautions to protect patient from injury from falling.
PATIENT TEACHING
•Instruct patient to take clidinium exactly as prescribed and not to stop taking it suddenly because it can cause withdrawal symptoms, such as vomiting, diaphoresis, and dizziness.
•Advise patient to take drug 30 to 60 minutes before meals.
•Tell patient not to store capsules in damp places, such as the bathroom.
•Teach patient how to prevent or relieve constipation and dry mouth.

•Instruct patient to avoid alcohol and other CNS depressants because they increase the drug's effects.
•Instruct patient to report constipation, vision changes, sore throat, difficulty urinating, and palpitations.

clindamycin hydrochloride

Cleocin, Dalacin C

clindamycin palmitate hydrochloride

Cleocin Pediatric, Dalacin C Flavored Granules (CAN)

clindamycin phosphate

Cleocin, Clindesse, Dalacin C Phosphate (CAN), Evoclin

Class and Category
Chemical class: Lincosamide
Therapeutic class: Antibacterial and antiprotozoal antibiotic
Pregnancy category: B

Indications and Dosages
➤ *To treat serious respiratory tract infections caused by anaerobes such as occur with anaerobic pneumonitis, empyema, and lung abscess and those caused by pneumococci, staphylococci, and streptococci; serious skin and soft-tissue infections caused by anaerobes, staphylococci, and streptococci; septicemia caused by anaerobes; intra-abdominal infections caused by anaerobes such as occur with intra-abdominal abscess and peritonitis; infections of the female pelvis and genital tract caused by anaerobes such as occur with endometritis, nongonococcal tubo-ovarian abscess, pelvic cellulitis, and postsurgical vaginal cuff infection; bone and joint infections caused by* Staphylococcus aureus; *as adjunct therapy in chronic bone and joint infections*
CAPSULES, ORAL SOLUTION
Adults and adolescents. For serious infections, 150 to 300 mg every 6 hr; for severe infections, 300 to 450 mg every 6 hr.

Children. For serious infections, 8 to 16 mg/kg daily in equally divided doses t.i.d. or q.i.d.; for severe infections, 16 to 20 mg/kg/day in equally divided doses t.i.d. or q.i.d.
I.V. INFUSION, I.M. INJECTION
Adults and adolescents age 16 and over. For serious infections, 600 to 1,200 mg daily in equally divided doses b.i.d. to q.i.d.; for severe infections, 1,200 to 2,700 mg daily in equally divided doses b.i.d. to q.i.d.; for life-threatening infections, 4,800 mg daily in equally divided doses b.i.d. to q.i.d.
Children ages 1 month to 16 years. 20 to 40 mg/kg daily in equally divided doses t.i.d. or q.i.d., depending on severity of infection.
Neonates less than age 1 month. 15 to 20 mg/kg daily in equally divided doses t.i.d. or q.i.d., depending on severity of infection.
➤ *To treat vaginal infections caused by* Gardnerella *or* Haemophilus
VAGINAL CREAM
Nonpregnant adults. 100 mg (1 applicatorful) into vagina daily, preferably at bedtime, for 3 to 7 consecutive days.
Pregnant adults in second or third trimester. 100 mg (1 applicatorful) into vagina daily, preferably at bedtime, for 7 consecutive days.
➤ *To treat acne vulgaris*
FOAM
Adults and adolescents. Apply to affected area daily.

Mechanism of Action
Inhibits protein synthesis in susceptible bacteria by binding to the 50S subunits of bacterial ribosomes and preventing peptide bond formation, which causes bacterial cells to die.

Incompatibilities
To prevent physical incompatibility, don't administer with aminophylline, ampicillin, barbiturates, calcium gluconate, magnesium sulfate, or phenytoin.

Contraindications
Hypersensitivity to clindamycin or lincomycin

Interactions
DRUGS
erythromycin: Possibly blocked access of

clindamycin to its site of action
kaolin-pectin antidiarrheals: Decreased absorption of oral clindamycin
neuromuscular blockers: Increased neuromuscular blockade

Adverse Reactions
CNS: Fatigue, headache
CV: Hypotension, thrombophlebitis (after I.V. injection)
EENT: Glossitis, metallic or unpleasant taste (with high I.V. doses), stomatitis
GI: Abdominal pain, diarrhea, esophagitis, nausea, pseudomembranous colitis, vomiting
GU: Cervicitis, vaginitis, and vulvar irritation (with vaginal form)
HEME: Agranulocytosis, eosinophilia, leukopenia, neutropenia, thrombocytopenic purpura
SKIN: Pruritus, rash, urticaria
Other: Anaphylaxis; induration, pain, or sterile abscess after injection; superinfection

Nursing Considerations
•Expect to obtain a specimen for culture and sensitivity testing before giving first dose.
•Use clindamycin cautiously in patients who have a history of asthma, significant allergies, or GI disease; in those with renal or hepatic dysfunction; and in elderly or atopic patients.
•**WARNING** Don't give 75- and 150-mg capsules to tartrazine-sensitive patients.
•Store oral solution for up to 2 weeks at room temperature or reconstituted parenteral solution for up to 24 hours at room temperature.
•Give I.V. dose by infusion only; don't give bolus dose. Dilute 300 mg of clindamycin in 50 ml of diluent and give over 10 minutes. Dilute 600 mg of clindamycin in 100 ml of diluent and give over 20 minutes. Dilute 900 mg of clindamycin in 100 ml of diluent and give over 30 minutes.
•**WARNING** Don't use diluents that contain benzyl alcohol when clindamycin is to be administered to neonates because a fatal toxic syndrome may occur.
•Give I.M. injection deep into large muscle mass, such as the gluteus maximus. Rotate injection sites, and avoid giving more than 600 mg by I.M. injection.
•Check I.V. site often for phlebitis and irritation.
•For topical foam, wash the affected area with mild soap, let it dry fully, and then apply foam to entire affected area.
•Monitor results of liver function tests, CBC, and platelet counts during prolonged therapy.
•Observe patient for signs and symptoms of superinfection, such as vaginal itching and sore mouth, which may occur 2 to 9 days after therapy begins.
•Assess patient's bowel pattern daily; severe diarrhea may indicate pseudomembranous colitis caused by *Clostridium difficile.* If diarrhea occurs, notify prescriber and expect to withhold clindamycin and treat with fluids, electrolytes, protein, and an antibiotic effective against *C. difficile.*

PATIENT TEACHING
•Tell patient to complete the prescribed course of therapy, even if he feels better before it's finished.
•Instruct patient to take oral clindamycin with at least 8 oz of water to prevent esophageal irritation.
•Advise patient to take oral drug with food, if needed, to reduce GI distress.
•Tell patient not to refrigerate reconstituted oral solution because it may become thick and difficult to pour and to discard unused drug after 14 days.
•If patient will use topical foam, tell him to wash affected area with mild soap, let it dry fully, and then apply foam to entire area. Caution against dispensing foam directly onto hands or face because foam will melt when it contacts warm skin. Instead, patient should dispense amount to be used into the cap or onto a cool surface. Tell patient to pick up a small amount with fingertips and gently massage into affected area until foam disappears. If foam feels warm or looks runny, tell patient to run the can under cold water before dispensing.
•Warn patient not to rely on latex or rubber condoms and diaphragms for 72 hours after vaginal treatment because mineral oil in the vaginal cream may weaken these items.
•Explain that having sexual intercourse after using vaginal cream can increase irritation.
•Inform patient that I.M. injection may be painful.
•Tell patient to immediately report an inflamed mouth or vagina, and rash or lesions.
•Urge patient to immediately report watery, bloody stools to prescriber, even if they occur up to 2 months after drug therapy has ended.

clofibrate

Abitrate, Atromid-S, Claripex (CAN),
Novofibrate (CAN)

Class and Category

Chemical class: Aryloxyisobutyric acid
derivative
Therapeutic class: Antihyperlipidemic
Pregnancy category: C

Indications and Dosages

➤ *To treat primary hyperlipidemia (type
III) that doesn't respond to diet, and
type IV and type V hyperlipidemia that
don't respond to diet in patients at risk
for abdominal pain and pancreatitis*

CAPSULES

Adults. 1.5 to 2 g daily in divided doses b.i.d.
to q.i.d.

Route	Onset	Peak	Duration
P.O.	2 to 5 days	3 wk	3 wk

Mechanism of Action

Increases the amount of cholesterol that's
secreted into bile and of bile that's excreted
in the feces. Clofibrate also may increase
the activity of lipoprotein lipase, which degrades VLDLs.

Contraindications

Hepatic dysfunction, hypersensitivity to clofibrate, lactation, peptic ulcer, pregnancy,
primary biliary cirrhosis, renal dysfunction

Interactions

DRUGS

chenodiol, ursodiol: Counteracted effectiveness of these drugs
dantrolene: Decreased plasma protein binding of dantrolene
furosemide: Increased furosemide and clofibrate effects
insulin, sulfonylureas: Increased antidiabetic
effect
oral anticoagulants: Increased bleeding tendency
oral contraceptives: Decreased effectiveness
of clofibrate
phenytoin: Displacement of phenytoin from
binding site
probenecid: Increased clofibrate effects
rifampin: Decreased clofibrate effects

Adverse Reactions

CNS: Dizziness, drowsiness, fatigue, head-
ache, weakness
CV: Angina, edema, phlebitis
EENT: Stomatitis
GI: Abdominal pain, bloating, diarrhea, flat-
ulence, nausea, vomiting
GU: Decreased libido, decreased urine out-
put, impotence, proteinuria
HEME: Eosinophilia
MS: Arthralgia, myalgia
SKIN: Alopecia, dry skin and hair, pruritus,
rash, urticaria
Other: Weight gain

Nursing Considerations

•Obtain baseline CBC, liver and renal function studies, and cholesterol profile, as ordered.
•Use clofibrate cautiously in patients with a
history of hepatic disease or jaundice and in
those with peptic ulcer disease.

PATIENT TEACHING

•Tell patient to take clofibrate with milk or
food to reduce GI distress.
•Tell patient that repeated laboratory tests
will be needed to evaluate serum cholesterol
and triglyceride levels.
•Stress the importance of diet, exercise, and
weight loss to control cholesterol.
•Tell patient to report ankle or leg swelling,
chest pain, decreased urine output, severe GI
reactions, and unusual weight gain.
•If patient takes an anticoagulant, tell him
to watch carefully for signs and symptoms of
abnormal bleeding.
•If patient takes antidiabetic drugs, instruct
him to stay alert for signs of hypoglycemia
from interactions with these drugs.
•Advise women of childbearing age to use
contraception during and for several months
after clofibrate therapy because of teratogenic effects.

clomipramine hydrochloride

Anafranil

Class and Category

Chemical class: Dibenzazepine derivative
Therapeutic class: Antiobsessional tricyclic
antidepressant
Pregnancy category: C

Indications and Dosages
➤ *To treat obsessive-compulsive disorder*
CAPSULES, TABLETS
Adults. *Initial:* 25 mg daily. Gradually increased to 100 mg daily in divided doses over 2 wk, then to maximum of 250 mg daily in divided doses over next few weeks. At maximum dose, total daily amount may be given at bedtime.
Children age 10 and over. *Initial:* 25 mg daily. Gradually increased to the lesser of 3 mg/kg daily or 100 mg daily in divided doses over 2 wk, then to maximum of 3 mg/kg daily or 200 mg daily, whichever is less. At maximum dose, total daily amount may be given at bedtime.

Route	Onset	Peak	Duration
P.O.	Unknown	2 to 4 wk	Unknown

Mechanism of Action
May inhibit neuronal reuptake of norepinephrine and serotonin, which may be a factor in normalizing neurotransmission in obsessive-compulsive behavior.

Contraindications
Acute recovery period after MI, hypersensitivity to clomipramine or its components, use of an MAO inhibitor within 14 days

Interactions
DRUGS
anticholinergics: Increased anticholinergic effects
barbiturates: Decreased level and effects of clomipramine; additive CNS depression
bupropion, cimetidine, haloperidol, H_2-receptor antagonists, selective serotonin reuptake inhibitors, valproic acid: Increased blood level and therapeutic and adverse effects of clomipramine
carbamazepine: Decreased blood clomipramine level; increased carbamazepine level
clonidine: Severely increased blood pressure and risk of hypertensive crisis
CNS depressants: Increased CNS depression
dicumarol: Increased anticoagulant effect
grepafloxacin, quinolones, sparfloxacin: Increased risk of life-threatening arrhythmias
guanethidine: Antagonized antihypertensive effect of guanethidine
levodopa: Delayed absorption and decreased bioavailability of levodopa
MAO inhibitors: Increased risk of seizures, coma, or death
rifamycins: Decreased clomipramine level
sympathomimetics: Possibly potentiated cardiovascular effects
thyroid drugs: Increased effects of thyroid drugs and clomipramine
ACTIVITIES
alcohol use: Increased CNS depression

Adverse Reactions
CNS: Anxiety, confusion, depersonalization, depression, dizziness, drowsiness, emotional lability, fatigue, headache, insomnia, panic reaction, paresthesia, somnolence, suicidal ideation (children and teens), syncope, tremor, unusual dreams, yawning
CV: Orthostatic hypotension, palpitations, tachycardia
EENT: Blurred vision, dry mouth, epistaxis, pharyngitis, rhinitis, sinusitis, unpleasant taste
GI: Abdominal pain, anorexia, constipation, diarrhea, flatulence, increased appetite, indigestion, nausea, vomiting
GU: Dysmenorrhea, ejaculation failure, impotence, urinary hesitancy, urine retention
RESP: Bronchospasm
SKIN: Abnormal skin odor, acne, dermatitis, dry skin, photosensitivity, rash, urticaria
Other: Weight gain

Nursing Considerations
•Be aware that stopping clomipramine abruptly may cause withdrawal symptoms and worsen disorder.
•**WARNING** Don't give drug within 14 days of an MAO inhibitor to avoid possible seizures, coma, or death.
•**WARNING** Monitor children and teens closely for evidence of suicidal ideation; clomipramine increases the risk in these groups.

PATIENT TEACHING
•Tell patient not to use alcohol, barbiturates, or other CNS depressants; clomipramine increases their effects.
•**WARNING** Urge parents to watch their child or teen closely for abnormal thinking or behavior or increased aggression or hostility. Stress the need to notify prescriber if they occur.
•Inform male patients about risk of sexual dysfunction while taking drug.

• Caution patient that drug may cause drowsiness, especially during initial dosage adjustment.

• Warn patient not to stop taking drug abruptly.

• Instruct patient to take a missed dose as soon as he remembers unless it's almost time for the next scheduled dose, in which case he should skip the missed dose. Warn against doubling the next dose.

• Teach patient how to prevent photosensitivity reactions.

• Tell patient to report difficulty urinating, dizziness, dry mouth, sedation, and mental changes.

• Caution patient to avoid hazardous activities until CNS effects of drug are known.

clonazepam

Apo-Clonazepam (CAN), Clonapam (CAN), Gen-Clonazepam (CAN), Klonopin, Rivotril (CAN)

Class, Category, and Schedule
Chemical class: Benzodiazepine
Therapeutic class: Anticonvulsant
Pregnancy category: D
Controlled substance schedule: IV

Indications and Dosages
➤ *To treat Lennox-Gastaut syndrome (type of absence seizure disorder) and akinetic and myoclonic seizures*

TABLETS

Adults and children over age 10. 1.5 mg daily in divided doses t.i.d. Increased by 0.5 to 1 mg every 3 days, if needed, until seizures are controlled. *Maximum:* 20 mg daily.

Children age 10 and under or weighing less than 30 kg (66 lb). 0.01 to 0.03 mg/kg daily in divided doses b.i.d. or t.i.d. Increased by 0.25 to 0.5 mg every third day up to maintenance dosage. *Maintenance:* 0.1 to 0.2 mg/kg daily, preferably in three equal doses, or if unequal, with largest dose given at bedtime. *Maximum:* 0.05 mg/kg daily.

➤ *To treat panic disorder*

TABLETS

Adults. *Initial:* 0.25 mg b.i.d. Increased, if needed, to 1 mg daily after 3 days. If more than 1 mg daily is required, dosage increased in increments of 0.125 to 0.25 mg

b.i.d. every 3 days until panic disorder is controlled or adverse reactions make further increases undesirable. This maintenance dosage may be given as a single dose at bedtime. *Maximum:* 4 mg daily.

Mechanism of Action

Prevents seizures by potentiating the effects of gamma-aminobutyric acid (GABA), which is an inhibitory neurotransmitter. Suppresses the spread of seizure activity caused by seizure-producing foci in the cortex, thalamus, and limbic structures.

Contraindications
Acute angle-closure glaucoma, hepatic disease, hypersensitivity to benzodiazepines or their components

Interactions
DRUGS
antianxiety drugs, barbiturates, MAO inhibitors, opioids, phenothiazines, tricyclic antidepressants: Increased CNS depression
ACTIVITIES
alcohol use: Increased CNS depression

Adverse Reactions
CNS: Ataxia, confusion, depression, dizziness, drowsiness, emotional lability, fatigue, headache, memory loss, nervousness, reduced intellectual ability
CV: Palpitations
EENT: Blurred vision, eyelid spasm, increased salivation, loss of taste, pharyngitis, rhinitis, sinusitis
GI: Abdominal pain, anorexia, constipation
GU: Difficult ejaculation, dysmenorrhea, dysuria, enuresis, impotence, nocturia, urine retention, UTI
HEME: Anemia, eosinophilia, leukopenia, thrombocytopenia
MS: Dysarthria, myalgia
RESP: Bronchitis, cough
Other: Allergic reaction

Nursing Considerations
• Use clonazepam cautiously in patients with renal failure, mixed seizure disorder (because drug can increase the risk of generalized tonic-clonic seizures), or respiratory disease and troublesome secretions (because clonazepam increases salivation) and in elderly

patients (because they're more sensitive to drug's CNS effects).
•Monitor blood drug level, CBC, and liver function test results during long-term or high-dose therapy, as ordered.
•**WARNING** Don't stop drug abruptly; expect to taper dosage gradually to avoid withdrawal symptoms and seizures.

PATIENT TEACHING
•Instruct patient to take drug exactly as prescribed. Explain that stopping abruptly can cause seizures and withdrawal symptoms.
•Advise patient to avoid alcohol and sleep-inducing drugs during therapy. Instruct him to consult prescriber before taking any OTC drugs.
•Urge patient to carry medical identification of his seizure disorder and drug therapy.
•Warn patient about possible drowsiness.
•Instruct patient to report severe dizziness, persistent drowsiness, palpitations, difficulty urinating, seizure activity, and other disruptive adverse reactions.
•Suggest that parents monitor child's performance in school because clonazepam can cause drowsiness or inattentiveness.

clonidine

Catapres-TTS

clonidine hydrochloride

Catapres, Dixarit (CAN), Duraclon

Class and Category
Chemical class: Imidazoline derivative
Therapeutic class: Analgesic, antihypertensive
Pregnancy category: C

Indications and Dosages
➤ *To manage hypertension*
TABLETS
Adults. *Initial:* 0.1 mg b.i.d. Dosage increased by 0.1 mg/wk to produce desired response. *Maintenance:* 0.2 to 0.6 mg daily in divided doses b.i.d. or t.i.d. *Maximum:* 2.4 mg daily.
TRANSDERMAL PATCH
Adults. *Initial:* 0.1-mg patch applied to hairless area of intact skin on upper arm or torso every 7 days. After 1 to 2 wk, if blood pressure isn't controlled, two 0.1-mg patches or one 0.2-mg patch applied to skin. Dosage adjusted, as needed, every 7 days. *Maximum:* Two 0.3-mg patches worn at same time.

➤ *To treat severe hypertension*
TABLETS
Adults. 0.2 mg, then 0.1 mg every 1 hr until diastolic blood pressure reaches acceptable range or 0.8 mg have been administered.
DOSAGE ADJUSTMENT Dosage individualized for patients with renal failure.

➤ *As adjunct to relieve severe pain (in cancer patients) that isn't adequately relieved by opioid analgesics alone*
CONTINUOUS EPIDURAL INFUSION
Adults. *Initial:* 30 mcg/hr. Titrated up or down, if needed, depending on comfort. *Maximum:* 40 mcg/hr.
Children old enough to tolerate placement and management of epidural catheter. *Initial:* 0.5 mcg/kg/hr. Then, titrated to achieve comfort.

Route	Onset	Peak	Duration
P.O.	30 to 60 min	2 to 4 hr	8 hr
Transdermal	2 to 3 days	Unknown	7 days

Mechanism of Action
Stimulates peripheral alpha-adrenergic receptors in the CNS to produce transient vasoconstriction and then stimulates central alpha-adrenergic receptors in the brain stem to reduce peripheral vascular resistance, heart rate, and systolic and diastolic blood pressure. May produce analgesia by preventing transmission of pain signals to the brain at presynaptic and postjunctional alpha$_2$-adrenoreceptors in the spinal cord. With epidural administration, clonidine produces analgesia in body areas innervated by the spinal cord segments in which the drug concentrates.

Contraindications
Anticoagulant therapy (epidural infusion); bleeding diathesis; hypersensitivity to clonidine or its components, including components of adhesive used in the transdermal patch; injection site infection (epidural infusion)

Interactions
DRUGS
barbiturates, other CNS depressants: In-

creased depressant effects of these drugs
*beta blockers, calcium channel blockers,
digoxin:* Additive effects, such as bradycardia and AV block; increased risk of worsened hypertensive response when clonidine is withdrawn (beta blockers only)
diuretics, other antihypertensive drugs: Increased hypotensive effect
epidural local anesthetics: Prolonged effects of epidural local anesthetics when used with epidural clonidine
levodopa: Decreased levodopa effectiveness
prazosin, tricyclic antidepressants: Decreased antihypertensive effect of clonidine

ACTIVITIES
alcohol use: Enhanced CNS depressant effects of alcohol

Adverse Reactions
CNS: Agitation, depression, dizziness, drowsiness, fatigue, headache, malaise, nervousness, sedation, weakness
CV: Chest pain, orthostatic hypotension
EENT: Blurred vision, burning eyes, dry eyes and mouth
GI: Constipation, mildly elevated liver function test results, nausea, vomiting
GU: Decreased libido, impotence, nocturia
SKIN: Rash
Other: Weight gain, withdrawal symptoms

Nursing Considerations
•Use clonidine cautiously in elderly patients, who may be more sensitive to its hypotensive effect.
•Monitor blood pressure and heart rate often during clonidine therapy.
•Expect transdermal clonidine to take 2 to 3 days to lower blood pressure.
•Remove patch before patient has an MRI to avoid possible burns at the patch site.
•Be aware that stopping drug abruptly can elevate serum catecholamine levels and cause such withdrawal symptoms as nervousness, agitation, headache, confusion, tremor, and rebound hypertension.
•Expect hypertension to return within 48 hours after drug is discontinued.

PATIENT TEACHING
•Advise patient to take drug exactly as prescribed and not to stop abruptly because withdrawal symptoms and severe hypertension may occur.
•Instruct patient to consult prescriber if dry mouth or drowsiness becomes a problem

during oral clonidine therapy. To minimize these effects, prescriber may suggest taking most of dosage at bedtime.
•If a transdermal patch loosens during the 7-day application period, tell patient to place the adhesive overlay directly over the patch to ensure adhesion.
•Tell patient to rotate transdermal sites.
•Instruct patient to remove patch and place a fresh one on another site if skin irritation, redness, or rash develops at the patch site.
•Advise patient to fold used transdermal patch in half with adhesive sides together and discard it out of the reach of children.
•Because of possible sedation, advise patient to avoid potentially hazardous activities until drug's CNS effects are known.
•Advise men that libido may decrease.
•Instruct patient to report chest pain, dizziness with position changes, excessive drowsiness, rash, urine retention, and vision changes. As needed, tell patient to rise slowly to avoid hypotensive effects.

clopidogrel bisulfate

Plavix

Class and Category
Chemical class: Thienopyridine derivative
Therapeutic class: Platelet aggregation inhibitor
Pregnancy category: B

Indications and Dosages
➤ *To reduce atherosclerotic events, such as stroke and MI, in patients with atherosclerosis documented by recent stroke, MI, or peripheral artery disease*
TABLETS
Adults. 75 mg daily.

➤ *To reduce atherosclerotic events, such as stroke and MI, in patients with acute coronary syndrome (unstable angina or non–Q-wave MI)*
TABLETS
Adults. *Loading dose:* 300 mg. *Maintenance:* 75 mg daily.

➤ *To reduce rate of death, reinfarction, or stroke in patients with ST-segment elevation acute MI*
TABLETS
Adults. 75 mg once daily. Or, loading dose of 300 mg followed by 75 mg once daily.

Route	Onset	Peak	Duration
P.O.	2 hr	3 to 7 days*	5 days

Mechanism of Action

Binds to adenosine diphosphate (ADP) receptors on the surface of activated platelets. This action blocks ADP, which deactivates nearby glycoprotein IIb/IIIa receptors and prevents fibrinogen from attaching to receptors. Without fibrinogen, platelets can't aggregate and form thrombi.

Contraindications

Active pathological bleeding, including peptic ulcer and intracranial hemorrhage; hypersensitivity to clopidogrel or its components

Interactions

DRUGS

aspirin: Increased risk of bleeding
fluvastatin, phenytoin, tamoxifen, tolbutamide, torsemide: Interference with metabolism of these drugs
NSAIDs: Increased risk of GI bleeding, interference with NSAID metabolism
warfarin: Prolonged bleeding time, interference with warfarin metabolism

Adverse Reactions

CNS: Confusion, depression, dizziness, fatigue, hallucinations, headache
CV: Chest pain, edema, hypercholesterolemia, hypertension, hypotension, vasculitis
EENT: Altered taste; conjunctival, ocular, or retinal bleeding; epistaxis; rhinitis; taste disorders
GI: Abdominal pain; acute liver failure; colitis; diarrhea; duodenal, gastric, or peptic ulcer; elevated liver function test results; gastritis; indigestion; nausea; noninfectious hepatitis; pancreatitis
GU: Elevated serum creatinine level, glomerulopathy, UTI
HEME: Agranulocytosis, aplastic anemia, neutropenia, pancytopenia, prolonged bleeding time, thrombocytopenic purpura, thrombotic thrombocytopenic purpura, unusual bleeding or bruising
MS: Arthralgia, back pain, myalgia

---

* With repeated doses.

RESP: Bronchitis, bronchospasm, cough, dyspnea, interstitial pneumonitis, upper respiratory tract infection
SKIN: Erythema multiforme, lichen planus, pruritus, purpura, rash, Stevens-Johnson syndrome, toxic epidermal necrolysis
Other: Anaphylaxis, angioedema, flulike symptoms, serum sickness

Nursing Considerations

• Use clopidogrel cautiously in patients with severe hepatic or renal disease, risk of bleeding from trauma or surgery, or conditions that predispose to bleeding (such as peptic ulcer disease or thrombotic thrombocytopenic purpura).
• In patient with acute coronary syndrome, expect to give aspirin with clopidogrel.
• **WARNING** Clopidogrel prolongs bleeding time; expect to stop it 5 days before elective surgery.
• Obtain blood cell count, as ordered, whenever signs and symptoms suggest a hematologic problem.
• Monitor patient who takes aspirin closely because risk of bleeding is increased.

PATIENT TEACHING

• Discourage the use of NSAIDs, including OTC preparations, during clopidogrel therapy because of potential for bleeding.
• Caution patient that bleeding may continue for longer than usual. Instruct him to notify prescriber about unusual bleeding or bruising.
• Because he has an increased risk of bleeding, urge patient to inform all other health care providers, including dentists, that he takes clopidogrel before having surgery or other procedures or taking a new drug.
• Instruct patient to inform his health care providers about his clopidogrel therapy.

clorazepate dipotassium

Apo-Clorazepate (CAN), Novo-Clopate (CAN), Tranxene (CAN), Tranxene-SD, Tranxene-SD Half Strength

Class, Category, and Schedule

Chemical class: Benzodiazepine
Therapeutic class: Alcohol withdrawal adjunct, antianxiety drug, anticonvulsant
Pregnancy category: Not rated
Controlled substance schedule: IV

Indications and Dosages

➤ *To relieve anxiety*

CAPSULES, TABLETS

Adults and adolescents. *Initial:* 15 mg at bedtime or 7.5 to 15 mg b.i.d. Dosage adjusted, as needed, to 15 to 60 mg daily in divided doses b.i.d. to q.i.d. *Maximum:* 90 mg daily.

E.R. TABLETS

Adults and adolescents. 11.25 mg daily as substitute for capsules or tablets in patients who were stabilized on 3.75 mg t.i.d. of those forms; 22.5 mg daily as substitute for capsules or tablets in patients who were stabilized on 7.5 mg t.i.d. of those forms.

➤ *To relieve symptoms of acute alcohol withdrawal*

CAPSULES, TABLETS

Adults. *Initial:* 30 mg followed by 15 mg b.i.d. to q.i.d. on day 1 of therapy; 15 mg three to six times on day 2; 7.5 to 15 mg t.i.d. on day 3; 7.5 mg b.i.d. to q.i.d. on day 4; and thereafter, 3.75 mg b.i.d. to q.i.d. *Maximum:* 90 mg daily.

➤ *As adjunct to treat partial seizure disorder*

CAPSULES, TABLETS

Adults and adolescents. *Initial:* Up to 7.5 mg t.i.d. Increased, if needed, by up to 7.5 mg/wk. *Maximum:* 90 mg daily.

Children ages 9 to 12. *Initial:* 7.5 mg b.i.d. Increased, if needed, by up to 7.5 mg/wk. *Maximum:* 60 mg daily.

E.R. TABLETS

Adults and adolescents. 11.25 mg daily as substitute for capsules or tablets in patients who were stabilized on 3.75 mg t.i.d. of those forms; 22.5 mg daily as substitute for capsules or tablets in patients who were stabilized on 7.5 mg t.i.d. of those forms.

DOSAGE ADJUSTMENT Initial dosage reduced to 3.75 to 15 mg daily to treat anxiety in elderly patients.

Contraindications

Angle-closure glaucoma, hypersensitivity to chlorazepate dipotassium or its components

Interactions

DRUGS

barbiturates, MAO inhibitors, narcotics, other antidepressants, phenothiazines: Potentiated effects of clorazepate

cimetidine, disulfiram, fluoxetine, isoniazid, ketoconazole, metoprolol, oral contraceptives, propoxyphene, propranolol, valproic acid: Increased blood clorazepate level

clozapine: Possibly increased risk of shock

ACTIVITIES

alcohol use: Potentiated clorazepate effects

Mechanism of Action

Potentiates action of gamma-aminobutyric acid (GABA) and other inhibitory neurotransmitters by binding to specific benzodiazepine receptor sites in the limbic and cortical areas of the CNS, which helps control emotional behavior and suppresses the spread of seizure activity. The drug also helps relieve symptoms of alcohol withdrawal by depressing the CNS.

Adverse Reactions

CNS: Anxiety, ataxia, confusion, depression, dizziness, drowsiness, fatigue, headache, insomnia, irritability, nervousness, psychosis, slurred speech, tremor

CV: Hypotension

EENT: Blurred vision, diplopia, dry mouth

GI: Anorexia, constipation, diarrhea, elevated liver function test results, nausea, vomiting

GU: Elevated BUN and serum creatinine levels, incontinence, libido changes, menstrual irregularities, urine retention

HEME: Decreased hematocrit

SKIN: Rash

Other: Drug dependence

Nursing Considerations

• WARNING Be aware that prolonged use of therapeutic doses can lead to dependence.

• Monitor liver function test results during therapy.

PATIENT TEACHING

• Tell patient to take clorazepate with food if GI distress occurs.

• Advise patient to avoid alcohol and other CNS depressants while taking drug.

• Urge patient to avoid potentially hazardous activities until CNS effects of clorazepate are known.

cloxacillin sodium

Apo-Cloxi (CAN), Cloxapen, Novo-Cloxin (CAN), Nu-Cloxi (CAN), Orbenin (CAN), Tegopen

Class and Category
Chemical class: Penicillinase-resistant
isoxazolyl penicillin derivative
Therapeutic class: Antibiotic
Pregnancy category: B

Indications and Dosages
➤ *To treat mild to moderate upper respiratory tract infections or localized skin and soft-tissue infections caused by penicillinase-producing staphylococci*

CAPSULES, ORAL SOLUTION, I.V. INFUSION, I.V. OR I.M. INJECTION

Adults and children weighing 20 kg (44 lb) or more. 250 mg every 6 hr. *Maximum:* 6 g daily.

Children and infants weighing less than 20 kg. 50 mg/kg daily in equally divided doses every 6 hr.

➤ *To treat severe lower respiratory tract infections or disseminated infections caused by penicillinase-producing staphylococci*

CAPSULES, ORAL SOLUTION, I.V. INFUSION, I.V. OR I.M. INJECTION

Adults and children weighing 20 kg or more. 500 mg every 6 hr. *Maximum:* 6 g daily.

Infants and children weighing less than 20 kg. 100 mg/kg daily in divided doses every 6 hr.

Mechanism of Action
Inhibits cell wall synthesis and causes cell lysis and death in bacteria that make rigid, cross-linked cell walls in several steps. Cloxacillin affects the final stage of cross-linking by binding with and inactivating penicillin-binding protein, the enzyme that causes linkage in cell wall strands.

Incompatibilities
Don't mix cloxacillin with aminoglycosides because of risk of mutual inactivation.

Contraindications
Hypersensitivity to cloxacillin, penicillin, or their components

Interactions
DRUGS
chloramphenicol, erythromycins, sulfonamides, tetracyclines: Decreased cloxacillin effects

hepatotoxic drugs, such as fluconazole: Increased risk of hepatotoxicity
methotrexate: Increased blood methotrexate level and risk of toxicity
probenecid: Increased and prolonged blood cloxacillin level

Adverse Reactions
CNS: Headache
EENT: Glossitis, oral candidiasis
GI: Abdominal pain, diarrhea, elevated liver function test results, nausea, pseudomembranous colitis, vomiting
GU: Hematuria, vaginal candidiasis
MS: Muscle twitching
SKIN: Pruritus, rash, urticaria
Other: Anaphylaxis

Nursing Considerations
•Use cloxacillin cautiously in patients hypersensitive to cephalosporins (allergic reaction may be delayed) and those with hypertension (drug is relatively high in sodium).
•For I.V. injection, reconstitute 250-mg vial with 4.9 ml of sterile water for injection, 500-mg vial with 4.8 ml, and 2,000-mg vial with 6.8 ml. Shake to dissolve.
•For direct I.V. injection, give over 2 to 4 minutes through the tubing of a compatible infusing I.V. solution. If giving by intermittent I.V. infusion, further dilute with a suitable diluent (see manufacturer's package insert) and administer over 30 to 40 minutes.
•For I.M. injection, reconstitute 250-mg vial with 1.9 ml of sterile water for injection and 500-mg vial with 1.7 ml of sterile water. Shake to dissolve.
•Be aware that parenteral solutions are stable for 24 hours at room temperature and for 72 hours if refrigerated.

PATIENT TEACHING
•Tell patient to finish full course of therapy, even if he feels better before drug is gone.
•Instruct patient to take oral cloxacillin 1 to 2 hours before meals.
•Tell patient to take oral form with a full glass of water (not fruit juice or soda).
•Instruct patient taking oral solution to refrigerate container and to discard unused portion after 14 days. Also instruct him to use a calibrated measuring device to ensure accurate doses.
•Advise patient to report signs or symptoms of allergic reaction.

clozapine

Clozaril, Fazaclo

Class and Category

Chemical class: Dibenzodiazepine derivative
Therapeutic class: Antipsychotic
Pregnancy category: B

Indications and Dosages

➤ *To treat severe schizophrenia unresponsive to standard drugs; to reduce risk of
recurrent suicidal behavior in schizophrenia or schizoaffective disorders*

ORALLY DISINTEGRATING TABLETS, TABLETS
Adults. *Initial:* 12.5 mg once or twice daily.
Increased by 25 to 50 mg daily to 300 to
450 mg daily by the end of 2 wk. Subsequent dosage adjustments shouldn't exceed
100 mg once or twice per wk. *Maximum:*
900 mg daily.

Route	Onset	Peak	Duration
P.O.	1 to 6 hr	Unknown	4 to 12 hr

Mechanism of Action

May produce antipsychotic effects by interfering with dopamine binding to dopamine—especially D_4—receptors in the limbic region of the brain and by antagonizing adrenergic, cholinergic, histaminic,
and serotoninergic receptors.

Contraindications

Angle-closure glaucoma, coma, history of
clozapine-induced agranulocytosis or severe
granulocytopenia, hypersensitivity to clozapine or its components, myeloproliferative
disorders, severe CNS depression, uncontrolled epilepsy, WBC count below 3,500/mm³

Interactions

DRUGS
anticholinergics: Potentiated anticholinergic
effects
benzodiazepines, psychotropics: Additive
hypotensive effects; increased risk of cardiopulmonary collapse
bone marrow depressants: Potentiated myelosuppressive effects
carbamazepine, phenytoin: Decreased blood
clozapine level
cimetidine, citalopram, erythromycin: Increased blood clozapine level

CNS depressants: Increased CNS depression
digoxin, warfarin: Increased blood level of
digoxin and warfarin; displacement of clozapine from its binding site
lithium: Increased risk of confusion, dyskinesia, neuroleptic malignant syndrome, and
seizures
selective serotonin reuptake inhibitors:
Markedly increased blood clozapine level;
increased risk of adverse effects and leukocytosis
ACTIVITIES
alcohol use: Increased CNS depression

Adverse Reactions

CNS: Agitation, akinesia, anxiety, ataxia,
confusion, depression, dizziness, drowsiness,
dystonia, fatigue, fever, headache, hyperkinesia, hypokinesia, insomnia, lethargy, myoclonic jerks, neuroleptic malignant syndrome, nightmares, restlessness, rigidity, sedation, seizures, sleep disturbance, slurred
speech, syncope, tardive dyskinesia, tremor,
vertigo, weakness
CV: Cardiac arrest, cardiomyopathy, chest
pain, deep vein thrombosis, ECG changes,
hypercholesterolemia, hypertension, hypertriglyceridemia, hypotension, myocarditis,
orthostatic hypotension, tachycardia
EENT: Blurred vision, dry mouth, increased
nasal congestion, increased salivation,
pharyngitis, tongue numbness or soreness
ENDO: Ketoacidosis, severe hyperglycemia
GI: Abdominal discomfort, anorexia, constipation, diarrhea, elevated liver function test
results, heartburn, nausea, vomiting
GU: Abnormal ejaculation; urinary frequency, urgency, and incontinence; urine retention
HEME: Agranulocytosis, eosinophilia,
leukopenia, neutropenia
MS: Back or leg pain, muscle spasm or
weakness, myalgia
RESP: Dyspnea, respiratory arrest
SKIN: Rash
Other: Weight gain

Nursing Considerations

• Use clozapine cautiously in patients with
hepatic, renal, or cardiovascular disease and
in elderly patients with dementia-related
psychosis because they have increased risk of
serious or fatal adverse reactions.
• **WARNING** Rarely, clozapine causes severe or
life-threatening adverse reactions, such as

agranulocytosis, cardiac or respiratory arrest, deep vein thrombosis, myocarditis (especially in first month), neuroleptic malignant syndrome, and severe hyperglycemia with ketoacidosis in nondiabetic patients. It also may cause seizures and tardive dyskinesia. Monitor patient closely.

•**WARNING** Check patient's baseline WBC count and absolute neutrophil count (ANC) before therapy and weekly for first 6 months. If WBC count is at least 3,500/mm³ and ANC at least 2,000/mm³, check every 2 weeks for next 6 months. If counts remain stable, expect to continue checking every 4 weeks thereafter.

•If patient develops mild leukopenia (WBCs 3,000 to 3,500/mm³) or granulocytopenia (ANC 1,500 to 2,000/mm³), expect to check counts twice weekly until normal. In moderate leukopenia (WBCs 2,000 to 3,000/mm³) or granulocytopenia (ANC 1,000 to 1,500/mm³), expect to stop drug temporarily and check counts daily until improved. Follow manufacturer's direction for resuming drug and monitoring. In severe leukopenia (WBCs less than 2,000/mm³) or granulocytopenia (ANC less than 1,000/mm³), expect to stop drug permanently and monitor counts daily, then as specified by manufacturer.

•Monitor temperature. A transient increase above 100.4° F (38° C) may occur, most often within the first 3 weeks of therapy.

•When therapy ends, expect to check WBC count and ANC weekly for at least 4 weeks or until WBC count is 3,500/mm³ or more and ANC is 2,000/mm³ or more.

•Monitor patienst, especially male patients and younger patients, for dystonia, particularly during the first few days of treatment. Be alert for complaints of neck spasms, which sometimes may progress to throat tightness, trouble swallowing or breathing, and tongue protrusion.

PATIENT TEACHING

•Tell patient that he'll receive only a 1-week supply at a time.

•Tell patient taking orally disintegrating tablets (Fazaclo) to leave tablet in blister pack until ready to take it. Tell him to peel foil back to remove tablet (rather than pushing tablet through foil) and then to immediately place tablet in mouth and let it dissolve before swallowing. Explain that no water is needed.

•Inform patient that he'll need weekly blood tests. Review evidence of dyscrasias (fatigue, fever, sore throat, weakness); urge patient to report them to prescriber if they occur.

•Instruct patient to avoid hazardous activities until drug's CNS effects are known.

•Advise patient to rise slowly from lying or sitting positions to minimize orthostatic hypotension.

•If patient stops drug for more than 2 days, stress need to contact prescriber for instructions; dosage will need to be changed.

•Tell patient to consult prescriber before using alcohol or taking OTC drugs.

•Advise female patients to notify prescriber if pregnancy occurs or is suspected.

coagulation factor VIIa (recombinant)

NovoSeven, NovoSeven RT

Class and Category

Chemical class: Vitamin K–dependent glycoprotein
Therapeutic class: Antihemophilic, hemostatic
Pregnancy category: C

Indications and Dosages

➤ *To treat bleeding episodes in patients with hemophilia A or B or with inhibitors to Factor VIII or Factor IX*

I.V. INJECTION
Adults. 90 mcg/kg as bolus injected over 2 to 5 min every 2 hr until hemostasis achieved; then every 3 to 6 hr, as needed.

➤ *To prevent bleeding in surgical intervention or invasive procedure in hemophilia A or B patients with inhibitors to factor VIII or factor IX*

I.V. INJECTION
Adults. 90 mcg/kg as bolus injected over 2 to 5 min immediately before surgery or procedure; then every 2 hr throughout surgery or procedure. *After minor surgery:* 90 mcg/kg injected over 2 to 5 min every 2 hr for 48 hr; then 90 mcg/kg injected over 2 to 5 min every 2 to 6 hr until healing has occurred. *After major surgery:* 90 mcg/kg over 2 to 5 min every 2 hr for 5 days; then 90 mcg/kg over 2 to 5 min every 4 hr until healing has occurred.

➤ *To treat or prevent bleeding episodes in patients with congenital factor VII deficiency*

I.V. INFUSION

Adults. 15 to 30 mcg/kg over 2 to 5 min every 4 to 6 hr until hemostasis occurs.

➤ *To treat patients with acquired hemophilia*

I.V. INFUSION

Adults. 70 to 90 mcg/kg over 2 to 5 min every 2 to 3 hr until hemostasis occurs.

Mechanism of Action

Activates the extrinsic pathway of coagulation by forming complexes with tissue factor to activate factors IX and X. Activated factor X complexes with other factors to convert prothrombin to thrombin. Thrombin then converts fibrinogen to fibrin, which leads to formation of a hemostatic plug to produce local hemostais. This process may also occur on the surface of activated platelets.

Contraindications

Hypersensitivity to recombinant coagulation factor VIIa, to its components, or to mouse, hamster, or bovine proteins

Interactions

DRUGS

activated and nonactivated prothrombin complex concentrates: Increased risk of thrombosis

warfarin: Possibly reversed warfarin effects

Adverse Reactions

CNS: Fever, headache

CV: Acute MI, bradyarrhythmia, chest tightness or pain, edema, hypertension, hypotension, supraventricular tachycardia, thrombosis

EENT: Epistaxis

GI: Nausea, vomiting

HEME: Disseminated intravascular coagulation, hemorrhage

MS: Arthralgia

RESP: Wheezing

SKIN: Pruritus, purpura, rash, urticaria

Other: Anaphylaxis, injection site reaction

Nursing Considerations

•Patients with disseminated intravascular

coagulation, advanced atherosclerotic disease, crush injury, septicemia, or concomitant treatment with activated or nonactivated prothrombin complex concentrate are at increased risk for a thrombotic event such as myocardial ischemia or infarction and cerebral ischemia or infarction.

•Monitor factor VII–deficient patient's PT and factor VII coagulant activity before and after administration of drug. If factor VIIa activity fails to reach the expected level, the PT isn't corrected, or bleeding isn't controlled, notify prescriber. Patient may have developed antibodies to the drug. Be prepared to obtain specimen for antibody analysis.

•Reconstitute drug with correct amount of sterile water (2.2 ml for 1.2-mg vial, 4.3 ml for 2.4-mg vial, and 8.5 ml for 4.8-mg vial). Clean the rubber stopper with alcohol, and insert syringe needle into the center of the stopper, aiming needle against the side of the vial so stream of sterile water runs down vial wall. Do not inject diluent directly onto powder. Gently swirl vial until powder is dissolved. Don't shake reconstituted solution. If solution is foamy, let it settle before giving the drug. Once reconstituted, use within 3 hours.

•Monitor patient's clotting status closely. If intravascular coagulation is confirmed by test results or if signs and symptoms occur, notify prescriber and expect to reduce dosage or stop drug.

PATIENT TEACHING

•Tell patient to immediately report any signs and symptoms of allergic reaction, such as hives, rash, chest tightness, or difficulty breathing.

•Inform patient that he'll need regular laboratory tests to determine effectiveness of drug.

codeine phosphate

codeine sulfate

Class, Category, and Schedule

Chemical class: Phenanthrene derivative

Therapeutic class: Antitussive, opioid analgesic

Pregnancy category: C

Controlled substance schedule: II

Indications and Dosages

➤ *To treat mild to moderate pain*

ORAL SOLUTION, TABLETS, I.M. OR SUBCUTANEOUS INJECTION

Adults. 15 to 60 mg (usual, 30 mg) every 4 hr, p.r.n.

Children age 1 year or over. 0.5 mg/kg every 4 to 6 hr, p.r.n.

I.V. INJECTION

Adults. 15 to 60 mg (usual, 30 mg) every 4 hr.

➤ *To treat cough from chemical or mechanical irritation of respiratory system*

ORAL SOLUTION, TABLETS

Adults and adolescents. 10 to 20 mg every 4 to 6 hr. *Maximum:* 120 mg daily.

Children ages 6 to 12. 5 to 10 mg every 4 to 6 hr. *Maximum:* 60 mg daily.

Children ages 2 to 6. 2.5 to 5 mg every 4 to 6 hr. *Maximum:* 30 mg daily.

Route	Onset	Peak	Duration
P.O.	30 to 45 min	1 to 2 hr	4 hr*
I.M.	10 to 30 min	30 to 60 min	4 hr*
SubQ	10 to 30 min	Unknown	4 hr*

Mechanism of Action

May produce analgesia through partial metabolism to morphine. Drug binds with mu, delta, and kappa receptors in the spinal cord and with mu_1 and $kappa_3$ receptors higher in the CNS, decreasing intracellular cAMP, which inhibits adenylate cyclase activity and prevents release of pain neurotransmitters, such as substance P and dopamine, and altering perception of and emotional response to pain. Drug also suppresses cough by acting on opiate receptors in the cough center.

Contraindications

Hypersensitivity to codeine, other opioids, or their components; significant respiratory depression

Interactions

DRUGS

anticholinergics, paregoric: Increased risk of

---

* For pain; 4 to 6 hr for cough.

severe constipation

antihypertensives, diuretics: Potentiated hypotensive effects

buprenorphine: Decreased codeine effectiveness

CNS depressants: Additive CNS effects

hydroxyzine: Increased analgesia; increased CNS depressant and hypotensive effects

MAO inhibitors: Increased risk of unpredictable, severe, and sometimes fatal reactions

metoclopramide: Antagonized effect of metoclopramide on GI motility

naloxone: Antagonized codeine effect

naltrexone: Precipitated withdrawal symptoms in codeine-dependent patients

neuromuscular blockers: Additive respiratory depressant effects

other opioids: Additive CNS, respiratory depressant, and hypotensive effects

ACTIVITIES

alcohol use: Additive CNS effects

Adverse Reactions

CNS: Coma, delirium, depression, disorientation, dizziness, drowsiness, euphoria, hallucinations, headache, lack of coordination, lethargy, light-headedness, mental and physical impairment, mood changes, restlessness, sedation, seizures, tremor

CV: Bradycardia, heart block, hypertension, orthostatic hypotension, palpitations, tachycardia

EENT: Altered taste, blurred vision, diplopia, dry mouth, laryngeal edema, laryngospasm, miosis

GI: Abdominal cramps and pain, anorexia, constipation, flatulence, gastroesophageal reflux, ileus, indigestion, nausea, vomiting

GU: Decreased libido, difficult ejaculation, dysuria, impotence, oliguria, ureteral spasm, urinary incontinence, urine retention

MS: Muscle rigidity

RESP: Apnea, bronchoconstriction, bronchospasm, depressed cough reflex, respiratory depression

SKIN: Diaphoresis, flushing, pallor, pruritus, rash, urticaria

Other: Anaphylaxis, facial edema, physical and psychological dependence

Nursing Considerations

•Evaluate patient for therapeutic response, including decreased pain, cough, and facial grimacing.

•Take safety precautions, if needed.

•Monitor respiratory depth, effort, and rate.

Notify prescriber immediately if respiratory rate drops below 10 breaths/min.
• Assess urine output to detect retention.
• **WARNING** Assess patient for evidence of physical and psychological dependence.
• Rotate sites for subcutaneous delivery. Tissue irritation, pain, and induration may occur with repeated injection into same site.

PATIENT TEACHING
• Advise patient to avoid alcohol or other CNS depressants while taking codeine.
• To minimize nausea, suggest that patient take drug with food.
• Advise patient to avoid hazardous activities until drug's CNS effects are known.
• Caution patient to get up slowly from a sitting or lying position.
• To prevent constipation, urge patient to consume plenty of fluids and high-fiber foods, if not contraindicated.
• Instruct patient to take codeine exactly as prescribed and not to adjust dose or frequency without consulting prescriber.
• Advise patient to report shortness of breath or difficulty breathing.
• Urge breastfeeding women to notify prescriber before taking codeine because drug appears in breast milk and could lead to overdose in infant.

colchicine

Class and Category

Chemical class: Colchicum alkaloid derivative
Therapeutic class: Antigout, anti-inflammatory
Pregnancy category: C (oral form), D (parenteral forms)

Indications and Dosages

➤ *To prevent gouty arthritis attacks*
TABLETS
Adults. 0.5 to 0.6 mg daily. Dosage increased to 0.5 to 0.6 mg b.i.d. or t.i.d., if needed.
I.V. INFUSION OR INJECTION
Adults. 0.5 to 1 mg once or twice daily. *Maximum:* 4 mg daily.

➤ *To prevent gouty arthritis attacks before, during, and after surgery*
TABLETS
Adults. 0.5 to 0.6 mg t.i.d. for 3 days before and 3 days after surgery.

➤ *To treat acute gouty arthritis*
TABLETS
Adults. *Initial:* 0.5 to 1.2 mg; then 0.5 to 0.6 mg every 1 to 2 hr, or 1 to 1.2 mg every 2 hr until pain decreases or adverse reactions occur. *Maximum:* 6 mg daily.
I.V. INFUSION OR INJECTION
Adults. 2 mg over 2 to 5 min; then 0.5 mg every 6 hr or 1 mg every 6 to 12 hr until pain decreases. *Maximum:* 4 mg daily.
DOSAGE ADJUSTMENT For elderly patients, maximum I.V. dosage reduced to 2 mg/24 hr; maximum oral dosage to 2 mg/24 hr. After initial I.V. course, elderly patient should receive no form of colchicine for 21 days.

Route	Onset	Peak	Duration
P.O.	In 12 hr	In 24 to 48 hr	Unknown
I.V.	In 6 to 12 hr	Unknown	Unknown

Contraindications

Blood dyscrasias; hypersensitivity to colchicine or its components; serious cardiac, GI, hepatic, or renal disorders

Incompatibilities

Don't combine colchicine with bacteriostatic agents, any solution or injection that contains D_5W, and any other solution that may change colchicine's pH because precipitation may occur.

Interactions

DRUGS
anticoagulants, such as heparin; platelet aggregation inhibitors, such as aspirin; thrombolytics, such as alteplase: Increased risk of GI ulcers or hemorrhage
antineoplastics: Possibly increased serum uric acid level and decreased therapeutic effectiveness of colchicine
cyclosporine: Increased blood cyclosporine level
NSAIDs, such as phenylbutazone: Possibly increased risk of bone marrow depression, GI bleeding, leukopenia, thrombocytopenia
vitamin B_{12}: Possibly impaired absorption of and increased dosage requirements for vitamin B_{12}

ACTIVITIES
alcohol use: Increased risk of adverse GI effects

Mechanism of Action

In gouty arthritis, leukocytes phagocytose urate crystals in affected joints, a process that releases chemotactic factors, degradation enzymes, and other inflammatory substances. Colchicine helps stop this process, probably by disrupting microtubules within leukocytes. Normally, microtubules contribute to cell structure and movement. When colchicine binds to tubulin (the protein from which microtubules are made), the microtubule falls apart, as shown. This process disrupts cell function and prevents leukocytes from invading joints and producing inflammation.

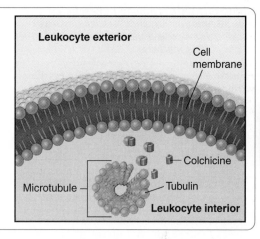

Adverse Reactions

CNS: Peripheral neuropathy
CV: Arrhythmias (I.V. form)
GI: Abdominal pain, anorexia, diarrhea, nausea, vomiting
HEME: Agranulocytosis, aplastic anemia, thrombocytopenia
MS: Myopathy
SKIN: Alopecia, rash
Other: Injection site pain and tenderness, median nerve neuritis in affected arm, and skin and soft-tissue necrosis if extravasation occurs (I.V. form)

Nursing Considerations

•**WARNING** Avoid subcutaneous or I.M. administration of colchicine because these routes may cause tissue necrosis and sloughing. To prevent extravasation, ensure that I.V. catheter is patent and correctly positioned before giving drug. Throughout therapy, check I.V. injection site often for pain, tenderness, and skin peeling. Consult prescriber about switching to oral form.
•**WARNING** To reduce the risk of toxicity, avoid giving colchicine by any route within 7 days after a full I.V. course (4 mg). Expect to wait 3 days after oral therapy before starting second oral course. Elderly or debilitated patients and those with a history of cardiac disease or impaired renal or hepatic function are at increased risk for cumulative toxicity.
•Dilute I.V. form with 10 to 20 ml of normal saline solution. Or, administer colchicine into a large vein through an I.V. line with normal saline solution infusion.
•Administer I.V. form over 2 to 5 minutes.
•Expect to monitor CBC and platelet and reticulocyte counts at baseline and every 3 months after therapy starts.
•Notify prescriber immediately and expect to stop colchicine if patient develops signs or symptoms of colchicine toxicity, such as abdominal pain, diarrhea, nausea, or vomiting.

PATIENT TEACHING
•Instruct patient to return for blood tests every 3 months, as ordered, while taking colchicine.
•Explain that gouty arthritis pain and swelling typically subside in 24 to 48 hours after therapy begins.
•Advise patient to notify prescriber immediately if abdominal pain, diarrhea, nausea, or vomiting occurs.

colesevelam hydrochloride

Welchol

Class and Category

Chemical class: Nonabsorbed hydrogel polymer
Therapeutic class: Bile acid sequestrant
Pregnancy category: B

Indications and Dosages

➤ *As adjunct to diet and exercise to reduce elevated LDL cholesterol levels in patients with primary hypercholesterolemia; as adjunct to diet and exercise to improve glycemic control in type 2 diabetes mellitus*

TABLETS
Adults. 3.75 g once daily or 1.875 g b.i.d. with a meal and a beverage.

Mechanism of Action
Binds with bile acids in the intestines, preventing their absorption and forming an insoluble complex that's excreted in feces. This action decreases the amount of bile acids returning through the entero-hepatic circulation to the liver. As a result, the liver must convert more cholesterol to bile acids, which increases the liver's demand for cholesterol. This, in turn, causes an increase in the production and activity of the hepatic enzyme hydroxymethyl-glutaryl-coenzyme A (HMG-CoA) reductase, which is necessary for cholesterol production. However, synthesis of cholesterol in the liver typically can't match the amount needed to synthesize bile acids. Because the cholesterol levels can't be sustained, LDLs, lipoproteins composed mostly of cholesterol, are increasingly removed from the blood, thereby decreasing the LDL level in the blood.

Contraindications
History of bowel obstruction or pancreatitis induce by hypertriglyceridemia, hypersensitivity to colesevelam or its components, serum triglyceride level greater than 500 mg/dl

Interactions
DRUGS
drugs with narrow therapeutic index, glyburide, levothyroxine, oral contraceptives, phenytoin: Possibly altered effectiveness of these drugs
warfarin: Reduced INR

Adverse Reactions
CNS: Asthenia
CV: Hypertension, hypertriglyceridemia
EENT: Oral blistering, pharyngitis, rhinitis
ENDO: Hypoglycemia, hypertriglyceridemia
GI: Abdominal distention or pain, bowel or

esophageal obstruction, constipation, dyspepsia, elevated liver enzymes, fecal impaction, indigestion, nausea, pancreatitis, worsening of hemorrhoids
MS: Myalgia
SKIN: Rash
Other: Flu syndrome

Nursing Considerations
• Colesevelam shouldn't be given to patients with gastroparesis or other GI motility disorders or to patients who had major GI tract surgery and are at risk for bowel obstruction because of its constipating effects.
• Use cautiously in patients with dysphagia or esophageal obstruction because the size of the tablet can cause dysphagia or esophageal obstruction.
• Use colesevelam cautiously in patients whose total triglycerides exceed 300 mg/dl because bile acid sequestrants can increase this level.
• Evaluate the patient's lipid levels before starting therapy to treat primary hyperlipidemia, again in 4 to 6 weeks, and then periodically, as ordered, throughout therapy. Expect drug to be discontinued if patient develops hypertriglyceridemia-induced pancreatitis or triglyceride level exceeds 500 mg/dl.
• Monitor diabetic patient's blood glucose level regularly, as ordered, to assess effectiveness of colesevelam therapy.
• When giving colesevelam with a drug that has a narrow therapeutic index, expect to give that drug at least 4 hours before colesevelam to prevent reduced effectiveness.
• Because colesevelam may decrease or delay absorption of other drugs, administer it separately if possible.
• Ensure that patient drinks enough fluids when taking drug.
• **WARNING** Monitor patients with preexisting constipation, who are at increased risk for developing fecal impaction.
• Monitor frequency of bowel movements and consistency of stools in patients with coronary artery disease or hemorrhoids because constipation may aggravate these conditions.

PATIENT TEACHING
• Instruct patient to take colesevelam with meals and to drink plenty of liquids when taking drug.
• Advise patient to protect tablets from moisture.

•Caution patient against changing prescribed dosage or stopping colesevelam abruptly because serum lipid level may increase significantly.
•Remind patient that drug therapy doesn't reduce the need for dietary changes.
•Urge patient to keep regularly scheduled appointments for follow-up blood tests.
•Instruct patient to take vitamin supplements at least 4 hours before taking colesevelam.

colestipol hydrochloride

Colestid

Class and Category
Chemical class: Diethylenetriamine and 1-chloro-2,3-epoxypropane copolymer, high-molecular-weight anion exchange resin
Therapeutic class: Antihyperlipidemic
Pregnancy category: Not rated

Indications and Dosages
➤ *To treat primary hypercholesterolemia*
GRANULES
Adults. 15 to 30 g daily in divided doses b.i.d. to q.i.d., before meals and at bedtime.
TABLETS
Adults. *Initial:* 2 g once daily or in divided doses b.i.d., increased every 1 to 2 mo in 2-g increments once or twice daily. *Maximum:* 16 g daily.

Mechanism of Action
Combines with bile acids in the intestine, preventing their absorption and forming an insoluble complex that's excreted in feces. Loss of bile acids increases hepatic production of cholesterol to form new bile acids and increases oxidation of cholesterol to bile acids. The depletion of cholesterol increases hepatic LDL receptor activity, which removes LDLs from the blood.

Contraindications
Complete biliary obstruction, hypersensitivity to colestipol or its components

Interactions
DRUGS
chenodiol, ursodiol: Possibly reduced therapeutic effects of colestipol
digitalis glycosides: Possibly increased risk of digitalis toxicity when colestipol is discontinued
furosemide, sulfonylureas, thyroid hormones: Decreased absorption and therapeutic effects of these drugs
oral anticoagulants: Possibly increased or decreased anticoagulant effect
penicillin G, propranolol, tetracyclines (oral), thiazide diuretics: Decreased absorption of these drugs
vancomycin (oral): Possibly markedly decreased antibacterial action of vancomycin
vitamins (fat-soluble): Possibly interference with vitamin absorption

Adverse Reactions
CNS: Headache
GI: Abdominal distention and pain, constipation, diarrhea, eructation, esophageal reaction, fecal impaction, heartburn, nausea, vomiting

Nursing Considerations
•Mix colestipol granules with at least 90 ml of fluid before administering it to prevent accidental inhalation or esophageal distress.
•Because colestipol may interact with various drugs, administer it on a separate schedule from other drugs when possible.
•Ensure that patient has adequate fluid intake, and obtain an order for a stool softener or laxative to prevent constipation. To prevent impaction, expect to decrease dosage or discontinue drug if constipation occurs or worsens.
•Expect to discontinue drug if no response occurs after 3 months.
•Monitor patient's serum cholesterol level as appropriate, usually at baseline, 4 to 6 weeks after starting therapy, and then every 3 months. Expect to reduce monitoring frequency to every 4 months if response is adequate.
•Be aware that HDL and serum triglyceride levels may increase or remain unchanged during colestipol therapy.
•Keep in mind that adverse GI reactions are more common in patients over age 60.
PATIENT TEACHING
•To help minimize adverse GI reactions, advise patient to mix granules thoroughly in fluid so that they're completely wet before drinking.

•Remind patient that colestipol doesn't reduce the importance of dietary changes.
•Caution patient not to increase or decrease the prescribed dosage or to suddenly stop taking drug. Inform him that abrupt discontinuation may significantly increase serum lipid levels.
•Instruct patient to keep appointments for follow-up blood tests.
•Teach patient how to prevent constipation, and advise him to contact prescriber if constipation occurs or worsens.

colistimethate sodium

Coly-Mycin M

Class and Category
Chemical class: Polypeptide
Therapeutic class: Antibiotic
Pregnancy category: C

Indications and Dosages
➤ *To treat acute or chronic gram-negative infections caused by* Enterobacter aerogenes, Escherichia coli, Klebsiella pneumoniae, *and* Pseudomonas aeruginosa

I.M. INJECTION, I.V. INJECTION, I.V. INFUSION
Adults. 2.5 to 5 mg/kg daily in 2 to 4 divided doses. *Maximum:* 5 mg/kg/day.
DOSAGE ADJUSTMENT For obese patients, dosage should be based on ideal body weight. For patients with severe renal impairment, dosage reduced to 1.5 mg/kg daily and interval reduced to every 36 hr. For patients with moderate renal impairment, interval shouldn't exceed twice daily and may need to be reduced to once daily or every 36 hr. For patients with mild renal impairment, interval shouldn't exceed twice daily.

Contraindications
Hypersensitivity to colistimethate or its components, renal disease

Interactions
DRUGS
aminoglycosides, vancomycin: Increased risk of developing nephrotoxicity
curaniform muscle relaxants, such as tubocurarine, decamethonium, ether, gallamine, succinylcholine: Potentiated neuromuscular blocking effect of these drugs
sodium cephalothin: Possibly enhanced nephrotoxicity

Mechanism of Action
Penetrates into and disrupts bacterial cell membrane, resulting in cell death. Colistimethate is an inactive pro-drug of the bioactive form colistin. Colistin binds to gram-negative bacterial cell membrane phospholipids, increasing cell membrane permeability and causing loss of metabolites essential to bacterial existence.

Adverse Reactions
CNS: Dizziness, fever, paresthesia, slurred speech, tingling of extremities, vertigo
GI: Nausea, vomiting
GU: Decreased creatinine clearance and urine output, increased BUN and serum creatinine, nephrotoxicity
MS: Muscle weakness
RESP: Apnea, respiratory distress
SKIN: Pruritus, rash, urticaria

Nursing Considerations
•Use colistimethate cautiously in patients with impaired renal function.
•Reconstitute each 150-mg vial with 2 ml sterile water for injection to yield 75 mg/ml. During reconstitution, swirl vial gently to avoid frothing.
•When giving by I.V. injection, slowly inject half of total daily dose over 3 to 5 minutes and repeat dose 12 hours later, as prescribed.
•When giving by I.V. infusion, slowly inject half of total daily dose over 3 to 5 minutes. Then add the remaining half of total daily dose to an appropriate solution, such as normal saline solution or D_5W, with type and amount of solution dictated by patient's fluid and electrolyte needs. Starting 1 to 2 hours after first dose, slowly infuse remaining drug over 22 to 23 hours. If patient has renal impairment, use a reduced infusion rate. Once the infusion is prepared, use within 24 hours.
•Notify prescriber if patient develops neurologic disturbances (paresthesia, tingling of limbs, pruritus, vertigo, dizziness, slurred speech). Dosage may need to be reduced.
•**WARNING** Monitor patient's BUN and serum creatinine levels, as ordered. If elevated, notify prescriber because drug may cause nephrotoxicity (usually reversible if drug is stopped) with possible renal shutdown. Toxic levels interfere with nerve transmission at neuromuscular junctions, resulting in apnea

and muscle weakness.
•Monitor patient receiving drug I.M. because apnea and neuromuscular blockade have occurred with this route, especially in patients with impaired renal function. Before giving drug I.M., make sure dose is appropriate for degree of renal function present.
•Monitor patient's bowel elimination. If diarrhea develops, obtain stool culture to check for pseudomembranous colitis. If confirmed, expect to stop drug and give fluid, electrolytes, and antibiotics effective against *Clostridium difficile.*

PATIENT TEACHING
•Caution patient to avoid performing hazardous activities, including driving, during colistimethate therapy.
•Tell patient to immediately report tingling in her extremities, vertigo, dizziness, generalized pruritus, or slurred speech because dosage may need to be decreased.
•Inform patient of need for frequent blood tests during drug therapy to monitor her kidney function.
•Instruct patient to immediately report severe diarrhea to prescriber.

conivaptan hydrochloride

Vaprisol

Class and Category
Chemical class: Arginine vasopressin antagonist (antidiuretic hormone)
Therapeutic class: Aquaretic (sodium/water stabilizer)
Pregnancy category: C

Indications and Dosages
➤ *To treat euvolemic and hypervolemic hyponatremia in hospitalized patients such as may occur in the syndrome of inappropriate antidiuretic hormone, hypothyroidism, adrenal insufficiency, or pulmonary disorders*

I.V. INFUSION
Adults. *Loading dose:* 20 mg over 30 minutes followed by 20 mg as a continuous infusion over 24 hours. An additional 20 mg daily may be given by continuous infusion for 1 to 3 days, as needed. *Maximum:* 40 mg daily with total duration of therapy, including loading dose, not to exceed 4 days.

Route	Onset	Peak	Duration
I.V.	Unknown	24 hr	Unknown

Mechanism of Action
Binds with arginine vasopressin V2 receptor sites in collecting ducts of the kidneys. By doing so, drug blocks the action of arginine vasopressin on the V2 receptor, decreasing water resorption in collecting ducts. This increases excretion of free water (urine output) and increases serum sodium concentration, thereby correcting water and sodium imbalance.

Incompatibilities
Don't mix with lactated Ringer's solution, normal saline solution, or other drugs.

Contraindications
Hypersensitivity to conivaptan or its components; patients with hypovolemic hyponatremia; use with potent CYP3A4 inhibitors such as clarithromycin, indinavir, itraconazole, ketoconazole, and ritonavir

Interactions
DRUGS
amphotericin B, cisplatin, corticosteroids: Possibly additive hypokalemic effects
clarithromycin, indinavir, itraconazole, ketoconazole, ritonavir, and other strong CYP3A4 inhibitors: Increased blood conivaptan level
digoxin: Possibly increased digoxin level and risk of digoxin toxicity
drugs metabolized by CYP3A4, such as HMG-CoA reductase inhibitors: Possibly increased risk of rhabdomyolysis

Adverse Reactions
CNS: Confusion, fever, headache, insomnia
CV: Atrial fibrillation, hypertension, hypotension, orthostatic hypotension, peripheral edema
EENT: Dry mouth, oral candidiasis, pharyngeal pain
ENDO: Hyperglycemia, hypoglycemia
GI: Constipation, diarrhea, nausea, thirst, vomiting
GU: Hematuria, pollakiuria, polyuria, UTI
HEME: Anemia
RESP: Pneumonia
SKIN: Erythema, pruritus
Other: Dehydration, hypokalemia, hypomag-

nesemia, hyponatremia, infusion site reactions (erythema, pain, phlebitis, swelling)

Nursing Considerations
•Conivaptan shouldn't be used to treat patients with heart failure.
•Use cautiously in patients with hepatic or renal dysfunction because levels remain elevated longer in these patients.
•Give drug only through large veins, and change infusion site every 24 hours. Drug may cause serious infusion site reactions even when diluted and infused correctly. Inspect site regularly; change immediately if reactions occur.
•Dilute 20-mg (4-ml) loading dose with 100 ml of 5% dextrose injection before administration. Gently invert the bag several times to mix thoroughly. Use mixture within 24 hours, infusing over 30 minutes.
•Dilute 20-mg (4-ml) or 40-mg (8-ml) continuous infusion dose with 250 ml of D_5W before administration. Gently invert the bag several times to mix thoroughly. Infuse immediately over 24 hours. If infusion is interrupted for any reason, discard any remaining solution 24 hours after mixing.
•Monitor neurologic status and serum sodium level closely during therapy because rapid increase in serum sodium level (more than 12 mEq/L/24 hr) may result in serious neurologic impairment. If serum sodium level rises faster than expected, stop infusion temporarily and notify prescriber. If it keeps rising, expect conivaptan to be discontinued. If hyponatremia persists or recurs and patient has no neurologic abnormalities, drug may be resumed at a reduced rate.
•Monitor vital signs, and assess patient regularly for evidence of hypovolemia. If patient develops hypovolemia or hypotension while receiving conivaptan, stop infusion, notify prescriber, and provide supportive care, as prescribed. After hypovolemia and hypotension have been corrected, drug may be resumed at a reduced rate.
•Store ampules in cardboard container, protected from light, until ready for use.

PATIENT TEACHING
•Instruct patient to report any infusion site discomfort immediately.
•Tell patient that frequent laboratory tests will be performed to monitor his serum sodium level and volume status.

cortisone acetate
Cortisone Acetate-ICN (CAN), Cortone (CAN), Cortone Acetate

Class and Category
Chemical class: Glucocorticoid
Therapeutic class: Anti-inflammatory, corticosteroid replacement, immunosuppressant
Pregnancy category: Not rated

Indications and Dosages
➤ *To treat allergic and inflammatory disorders, collagen disorders, congenital adrenal hyperplasia, dermatologic disorders, edema (from systemic lupus erythematosus or nephrotic syndrome), GI disorders, hematologic disorders, multiple sclerosis (acute exacerbations), neoplastic diseases, primary or secondary adrenocortical insufficiency, respiratory disorders, rheumatic disorders, trichinosis with myocardial or neurologic involvement, and tuberculous meningitis*

TABLETS
Adults and adolescents. *Initial:* 25 to 300 mg before 9 a.m. daily. *Maintenance:* Dosage adjusted based on patient response.
Children. 2.5 to 10 mg/kg daily before 9 a.m. For adrenocortical insufficiency, 0.7 mg/kg/day before 9 a.m.

I.M. INJECTION
Adults and adolescents. *Initial:* 25 to 300 mg daily. *Maintenance:* Dosage adjusted based on patient response.
Children. 0.83 to 5 mg/kg every 12 to 24 hr. For adrenocortical insufficiency, 0.7 mg/kg daily or every third day, or 0.23 to 0.35 mg/kg daily.

Route	Onset	Peak	Duration
P.O.	Rapid	2 hr	1.25 to 1.5 days
I.M.	Slow	20 to 48 hr	1.25 to 1.5 days

Contraindications
Hypersensitivity to cortisone or its components, idiopathic thrombocytopenic purpura (parenteral form), live-virus vaccine administration, systemic fungal infection

Mechanism of Action

Binds to intracellular glucocorticoid receptors and suppresses the inflammatory and immune responses by:
• inhibiting neutrophil and monocyte accumulation at the inflammation site and suppressing their phagocytic and bactericidal activity
• stabilizing lysosomal membranes
• suppressing the antigen response of macrophages and helper T cells
• inhibiting the synthesis of cellular mediators of the inflammatory response, such as cytokines, interleukins, and prostaglandins.

Interactions

DRUGS

anticholinesterases: Possibly antagonized anticholinesterase effects in myasthenia gravis
barbiturates: Decreased cortisone effectiveness, increased cortisol clearance
digitalis glycosides: Possibly digitalis toxicity
estrogens, oral contraceptives: Increased cortisone effects and risk of toxicity
hydantoins, rifampin: Increased metabolism and decreased effects of cortisone
isoniazid: Decreased blood isoniazid level
neuromuscular blockers: Possibly enhanced blockade of neuromuscular blockers, leading to increased or prolonged respiratory depression or apnea
oral anticoagulants: Possibly obstructed anticoagulant effects
potassium-wasting diuretics: Possibly hypokalemia
salicylates: Decreased effectiveness and blood level of salicylates
somatrem: Decreased growth-promoting effect

Adverse Reactions

CNS: Ataxia, behavior changes, depression, dizziness, euphoria, fatigue, headache, increased ICP with papilledema, insomnia, lassitude, malaise, mood swings, paresthesia, seizures, steroid psychosis, syncope, vertigo
CV: Arrhythmias (from hypokalemia), fat embolism, heart failure, hypertension, hypotension, thromboembolism, thrombophlebitis
EENT: Exophthalmos, glaucoma, increased intraocular pressure, nystagmus, posterior subcapsular cataracts
ENDO: Adrenal insufficiency during stress, Cushing's syndrome, diabetes mellitus, growth

uppression in children, hyperglycemia, negative nitrogen balance from protein catabolism
GI: Abdominal distention, hiccups, increased appetite, nausea, pancreatitis, peptic ulcer, ulcerative esophagitis, vomiting
GU: Glycosuria, menstrual irregularities, perineal burning or tingling
HEME: Leukocytosis
MS: Arthralgia; aseptic necrosis of femoral and humeral heads; compression fractures; muscle atrophy, weakness, and twitching; myalgia; osteoporosis; spontaneous fractures; steroid myopathy; tendon rupture
SKIN: Acne; diaphoresis; ecchymosis; erythema; hirsutism; hyperpigmentation; hypopigmentation; necrotizing vasculitis; petechiae; purpura; rash; scarring; sterile abscesses; striae; subcutaneous fat atrophy; thin, fragile skin; urticaria
Other: Anaphylaxis, hypocalcemia, hypokalemia, hypokalemic alkalosis, impaired wound healing, masking of infection, metabolic alkalosis, suppressed skin test reaction, weight gain

Nursing Considerations

• Use cortisone cautiously in patients with ocular herpes simplex because corneal perforation may occur.
• Expect prescriber to order baseline ophthalmologic examination before beginning therapy because prolonged use of cortisone may result in glaucoma, increased intraocular pressure, and damage to optic nerve.
• Assess patient for signs and symptoms of infection before giving cortisone because drug may mask them. Be aware that new infections may develop during therapy because of risk of immunosuppression. If a new infection develops, expect to administer appropriate antibiotics.
• Obtain serum electrolyte levels before beginning therapy, as ordered, and monitor results frequently during therapy to detect electrolyte imbalances. Increased calcium excretion, potassium depletion, and sodium and water retention may occur with large doses of cortisone. Anticipate the need for potassium and calcium supplementation and sodium restriction, if indicated.
• Keep in mind that prescriber will order lowest effective dose.
• To avoid peptic ulcer formation from cortisone, expect patient to receive concurrent antacid or antihistamine therapy.

•**WARNING** Be aware that live-virus vaccines shouldn't be given during cortisone therapy because patient may become immunosuppressed and develop the viral infection.

•**WARNING** Assess for adrenal suppression or insufficiency (fatigue, hypotension, lassitude, nausea, vomiting, and weakness) in patient exposed to stress or receiving prolonged cortisone therapy. Notify prescriber immediately if patient exhibits signs or symptoms of this life-threatening adverse reaction.

•Watch for signs and symptoms of steroid psychosis (confusion, delirium, euphoria, insomnia, mood swings, personality changes, severe depression), which may develop 15 to 30 days after starting drug. Be prepared to stop drug if such signs occur. If stopping isn't possible, expect to administer a psychotropic drug.

•Watch for cushingoid signs, such as acne, buffalo hump, central obesity, ecchymosis, moon face, striae, and weight gain. Notify prescriber at once if they occur.

•Expect to taper oral cortisone dosage slowly to prevent withdrawal syndrome (abdominal or back pain, anorexia, dizziness, fever, headache, and syncope).

PATIENT TEACHING

•Instruct patient to take oral cortisone exactly as prescribed, every morning before 9 a.m. Advise him to take it with food if GI distress occurs.

•Caution patient not to stop drug abruptly because doing so may lead to adrenal insufficiency, withdrawal symptoms, or both.

•Inform patient about adrenal insufficiency and need for possible dosage increases during stress. Advise him to notify prescriber immediately if signs or symptoms develop or if he's exposed to stress.

•Caution patient to avoid exposure to people with infections because cortisone can cause immunosuppression. Also, teach him to recognize and immediately report signs and symptoms of infection.

•Teach patient to recognize and report adverse reactions, including Cushing's syndrome.

•Urge patient receiving long-term cortisone therapy to carry medical identification.

•Recommend regular eye examinations.

•Urge him to keep follow-up appointments with prescriber, which may include laboratory tests, to evaluate effects of therapy.

cromolyn sodium
(disodium cromoglycate, sodium cromoglycate)

Apo-Cromolyn (CAN), Gastrocrom, Intal, Intal Syncroner (CAN), Nalcrom (CAN), Nasalcrom, Novo-cromolyn (CAN)

Class and Category

Chemical class: Disodium chromoglycate
Therapeutic class: Antiasthmatic, anti-inflammatory
Pregnancy category: B

Indications and Dosages

➤ *To prevent bronchial asthma attacks*

AEROSOL (METERED-DOSE INHALER)

Adults and children over age 5. 2 metered sprays (1.6 to 2 mg) every 4 to 6 hr. *Maximum:* 16 sprays (12.8 to 16 mg) daily.

CAPSULES FOR INHALATION

Adults and children over age 2. 1 capsule (20 mg) every 4 to 6 hr. *Maximum:* 8 capsules (160 mg) daily.

SOLUTION FOR NEBULIZATION

Adults and children over age 2. 20 mg every 4 to 6 hr. *Maximum:* 160 mg daily.

➤ *To prevent bronchospasm caused by environmental exposure or exercise*

AEROSOL (METERED-DOSE INHALER)

Adults and children over age 5. 2 metered sprays (1.6 to 2 mg) as a single dose at least 10 to 15 min (no longer than 1 hr) before exposure or exercise. *Maximum:* 16 sprays (12.8 to 16 mg) daily.

CAPSULES FOR INHALATION

Adults and children over age 2. 1 capsule (20 mg) as a single dose inhaled at least 10 to 15 min (no longer than 1 hr) before exposure or exercise. *Maximum:* 8 capsules (160 mg) daily.

SOLUTION FOR NEBULIZATION

Adults and children over age 2. *Initial:* 20 mg inhaled 10 to 15 min (no longer than 1 hr) before exposure or exercise. Repeated p.r.n. during prolonged exercise. *Maximum:* 160 mg daily.

➤ *To treat allergic rhinitis*

NASAL SOLUTION

Adults and children over age 2. 1 spray (5.2 mg) in each nostril at regular intervals t.i.d. or q.i.d. *Maximum:* 1 spray (5.2 mg) in each nostril 6 times daily.

Mechanism of Action

In asthma, inflammation results when antigen reexposure causes mast cells to degranulate and release histamine and chemical mediators. Cromolyn helps reduce inflammation by preventing mast cells from degranulating. After exposure to an antigen, mast cells become sensitized to it, and immunoglobulin E (IgE) antibodies appear on their surfaces. When the antigen returns, it attaches to IgE antibodies (1) and triggers events that lead to degranulation (2). By preventing granules from opening on the cells' surfaces (3), cromolyn blocks the release of histamine and chemical mediators.

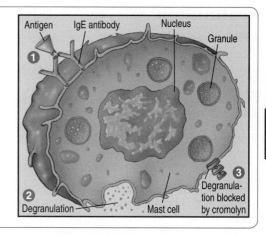

➤ *To prevent systemic mastocytosis*

CAPSULES, ORAL CONCENTRATE
Adults and adolescents. 200 mg q.i.d., 30 min before meals and at bedtime.
Children ages 2 to 12. 100 mg q.i.d., 30 min before meals and at bedtime. *Maximum:* 40 mg/kg/day.
Children under age 2. 5 mg/kg q.i.d. *Maximum:* 40 mg/kg daily.

Route	Onset	Peak	Duration
Aerosol	In minutes	Unknown	Up to 2 hr
Nasal solution	In 1 wk	1 to 4 wk	Unknown
Nebulizer solution	In minutes	Unknown	3 to 6 hr

Contraindications

Arrhythmias, coronary artery disease (aerosol); hypersensitivity to cromolyn or its components, status asthmaticus (all forms); nasal polyps (nasal solution)

Adverse Reactions

CNS: Dizziness, headache, neuritis
EENT: Burning eyes, hoarseness, laryngeal edema, nasal congestion, and swollen parotid glands (all forms); increased sneezing, nasal stinging, and throat irritation (nasal solution); taste perversion (aerosol)
GI: Anorexia, diarrhea (capsules and oral concentrate), nausea, vomiting
GU: Dysuria, urinary frequency
MS: Arthralgia, joint swelling

RESP: Cough, wheezing
SKIN: Rash, urticaria

Nursing Considerations

•**WARNING** Be aware that cromolyn sodium shouldn't be used to relieve acute asthma attack or severe bronchospasm; it should be used only for prevention.
•Don't give cromolyn sodium through handheld nebulizer. Instead, administer via power-operated nebulizer with a face mask or mouthpiece.
•Evaluate patient for effective inhalation; patient must be able to inhale adequately for nebulizer solution to be effective.
•Thoroughly mix oral concentrate or capsule contents into half a glass of hot water (not fruit juice, milk, or food), and let cool before administering.
•Give drug at regular intervals to maximize effectiveness.

PATIENT TEACHING
•Teach patient how to use power-operated nebulizer; warn against using handheld nebulizer.
•Advise patient to use cromolyn sodium 10 to 15 minutes before exercising or exposing himself to other precipitating factors.
•Instruct patient to thoroughly mix oral concentrate with hot water (not fruit juice, milk, or food) and let it cool before drinking.
•Inform patient that nasal spray may cause minor nasal irritation.
•Explain that cromolyn sodium may take up to 1 month to reach full therapeutic effects.

crotamiton

Eurax

Class and Category
Chemical class: Synthetic chloroformate salt
Therapeutic class: Antipruritic, scabicide
Pregnancy category: C

Indications and Dosages
➤ *To treat scabies*
CREAM, LOTION
Adults. 30 to 60 g (thin layer) massaged into skin from chin down and repeated in 24 hr. Applied p.r.n. to skin folds, creases, and areas of intense pruritus for up to 48 hr.
➤ *To relieve pruritus caused by scabies*
CREAM, LOTION
Adults. 30 to 60 g (thin layer) massaged gently into affected areas until drug is completely absorbed. Repeated p.r.n.

> ### Mechanism of Action
> Exerts a toxic effect on *Sarcoptes scabiei* by an unknown mechanism.

Contraindications
Abrasions, application to mucous membranes, breaks in skin, hypersensitivity to crotamiton or its components, inflammation

Adverse Reactions
SKIN: Contact dermatitis, irritation, pruritus, rash

Nursing Considerations
•Expect pruritus to continue for 4 to 6 weeks after treatment.
PATIENT TEACHING
•Advise patient to shake lotion bottle well before applying.
•Warn him to keep drug away from eyes, nose, mouth, and inflamed skin.
•Advise patient to use a topical corticosteroid for dermatitis and an antihistamine for pruritus, as prescribed.
•Instruct patient to change clothing and bed linens the morning after final application and to take a cleansing bath 48 hours after final application.
•Inform patient that pruritus may continue for 4 to 6 weeks after treatment.
•Advise patient to notify prescriber if skin irritation or rash occurs.

cyclizine hydrochloride

Marezine

cyclizine lactate

Marzine (CAN)

Class and Category
Chemical class: Piperazine derivative
Therapeutic class: Anticholinergic, antiemetic
Pregnancy category: B

Indications and Dosages
➤ *To prevent postoperative vomiting*
I.M. INJECTION
Adults and adolescents. 50 mg 15 to 30 min before surgery ends, then every 4 to 6 hr, p.r.n., during first few postoperative days.
Children ages 6 to 12. 25 mg 15 to 30 min before surgery ends, then t.i.d., p.r.n., during first few postoperative days.
Children up to age 6. 12.5 mg 15 to 30 min before surgery ends, then t.i.d., p.r.n., during first few postoperative days.
➤ *To prevent and treat motion sickness*
TABLETS
Adults and adolescents. 50 mg 30 min before travel, then every 4 to 6 hr, p.r.n. *Maximum:* 200 mg daily.
Children ages 6 to 12. 25 mg 30 min before travel, then every 6 to 8 hr, p.r.n. *Maximum:* 75 mg daily.
I.M. INJECTION
Adults and adolescents. 50 mg every 4 to 6 hr, p.r.n.
Children. 1 mg/kg t.i.d., p.r.n.

Route	Onset	Peak	Duration
P.O., I.M.	30 to 60 min	Unknown	4 to 6 hr

> ### Mechanism of Action
> May act centrally on the vomiting center by blocking chemoreceptor trigger zones. Cyclizine also may reduce the sensitivity of the labyrinthine apparatus in the inner ear.

Contraindications
Hypersensitivity to cyclizine or its components, shock

Interactions
DRUGS
anticholinergics: Possibly potentiated anti-

cholinergic effects

apomorphine: Possibly decreased emetic response of apomorphine

CNS depressants: Possibly potentiated CNS depression

ACTIVITIES

alcohol use: Possibly potentiated CNS depression

Adverse Reactions

CNS: Dizziness, drowsiness, euphoria, excitation, hallucinations, insomnia, nervousness, restlessness, seizures (in children), vertigo

CV: Hypotension, palpitations, tachycardia

EENT: Blurred vision; diplopia; dry mouth, nose, and throat; tinnitus

GI: Anorexia, constipation, diarrhea, nausea, vomiting

GU: Urinary frequency and hesitancy, urine retention

SKIN: Jaundice, rash, urticaria

Nursing Considerations

• Help patient with ambulation and take safety precautions to prevent injury from falls if drowsiness or dizziness occurs.

• Don't schedule allergen skin tests until at least 5 days after cyclizine therapy stops because drug may interfere with test results.

PATIENT TEACHING

• Urge patient to avoid alcohol and other CNS depressants during cyclizine therapy.

• Advise patient to ask for help with ambulation if he feels drowsy or dizzy.

cyclobenzaprine hydrochloride

Flexeril

Class and Category

Chemical class: Tricyclic amine salt

Therapeutic class: Skeletal muscle relaxant

Pregnancy category: B

Indications and Dosages

➤ *As adjunct to rest and physical therapy for relief of muscle spasm associated with acute, painful musculoskeletal conditions*

TABLETS

Adults and adolescents. 5 mg t.i.d., increased as needed to 10 mg t.i.d. *Maximum:* 30 mg daily for 3 wk.

DOSAGE ADJUSTMENT Dosage frequency reduced in elderly patients and those with hepatic impairment.

Route	Onset	Peak	Duration
P.O.	1 hr	1 to 2 wk	12 to 24 hr

Mechanism of Action

Acts in the brain stem to reduce or abolish tonic muscle hyperactivity. Because cyclobenzaprine doesn't act at the neuromuscular junction or directly on skeletal muscle, it relieves muscle spasm without disrupting muscle function.

Contraindications

Acute recovery phase of MI; age less than 12; arrhythmias, including heart block and other conduction disturbances; heart failure; hypersensitivity to cyclobenzaprine or its components; hyperthyroidism; MAO inhibitor use within 14 days

Interactions

DRUGS

anticholinergics, antidyskinetics: Possibly potentiated anticholinergic effects of these drugs

CNS depressants, tricyclic antidepressants: Possibly additive CNS depressant effects of these drugs, increased risk of adverse effects of antidepressants and cyclobenzaprine

guanadrel, guanethidine: Possibly decreased or blocked antihypertensive effects of these drugs

MAO inhibitors: Possibly hyperpyretic crisis, severe seizures, and death

ACTIVITIES

alcohol use: Possibly additive CNS depression

Adverse Reactions

CNS: Asthenia, confusion, depression, dizziness, drowsiness, fatigue, fever, headache, insomnia, irritability, nervousness, paresthesia, seizures, tremor, weakness

CV: Arrhythmias, including tachycardia; orthostatic hypotension; palpitations; vasodilation

EENT: Blurred vision, diplopia, dry mouth, transient vision loss, unpleasant taste

GI: Constipation, hiccups, indigestion, nausea, vomiting

GU: Libido changes, urinary frequency, urine retention

SKIN: Diaphoresis, facial flushing, pruritus, rash

Nursing Considerations
• Use cyclobenzaprine cautiously in patients with history of low seizure threshold.
• If possible, avoid giving drug to elderly patients because of its anticholinergic effects.
• To prevent falls, take safety precautions if patient is confused, dizzy, or weak.

PATIENT TEACHING
• Urge patient to avoid alcohol and other CNS depressants during therapy.
• Inform patient about possible lack of alertness and dexterity.
• Advise patient to ask for assistance with walking, driving, or hazardous activities if he experiences dizziness or weakness.

cycloserine

Seromycin

Class and Category
Chemical class: D-alanine analogue, *Streptomyces garyphalus* or *Streptomyces orchidaceus* derivative
Therapeutic class: Antitubercular
Pregnancy category: C

Indications and Dosages
➤ *To treat tuberculosis with other antituberculotics after failure of primary drugs, including ethambutol, isoniazid, pyrazinamide, rifampin, streptomycin*

CAPSULES
Adults and adolescents. 250 mg every 12 hr for 2 wk, then every 6 to 8 hr for 2 wk. Dosage increased gradually to maintain blood cycloserine level below 30 mcg/ml. *Maximum:* 1 g daily.
Children. 10 to 20 mg/kg daily in divided doses every 12 hr. *Maximum:* 1 g daily.

Contraindications
Chronic alcoholism, depression, hypersensitivity to cycloserine or its components, psychosis, renal disease, seizure disorder, severe anxiety

Interactions
DRUGS
ethionamide: Possibly increased risk of seizures
isoniazid: Possibly increased risk of adverse CNS effects
phenytoin: Possibly increased blood phenytoin level
pyridoxine: Possibly anemia or peripheral neuritis

ACTIVITIES
alcohol use: Possibly increased risk of seizures

> ### Mechanism of Action
> Inhibits bacterial cell wall synthesis in gram-positive organisms, including *Mycobacterium tuberculosis*. In early stages of bacterial cell wall synthesis, cycloserine inhibits two enzymes that help form peptidoglycan, which is needed to make the cell membrane rigid and protective.

Adverse Reactions
CNS: Aggression, anxiety, coma, confusion, depression, dizziness, drowsiness, headache, irritability, lethargy, memory loss, nervousness, nightmares, psychosis, restlessness, seizures, suicidal tendencies, tremor, vertigo
CV: Heart failure
HEME: Leukocytosis, megaloblastic anemia
MS: Dysarthria, hyperreflexia
SKIN: Dermatitis, photosensitivity
Other: Folic acid deficiency, vitamin B$_{12}$ deficiency

Nursing Considerations
• Monitor blood cycloserine level, as appropriate. Blood level should be maintained at 25 to 30 mcg/ml.
• Monitor mental status, mood, and affect for aggression or depression.
• Monitor CBC to detect blood dyscrasias.
• To prevent injury from falls, take safety precautions if adverse CNS reactions, such as dizziness or drowsiness, develop.

PATIENT TEACHING
• Urge patient to avoid alcohol while taking cycloserine.
• Instruct patient to seek help immediately if he has suicidal thoughts.
• Advise patient to avoid driving and to ask for assistance with walking or hazardous activities if he develops adverse CNS reactions, such as dizziness and drowsiness.
• Tell patient to contact prescriber if symptoms haven't improved after 2 to 3 weeks.

•Emphasize the importance of complying with drug therapy because effective treatment may take years to complete.

cyclosporine
(cyclosporin A)

Neoral, Sandimmune, SangCya

Class and Category

Chemical class: Tolypocladium inflatum Gams– or Cylindrocarpon lucidum Booth–derived polypeptide
Therapeutic class: Antipsoriatic, antirheumatic, immunosuppressant
Pregnancy category: C

Indications and Dosages

➤ *To prevent or treat organ rejection in kidney, liver, and heart allogenic transplantation*
CAPSULES, MODIFIED CAPSULES, MODIFIED ORAL SOLUTION, ORAL SOLUTION

Adults and children. *Initial:* 12 to 15 mg/kg daily in divided doses every 12 hr starting 4 to 12 hr before surgery and continuing 1 to 2 wk afterward. Then, dosage reduced by 5% every wk to maintenance dose. *Maintenance:* 5 to 10 mg/kg daily in divided doses every 12 hr.

I.V. INFUSION

Adults. 2 to 6 mg/kg daily starting 4 to 12 hr before surgery and continuing afterward until patient can tolerate oral form of drug.

➤ *To treat severe rheumatoid arthritis*
MODIFIED CAPSULES, MODIFIED ORAL SOLUTION

Adults. 2.5 mg/kg daily in divided doses every 12 hr, increased by 0.5 to 0.75 mg/kg daily after 8 wk and again after 12 wk. *Maximum:* 4 mg/kg daily.

➤ *To treat psoriasis*
MODIFIED CAPSULES, MODIFIED ORAL SOLUTION

Adults. *Initial:* 2.5 mg/kg daily in divided doses b.i.d., increased by 0.5 mg/kg daily after 4 wk. Then dosage increased every 2 wk, if needed. *Maximum:* 4 mg/kg daily.

Contraindications

Abnormal renal function, neoplastic diseases, and uncontrolled hypertension in patients with psoriasis or rheumatoid arthritis (modified capsules and oral solution); hypersensitivity to cyclosporine, its components, or polyoxyethylated castor oil (I.V. infusion)

Mechanism of Action

Causes immunosuppression by inhibiting the proliferation of T lymphocytes, the production and release of lymphokines, and the release of interleukin-2.

Interactions
DRUGS

ACE inhibitors, angiotensin II receptor antagonists, potassium-sparing diuretics, potassium supplements: Increased risk of hyperkalemia
allopurinol, amiodarone, azithromycin, bromocriptine, clarithromycin, colchicine, danazol, diltiazem, erythromycin, fluconazole, hormonal contraceptives, imatinib, itraconazole, ketoconazole, methylprednisolone, metoclopromide, nicardipine, oral contraceptives, quinupristin and dalfopristin, verapamil, voriconazole: Increased cyclosporine level
amphotericin B, azapropazon, cimetidine, ciprofloxacin, colchicine, co-trimoxazole, fibric acid derivatives (bezafibrate, fenofibrate), gentamicin, ketoconazole, melphalan, NSAIDs, ranitidine, tacrolimus, tobramycin, vancomycin: Increased risk of nephrotoxicity
atorvastatin, fluvastatin, lovastatin, pravastatin, simvastatin: Risk of myotoxicity
bosentan, carbamazepine, nafcillin, octreotide, orlistat, oxcarbazepine, phenobarbital, phenytoin, rifampin, St. John's wort, sulfinpyrazone, terbinafine, ticlopidine: Decreased blood cyclosporine level and therapeutic response
digoxin: Increased blood digoxin level and risk of digitalis toxicity
indinavir, nelfinavir, ritonavir, saquinavir: Possibly increased blood cyclosporine level
methotrexate: Increased blood methotrexate level and risk of renal dysfunction
methylprednisolone (high dose): Increased risk of seizures
other immunosuppressants: Possibly excessive immunosuppression
prednisolone: Increased prednisolone level
sirolimus: Increased blood sirolimus level
vaccines (killed or live virus): Possibly suppressed immune response and increased adverse effects of vaccine
FOODS

Grapefruit, grapefruit juice: Increased risk of nephrotoxicity
Potassium-rich foods: Increased risk of hyperkalemia

Adverse Reactions

CNS: Altered level of consciousness, confusion, headache, intracranial hypertension, loss of motor function, paresthesia, psychiatric disturbances, seizures, tremor
CV: Chest pain, hypertension
EENT: Gingival hyperplasia, optic disc edema, oral candidiasis, visual impairment
ENDO: Gynecomastia
GI: Diarrhea, nausea, pancreatitis, vomiting
GU: Albuminuria, hematuria, proteinuria, renal failure
HEME: Anemia, leukopenia, thrombocytopenia
SKIN: Acne, flushing, hirsutism, rash
Other: Anaphylaxis, hyperkalemia, hypomagnesemia, life-threatening infections, lymphoma

Nursing Considerations

•Be aware that capsules and oral solution aren't interchangeable with modified capsules and modified oral solution. Modified forms have greater bioavailability.
•Prepare I.V. infusion by diluting each milliliter of concentrate in 20 to 100 ml of normal saline solution or D$_5$W. Use glass containers because of possible leaching of diethylhexyphthalate from polyvinyl chloride bags into cyclosporine solution.
•Administer I.V. infusion over 2 to 6 hr. If needed, the drug may be infused over 24 hr.
•**WARNING** Closely monitor for anaphylaxis at least during first 30 minutes of I.V. administration. Make sure emergency equipment and drugs are immediately available.
•**WARNING** Be aware that rapid I.V. infusion may cause acute nephrotoxicity.
•Don't draw blood to measure cyclosporine level through same I.V. tubing used to give drug, even if line was flushed after administration. Blood level may be falsely elevated.
•Discard diluted solution after 24 hours.
•Be aware that oral solution contains alcohol and shouldn't be administered to patient who drinks heavily or has a history of alcohol dependence.
•Don't add water to oral solution because it will alter drug's effectiveness.
•Avoid giving oral cyclosporine with grapefruit juice, which may raise trough level, increasing risk of nephrotoxicity.
•Monitor blood pressure, especially in patients with a history of hypertension, because

drug can worsen this condition. Expect to decrease dosage if hypertension develops.
•Monitor liver and renal function tests, as ordered, to detect decreased function.
•Although uncommon, cyclosporine may cause neurotoxicity, especially after liver transplantation. Watch for evidence of encephalopathy, such as impaired consciousness, loss of motor function, psychiatric disturbance, seizures, and visual disturbance.
•Be aware that cyclosporine use may result in increased serum cholesterol levels.
•Be aware that St. John's wort may decrease blood cyclosporine level.
•Store capsules at 77° F (25° C) in prepackaged foil wrap to protect them from light.
•Expect about 50% of patients treated for psoriasis to relapse about 4 months after therapy stops.

PATIENT TEACHING
•Instruct patient to take drug at same time each day and in same relation to type and timing of food intake to help increase compliance and maintain steady blood level.
•Advise patient to mix oral solution in a glass—not plastic—container with room-temperature orange or apple juice to improve flavor. Also advise him to avoid grapefruit juice because it alters drug metabolism.
•Instruct patient to use accompanying syringe supplied by manufacturer to ensure accurate measurement of oral solution dose and to wipe syringe—not rinse it—after use to prevent cloudiness.
•Advise patient not to stop taking drug without consulting prescriber.
•Instruct patient to avoid virus vaccines during therapy and people who have received such vaccines. Or, suggest wearing a protective mask when he's around them.
•Caution patient to avoid people who have infections during therapy because cyclosporine causes immunosuppression.
•Advise good dental hygiene because of risk of gingival hyperplasia.
•Advise patient to discard oral solution after it has been opened for 2 months.
•Inform patient with rheumatoid arthritis that drug effects may not appear for 4 to 6 weeks.
•Caution patient to avoid excessive exposure to ultraviolet light.

daclizumab
(dacliximab)

Zenapax

Class and Category

Chemical class: Monoclonal antibody
Therapeutic class: Immunosuppressant
Pregnancy category: C

Indications and Dosages

➤ *To prevent acute organ rejection after kidney transplantation*

I.V. INFUSION

Adults and children. 1 mg/kg given in 5 doses: dose 1 given no more than 24 hr before transplantation; doses 2 through 5, at 14-day intervals.

Mechanism of Action

Inhibits interleukin-2–mediated activation of lymphocytes, which prevents WBCs from attacking the transplanted kidney. Daclizumab also reduces the body's infection-fighting ability.

Contraindications

Hypersensitivity to daclizumab or its components

Adverse Reactions

CNS: Anxiety, chills, depression, dizziness, fatigue, fever, headache, insomnia, prickly sensation, tremor, weakness
CV: Chest pain, edema, hypertension, hypotension, tachycardia, thrombosis
EENT: Blurred vision, pharyngitis, rhinitis
ENDO: Hyperglycemia
GI: Abdominal distention and pain, constipation, diarrhea, flatulence, gastritis, heartburn, hemorrhoids, indigestion, nausea, vomiting
GU: Dysuria, hematuria, hydronephrosis, oliguria, renal insufficiency, renal tubular necrosis, urine retention
HEME: Bleeding
MS: Arthralgia, back pain, leg cramps, myalgia

RESP: Atelectasis, cough, crackles, dyspnea, hypoxia, lung congestion, pleural effusion, pulmonary edema
SKIN: Acne, diaphoresis, hirsutism, impaired wound healing, night sweats, pruritus, rash
Other: Dehydration, fluid overload, injection site pain and redness, lymphocele

Nursing Considerations

• Dilute calculated dose of daclizumab in 50 ml of normal saline solution. Gently invert bag to mix; to prevent foaming, don't shake it.
• Use room temperature solution within 4 hours or refrigerate it for up to 24 hours. Discard unused solution.
• Because daclizumab's compatibility with other drugs isn't known, don't add or simultaneously infuse other drugs through same I.V. line.
• Monitor blood glucose level for increases during therapy.
• **WARNING** Although daclizumab seldom causes severe hypersensitivity reactions, keep drugs to treat such a reaction nearby for immediate use.

PATIENT TEACHING

• Urge patient to complete the course of therapy and return for follow-up visits.

dalteparin sodium
(tedelparin)

Fragmin

Class and Category

Chemical class: Low-molecular-weight heparin
Therapeutic class: Anticoagulant, antithrombotic
Pregnancy category: B

Indications and Dosages

➤ *To prevent ischemic complications in patients who receive aspirin as part of treatment for unstable angina and non–Q-wave MI*

SUBCUTANEOUS INJECTION

Adults. 120 international units/kg every 12 hr with aspirin (75 to 165 mg daily) until patient is stable, usually 5 to 8 days. *Maximum:* 10,000 international units/dose.

➤ *To prevent blood clots in patients undergoing hip replacement surgery*

SUBCUTANEOUS INJECTION

Adults. *Initial:* 2,500 international units 1 to 2 hr before surgery, repeated in 8 to 12 hr and again 8 to 12 hr later. *Maintenance:* 5,000 international units every morning for 5 to 10 days postoperatively or until patient is fully ambulatory. *Alternate:* 5,000 international units the evening before surgery followed by 5,000 international units daily (starting the next evening) for 5 to 10 days or until patient is fully ambulatory.

➤ *To prevent blood clots in patients undergoing abdominal surgery who are at risk for thromboembolic complications*

SUBCUTANEOUS INJECTION

Adults. 2,500 international units daily, starting 1 to 2 hr before surgery and repeated for 5 to 10 days. For patients at high risk (those with cancer), 5,000 international units the evening before surgery, repeated daily for 5 to 10 days; or 2,500 international units 1 to 2 hr before surgery followed by 2,500 international units 12 hr later and then 5,000 international units daily for 5 to 10 days.

➤ *To prevent blood clots in patients with severe mobility restrictions during acute illness*

SUBCUTANEOUS INJECTION

Adults. 5,000 international units daily.

➤ *To treat symptomatic venous thromboembolism and prevent recurrence in patients with cancer*

SUBCUTANEOUS INJECTION

Adults. 200 international units/kg (not to exceed 18,000 international units) once daily for 30 days. Then 150 international units/kg once daily for 5 more mo.

Mechanism of Action

Binds to and accelerates the activity of antithrombin III, thus inhibiting thrombin and blocking the formation of fibrin clots.

Incompatibilities

Don't mix dalteparin with other drugs.

Contraindications

Active major bleeding; hypersensitivity to low-molecular-weight heparins, heparin, or pork products; thrombocytopenia associated with positive laboratory tests for antiplatelet antibodies in the presence of dalteparin

Interactions

DRUGS

NSAIDs, oral anticoagulants, platelet aggregation inhibitors, thrombolytics: Possibly increased risk of hemorrhage

Adverse Reactions

GI: Elevated liver emzymes
HEME: Hemorrhage, thrombocytopenia
SKIN: Alopecia, bullous eruption, necrosis, pruritus, rash
Other: Anaphylaxis, injection site hematoma and pain

Nursing Considerations

• Use dalteparin with extreme caution in patients with a history of heparin-induced thrombocytopenia; those at increased risk for hemorrhage (such as those who use a platelet inhibitor or have bacterial endocarditis, bleeding disorders, active ulcerative GI disease, uncontrolled hypertension, or hemorrhagic stroke); and those who have recently had brain, eye, or spinal surgery.

• Use drug cautiously in patients with bleeding diathesis, diabetic retinopathy, platelet defects, recent GI bleeding, severe hepatic or renal insufficiency, or thrombocytopenia.

• Before giving first dose, tell Jewish patients that drug comes from porcine intestine.

• Be aware that risk factors for thromboembolic events include age over 40, cancer, history of deep vein thrombosis or pulmonary embolism, obesity, and planned use of anesthesia for more than 30 minutes.

• Don't give drug by I.M. or I.V. injection.

• With the patient seated or supine, administer drug deep into subcutaneous tissue in U-shaped area around navel, upper outer thigh, or upper outer quadrant of buttocks. If using area around navel or on thigh, lift skin fold with thumb and forefinger while giving injection. Insert entire length of needle at a 45-to 90-degree angle. Rotate sites daily.

• Be aware that routine coagulation tests and dosage adjustments usually aren't required.

PATIENT TEACHING

• If therapy will continue at home, teach patient or caregiver to select injeciton sites, give subcutaneous injections, and rotate sites daily. Tell patient to discard drug if it's discolored or contains particles. Review safe

handling and disposal of syringes and needles.
•Teach patient to store drug at room temperature, away from moisture and heat.
•Urge patient to report adverse reactions, especially bleeding, and to seek help immediately if signs of thromboembolism develop, such as severe dyspnea (pulmonary embolism) or neurologic deficits (cerebral embolism).
•Stress the importance of follow-up visits.

danaparoid sodium

Orgaran

Class and Category

Chemical class: Glycosaminoglycan heparinoid, low-molecular-weight heparin
Therapeutic class: Anticoagulant, antithrombotic
Pregnancy category: B

Indications and Dosages

➤ *To prevent deep vein thrombosis after hip replacement surgery*
SUBCUTANEOUS INJECTION
Adults. 750 anti-factor Xa units b.i.d. (first dose 1 to 4 hr preoperatively; second dose no sooner than 2 hr after surgery) for 7 to 14 days, as indicated.

Mechanism of Action

Inhibits thrombin generation in coagulation pathway, thus preventing fibrin formation and clotting.

Contraindications

Active major bleeding (including hemorrhagic stroke); hypersensitivity to low-molecular-weight heparins, heparin, or pork products; severe hemorrhagic disorders, such as hemophilia and thrombocytopenic purpura; sulfite sensitivity; type II thrombocytopenia associated with positive laboratory tests for antiplatelet antibodies in the presence of danaparoid

Interactions

DRUGS
NSAIDs, oral anticoagulants, platelet aggregation inhibitors: Possibly increased risk of bleeding

Adverse Reactions

CNS: Asthenia, dizziness, fever, headache, insomnia
CV: Chest pain, edema
GI: Abdominal pain, constipation, nausea, vomiting
GU: Urine retention, UTI
HEME: Anemia, excessive bleeding
MS: Arthralgia, myalgia
SKIN: Pruritus, rash
Other: Anaphylaxis, injection site pain

Nursing Considerations

•Use danaparoid with extreme caution in patients who are at increased risk for hemorrhage (such as those with severe uncontrolled hypertension, acute bacterial endocarditis, bleeding disorders, active ulcerative GI disease, severe renal dysfunction, or nonhemorrhagic stroke); those with a postoperative indwelling epidural catheter; and those who have recently had brain, eye, or spinal surgery.
•Don't give drug by I.M. or I.V. injection.
•Administer drug with patient lying down. Use a 25G or 26G needle to minimize tissue trauma. Select site on left or right anterolateral or posterolateral abdominal wall. Hold skin fold gently between thumb and forefinger, and insert entire length of needle deep into subcutaneous tissue at a 45- to 90-degree angle. Don't pinch or rub site afterward. Rotate sites.
•Expect to monitor results of CBCs and fecal occult blood tests during therapy. Typical coagulation tests, such as PT, APTT, clotting time, whole blood clotting time, and thrombin time, aren't useful for monitoring danaparoid's anticoagulant effect.

PATIENT TEACHING
•Before administering first dose, inform Jewish patients that drug comes from porcine intestinal mucosa.
•If therapy must continue at home, teach patient or caregiver how to administer subcutaneous injections. Review appropriate injection sites, and instruct her to rotate them daily. Also instruct her to discard drug if it's discolored or contains particles. Review safe handling and disposal of syringes and needles.
•Teach patient to store drug at room temperature, away from moisture and heat.
•Instruct patient to consult prescriber before using aspirin, ibuprofen, indomethacin, ketoprofen, naproxen, and other NSAIDs because

D

they may increase the risk of bleeding.
•Advise patient to stop taking drug and seek help immediately if she experiences severe dizziness, fever, rash, wheezing, or prolonged or unexplained bleeding and pain at the injection site.

dantrolene sodium

Dantrium, Dantrium Intravenous

Class and Category

Chemical class: Hydantoin derivative, imidazolidinedione sodium salt
Therapeutic class: Antispastic, malignant hyperthermia therapy adjunct
Pregnancy category: C (parenteral), Not rated (oral)

Indications and Dosages

➤ *To treat chronic spastic conditions caused by severe chronic disorders, such as cerebral palsy, stroke, multiple sclerosis, and spinal cord injury*

CAPSULES

Adults and adolescents. *Initial:* 25 mg daily for 7 days. Then dosage increased to 25 mg/day every 4 to 7 days until desired response occurs or dosage reaches 100 mg q.i.d. *Maximum:* 400 mg daily.
Children. *Initial:* 0.5 mg/kg b.i.d. for 7 days. Then increased by 0.5 mg/kg daily every 4 to 7 days until desired response occurs or dosage reaches 3 mg/kg q.i.d. *Maximum:* 400 mg daily.

➤ *To prevent malignant hyperthermia before surgery*

CAPSULES

Adults and children. 4 to 8 mg/kg daily in divided doses t.i.d. or q.i.d. 1 or 2 days before surgery, with last dose given 3 to 4 hr before surgery.

I.V. INFUSION

Adults and children. *Initial:* 2.5 mg/kg 60 to 75 min before anesthesia and infused over 1 hr. Additional individualized doses given as needed during surgery.

➤ *To treat malignant hyperthermic crisis*

I.V. INJECTION

Adults and adolescents. *Initial:* 1 mg/kg by rapid bolus; repeated, p.r.n., until symptoms subside or cumulative dose of 10 mg/kg has been reached and if symptoms reappear.

➤ *To treat postmalignant hyperthermic crisis*

CAPSULES

Adults and children. 4 to 8 mg/kg daily in divided doses q.i.d. for 1 to 3 days.

I.V. INJECTION

Adults and children: *Initial:* Individualized dosage beginning with 1 mg/kg or more as needed if oral therapy can't be used. *Maximum:* 10 mg/kg total dose.

Route	Onset	Peak	Duration
P.O.	1 wk*	Unknown	Unknown

Mechanism of Action

Acts directly on skeletal muscle to reduce the force of reflex muscle contraction. This in turn reduces hyperreflexia, spasticity, involuntary movements, and clonus, probably by preventing calcium release from the sarcoplasmic reticulum of skeletal muscle cells. Blocked calcium release also inhibits the activation of acute catabolism associated with malignant hyperthermic crisis syndrome.

Incompatibilities

Don't administer parenteral dantrolene with acidic solutions, including D₅W and normal saline solution.

Contraindications

For oral drug only: Active hepatic disease (such as cirrhosis and hepatitis), conditions in which spasticity helps maintain upright posture and improve balance or function, skeletal muscle spasms caused by rheumatic disorders

Interactions

DRUGS

calcium channel blockers (especially verapamil): Possibly hyperkalemia, life-threatening arrhythmias, shock
hepatotoxic drugs: Increased risk of hepatotoxicity with long-term oral dantrolene use
sedatives: Possibly profound sedation

ACTIVITIES

alcohol use: Possibly increased CNS depression

---

* For spasticity; unknown for malignant hyperthermia.

Adverse Reactions

CNS: Chills, confusion, depression, dizziness, drowsiness, fatigue, fever, headache, insomnia, light-headedness, malaise, nervousness, seizures, slurred speech or other speech problems, weakness
CV: Heart failure (I.V.), labile blood pressure, pericarditis, phlebitis, tachycardia
EENT: Abnormal vision, altered taste, diplopia, lacrimation
GI: Abdominal cramps, anorexia, constipation, diarrhea, dysphagia, gastric irritation, GI bleeding, hepatitis, hepatotoxicity
GU: Crystalluria, dysuria, erectile dysfunction, hematuria, nocturia, urinary frequency, urinary incontinence, urine retention
MS: Backache, myalgia
RESP: Feeling of suffocation, pleural effusion
SKIN: Acne, diaphoresis, eczematoid eruption, erythema (I.V.), extravasation with tissue damage, hirsutism, pruritus, rash, urticaria

Nursing Considerations

•Use dantrolene cautiously in patients with impaired pulmonary function, especially those with COPD, and in those with severe cardiac or hepatic dysfunction.
•Reconstitute drug with 60 ml of sterile water for injection. Shake vial until clear. Store reconstituted solution at room temperature, protected from direct sunlight. Discard after 6 hours.
•To prevent precipitation, transfer reconstituted drug to a plastic I.V. bag, rather than a glass bottle, for infusion.
•Because drug has a high pH, infuse into a central vein, if possible, to avoid tissue damage from extravasation.
•Monitor blood pressure and heart rate frequently during drug administration to detect tachycardia and blood pressure changes.
•Notify prescriber if persistent diarrhea develops with oral therapy; drug may need to be stopped.
•Monitor results of liver function tests—especially ALT, AST, alkaline phosphatase, and total bilirubin levels—to detect hepatotoxicity. Expect to stop drug after 45 days if benefits aren't sufficient because the risk of hepatotoxicity increases with dose and time, especially for women and patients over age 35.

PATIENT TEACHING

•Advise patient to take dantrolene with food if gastric irritation develops.

•Inform patient that drug may weaken muscles used for walking and climbing stairs.
•Warn patient about drug's sedating effects. Caution her to avoid sedatives, unless prescribed, and other sedating substances, such as alcohol.
•Advise patient to report yellow skin or sclerae, itching, anorexia, and fatigue.
•Advise patient that if she misses a dose, she should wait until the next scheduled dose if more than 2 hours have passed since the missed dose. Instruct her not to double the dose.
•Caution patient not to stop taking drug without consulting prescriber. Gradual dosage reduction may be required, especially after long-term use.

daptomycin

Cubicin

Class and Category

Chemical class: Cyclic lipopeptide
Therapeutic class: Antibiotic
Pregnancy category: B

Indications and Dosages

➤ *To treat complicated skin and skin structure infections caused by* Staphylococcus aureus *(including methicillin-resistant isolates),* Streptococcus pyogenes, Streptococcus agalactiae, Streptococcus dysgalactiae *subspecies* Equisimilis, *and* Enterococcus faecalis *(vancomycin-susceptible isolates only)*

I.V. INFUSION

Adults. 4 mg/kg administered over 30 min daily for 7 to 14 days. *Maximum:* 6 mg/kg I.V. every 24 hr.

DOSAGE ADJUSTMENT For patients with creatinine clearance of less than 30 ml/min, 4 or 6 mg/kg (depending on infection type) once every 48 hr.

➤ *To treat* Staphylococcus aureus *bloodstream infections, including right-sided infective endocarditis, caused by methicillin-susceptible and methicillin-resistant isolates*

I.V. INFUSION

Adults. 6 mg/kg administered over 30 min daily for 2 to 6 wk. *Maximum:* 6 mg/kg I.V. every 24 hr.

DOSAGE ADJUSTMENT For patients with creatinine clearance of less than 30 ml/min/ 1.73 m^2, dosage is 4 or 6 mg/kg (depending on infection) once every 48 hr.

Mechanism of Action

Binds to bacterial membranes to cause rapid depolarization of membrane potential. This loss of membrane potential inhibits protein, DNA, and RNA synthesis, which results in bacterial cell death.

Contraindications

Hypersensitivity to daptomycin or its components

Interactions

DRUGS

HMG-CoA reductase inhibitors: Possibly increased CK level and increased risk of myopathy

Adverse Reactions

CNS: Anxiety, asthenia, confusion, dizziness, fever, headache, insomnia, peripheral neuropathy

CV: Cardiac failure, chest pain, hypertension, hypotension, peripheral edema, supraventricular tachycardia

EENT: Pharyngolaryngeal pain, oral candidiasis, sore throat

ENDO: Hyperglycemia, hypoglycemia

GI: Abdominal pain, anorexia, constipation, diarrhea, dyspepsia, dysphagia, elevated liver enzymes, GI hemorrhage, nausea, pseudomembranous diarrhea, vomiting

GU: Renal failure, UTI, vaginal candidiasis

HEME: Anemia, eosinophilia, increased INR, leukocytosis, thrombocytopenia, thrombocytosis

MS: Arthralgia, back or limb pain, elevated myoglobin level, myopathy, rhabdomyolysis, osteomyelitis

RESP: Cough, dyspnea, pleural effusion, pneumonia, pulmonary eosinophilia, shortness of breath

SKIN: Cellulitis, diaphoresis, erythema, pruritus, rash, urticaria, vesiculobullous rash

Other: Anaphylaxis, bacteremia, elevated alkaline phosphatase level, elevated serum sodium bicarbonate level, fungal infection, hyperkalemia, hypokalemia, hypomagnesemia, injection site reactions, sepsis

Nursing Considerations

• Obtain blood samples for culture and sensitivity testing before starting daptomycin therapy.

• Reconstitute daptomycin powder by slowly transferring 10 ml of normal saline for injection into vial and pointing needle toward the wall of the vial to minimize foaming. Then gently rotate vial until all powder is wet. Don't agitate or shake the vial. Let vial stand undisturbed for 10 minutes, and then gently rotate or swirl contents for a few minutes, as needed, to obtain a completely reconstituted solution.

• Further dilute reconstituted daptomycin solution with normal saline for injection, and give by I.V. infusion over 30 minutes. Reconstituted drug is stable in infusion bag for 12 hours at room temperature or 48 hours refrigerated.

• Daptomycin may cause a significant false increase in PT and INR. If this occurs during daptomycin therapy, draw blood sample just before next daptomycin dose and evaluate patient for other causes of the increase.

• Monitor patient closely for diarrhea, which may herald pseudomembranous colitis caused by *Clostridium difficile*. If diarrhea occurs, notify prescriber. If pseudomembranous colitis develops, expect to discontinue drug and give fluids, electrolytes, protein, and antibiotic effective against *C. difficile*.

• Monitor patient for evidence of superinfection, and inform prescriber if present. Expect to stop datomycin and give appropriate care.

• Assess patient for muscle pain or weakness, especially of the distal limbs. Expect to monitor CK level weekly or more often in patients recently or currently taking an HMG-CoA reductase inhibitor. Expect to discontinue daptomycin, as ordered, if patient has myopathy or marked elevation in CK level.

• Monitor patient's BUN and serum creatinine levels closely, especially if renal insufficiency is already present.

PATIENT TEACHING

• Inform patient that diarrhea may occur 2 months or longer after daptomycin therapy stops. If severe or prolonged, advise patient to notify prescriber as soon as possible because additional treatment may be needed.

• Urge patient to immediately report muscle pain, tenderness, or weakness and other symptoms of myopathy.

darbepoetin alfa

Aranesp

Class and Category

Chemical class: 165-amino acid glycoprotein identical to human erythropoietin
Therapeutic class: Antianemic
Pregnancy category: C

Indications and Dosages

➤ *To treat anemia from chronic renal failure*

I.V. OR SUBCUTANEOUS INJECTION

Adults. *Initial:* 0.45 mcg/kg as a single dose every wk. *Maintenance:* Dosage individualized and increased once a month to maintain a hemoglobin level not to exceed 12 g/dl.

DOSAGE ADJUSTMENT Dosage reduced by about 25% if hemoglobin level increases and approaches 12 g/dl. If hemoglobin level continues to increase, doses temporarily withheld until hemoglobin level begins to decrease; then therapy is restarted at a dose about 25% below previous dose. Dosage reduced by about 25% if hemoglobin level increases by more than 1 g/dl in a 2-wk period. Dosage increased by about 25% of previous dose if hemoglobin level increases less than 1 g/dl over 4 wk but only if serum ferritin level is 100 mcg/L or greater and serum transferrin saturation is 20% or greater. Further increases made at 4-wk intervals until specified hemoglobin level is obtained.

DOSAGE ADJUSTMENT For conversion from epoetin alfa to darbepoetin alfa, dosage administered every wk for patient who previously received epoetin alfa 2 to 3 times/wk and once every 2 wk for patient who previously received epoetin alfa once/wk. For patients being converted from epoetin alfa, 6.25 mcg/wk darbepoetin alfa given every wk for patients who received less than 2,500 units/wk of epoetin alfa; 12.5 mcg/wk darbepoetin alfa given every wk for patients who received 2,500 to 4,999 units/wk of epoetin alfa; 25 mcg/wk darbepoetin alfa given every wk for patients who received 5,000 to 10,999 units/wk of epoetin alfa; 40 mcg/wk darbepoetin alfa given every wk for patients who received 11,000 to 17,999 units/wk of epoetin alfa; 60 mcg/wk darbepoetin alfa given every wk for patients who received 18,000 to 33,999 units/wk of epoetin alfa; 100 mcg/wk darbepoetin alfa given every wk for patients who received 34,000 to 89,999 units/wk of epoetin alfa; 200 mcg/wk darbepoetin alfa given every wk for patients who received 90,000 or more units/wk of epoetin alfa.

➤ *To treat chemotherapy-induced anemia in patients with nonmyeloid malignancies who have a hemoglobin level less than 10 g/dl*

SUBCUTANEOUS INJECTION

Adults. *Initial:* 2.25 mcg/kg as a single dose every wk. *Maintenance:* Dosage individualized to maintain a target hemoglobin level.

DOSAGE ADJUSTMENT Dosage increased up to 4.5 mcg/kg if hemoglobin level increases less than 1.0 g/dl after 6 wk of therapy. If hemoglobin level increases by more than 1.0 g/dl over 2 wk or if it exceeds 12 g/dl, dosage reduced by about 25%. If hemoglobin level exceeds 13 g/dl, doses temporarily withheld until it falls to 12 g/dl. Then darbepoetin alfa therapy is restarted at a dose about 25% less than last dose given.

Route	Onset	Peak	Duration
I.V., SubQ	In 2 to 6 wk	Unknown	Unknown

Mechanism of Action

Stimulates the release of reticulocytes from the bone marrow into the bloodstream, where they develop into mature RBCs.

Incompatibilities

Don't mix darbepoetin alfa with any other drug.

Contraindications

Hypersensitivity to human albumin or products made from mammal cells; uncontrolled hypertension

Interactions

DRUGS

None known

Adverse Reactions

CNS: Asthenia, dizziness, fatigue, fever, headache, seizures, stroke, transient ischemic attack
CV: Acute MI, angina, arrhythmias, cardiac arrest, chest pain, congestive heart failure, hypertension, hypotension, peripheral edema,

vascular access hemorrhage, vascular access thrombosis

GI: Abdominal pain, constipation, diarrhea, nausea, vomiting

MS: Arthralgia, back pain, limb pain, muscle spasm, myalgia

RESP: Bronchitis, cough, dyspnea, pneumonia, pulmonary embolism, upper respiratory tract infection

SKIN: Pruritus, rash, urticaria

Other: Dehydration, fluid overload, infection, flulike symptoms, injection site pain, sepsis

Nursing Considerations

• Before starting darbepoetin alfa therapy, expect to correct folic acid or vitamin B$_{12}$ deficiencies because these conditions may interfere with drug's effectiveness.

• Darbepoetin alfa shouldn't be given to cancer patients when a cure is anticipated because drug may decrease survival rate and increase tumor progression in patients with certain types of cancers, such as breast, non-small cell lung, head and neck, lymphoid, and cervical cancers.

• To ensure effective drug response, expect to obtain serum ferritin level and serum transferrin saturation before beginning and during therapy, as ordered. If serum ferritin level is less than 100 mcg/L or serum transferrin saturation is less than 20%, expect to begin supplemental iron therapy.

• Don't shake vial during preparation to avoid denaturing drug and rendering it biologically inactive.

• Discard drug if you see particulate matter or discoloration.

• Don't dilute drug before giving it.

• Be aware that needle cover on prefilled syringe contains dry natural rubber and may cause allergic reaction in those with latex sensitivity.

• Discard unused portion of drug because it contains no preservatives.

• Monitor blood pressure frequently during therapy for hypertension. Expect to reduce dosage or withhold drug if blood pressure is poorly controlled with antihypertensive and dietary measures.

• Monitor hemoglobin level weekly, as ordered, until hemoglobin stabilizes and maintenance dosage has been achieved. Thereafter, monitor hemoglobin level regularly, as ordered. After each dosage adjustment, expect to monitor hemoglobin level weekly for 4 weeks until hemoglobin level stabilizes in response to dosage change.

• **WARNING** If hemoglobin level increases more than about 1 g/dl during any 2-week period or it exceeds 12 g/dl, the risk of cardiac arrest, seizures, stroke, worsened hypertension, congestive heart failure, vascular thrombosis, vascular ischemia, vascular infarction, acute MI, fluid overload with peripheral edema, tumor prgression, and shortened survival increases. Expect to decrease darbepoetin dosage if this occurs.

• Expect to discontinue darbepoetin in cancer patients if hemoglobin level hasn't increased after 8 weeks of therapy or if patient continues to need transfusions despite therapy.

• Institute seizure precautions according to facility policy.

• For patients with chronic renal failure who aren't receiving dialysis, expect to administer doses lower than those given to patients receiving dialysis. Also, monitor renal function test results and fluid and electrolyte balance in these patients for signs of deteriorating renal function. If patient is transitioned to dialysis, monitor hemoglobin and blood pressure closely and expect maintenance dosage to be adjusted, as needed.

• Store drug at 2° to 8° C (36° to 46° F). Don't freeze, and do protect from light.

PATIENT TEACHING

• Advise patient that the risk of seizures is highest during the first 90 days of drug therapy. Discourage her from engaging in hazardous activities during this time.

• Stress the importance of complying with the dosage regimen and keeping follow-up medical and laboratory appointments.

• Advise patient to follow up with her prescriber for blood pressure monitoring.

• Encourage patient to eat adequate quantities of iron-rich foods.

• If patient will self-administer darbepoetin, teach her and her caregiver the proper administration technique.

• Caution patient and her caregiver not to reuse needles, syringes, or drug product. Thoroughly instruct them in proper needle and syringe disposal using a puncture-resistant container.

• Explain that needle cover on prefilled syringe contains dry natural rubber and may cause allergic reaction in those with latex sensitivity.

• Review possible adverse reactions, and urge patient to notify prescriber if she experiences chest pain, headache, rash, seizures, shortness of breath, or swelling.

darifenacin

Enablex

Class and Category

Chemical class: Muscarinic receptor antagonist
Therapeutic class: Bladder antispasmodic
Pregnancy category: C

Indications and Dosages

➤ *To treat overactive urinary bladder with symptoms of urge incontinence, including urgency and frequency*

E.R. TABLETS

Adults. *Initial:* 7.5 mg daily, increased to 15 mg daily after 2 wk as needed.

DOSAGE ADJUSTMENT For patients with moderate hepatic impairment and patients taking potent CYP3A4 inhibitors (such as clarithromycin, itraconazole, ketoconazole, nefazodone, nelfinavir, and ritonavir) daily dosage should not exceed 7.5 mg.

Route	Onset	Peak	Duration
P.O.	Unknown	7 hr	Unknown

Mechanism of Action

Antagonizes effect of acetylcholine on muscarinic receptors in detrusor muscle, decreasing muscle spasms that cause inappropriate bladder emptying. This action increases bladder capacity and volume, which relieves sensations of urgency and frequency and enhances bladder control.

Contraindications

Gastric retention, hypersensitivity to darifenacin or its components, uncontrolled narrow-angle glaucoma, urine retention, and patients at risk for these conditions

Interactions

DRUGS

anticholinergics: Increased frequency and severity of anticholinergic adverse reactions
flecainide, thioridazine, tricyclic antidepressants: Increased risk of toxicity of these drugs
potent CYP3A4 inhibitors (such as clarithromycin, itraconazole, ketoconazole, nefazodone, nelfinavir, and ritonavir): Decreased metabolism and increased effects of darifenacin, possibly increasing the risk of adverse reactions

Adverse Reactions

CNS: Asthenia, confusion, dizziness, hallucinations
CV: Hypertension, peripheral edema
EENT: Abnormal vision, dry eyes or mouth, pharyngitis, rhinitis, sinusitis
GI: Abdominal pain, constipation, diarrhea, indigestion, nausea, vomiting
GU: Urine retention, UTI, vaginitis
MS: Arthralgia, back pain
RESP: Bronchitis
SKIN: Dry skin, pruritus, rash
Other: Angioedema, flulike symptoms, hypersensitivity reactions, weight gain

Nursing Considerations

• Administer darifenacin cautiously to patients with significant bladder outflow obstruction because they have an increased risk of urine retention.
• Use darifenacin cautiously in patients with severe constipation, ulcerative colitis, or myasthenia gravis because darifenacin may decrease GI motility. Also use darifenacin cautiously in patients with obstructive GI disorders because drug increases the risk of gastric retention.

PATIENT TEACHING

• Tell patient to swallow tablets with liquid and not to crush, split, or break them.
• Advise patient to avoid exercising in hot weather because darifenacin decreases sweating, increasing the risk of heatstroke.
• Caution patient to avoid hazardous activities until drug's CNS effects are known.

decitabine

Dacogen

Class and Category

Chemical class: Analogue of natural nucleoside 2′-deoxycytidine
Therapeutic class: Antineoplastic
Pregnancy category: D

Indications and Dosages

➤ *To treat myelodysplastic syndromes (MDS) including secondary MDS of all French-American-British subtypes and intermediate 1 and 2 and high-risk International Prognostic Scoring System groups*

I.V. INFUSION

Adults. 15 mg/m² over 3 hr, repeated every 8 hr for 3 days with cycle repeated every 6 wk for at least four cycles.

DOSAGE ADJUSTMENT For hematologic recovery that requires more than 6 wk but less than 8 wk, doses delayed for up to 2 wk and temporarily reduced to 11 mg/m² every 8 hr. For hematologic recovery that requires more than 8 wk but less than 10 wk, doses delayed up to 2 more wk and reduced to 11 mg/m² every 8 hr, maintained or increased in subsequent cycles as clinically indicated.

Mechanism of Action

Inhibits DNA methyltransferase after phosphorylation and direct incorporation into DNA, resulting in hypomethylation of the DNA and cellular differentiation. In neoplastic cells, hypomethylation may restore normal function to genes essential for controlling cellular differentiation and proliferation. In rapidly dividing cells, decitabine also may cause cell death by forming covalent adducts between DNA methyltransferase and decitabine-saturated DNA.

Contraindications

Hypersensitivity to decitabine or its components

Adverse Reactions

CNS: Anxiety, confusion, dizziness, fatigue, fever, headache, hypoesthesia, insomnia, lethargy, malaise, rigors
CV: Chest discomfort or pain, hypotension, peripheral edema
EENT: Bleeding gums, blurred vision, lip or tongue ulceration, oral mucous petechiae, oral candidasis, pharyngitis, postnasal drip, sinusitis, stomatitis
ENDO: Hyperglycemia
GI: Abdominal distention or pain, anorexia, ascites, abdominal pain, constipation, decreased appetite, diarrhea, dysphagia, dyspepsia, gastroesophageal reflux disease, hyperbilirubinemia, nausea, vomiting
GU: Dysuria, urinary frequency, UTI
HEME: Anemia, leukopenia, neutropenia, thrombocytopenia, thrombocythemia
MS: Arthralgia, back or limb pain, myalgia
RESP: Decreased breath sounds, cough, crackles, hypoxia, pneumonia, pulmonary edema
SKIN: Alopecia, cellulites, ecchymosis, erythema, hematoma, pallor, petechiae, pruritus, rash, urticaria
Other: Bacteremia; candidal infection; dehydration; facial edema; hyperkalemia; hypoalbuminemia; hypokalemia; hypomagnesemia; hyponatremia; injection site swelling, pain, and redness; lymphodenpathy

Nursing Considerations

• Use cautiously in patients with liver or renal impairment.
• Follow facility protocols for preparing and handling antineoplastic drugs and for disposing of used equipment.
• Reconstitute with 10 ml sterile water using aseptic technique; each milliliter contains about 5 mg of decitabine. Immediately after reconstitution, further dilute with normal saline solution, dextrose 5%, or lactated Ringer's solution to a final concentration of 0.1 to 1 mg/ml. Use within 15 minutes. If delay is expected, reconstitute drug using cold dilution solution and store in refrigerator for up to 7 hours.
• Monitor CBC, including hematocrit, platelet count, and WBC with differential as well as electrolyte, liver enzyme, and serum creatinine levels before and intermittently during decitabine therapy, as ordered.
• If patient develops leukopenia, look for evidence of infection, such as fever. Expect to obtain appropriate specimens for culture and sensitivity testing.
• **WARNING** Monitor patient closely for nonhematological toxicities, such as active or uncontrolled infection, serum creatinine level greater than 2 mg/dl, or serum glutamic pyruvic transaminase or total bilirubin 2 or more times the upper limit of normal. If present, notify prescriber and expect decitabine therapy to be withheld until resolved.

PATIENT TEACHING

• Advise male patients not to father a child

during decitabine therapy and for 2 months after. Also urge female patients to use contraception to avoid pregnancy during therapy and to notify prescriber immediately if pregnancy occurs.

•Urge patient to have needed dental work completed before starting decitabine therapy, if possible, or to defer such work until blood counts return to normal because decitabine can delay healing and cause gingival bleeding. Teach patient proper oral hygiene, and advise him to use a soft-bristled toothbrush.

•If patient develops bone marrow depression, instruct him to avoid people with infections and to report fever, cough, or lower back or side pain; they may indicate infection.

•Stress the need to avoid accidental cuts from sharp objects, such as razor blades or fingernail clippers, because excessive bleeding or infection may occur.

•Advise patient with stomatitis to eat bland, soft foods served cold or at room temperature to decrease irritation.

•Stress the need to comply with the dosage regimen and to keep follow-up medical and laboratory appointments.

deferasirox

Exjade

Class and Category
Chemical class: Benzoic acid
Therapeutic class: Iron chelator
Pregnancy category: B

Indications and Dosages
➤ *To treat chronic iron overload caused by blood transfusions*

TABLETS
Adults and children age 2 and over. *Initial:* 20 mg/kg/day; then increased by 5 to 10 mg/kg every 3 to 6 months. Maximum: 30 mg/kg/day.

Route	Onset	Peak	Duration
P.O.	Unknown	1.5 to 4 hr	Unknown

Contraindications
Hypersensitivity to deferasirox or its components, hearing impairment

Interactions
DRUGS
aluminum-containing antacids: Possibly de-

creased effectiveness of deferasirox
other iron chelators: Possibly combined effect
anticoagulants, corticosteroids, NSAIDs, oral bisphosphonates: Increased risk of GI ulceration or hemorrhage
cyclosporine, hormonal contraceptives, midazolam, simvastatin: Possibly decreased effectiveness of these drugs

FOODS
all foods: increased bioavailability of deferasirox

Mechanism of Action
Binds iron with high affinity and removes it from the body in feces. Deferasirox is a tridentate ligan.

Adverse Reactions
CNS: Dizziness, fatigue, fever, headache, hyperactivity, insomnia
EENT: Acute tonsillitis, cataracts, decreased hearing, ear infection, elevated intraocular pressure, high-frequency hearing loss, lens opacities, nasopharyngitis, pharyngolaryngeal pain, pharyngitis, retinal disturbances, rhinitis
GI: Abdominal pain, diarrhea, elevated liver enzymes, gallstones, hepatic failure, hepatitis, nausea, pancreatitis, upper GI ulceration and hemorrhage, vomiting
GU: Acute renal failure, glycosuria, increased creatinine level, proteinuria, renal tubulopathy
HEME: Agranulocytosis, neutropenia, thrombocytopenia
MS: Arthralgia, back pain
RESP: Bronchitis, cough, respiratory tract infection
SKIN: Leukocytoclastic vascultitis, purpura, rash, urticaria
Other: Anaphylaxis, angioedema, drug fever, influenza

Nursing Considerations
•Because deferasirox can cause renal failure, obtain a baseline assessment of patient's renal function by collecting blood samples to measure serum creatinine level twice before starting deferasirox therapy. When therapy starts, monitor serum creatinine level, as ordered, especially in elderly patients, patients taking other drugs that depress renal func-

tion, and patients with increased risk of complications, pre-existing renal conditions, or comorbid conditions. For patients at increased risk for renal failure, expect to monitor serum creatinine level weekly for the first month of therapy and then monthly thereafter. Report increased serum creatinine level, and expect deferasirox dosage to be decreased.

•Obtain auditory and ophthalmic testing (including slit lamp examination and dilated fundoscopy) before deferasirox therapy begins and yearly thereafter, as ordered, because drug infrequently causes auditory or visual disturbances.

•Monitor patient's blood counts regularly, as ordered, because deferasirox can cause cytopenias. If cytopenia occurs, expect drug to be discontinued until blood counts return to normal.

•Monitor patient's liver enzymes monthly, as ordered, because deferasirox may cause liver impairment. Notify prescriber if elevations occur, and expect to decrease dose for severe or persistent elevations.

•Especially in the first month of therapy, assess patient closely for hypersensitivity reactions, such as anaphylaxis or angioedema. Notify prescriber immediately if present, and expect drug to be discontinued. Provide appropriate medical intervention, as needed.

•Inspect patient's skin regularly for rash. If it occurs and becomes severe, drug may be withheld temporarily.

PATIENT TEACHING

•Instruct patient to take deferasirox 30 minutes before eating. Tell her to completely disperse the tablet in water, orange juice, or apple juice; drink the suspension immediately; and then add liquid to any remaining residue and drink again.

•Tell patient to avoid taking aluminum-based antacids at the same time as deferasirox and to seek prescriber advice before taking other drugs, including OTC preparations such as NSAIDs, because of potential interactions.

•Advise her to report any hearing or visual disturbances.

•If patient has diarrhea or vomiting, tell her to notify prescriber and to maintain adequate hydration.

•Caution her to avoid hazardous activities, such as driving, if she becomes dizzy.

demeclocycline hydrochloride

Declomycin

Class and Category

Chemical class: Tetracycline derivative
Therapeutic class: Antibiotic
Pregnancy category: D

Indications and Dosages

➤ *To treat Rocky Mountain spotted fever, typhus infections, Q fever, and rickettsialpox and tick fevers caused by* Rickettsieae; *psittacosis (ornithosis), lymphogranuloma venereum, granuloma inguinale, and* Mycoplasma pneumoniae *or* Borrelia recurrentis *infections; infections caused by gram-negative organisms, such as* Bacteroides *species,* Bartonella bacilliformis, Brucella *species,* Campylobacter fetus, Francisella tularensis, Haemophilus ducreyi, Vibrio cholerae, *and* Yersinia pestis; *infections caused by susceptible strains of* Acinetobacter calcoaceticus, Enterobacter aerogenes, Escherichia coli, Haemophilus influenzae *(respiratory tract infections),* Herellea *species,* Klebsiella *species (respiratory tract infections and UTIs), and* Shigella *species; infections caused by susceptible strains of* Staphylococcus aureus *(skin and soft-tissue infections) and* Streptococcus *species; infections caused by* Actinomyces *species,* Bacillus anthracis, Clostridium *species,* Fusobacterium fusiforme, Listeria monocytogenes, Treponema pallidum, *and* Treponema pertenue; *and acute intestinal amebiasis*

CAPSULES, TABLETS

Adults and adolescents. 150 mg every 6 hr or 300 mg every 12 hr.

Children ages 8 to 12. 6 to 12 mg/kg daily in divided doses every 6 to 12 hr.

➤ *To treat gonorrhea*

CAPSULES, TABLETS

Adults and adolescents. 600 mg followed by 300 mg every 12 hr for 4 days for total dose of 3,000 mg.

Contraindications

Hypersensitivity to demeclocycline or other tetracyclines

Mechanism of Action

Binds with ribosomal subunits of susceptible bacteria and alters the cytoplasmic membrane, inhibiting bacterial protein synthesis and rendering the organism ineffective.

Interactions

DRUGS

antacids, calcium supplements, cholestyramine, choline, colestipol, iron supplements, magnesium-containing laxatives, magnesium salicylate, sodium bicarbonate: Decreased demeclocycline absorption
digoxin: Possibly increased blood digoxin level and risk of digitalis toxicity
methoxyflurane: Increased nephrotoxic effect
oral anticoagulants: Increased anticoagulant effects
oral contraceptives: Decreased contraceptive effectiveness
penicillins: Decreased bactericidal action of penicillins
vitamin A: Possibly benign intracranial hypertension

FOODS

milk, other dairy products: Decreased drug absorption

Adverse Reactions

CNS: Dizziness, headache, light-headedness, vertigo
EENT: Tinnitus, vision changes
GI: Abdominal cramps, diarrhea, nausea, pseudomembranous colitis, vomiting
GU: Elevated BUN level, nephrogenic diabetes insipidus
HEME: Eosinophilia, hemolytic anemia, neutropenia, thrombocytopenia
SKIN: Photosensitivity, pruritus, rash, urticaria
Other: Anaphylaxis, angioedema

Nursing Considerations

•Monitor results of renal and liver function tests during demeclocycline therapy, as indicated.
•**WARNING** Watch for development of nephrogenic diabetes insipidus during long-term therapy.
•Assess patient's bowel pattern daily; severe diarrhea may indicate pseudomembranous colitis caused by *Clostridium difficile.* If diarrhea occurs, notify prescriber and expect to withhold clindamycin and treat with fluids, electrolytes, protein, and an antibiotic effective against *C. difficile.*

PATIENT TEACHING

•Stress the importance of completing therapy as prescribed, even if symptoms improve before it's completed.
•Advise patient not to take demeclocycline within 3 hours of other drugs or dairy products; they may decrease its absorption.
•Instruct patient to avoid taking antacids while taking demeclocycline because of impaired absorption.
•Advise patient to avoid direct sunlight, use sunscreen, and wear protective clothing outdoors; among tetracyclines, demeclocycline causes the most photosensitivity.
•Urge patient to immediately report edema, rash, or other hypersensitivity reactions.
•Urge patient to report watery, bloody stools to prescriber immediately, even up to 2 months after drug therapy has ended.
•Advise patient to avoid hazardous activities if light-headedness, dizziness, or vertigo occurs.
•Instruct woman of childbearing age to notify prescriber if she may be pregnant; demeclocycline may need to be discontinued.

desipramine hydrochloride

Norpramin, Pertofrane (CAN)

Class and Category

Chemical class: Dibenzazepine derivative
Therapeutic class: Antidepressant
Pregnancy category: C

Indications and Dosages

➤ *To treat depression*

TABLETS

Adults. *Initial:* 100 to 200 mg daily as a single dose or in divided doses. Increased gradually to 300 mg daily, if needed. *Maximum:* 300 mg daily.
Adolescents. *Initial:* 25 to 50 mg daily in divided doses. Increased gradually, if needed. *Maximum:* 100 mg daily.
Children ages 6 to 12. *Initial:* 10 to 30 mg daily, or 1 to 5 mg/kg, in divided doses.
DOSAGE ADJUSTMENT For elderly patients, initial dosage decreased to 25 to 50 mg daily

in divided doses; increased gradually if needed to maximum of 150 mg daily.

Route	Onset	Peak	Duration
P.O.	2 to 3 wk	Unknown	Unknown

Mechanism of Action
Blocks serotonin and norepinephrine reuptake by adrenergic nerves, which normally release these neurotransmitters from their storage sites when activated by a nerve impulse. By blocking reuptake, this tricyclic antidepressant increases serotonin and norepinephrine levels at nerve synapses, which may elevate mood and reduce depression.

Contraindications
Acute recovery phase of MI; hypersensitivity to desipramine, other tricyclic antidepressants, or their components; MAO inhibitor therapy within 14 days

Interactions
DRUGS
activated charcoal: Prevention of desipramine absorption, reduced therapeutic effects
barbiturates: Decreased blood desipramine level, increased CNS depression
bupropion, haloperidol, H₂-receptor antagonists, valproic acid: Increased blood level and adverse effects of desipramine
carbamazepine: Increased blood carbamazepine level, decreased blood desipramine level
cimetidine: Increased blood desipramine level and anticholinergic effects (dry mouth, urine retention, blurred vision)
clonidine: Increased risk of hypertensive crisis
dicumarol: Increased anticoagulant effect
grepafloxacin, quinolones, sparfloxacin: Increased risk of arrhythmias, including torsades de pointes
guanethidine: Antagonized antihypertensive effect of guanethidine
levodopa: Delayed levodopa absorption, increased risk of hypotension
MAO inhibitors: Increased risk of life-threatening adverse effects, such as hyperpyretic or hypertensive crisis and severe seizures
phenothiazines: Increased desipramine level, risk of inhibited phenothiazine metabolism and neuroleptic malignant syndrome

quinidine: Increased blood quinidine level
rifamycins: Decreased desipramine effects
selective serotonin reuptake inhibitors: Increased desipramine effects
sympathomimetics: Possibly arrhythmias, possibly increased or decreased vasopressor effects of sympathomimetics
ACTIVITIES
alcohol use: Possibly increased CNS or respiratory depression, hypotension, alcohol effects

Adverse Reactions
CNS: Agitation, akathisia, anxiety, ataxia, confusion, delusions, disorientation, dizziness, drowsiness, exacerbation of psychosis, extrapyramidal reactions, fatigue, headache, hypomania, insomnia, lack of coordination, nervousness, nightmares, paresthesia, peripheral neuropathy, restlessness, seizures, sleep disturbance, stroke, suicidal ideation (children and teens), tremor, weakness
CV: Arrhythmias, including heart block; hypertension; hypotension; palpitations
EENT: Black tongue, blurred vision, dry mouth, mydriasis, stomatitis, taste perversion, tinnitus
ENDO: Breast enlargement and galactorrhea (in women), gynecomastia (in men), hyperglycemia, hypoglycemia, syndrome of inappropriate ADH secretion
GI: Abdominal cramps, anorexia, constipation, diarrhea, elevated liver function test results, elevated pancreatic enzyme levels, epigastric distress, hepatitis, ileus, increased appetite, nausea, vomiting
GU: Acute renal failure, impotence, libido changes, nocturia, painful ejaculation, testicular swelling, urinary frequency and hesitancy, urine retention
HEME: Agranulocytosis, eosinophilia, thrombocytopenia
SKIN: Acne, alopecia, dermatitis, diaphoresis, dry skin, flushing, petechiae, photosensitivity, pruritus, purpura, rash, urticaria
Other: Angioedema, drug fever, weight gain

Nursing Considerations
•Use desipramine with extreme caution in patients with cardiovascular disease, glaucoma, seizure disorder, thyroid disease, or urine retention.
•**WARNING** Desipramine increases the risk of suicidal ideation in children and teens; monitor them closely for evidence.
•**WARNING** Expect drug to produce sedation and possibly to lower seizure threshold. Take

safety and seizure precautions.
•Monitor blood glucose level frequently.
•Be prepared to obtain blood sample for leukocyte and differential counts from patients in whom fever develops during therapy.
•Expect to discontinue drug as soon as possible before elective surgery because of its possible adverse cardiovascular effects.

PATIENT TEACHING
•**WARNING** Urge parents to watch their child or teen closely and report abnormal thinking or behavior, aggression, and hostility.
•Urge patient to use sunscreen when outdoors and to avoid sunlamps and tanning beds.
•Instruct patient to notify prescriber immediately about a fast and pounding heartbeat, fainting, severe agitation or restlessness, and strange behavior or thoughts.
•Caution patient not to stop drug abruptly; doing so may cause dizziness, headache, hyperthermia, irritability, malaise, nausea, sleep disturbances, and vomiting.
•Advise against drinking alcohol because of increased risk of adverse CNS reactions.
•Advise patient to avoid hazardous activities until drug's CNS effects are known.
•Urge diabetic patient to monitor blood glucose level often.

desmopressin acetate

DDAVP Injection, DDAVP Nasal Spray, DDAVP Rhinal Tube, DDAVP Rhinyle Nasal Solution (CAN), DDAVP Tablets, Octostim (CAN), Stimate, Stimate Nasal Spray

Class and Category

Chemical class: Synthetic ADH analogue
Therapeutic class: Antidiuretic, antihemorrhagic
Pregnancy category: B

Indications and Dosages

➤ *To manage primary nocturnal enuresis*
TABLETS
Adults and children age 6 and over. *Initial:* 0.2 mg at bedtime, increased as needed. *Maximum:* 0.6 mg daily.

➤ *To control symptoms of central diabetes insipidus*
TABLETS
Adults and children age 6 and over. *Initial:* 0.05 mg b.i.d., increased as needed. *Usual:* 0.1 to 0.8 mg in divided doses b.i.d. or t.i.d.

Maximum: 1.2 mg daily.
I.V. INFUSION, I.M. OR SUBCUTANEOUS INJECTION
Adults. 2 to 4 mcg daily in divided doses b.i.d. Dosage adjusted as needed.
NASAL SOLUTION
Adults and adolescents. 0.1 to 0.4 ml daily (10 to 40 mcg daily) as a single dose or in divided doses b.i.d. or t.i.d. Dosage adjusted as needed. If daily dose is divided, each dose adjusted separately.
Children ages 3 months to 12 years. 0.25 mcg/kg daily as a single dose or in divided doses b.i.d. Dosage adjusted as needed. If daily dose is divided, each dose adjusted separately.

➤ *To prevent or manage bleeding episodes in hemophilia A or mild to moderate type I von Willebrand's disease*
I.V. INFUSION
Adults and children weighing more than 10 kg (22 lb). 0.3 mcg/kg diluted in 50 ml of normal saline solution and infused over 15 to 30 min. If used preoperatively, give 30 min before procedure.
Children weighing 10 kg or less. 0.3 mcg/kg diluted in 10 ml normal saline solution and infused over 15 to 30 min. If used preoperatively, given 30 min before procedure.
NASAL SOLUTION (STIMATE NASAL SPRAY)
Adults and children weighing more than 50 kg (110 lb). 150 mcg in each nostril. If used preoperatively, dose is given 2 hr before procedure.
Adults and children weighing 50 kg or less. 150 mcg in one nostril. If used preoperatively, dose is given 2 hr before procedure.

Route	Onset	Peak	Duration
P.O.	1 hr*	4 to 7 hr*	8 to 12 hr*
I.V.	15 to 30 min†	30 to 60 min†	3 hr‡
Nasal	In 1 hr*	1 to 5 hr*	8 to 20 hr*

Contraindications

Hypersensitivity to desmopressin or its components, moderate to severe renal impairment (creatinine clearance below 50 ml/min/1.73 m^2), previous or current hyponatremia

---

* For antidiuretic effect.
† For antihemorrhagic effect.
‡ For von Willebrand disease; 4 to 20 hr for mild hemophilia A.

D

Mechanism of Action

Exerts an antidiuretic effect similar to that of vasopressin by increasing cellular permeability of renal collecting ducts and distal tubules, thus enhancing water reabsorption, reducing urine flow, and increasing osmolality. As an antihemorrhagic, drug increases blood level of clotting factor VIII (antihemophilic factor) and activity of von Willebrand factor (factor VII$_{VWF}$). It also may increase platelet aggregation and adhesion at injury sites by directly affecting blood vessel walls.

Interactions

DRUGS

carbamazepine, chlorpromazine, lamotrigine, NSAIDs, opioid analgesics, selective serotonin reuptake inhibitors, tricyclic antidepressants: Possibly increased risk of water intoxication with hyponatremia
demeclocycline, lithium: Possibly decreased antidiuretic effect of desmopressin
imipramine, oxybutinin: Increased risk of hyponatremic seizures
vasopressor drugs: Possibly potentiated vasopressor effect of desmopressin

Adverse Reactions

CNS: Asthenia, chills, dizziness, headache, stroke
CV: Hypertension (with high doses), MI, thrombosis, transient hypotension
EENT: Conjunctivitis, epistaxis, lacrimation, nasal congestion (nasal form), ocular edema, pharyngitis, rhinitis
GI: Nausea
GU: Vulvar pain (parenteral form)
SKIN: Flushing
Other: Anaphylaxis, hyponatremia, injection site pain and redness; water intoxication

Nursing Considerations

• Use desmopressin cautiously in patients with conditions associated with fluid and electrolyte imbalance, such as cystic fibrosis, heart failure, and renal disorders; these patients are prone to hyponatremia.
• Also use cautiously in patients with habitual or psychogenic polydipsia; they may be more likely to drink excessive amounts of water, raising the risk of hyponatremia.
• Be aware that nasal cavity scarring, edema, and other abnormalities may cause erratic absorption and require the use of a different administration route.
• Monitor blood pressure often during therapy.
• **WARNING** Monitor patient closely for evidence of hyponatremia, such as headache, nausea, vomiting, restlessness, fatigue, lethargy, depressed reflexes, and changes in mental status. If left undetected, seizures, coma, and respiratory arrest may occur. Monitor patient's serum sodium level, and notify prescriber of abnormalities.

PATIENT TEACHING

• To prevent hyponatremia and water intoxication in a child or an elderly patient, instruct the family to restrict the patient's fluids as prescribed.
• Tell patient to refrigerate nasal solution.
• Teach patient to prime nasal spray pump (only once) and spray dose into one or both nostrils, as prescribed, while inhaling briskly. Instruct her to clean tip of sprayer with hot water and dry it with clean tissue. Advise her to keep track of doses given and to discard bottle after 50 doses.
• Instruct patient who uses Stimate Nasal Spray to prime pump before first use by pressing down four times. Advise her to discard pump after 25 or 50 doses, depending on bottle, because delivery of an accurate dose can't be assured.
• For nasal tube delivery, teach patient to draw prescribed amount of solution into calibrated flexible plastic tube, insert one end of tube into a nostril and the other end into her mouth, and gently blow into tube to deposit solution deep into nasal cavity. Caution her not to let drug drain into her mouth.
• Teach patient or caregiver how to administer subcutaneous injection, if appropriate.
• Urge patient to report adverse reactions.

dexamethasone

Decadron, Decadron Elixir, Deronil (CAN), Dexamethasone Intensol, Dexasone (CAN), Dexone, Hexadrol, Oradexon (CAN)

dexamethasone acetate

Cortastat LA, Dalalone D.P., Dalalone L.A., Decadron-LA, Decaject L.A., Dexacen LA-8, Dexacorten-LA, Dexasone L.A., Dexone LA, Solurex LA

dexamethasone sodium phosphate

Cortastat, Dalalone, Decadrol, Decadron Respihaler, Decaject, Dexacen-4, Dexacorten, Dexacort Turbinaire, Dexasone, Dexone, Hexadrol Phosphate, Primethasone, Solurex

Class and Category

Chemical class: Synthetic adrenocortical steroid
Therapeutic class: Anti-inflammatory, diagnostic aid, immunosuppressant
Pregnancy category: C

Indications and Dosages

➤ *To treat endocrine disorders, such as congenital adrenal hyperplasia, hypercalcemia associated with cancer, and nonsuppurative thyroiditis; acute episodes or exacerbations of rheumatic disorders; collagen diseases, such as systemic lupus erythematosus and acute rheumatic carditis; severe dermatologic diseases; severe allergic conditions, such as seasonal or perennial allergic rhinitis, bronchial asthma, serum sickness, and drug hypersensitivity reactions; respiratory diseases, such as symptomatic sarcoidosis, Löffler's syndrome, berylliosis, fulminating or disseminated pulmonary tuberculosis, and aspiration pneumonitis; hematologic disorders, such as idiopathic thrombocytopenic purpura and secondary thrombocytopenia in adults, autoimmune hemolytic anemia, aplastic crisis, and congenital hypoplastic anemia; tuberculous meningitis and trichinosis with neurologic or myocardial involvement*

➤ *To manage leukemias and lymphomas in adults and acute leukemia in children; to induce diuresis or remission of proteinuria in idiopathic nephrotic syndrome without uremia or nephrotic syndrome caused by systemic lupus erythematosus*

➤ *To provide palliative therapy during acute exacerbations of GI diseases, such as ulcerative colitis and regional enteritis*

ELIXIR, ORAL SOLUTION, TABLETS, I.V. OR I.M. INJECTION
Adults. Highly individualized dosage based

on severity of disorder. *Usual:* 0.75 to 9 mg/day as a single dose or in divided doses.

ELIXIR, ORAL SOLUTION, TABLETS
Children. Highly individualized dosage based on severity of disorder. *Usual:* 83.3 to 333.3 mcg/kg daily in divided doses t.i.d. or q.i.d.

I.M. INJECTION
Children. Highly individualized dosage based on severity of disorder. *Usual:* 27.76 to 166.65 mcg/kg every 12 to 24 hr.

➤ *To manage adrenocortical insufficiency*

ELIXIR, ORAL SOLUTION, TABLETS, I.V. OR I.M. INJECTION
Adults. 0.5 to 9 mg daily as a single dose or in divided doses.

ELIXIR, ORAL SOLUTION, TABLETS
Children. 23.3 mcg/kg daily in divided doses t.i.d.

I.M. INJECTION
Children. 23.3 mcg/kg daily in divided doses t.i.d. given every third day; alternatively, 7.76 to 11.65 mcg/kg daily.

➤ *To test for Cushing's syndrome*

ELIXIR, ORAL SOLUTION, TABLETS
Adults. 0.5 mg every 6 hr for 48 hr followed by collection of 24-hr urine specimen to determine 17-hydroxycorticosteroid level. Or, 1 mg at 11 p.m. followed by plasma cortisol test performed at 8 a.m. the next day.

➤ *To distinguish Cushing's syndrome related to pituitary corticotropin excess from Cushing's syndrome related to other causes*

ELIXIR, ORAL SOLUTION, TABLETS
Adults. 2 mg every 6 hr for 48 hr followed by collection of 24-hr urine specimen to determine 17-hydroxycorticosteroid level.

➤ *To decrease cerebral edema*

ELIXIR, ORAL SOLUTION, TABLETS
Adults. 2 mg every 8 to 12 hr as maintenance after parenteral form has controlled initial symptoms.

I.V. OR I.M. INJECTION
Adults. 10 mg I.V. followed by 4 mg I.M. every 6 hr. Decreased after 2 to 4 days, if needed, gradually tapering off over 5 to 7 days unless inoperable or recurring brain tumor is present. If such a tumor is present, dosage gradually decreased after 2 to 4 days to maintenance dosage of 2 mg I.M. every 8 to 12 hr and switched to P.O. regimen as soon as possible.

D

➤ *To treat unresponsive shock*

I.V. INFUSION AND INJECTION

Adults. 20 mg as a single dose followed by 3 mg/kg over 24 hr as a continuous infusion; 40 mg as a single dose followed by 40 mg every 2 to 6 hr, as needed; or 1 mg/kg as a single dose. All regimens used no more than 3 days.

➤ *To decrease localized inflammation*

INTRA-ARTICULAR INJECTION

Adults. 2 to 4 mg for large joint; 0.8 to 1 mg for small joint; 2 to 3 mg for bursae; 0.4 to 1 mg for tendon sheaths.

SOFT-TISSUE INJECTION

Adults. 2 to 6 mg; 1 to 2 mg for ganglia.

INTRALESIONAL INJECTION

Adults. 0.8 to 1.6 mg/injection site.

➤ *To decrease inflammation in allergic conditions or nasal polyps (except in sinuses)*

NASAL AEROSOL

Adults and children age 12 and over. 2 sprays (0.2 mg) in each nostril b.i.d. or t.i.d. *Maximum:* 12 sprays (1.2 mg) daily.
Children ages 6 to 12. 1 or 2 sprays (0.1 to 0.2 mg) in each nostril b.i.d. *Maximum:* 8 sprays (0.8 mg) daily.

Mechanism of Action

Binds to intracellular glucocorticoid receptors and suppresses inflammatory and immune responses by:

• inhibiting neutrophil and monocyte accumulation at inflammation site and suppressing their phagocytic and bactericidal activity
• stabilizing lysosomal membranes
• suppressing antigen response of macrophages and helper T cells
• inhibiting synthesis of inflammatory response mediators, such as cytokines, interleukins, and prostaglandins.

Contraindications

Administration of live-virus vaccine to patient or family member, hypersensitivity to dexamethasone or its components (including sulfites), idiopathic thrombocytopenic purpura (I.M. administration), systemic fungal infections

Interactions

DRUGS

aminoglutethimide, antacids, barbiturates, carbamazepine, hydantoins, mitotane, rifampin: Decreased dexamethasone effectiveness

amphotericin B (parenteral), carbonic anhydrase inhibitors: Risk of hypokalemia

anticholinesterases: Decreased anticholinesterase effectiveness in myasthenia gravis

aspirin, NSAIDs: Increased risk of adverse GI effects

cholestyramine: Increased dexamethasone clearance

cyclosporine: Increased activity of both drugs, possibly resulting in seizures

digoxin: Increased risk of digitalis toxicity related to hypokalemia

ephedrine: Decreased half-life and increased clearance of dexamethasone

erythromycin, indinavir: Increased clearance and decreased plasma concentrations of these drugs

estrogens, ketoconazole, macrolide antibiotics: Decreased dexamethasone clearance

isoniazid: Decreased blood isoniazid level

neuromuscular blockers: Possibly potentiated or counteracted neuromuscular blockade

oral anticoagulants: Altered coagulation times, requiring reduced anticoagulant dosage

oral contraceptives: Increased half-life and concentration of dexamethasone

phenytoin: Increased risk of seizures

potassium-wasting diuretics: Increased potassium loss and risk of hypokalemia

salicylates: Decreased blood level and effectiveness of salicylates

somatrem: Possibly inhibition of somatrem's growth-promoting effect

thalidomide: Increased risk of toxic epidermal necrolysis

theophyllines: Altered effects of either drug

toxoids, vaccines: Decreased antibody response

ACTIVITIES

alcohol use: Increased risk of GI bleeding

Adverse Reactions

CNS: Depression, emotional lability, euphoria, fever, headache, increased ICP with papilledema, insomnia, light-headedness, malaise, neuritis, neuropathy, paresthesia, psychosis, seizures, syncope, tiredness, vertigo, weakness

CV: Arrhythmias, bradycardia, edema, fat embolism, heart failure, hypercholesterolemia, hyperlipidemia, hypertension, myocardial rupture, tachycardia, thromboembolism, thrombophlebitis, vasculitis
EENT: Cataracts, glaucoma, vision changes (all forms); epistaxis, loss of smell and taste, nasal burning and dryness, oral candidiasis, perforated nasal septum, pharyngitis, rebound nasal congestion, rhinorrhea, sneezing (nasal aerosol)
ENDO: Cushingoid symptoms, decreased iodine uptake, growth suppression in children, hyperglycemia, menstrual irregularities, secondary adrenocortical and pituitary unresponsiveness
GI: Abdominal distention, bloody stools, elevated liver function test results, heartburn, hepatomegaly, increased appetite, indigestion, intestinal perforation, melena, nausea, pancreatitis, peptic ulcer with possible perforation, ulcerative esophagitis, vomiting
GU: Glycosuria, increased or decreased number and motility of spermatozoa, perineal irritation, urinary frequency
HEME: Leukocytosis, leukopenia
MS: Aseptic necrosis of femoral and humeral heads; muscle atrophy, spasms, or weakness; myalgia; osteoporosis; pathologic fracture of long bones; tendon rupture (intra-articular injection); vertebral compression fracture
RESP: Bronchospasm
SKIN: Acne, allergic dermatitis, diaphoresis, ecchymosis, erythema, hirsutism, necrotizing vasculitis, petechiae, subcutaneous fat atrophy, striae, thin and fragile skin, urticaria
Other: Aggravated or masked signs of infection, anaphylaxis, angioedema, hypernatremia, hypocalcemia, hypokalemia, hypokalemic alkalosis, impaired wound healing, metabolic acidosis, sodium and fluid retention, suppressed skin test reaction, weight gain

Nursing Considerations

• Use dexamethasone cautiously in patients with congestive heart failure, hypertension, or renal insufficiency because drug can cause sodium retention, which may lead to edema and hypokalemia.
• Also use cautiously in patients who have had intestinal sugery and in those with peptic ulcer, diverticulitis, or ulcerative colitis because of the risk of perforation.
• Give once-daily dose of dexamethasone in the morning to coincide with the body's natural cortisol secretion.
• Give oral drug with food to decrease GI distress.
• Be aware that dosage forms with a concentration of 24 mg/ml are for I.V. use only.
• Shake I.M. solution before injecting deep into large muscle mass.
• **WARNING** Avoid subcutaneous injection; it may cause atrophy and sterile abscess.
• Inject undiluted I.V. dose directly into I.V. tubing of infusing compatible solution over 30 seconds or less, as prescribed.
• **WARNING** Don't give acetate form by I.V. injection.
• Shake nasal aerosol container well, and hold it upright about 6″ (15 cm) from area being treated. Keep spray out of patient's eyes, and advise her not to inhale it.
• Expect to taper drug rather than stopping it abruptly; prolonged use can cause adrenal suppression.
• Monitor fluid intake and output and daily weight, and watch for crackles, dyspnea, peripheral edema, and steady weight gain.
• Evaluate growth if patient is a child.
• Test stool for occult blood.
• Monitor results of hematology studies and blood glucose, serum electrolyte, cholesterol, and lipid levels. Dexamethasone may cause hyperglycemia, hypernatremia, hypocalcemia, hypokalemia, or leukopenia. It also may increase serum cholesterol and lipid levels, and it may decrease iodine uptake by the thyroid.
• Assess patient for evidence of osteoporosis, Cushing's syndrome, and other systemic effects during long-term use.
• Monitor neonate for signs of hypoadrenocorticism if mother received dexamethasone during pregnancy. Be aware that some preparations contain benzyl alcohol, which may cause a fatal toxic syndrome in neonates and immature infants.
• Watch for hypersensitivity reactions after giving acetate or sodium phosphate form; both may contain bisulfites or parabens, inactive ingredients to which some people are allergic.

PATIENT TEACHING

• Instruct patient not to store drug in damp or hot places and to protect liquid form from freezing.
• Instruct patient to take once-daily oral dose in the morning with food to help prevent GI distress.

D

•Caution patient to avoid consuming alcohol during dexamethasone therapy because they increase the risk of GI bleeding.

•Advise patient to follow a low-sodium, high-potassium, high-protein diet, if prescribed, to help minimize weight gain, which is common with dexamethasone therapy. Instruct her to inform prescriber if she's on a special diet.

•Instruct patient not to stop using drug abruptly.

•Advise patient to notify prescriber if condition recurs or worsens after dosage is reduced or therapy stops.

•Urge patient to have regular eye examinations during long-term use.

•Advise patient on long-term therapy to carry medical identification and to notify all health care providers that she takes dexamethasone.

•Instruct patient (especially a child) to avoid close contact with anyone who has chickenpox or measles and to notify prescriber immediately if exposure occurs.

•Advise patient and family members to avoid live virus vaccinations, such as oral polio vaccine, during therapy unless prescriber approves.

•Inform diabetic patient that drug may affect her blood glucose level.

•If drug is injected into a joint, instruct patient to avoid putting excessive pressure on it and to notify prescriber if it becomes red or swollen.

•Tell patient to notify prescriber about anorexia, depression, light-headedness, malaise, muscle pain, nausea, vomiting, and early hyperadrenocorticism (abdominal distention, amenorrhea, easy bruising, extreme weakness, facial hair, increased appetite, moon face, weight gain). Tell patient and family about possible changes in appearance.

•Urge patient to notify prescriber about illness, surgery, or changes in stress level.

dexchlorpheniramine maleate

Dexchlor, Polaramine, Polaramine Repetabs

Class and Category

Chemical class: Propylamine derivative
Therapeutic class: Antihistamine
Pregnancy category: B

Indications and Dosages

➤ *To treat allergic conjunctivitis; transfusion reaction; dermographism; mild, uncomplicated allergic skin reactions, such as urticaria and angioedema; perennial and seasonal allergic rhinitis; and vasomotor rhinitis and as adjunct to treat anaphylaxis*

E.R. TABLETS

Adults and adolescents. 4 to 6 mg daily at bedtime or every 8 to 10 hr, p.r.n.

SYRUP, TABLETS

Adults and adolescents. 2 mg every 4 to 6 hr, p.r.n.

Children ages 6 to 12. 1 mg every 4 to 6 hr or 150 mcg/kg in divided doses q.i.d., p.r.n.

Children ages 2 to 6. 0.5 mg every 4 to 6 hr, p.r.n.

Route	Onset	Peak	Duration
P.O.	15 to 60 min*	Unknown*	4 to 8 hr*

Mechanism of Action

Binds to central and peripheral H_1 receptors, competing with histamine for these sites and preventing histamine from reaching its site of action. By blocking histamine, dexchlorpheniramine:
• inhibits respiratory, vascular, and GI smooth-muscle contraction, which prevents wheezing
• decreases capillary permeability, which reduces itching, flares, and wheals
• decreases lacrimal and salivary gland secretions, reducing nasal secretions, itching, sneezing, and watery eyes.

Contraindications

Angle-closure glaucoma; benign prostatic hyperplasia; bladder neck obstruction; hypersensitivity to dexchlorpheniramine or other antihistamines; lower respiratory tract disorders, such as asthma; MAO inhibitor therapy within 14 days; pyloroduodenal obstruction; stenosing peptic ulcer

Interactions

DRUGS

anticholinergics: Potentiated anticholinergic effects

---

* For syrup and tablets; unknown for E.R. tablets.

CNS depressants: Increased CNS depression
MAO inhibitors: Possibly severe hypotension and prolonged and intensified anticholinergic and sedative effects of dexchlorpheniramine

ACTIVITIES
alcohol use: Increased CNS depression

Adverse Reactions

CNS: Ataxia, confusion, dizziness, drowsiness, euphoria, excitement, headache, insomnia, irritability, nervousness, neuritis, nightmares, paresthesia, restlessness, vertigo, weakness
CV: Hypotension, palpitations, tachycardia
EENT: Acute labyrinthitis, blurred vision, dry mouth, tinnitus, vision changes
GI: Anorexia, constipation, diarrhea, indigestion, nausea, vomiting
GU: Urinary hesitancy, urine retention
RESP: Tenacious bronchial secretions
SKIN: Diaphoresis, photosensitivity, rash

Nursing Considerations

•Use dexchlorpheniramine cautiously in elderly patients and those with CV disease, hyperthyroidism, increased intraocular pressure, prostatic hypertrophy, or renal disease.
•Monitor patient for adverse reactions, especially in elderly patients and children.
•Assess patient for signs of overdose, including clumsiness; drowsiness; dry mouth, nose, or throat; dyspnea; flushed or red face; hallucinations; insomnia; light-headedness; seizures; and unsteadiness.

PATIENT TEACHING
•Inform patient that drug provides temporary relief of symptoms.
•Advise patient to take drug with food, water, or milk to reduce GI irritation. Inform her that she can crush regular (not E.R.) tablets and mix with food or fluid.
•For E.R. tablets, tell patient not to break, crush, or chew them before swallowing.
•Advise patient to take missed dose as soon as possible unless it's almost time for next dose.
•Because drug may cause drowsiness, caution patient to avoid potentially hazardous activities until its CNS effects are known.
•Instruct her to avoid prolonged sun exposure and to use a sunscreen.
•Suggest that patient use sugarless candy or gum, ice chips, or saliva substitute to relieve dry mouth. If dryness lasts longer than

2 weeks, advise her to notify prescriber.
•Caution patient to avoid alcohol and CNS depressants, such as sedatives, sleepng pills, and tranquilizers, while taking dexchlorpheniramine.
•If patient takes high doses of aspirin, urge her to inform prescriber because antihistamines may mask adverse reactions to aspirin overdose, such as tinnitus.
•Inform patient that drug needs to be discontinued 3 to 4 days before skin tests for allergies are performed.

dexmethylphenidate hydrochloride

Focalin, Focalin XR

Class, Category, and Schedule

*Chemical class: d-threo-*enantiomer of methylphenidate
Therapeutic class: CNS stimulant
Pregnancy category: C
Controlled substance schedule: II

Indications and Dosages

➤ *To treat attention deficit hyperactivity disorder (ADHD)*

TABLETS
Adults and children age 6 and over who are new to methylphenidate. 2.5 mg b.i.d. at least 4 hr apart, increased in weekly increments of 2.5 to 5 mg. *Maximum:* 10 mg b.i.d.
Adults and children age 6 and over who take methylphenidate. One-half of racemic methylphenidate dosage. *Maximum:* 10 mg b.i.d. at least 4 hr apart.
DOSAGE ADJUSTMENT Drug stopped if no improvement within 1 mo after appropriate dosage adjustments. Dosage decreased or drug stopped for paradoxical aggravation of symptoms or adverse reactions.

E.R. CAPSULES, E.R. TABLETS
Adults who are new to methylphenidate. 10 mg daily, increased after 1 wk as needed to 20 mg daily.
Children age 6 and over who are new to methylphenidate. 5 mg daily, increased as needed in weekly intervals by 5-mg increments. *Maximum:* 20 mg daily.
Adults and children age 6 and over who take methylphenidate. Half of racemic methylphenidate dosage. *Maximum:* 20 mg daily.

Mechanism of Action

May block the reuptake of norepinephrine and dopamine into presynaptic neurons in the cerebral cortex, which increases the availability of norepinephrine and dopamine in the extraneuronal space.

Contraindications

Diagnosis or family history of Tourette's syndrome; glaucoma; hypersensitivity to dexmethylphenidate, methylphenidate, or their components; marked anxiety, tension, and agitation; motor tics; use within 14 days of MAO inhibitor therapy

Interactions

DRUGS

anticoagulants (oral), anticonvulsants, antidepressants (tricyclic and selective serotonin reuptake inhibitors): Possibly decreased metabolism of these drugs
antihypertensives: Decreased therapeutic effect of these drugs
dopamine and other vasopressors: Increased therapeutic effect of these drugs
MAO inhibitors: Increased adverse effects, risk of hypertensive crisis

Adverse Reactions

CNS: Cerebral arteritis or occlusion, dizziness, drowsiness, dyskinesia, fever, headache, insomnia, motor or vocal tics, nervousness, seizures, Tourette's syndrome, toxic psychosis
CV: Angina, arrhythmias, hypertension, hypotension, increased or decreased pulse rate, palpitations, tachycardia
EENT: Accommodation abnormality, blurred vision
GI: Abdominal pain, anorexia, nausea
HEME: Thrombocytopenic purpura
MS: Arthralgia
SKIN: Erythema multiforme, exfoliative dermatitis, necrotizing vasculitis, rash, urticaria
Other: Weight loss (with prolonged dexmethylphenidate therapy)

Nursing Considerations

•**WARNING** Be aware that dexmethylphenidate may induce CNS stimulation, mania, and psychosis and may worsen behavior disturbances and thought disorders. Use drug cautiously in children with psychosis or mania. Be aware that withdrawal symptoms may occur with long-term use.

•Also know that dexmethylphenidate should be used cautionly in patients with serious structural cardiac abnormalities, cardiomyopathy, serious heart rhythm abnormalities, or other serious cardiac problems because drug may increase the risk of sudden death from these conditions.

•Monitor patient's blood pressure and pulse rate to detect hypertension and signs of excessive stimulation. Notify prescriber if you detect such signs.

•Be aware that dexmethylphenidate shouldn't be used to treat severe depression or to prevent or treat normal fatigue.

•**WARNING** Monitor patient for signs of physical or psychological dependence. Use drug cautiously in patients with a history of drug abuse, including alcoholism.

•Monitor CBC and differential and platelet counts, as ordered, during prolonged therapy.

•Expect to stop drug if seizures occur. Drug may lower seizure threshold, especially in patients with a history of seizures or EEG abnormalities.

•Monitor children on long-term dexmethylphenidate therapy for signs of growth suppression, which has been noted during long-term use of stimulants.

•Be aware that the dosages of drugs affected by dexmethylphenidate, such as anticoagulants and antihypertensives, may need adjustment.

PATIENT TEACHING

•Tell patient that extended-release capsules should either be taken whole, without being chewed, crushed, or divided, or capsule contents should be sprinkled on a small amount of applesauce.

•Encourage patient to notify her prescriber if she experiences excessive nervousness, fever, insomnia, nausea, palpitations, or rash while undergoing dexmethylphenidate therapy.

•Caution patient with seizure disorder that drug may cause seizures.

•Advise patient to protect drug from light and moisture.

•Teach patient (or parent) to watch for improvement in signs and symptoms of ADHD, such as decreased impulsiveness and increased attention. Stress the need for continued follow-up care, and suggest participation in an ADHD program.

dexrazoxane

Zinecard

Class and Category

Chemical class: Piperazinedione
Therapeutic class: Cardioprotective agent, chelating agent
Pregnancy category: C

Indications and Dosages

➤ *To prevent or reduce severity of cardiomyopathy associated with doxorubicin therapy in women with metastatic breast cancer*

I.V. INJECTION

Adults. *Initial:* 500 mg/m^2 for every 50 mg/m^2 of doxorubicin every 3 wk.

DOSAGE ADJUSTMENT In patients with hyperbilirubinemia, dosage proportionately reduced (depending on severity) to maintain a dexrazoxane-to-doxorubicin ratio of 10:1. In patients with creatinine clearance of less than 40 ml/min, dosage decreased 50%.

Mechanism of Action

Rapidly enters cardiac cells and acts as an intracellular heavy metal chelator. In cardiac tissues, anthracyclines, such as doxorubicin, form complexes with iron or copper, damaging cardiac cell membranes and mitochondria. Dexrazoxane combines with intracellular iron and protects against anthracycline-induced free radical damage to the myocardium. It also prevents conversion of ferrous ions back to ferric ions for use by free radicals.

Incompatibilities

Don't mix dexrazoxane in same I.V. line with other drugs.

Contraindications

Hypersensitivity to dexrazoxane or its components; use with chemotherapy regimens that do not contain an anthracycline, such as daunorubicin, doxorubicin, epirubicin, idarubicin, or mitoxantrone

Interactions

bone marrow depressants: Possibly enhanced bone marrow depression

Adverse Reactions

HEME: Myelosuppression including granulocytopenia, leukopenia, or thrombocytopenia
Other: Injection site pain

Nursing Considerations

•WARNING Use gloves when preparing reconstituted solution. If dexrazoxane powder or solution comes in contact with your skin or mucosa, immediately and thoroughly wash with soap and water.

•Reconstitute drug by mixing with 25 or 50 ml of 0.167 molar sodium lactate, supplied by the manufacturer, to produce a final concentration of 10 mg/ml. Administer reconstituted solution by slow I.V. push, or further dilute with either normal saline solution or D$_5$W to a concentration of 1.3 to 5 mg/ml, as prescribed, for rapid I.V. infusion.

•Be aware that dexrazoxane may interfere with tumor response to doxorubicin, especially in patients receiving drug at start of fluorouracil-doxorubicin-cyclophosphamide therapy.

•Monitor patient with immunosuppression or decreased bone marrow reserves resulting from prior chemotherapy or radiation therapy to prevent worsening of her condition. Notify prescriber if condition deteriorates.

PATIENT TEACHING

•Inform patient that dexrazoxane protects the heart from damage caused by myelosuppression and that she'll be given the drug by a health care professional in the hospital or clinic before receiving chemotherapy.

•Inform patient that dexrazoxane and chemotherapy may make her feel generally unwell, but urge her to continue treatment unless prescriber tells her to stop.

•Instruct patient to report chills, fever, mouth sores, pain at injection site, sore throat, unusual bleeding or bruising, unusual tiredness or weakness, and vomiting. Dosage may need to be changed or therapy stopped.

•Inform patient that drug may exacerbate symptoms of bone marrow suppression caused by anthracycline chemotherapy, including increased risk of infection.

•Teach patient importance of avoiding injury and infection during dexrazoxane therapy. For example, advise her to use a soft-bristled toothbrush to prevent damage to teeth and gums; to avoid people with colds, the flu, or bronchitis; and to avoid anyone who has recently had oral polio vaccine because of the increased risk of infection from live virus.

dextrose
(d-glucose)
B-D Glucose, Glutose, Insta-Glucose, Insulin Reaction

glucose
2.5% Dextrose Injection, 5% Dextrose Injection, 10% Dextrose Injection, 20% Dextrose Injection, 25% Dextrose Injection, 50% Dextrose Injection, 60% Dextrose Injection, 70% Dextrose Injection

Class and Category
Chemical class: Monosaccharide
Therapeutic class: Antidiabetic, nutritional supplement
Pregnancy category: C

Indications and Dosages
➤ *To treat insulin-induced hypoglycemia*
CHEWABLE TABLETS, ORAL GEL
Adults and children. *Initial:* 10 to 20 g. Repeated in 10 to 20 min, if needed, based on serum glucose level.
I.V. INFUSION OR INJECTION
Adults and children. *Initial:* 20 to 50 ml of 50% solution given at 3 ml/min. *Maintenance:* 10% to 15% solution by continuous infusion until blood glucose level reaches therapeutic range.
Infants and neonates. 2 ml/kg of 10% to 25% solution until blood glucose level reaches therapeutic range.
➤ *To replace calories*
I.V. INFUSION
Adults and children. Individualized dosage of 2.5%, 5%, or 10% solution, based on need for fluids or calories and given by peripheral I.V. line. Or a 10% to 70% solution given by large central vein, if needed, typically mixed with amino acids or other solutions.

Route	Onset	Peak	Duration
P.O.	10 to 20 min	40 min	Unknown
I.V.	2 to 3 min	Unknown	Unknown

Incompatibilities
Don't give dextrose through same infusion set as blood or blood products because pseudoagglutination of RBCs may occur.

> ### Mechanism of Action
> Prevents protein and nitrogen loss, promotes glycogen deposition, prevents or decreases ketosis, and, in large amounts, acts as an osmotic diuretic. Dextrose is readily metabolized and undergoes oxidation to carbon dioxide and water. The oral form—glucose—is absorbed directly into the bloodstream from the intestines and is distributed, used, or stored in the liver.

Contraindications
For all solutions: Diabetic coma with excessively elevated blood glucose level
For concentrated solutions: Anuria, alcohol withdrawal syndrome in dehydrated patient, glucose-galactose malabsorption syndrome, hepatic coma, hypersensitivity to corn or corn products, intracranial or intraspinal hemorrhage, overhydration

Interactions
DRUGS
corticosteroids, corticotropin: Increased risk of fluid and electrolyte imbalance if dextrose solution contains sodium ions

Adverse Reactions
CNS: Confusion, fever
GU: Glycosuria
Other: Dehydration; hyperosmolar coma; hypervolemia; hypovolemia; injection site extravasation with tissue necrosis, infection, phlebitis, and venous thrombosis

Nursing Considerations
•Use dextrose cautiously in patients with renal impairment because dextrose solutions contain aluminum that could be toxic if patients receive prolonged parenteral therapy.
•Give highly concentrated dextrose solution by central venous catheter—not by subcutaneous or I.M. route.
•**WARNING** Avoid rapid or excessive delivery of dextrose solution in a very low–birth-weight infant; it may increase serum osmolality and cause intracerebral hemorrhage.
•Assess infusion site regularly for signs of infiltration, such as pain or swelling.
•Assess patient for glucosuria by using a

urine reagent strip or collecting a urine sample and reviewing urinalysis results.
•When discontinuing a concentrated solution, expect to give a 5% to 10% dextrose infusion to avoid rebound hypoglycemia.
•Monitor patient for signs of hypervolemia, such as jugular vein distention and crackles.

PATIENT TEACHING
•Advise patient to swallow oral dextrose because it isn't absorbed from the buccal cavity.
•Instruct patient to monitor her blood glucose level as directed.
•Stress the importance of reporting discomfort, pain, or signs of infection at I.V. site.

dezocine

Dalgan

Class and Category
Chemical class: Aminotetralin, synthetic opioid
Therapeutic class: Analgesic
Pregnancy category: C

Indications and Dosages
➤ *To relieve pain*
I.V. INJECTION
Adult. *Initial:* 5 mg followed by 2.5 to 10 mg every 2 to 4 hr, p.r.n. *Maximum:* 120 mg daily.
I.M. INJECTION
Adult. *Initial:* 10 mg followed by 5 to 20 mg every 3 to 6 hr, p.r.n. *Maximum:* 20 mg/dose, 120 mg daily.

Route	Onset	Peak	Duration
I.V.	In 15 min	30 min	2 to 4 hr
I.M.	In 30 min	1 to 2 hr	2 to 4 hr

Mechanism of Action
Binds with opiate receptors at many CNS sites. This affects the perception of and emotional response to pain.

Contraindications
Hypersensitivity to dezocine or its components

Interactions
DRUGS
CNS depressants, general anesthetics, hyp-

notics, sedatives, tranquilizers: Increased CNS depressant effects
opioids: Possibly decreased therapeutic effects of opioid and withdrawal symptoms in patient receiving long-term opioid therapy
ACTIVITIES
alcohol use: Increased CNS depressant effects

Adverse Reactions
CNS: Dizziness, sedation, vertigo
GI: Nausea, vomiting
Other: Injection site redness and swelling

Nursing Considerations
•Use dezocine cautiously and in low doses in elderly patients and those who have common bile duct, hepatic, renal, or respiratory disease.
•Discard solution if it contains precipitate.
•Frequently monitor blood pressure and pulse and respiratory rates after giving first dose, especially if given by I.V. route.
•**WARNING** Avoid administering dezocine to a patient who is opioid-dependent. Doing so may precipitate withdrawal symptoms because dezocine can antagonize the effects of opioids.
•Assess patient for pain relief frequently, and document findings.

PATIENT TEACHING
•Instruct patient to notify prescriber if pain isn't relieved within 1 hour.
•Advise patient to avoid hazardous activities until drug's CNS effects are known.

diazepam

Apo-Diazepam (CAN), Diastat, Diazepam Intensol, Dizac, Novo-Dipam (CAN), Valium, Vivol (CAN)

Class, Category, and Schedule
Chemical class: Benzodiazepine
Therapeutic class: Anticonvulsant, anxiolytic, sedative-hypnotic, skeletal muscle relaxant
Pregnancy category: D
Controlled substance schedule: IV

Indications and Dosages
➤ *To relieve anxiety*
ORAL SOLUTION, TABLETS
Adults. 2 to 10 mg b.i.d. to q.i.d.
DOSAGE ADJUSTMENT Dosage reduced to 2 to

2.5 mg daily or b.i.d. and increased gradually as needed and tolerated for elderly or debilitated patients.

Children age 6 months and over. *Initial:* 1 to 2.5 mg t.i.d. or q.i.d. Increased gradually as needed and tolerated.

I.V. OR I.M. INJECTION

Adults. 2 to 5 mg every 3 to 4 hr, p.r.n., for moderate anxiety; 5 to 10 mg every 3 to 4 hr, p.r.n., for severe anxiety.

Children. Individualized dosage. *Maximum:* 0.25 mg/kg given over 3 min and repeated after 15 to 30 min if needed and after another 15 to 30 min if needed.

➤ *To treat symptoms of acute alcohol withdrawal*

ORAL SOLUTION, TABLETS

Adults. 10 mg t.i.d. or q.i.d. during first 24 hr. Then 5 mg t.i.d. or q.i.d., if needed.

I.V. OR I.M. INJECTION

Adults. 10 mg and then 5 to 10 mg in 3 to 4 hr, if needed.

➤ *To provide muscle relaxation, to provide sedation*

ORAL SOLUTION, TABLETS

Adults. 2 to 10 mg t.i.d. or q.i.d.

DOSAGE ADJUSTMENT Dosage reduced to 2 to 2.5 mg once or twice daily and increased gradually as needed and tolerated for elderly or debilitated patients.

Children age 6 months and over. *Initial:* 1 to 2.5 mg t.i.d. or q.i.d. Increased gradually as needed and tolerated.

I.V. OR I.M. INJECTION

Adults. 2 to 5 mg every 3 to 4 hr, p.r.n., for moderate anxiety; 5 to 10 mg every 3 to 4 hr, p.r.n., for severe anxiety.

Children. Individualized dosage. *Maximum:* 0.25 mg/kg given over 3 min and repeated after 15 to 30 min if needed and after another 15 to 30 min if needed.

➤ *To treat seizures*

ORAL SOLUTION, TABLETS

Adults. 2 to 10 mg b.i.d. to q.i.d.

DOSAGE ADJUSTMENT Dosage reduced to 2 to 2.5 mg once or twice daily and increased gradually as needed and tolerated for elderly or debilitated patients.

Children age 6 months and over. *Initial:* 1 to 2.5 mg t.i.d. or q.i.d. Increased gradually as needed and tolerated.

➤ *To treat status epilepticus and severe recurrent seizures*

I.V. INJECTION

Adults. 5 to 10 mg repeated every 10 to 15 min, as needed, up to a cumulative dose of 30 mg. Regimen repeated, if needed, in 2 to 4 hr. (Use I.M. route if I.V. access is impossible.)

Children age 5 and over. 1 mg repeated every 2 to 5 min, as needed, up to a cumulative dose of 10 mg. Regimen repeated, if needed, in 2 to 4 hr.

Children ages 1 month to 5 years. 0.2 to 0.5 mg repeated every 2 to 5 min, as needed, up to a cumulative dose of 5 mg. Regimen repeated, if needed, in 2 to 4 hr.

RECTAL GEL

Adults and adolescents. 0.2 mg/kg rounded up to next available unit dose (or rounded down for elderly or debilitated patient). Repeated in 4 to 12 hr, if needed.

Children ages 6 to 12. 0.3 mg/kg rounded up to next available unit dose. Repeated in 4 to 12 hr, if needed.

Children ages 2 to 6. 0.5 mg/kg rounded up to next available unit dose. Repeated in 4 to 12 hr, if needed.

➤ *To provide preoperative sedation*

I.V. OR I.M. INJECTION

Adults. 5 to 10 mg 30 min before surgery.

➤ *To reduce anxiety before cardioversion*

I.V. INJECTION

Adults. 5 to 15 mg 5 to 10 min before procedure.

➤ *To reduce anxiety before endoscopic procedures*

I.V. INJECTION

Adults. Up to 20 mg titrated to desired sedation and administered immediately before procedure.

I.M. INJECTION

Adults. 5 to 10 mg 30 min before procedure.

➤ *To treat tetanus*

I.V. OR I.M. INJECTION

Adults and children age 5 and over. *Initial:* 5 to 10 mg repeated every 3 to 4 hr, if needed. Sometimes larger doses are needed for adults.

DOSAGE ADJUSTMENT Initial dose reduced to 2 to 5 mg and increased gradually as needed and tolerated for debilitated patients.

Children ages 1 month to 5 years. 1 to 2 mg repeated every 3 to 4 hr, as needed.

Incompatibilities

Don't mix diazepam injection with aqueous

solutions. Don't mix diazepam emulsion for I.M. injection with morphine or glycopyrrolate or administer it through an infusion set that contains polyvinyl chloride.

Mechanism of Action

May potentiate the effects of gamma-aminobutyric acid (GABA) and other inhibitory neurotransmitters by binding to specific benzodiazepine receptors in the limbic and cortical areas of the CNS. GABA inhibits excitatory stimulation, which helps control emotional behavior. The limbic system contains a highly dense area of benzodiazepine receptors, which may explain the drug's antianxiety effects. Diazepam suppresses the spread of seizure activity caused by seizure-producing foci in the cortex, thalamus, and limbic structures.

Contraindications

Acute angle-closure glaucoma, hypersensitivity to diazepam or its components, untreated open-angle glaucoma

Interactions

DRUGS

antacids: Altered rate of diazepam absorption

anticonvulsants: Decreased effectiveness of these drugs

cimetidine, disulfiram, fluoxetine, fluvoxamine, isoniazid, itraconazole, ketoconazole, metoprolol, omeprazole, oral contraceptives, propoxyphene, propranolol, valproic acid: Decreased diazepam metabolism, increased blood level and risk of adverse effects of diazepam

CNS depressants: Increased CNS depressant effects

digoxin: Increased serum digoxin level and risk of digitalis toxicity

levodopa: Decreased antidyskinetic effect of levodopa

phenytoin: Decreased metabolic elimination of phenytoin, increased risk of adverse reactions

probenecid: Faster onset or more prolonged effects of diazepam

ranitidine: Delayed elimination and increased blood level of diazepam

rifampin: Decreased blood diazepam level

theophyllines: Antagonized sedative effect of diazepam

ACTIVITIES

alcohol use: Increased CNS depression

Adverse Reactions

CNS: Anterograde amnesia, anxiety, ataxia, confusion, depression, dizziness, drowsiness, fatigue, headache, insomnia, lethargy, light-headedness, paradoxical reactions, psychiatric effects, sedation, sleepiness, slurred speech, suicidal ideation, tremor, vertigo

CV: Hypotension, palpitations, tachycardia

EENT: Blurred vision, diplopia, dry mouth, increased salivation

GI: Anorexia, constipation, diarrhea, elevated liver enzymes, jaundice, nausea, vomiting

GU: Libido changes, urinary incontinence, urine retention

HEME: Neutropenia

MS: Dysarthria, muscle weakness

RESP: Respiratory depression

SKIN: Dermatitis

Other: Physical and psychological dependence

Nursing Considerations

• Use diazepam with extreme caution in patients with a history of alcohol or drug abuse, because drug can cause physical and psychological dependence, and in patients with hepatic disorders such as hepatic fibrosis and hepatitis because of potentially significant increase in drug's half-life.

• Use diazepam cautiously in patients with hepatic or renal impairment. Severe hepatic impairment is a contraindication to use.

• Expect to give a lower dose of diazepam in a patient with chronic respiratory insufficiency because of the risk of respiratory depression.

• Mix concentrated oral solution (Intensol) with liquid or semisolid food. Use supplied calibrated dropper for accurate dosing.

• Protect diazepam injection from light. Don't use solution that's more than slightly yellow or that contains precipitate.

• Give I.M. injection into deltoid muscle for rapid and complete absorption. Using other sites may cause slow, erratic absorption.

• Before administering emulsion form, ask if patient is allergic to soybeans because this form contains soybean oil.

•For an infant or a child, administer I.V. injection slowly over 3 minutes in a dose not to exceed 0.25 mg/kg.

•Give emulsion form within 6 hours of opening ampule because it contains no preservatives and allows rapid microbial growth. Use polyethylene-lined or glass infusion sets and polyethylene or polypropylene plastic syringes for administration. Don't use a filter with a pore size less than 5 microns because a smaller size may break down the emulsion.

•Don't mix emulsion form with anything other than its emulsion base. Otherwise, it may become unstable and increase the risk of serious adverse reactions.

•Monitor patient for adverse reactions, especially if she has hypoalbuminemia, which increases the risk of sedation.

•**WARNING** Watch for signs of physical and psychological dependence: a strong desire or need to continue taking diazepam, a need to increase the dose to maintain drug effects, and posttherapy withdrawal symptoms, such as abdominal cramps, insomnia, irritability, nervousness, and tremor.

•Monitor patient closely for increase in frequency or severity of grand mal seizures when diazepam is used with standard anticonvulsant therapy. Dosage of other anticonvulsants may need to be increased.

•Avoid abrupt withdrawal of diazepam, as ordered, when used as part of the patient's seizure control regimen because a transient increase in frequency or severity of seizures may occur.

•Monitor severely depressed patient or patient with depression-related anxiety for suicidal tendencies, particularly when therapy starts and dosage changes, because depression may worsen temporarily during these times.

•Watch for psychiatric and paradoxical reactions to diazepam, especially in children and the elderly. If reations occur, notify prescriber and expect drug to be discontinued.

•Monitor patient for decreased drug effectiveness, which can occur with prolonged use.

•Check patient's blood counts and liver function periodically, as ordered, because prolonged diazepam therapy rarely causes neutropenia and jaundice.

PATIENT TEACHING

•Instruct patient not to take more drug than prescribed, more often, or for a longer time.

Warn her that physical and psychological dependence can occur, and teach her to recognize signs of dependence.

•Advise patient not to take drug to relieve everyday stress.

•Advise patient to avoid hazardous activities until drug's CNS effects are known.

•Advise patient to avoid CNS depressants and alcohol during therapy.

•Instruct patient not to stop taking drug abruptly without prescriber's supervision. If patient has a history of seizures, warn that abrupt drug withdrawal may trigger them.

•Instruct patient to mix Diazepam Intensol with water, soda, or a similar beverage; applesauce; or pudding just before taking it. Caution her not to save the mixture for later. Also tell patient to use calibrated dropper that's provided to measure each dose.

•Teach patient how to self-administer a rectal form, if prescribed.

•Instruct female patient of childbearing age to notify prescriber immediately if she is or could be pregnant because diazepam therapy will need to be discontinued.

•Urge family or caregiver to watch patient closely for suicidal tendencies, especially when therapy starts or dosage changes.

diazoxide

Hyperstat, Proglycem

Class and Category

Chemical class: Benzothiadiazine derivative
Therapeutic class: Antihypertensive, antihypoglycemic
Pregnancy category: C

Indications and Dosages

➤ *To manage hypoglycemia caused by hyperinsulinism*

CAPSULES, ORAL SUSPENSION

Adults and children. *Initial:* 1 mg/kg every 8 hr. *Maintenance:* 3 to 8 mg/kg daily in 2 or 3 equal doses given every 8 or 12 hr. *Maximum:* 15 mg/kg daily.

Infants and neonates. *Initial:* 3.3 mg/kg every 8 hr. *Maintenance:* 8 to 15 mg/kg daily in 2 or 3 equal doses given every 8 or 12 hr.

➤ *To treat severe hypertension in hospitalized patients*

I.V. INJECTION

Adults and children. *Initial:* 1 to 3 mg/kg by

rapid bolus, repeated every 5 to 15 min until diastolic pressure falls below 100 mm Hg. Repeated in 4 hr and again in 24 hr, if needed, until oral antihypertensive therapy begins. *Maximum:* 150 mg/dose, 1.2 g daily.

Route	Onset	Peak	Duration
P.O.	In 1 hr	Unknown	8 hr
I.V.	1 min	2 to 5 min	2 to 12 hr

Mechanism of Action
Directly affects smooth muscle cells of peripheral arteries and arterioles, causing them to dilate. This action decreases peripheral resistance, which helps reduce blood pressure. Diazoxide also inhibits insulin release from the pancreas, stimulates catecholamine release, and increases hepatic glucose release.

Contraindications
Acute aortic dissection; hypersensitivity to diazoxide, thiazides, other sulfonamide derivatives, or their components; treatment of compensatory hypertension, as occurs with aortic coarctation

Interactions
DRUGS
allopurinol, colchicine, probenecid, sulfinpyrazone: Increased serum uric acid level
antihypertensives: Additive hypotensive effects
beta blockers: Increased hypotensive effects of diazoxide
diuretics, especially thiazides: Potentiated hyperglycemic, hyperuricemic, and antihypertensive effects of diazoxide
estrogens, NSAIDs, sympathomimetics: Antagonized hypotensive effects of diazoxide
insulin, oral antidiabetic drugs: Possibly decreased effectiveness of these drugs
oral anticoagulants: Increased anticoagulant effects
peripheral vasodilators, ritodrine (I.V.): Additive, possibly severe, hypotensive effects

Adverse Reactions
CNS: Anxiety, apprehension, cerebral ischemia, dizziness, euphoria, headache, insomnia, light-headedness, malaise, somnolence, weakness

CV: Bradycardia, chest pain, hypotension, palpitations, tachycardia, transient hypertension
EENT: Blurred vision, dry mouth, increased salivation, taste perversion, tinnitus, transient hearing loss
ENDO: Transient hyperglycemia
GI: Abdominal pain, anorexia, constipation, diarrhea, ileus, nausea, vomiting
MS: Gout
SKIN: Diaphoresis, flushing, pruritus, rash, sensation of warmth
Other: Extravasation with injection site cellulitis and pain; fluid and sodium retention

Nursing Considerations
• Use diazoxide cautiously in patients with uncompensated heart failure (because it can cause fluid retention and heart failure) and in patients with impaired cardiac or cerebral circulation in whom abrupt blood pressure reduction, mild tachycardia, and decreased blood perfusion may be harmful.
• Give I.V. drug undiluted over 10 to 30 seconds. Don't give it I.M. or subcutaneously.
• Keep patient supine during I.V. injection and for 1 hour afterward.
• Monitor blood pressure throughout treatment to check for hypertension. Before ending surveillance, measure patient's standing blood pressure if she's ambulatory.
• Frequently assess I.V. site for extravasation because the drug is alkaline and can irritate tissue.
• Expect to adjust dosage as prescribed if patient switches from oral suspension to capsules; suspension produces a higher blood diazoxide level.
• If diabetic patient receives I.V. diazoxide to treat hypertension, monitor for signs and symptoms of hyperglycemia because parenteral form commonly causes transient hyperglycemia.
• Monitor the blood glucose level of all patients who receive oral diazoxide to determine if drug has raised the blood glucose level to normal.

PATIENT TEACHING
• For patient receiving I.V. diazoxide, explain that she'll be on bed rest until oral therapy starts.
• Advise patient to protect oral suspension from light.

D

•Tell patient to take oral drug on a regular schedule and not to skip or double doses.
•Instruct patient to check her blood glucose level regularly if she takes oral diazoxide to treat hypoglycemia.
•Caution patient not to take antidiabetic drugs unless prescribed.
•Advise patient to notify prescriber if she experiences signs of hyperglycemia, such as increased urinary frequency, increased thirst, and fruity breath.

dichloralphenazone

(all contain 325 mg of acetaminophen, 100 mg of dichloralphenazone, and 65 mg of isometheptene mucate)

Amidrine, I.D.A., Iso-Acetozone, Isocom, Midchlor, Midrin, Migquin, Migragap, Migratine, Migrazone, Migrend, Migrex, Mitride

Class and Category
Chemical class: Sympathomimetic amine
Therapeutic class: Analgesic
Pregnancy category: Not rated

Indications and Dosages
➤ *To relieve tension headache*
CAPSULES
Adults. 1 to 2 caps every 4 hr. *Maximum:* 8 capsules daily.
➤ *To relieve migraine headache*
CAPSULES
Adults. 2 caps followed by 1 cap every hr until relief occurs. *Maximum:* 5 capsules every 12 hr.

Route	Onset	Peak	Duration
P.O.	30 to 60 min	1 to 3 hr	3 to 4 hr

Mechanism of Action
Acetaminophen raises the pain threshold by acting on the hypothalamus. Dichloralphenazone reduces the patient's emotional reaction to pain through its mild sedative effect. Isometheptene constricts dilated cranial and cerebral arterioles through sympathomimetic action, which reduces stimuli that lead to vascular headaches.

Contraindications
Heart disease, hepatic disease, hypersensitivity to acetaminophen or isometheptene, MAO inhibitor therapy within 14 days, severe renal disease, uncontrolled glaucoma, uncontrolled hypertension

Interactions
DRUGS
CNS depressants: Additive sedative effects
hepatic enzyme inducers, other hepatotoxic drugs: Increased risk of hepatotoxicity
MAO inhibitors: Increased risk of severe hypertension and hyperpyrexia
ACTIVITIES
alcohol use: Additive sedative effects, increased risk of hepatotoxicity

Adverse Reactions
CNS: Dizziness, drowsiness
SKIN: Rash

Nursing Considerations
•Because dichloralphenazone has vasoconstrictive and sympathomimetic actions, assess patients with peripheral vascular disease or recent angina pectoris or MI for signs and symptoms indicating aggravation or deterioration of these conditions.
•Institute safety precautions to prevent injury from falls.
PATIENT TEACHING
•**WARNING** Caution patient not to take dichloralphenazone within 14 days of an MAO inhibitor; doing so can cause severe hypertension or hyperpyrexia.
•Advise patient to take drug only after a headache or migraine warning sign occurs. Too-frequent use may make drug less effective and may worsen headaches.
•Instruct patient to lie down in a quiet, dark room after taking drug.
•Because of possible dizziness or drowsiness, caution patient to avoid hazardous activities until drug's CNS effects are known.
•Caution patient to avoid alcohol and CNS depressants during therapy because they increase dizziness, drowsiness, and the risk of hepatotoxicity.
•Advise patient to notify prescriber if drug becomes less effective or if headaches occur more frequently.
•Teach patient how to read drug labels, and stress the need to avoid taking too much acetaminophen, which can cause hepatic or renal damage.
•Explain that decreasing dichloralphenazone

dose may prevent transient dizziness or rash.
•Instruct patient to store drug away from heat, moisture, and direct light.

dichlorphenamide

Daranide

Class and Category
Chemical class: Sulfonamide derivative
Therapeutic class: Antiglaucoma drug
Pregnancy category: C

Indications and Dosages
➤ *To manage chronic open-angle glaucoma, secondary glaucoma, and acute angle-closure glaucoma (pre-operatively)*

TABLETS
Adults. *Initial:* 100 to 200 mg followed by 100 mg every 12 hr. *Maintenance:* 25 to 50 mg once daily to t.i.d.

Route	Onset	Peak	Duration
P.O.	30 to 60 min	2 to 4 hr	6 to 12 hr

Mechanism of Action
Inhibits the enzyme carbonic anhydrase, which normally exists in renal proximal tubule cells, choroid plexes of the brain, and ciliary processes of the eyes. In the eyes, enzyme inhibition decreases aqueous humor secretion, which reduces intraocular pressure.

Contraindications
Adrenocortical insufficiency, hepatic insufficiency, hyperchloremic acidosis, hypersensitivity to dichlorphenamide or sulfa drugs, hypokalemia, hyponatremia, renal failure, severe obstructive pulmonary disease

Interactions
DRUGS
diflunisal: Increased adverse effects of dichlorphenamide, significantly decreased intraocular pressure
salicylates: Increased risk of dichlorphenamide toxicity, including CNS depression and metabolic acidosis

Adverse Reactions
CNS: Depression, disorientation, dizziness, drowsiness, lassitude, paresthesia
CV: Arrhythmias
EENT: Metallic taste, pharyngitis
ENDO: Hyperglycemia
GI: Anorexia, diarrhea, hepatic dysfunction, nausea, vomiting
GU: Phosphaturia, renal calculi, renal colic, urinary frequency
HEME: Hemolytic anemia, leukopenia, pancytopenia, thrombocytopenia
SKIN: Photosensitivity
Other: Hyperchloremia, hyperuricemia, weight loss

Nursing Considerations
•Use dichlorphenamide cautiously in patients who have emphysema, pulmonary obstruction, or severe respiratory acidosis.
•Frequently monitor serum potassium level (especially in elderly patients and those taking digoxin) because diuresis may cause hypokalemia.

PATIENT TEACHING
•Instruct patient to take dichlorphenamide with food or full glass of water to decrease GI distress.
•Advise patient to avoid hazardous activities until drug's CNS effects are known.
•**WARNING** Urge patient to immediately report evidence of blood dyscrasias, such as fever, numbness or tingling, rash, sore throat, and unusual bleeding or bruising.
•Advise patient to avoid prolonged exposure to sunlight, to apply sunscreen, and to wear protective clothing outdoors.
•Instruct patient to take a missed dose as soon as she remembers it, unless it's almost time for the next dose.
•Advise patient to store drug at room temperature and to protect it from moisture and heat.

diclofenac potassium

Cataflam, Voltaren Rapide (CAN)

diclofenac sodium

Apo-Diclo (CAN), Novo-Difenac (CAN), Nu-Diclo (CAN), Voltaren, Voltaren SR (CAN)

Class and Category
Chemical class: Phenylacetic acid derivative
Therapeutic class: Analgesic, anti-inflammatory

Pregnancy category: B

Indications and Dosages

➤ *To relieve pain and inflammation in rheumatoid arthritis*

DELAYED-RELEASE TABLETS, TABLETS

Adults. *Initial:* 150 to 200 mg daily in divided doses t.i.d. or q.i.d. *Maintenance:* 75 to 100 mg/ day, divided, t.i.d. *Maximum:* 225 mg daily.

E.R. TABLETS

Adults. *Initial:* 75 or 100 mg daily in the morning or evening, or 75 mg b.i.d. in the morning and evening.

RECTAL SUPPOSITORIES

Adults. 50 or 100 mg as substitute for last P.O. dose of day.

➤ *To relieve pain and inflammation in osteoarthritis*

DELAYED-RELEASE TABLETS, TABLETS

Adults. 100 to 150 mg daily in divided doses b.i.d. or t.i.d. *Maximum:* 150 mg daily.

➤ *To relieve pain in patients with ankylosing spondylitis*

DELAYED-RELEASE TABLETS, TABLETS

Adults. 100 to 125 mg daily in 4 or 5 divided doses.

➤ *To relieve pain and dysmenorrhea*

TABLETS

Adults. 50 mg t.i.d., p.r.n.; if needed, 100 mg for first dose only.

DOSAGE ADJUSTMENT Dosage reduced, if needed, for elderly patients and those with serious renal dysfunction.

Route	Onset	Peak	Duration
P.O.*	30 min	Unknown	8 hr

Contraindications

Active GI bleeding or ulcers; asthmatic attacks, rhinitis, or urticaria precipitated by aspirin or other NSAIDs; hypersensitivity to diclofenac or NSAIDs; treatment of perioperative pain after coronary artery bypass grafting

Interactions

DRUGS

acetaminophen: Increased risk of adverse renal effects with long-term concurrent use
anticoagulants, thrombolytics: Prolonged PT,

---

* For tablets; unknown for delayed-release and E.R. tablets.

increased risk of bleeding
antihypertensives: Decreased antihypertensive effectiveness
aspirin, other NSAIDs, salicylates: Increased GI irritability and bleeding, decreased diclofenac effectiveness
beta blockers: Impaired antihypertensive effect
cefamandole, cefoperazone, cefotetan, plicamycin, valproic acid: Increased risk of hypoprothrombinemia
cimetidine: Altered blood diclofenac level
colchicine, corticotropin (long-term use), glucocorticoids, potassium supplements: Increased GI irritability and bleeding
cyclosporine, gold compounds, nephrotoxic drugs: Increased risk of nephrotoxicity
digoxin: Increased blood digoxin level
insulin, oral antidiabetic drugs: Decreased effects of these drugs
lithium: Increased risk of lithium toxicity
loop diuretics: Decreased loop diuretic effectiveness
methotrexate: Increased risk of methotrexate toxicity
phenytoin: Increased blood phenytoin level
potassium-sparing diuretics: Increased risk of hyperkalemia
probenecid: Increased diclofenac toxicity

FOODS

food: Delayed absorption of delayed-release tablets

ACTIVITIES

alcohol use: Increased risk of GI irritability and bleeding

Mechanism of Action

Blocks the activity of cyclooxygenase, the enzyme needed to synthesize prostaglandins, which mediate the inflammatory response and cause local pain, swelling, and vasodilation. By blocking cyclooxygenase and inhibiting prostaglandins, diclofenac reduces inflammatory symptoms. This mechanism also relieves pain because prostaglandins promote pain transmission from the periphery to the spinal cord.

Adverse Reactions

CNS: Aseptic meningitis, cerebral hemorrhage, dizziness, drowsiness, headache
CV: Bradycardia and other arrhythmias,

hypotension, vasculitis
EENT: Glaucoma, hearing loss, tinnitus
ENDO: Hypoglycemia
GI: Abdominal pain, constipation, diarrhea, dysphagia, elevated liver function test results, esophageal ulceration, flatulence, GI bleeding or ulceration, hepatic failure, hepatitis, indigestion, jaundice, nausea, perforation of stomach or intestine
GU: Acute renal failure, interstitial nephritis
HEME: Agranulocytosis, aplastic anemia, eosinophilia, leukocytosis, leukopenia, pancytopenia, porphyria, thrombocytopenia
SKIN: Erythema multiforme, exfoliative dermatitis, pruritus, rash, Stevens-Johnson syndrome, toxic epidermal necrolysis
Other: Anaphylaxis, angioedema, fluid retention, hyperkalemia, hyperuricemia, hyponatremia, lymphadenopathy

Nursing Considerations
• Use diclofenac with extreme caution in patients who have a history of GI bleeding or ulcer disease because NSAIDs increase the risk of GI bleeding and ulceration. Use diclofenac for shortest possible time in these patients.
• Be aware that serious GI tract ulceration and bleeding, as well as perforation of stomach or intestine, can occur without warning or symptoms. Elderly patients are at greater risk. Monitor patient for signs of GI irritation and ulceration, especially if patient has a predisposing condition (such as a history of GI bleeding); takes an oral corticosteroid, anticoagulant, or NSAID (long-term); smokes; is an alcoholic; is over age 60; has poor general health; or tests positive for *Helicobacter pylori*. To minimize risk, give diclofenac with food. If patient develops GI distress, withhold diclofenac and notify prescriber immediately.
• Use diclofenac cautiously in patients with hypertension, and monitor blood pressure closely during therapy; drug can cause or worsen hypertension.
• Assess for hypotension. If patient takes a potassium-sparing diuretic, check for elevated serum potassium level.
• **WARNING** Monitor patient closely for thrombotic events, including MI and stroke, because NSAIDs such as diclofenac increase the risk for such events.
• Report signs of bleeding, such as bleeding

gums, bloody or cloudy urine, ecchymoses, melena, and petechiae.
• Monitor BUN and serum creatinine levels in elderly patients, patients taking ACE inhibitors or diuretics, and patients with heart failure or impaired renal or hepatic function. These patients may have an increased risk of renal failure.
• Assess patient's skin routinely for rash or other signs of hypersensitivity reaction; drug may cause serious skin reactions without warning. At first sign of reaction, stop drug and notify prescriber.
• Monitor liver function test results and serum uric acid level. Liver enzyme elevations usually occur within 2 months of starting diclofenac therapy.
• Report weight gain of more than 1 kg (2 lb) in 24 hours because it suggests fluid retention.

PATIENT TEACHING
• Advise patient not to chew, crush, or dissolve diclofenac tablet, but to swallow it whole.
• Instruct patient to take drug with food to minimize GI distress.
• To decrease risk of esophageal ulceration, instruct patient not to lie down for 15 to 30 minutes after taking drug.
• Warn patient to avoid potentially hazardous activities until diclofenac's CNS effects are known.
• Instruct patient to notify prescriber if she experiences ringing or buzzing in the ears, impaired hearing, dizziness, or GI distress or bleeding.
• Advise patient to consult prescriber before taking aspirin or other OTC analgesics or drinking alcohol.
• Explain that diclofenac may increase the risk of serious adverse cardiovascular reactions; urge patient to seek immediate medical attention for signs and symptoms such as chest pain, shortness of breath, weakness, and slurred speech.
• Tell patient that diclofenac also may increase the risk of serious adverse GI reactions; stress the need to seek immediate medical attention for such signs and symptoms as epigastric or abdominal pain, indigestion, black or tarry stools, and vomiting blood or material that looks like coffee grounds.
• Alert patient about possibly serious skin reactions and the need to seek immediate me-

dial attention for such as problems as blisters, fever, itching, rash, and other signs of hypersensitivity.

dicloxacillin sodium

Dycill, Dynapen, Pathocil

Class and Category

Chemical class: Isoxazolyl penicillin derivative
Therapeutic class: Antibiotic
Pregnancy category: B

Indications and Dosages

➤ *To treat mild to moderate upper respiratory tract and localized skin and soft-tissue infections caused by penicillinase-producing staphylococci*

CAPSULES, ORAL SOLUTION

Adults and children weighing 40 kg (88 lb) or more. 125 mg every 6 hr.
Children weighing less than 40 kg. 12.5 mg/kg daily divided into four equal doses and given every 6 hr.

➤ *To treat severe infections, such as lower respiratory tract or disseminated infections, caused by penicillinase-producing staphylococci*

CAPSULES, ORAL SOLUTION

Adults and children weighing 40 kg or more. 250 mg every 6 hr, or higher doses, if needed. *Maximum:* 6 g daily.
Children over age 1 month weighing less than 40 kg. 25 mg/kg daily divided into 4 equal doses and given every 6 hr, or higher doses if needed.

Contraindications

Hypersensitivity to dicloxacillin, other penicillins, beta-lactamase inhibitors (such as piperacillin/tazobactam), cephalosporins, imipenem, or their components

Mechanism of Action

Inhibits cell wall synthesis in susceptible bacteria, which assemble rigid, cross-linked cell walls in several steps. Dicloxacillin affects final cross-linking by inactivating penicillin-binding protein (the enzyme needed to link cell wall strands). This action inhibits cell wall synthesis and causes cell lysis and death.

Interactions

DRUGS

hepatotoxic drugs: Increased risk of hepatotoxicity
methotrexate: Decreased methotrexate clearance and increased risk of methotrexate toxicity
oral contraceptives: Decreased contraceptive action
probenecid: Increased and prolonged blood dicloxacillin level
tetracyclines: Decreased dicloxacillin effectiveness

FOODS

All foods: Possibly delayed absorption

Adverse Reactions

CNS: Dizziness, fatigue, fever, insomnia
EENT: Black "hairy" tongue, dry mouth, glossitis, laryngeal edema, laryngospasm, stomatitis, taste perversion
GI: Abdominal pain, anorexia, diarrhea, flatulence, nausea, pseudomembranous colitis, transient hepatitis, vomiting
GU: Nephropathy, vaginitis
MS: Prolonged muscle relaxation
SKIN: Dermatitis, erythema multiforme, pruritus, rash, urticaria, vesicular eruptions
Other: Anaphylaxis, serum sicknesslike reaction, superinfection

Nursing Considerations

•Before dicloxacillin therapy begins, expect to obtain body fluid and tissue samples for culture and sensitivity tests, as ordered, and review the results, if possible. Also check for history of sensitivity to cephalosporins, penicillins, and other substances.
•If diarrhea develops, notify prescriber; it could be of pseudomembranous colitis.

PATIENT TEACHING

•Instruct patient to take dicloxacillin 1 hour before or 2 hours after meals.
•Instruct patient to take drug around the clock, not to miss a dose, and to complete the entire prescription unless directed otherwise by prescriber.
•Advise patient to take oral solution with a cold beverage but not acidic juice, such as orange juice. Explain that solution is effective for 7 days at room temperature and for 14 days if refrigerated.
•Caution patient not to open capsules and mix contents with food or liquids because an unpleasant taste and decreased drug absorp-

tion will result.
•Instruct parent to shake oral solution thoroughly and measure doses with a calibrated device for accuracy.
•Advise patient to notify prescriber if she experiences adverse GI reactions or signs of hypersensitivity or superinfection.
•If patient takes an oral contraceptive, advise her to use an additional form of contraception during therapy.
•Instruct patient to store drug away from heat, moisture, and direct light and to refrigerate—but not freeze—oral solution.

dicumarol

Class and Category
Chemical class: Coumarin derivative
Therapeutic class: Anticoagulant
Pregnancy category: X

Indications and Dosages
➤ *To prevent and treat pulmonary embolus, thromboembolus, and venous thrombus; to prevent thromboembolism related to atrial fibrillation and mechanical heart valves*
TABLETS
Adults. *Initial:* 200 to 300 mg on the first day. *Maintenance:* 25 to 200 mg daily.
DOSAGE ADJUSTMENT Dosage reduced for elderly patients and those with hepatic or renal impairment.

Route	Onset	Peak	Duration
P.O.	1 to 5 days	Unknown	5 to 6 days

Mechanism of Action
Prevents coagulation by interfering with the liver's ability to synthesize vitamin K–dependent clotting factors. This in turn depletes clotting factors II (prothrombin), VII, IX, and X. Normally, clots result from a cascade of proteolytic reactions that involve several clotting factors, including vitamin K–dependent factors. These clotting factors must be converted to an activated form before the clotting cascade can continue. By depleting vitamin K–dependent clotting factors, dicumarol interferes with the clotting cascade and prevents coagulation.

Contraindications
Active bleeding; aneurysm; ascorbic acid deficiency; bacterial endocarditis; blood dyscrasia; continuous tube drainage of small intestine; diverticulitis; eclampsia or preclampsia; emaciation; hemophilia; hemorrhagic tendency; history of bleeding diathesis or warfarin-induced necrosis; leukemia; major regional lumbar block anesthesia; malnutrition; pericardial effusion; pericarditis; polyarthritis; pregnancy; prostatectomy; recent surgery on brain, eye, GI tract, or prostate; recovery from spinal puncture; severe hepatic or renal impairment; stroke; surgery resulting in large, open surfaces; threatened abortion; thrombocytopenic purpura; uncontrolled or malignant hypertension; visceral cancer; vitamin K deficiency

Interactions
DRUGS
acetaminophen, androgens, beta blockers, chlorpropamide, clofibrate, corticosteroids, cyclophosphamide, dextrothyroxine, disulfiram, erythromycin, fluconazole, gemfibrozil, glucagon, hydantoins, influenza virus vaccine, isoniazid, ketoconazole, miconazole, moricizine, propoxyphene, quinolones, streptokinase, sulfonamides, tamoxifen, thioamines, thyroid drugs, urokinase: Increased effects of dicumarol and risk of bleeding

Adverse Reactions
CNS: Fever, malaise
ENDO: Adrenal hemorrhage
GI: Abdominal cramps and distention, anorexia, diarrhea, flatulence, nausea, vomiting
GU: Menorrhagia, priapism
HEME: Hemorrhage, leukopenia
SKIN: Alopecia, pruritus, rash, urticaria
Other: Allergic reaction, purple toes syndrome

Nursing Considerations
•Use dicumarol cautiously in elderly patients and those with hepatic or renal impairment.
•Monitor results of serial tests for PT and INR and expect to adjust dosage accordingly.
•If patient also receives heparin, expect heparin therapy to continue until INR reaches desired level: 2 to 3 times the control value for pulmonary embolus, thromboembolus, or venous thrombus; or 3 to 4.5 times the control value for thromboembolism related to atrial fibrillation or mechanical valves.

•If PT or INR are prolonged, withhold one dicumarol dose, as prescribed, and, to reverse anticoagulation, give vitamin K. If patient has severe bleeding, expect to give blood to offset vitamin K's delayed onset.
•Assess patient for signs of hemorrhage, such as ecchymosis, epistaxis, gingival bleeding, hematuria, and melena.
•To reduce bleeding, apply pressure to I.M. or venipuncture sites for up to 5 minutes.

PATIENT TEACHING
•Instruct patient to take dicumarol at the same time every day.
•Inform patient that drug's full effects may not occur for 2 to 7 days.
•Instruct patient to have frequent coagulation tests, as prescribed.
•Advise patient to stabilize her intake of foods high in vitamin K. Urge her to consult prescriber before starting a weight-loss diet, altering eating habits, or taking new vitamins or other nutritional supplements; these activities may alter her vitamin K intake.
•Caution patient to avoid activities that may cause bleeding. Advise the use of a soft toothbrush and an electric razor.
•Urge patient to consult prescriber before taking OTC drugs, including herbs, which may affect dicumarol's anticoagulant effect.
•Instruct patient to take a missed dose as soon as she remembers unless it's nearly time for the next dose. Urge her to report missed doses to prescriber.
•Caution patient to immediately notify prescriber if signs of bleeding occur, such as abdominal pain or swelling; back pain; bloody or black stools; bloody urine; coughing up blood; joint pain, swelling, or stiffness; severe or continuing headache; and vomiting blood or material that looks like coffee grounds.
•Urge patient to carry medical identification and tell all health care providers that she takes dicumarol.
•Explain that coagulation will gradually return to normal after therapy stops. Remind patient to keep watching for bleeding.

dicyclomine hydrochloride

Bentyl, Bentylol (CAN), Formulex (CAN), Spasmoban (CAN)

Class and Category
Chemical class: Tertiary amine
Therapeutic class: Anticholinergic, antispasmodic
Pregnancy category: Not rated

Indications and Dosages
➤ *To control diarrhea and GI tract spasms*
CAPSULES, TABLETS
Adults and adolescents. 10 to 20 mg t.i.d. or q.i.d., increased as needed and tolerated. *Maximum:* 160 mg daily.
Children ages 6 to 12. 10 mg t.i.d. or q.i.d.
E.R. TABLETS
Adults and adolescents. 30 mg b.i.d.
SYRUP
Adults and adolescents. 10 to 20 mg t.i.d. or q.i.d., increased as needed and tolerated. *Maximum:* 60 mg daily.
Children ages 2 to 13. 10 mg t.i.d. or q.i.d.
Children ages 6 months to 2 years. 5 to 10 mg t.i.d. or q.i.d.
I.M. INJECTION
Adults. 20 mg every 4 to 6 hr. Dosage adjusted as needed and tolerated.

Mechanism of Action
Inhibits acetylcholine's muscarinic actions at postganglionic parasympathetic receptors in smooth muscles, secretory glands, and the CNS. These actions relax smooth muscles and diminish GI, GU, and biliary tract secretions.

Contraindications
Adhesions between iris and lens, angle-closure glaucoma, GI obstruction, hemorrhagic shock, hepatic disease, hiatal hernia, hypersensitivity to any anticholinergic, ileus, intestinal atony in elderly or debilitated patients, myasthenia gravis, myocardial ischemia, obstructive uropathy, renal disease, severe ulcerative colitis, tachycardia, toxic megacolon

Interactions
DRUGS
adsorbent antidiarrheals, antacids: Decreased dicyclomine absorption
amantadine, anticholinergics, phenothiazines, tricyclic antidepressants: Increased dicyclomine effects
antimyasthenics: Reduced intestinal motility

atenolol: Increased atenolol effects
cyclopropane: Risk of ventricular arrhythmias
haloperidol: Decreased antipsychotic effect of haloperidol
ketoconazole: Decreased ketoconazole absorption
metoclopramide: Decreased effect of metoclopramide on GI motility
opioid analgesics: Increased risk of ileus, severe constipation, and urine retention
potassium chloride, especially wax-matrix preparations: Possibly GI ulceration
urinary alkalinizers (antacids that contain calcium or magnesium, carbonic anhydrase inhibitors, citrates, sodium bicarbonate): Delayed excretion and increased risk of adverse effects of dicyclomine

Adverse Reactions
CNS: Agitation, dizziness, drowsiness, dyskinesia, excitement, fever, insomnia, lethargy, light-headedness (with I.M. use), nervousness, paresthesia, syncope
CV: Palpitations, tachycardia
EENT: Blurred vision, cycloplegia, dry mouth, loss of taste, mydriasis, nasal congestion, photophobia
GI: Constipation, dysphagia, heartburn, ileus, vomiting
GU: Impotence, urine retention
SKIN: Decreased sweating, flushing, pruritus
Other: Heatstroke; injection site pain, redness, and swelling

Nursing Considerations
• Assess patient for tachycardia before giving dicyclomine; it may increase heart rate.
• Don't give drug by I.V. route.
• Watch for symptoms of hypersensitivity, such as agitation and pruritus. They usually resolve within 48 hours after stopping drug.
• During long-term use, assess patient for chronic constipation and fecal impaction, and take corrective measures, as prescribed.
PATIENT TEACHING
• Instruct patient to store dicyclomine in a tightly sealed container at room temperature, protected from moisture and direct light. Advise her not to refrigerate syrup.
• Inform patient that dicyclomine relieves symptoms but doesn't cure the disorder.
• For best results, instruct patient to take drug 30 to 60 minutes before eating.
• Advise patient not to take antacid or antidiarrheal within 2 hours of dicyclomine.

• Inform patient that blurred vision, dizziness, or drowsiness may occur.
• To prevent constipation, advise patient to eat high-fiber foods and drink at least eight glasses of water daily.
• **WARNING** Urge patient to avoid getting overheated during exercise or in hot weather because heatstroke may result. Inform patient that hot baths or saunas may cause dizziness or fainting.
• Instruct patient to change position slowly to avoid light-headedness.
• Inform patient that stopping drug abruptly may cause dizziness and vomiting.
• Tell patient to take a missed dose as soon as she remembers unless it's nearly time for the next dose. Caution against doubling it.

diflunisal
Apo-Diflunisal (CAN), Dolobid, Novo-Diflunisal (CAN)

Class and Category
Chemical class: Difluorophenyl, salicylic acid derivative
Therapeutic class: Analgesic, anti-inflammatory
Pregnancy category: C (first trimester), Not rated (later trimesters)

Indications and Dosages
➤ *To relieve mild to moderate pain*
TABLETS
Adults. 1 g followed by 0.5 g every 8 to 12 hr. *Maximum:* 1.5 g daily.

➤ *To reduce inflammation in osteoarthritis or rheumatoid arthritis*
TABLETS
Adults. 0.5 to 1 g daily in divided doses b.i.d. *Maximum:* 1.5 g daily.
DOSAGE ADJUSTMENT Dosage reduced for elderly patients and those who use diuretics; who could be harmed by prolonged bleeding time; or who have compromised cardiac function, conditions that cause fluid retention, hepatic or renal impairment, hypertension, or upper GI disease.

Route	Onset	Peak	Duration
P.O.*	1 hr	2 to 3 hr	8 to 12 hr

* For analgesia; unknown for anti-inflammatory effects.

Mechanism of Action

Blocks the activity of cyclooxygenase, the enzyme needed to synthesize prostaglandins, which mediate the inflammatory response and cause local vasodilation, swelling, and pain. By blocking cyclooxygenase and inhibiting prostaglandins, this NSAID reduces inflammatory symptoms. This mechanism also relieves pain because prostaglandins promote pain transmission from the periphery to the spinal cord.

Contraindications

Asthma attacks, rhinitis, or urticaria precipitated by aspirin or other NSAIDs; hypersensitivity to diflunisal; treatment of perioperative pain after coronary artery bypass graft surgery

Interactions

DRUGS

acetaminophen: Increased risk of adverse renal effects with long-term use of both drugs
antacids: Decreased blood diflunisal level
antihypertensives: Decreased antihypertensive effects
aspirin, other NSAIDs, salicylates: Increased GI irritability and bleeding, decreased diflunisal effectiveness
beta blockers: Impaired antihypertensive effects of beta blocker
cefamandole, cefoperazone, cefotetan, plicamycin, valproic acid: Increased risk of hypoprothrombinemia
colchicine, corticotropin (long-term use), glucocorticoids, potassium supplements: Increased GI irritability and bleeding
cyclosporine, gold compounds, nephrotoxic drugs: Increased risk of nephrotoxicity
digoxin: Increased blood digoxin level
heparin, oral anticoagulants, thrombolytics: Prolonged PT, increased risk of bleeding
hydrochlorothiazide: Increased blood hydrochlorothiazide level
insulin, oral antidiabetic drugs: Increased hypoglycemic effects
loop diuretics: Decreased loop diuretic effectiveness
methotrexate: Increased risk of methotrexate toxicity
phenytoin: Increased blood phenytoin level
probenecid: Increased diflunisal toxicity

ACTIVITIES

alcohol use: Increased GI irritability and bleeding

Adverse Reactions

CNS: Aseptic meningitis, cerebral hemorrhage, dizziness, drowsiness, headache, insomnia
CV: Vasculitis
EENT: Tinnitus
ENDO: Hypoglycemia
GI: Abdominal pain, constipation, diarrhea, esophageal irritation, GI bleeding or ulceration, hepatic failure, hepatitis, indigestion, jaundice, nausea, perforation of stomach or intestine, vomiting
GU: Acute renal failure, interstitial nephritis
HEME: Agranulocytosis, aplastic anemia, leukopenia, pancytopenia, thrombocytopenia
SKIN: Erythema multiforme, exfoliative dermatitis, rash, Stevens-Johnson syndrome, toxic epidermal necrolysis
Other: Anaphylaxis, angioedema, hyponatremia

Nursing Considerations

•Use diflunisal with extreme caution in patients with a history of GI bleeding or ulcer disease because NSAIDs such as diflunisal increase the risk. Use drug for the shortest time possible in these patients.
•Be aware that serious GI tract ulceration and bleeding, as well as perforation of stomach or intestine, can occur without warning or symptoms. Elderly patients are at greater risk. To minimize risk, give diflunisal with food. If patient develops GI distress, withhold drug and notify prescriber immediately.
•Use diflunisal cautiously in patients with hypertension, and monitor blood pressure closely during therapy; drug can cause or worsen hypertension.
•Use diflunisal cautiously in elderly patients, those with renal dysfunction, and those who should avoid a prolonged bleeding time.
•WARNING Monitor patient closely for thrombotic events, including stroke and MI, because NSAIDs such as diflunisal increase the risk of these events.
•Monitor BUN and serum creatinine levels in elderly patients, patients taking ACE inhibitors or diuretics, and patients with heart falure or impaired hepatic or renal function. These patients may have an increased risk of renal failure.

•Assess patient's skin routinely for rash or other signs of hypersensitivity reaction; drug may cause serious skin reactions without warning. At first sign of reaction, stop drug and notify prescriber.

•Assess type, location, and intensity of pain before and 1 to 2 hours after giving drug.

•Assess patient carefully because long-term or high-dose therapy may mask fever.

PATIENT TEACHING

•Teach patient not to crush or chew diflunisal tablets.

•Instruct patient to take tablet with a full glass of water and not to lie down for 30 minutes afterward to avoid esophageal irritation.

•Inform patient that drug will start working in about 1 week but that full effects may not occur for several weeks.

•Explain that diflunisal may increase the risk of serious adverse cardiovascular reactions; urge patient to seek immediate medical attention for such signs and symptoms as chest pain, shortness of breath, slurred speech, and weakness.

•Tell patient that diflunisal also may increase the risk of serious adverse GI reactions; stress the need to seek immediate medical attention for signs and symptoms such as abdominal or epigastric pain, black or tarry stools, indigestion, and vomiting blood or material that resembles coffee grounds.

•Alert patient about possibly serious skin reactions and the need to seek immediate medial attention for such as problems as blisters, fever, itching, rash, and other signs of hypersensitivity.

•Caution patient to avoid acetaminophen, alcohol, aspirin, and other salicylates during diflunisal therapy, unless directed otherwise by prescriber.

•Advise patient to avoid potentially hazardous activities until drug's CNS effects are known.

•Advise patient to tell health care providers about diflunisal therapy before surgery, including dental surgery. Therapy should stop for 1 week before procedure.

digoxin

Lanoxicaps, Lanoxin, Lanoxin Elixir Pediatric, Lanoxin Injection, Lanoxin Injection Pediatric, Novo-Digoxin (CAN)

Class and Category

Chemical class: Digitalis glycoside
Therapeutic class: Antiarrhythmic, cardiotonic
Pregnancy category: C

Indications and Dosages

➤ *To treat heart failure, atrial flutter, atrial fibrillation, and paroxysmal atrial tachycardia with rapid digitalization*

CAPSULES, I.V. INJECTION

Adults. *Loading:* 10 to 15 mcg/kg in 3 divided doses every 6 to 8 hr, with first dose equal to 50% of total dose. *Maintenance:* 125 to 350 mcg daily once or twice daily.

Children over age 10. *Loading:* 8 to 12 mcg/kg in 3 or more divided doses, with first dose equal to 50% of total dose. Subsequent doses given every 6 to 8 hr. *Maintenance:* 2 to 3 mcg/kg once daily.

Children ages 6 to 10. *Loading:* 15 to 30 mcg/kg in 3 or more divided doses, with first dose equal to 50% of total dose. Subsequent doses given every 6 to 8 hr. *Maintenance:* 4 to 8 mcg/kg daily in 2 divided doses.

Children ages 2 to 5. *Loading:* 25 to 35 mcg/kg in 3 or more divided doses, with first dose equal to 50% of total dose. Subsequent doses given every 6 to 8 hr. *Maintenance:* 6 to 9 mcg/kg daily in 2 divided doses.

Infants ages 1 to 24 months. *Loading:* 30 to 50 mcg/kg in 3 or more divided doses, with first dose equal to 50% of total dose. Subsequent doses every 6 to 8 hr. *Maintenance:* 7.5 to 12 mcg/kg daily in 2 divided doses.

Full-term neonates. *Loading:* 20 to 30 mcg/kg in 3 or more divided doses, with first dose equal to 50% of total dose. Subsequent doses given every 6 to 8 hr. *Maintenance:* 5 to 8 mcg/kg daily in 2 divided doses.

Premature neonates. *Loading:* 15 to 25 mcg/kg in 3 or more divided doses, with first dose equal to 50% of total dose. Subsequent doses given every 6 to 8 hr. *Maintenance:* 4 to 6 mcg/kg daily in 2 divided doses.

ELIXIR, TABLETS

Adults. *Loading:* 10 to 15 mcg/kg total dose given in 3 divided doses every 6 to 8 hr, with first dose equal to 50% of total dose. *Maintenance:* 125 to 500 mcg daily.

Children over age 10. *Loading:* 10 to 15 mcg/kg total given in 3 divided doses every 6 to 8 hr, with first dose equal to 50% of total dose. *Maintenance:* 2.5 to 5 mcg/kg daily.

D

Children ages 5 to 10. *Loading:* 20 to 35 mcg/kg in 3 divided doses every 6 to 8 hr. *Maintenance:* 5 to 10 mcg/kg daily in 2 divided doses.

Children ages 2 to 5. *Loading:* 30 to 40 mcg/kg in 3 divided doses every 6 to 8 hr. *Maintenance:* 7.5 to 10 mcg/kg daily in 2 divided doses.

Infants ages 1 to 24 months. *Loading:* 35 to 60 mcg/kg in 3 divided doses every 6 to 8 hr. *Maintenance:* 10 to 15 mcg/kg daily in 2 divided doses.

Full-term neonates. *Loading:* 25 to 35 mcg/kg in 3 divided doses every 6 to 8 hr. *Maintenance:* 6 to 10 mcg/kg daily in 2 divided doses.

Premature neonates. *Loading:* 20 to 30 mcg/kg in 3 divided doses every 6 to 8 hr. *Maintenance:* 5 to 7.5 mcg/kg daily in 2 divided doses.

DOSAGE ADJUSTMENT Dosage carefully adjusted for patients who are elderly or debilitated or have implanted pacemakers because toxicity may develop at doses tolerated by most patients.

Route	Onset	Peak	Duration
P.O.	30 to 120 min	6 to 8 hr	3 to 4 days
I.V.	5 to 30 min	1 to 5 hr	3 to 4 days

Mechanism of Action
Increases the force and velocity of myocardial contraction, resulting in positive inotropic effects. Digoxin produces antiarrhythmic effects by decreasing the conduction rate and increasing the effective refractory period of the AV node.

Contraindications
Hypersensitive carotid sinus syndrome, hypersensitivity to digoxin, presence or history of digitalis toxicity or idiosyncratic reaction to digoxin, ventricular fibrillation, ventricular tachycardia unless heart failure occurs unrelated to digoxin therapy

Interactions
DRUGS
adsorbent antidiarrheals, such as kaolin and pectin; bulk laxatives; cholestyramine; colestipol; oral neomycin; sulfasalazine: Inhibited digoxin absorption

amiodarone, propafenone: Elevated blood digoxin level, possibly to toxic level
antacids: Inhibited digoxin absorption
antiarrhythmics, pancuronium, parenteral calcium salts, rauwolfia alkaloids, sympathomimetics: Increased risk of arrhythmias
diltiazem, verapamil: Increased blood digoxin level, possibly excessive bradycardia
edrophonium: Excessive slowing of heart rate
erythromycin, neomycin, tetracycline: Possibly increased blood digoxin level
hypokalemia-causing drugs, potassium-wasting diuretics: Increased risk of digitalis toxicity from hypokalemia
indomethacin: Decreased renal clearance and increased blood level of digoxin
magnesium sulfate (parenteral): Possibly cardiac conduction changes and heart block
quinidine, quinine: Increased blood digoxin level
spironolactone: Increased half-life and risk of adverse effects of digoxin
succinylcholine: Increased risk of digoxin-induced arrhythmias
sucralfate: Decreased digoxin absorption
FOODS
high-fiber food: Inhibited digoxin absorption

Adverse Reactions
CNS: Confusion, depression, drowsiness, extreme weakness, headache, syncope
CV: Arrhythmias, heart block
EENT: Blurred vision, colored halos around objects
GI: Abdominal discomfort or pain, anorexia, diarrhea, nausea, vomiting
Other: Electrolyte imbalances

Nursing Considerations
•Administer parenteral digoxin undiluted, or dilute with a fourfold or greater volume of sterile water for injection, normal saline solution, or D_5W for I.V. administration. Once diluted, administer immediately. Discard if solution is markedly discolored or contains precipitate.
•Before giving each dose, take patient's apical pulse and notify prescriber if pulse is below 60 beats/minute (or other specified level).
•Monitor patient closely for signs of digitalis toxicity, such as altered mental status, arrhythmias, heart block, nausea, vision disturbances, and vomiting. If they appear, notify prescriber, check serum digoxin level as or-

dered, and expect to withhold drug until level is known. Monitor ECG tracing continuously.

•If patient has acute or unstable chronic atrial fibrillation, assess for drug effectiveness. Ventricular rate may not normalize even when serum drug level falls within therapeutic range; raising the dosage probably won't produce a therapeutic effect and may lead to toxicity.

•Frequently obtain ECG tracings as ordered in elderly patients because of their smaller body mass and reduced renal clearance. Elderly patients, especially those with coronary insufficiency, are more susceptible to arrhythmias—particularly ventricular fibrillation—if digitalis toxicity occurs.

•Monitor paptient's serum potassium level regularly because hypokalemia predisposes to digitalis toxicity and serious arrhythmias. Also monitor potassium level frequently when giving potassium salts because hyperkalemia in patients receiving digoxin can be fatal.

PATIENT TEACHING

•Stress the importance of taking digoxin exactly as prescribed. Warn patient about possible toxicity from taking too much and decreased effectiveness from taking too little.

•Instruct patient to take digoxin at the same time each day to help increase compliance.

•Teach patient how to take her pulse, and instruct her to do so before each dose. Urge her to notify prescriber if pulse falls below 60 beats/minute or suddenly increases.

•Inform patient that small, white 0.25-mg tablets can easily be confused with other drugs. Caution against carrying digoxin in anything other than its original labeled container.

•Emphasize the need to use the special dropper supplied with elixir to ensure accurate dose measurement.

•Instruct patient to take a missed dose as soon as she remembers if within 12 hours of scheduled dose. If not, urge her to notify prescriber immediately.

•Urge patient to notify prescriber if she experiences adverse reactions, such as GI distress or pulse changes.

•Instruct patient to carry medical identification that indicates her need for digoxin.

•Advise patient to consult prescriber before using other drugs, including OTC products.

digoxin immune Fab (ovine)

Digibind

Class and Category

Chemical class: Digoxin-specific antigen-binding fragments
Therapeutic class: Digitalis glycoside antidote
Pregnancy category: C

Indications and Dosages

➤ *To treat acute toxicity from a known amount of digoxin elixir or tablets*

I.V. INJECTION

Adults and children. Individualized dosage based on amount ingested. Dose (mg) = dose ingested (mg) multiplied by 0.8 and then divided by 0.5, multiplied by 38, and rounded up to next whole vial.

➤ *To treat acute toxicity from a known amount of digoxin capsules, digitoxin tablets, or I.V. injection of digoxin or digitoxin*

I.V. INJECTION

Adults and children. Individualized dosage based on amount ingested. Dose (mg) = dose ingested (mg) divided by 0.5, then multiplied by 38 and rounded up to next whole vial.

➤ *To treat acute toxicity from an unknown amount of digoxin or digitoxin during long-term therapy*

I.V. INJECTION

Adults and children. Individualized dosage for digoxin toxicity: dose (mg) = serum digoxin level (ng/ml) multiplied by body weight (kg), then divided by 100, and then multiplied by 38. Individualized dosage for digitoxin toxicity: dose (mg) = serum digitoxin level (ng/ml) multiplied by body weight (kg) and then divided by 1,000, multiplied by 38, and rounded up to next whole vial.

DOSAGE ADJUSTMENT Higher dose administered, as prescribed, if the dose based on ingested amount differs substantially from the dose based on serum digoxin or digitoxin level. Dose repeated after several hours, if needed.

Route	Onset	Peak	Duration
I.V.	15 to 30 min	Unknown	8 to 12 hr

Mechanism of Action
Binds with digoxin or digitoxin molecules. The resulting complex is excreted through the kidneys. As the free serum digoxin level declines, tissue-bound digoxin enters the serum and also is bound and excreted.

Contraindications
Hypersensitivity to digoxin immune Fab

Adverse Reactions
CV: Increased ventricular rate (in atrial fibrillation), worsening of heart failure or low cardiac output
Other: Allergic reaction (difficulty breathing, urticaria), febrile reaction, hypokalemia

Nursing Considerations
• Expect each 38-mg vial of purified digoxin immune Fab to bind about 0.5 mg of digoxin or digitoxin.
• To reconstitute for I.V. use, dissolve 38 mg in 4 ml of sterile water for injection to yield 9.5 mg/ml. Mix gently. Further dilute with normal saline solution to proper volume for I.V. infusion. For very small doses, reconstituted 38-mg vial may be diluted with 34 ml of normal saline solution to yield 1 mg/ml.
• **WARNING** Before administering digoxin immune Fab to high-risk patient, test for allergic reaction as prescribed by diluting 0.1 ml of reconstituted drug in 9.9 ml of sodium chloride for injection and then injecting 0.1 ml (9.5 mcg/0.1 ml) intradermally. After 20 minutes, observe for an urticarial wheal surrounded by erythema. Alternatively, perform a scratch test by placing one drop of 9.5 mcg/0.1 ml dilution on patient's skin and making a ¼" scratch through the drop with a sterile needle. Inspect site in 20 minutes. Test is considered positive if it produces a wheal surrounded by erythema. If test causes a systemic reaction, apply tourniquet above test site, notify prescriber, and prepare to respond to anaphylaxis. Be aware that if a skin or systemic reaction occurs, additional drug shouldn't be given unless essential; if more of the drug must be given, expect prescriber to pretreat patient with corticosteroids and diphenhydramine. Prescriber should be on standby to treat anaphylaxis.
• For an infant, reconstitute digoxin immune Fab as ordered and administer with a tuberculin syringe.
• When administering to a child, watch for fluid volume overload.
• When giving a large dose, expect a faster onset but watch closely for febrile reaction.
• Give I.V. infusion through a 0.22-micron membrane filter over 30 minutes. Keep in mind that drug may be given by rapid I.V. injection if cardiac arrest is imminent.
• Monitor serum potassium level often, especially during first few hours of therapy. The potassium level may drop rapidly.

PATIENT TEACHING
• Inform patient of the purpose of digoxin immune Fab and how it will be given.
• Advise patient to notify you immediately if she experiences adverse reactions, especially difficulty breathing and urticaria.

dihydroergotamine mesylate
D.H.E. 45, Dihydroergotamine-Sandoz (CAN), Migranal

Class and Category
Chemical class: Semisynthetic ergot alkaloid
Therapeutic class: Antimigraine
Pregnancy category: X

Indications and Dosages
➤ *To treat acute migraine with or without aura*

I.V. INJECTION
Adults. 1 mg, repeated in 1 hr, if needed. *Maximum:* 6 mg/wk.

I.M. INJECTION
Adults. 1 mg at first sign of headache, repeated every hr up to 3 mg, if needed. *Maximum:* 3 mg/24 hr, 6 mg/wk.

NASAL SPRAY
Adults. 1 spray (0.5 mg) in each nostril, repeated in 15 min for a total dose of 2 sprays in each nostril or 2 mg. *Maximum:* 3 mg/ 24 hr, 4 mg/wk.

Route	Onset	Peak	Duration
I.V.	In 5 min	15 min to 2 hr	About 8 hr
I.M.	15 to 30 min	15 min to 2 hr	3 to 4 hr
Nasal	In 30 min	30 to 60 min	Unknown

Mechanism of Action
Produces intracranial and peripheral vasoconstriction by binding to all known 5-hydroxytryptamine$_1$ (5-HT$_1$) receptors, alpha$_1$- and alpha$_2$-adrenergic receptors, and dopaminergic receptors. Activation of 5-HT$_1$ receptors on intracranial blood vessels probably constricts large intracranial arteries and closes arteriovenous anastomoses to relieve migraine headache. Activation of 5-HT$_1$ receptors on sensory nerves in the trigeminal system also may inhibit the release of pro-inflammatory neuropeptides.

Peripherally, dihydroergotamine causes vasoconstriction by stimulating alpha-adrenergic receptors. At therapeutic doses, it inhibits norepinephrine reuptake, increasing vasoconstriction. The drug constricts veins more than arteries, increasing venous return while decreasing venous stasis and pooling.

Contraindications
Coronary artery disease, including vasospasm; hemiplegic or basilar migraine; hypersensitivity to dihydroergotamine or other ergot alkaloids; malnutrition; peripheral vascular disease or after vascular surgery; pregnancy; sepsis; severe hepatic or renal impairment; severe pruritus; uncontrolled hypertension; use of macrolide antibiotics or protease inhibitors; use within 24 hours of 5-HT$_1$ agonist, ergotamine-containing or ergot-type drug, or methysergide

Interactions
DRUGS
beta blockers: Possibly peripheral vasoconstriction and peripheral ischemia, increased risk of gangrene
macrolides, protease inhibitors: Possibly increased risk of vasospasm, acute ergotism with peripheral ischemia
nitrates: Decreased antianginal effects of nitrates
other ergot drugs, including ergoloid mesylates, ergonovine, methylergonovine, methysergide, and sumatriptan: Increased risk of serious adverse effects from nasal dihydroergotamine
systemic vasoconstrictors: Risk of severe hypertension
ACTIVITIES

smoking: Possibly increased ischemic response to ergot therapy

Adverse Reactions
CNS: Anxiety, confusion, dizziness, fatigue, headache, paresthesia, somnolence, weakness
CV: Bradycardia, chest pain, peripheral vasospasm (calf or heel pain with exertion, cool and cyanotic hands and feet, leg weakness, weak or absent pulses), tachycardia
EENT: Abnormal vision; dry mouth; epistaxis, nasal congestion or rhinitis, and sore nose (nasal spray); miosis; pharyngitis; sinusitis; taste perversion
GI: Diarrhea, nausea, vomiting
MS: Muscle stiffness
SKIN: Localized edema of face, feet, fingers, and lower legs; sensation of heat or warmth; sudden diaphoresis

Nursing Considerations
•**WARNING** Monitor for signs of dihydroergotamine overdose, such as abdominal pain, confusion, delirium, dizziness, dyspnea, headache, nausea, pain in legs or arms, paresthesia, seizures, and vomiting.
•Assess peripheral pulses, skin sensation, warmth, and capillary refill. After giving nasal dihydroergotamine, monitor for signs of widespread blood vessel constriction and adverse reactions caused by decreased circulation to many body areas.
PATIENT TEACHING
•Instruct patient to use nasal spray when headache pain—not aura—begins.
•Teach her to prime spray pump by squeezing it four times.
•Advise patient to wait 15 minutes between each set of nasal sprays.
•Encourage patient to lie down in a quiet, dark room after using drug.
•Instruct patient to use more drug if headache returns or worsens but not to exceed maximum prescribed amount or frequency.
•Remind patient to take drug only as needed, not on a daily basis.
•Instruct patient to discard residual nasal spray in an open ampule after 8 hours.
•If patient has a headache different from her usual migraines, caution her not to use dihydroergotamine and to notify prescriber.
•Inform patient that nasal drug won't relieve pain other than throbbing headaches.
•Advise patient to avoid alcohol, which can cause or worsen headaches, and to avoid

D

smoking, which may cause an ischemic response.
•Warn patient about possible dizziness during or after a migraine for which she took dihydroergotamine.

dihydrotachysterol

DHT, DHT Intensol, Hytakerol

Class and Category

Chemical class: Sterol derivative, vitamin D analogue
Therapeutic class: Antihypocalcemic, antihypoparathyroid
Pregnancy category: C

Indications and Dosages

➤ *To treat hypocalcemic and idiopathic tetany*

CAPSULES, ORAL SOLUTION, TABLETS

Adults and adolescents. *Initial:* 0.75 to 2.5 mg daily for 3 days for acute cases; 0.25 to 0.5 mg daily for 3 days for less acute cases. *Maintenance:* 0.25 mg/wk to 1 mg daily, as needed to maintain normal serum calcium level.

➤ *To treat hypoparathyroidism*

CAPSULES, ORAL SOLUTION, TABLETS

Adults and adolescents. *Initial:* 0.75 to 2.5 mg daily for several days. *Maintenance:* 0.2 to 1 mg daily.
Children. *Initial:* 1 to 5 mg daily for 4 days; then continued or decreased to one-quarter the dose. *Maintenance:* 0.5 to 1.5 mg daily.

Route	Onset	Peak	Duration
P.O.	Several hr	Unknown	Up to 9 wk

Mechanism of Action

Stimulates intestinal calcium absorption and mobilizes bone calcium when parathyroid hormone and renal tissue fail to raise the serum calcium level.

Contraindications

Hypercalcemia, hypersensitivity to vitamin D, hypervitaminosis D, malabsorption syndrome, renal dysfunction

Interactions

DRUGS

aluminum-containing antacids: Possibly increased serum aluminum level, leading to toxicity
barbiturates, phenytoin: Decreased half-life and therapeutic effects of vitamin D
calcium-containing drugs, thiazide diuretics: Risk of hypercalcemia in patients with hypoparathyroidism
cholestyramine, colestipol, mineral oil: Decreased vitamin D absorption
digitalis glycosides: Possibly hypercalcemia; possibly potentiated effects of digitalis glycosides, resulting in arrhythmias
magnesium-containing antacids: Risk of hypermagnesemia, especially in patients with chronic renal failure
phosphorus-containing drugs: Increased risk of hyperphosphatemia
vitamin D analogues: Increased risk of vitamin D toxicity

Adverse Reactions

Other: Vitamin D toxicity (long-term, high-dose therapy)

Nursing Considerations

•After thyroid surgery, expect to give 0.25 mg once daily with 6 g of oral calcium lactate until danger of tetany has passed.
•Monitor serum calcium level regularly to determine dosage schedule and detect or prevent hypercalcemia. The difference between therapeutic and toxic doses may be small.
•Monitor closely for signs of vitamin D toxicity: abdominal cramps, amnesia, anorexia, ataxia, coma, constipation, depression, diarrhea, disorientation, hallucinations, headache, hypotonia, lethargy, nausea, syncope, tinnitus, vertigo, vomiting, and weakness. Renal impairment may cause albuminuria, polydipsia, and polyuria. Delayed treatment can result in death from cardiac and renal failure caused by widespread calcification of soft tissues, including the heart, blood vessels, kidneys, and lungs.
•If toxicity occurs, notify prescriber and expect to stop dihydrotachysterol immediately. Place patient on bed rest, administer fluids and a laxative, and place her on a low-calcium diet as ordered. For hypercalcemic crisis with dehydration, prepare to give I.V. normal saline solution and a loop diuretic (such as furosemide or ethacrynic acid) to increase urinary calcium excretion.

PATIENT TEACHING

•Stress the importance of not exceeding pre-

scribed dihydrotachysterol dosage because of the risk of vitamin D toxicity.
•If patient detects signs of toxicity, caution her not to take the next dose and to notify prescriber immediately.
•Advise patient to drop solution directly into her mouth or to mix it with fruit juice, cereal, or other food.
•Tell patient to take a missed dose as soon as she remembers unless it's nearly time for the next dose. Warn her not to double it.
•Advise patient to avoid OTC drugs and dietary supplements that contain aluminum, calcium, phosphorus, or vitamin D, unless directed by prescriber. Also advise her to avoid antacids that contain magnesium.
•Urge patient to keep follow-up appointments and to have her serum calcium level measured periodically.

diltiazem hydrochloride

Apo-Diltiaz (CAN), Cardizem, Cardizem CD, Cardizem LA, Cardizem SR, Dilacor XR, Novo-Diltiazem (CAN), Nu-Diltiaz (CAN)

Class and Category
Chemical class: Benzothiazepine derivative
Therapeutic class: Antianginal, antiarrhythmic, antihypertensive
Pregnancy category: C

Indications and Dosages
➤ *To treat Prinzmetal's (variant) angina and chronic stable angina*
TABLETS
Adults and adolescents. *Initial:* 30 mg t.i.d. or q.i.d. before meals and at bedtime, increased every 1 or 2 days as appropriate. *Maximum:* 360 mg daily in divided doses t.i.d. or q.i.d.
E.R. TABLETS
Adults and adolescents. *Initial:* 180 mg daily, increased every 7 to 14 days as needed. *Maximum:* 360 mg daily.

➤ *To control hypertension*
E.R. CAPSULES
Adults and adolescents. *Initial:* 180 to 240 mg daily, adjusted after 14 days as appropriate. *Maximum:* 360 mg daily.
S.R. CAPSULES
Adults and adolescents. *Initial:* 60 to 120 mg b.i.d., adjusted after 14 days as appropriate. *Maximum:* 360 mg daily.

TABLETS
Adults and adolescents. *Initial:* 30 mg t.i.d. or q.i.d. before meals and at bedtime, increased every 1 or 2 days as appropriate. *Maximum:* 360 mg daily in divided doses t.i.d. or q.i.d.
E.R. TABLETS
Adults. *Initial:* 180 to 240 mg daily, adjusted after 14 days, as needed. *Maximum:* 540 mg daily.

➤ *To treat atrial fibrillation, atrial flutter, and paroxysmal supraventricular tachycardia*
I.V. INFUSION OR INJECTION
Adults and adolescents. 0.25 mg/kg given by bolus over 2 min. If response is inadequate after 15 min, 0.35 mg/kg given by bolus over 2 min. Then 10 mg/hr for continued reduction of heart rate after bolus, increased by 5 mg/hr, as needed. *Maximum:* 15 mg/hr for up to 24 hr.

Route	Onset	Peak	Duration
P.O.	30 to 60 min	In 2 wk	Unknown
P.O. (E.R.)	2 to 3 hr	In 2 wk	Unknown
P.O. (S.R.)	Unknown	In 2 wk	Unknown
I.V.	In 3 min	2 to 7 min	30 min to 10 hr*

Incompatibilities
Don't give diltiazem through same I.V. line as acetazolamide, acyclovir, aminophylline, ampicillin sodium/sulbactam sodium, cefamandole, cefoperazone, diazepam, furosemide, heparin, hydrocortisone sodium succinate, methylprednisolone sodium succinate, mezlocillin, nafcillin, phenytoin, rifampin, or sodium bicarbonate.

Contraindications
Acute MI; cardiogenic shock; Lown-Ganong-Levine or Wolff-Parkinson-White syndrome, second- or third-degree AV block, and sick sinus syndrome, unless artificial pacemaker is in place; pulmonary edema; systolic blood pressure below 90 mm Hg; ventricular tachycardia (wide complex)

---

*For infusion; 1 to 3 hr for injection.

Mechanism of Action

Diltiazem inhibits calcium movement into coronary and vascular smooth-muscle cells by blocking slow calcium channels in cell membranes, as shown. This action decreases intracellular calcium, which:

• inhibits smooth-muscle cell contractions
• decreases myocardial oxygen demand by relaxing coronary and vascular smooth muscle, reducing peripheral vascular resistance and systolic and diastolic blood pressures
• slows AV conduction time and prolongs AV nodal refractoriness
• interrupts the reentry circuit in AV nodal reentrant tachycardias.

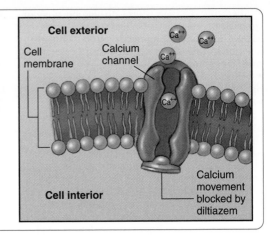

Interactions

DRUGS

anesthetic: Additive hypotension; possibly decreased cardiac contractility, conductivity, and automaticity
benzodiazepines: Increased risk of prolonged sedation
beta blockers: Possibly increased risk of adverse cardiovascular effects
buspirone: Increased effects and risk of buspirone toxicity
carbamazepine, cyclosporine, lovastatin, quinidine, theophyllines: Decreased hepatic clearance and increased serum levels of these drugs, leading to toxicity
cimetidine: Decreased diltiazem metabolism, increased blood diltiazem level
digoxin: Increased blood digoxin level
lithium: Possibly neurotoxicity
NSAIDs: Possibly antagonized antihypertensive effect of diltiazem
prazocin: Possibly increased risk of hypotension
procainamide: Possibly increased risk of prolonged QT interval
quinidine: Increased risk of adverse quinidine effects
rifampin: Decreased blood diltiazem level to undetectable amounts

Adverse Reactions

CNS: Abnormal gait, amnesia, asthenia, depression, dizziness, dream disturbances, extrapyramidal reactions, fatigue, hallucinations, headache, insomnia, nervousness, paresthesia, personality change, somnolence, syncope, tremor, weakness
CV: Angina, atrial flutter, AV block (first-, second-, and third-degree), bradycardia, bundle-branch block, heart failure, hypotension, palpitations, peripheral edema, PVCs, sinus arrest, sinus tachycardia, 12-lead ECG abnormalities, ventricular fibrillation, ventricular tachycardia
EENT: Amblyopia, dry mouth, epistaxis, eye irritation, gingival bleeding and hyperplasia, gingivitis, nasal congestion, retinopathy, taste perversion, tinnitus
ENDO: Hyperglycemia
GI: Anorexia, constipation, diarrhea, elevated liver function test results, indigestion, nausea, thirst, vomiting
GU: Acute renal failure, impotence, nocturia, polyuria, sexual dysfunction
HEME: Hemolytic anemia, leukopenia, prolonged bleeding time, thrombocytopenia
MS: Arthralgia, muscle spasms, myalgia
RESP: Cough, dyspnea
SKIN: Alopecia, diaphoresis, erythema multiforme, exfoliative dermatitis, flushing, leukocytoclastic vasculitis, petechiae, photosensitivity, pruritus, purpura, rash, Stevens-Johnson syndrome, toxic epidermal necrolysis, urticaria
Other: Angioedema, hyperuricemia, weight gain

Nursing Considerations

• Use diltiazem cautiously in patients with impaired hepatic or renal function, and monitor liver and renal function test results, as appropriate; diltiazem is metabolized mainly in the liver and excreted by the kidneys.

•**WARNING** Monitor patient's blood pressure, pulse rate, and heart rate and rhythm by continuous ECG as appropriate during therapy. Keep emergency equipment and drugs available.

•Assess patient for signs and symptoms of heart failure.

•If patient takes digoxin, watch for signs of digitalis toxicity, such as nausea, vomiting, halo vision, and elevated serum digoxin level.

•Administer sublingual nitroglycerin, as prescribed, during diltiazem therapy.

•Expect to discontinue drug if adverse skin reactions, usually transient, persist.

PATIENT TEACHING

•Explain that regular tablets can be crushed but that capsules and E.R. tablets must be swallowed whole.

•**WARNING** Tell patient that stopping drug suddenly may cause life-threatening effects.

•Advise patient to monitor blood pressure and pulse rate regularly and to report significant changes to prescriber.

•Urge patient to report chest pain, difficulty breathing, dizziness, fainting, irregular heartbeat, rash, or swollen ankles.

•Instruct patient to maintain good oral hygiene, perform gum massage, and see a dentist every 6 months to prevent gingival bleeding and hyperplasia and gingivitis.

dimenhydrinate

Dinate, Dramanate, Gravol (CAN), Hydrate

Class and Category

Chemical class: Ethanolamine derivative
Therapeutic class: Antiemetic, antivertigo
Pregnancy category: B

Indications and Dosages

➤ *To treat nausea, vomiting, dizziness, or vertigo associated with motion sickness*

CHEWABLE TABLETS, ORAL SOLUTION, SYRUP, TABLETS

Adults and adolescents. 50 to 100 mg every 4 to 6 hr, p.r.n. *Maximum:* 400 mg/24 hr.

Children ages 6 to 12. 25 to 50 mg every 6 to 8 hr, p.r.n. *Maximum:* 150 mg/24 hr.

Children ages 2 to 6. 12.5 to 25 mg every 6 to 8 hr, p.r.n. *Maximum:* 75 mg/24 hr.

I.M. INJECTION

Adults and adolescents. 50 mg every 4 hr, p.r.n.

Children. 1.25 mg/kg or 37.5 mg/m² every 6 hr, p.r.n. *Maximum:* 300 mg daily.

I.V. INFUSION OR INJECTION

Adults and adolescents. 50 mg in 10 ml of normal saline solution administered slowly, over at least 2 min, every 4 hr, p.r.n.

Children. 1.25 mg/kg or 37.5 mg/m² in 10 ml of normal saline solution administered slowly, over at least 2 min, every 6 hr, p.r.n. *Maximum:* 300 mg daily.

Route	Onset	Peak	Duration
P.O.	Unknown	Unknown	3 to 6 hr
I.M.	20 to 30 min	Unknown	3 to 6 hr
I.V.	Immediate	Unknown	3 to 6 hr

Mechanism of Action
May inhibit vestibular stimulation and labyrinthine stimulation and function by acting on the otolith system and, with larger doses, on the semicircular canals.

Contraindications

Age less than 1 month, hypersensitivity to dimenhydrinate or its components

Interactions

DRUGS

aminoglycosides, other ototoxic drugs: Masked symptoms of ototoxicity
anticholinergics, drugs with anticholinergic activity: Potentiated anticholinergic effects of dimenhydrinate
apomorphine: Possibly decreased emetic response to apomorphine in treatment of poisoning
barbiturates, other CNS depressants: Possibly increased CNS depression
MAO inhibitors: Increased anticholinergic and CNS depressant effects of dimenhydrinate

ACTIVITIES

alcohol use: Possibly increased CNS depression

Adverse Reactions

CNS: Confusion, drowsiness, hallucinations, nervousness, paradoxical stimulation
CV: Hypotension, palpitations, tachycardia
EENT: Blurred vision, diplopia, dry eyes, dry mouth, nasal congestion

GI: Anorexia, constipation, diarrhea, epigastric discomfort, nausea, vomiting
GU: Dysuria
HEME: Hemolytic anemia
RESP: Thickening of bronchial secretions, wheezing
SKIN: Photosensitivity, rash, urticaria
Other: Anaphylaxis

Nursing Considerations

•**WARNING** Be aware that I.V. dimenhydrinate shouldn't be administered to premature or full-term neonates. Some I.V. preparations may contain benzyl alcohol, which can cause a fatal toxic syndrome characterized by CNS, respiratory, circulatory, and renal impairment and metabolic acidosis.
•**WARNING** Be aware that 50-mg/ml concentration of dimenhydrinate is intended for I.M. use. For I.V. use, the solution must be diluted further with at least 10 ml of diluent, such as D_5W or normal saline solution, for each milliliter of dimenhydrinate.
•Monitor patients with prostatic hyperplasia, stenosing peptic ulcer, pyloroduodenal obstruction, bladder neck obstruction, angle-closure glaucoma, bronchial asthma, or cardiac arrhythmias for worsening of these conditions caused by anticholinergic effects.
•Monitor elderly patients for increased sensitivity to dimenhydrinate, such as excessive drowsiness, confusion, and restlessness.
•Assess patients, especially children and elderly patients, for evidence of paradoxical stimulation, such as nightmares, unusual excitement, nervousness, restlessness, or irritability.
•Store parenteral drug at 15° to 30° C (59° to 86° F); don't freeze.

PATIENT TEACHING

•Because dimenhydrinate may cause drowsiness, instruct patient to avoid potentially hazardous activities until drug's CNS effects are known.
•Advise patient to inform health care providers about dimenhydrinate therapy, especially if she's being evaluated for medical conditions that are affected by this drug, such as appendicitis.
•Instruct patient to avoid alcohol, sedatives, and tranquilizers while taking dimenhydrinate.
•Encourage patient to use sunscreen to prevent photosensitivity reactions.

diphenhydramine hydrochloride

Allerdryl (CAN), Banophen, Benadryl, Benadryl Allergy, Diphenhist CapTabs, Genahist, Hyrexin, Nytol QuickCaps, Siladryl, Sleep-Eze D Extra Strength, Unisom SleepGels Maximum Strength

Class and Category

Chemical class: Ethanolamine derivative
Therapeutic class: Antianaphylactic adjunct, antidyskinetic, antiemetic, antihistamine, antitussive (syrup), antivertigo, sedative-hypnotic
Pregnancy category: B

Indications and Dosages

➤ *To treat hypersensitivity reactions, such as perennial and seasonal allergic rhinitis, vasomotor rhinitis, allergic conjunctivitis, uncomplicated allergic skin eruptions, and transfusion reactions*

CAPSULES, TABLETS

Adults and adolescents. 25 to 50 mg every 4 to 6 hr, p.r.n. *Maximum:* 300 mg daily.
Children ages 6 to 12. 12.5 to 25 mg every 4 to 6 hr. *Maximum:* 150 mg daily.
Children up to age 6. 6.25 to 12.5 mg every 4 to 6 hr.

ELIXIR

Adults and adolescents. 25 to 50 mg every 4 to 6 hr, p.r.n. *Maximum:* 300 mg daily.
Children. 1.25 mg/kg every 4 to 6 hr. *Maximum:* 300 mg daily.

I.V. OR I.M. INJECTION

Adults and adolescents. 10 to 50 mg every 4 to 6 hr up to 100 mg/dose, if needed. *Maximum:* 400 mg daily.
Children. 1.25 mg/kg every 4 to 6 hr. *Maximum:* 300 mg daily.

➤ *To treat sleep disorders*

CAPSULES, TABLETS

Adults and adolescents. 50 mg 20 to 30 min before bedtime.

➤ *To provide antitussive effects*

ELIXIR

Adults and adolescents. 25 mg every 4 hr. *Maximum:* 100 mg/24 hr.
Children ages 6 to 12. 12.5 mg every 4 to 6 hr. *Maximum:* 75 mg daily.
Children ages 2 to 6. 6.25 mg every 4 to 6 hr. *Maximum:* 25 mg daily.

> *To prevent motion sickness or treat vertigo*

CAPSULES, ELIXIR, TABLETS
Adults and adolescents. 25 to 50 mg every 4 to 6 hr, p.r.n. *Maximum:* 300 mg daily.
Children. 1 to 1.5 mg/kg every 4 to 6 hr, p.r.n. *Maximum:* 300 mg daily.
I.V. OR I.M. INJECTION
Adults and adolescents. *Initial:* 10 mg. Increased to 20 to 50 mg every 2 to 3 hr, if needed. *Maximum:* 100 mg/dose, 400 mg daily.
Children. 1 to 1.5 mg/kg I.M. every 4 to 6 hr, p.r.n. *Maximum:* 300 mg daily.

> *To treat symptoms of Parkinson's disease and drug-induced extrapyramidal reactions in elderly patients who can't tolerate more potent antidyskinetic drugs*

CAPSULES, ELIXIR, TABLETS
Adults. 25 mg t.i.d. increased gradually to 50 mg q.i.d., if needed. *Maximum:* 300 mg daily.
I.V. OR I.M. INJECTION
Adults and adolescents. 10 to 50 mg q.i.d., as needed. *Maximum:* 100 mg/dose, 400 mg daily.

Route	Onset	Peak	Duration
P.O.	15 to 60 min	1 to 3 hr	6 to 8 hr
I.V.	Immediate	1 to 3 hr	6 to 8 hr
I.M.	30 min	1 to 3 hr	6 to 8 hr

Contraindications
Bladder neck obstruction, hypersensitivity to diphenhydramine or its components, lower respiratory tract symptoms (including asthma), MAO inhibitor therapy, narrow-angle glaucoma, pyloroduodenal obstruction, stenosing peptic ulcer, symptomatic benign prostatic hyperplasia

Interactions
DRUGS
apomorphine: Possibly decreased emetic response in treatment of poisoning
barbiturates, other CNS depressants: Possibly increased CNS depression
MAO inhibitors: Increased anticholinergic and CNS depressant effects of diphenhydramine
ACTIVITIES
alcohol use: Possibly increased CNS depression

Mechanism of Action
Binds to central and peripheral H_1 receptors, competing with histamine for these sites and preventing it from reaching its site of action. By blocking histamine, diphenhydramine produces antihistamine effects, inhibiting respiratory, vascular, and GI smooth-muscle contraction; decreasing capillary permeability, which reduces wheals, flares, and itching; and decreasing salivary and lacrimal gland secretions.

Diphenhydramine produces antidyskinetic effects, possibly by inhibiting acetylcholine in the CNS. It also produces antitussive effects by directly suppressing the cough center in the medulla oblongata in the brain. Diphenhydramine's antiemetic and antivertigo effects may be related to its ability to bind to CNS muscarinic receptors and depress vestibular stimulation and labyrinthine function. Its sedative effects are related to its CNS depressant action.

Adverse Reactions
CNS: Confusion, dizziness, drowsiness
CV: Arrhythmias, palpitations, tachycardia
EENT: Blurred vision, diplopia
GI: Epigastric distress, nausea
HEME: Agranulocytosis, hemolytic anemia, thrombocytopenia
RESP: Thickened bronchial secretions
SKIN: Photosensitivity

Nursing Considerations
•Expect to give parenteral form of diphenhydramine only when oral ingestion isn't possible.
•Keep elixir container tightly closed. Protect elixir and parenteral forms from light.
•Expect to discontinue drug at least 72 hours before skin tests for allergies because drug may inhibit cutaneous histamine response, thus producing false-negative results.
PATIENT TEACHING
•Instruct patient to take diphenhydramine at least 30 minutes before exposure to situations that may cause motion sickness.
•Advise her to take drug with food to minimize GI distress.
•Urge patient to avoid alcohol while taking

diphenhydramine.
•Instruct her to use sunscreen to prevent photosensitivity reactions.
•Advise patient to avoid taking other OTC drugs that contain diphenhydramine to prevent additive effects.

dipyridamole

Apo-Dipyridamole FC (CAN), Apo-Dipyridamole SC (CAN), Novo-Dipiradol (CAN), Persantine

Class and Category

Chemical class: Pyrimidine
Therapeutic class: Coronary vasodilator, diagnostic aid, platelet aggregation inhibitor
Pregnancy category: B

Indications and Dosages

➤ *To prevent thromboembolic complications of cardiac valve replacement*
TABLETS
Adults. 75 to 100 mg q.i.d. with coumarin or indanedione derivative anticoagulant.

➤ *To aid diagnosis during thallium perfusion imaging of myocardium*
I.V. INFUSION
Adults. 0.57 mg/kg in 50 ml of D_5W infused over 4 min. *Maximum:* 60 mg.

Route	Onset	Peak	Duration
I.V.	Unknown	3.8 to 8.7 min*	Unknown

Contraindications

Asthma (I.V.), hypersensitivity to dipyridamole or its components, hypotension, unstable angina pectoris

Interactions

DRUGS
adenosine: Potentiated effects of adenosine
cefamandole, cefoperazone, cefotetan, plicamycin, valproic acid: Possibly hypoprothrombinemia and increased risk of bleeding
heparin, NSAIDs, thrombolytics: Possibly increased risk of bleeding
theophylline: Reversal of coronary vasodilation caused by dipyridamole, possibly false-negative thallium imaging result

---

* After start of infusion, for increased velocity of coronary artery blood flow.

Mechanism of Action

May increase the intraplatelet level of adenosine, which causes coronary vasodilation and inhibits platelet aggregation. Dipyridamole also may increase the intraplatelet level of cyclic adenosine monophosphate (cAMP) and may inhibit formation of the potent platelet activator stimulant thromboxane A_2, which decreases platelet activation. Vasodilation and increased blood flow occur preferentially in nondiseased coronary vessels, which results in redistribution of blood away from significantly diseased vessels. These changes in perfusion are observed during thallium imaging studies.

Adverse Reactions

CNS: Dizziness, headache
CV: Angina, arrhythmias, ECG changes (specifically, ST-segment and T-wave changes)
GI: Abdominal pain, diarrhea, nausea, vomiting
RESP: Dyspnea
SKIN: Flushing, pruritus, rash

Nursing Considerations

•Protect I.V. form of dipyridamole from direct light and freezing.
•Monitor blood pressure, pulse rate and rhythm, and breath sounds every 10 to 15 minutes during I.V. infusion.
•Keep parenteral aminophylline available to relieve adverse reactions to dipyridamole infusion.
•At therapeutic doses, expect adverse reactions to be minimal and transient. They typically resolve with long-term use.

PATIENT TEACHING
•Urge patient to take dipyrinamole at least 1 hour before or 2 hours after meals for faster absorption. If she experiences GI distress, advise her to take drug with meals or milk.
•Advise patient to take drug at evenly spaced intervals.
•Inform patient that drug commonly is taken with other anticoagulants.
•Urge her to keep appointments for coagulation tests.
•Instruct patient to seek immediate emergency treatment if chest pain occurs.

•Caution patient to consult prescriber before taking aspirin and other OTC NSAIDs because of the possible increased risk of bleeding.
•Advise patient to notify all health care providers about dipyridamole use.

dirithromycin

Dynabac

Class and Category
Chemical: Semisynthetic macrolide
Therapeutic: Antibiotic
Pregnancy category: C

Indications and Dosages
➤ *To treat acute bacterial exacerbations and secondary bacterial infections in patients with bronchitis caused by* Moraxella catarrhalis *or* Streptococcus pneumoniae, *and uncomplicated skin and soft-tissue infections caused by methicillin-susceptible* Staphylococcus aureus
TABLETS
Adults and adolescents. 500 mg daily for 7 days.
➤ *To treat streptococcal pharyngitis*
TABLETS
Adults and adolescents. 500 mg daily for 10 days.
➤ *To treat community-acquired pneumonia caused by* Legionella pneumophila, Mycoplasma pneumoniae, *or* S. pneumoniae
TABLETS
Adults and adolescents. 500 mg daily for 14 days.

Mechanism of Action
Binds with the 50S ribosomal subunit of the 70S ribosome in susceptible bacteria. This action inhibits RNA-dependent protein synthesis in bacterial cells, causing them to die.

Contraindications
Concurrent use of astemizole, cisapride, or pimozide; hypersensitivity to dirithromycin, erythromycin, other macrolide antibiotics, or their components; known, potential, or suspected bacteremia

Interactions
DRUGS
antacids, H₂-receptor antagonists: Increased dirithromycin absorption
astemizol, terfenadine: Possibly life-threatening arrhythmias
theophylline: Possibly increased serum theophylline level

Adverse Reactions
CNS: Dizziness, headache, weakness
GI: Abdominal pain, diarrhea, nausea, pseudomembranous colitis, vomiting
SKIN: Pruritus, rash, urticaria

Nursing Considerations
•Use dirithromycin cautiously in patients with impaired hepatic function. Monitor liver function test results as indicated because drug is metabolized in liver.
PATIENT TEACHING
•Instruct patient to take dirithromycin at the same time each day with food or within 1 hour of eating.
•Caution patient not to cut, chew, or crush tablets.
•Advise patient to store drug at room temperature in a dry place.
•Instruct patient to complete the full course of prescribed therapy, even if she feels better before the drug is gone.
•Advise patient to notify prescriber immediately if GI problems persist.

disopyramide

Rythmodan (CAN)

disopyramide phosphate

Norpace, Norpace CR, Rythmodan-LA (CAN)

Class and Category
Chemical class: Substituted pyramide derivative
Therapeutic class: Class IA antiarrhythmic
Pregnancy category: C

Indications and Dosages
➤ *To rapidly control ventricular arrhythmias*
CAPSULES
Adults. *Loading:* 300 mg (200 mg if patient weighs less than 50 kg [110 lb]). If no response to loading dose within 6 hr, 200 mg given every 6 hr. If no response within 48 hr,

drug discontinued or dosage carefully increased to 250 to 300 mg every 6 hr.

➤ *To treat ventricular arrhythmias*

CAPSULES

Adults. 400 to 800 mg daily in divided doses every 6 hr, limited to 400 mg daily if patient weighs less than 50 kg. *Maximum:* 800 mg daily.

Children ages 12 to 18. 6 to 15 mg/kg daily in divided doses every 6 hr.

Children ages 4 to 12. 10 to 15 mg/kg daily in divided doses every 6 hr.

Children ages 1 to 4. 10 to 20 mg/kg daily in divided doses every 6 hr.

Children under age 1. 10 to 30 mg/kg daily in divided doses every 6 hr.

DOSAGE ADJUSTMENT Initial dosage reduced to 100 mg every 6 to 8 hr for adults with cardiomyopathy or possible cardiac decompensation. In patients with renal insufficiency, dosage reduced to 100 mg every 6 hr if creatinine clearance exceeds 40 ml/min/1.73 m^2 or hepatic function is impaired; to 100 mg every 8 hr if creatinine clearance is 30 to 40 ml/min/1.73 m^2; to 100 mg every 12 hr if creatinine clearance is 15 to 29 ml/min/1.73 m^2; and to 100 mg every 24 hr if creatinine clearance is less than 15 ml/min/1.73 m^2.

E.R. CAPSULES, E.R. TABLETS

Adults. 400 to 800 mg daily in divided doses every 12 hr, limited to 200 mg every 12 hr if patient weighs less than 50 kg. *Maximum:* 800 mg daily.

Mechanism of Action

Inhibits sodium influx through fast channels of myocardial cell membranes, thus increasing the recovery period after repolarization. Disopyramide decreases automaticity in the His-Purkinje system and conduction velocity in the atria, ventricles, and accessory pathways. It prolongs the QRS and QT intervals in normal sinus rhythm and atrial arrhythmias. The drug has a potent negative inotropic effect. It also acts as an anticholinergic and increases peripheral vascular resistance.

Contraindications

Cardiogenic shock, congenital QT-interval prolongation, hypersensitivity to disopyramide or its components, second- or third-degree AV block (without pacemaker), sick sinus syndrome

Interactions

DRUGS

antiarrhythmics: Widened QRS complex, prolonged QT interval, risk of arrhythmias, serious negative inotropic effects
anticholinergics: Possibly additive anticholinergic effects
cisapride: Possibly increased risk of prolonged QT interval
clarithromycin, erythromycin: Increased blood disopyramide level
digoxin: Increased serum digoxin level
hydantoins, rifampin: Decreased blood disopyramide level
insulin, oral antidiabetic drugs: Possibly intensified antidiabetic effects
quinidine: Increased blood disopyramide level, decreased blood quinidine level, or both
verapamil: Widened QRS complex, prolonged QT interval, possibly death

Adverse Reactions

CNS: Depression, dizziness, fatigue, fever, headache, insomnia, nervousness, syncope
CV: Chest pain; conduction disturbances; edema; heart failure (new or worsened); hypercholesterolemia; hypertriglyceridemia; hypotension; palpitations; proarrhythmias, including torsades de pointes; ventricular fibrillation; ventricular tachycardia
EENT: Blurred vision; dry eyes, mouth, nose, and throat
ENDO: Gynecomastia, hypoglycemia
GI: Abdominal distention, anorexia, constipation, diarrhea, vomiting
GU: Impotence, urinary frequency and urgency, urine retention
HEME: Reversible agranulocytosis (rare), thrombocytopenia
MS: Muscle weakness
RESP: Dyspnea
SKIN: Decreased sweating, pruritus, rash, reversible cholestatic jaundice
Other: Hypokalemia, lupus erythematosus–like symptoms

Nursing Considerations

•**WARNING** Because of disopyramide's anticholinergic activity, avoid using drug in patients with glaucoma, myasthenia gravis, or

urine retention.
• Use disopyramide cautiously and expect to reduce dosage in patients with impaired hepatic or renal function. Monitor hepatic and renal function, as ordered. Be aware that E.R. form shouldn't be given to patients with severe renal insufficiency.
• When changing from immediate-release to E.R. form, expect to start maintenance schedule 6 hours after last immediate-release dose.
• At therapeutic doses in hemodynamically uncompromised patients, expect drug to reduce cardiac output without decreasing resting sinus rate or affecting blood pressure. Keep in mind, however, that 2 mg/kg given I.V. over 3 minutes can increase heart rate and total peripheral resistance.
• Monitor heart rate and rhythm by continuous ECG.
• Assess serum electrolyte levels, especially the potassium level, because drug may be ineffective in hypokalemia and its toxic effects enhanced in hyperkalemia.
• If patient takes quinidine, expect to start disopyramide 6 to 12 hours after last dose of quinidine. If patient takes procainamide, expect to start disopyramide 3 to 6 hours after the last dose of procainamide. A loading dose may not be required in either case.

PATIENT TEACHING
• Warn patient not to stop taking disopyramide abruptly; doing so may cause life-threatening cardiac problems.
• Advise patient to take a missed dose as soon as possible after she remembers, unless it's nearly time for the next dose. Caution her against doubling the dose. Urge her to notify prescriber if she misses more than one dose.
• Instruct patient to store drug at room temperature in a dry place.
• Instruct patient to check her pulse rate regularly and report significant changes to prescriber.
• Urge patient to report blurred vision, constipation, difficulty urinating, dizziness, dry mouth, and trouble breathing.
• Advise patient to avoid potentially hazardous activities until drug's CNS effects are known.
• Instruct patient to rise slowly from a lying or sitting position to reduce dizziness.
• Urge patient to avoid becoming overheated during hot weather or exercise because of risk of heatstroke.

disulfiram
Antabuse

Class and Category
Chemical class: Thiuram derivative
Therapeutic class: Alcohol abuse deterrent
Pregnancy category: Not rated

Indications and Dosages
➤ *As adjunct to maintain sobriety in treatment of chronic alcoholism*
TABLETS
Adults. *Initial:* Up to 500 mg daily for 1 to 2 wk. *Maintenance:* 125 to 500 mg daily. *Maximum:* 500 mg daily.

Route	Onset	Peak	Duration
P.O.	In 1 to 2 hr	Unknown	Up to 14 days

Mechanism of Action
Interferes with the enzyme responsible for hepatic oxidation of acetaldehyde to acetate, which occurs during alcohol catabolism. Ingestion of even a small amount of alcohol after taking disulfiram raises the blood acetaldehyde level to 5 to 10 times normal. Disulfiram doesn't alter the rate of alcohol elimination. Its major metabolite, diethyldithiocarbamate, inhibits norepinephrine synthesis and may be responsible for the drug's hypotensive effect.

Contraindications
Alcohol intoxication; coronary artery occlusion; hypersensitivity to disulfiram, its components, rubber, pesticides, or fungicides; psychosis; recent use of alcohol, alcohol-containing preparations, metronidazole, or paraldehyde; severe myocardial disease

Interactions
DRUGS
alfentanil: Decreased plasma clearance and prolonged duration of action of alfentanil
amoxicillin-clavulanate, bacampicillin: Possibly disulfiram-alcohol reaction
ascorbic acid: Possibly interference with disulfiram-alcohol reaction

CNS depressants: Possibly increased CNS depressant effects of either drug
isoniazid: Increased risk of additive neurotoxic effect of disulfiram; possibly increased adverse CNS effects
metronidazole: Risk of CNS toxicity, resulting in confusion and psychosis
oral anticoagulants: Possibly increased anticoagulant effects
paraldehyde: Decreased paraldehyde metabolism, increased blood paraldehyde level
phenytoin: Possibly increased blood phenytoin level and risk of phenytoin toxicity
tricyclic antidepressants: Possibly temporary delirium

FOODS
caffeine: Possibly increased cardiovascular and CNS effects of caffeine

ACTIVITIES
alcohol use: Disulfiram-alcohol reaction (if used within 14 days of disulfiram therapy)

Adverse Reactions
CNS: Drowsiness, headache, peripheral neuropathy, psychotic reaction, tiredness
EENT: Blurred vision, garlic or metallic taste, optic atrophy, optic neuritis
GU: Impotence
SKIN: Rash

Nursing Considerations
• Know that disulfiram is given only to patients who are highly motivated to stop drinking and who are receiving psychotherapy or substance abuse counseling.
• Be aware that alcohol content of patient's other drugs should be checked before starting therapy.
•**WARNING** Never give drug to patient without her knowledge or who is intoxicated.
• If needed, crush tablet and mix with fluids before administration.
• Don't give drug within 14 days of patient's ingestion of a substance that contains alcohol.
• Expect alcohol ingestion during disulfiram therapy to produce a severe reaction that lasts from 30 minutes to several hours. Symptoms may include angina, anxiety, blurred vision, confusion, diaphoresis, dyspnea, heart failure, hypotension, nausea, palpitations, sinus tachycardia, syncope, thirst, throbbing headache, throbbing in neck, vertigo, vomiting, and weakness. A deep sleep usually follows.

•**WARNING** Be aware that ingestion of three or more alcoholic beverages with a disulfiram dose greater than 500 mg daily may cause respiratory depression, arrhythmias, and cardiac arrest.
• If patient takes phenytoin, monitor blood phenytoin level before and during disulfiram therapy, and adjust dosage of either drug as prescribed. Interactions may not occur if disulfiram therapy starts before phenytoin therapy. A subtherapeutic phenytoin level may result if disulfiram therapy stops.
• If patient takes an oral anticoagulant, monitor PT before and during disulfiram therapy, and adjust anticoagulant dosage as prescribed. Drug interactions may not occur if disulfiram therapy starts before warfarin therapy. If disulfiram therapy stops, be prepared to adjust warfarin dosage to avoid loss of hypoprothrombinemic effects.
• Expect some adverse reactions, such as drowsiness, headache, and impotence, to subside over time or with a brief dosage reduction.
• Because one-fifth of a disulfiram dose may stay in the body for 1 week or longer, know that alcohol ingestion may continue to produce unpleasant symptoms for up to 2 weeks after therapy stops.
• Expect therapy to last months to years, depending on patient's ability to abstain from alcohol.

PATIENT TEACHING
• Teach patient's household and family members about precautions needed and risks associated with disulfiram therapy.
• Inform patient that drug doesn't cure alcoholism but does help deter alcohol consumption.
• If patient reports daytime drowsiness, advise her to take drug in the evening.
• Warn patient to avoid alcohol-containing substances, such as vinegar, cough syrup, and sauces, during therapy because a disulfiram-alcohol reaction may occur after ingesting as little as 15 ml of 100-proof alcohol. Encourage patient to avoid alcohol-containing liniments and lotions as well.
• Teach patient what to expect if a disulfiram-alcohol reaction occurs. Inform her that a deep sleep usually follows the reaction.
• Advise patient that a reaction can occur up to 14 days after therapy stops and that a severe reaction may cause respiratory depression, arrhythmias, and cardiac arrest.

•Instruct patient to carry medical identification that indicates drug, describes possible reactions, and lists someone to notify in case of emergency.

dobutamine hydrochloride

Dobutrex

Class and Category
Chemical class: Synthetic catecholamine
Therapeutic class: Cardiac stimulant
Pregnancy category: Not rated

Indications and Dosages
➤ *To treat low cardiac output and heart failure*

I.V. INFUSION
Adults. 2.5 to 10 mcg/kg/min as continuous infusion adjusted according to hemodynamic response.
Children. 5 to 20 mcg/kg/min as continuous infusion adjusted according to hemodynamic response.

Route	Onset	Peak	Duration
I.V.	1 to 2 min	Unknown	Under 5 min

Mechanism of Action
Primarily stimulates beta$_1$-adrenergic receptors, and mildly stimulates beta$_2$- and alpha$_1$-adrenergic receptors. Beta$_1$-receptor stimulation produces a positive inotropic effect on the myocardium. This increases cardiac output by boosting myocardial contractility and stroke volume. Increased myocardial contractility raises coronary blood flow and myocardial oxygen consumption. Systolic blood pressure typically rises as a result of increased stroke volume. Other hemodynamic effects include decreased systemic vascular resistance, which reduces afterload, and decreased ventricular filling pressure, which reduces preload.

Incompatibilities
Don't combine dobutamine with cefamandole, cefazolin, hydrocortisone sodium succinate, cephalothin, penicillin, sodium ethycrynate, and sodium heparin because of incom-

patibility. Don't mix dobutamine with alkaline solutions, such as sodium bicarbonate, because of possible physical incompatibility. Don't use diluents that contain sodium bisulfite or ethanol.

Contraindications
Hypersensitivity to dobutamine or its components, idiopathic hypertrophic subaortic stenosis

Interactions
DRUGS
beta blockers: Possibly increased alpha-adrenergic activity and peripheral resistance
bretylium: Potentiated vasopressor activity, possibly arrhythmias
cyclopropane, halothane: Possibly serious arrhythmias
guanethidine: Decreased hypotensive effect of guanethidine, possibly resulting in severe hypertension
thyroid hormones: Increased cardiovascular effects of thyroid hormones or dobutamine
tricyclic antidepressants: Possibly potentiated cardiovascular and vasopressor effects of dobutamine, resulting in arrhythmias, hyperpyrexia, or severe hypertension

Adverse Reactions
CNS: Fever, headache, nervousness, restlessness
CV: Angina, bradycardia, hypertension, hypotension, palpitations, PVCs, tachycardia
GI: Nausea, vomiting
RESP: Dyspnea
SKIN: Extravasation with tissue necrosis and sloughing, rash
Other: Hypokalemia

Nursing Considerations
•Avoid giving dobutamine to patients with uncorrected hypovolemia. Expect prescriber to order whole blood or plasma volume expanders to correct hypovolemia. Also avoid giving dobutamine to patients with acute MI because it can intensify or extend myocardial ischemia.
•Use drug cautiously in patients who are allergic to sulfites because drug may cause anaphylactic-like signs and symptoms; commercially available dobutamine injections contain sodium bisulfite. Also use drug cautiously in patients with atrial fibrillation because drug increases AV conduction. Keep in mind that patient should be adequately digitalized before administration.

•Dilute concentrate with at least 50 ml of compatible I.V. solution. A common dilution is 500 mg (40 ml from 250-ml bag) in 210 ml of D$_5$W or normal saline solution to yield 2,000 mcg/ml. Or dilute 1,000 mg (80 ml from 250-ml bag) in 170 ml of D$_5$W or normal saline solution to yield 4,000 mcg/ml. Adjust maximum concentration according to patient's fluid requirements as prescribed. Don't exceed a concentration of 5,000 mcg/ml. Discard solution after 24 hours.

•Inspect parenteral solution for particles and discoloration before administering it.

•Give I.V. drug using an infusion pump.

•Monitor blood pressure frequently during therapy, preferably by continuous intra-arterial monitoring; a systolic pressure increase of 10 to 20 mm Hg may indicate a dobutamine-induced increase in cardiac output.

•If hypotension develops, expect to reduce dosage or discontinue drug.

•Monitor heart rate and rhythm continuously for PVCs, which may result from drug's stimulatory effect on the heart's conduction system, and sinus tachycardia, which results from positive chronotropic effect of beta stimulation and may increase the heart rate by 5 to 15 beats/minute.

•Monitor hemodynamic parameters, such as central venous pressure, pulmonary artery wedge pressure, and cardiac output, as indicated, to assess drug's effectiveness.

•**WARNING** Monitor serum potassium level to check for hypokalemia, a rare result of beta$_2$ stimulation that causes electrolyte imbalance.

•Monitor urine output hourly, as appropriate, to assess for improved renal blood flow.

•Be aware that dobutamine isn't indicated for long-term treatment of heart failure because it may not be effective and may increase the risk of hospitalization and death.

PATIENT TEACHING
•Explain the need for frequent hemodynamic monitoring.

docusate calcium
(dioctyl calcium sulfosuccinate)

Albert Docusate (CAN), DC Softgels, Docucal-P, Doxidan (CAN), Pro-Cal-Sof, Sulfolax, Surfak

docusate potassium
(dioctyl potassium sulfosuccinate)

Diocto-K, Kasof

docusate sodium
(dioctyl sodium sulfosuccinate)

Afko-Lube, Afko-Lube Lax, Bilax, Colace, Colax, Correctol Stool Softener Soft Gels, Dialose, Diocto, Dioeze, DOK, D.O.S. Softgels, Ex-Lax Light Formula (CAN), Modane Soft, Regulax SS, Silace

Class and Category
Chemical class: Anionic surfactant
Therapeutic class: Laxative, stool softener
Pregnancy category: C

Indications and Dosages
➤ *To treat constipation*
CAPSULES (DOCUSATE CALCIUM)
Adults and adolescents. 240 mg at bedtime until bowel movements are normal.
Children age 6 and over. 50 to 150 mg at bedtime.
CAPSULES, LIQUID, SYRUP, TABLETS (DOCUSATE SODIUM)
Adults and adolescents. 50 to 500 mg at bedtime.
Children ages 6 to 12. 40 to 120 mg at bedtime.
Children ages 3 to 6. 20 to 60 mg at bedtime.
Children under age 3. 10 to 40 mg at bedtime.
CAPSULES, TABLETS (DOCUSATE POTASSIUM)
Adults and adolescents. 100 mg t.i.d. until bowel movements are normal.
Children age 6 and over. 100 mg at bedtime.

Route	Onset	Peak	Duration
P.O.	24 to 72 hr	Unknown	Unknown

Mechanism of Action
Acts as a surfactant that softens stool by decreasing the surface tension between the oil and water in fecal matter. This action lets more fluid penetrate the stool, thus forming a softer fecal mass.

Contraindications
Fecal impaction; hypersensitivity to docu-

sate salts or their components; intestinal obstruction; nausea, vomiting, or other symptoms of appendicitis; undiagnosed abdominal pain

Interactions
DRUGS
mineral oil: Increased mineral oil absorption, increased risk of toxicity
tetracycline: Decreased tetracycline absorption

Adverse Reactions
CNS: Dizziness, syncope
CV: Palpitations
GI: Abdominal cramps and distention, diarrhea, nausea, perianal irritation, vomiting
MS: Muscle weakness

Nursing Considerations
•**WARNING** Expect long-term or excessive use of docusate to cause dependence on laxatives for bowel movements, electrolyte imbalances, osteomalacia, steatorrhea, and vitamin and mineral deficiencies.
•Assess for laxative abuse syndrome, especially in women with depression, personality disorders, or anorexia nervosa.
PATIENT TEACHING
•Tell patient not to use docusate when she's has abdominal pain, nausea, or vomiting.
•Advise patient to take docusate with a full glass of water or milk.
•To help prevent constipation, encourage patient to increase her fiber intake, exercise regularly, and drink 6 to 8 glasses (240 ml/glass) of water daily.
•Instruct patient to notify prescriber about rectal bleeding; symptoms of electrolyte imbalances, such as dizziness, light-headedness, muscle cramping, and weakness; and unrelieved constipation.

dofetilide

Tikosyn

Class and Category
Chemical class: Methanesulfonanilide derivative
Therapeutic class: Class III antiarrhythmic
Pregnancy category: C

Indications and Dosages
➤ *To convert symptomatic atrial fibrilla-tion or flutter to normal sinus rhythm or to maintain normal sinus rhythm in patients converted from symptomatic atrial fibrillation or flutter*
CAPSULES
Adults. *Initial:* 500 mcg b.i.d. for patients with creatinine clearance greater than 60 ml/min/1.73 m². *Maintenance:* Dosage based on QTc interval. If, 2 to 3 hr after initial dose, QTc interval increase is 15% of baseline or less, initial dose given b.i.d. *Maximum:* 500 mcg b.i.d.
DOSAGE ADJUSTMENT Initial dose reduced to 250 mcg b.i.d. for patients with creatinine clearance of 40 to 60 ml/min/1.73 m² and to 125 mcg b.i.d. for clearance of 20 to 39 ml/min/1.73 m², as prescribed. If, 2 to 3 hr after initial dose, QTc interval has increased by at least 15% or is more than 500 milliseconds (msec) (550 msec in patients with ventricular conduction abnormalities), dosage decreased by 50%, as prescribed. However, for patients receiving lowest initial dose of 125 mcg b.i.d., dosage is reduced to 125 mcg daily, as prescribed. During next four doses (given every 2 to 3 hr, as prescribed), if QTc interval increases to more than 500 msec (550 msec in patients with ventricular conduction abnormalities), expect to discontinue therapy, as prescribed.

Route	Onset	Peak	Duration
P.O.	Unknown	2 hr	4 hr

Mechanism of Action
Selectively blocks potassium channels in myocardial cell membranes involved in cardiac repolarization. By blocking potassium channels, dofetilide prolongs ventricular refractoriness (widens QT interval), effective refractory period, and action potential duration. These actions terminate or prevent reentrant tachyarrhythmias, such as atrial fibrillation, atrial flutter, and ventricular tachycardia.

Contraindications
Cardiac conduction disturbances without an artificial pacemaker; congenital or acquired QT prolongation syndrome; concurrent therapy with cimetidine, hydrochlorothiazide,

ketoconazole, trimethoprim, or verapamil; hypersensitivity to dofetilide or its components; severe renal impairment (creatinine clearance less than 20 ml/min/1.73 m^2)

Interactions
DRUGS
amiloride, cimetidine, co-trimoxazole, ketoconazole, megestrol, metformin, triamterene, trimethoprim: Possibly increased blood dofetilide level
azole antifungals, diltiazem, nefazodone, norfloxacin, protease inhibitors, quinine, selective serotonin reuptake inhibitors, zafirlukast: Possibly increased blood dofetilide level and risk of dofetilide toxicity
bepridil, cisapride, macrolide antibiotics, phenothiazines, tricyclic antidepressants: Possibly prolonged QT interval
class I and III antiarrhythmics, especially amiodarone: Possibly prolonged QT interval and increased risk of dofetilide-induced proarrhythmias
diuretics (potassium-depleting): Increased risk of torsades de pointes in patients with hypokalemia or hypomagnesemia
hydrochlorothiazide, verapamil: Possibly increased blood dofetilide level and increased risk of torsades de pointes
FOODS
grapefruit juice: Increased blood dofetilide level
ACTIVITIES
marijuana use: Increased blood dofetilide level

Adverse Reactions
CNS: Cerebral ischemia, dizziness, facial or flaccid paralysis, headache, insomnia, paresthesia, slurred speech, stroke, syncope
CV: AV block, bradycardia, cardiac arrest, chest pain, edema, MI, tachycardia, ventricular arrhythmias (including torsades de pointes and ventricular tachycardia)
GI: Abdominal pain, diarrhea, hepatic dysfunction, nausea
MS: Back pain, muscle weakness
RESP: Cough, dyspnea, respiratory tract infection
SKIN: Jaundice, rash
Other: Angioedema, flulike symptoms, weight gain

Nursing Considerations
•**WARNING** If patient has previously received amiodarone drug therapy, be aware that dofetilide therapy should not be initiated until blood amiodarone level is less than 0.3 mcg/ml or until amiodarone has been withdrawn for at least 3 months.
•Evaluate and document QTc interval before and during dofetilide therapy.
•Place patient on continuous ECG monitoring for at least 3 days, as ordered, during dofetilide therapy.
•**WARNING** If patient does not convert to normal sinus rhythm within 24 hours of starting dofetilide, expect to prepare her for possible synchronized electrical cardioversion.
•Be prepared to reevaluate renal function and QTc every 3 months, as ordered, during dofetilide therapy.
•When switching to dofetilide from class I or class III antiarrhythmics, or after withdrawing antiarrhythmic treatment, monitor continuous ECG for at least 30 hours, as ordered.
•If patient requires a drug that may interact with dofetilide, expect to discontinue dofetilide, as prescribed, for 2 or more days before starting the other drug.
•**WARNING** Monitor laboratory test results for hypokalemia or hypomagnesemia, especially in patients who are taking diuretics, because of the increased risk of dofetilide-induced torsades de pointes.
•Monitor women often for adverse reactions, including prolonged QTc interval and torsades de pointes; they have 12% to 18% lower renal clearance of drug than men and therefore a greater risk of adverse drug reactions.
PATIENT TEACHING
•Advise patient to swallow dofetilide capsules with water.
•Instruct patient to avoid drinking grapefruit juice while taking this drug.
•Inform patient that she may be hospitalized for at least 3 days if dofetilide dosage is increased.
•Teach patient how to measure pulse rate and blood pressure during dofetilide therapy.
•Urge patient to report chest discomfort, fluttering, or palpitations immediately.
•Advise patient to consult prescriber before using any OTC drugs, nutritional supplements, or herbal products.
•Instruct patient to keep follow-up appointments to monitor heart rhythm.

dolasetron mesylate

Anzemet

Class and Category

Chemical class: Carboxylate monomethane-sulfonate
Therapeutic class: Antiemetic
Pregnancy category: B

Indications and Dosages

➤ *To prevent nausea and vomiting due to chemotherapy*

ORAL SOLUTION, TABLETS
Adults and children over age 16. 100 mg within 1 hr before chemotherapy.
Children ages 2 to 16. 1.8 mg/kg within 1 hr before chemotherapy. *Maximum:* 100 mg.

I.V. INJECTION
Adults and children over age 16. 1.8 mg/kg or 100 mg as a single dose within 30 min before chemotherapy.
Children ages 2 to 16. 1.8 mg/kg as a single dose within 30 min before chemotherapy. *Maximum:* 100 mg.

➤ *To prevent postoperative nausea and vomiting*

ORAL SOLUTION, TABLETS
Adults and children over age 16. 100 mg within 2 hr before surgery.
Children ages 2 to 16. 1.2 mg/kg within 2 hr before surgery. *Maximum:* 100 mg.

I.V. INJECTION
Adults and children over age 16. 12.5 mg 15 min before end of anesthesia.
Children ages 2 to 16. 0.35 mg/kg 15 min before end of anesthesia. *Maximum:* 12.5 mg/dose.

➤ *To treat postoperative nausea and vomiting*

I.V. INJECTION
Adults and children over age 16. 12.5 mg as a single dose as soon as symptoms develop.
Children ages 2 to 16. 0.35 mg/kg as a single dose as soon as symptoms develop. *Maximum:* 12.5 mg/dose.

Contraindications

Hypersensitivity to dolasetron or components

Interactions

DRUGS
atenolol: Possibly decreased dolasetron clearance
cimetidine: Possibly increased blood

dolasetron level
rifampin: Possibly decreased blood dolasetron level

Mechanism of Action

With its active metabolite hydrodolasetron, prevents activation of the serotonin 5-HT$_3$ receptors located peripherally on the vagal nerve terminals and centrally in the chemoreceptor trigger zone, thereby decreasing the vomiting reflex.

Adverse Reactions

CNS: Headache
CV: Cardiac arrest, hypertension, hypotension, MI, ventricular fibrillation and tachycardia, wide-complex tachycardia
GI: Diarrhea
SKIN: Rash
Other: Injection site pain

Nursing Considerations

• Expect to give up to 100 mg of dolasetron I.V. in 30 seconds or to dilute it in normal saline solution, D$_5$W, dextrose 5% in half-normal (0.45) saline solution, or lactated Ringer's solution and infuse for up to 15 minutes, as prescribed.
• Flush I.V. line with compatible solution before and after drug administration.
• Expect to prepare an oral solution of dolasetron for patients unable to swallow tablets by diluting injection solution with apple or apple-grape juice.
• **WARNING** Monitor patient for ECG changes, including prolonged PR, QTc, and QT intervals and widened QRS complex.

PATIENT TEACHING
• For children or patients who have trouble swallowing, explain that oral solution can be prepared by diluting injection form of drug with apple or apple-grape juice.
• Inform patient that oral solution may be refrigerated for up to 48 hours but should be discarded after 2 hours at room temperature.

donepezil hydrochloride

Aricept

Class and Category

Chemical class: Piperidine derivative
Therapeutic class: Antidementia

Pregnancy category: C

Indications and Dosages

➤ *To treat dementia of the Alzheimer's type*

ORAL SOLUTION, TABLETS

Adults. *Initial:* 5 mg at bedtime. After 4 to 6 wk, dosage increased to 10 mg at bedtime, as indicated. *Maximum:* 10 mg daily.

Mechanism of Action

Reversibly inhibits acetylcholinesterase and improves acetylcholine's concentration at cholinergic synapses. Raising the acetylcholine level in the cerebral cortex may improve cognition. Donepezil becomes less effective as Alzheimer's disease progresses and the number of intact cholinergic neurons declines.

Contraindications

Hypersensitivity to donepezil, piperidine derivatives, or their components

Interactions

DRUGS

anticholinergics: Possibly interference with activity of these drugs
carbamazepine, dexamethasone, phenobarbital, phenytoin, rifampin: Increased donepezil elimination rate
cholinergic agonists, neuromuscular blockers: Possibly synergistic effects of these drugs
ketoconazole, quinidine: Inhibited donepezil metabolism
NSAIDs: Possibly increased gastric acid secretion and increased risk of GI bleeding

Adverse Reactions

CNS: Abnormal gait, agitation, anxiey, asthenia, depression, dizziness, dream disturbances, fatigue, fever, headache, hostility, insomnia, nervousness, seizures, somnolence, syncope, tremor
CV: Abnormal ECG, bradycardia, chest pain, edema, heart failure, hypertension, hypotension
EENT: Pharyngitis
ENDO: Hyperglycemia
GI: Abdominal pain, anorexia, constipation, diarrhea, dyspepsia, gastroenteritis, fecal incontinence, nausea, vomiting
GU: Cystitis, glycosuria, hematuria, urinary frequency or incontinence, UTI
HEME: Anemia, hemorrhage
MS: Arthralgia, back pain, elevated creatine kinase level, muscle spasms
RESP: Bronchitis, increased cough, pneumonia
SKIN: Ecchymosis, eczema, pruritus, rash, ulceration
Other: Angioedema, dehydration, elevated alkaline phosphatase or lactate dehydrogenase level, flu syndrome, weight loss

Nursing Considerations

•Use donepezil cautiously in patients with bladder obstruction because drug's weak peripheral cholinergic effect could obstruct outflow.
•Use donepezil cautiously in patients with asthma, COPD, or other pulmonary disorders because this drug has a weak affinity for peripheral cholinesterase, which may increase bronchoconstriction and bronchial secretions.
•If patient has cardiac disease, monitor heart rate and rhythm for bradycardia, which may result from increased vagal tone caused by drug's inhibition of peripheral cholinesterase. Reduced heart rate may be especially significant if patient has sick sinus syndrome, bradycardia, or other supraventricular arrhythmia.
•Take safety precautions if patient is dizzy or has other adverse CNS reactions.

PATIENT TEACHING

•Advise patient to take donepezil just before going to bed.
•Inform her that drug may be taken with or without food.
•Instruct patient to avoid hazardous activities, such as driving, until drug's CNS effects are known. Encourage her to take safety precautions to prevent falling if she experiences adverse reactions, such as dizziness.
•If patient has history of peptic ulcer disease or gastric irritation, explain that drug may aggravate these conditions by increasing gastric acid secretion.
•Caution patient to avoid NSAIDs during therapy because of risk of GI bleeding. Urge her to notify prescriber immediately if she notices black, tarry stools.

dopamine hydrochloride

Intropin, Revimine (CAN)

Class and Category
Chemical class: Catecholamine
Therapeutic class: Cardiac stimulant, vasopressor
Pregnancy category: C

Indications and Dosages
➤ *To correct hypotension that is unresponsive to adequate fluid volume replacement or occurs as part of shock syndrome caused by bacteremia, chronic cardiac decompensation, drug overdose, MI, open-heart surgery, renal failure, trauma, or other major systemic illnesses; to improve low cardiac output*

I.V. INFUSION

Adults. 0.5 to 3 mcg/kg/min for vasodilation of renal arteries; 2 to 10 mcg/kg/min for positive inotropic effects and increased cardiac output; 10 mcg/kg/min, increased gradually according to patient's response, for increased systolic and diastolic blood pressures.

DOSAGE ADJUSTMENT Initial dosage reduced to 10% of usual amount if patient has received MAO inhibitor in previous 2 to 3 wk.

Children. 1 to 5 mcg/kg/min increased gradually in increments of 2.5 to 5 mcg/kg/min to achieve desired results. *Maximum:* 20 mcg/kg/min.

Route	Onset	Peak	Duration
I.V.	In 5 min	Unknown	Up to 10 min

Incompatibilities
Don't add dopamine to 5% sodium bicarbonate, alkaline I.V. solutions, oxidizing agents, or iron salts.

Contraindications
Pheochromocytoma, uncorrected ventricular fibrillation, ventricular tachycardia, and other tachyarrhythmias

Interactions
DRUGS
alpha blockers, haloperidol, loxapine, phenothiazines, thioxanthenes: Antagonized peripheral vasoconstriction with high doses of dopamine
anesthetics, such as chloroform, enflurane, halothane, isoflurane, and methoxyflurane: Increased risk of severe atrial and ventricular arrhythmias
antihypertensives, diuretics used as antihypertensives: Possibly decreased antihypertensive effects of these drugs
beta blockers: Antagonized beta receptor–mediated inotropic effects of dopamine
digitalis glycosides: Possibly increased risk of arrhythmias and additive inotropic effects
diuretics: Possibly increased diuretic effects of dopamine or diuretic
doxapram: Possibly increased vasopressor effects of dopamine or doxapram
ergot alkaloids: Enhanced peripheral vasoconstriction
guanadrel, guanethidine: Possibly decreased hypotensive effects of these drugs and potentiated vasopressor response to dopamine, resulting in hypertension and arrhythmias
levodopa: Increased risk of arrhythmias
MAO inhibitors: Prolonged and intensified cardiac stimulation and vasopressor effect
maprotiline, tricyclic antidepressants: Possibly potentiated cardiovascular and vasopressor effects of dopamine, resulting in arrhythmias, hyperpyrexia, or severe hypertension
mecamylamine, methyldopa: Possibly decreased hypotensive effects of these drugs and enhanced vasopressor effect of dopamine
methylphenidate: Possibly potentiated vasopressor effect of dopamine
nitrates: Possibly decreased antianginal effects of nitrates; possibly decreased vasopressor effect of dopamine, resulting in hypotension
oxytocic drugs: Possibly severe hypertension
phenoxybenzamine: Possibly antagonized peripheral vasoconstriction of dopamine, causing hypotension and tachycardia
phenytoin: Possibly sudden bradycardia and hypotension
rauwolfia alkaloids: Possibly decreased hypotensive effects of these drugs
sympathomimetics: Possibly increased adverse cardiovascular and other effects
thyroid hormones: Increased risk of coronary insufficiency

Adverse Reactions
CNS: Headache
CV: Angina, bradycardia, hypertension, hypotension, palpitations, peripheral vasoconstriction, sinus tachycardia, ventricular arrhythmias
GI: Nausea, vomiting
RESP: Dyspnea
SKIN: Extravasation with tissue necrosis

Mechanism of Action

Stimulates dopamine$_1$ (D$_1$) and dopamine$_2$ (D$_2$) postsynaptic receptors. D$_1$ receptors mediate vasodilation in renal, mesenteric, coronary, and cerebral blood vessels. D$_2$ receptors, when stimulated, inhibit norepinephrine release. In higher doses, dopamine also stimulates alpha$_1$ and alpha$_2$ receptors, causing vascular smooth-muscle contraction.

At doses of 0.5 to 3 mcg/kg/min, this naturally occurring catecholamine mainly affects dopaminergic receptors in renal, mesenteric, coronary, and cerebral vessels, resulting in vasodilation, increased renal blood flow, improved GFR, and increased urine output. At doses of 2 to 10 mcg/kg/min, dopamine stimulates beta$_1$-adrenergic receptors, increasing cardiac output while maintaining dopaminergic-induced vasodilation. At doses of 10 mcg/kg/min or more, alpha-adrenergic agonism takes over, causing increased peripheral vascular resistance and renal vasoconstriction.

Nursing Considerations

•If possible, avoid giving dopamine to patients with occlusive vascular disease, such as atherosclerosis, Buerger's disease, diabetic endarteritis, or Raynaud's disease, because of the risk of decreased peripheral circulation.
•Use drug cautiously in patients with cardiac disease, particularly coronary artery disease, because dopamine increases myocardial oxygen demand. Also use drug cautiously in patients who are allergic to sulfites, which are contained in some forms of dopamine.
•Inspect parenteral solution for particles and discoloration before administration.
•Dilute dopamine concentrate with a compatible I.V. solution before administering. Typical dilution is 400 mg in 250 ml to yield 1.6 mg/ml. Don't exceed 3.2 mg/ml.
•If patient has hypovolemia, ensure adequate fluid resuscitation before giving drug.
•Give drug by I.V. infusion using an infusion pump.
•**WARNING** When the infusion rate exceeds 20 mcg/kg/min, monitor patient for excessive vasoconstriction and loss of renal vasodilating effects. Avoid using an infusion rate above 50 mcg/kg/min.

•If you must infuse more than 20 mcg/kg/min of dopamine to maintain blood pressure, expect to infuse norepinephrine as prescribed.
•To avoid extravasation and tissue necrosis, administer infusion through a central catheter. If you must administer drug through a peripheral line, inspect site frequently for signs of extravasation and necrosis. If you detect such signs, start a new I.V. line for dopamine infusion, discontinue previous I.V. line, and notify prescriber immediately.
•If drug extravasates, expect to give 5 to 10 mg of phentolamine diluted in 10 to 15 ml of normal saline solution, as prescribed. Phentolamine infiltrates directly into area to antagonize vasoconstriction and minimize sloughing and tissue necrosis.
•Titrate dopamine gradually to minimize hypotension, especially after a high infusion rate.
•Monitor blood pressure continuously with an intra-arterial line, as indicated.
•Place patient on continuous ECG monitoring, and assess heart rate and rhythm for arrhythmias.
•Monitor patient's hemodynamic parameters, such as central venous pressure, pulmonary artery wedge pressure, and cardiac output, as indicated, to assess effectiveness of dopamine therapy.
•Monitor urine output hourly as appropriate to assess patient for improved renal blood flow.

PATIENT TEACHING
•Explain the need for frequent hemodynamic monitoring.

doripenem

Doribax

Class and Category

Chemical class: Carbapenem
Therapeutic class: Antibiotic
Pregnancy category: B

Indications and Dosages

➤ *To treat complicated intra-abdominal infections caused by* Escherichia coli, Klebsiella pneumoniae, Pseudomonas aeruginosa, Bacteroides caccae, B. fragilis, B. thetaiotaomicron, B. uniformis, B. vulgatus, Streptococcus intermedius,

S. constellatus *and* Peptostreptococcus micros *and complicated UTIs, including pyelonephritis caused by* E. coli, K. pneumoniae, Proteus mirabilis, P. aeruginosa, *and* Acinetobacter baumannii

I.V. INFUSION

Adults. 500 mg infused over 1 hr every 8 hr for 5 to 14 days. May switch to oral therapy if improvement after 3 days.

DOSAGE ADJUSTMENT For patients with impaired renal function or creatinine clearance of 30 to 50 ml/min/1.73 m^2, dosage reduced to 250 mg infused over 1 hr every 8 hr. For patients with creatinine clearance of 10 to 30 ml/min/1.73 m^2, dosage reduced to 250 mg infused over 1 hr every 12 hr.

Route	Onset	Peak	Duration
I.V.	Unknown	1 hr	8 hr

Mechanism of Action

Inhibits cell wall synthesis in susceptible bacteria. Doripenem inactivates multiple essential penicillin-binding proteins involved in cell wall synthesis to cause cell death.

Incompatibilities

Don't mix doripenem with other drugs or add to solutions containing other drugs because of potential for incompatibility.

Contraindications

History of anaphylactic reactions to beta-lactams; hypersensitivity to doripenem, its components or other carbapenems

Interactions

DRUGS

divalproex sodium, valproic acid: Decreased effectiveness of valproic acid with possible loss of seizure control
probenecid: Increased plasma concentrations of doripenem

Adverse Reactions

CNS: Headache, seizure
CV: Phlebitis
EENT: Oral candidiasis
GI: Diarrhea, liver enzyme elevation, nausea
GU: Vaginitis
HEME: Neutropenia
SKIN: Dermatitis, erythema, erythema multiforme, macular or papular eruptions, pruritus, rash, Stevens Johnson Syndrome, toxic epidermal necrolysis, urticaria
Other: Anaphylaxis

Nursing Considerations

• Use cautiously in patients with a history of hypersensitivity to cephaloporins or penicillins because cross sensitivity may occur.

• Constitute vial with 10 ml sterile water for injection or normal saline solution, and gently shake to form a suspension. Withdraw suspension using a syringe with a 21G needle and add it to an infusion bag containing 100 ml of normal saline solution or 5% dextrose. Gently shake until clear. If administering a reduced dosage of 250 mg, remove 55 ml of prepared solution from the infusion bag and discard prior to infusion.

• Be aware that upon constitution, suspension in the vial must be diluted within 1 hour. Once drug is diluted in infusion solution, drug stored at room temperature must be used within 8 hours if mixed in normal saline solution and within 4 hours if mixed in 5% dextrose. If infusion solution is refrigerated, it must be used within 24 hours or discarded.

• Monitor patient closely for evidence of hypersensitivity, especially if patient has multiple allergies, because serious and occasionally fatal hypersensitivity reactions have occurred in patients receiving beta-lactam antibiotics. If an allergic reaction occurs, discontinue drug immediately, notify prescriber, and expect to administer emergency treatment such as epinephrine, oxygen, I.V. fluids, I.V. antihistamines, corticosteroids, and pressor amines, as ordered, and provide airway management.

• Assess patient's bowel pattern daily; severe diarrhea may be caused by *Clostridium difficile*. If suspected, stop drug, as ordered, and provide treatment as prescribed.

PATIENT TEACHING

• Instruct patient to report any evidence of allergic reaction, such as rash, hives, itching or trouble breathing.

• Advise patient to report diarrhea if severe or persistent.

doxapram hydrochloride

Dopram

Class and Category
Chemical class: Pyrrolidinone derivative
Therapeutic class: Respiratory stimulant
Pregnancy category: B

Indications and Dosages
➤ *To stimulate respiration in COPD-related acute respiratory insufficiency*

I.V. INFUSION

Adults and adolescents. 1 to 2 mg/min titrated according to respiratory response. *Maximum:* 3 mg/min for up to 2 hr.

➤ *To treat respiratory depression after anesthesia*

I.V. INFUSION

Adults and adolescents. 5 mg/min until desired response occurs and then reduced to 1 to 3 mg/min. *Maximum:* Cumulative dose of 4 mg/kg or 300 mg.

I.V. INJECTION

Adults and adolescents. 0.5 to 1 mg/kg, repeated every 5 min, if needed. *Maximum:* 1.5 mg/kg as a single dose or 2 mg/kg every 5 min.

Route	Onset	Peak	Duration
I.V.	20 to 40 sec	1 to 2 min	5 to 12 min

Mechanism of Action
Activates peripheral carotid, aortic, and other chemoreceptors to stimulate respiration, resulting in increased tidal volume and respiratory rate. Doxapram also may increase respiratory rate and tidal volume by directly stimulating the respiratory center in the medulla oblongata.

Incompatibilities
To avoid precipitation and gas formation, don't mix doxapram with alkaline solutions, such as aminophylline, sodium bicarbonate, or 2.5% thiopental.

Contraindications
Age less than 1 month; cerebral edema; head injury; hypersensitivity to doxapram or its components; mechanical disorders of ventilation, including acute bronchial asthma, flail chest, muscle paresis, obstruction, pneumothorax, and pulmonary fibrosis; pulmonary embolism; seizure disorder; severe cardiovascular disorder; severe hypertension; stroke; uncompensated heart failure

Interactions
DRUGS

chloroform, cyclopropane, enflurane, halothane, isoflurane, methoxyflurane, trichloroethylene: Possibly adverse myocardial effects if doxapram given within 10 minutes of these drugs
CNS stimulants: Possibly excessive CNS stimulation, resulting in arrhythmias, insomnia, irritability, nervousness, or seizures
MAO inhibitors, sympathomimetics: Additive vasopressor effects
skeletal muscle relaxants: Masked residual effects of muscle relaxants

Adverse Reactions
CNS: Disorientation, dizziness, headache
CV: Arrhythmias, including sinus tachycardia; hypertension
GI: Diarrhea, hiccups, nausea, vomiting
GU: Urine retention
RESP: Bronchospasm, cough, dyspnea
SKIN: Diaphoresis
Other: Injection site pain, redness, swelling, and thrombophlebitis

Nursing Considerations
• Avoid giving doxapram to patients receiving mechanical ventilation.
• Maintain a patent airway, and assess for optimal oxygenation before giving drug.
• Monitor I.V. insertion site for extravasation and signs of thrombophlebitis or local skin irritation.
• If hypertension or dyspnea develops suddenly, stop infusion as directed.
• Assess patient for early signs and symptoms of overdose, including enhanced deep tendon reflexes, skeletal muscle hyperactivity, and tachycardia.

PATIENT TEACHING

• Explain the need for frequent pulse and blood pressure monitoring.

doxazosin mesylate

Cardura, Cardura-1 (CAN), Cardura-2 (CAN), Cardura-4 (CAN)

Class and Category
Chemical class: Quinazoline derivative
Therapeutic class: Antihypertensive, benign prostatic hyperplasia therapeutic agent
Pregnancy category: C

Indications and Dosages

➤ *To manage hypertension*

TABLETS

Adults. *Initial:* 1 mg daily. Doubled every 1 to 2 wk, if needed to achieve desired blood pressure. *Maximum:* 16 mg daily.

➤ *To treat benign prostatic hyperplasia (BPH)*

TABLETS

Adults. *Initial:* 1 mg daily. Doubled every 1 to 2 wk, if needed, based on signs and symptoms. *Maximum:* 8 mg daily.

Route	Onset	Peak	Duration
P.O.	1 to 2 hr*	2 to 6 hr†	24 hr†

Mechanism of Action

Competitively inhibits alpha$_1$-adrenergic receptors in the sympathetic nervous system, causing peripheral vasodilation and reduced peripheral vascular resistance. This action increases heart rate and decreases blood pressure, especially when the patient stands. Doxazosin also relaxes smooth muscle of the bladder neck, prostate, and prostate capsule, which reduces urethral resistance and pressure and urinary outflow resistance.

Contraindications

Hypersensitivity to doxazosin, prazosin, terazosin, or their components

Interactions

DRUGS

antihypertensives, diuretics: Enhanced hypotensive effects

cimetidine: Possibly increased blood doxazosin level

dopamine: Antagonized vasopressor effect of high-dose dopamine

ephedrine, metaraminol, methoxamine, phenylephrine: Possibly decreased vasopressor effects of these drugs

epinephrine: Possibly severe hypotension and tachycardia

NSAIDs: Possibly loss of hypotensive activity from sodium or fluid accumulation

---

* For hypertension; in 2 wk for BPH.
† For hypertension; unknown for BPH.

Adverse Reactions

CNS: Dizziness, drowsiness, headache, nervousness, restlessness, vertigo

CV: Arrhythmias, including sinus tachycardia; first-dose orthostatic hypotension; palpitations; peripheral edema

EENT: Intraoperative floppy iris syndrome, rhinitis

GI: Nausea

RESP: Dyspnea

Nursing Considerations

• Don't give drug to hypotensive patients.

• Use doxazosin cautiously in patients with hepatic disease (because normal dosage may cause exaggerated effects) and in elderly patients (because hypotensive response may be more pronounced).

• **WARNING** Monitor patient for orthostatic hypotension (which may cause syncope) early in therapy, especially after exercise and in patients with hypovolemia.

• Monitor blood pressure for 2 to 6 hours after first dose and with each increase because orthostatic hypotension commonly occurs during this time. Adjust dose as prescribed, based on standing blood pressure.

• Carefully monitor patients with renal disease for exaggerated effects, such as first-dose orthostatic hypotension.

• Monitor urination, checking for difficulty urinating and urine retention, to assess drug's effects on BPH.

PATIENT TEACHING

• Inform patient that she may take doxazosin in the morning or evening and with food, if desired.

• Instruct patient to change position slowly to minimize orthostatic hypotension.

• Advise patient to avoid standing for long periods, exercising, using alcohol, and going outside in hot weather; these activities may exacerbate orthostatic hypotension.

• Advise patient to avoid hazardous activities until drug's CNS effects are known.

doxepin hydrochloride

Novo-Doxepin (CAN), Sinequan, Triadapin (CAN)

Class and Category

Chemical class: Dibenzoxepin derivative
Therapeutic class: Antidepressant

Pregnancy category: Not rated

Indications and Dosages

➤ *To treat mild to moderate depression or anxiety*

CAPSULES, ORAL SOLUTION

Adults and adolescents. 75 to 150 mg daily at bedtime. *Maximum:* 150 mg daily.

➤ *To treat mild to moderate depression or anxiety with organic disease*

CAPSULES, ORAL SOLUTION

Adults and adolescents. 25 to 50 mg daily.

➤ *To treat severe depression or anxiety*

CAPSULES, ORAL SOLUTION

Adults and adolescents. 50 mg t.i.d., gradually increased to 300 mg daily, as indicated.

Route	Onset	Peak	Duration
P.O.	2 to 3 wk	Unknown	Unknown

Mechanism of Action

May block serotonin and norepinephrine reuptake by adrenergic nerves. In this way, the tricyclic antidepressant raises serotonin and norepinephrine levels at nerve synapses, which may elevate mood and reduce depression.

Incompatibilities

Don't mix doxepin solution with carbonated beverages or grape juice.

Contraindications

Acute recovery phase of MI; concurrent use of MAO inhibitor; glaucoma; hypersensitivity to doxepin, other tricyclic antidepressants, or their components; urine retention

Interactions

DRUGS

amantadine, anticholinergics, antidyskinetics, antihistamines: Possibly intensified anticholinergic effects, causing confusion, hallucinations, and nightmares

anticonvulsants: Possibly lowered seizure threshold and decreased effects of these drugs

antithyroid drugs: Possibly increased risk of agranulocytosis

barbiturates, carbamazepine: Increased doxepin metabolism, decreased blood doxepin level, possibly lowered seizure threshold

bupropion, clozapine, cyclobenzaprine, hal-operidol, loxapine, maprotiline, molindone, phenothiazines, thioxanthenes: Possibly prolonged and intensified sedative and anticholinergic effects of either drug, possibly increased risk of seizures

cimetidine, flecainide, phenothiazines, propafenone, quinidine, selective serotonin reuptake inhibitors, tricyclic antidepressants: Increased blood doxepin level from inhibited systemic clearance, resulting in increased risk of toxicity

clonidine, guanadrel, guanethidine: Increased risk of hypertension, especially during second week of doxepin therapy

CNS depressants: Possibly potentiated CNS depression, hypotension, and respiratory depression

corticosteroids: Possibly worsened depression

direct-acting sympathomimetics, such as epinephrine and norepinephrine: Potentiated effects of these drugs

disulfiram: Possibly transient delirium

fluoxetine: Possibly increased blood doxepin level

MAO inhibitors: Possibly hyperpyrexia, hypertension, seizures, and death

oral anticoagulants: Possibly increased anticoagulant effects of these drugs

pimozide: Increased risk of arrhythmias

probucol: Possibly prolonged QT interval and increased risk of ventricular tachycardia

thyroid hormones: Possibly increased therapeutic and toxic effects of both drugs

tolazamide: Possibly severe hypoglycemia

ACTIVITIES

alcohol use: Possibly enhanced CNS depression, hypotension, and respiratory depression

Adverse Reactions

CNS: Confusion, delirium, dream disturbances, drowsiness, fatigue, hallucinations, headache, nervousness, parkinsonism, restlessness, sedation, seizures, suicidal ideation (children and teens), tremor

CV: ECG changes, orthostatic hypotension, palpitations

EENT: Blurred vision, dry mouth, taste perversion

GI: Constipation, diarrhea, heartburn, ileus, increased appetite, nausea, vomiting,

GU: Decreased libido, ejaculation disorders

SKIN: Diaphoresis, jaundice

Other: Weight gain

Nursing Considerations

•If desired, mix oral solution in 120 ml of water; milk; or orange, grapefruit, tomato, or pineapple juice.

•Expect to observe adverse reactions within a few hours after giving drug.

•Evaluate patient for therapeutic response, such as decreased anxiety, apprehension, depression, fear, guilt, somatic symptoms, and worry; increased energy; and more restful sleep.

•**WARNING** Monitor children and teens closely for evidence of suicidal thinking and behavior because doxepin increases the risk in these groups.

•Keep in mind that abrupt withdrawal of doxepin after prolonged therapy can cause cholinergic rebound effects, including diarrhea, nausea, and vomiting.

•Plan to discontinue drug, as prescribed, several days before elective surgery to avoid hypertension.

•Monitor elderly patients for signs of parkinsonism, especially with high-dose therapy.

•Be alert for seizures. Patients who have a seizure disorder may need an increased anticonvulsant dosage to maintain seizure control.

•For patients with asthma or sulfite sensitivity, know that doxepin tablets may aggravate asthma or cause allergic reactions because they contain sulfites.

•Follow diabetic patient's serum glucose level closely; drug may alter glucose metabolism.

•If patient takes a thyroid hormone, be alert for increased responses to both drugs and, possibly, exaggerated drug-induced effects, such as arrhythmias and CNS stimulation. Untreated hypothyroidism prevents adequate response to therapy.

PATIENT TEACHING

•**WARNING** Alert parents to watch their child or teen closely for abnormal thinking or behavior and increased aggression or hostility. Stress importance of notifying prescriber about unusual changes.

•Instruct patient to avoid alcohol during doxepin therapy because mental alertness may decrease.

•Advise diabetic patient to measure her serum glucose level more frequently than usual.

doxercalciferol

Hectorol

Class and Category

Chemical class: Fat-soluble vitamin D analogue
Therapeutic class: Antihyperparathyroid drug
Pregnancy category: B

Indications and Dosages

➤ *To reduce elevated intact parathyroid hormone (iPTH) serum level when managing secondary hyperparathyroidism in patients undergoing chronic hemodialysis*

CAPSULES

Adults. *Initial:* 10 mcg 3 times/wk (about every other day) before, during, or after dialysis. *Maintenance:* If iPTH level is decreased by 50% and above 300 picograms (pg)/ml, dosage increased by 2.5 mcg at 8-wk intervals, as needed. If iPTH level is between 150 and 300 pg/ml, initial dosage maintained. If iPTH level is less than 100 pg/ml, drug stopped for 1 wk and then restarted at a dose that's at least 2.5 mcg less than previous dose. *Maximum:* 20 mcg 3 times/wk for a total of 60 mcg/wk.

➤ *To reduce elevated iPTH blood level when managing secondary hyperparathyroidism in patients with stage 3 or 4 chronic renal disease*

CAPSULES

Adults. 1 mcg daily. *Maintenance:* If iPTH level exceeds 70 pg/ml for stage 3 or 110 pg/ml for stage 4, dosage increased by 0.5 mcg at 2-wk intervals, as needed. If iPTH level is 35 to 70 pg/ml for stage 3 or 70 to 110 pg/ml for stage 4, dosage is maintained. If iPTH is less than 35 pg/ml for stage 3 or less than 70 pg/ml for stage 4, drug is stopped for 1 wk and then restarted with a dose that's at least 0.5 mcg lower than previous dose. *Maximum:* 3.5 mcg daily.

Contraindications

Evidence of vitamin D toxicity, hypersensitivity to doxercalciferol or its components, risk or history of hypercalcemia or hyperphosphatemia

Interactions

DRUGS

antacids that contain magnesium: Possibly additive drug effects and increased risk of

Mechanism of Action

Undergoes hepatic conversion to an active metabolite (1,25-dihydroxyvitamin D_2 [1,25-dihydroxyergocalciferol]), which increases intestinal absorption of dietary calcium and renal tubular reabsorption of urinary calcium. Together with parathyroid hormone, doxercalciferol also mobilizes calcium from bone. These effects serve to maintain the blood calcium levels in patients with chronic renal failure, which in turn prevents hyperparathyroidism.

In patients with renal failure, decreased metabolic activation of vitamin D in the kidneys leads to chronic hypocalcemia. The parathyroid gland compensates by increasing PTH secretion, but renal failure prevents it from achieving a normal serum calcium level. Thus, secondary hyperparathyroidism develops. Because doxercalciferol doesn't require renal conversion to form its active metabolite, it can regulate the serum calcium level and thus suppress PTH secretion and reduce its serum level in patients with chronic renal failure. An elevated PTH level in these patients leads to metabolic bone disease, such as renal osteodystrophy.

hypermagnesemia

cholestyramine, mineral oil, orlistat, and other drugs that affect lipid absorption: Possibly decreased doxercalciferol absorption
glutethimide, phenobarbital: Possibly increased doxercalciferol metabolism and risk of adverse reactions
erythromycin, ketoconazole: Possibly inhibited doxercalciferol metabolism and decreased effectiveness
vitamin D and its analogues: Possibly additive effects, resulting in increased adverse effects, such as hypercalcemia

Adverse Reactions

CNS: Depression, dizziness, headache, insomnia, malaise, paresthesia
CV: Bradycardia, chest pain, peripheral edema
EENT: Rhinitis
ENDO: Oversuppression of iPTH
GI: Anorexia, constipation, indigestion, nausea, vomiting
HEME: Anemia
MS: Hypertonia
RESP: Cough, dyspnea
SKIN: Pruritus
Other: Dehydration, hypercalcemia, hypercalciuria, hyperphosphatemia, weight gain

Nursing Considerations

•WARNING Be aware that patients who take vitamin D also should not take doxercalciferol because they may develop severe vitamin D toxicity and hypercalcemia.
•Be alert for signs and symptoms of vitamin D toxicity and hypercalcemia in patients receiving high-dose or long-term doxercalciferol therapy. Early signs and symptoms include bone pain, constipation, dry mouth, headache, metallic taste, myalgia, nausea, somnolence, vomiting, and weakness. Late signs and symptoms include albuminuria, anorexia, arrhythmias, azotemia, conjunctivitis (calcific), decreased libido, elevated AST and ALT levels, elevated BUN level, generalized vascular calcification, hypercholesterolemia, hypertension, hyperthermia, irritability, mild metabolic acidosis, nephrocalcinosis, nocturia, pancreatitis, photophobia, polydipsia, polyuria, pruritus, rhinorrhea, and weight loss.
•Keep emergency equipment readily available in case patient develops toxicity.
•Expect to monitor patient's blood iPTH, calcium, and phosphorus levels before starting drug therapy and weekly during early treatment.
•For patients with renal failure who are undergoing hemodialysis, be aware that oral calcium-based or other non–aluminum-containing phosphate binders and a low-phosphate diet typically are used to control the serum phosphorus level. An elevated serum phosphorus level worsens secondary hyperparathyroidism and may decrease doxercalciferol's effectiveness in reducing the blood iPTH level.
•After doxercalciferol therapy starts, expect to decrease dosage of phosphate binders to correct persistent mild hypercalcemia. Expect to increase dosage to correct persistent mild hyperphosphatemia.
•Avoid giving magnesium-containing

antacids with doxercalciferol if patient receives long-term hemodialysis because doing so may lead to hypermagnesemia.

PATIENT TEACHING
•Encourage patient who takes doxercalciferol to strictly follow a low-phosphorus diet and to take calcium supplement, as prescribed, to maintain serum calcium level. Stress that diet and calcium-based phosphate binder should provide 1.5 to 2 g of calcium daily.
•Explain the importance of having periodic follow-up blood work to measure drug effectiveness. Tell the patient that it may take several months to achieve optimal PTH suppression.
•Warn patient not to take other forms of vitamin D while taking doxercalciferol and to consult prescriber before taking any OTC drugs.
•Advise patient to contact prescriber immediately if early signs or symptoms of toxicity, such as headache or nausea, develop.

doxycycline calcium

(contains 50 mg of base per 5 ml of oral suspension)

Vibramycin

doxycycline hyclate

(contains 50 or 100 mg of base per capsule, 100 mg of base per delayed-release capsule, 100 mg of base per tablet, and 100 or 200 mg of base per injection vial)

Alti-Doxycycline (CAN), Apo-Doxy (CAN), Doryx, Doxycin (CAN), Vibramycin, Vibra-Tabs

doxycycline monohydrate

(contains 50 or 100 mg of base per capsule and 25 mg of base per 5 ml of oral suspension)

Monodox, Vibramycin

Class and Category
Chemical class: Oxytetracycline derivative
Therapeutic class: Antibiotic
Pregnancy category: D

Indications and Dosages
➤ *To treat cutaneous, GI, or inhalation anthrax*

CAPSULES, DELAYED-RELEASE CAPSULES, ORAL SUSPENSION, TABLETS, I.V. INFUSION
Adults, adolescents, and children weighing more than 45 kg (99 lb). 100 mg (base) every 12 hr for 60 days.
Children weighing less than 45 kg. 2.2 mg/kg (base) every 12 hr for 60 days.

➤ *To treat inflammatory lesions (papules and pustules) of rosacea*
Adults. 40 mg once daily in morning

➤ *To treat endocervical, rectal, and urethral infections caused by* Chlamydia trachomatis
CAPSULES, DELAYED-RELEASE CAPSULES, ORAL SUSPENSION, TABLETS
Adults and children over age 8 weighing more than 45 kg. 100 mg (base) b.i.d. for 7 days. *Maximum:* 300 mg (base) daily.
Children weighing 45 kg or less. 2.2 mg (base)/kg b.i.d. on day 1 and then 2.2 to 4.4 mg (base)/kg daily or 1.1 to 2.2 mg (base)/kg b.i.d.
I.V. INFUSION
Adults and children over age 8 weighing more than 45 kg. 200 mg (base) once daily or 100 mg (base) every 12 hr on day 1 and then 100 to 200 mg (base) once daily or 50 to 100 mg (base) every 12 hr. *Maximum:* 300 mg (base) daily.
Children weighing 45 kg or less. 4.4 mg (base)/kg once daily or 2.2 mg (base)/kg every 12 hr on day 1 and then 2.2 to 4.4 mg (base)/kg once daily or 1.1 to 2.2 mg (base)/kg every 12 hr.

➤ *To treat epididymo-orchitis caused by* C. trachomatis *or* Neisseria gonorrhoeae *or nongonococcal urethritis caused by* C. trachomatis *or* Ureaplasma urealyticum
CAPSULES, DELAYED-RELEASE CAPSULES, ORAL SUSPENSION, TABLETS
Adults and children over age 8 weighing more than 45 kg. 100 mg (base) b.i.d. for at least 10 days. *Maximum:* 300 mg (base) daily.
Children weighing 45 kg or less. 2.2 mg (base)/kg b.i.d. on day 1 and then 2.2 to 4.4 mg (base)/kg once daily or 1.1 to 2.2 mg (base)/kg b.i.d.
I.V. INFUSION
Adults and children over age 8 weighing more than 45 kg. 200 mg (base) once daily or 100 mg (base) every 12 hr on day 1 and then 100 to 200 mg (base) once daily or 50 to

100 mg (base) every 12 hr. *Maximum:* 300 mg (base) daily.

Children weighing 45 kg or less. 4.4 mg (base)/kg once daily or 2.2 mg (base)/kg every 12 hr on day 1 and then 2.2 to 4.4 mg (base)/kg once daily or 1.1 to 2.2 mg (base)/kg every 12 hr.

➤ *To prevent malaria*

CAPSULES, DELAYED-RELEASE CAPSULES, ORAL SUSPENSION, TABLETS

Adults and children over age 8 weighing more than 45 kg. 100 mg (base) daily beginning 1 to 2 wk before travel, continued daily during travel, and then daily for 4 wk after travel ends. *Maximum:* 300 mg (base) daily.

Children over age 8. 2 mg (base)/kg daily beginning 1 to 2 days before travel, continued daily during travel, and then daily for 4 wk after travel ends. *Maximum:* 100 mg (base) daily.

➤ *To treat early syphilis in penicillin-allergic patients*

CAPSULES, DELAYED-RELEASE CAPSULES, ORAL SUSPENSION, TABLETS

Adults and children over age 8 weighing more than 45 kg. 100 mg (base) b.i.d. for 2 wk. *Maximum:* 600 mg (base) daily.

Children weighing 45 kg or less. 2.2 mg (base)/kg b.i.d. on day 1 and then 2.2 to 4.4 mg (base)/kg once daily or 1.1 to 2.2 mg (base)/kg b.i.d.

I.V. INFUSION

Adults and children over age 8 weighing more than 45 kg. 150 mg (base) every 12 hr for at least 10 days. *Maximum:* 300 mg (base) daily.

Children weighing 45 kg or less. 4.4 mg (base)/kg once daily or 2.2 mg (base)/kg every 12 hr on day 1 and then 2.2 to 4.4 mg (base)/kg once daily or 1.1 to 2.2 mg (base)/kg every 12 hr.

➤ *To treat syphilis of more than 1 year's duration in penicillin-allergic patients*

CAPSULES, DELAYED-RELEASE CAPSULES, ORAL SUSPENSION, TABLETS

Adults and children over age 8 weighing more than 45 kg. 100 mg (base) b.i.d. for 4 wk. *Maximum:* 300 mg (base) daily.

I.V. INFUSION

Adults and children over age 8 weighing more than 45 kg. 150 mg (base) every 12 hr for at least 10 days. *Maximum:* 300 mg (base) daily.

Children weighing 45 kg or less. 4.4 mg (base)/kg once daily or 2.2 mg (base)/kg every 12 hr on day 1 and then 2.2 to 4.4 mg (base)/kg once daily or 1.1 to 2.2 mg (base)/kg every 12 hr.

➤ *To treat all other infections caused by susceptible organisms*

CAPSULES, DELAYED-RELEASE CAPSULES, ORAL SUSPENSION, TABLETS

Adults and children over age 8 weighing more than 45 kg. 100 mg (base) every 12 hr on day 1 and then 100 mg (base) once daily or 50 mg (base) b.i.d. For severe infections, 100 mg (base) continued every 12 hr. *Maximum:* 300 mg (base) daily.

Children weighing 45 kg or less. 2.2 mg (base)/kg b.i.d. on day 1 and then 2.2 to 4.4 mg (base)/kg once daily or 1.1 to 2.2 mg (base)/kg b.i.d.

I.V. INFUSION

Adults and children over age 8 weighing more than 45 kg. 200 mg (base) once daily or 100 mg (base) every 12 hr on day 1 and then 100 to 200 mg (base) once daily or 50 to 100 mg (base) every 12 hr. *Maximum:* 300 mg (base) daily.

Children weighing 45 kg or less. 4.4 mg (base)/kg once daily or 2.2 mg (base)/kg every 12 hr on day 1 and then 2.2 to 4.4 mg (base)/kg once daily or 1.1 to 2.2 mg (base)/kg every 12 hr.

Mechanism of Action

Exerts a bacteriostatic effect against a wide variety of gram-positive and gram-negative organisms. Doxycycline is more lipophilic than other tetracyclines, which allows it to pass more easily through the bacterial lipid bilayer, where it binds reversibly to 30S ribosomal subunits. Bound doxycycline blocks the binding of amino-acyl transfer RNA to messenger RNA, thus inhibiting bacterial protein synthesis.

Contraindications

Hypersensitivity to any tetracycline

Interactions

DRUGS

antacids that contain aluminum, calcium, magnesium, or zinc; calcium supplements; choline and magnesium salicylates; iron

salts; laxatives that contain magnesium: Decreased doxycycline absorption and therapeutic effects
barbiturates, carbamazepine, phenytoin: Increased clearance and decreased effects of doxycycline
cholestyramine, colestipol: Decreased doxycycline absorption
digoxin: Increased bioavailability of digoxin, possibly leading to digitalis toxicity
oral anticoagulants: Possibly increased hypoprothrombinemic effects of these drugs
oral contraceptives: Decreased effectiveness of estrogen-containing oral contraceptives, increased risk of breakthrough bleeding
penicillins: Inhibited bactericidal action
penthrane: Possibly increased risk of fatal renal toxicity
sodium bicarbonate: Altered doxycycline absorption from increased gastric pH
FOODS
dairy products, other foods high in calcium or iron: Decreased doxycycline absorption

Adverse Reactions
CNS: Paresthesia
CV: Phlebitis
EENT: Black "hairy" tongue, glossitis, hoarseness, oral candidiasis, pharyngitis, stomatitis, tooth discoloration
GI: Anorexia; bulky, loose stools; diarrhea; dysphagia; enterocolitis; epigastric distress; esophageal ulceration; hepatotoxicity; nausea; pseudomembranous colitis; rectal candidiasis; vomiting
GU: Anogenital lesions, dark yellow or brown urine, elevated BUN level, vaginal candidiasis
HEME: Eosinophilia, hemolytic anemia, neutropenia, thrombocytopenia, thrombocytopenic purpura
SKIN: Dermatitis, photosensitivity, rash, urticaria
Other: Anaphylaxis, injection site phlebitis

Nursing Considerations
• Avoid giving doxycycline to breastfeeding women because of the risk of enamel hypoplasia, inhibited linear skeletal growth, oral and vaginal candidiasis, photosensitivity reactions, and tooth discoloration in breastfeeding infant.
• Avoid giving drug to children under age 8, if possible; drug may cause permanent discoloration and enamel hypoplasia of developing teeth.

• Use oral suspension cautiously in patients who are allergic to sulfites because it contains sodium metabisulfite.
• Expect to adjust dosage for patients who have hepatic disease to avoid drug accumulation.
•**WARNING** Don't give doxycycline by I.M. or subcutaneous route.
• Give doxycycline without regard to meals. Although food and milk may delay absorption, they don't significantly reduce it.
• Observe patient frequently for injection site phlebitis, a common adverse reaction to I.V. administration.
• Monitor liver function test results as appropriate to detect hepatotoxicity.
• Expect oral or parenteral doxycycline to increase risk of oral, rectal, or vaginal candidiasis—especially in elderly or debilitated patients and those on prolonged therapy—by changing the normal balance of microbial flora.
• Monitor patient closely for diarrhea, which may indicate pseudomembranous colitis. If diarrhea occurs, notify prescriber and expect to withhold doxycycline. Expect to treat pseudomembranous colitis with fluids, electrolytes, protein, and an antibiotic effective against *Clostridium difficile.*

PATIENT TEACHING
• Instruct patient to avoid taking doxycycline just before bed because it may not dissolve properly when she's recumbent and may cause esophageal burning and ulceration.
• Instruct patient taking doxycycline for rosacea to take the capsule in the morning on an empty stomach.
• Advise patient to avoid dairy products; foods high in calcium or iron; antacids containing aluminum, calcium, or magnesium; bismuth subsalicylate; and iron-containing products during therapy.
• Caution patient not to take bismuth subsalicylate while taking doxycycline because doxycycline absorption will be reduced.
• Instruct patient to drink plenty of fluids while taking doxycycline to reduce the risk of esophageal burning and ulceration.
• Inform patient that her urine may become dark yellow or brown during therapy.
• Urge patient to avoid sun exposure and ultraviolet light as much as possible during therapy and to use sunscreen or sunblock as needed. If patient develops evidence of phototoxicity, such as skin eruption, tell her to

stop drug and notify prescriber.

• Advise patients who take an oral contraceptive to use an additional contraceptive method during therapy.

• If patient is being treated for a sexually transmitted disease, explain that her partner may need treatment as well.

• Tell patient to notify prescriber immediately if she develops anorexia, epigastric distress, nausea, or vomiting during therapy.

• Urge patient to report watery, bloody stools to prescriber immediately, even up to 2 months after drug therapy has ended.

• Alert female patients that doxycycline may increase the risk of vaginal candidiasis. Tell her to notify prescriber if she develops vaginal itching or discharge.

• Advise patient taking doxycycline for malaria prevention to start taking drug 1 to 2 days before traveling to the region and continue it for 4 weeks after leaving the area. Note that the total length of therapy shouldn't exceed 4 months.

dronabinol
(delta-9-tetrahydrocannabinol, THC)
Marinol

Class, Category, and Schedule
Chemical class: Synthetic tetrahydrocannabinol
Therapeutic class: Antiemetic, appetite stimulant
Pregnancy category: C
Controlled substance schedule: II

Indications and Dosages
➤ *To prevent nausea and vomiting caused by chemotherapy and unresponsive to other antiemetics*
CAPSULES
Adults. 5 mg/m^2 1 to 3 hr before and 2 to 4 hr after chemotherapy, increased by 2.5 mg/m^2, p.r.n. *Maximum:* 15 mg/m^2/dose or a total of 4 to 6 doses daily.

➤ *To stimulate appetite in cancer and AIDS patients*
CAPSULES
Adults. *Initial:* 2.5 mg b.i.d. before lunch and supper, increased p.r.n. *Maximum:* 20 mg

daily in divided doses.

DOSAGE ADJUSTMENT Dosage reduced to 2.5 mg before supper or at bedtime for patients who can't tolerate 5 mg daily.

Route	Onset	Peak	Duration
P.O.	Unknown	Unknown	24 hr or longer*

Mechanism of Action
May exert antiemetic effect by inhibiting the vomiting control mechanism in the medulla oblongata. As the main psychoactive substance in marijuana (*Cannabis sativa* L.), dronabinol's effects may be mediated by cannabinoid receptors in neural tissues.

Contraindications
Hypersensitivity to dronabinol, its components, sesame oil, or marijuana

Interactions
DRUGS
anticholinergics, antihistamines: Possibly increased risk of tachycardia
apomorphine: Possibly potentiated CNS depression, possibly decreased emetic response with prior use of dronabinol
CNS stimulants (such as amphetamines), and CNS depressants (such as benzodiazepines): Additive CNS effects
sympathomimetics: Possibly enhanced hypertension, tachycardia, and other adverse cardiovascular effects
ACTIVITIES
alcohol use: Additive CNS depressant effects

Adverse Reactions
CNS: Amnesia, anxiety, ataxia, confusion, delusions, depression, dizziness, drowsiness, euphoria, fatigue, hallucinations, irritability, mood changes, nervousness, seizures, sleep disturbance
CV: Orthostatic hypotension, palpitations, sinus tachycardia
GI: Nausea, vomiting
Other: Physical and psychological dependence

---

* For appetite stimulant effects; unknown for antiemetic effects.

Nursing Considerations
•**WARNING** Be aware that drug shouldn't be discontinued abruptly; otherwise, withdrawal syndrome may occur.
•Use cautiously in patients with a history of seizures because dronabinol may lower the seizure threshold. Notify prescriber immediately if seizures occur, and expect drug to be discontinued.
•Know that patients under age 45 may tolerate drug better than those over age 45.
•Watch for adverse reactions that mimic psychosis, such as hallucinations and, possibly, acute anxiety, especially with high doses.
•Anticipate higher risk of cardiovascular reactions, such as increased heart rate and blood pressure changes (especially orthostatic hypotension), at higher doses.
•**WARNING** Expect tolerance to drug to develop over time, especially if patient has smoked marijuana.
•Be aware that short-term, low-dose therapy doesn't typically lead to physical and psychological dependence, which may occur with long-term, high-dose therapy.
•Expect drug to alter REM sleep pattern, even after therapy stops.
PATIENT TEACHING
•Caution patient not to stop drug abruptly because withdrawal symptoms may occur.
•Urge patient not to use alcohol while taking dronabinol because it may enhance CNS depression.
•Instruct patient to rise slowly to sitting or standing position to minimize effects of orthostatic hypotension.
•Advise patient to avoid potentially hazardous activities until drug's CNS effects are known.
•Inform patient that sleep pattern may be adversely affected during therapy and for sometime afterward.

droperidol

Inapsine

Class and Category
Chemical class: Butyrophenone derivative
Therapeutic class: Antiemetic
Pregnancy category: C

Indications and Dosages
➤ *To reduce nausea and vomiting after surgery or diagnostic procedures when other treatments are ineffective*
I.V. OR I.M. INJECTION
Adults and adolescents. Dosage individualized up to a maximum initial dose of 2.5 mg I.M. or slow I.V. Additional 1.25 mg may be administered to achieve desired effect if potential benefit outweighs potential risk.
Children ages 2 to 12. Dosage individualized up to a maximum initial dose of 0.1 mg/kg. Additional dose may be administered to achieve desired effect if potential benefit outweighs potential risk.
DOSAGE ADJUSTMENT Initial dosage reduced for elderly, debilitated, or critically ill patients because of the increased risk of hypotension and excessive sedation.

Route	Onset	Peak	Duration
I.V., I.M.	3 to 10 min	In 30 min	2 to 4 hr

Mechanism of Action
Produces sedation by blocking postsynaptic dopamine receptors in the limbic system. Droperidol may reduce nausea by blocking dopamine receptors in the chemoreceptor trigger zone in the reticular formation of the medulla oblongata. It also may produce antiemetic effects by attaching to postsynaptic gamma-aminobutyric acid (GABA) receptors in the chemoreceptor trigger zone.

Contraindications
Hypersensitivity to droperidol or its components, known or suspected prolonged QT interval (including congenital long QT syndrome)

Interactions
DRUGS
amoxapine, haloperidol, loxapine, metoclopramide, metyrosine, molindone, olanzapine, phenothiazines, pimozide, rauwolfia alkaloids, risperidone, tacrine, thioxanthenes: Possibly increased risk of severe extrapyramidal reactions
anesthetics: Possibly hypotension and peripheral vasodilation
antiarrhythmics (class I or III), antidepressants, antimalarials, benzodiazepines, diuretics, I.V. opioids, laxatives, MAO inhibitors,

volatile anesthetics, and other drugs that prolong QT interval (such as some antihistamines): Increased risk of serious adverse effects of droperidol, such as prolonged QT interval and arrhythmias
antihypertensives: Possibly orthostatic hypotension
bromocriptine, levodopa: Possibly inhibited actions of these drugs
CNS depressants: Additive CNS depression
epinephrine: Possibly paradoxical reduction of blood pressure
propofol: Possibly decreased antiemetic effect of both drugs

ACTIVITIES
alcohol use: Additive CNS depression

Adverse Reactions
CNS: Anxiety, drowsiness, dystonia, restlessness
CV: Cardiac arrest, hypertension, hypotension, potentially fatal arrhythmias (such as torsades de pointes and ventricular tachycardia), prolonged QT interval, sinus tachycardia
EENT: Fixed upward position of eyeballs, laryngospasm
MS: Spasms of tongue, face, neck, and back muscles
RESP: Bronchospasm

Nursing Considerations
•**WARNING** Use droperidol cautiously in patients over age 65 and in patients with alcoholism, bradycardia, heart failure, hypokalemia, hypomagnesemia, parkinsonism, or preexisting QT-interval prolongation because they're at increased risk for prolonged QT interval and potentially fatal adverse reactions. Patients who take drugs that prolong the QT interval, such as some antiarrhythmics and benzodiazepines, and patients who take drugs that may cause an electrolyte imbalance, such as diuretics and laxatives, are also at increased risk.
•Expect a 12-lead ECG to be performed on all patients before droperidol administration to verify the absence of prolonged QT interval. Monitor ECG continuously for 2 to 3 hours after administering drug. Also monitor serum electrolyte levels to detect electrolyte imbalances.
•Use droperidol cautiously in patients with cardiac disease, who may not be able to compensate for drug's hypotensive effect.

Monitor vital signs, including blood pressure, frequently. Be aware that hypertension and tachycardia may occur in patients with a history of pheochromocytoma.
•Expect altered level of consciousness to last up to 12 hours after drug is given. Expect dosage to be reduced if patient is taking an opioid analgesic.
•If drug causes extrapyramidal reactions, such as restlessness, dystonia, and oculogyric crisis, expect to administer an anticholinergic, such as benztropine or diphenhydramine. Be sure to maintain a patent airway and oxygenation.
•If patient develops severe hypotension, expect to give phenylephrine. If hypotension is related to hypovolemia, expect to administer fluids.

PATIENT TEACHING
•Advise patient to immediately report palpitations or faintness, which may indicate an abnormal cardiac rhythm.
•Instruct patient to ask for help with ambulation on first postoperative day because altered consciousness may last up to 12 hours.
•Caution patient to avoid drinking alcohol, taking CNS depressants, driving, and operating machinery for 24 hours after receiving droperidol.

drotrecogin alfa (activated)
(recombinant human activated protein C)

Xigris

Class and Category
Chemical class: Serine protease glycoprotein
Therapeutic class: Anti-inflammatory, anti-thrombolytic
Pregnancy category: C

Indications and Dosages
➤ *To reduce risk of death in patients with severe sepsis in acute organ dysfunction*
I.V. INFUSION
Adults. 24 mcg/kg/hr for 96 hr.

Incompatibilities
Don't infuse any drugs or solutions except D_5W, normal saline solution, lactated

Ringer's solution, or dextrose and saline mixtures through the drotrecogin alfa I.V. line.

Mechanism of Action
Interferes with a number of the body's responses to severe sepsis, including increased thrombin generation and fibrin formation, impaired fibrinolysis, and systemic inflammation. Drotrecogin alfa produces its antithrombotic effect by inhibiting factors Va and VIIIa and has indirect profibrinolytic effect by inhibiting plasminogen activator inhibitor-1 and limiting the generation of activated thrombin-activatable fibrinolysis inhibitor.

Drotrecogin may produce its anti-inflammatory effect by inhibiting production of human tumor necrosis factor and other cytokines, preventing leukocyte adhesion to selectins, and limiting thrombin-induced inflammatory responses in the microvascular endothelium.

Contraindications
Active internal bleeding; evidence of cerebral herniation; hemorrhagic stroke within the past 3 months; hypersensitivity to drotrecogin alfa or its components; intracranial or intraspinal surgery or severe head trauma within the past 2 months; intracranial neoplasm or lesion; presence of epidural catheter; trauma with an increased risk of life-threatening bleeding

Interactions
DRUGS
abciximab, eptifibatide, and other glycoprotein IIb/IIIa inhibitors; aspirin and other platelet inhibitors; heparin; oral anticoagulants; thrombolytics: Increased risk of bleeding

Adverse Reactions
CNS: Intracranial hemorrhage
CV: Intrathoracic bleeding
GI: GI, intra-abdominal, or retroperitoneal bleeding
GU: Genitourinary bleeding
HEME: Prolonged APTT
SKIN: Ecchymosis

Nursing Considerations
•Be aware that drotrecogin alfa is used only for patients with severe sepsis who are at high risk for death, as determined by an Acute Physiology and Chronic Health Evaluation (APACHE) II score, a method of assessing mortality risk. Patients with only single-organ dysfunction who are recovering from recent surgery may not be candidates for drotrecogin alfa despite an adequate APACHE II score.
•Reconstitute 5-mg and 20-mg vials by slowly adding 2.5 ml or 10 ml of sterile water for injection, respectively, to yield a concentration of 2 mg/ml. Gently swirl—don't shake—vial until powder is completely dissolved. Use immediately or store for up to 3 hours at 15° to 30° C (59° to 86° F).
•Add reconstituted drug to normal saline solution by directing stream to side of bag to minimize agitation. Gently invert bag to mix; don't shake. Dilute to final concentration of 100 to 200 mg/ml if drug will be given by I.V. infusion pump or 100 to 1,000 mg/ml if by syringe pump. Be aware that infusion bag shouldn't be transported by a mechanical delivery system, such as a tube delivery system, between pharmacy and nursing unit.
•Prime infusion set for 15 minutes at a flow rate of 5 ml/hour when infusing less than 200 mg/ml at less than 5 ml/hour. Use prepared I.V. solution within 12 hours.
•Give drotrecogin alfa through a dedicated I.V. line or lumen of a multilumen central venous catheter. Don't infuse any drugs or solutions except D_5W, normal saline solution, lactated Ringer's solution, or dextrose and saline mixtures through the same line.
•Be aware that total duration of the drotrecogin alfa infusion must equal 96 hours, even if you need to interrupt it for a period. For example, if you calculate that infusion should end on 5 p.m. Friday, but then have to stop to give the patient blood for 2 hours on Thursday, add those 2 hours to your estimated completion time, which would then be 7 p.m. Friday.
•**WARNING** Monitor patient closely for bleeding; if it occurs, stop drotrecogin alfa infusion immediately and notify prescriber. Patients at increased risk include those with chronic severe hepatic disease, intracranial arteriovenous malformation or aneurysm, known bleeding diathesis, GI bleeding in previous 6 weeks, or ischemic stroke in previous 3 months; those receiving concurrent

D

therapeutic heparin (15 units/kg/hour or more); those who have received thrombolytic therapy in previous 3 days, aspirin at more than 650 mg daily, other platelet inhibitors in previous 7 days, or oral anticoagulants or glycoprotein IIb/IIIa inhibitors in previous 7 days); those with any other condition in which bleeding would constitute a significant hazard or be difficult to manage because of its location; and those with a platelet count less than $30,000 \times 10^6$/L or PT (as INR) greater than 3.0.

•Expect to discontinue drotrecogin alfa 2 hours before an invasive surgical or other procedure that poses a risk of bleeding and to resume administration immediately after uncomplicated, less-invasive procedures or 12 hours after major invasive procedures or surgery at the same rate of 24 mg/kg/hour, as prescribed.

•Be aware that drotrecogin alfa may prolong APTT during administration; PT may need to be used to monitor coagulopathy status during treatment.

•Before using drotrecogin alfa, refrigerate it at 2° to 8° C (36° to 46° F); don't freeze it. Protect from heat and direct sunlight.

PATIENT TEACHING

•Teach patient about adverse reactions to drotrecogin alfa, including bleeding from gums or nose and increased bruising. Instruct her to immediately report any signs of bleeding.

•Reassure patient that she'll be monitored closely throughout therapy.

duloxetine hydrochloride

Cymbalta

Class and Category

Chemical: Selective serotonin and norepinephrine reuptake inhibitor
Therapeutic: Antidepressant, neuropathic pain reliever
Pregnancy category: C

Indications and Dosages

➤ *To treat major depressive disorder*
E.R. CAPSULES
Adults. 20 mg b.i.d. Alternatively, 60 mg once daily or 30 mg b.i.d.

➤ *To relieve neuropathic pain associated with diabetic peripheral neuropathy*

E.R. CAPSULES
Adults. 60 mg daily.

➤ *To treat generalized anxiety disorder*
E.R. CAPSULES
Adults. *Initial:* 30 or 60 mg once daily, increased in 30-mg increments weekly, as needed. *Maximum:* 120 mg once daily.

➤ *To treat fibromyalgia*
E.R. CAPSULES
Adults. *Initial:* 30 mg daily for 1 wk; then increased to 60 mg daily.

Route	Onset	Peak	Duration
P.O.	Unknown	6 hr	Unknown

Mechanism of Action

Inhibits neuronal serotonin, norepinephrine, and dopamine reuptake to potentiate serotonergic and noradrenergic activity in the CNS. These activities may elevate mood and inhibit pain signals stemming from peripheral nerves adversely affected by chronically elevated serum glucose level.

Contraindications

Hepatic insufficiency, hypersensitivity to duloxetine or its components, uncontrolled angle-closure glaucoma, use within 14 days of MAO inhibitor therapy

Interactions
DRUGS

amiodarone, celecoxib, cimetidine, erythromycin, fluoxetine, fluvoxamine, haloperidol, ketoconazole, methadone, paroxetine, quinidine, quinolones, ritonavir: Increased blood duloxetine level
amiodarone, amitriptyline, desipramine, flecainide, haloperidol, imipramine, methadone, nortriptyline, phenothiazines, propafenone, ritonavir, thioridazine: Increased blood levels of these drugs
aspirin, NSAIDs, warfarin: Possibly increased risk of bleeding
CNS drugs: Increased effect of duloxetine
MAO inhibitors: Serious, sometimes fatal, autonomic instability, hyperthermia, myoclonus, rigidity
plasma protein binders (warfarin, phenytoin): Increased free concentration of these drugs and increased risk of adverse reactions

serotonergic drugs: Increased risk of serotonin syndrome

ACTIVITIES
alcohol use: Increased risk of hepatotoxicity

Adverse Reactions

CNS: Abnormal dreams, agitation, anxiety, asthenia, chills, dizziness, extrapyramidal disorder, fatigue, fever, hallucinations, headache, insomnia, migraine, nervousness, neuroleptic malignant syndrome, parasthesia, serotonin syndrome, somnolence, suicidal ideation, syncope, tremor, vertigo
CV: Hypertension, hypertensive crisis, orthostatic hypotension, palpitations, paresthesia, peripheral edema, supraventricular arrhythmia
EENT: Blurred vision, dry mouth, glaucoma, nasopharyngitis, pharyngitis, taste alteration
ENDO: Hot flashes, hyperglycemia
GI: Abdominal pain, anorexia, cholestatic jaundice, constipation, diarrhea, elevated liver enzymes, flatulence, hepatitis, hepatotoxicity, indigestion, jaundice, nausea, upper abdominal pain, vomiting
GU: Abnormal orgasm, decreased libido, erectile or ejaculatory dysfunction, urinary frequency, UTI
HEME: Bleeding episodes, leukopenia, thrombocytopenia
MS: Arthralgia, back pain, extremity pain, muscle cramp, myalgia
RESP: Cough, upper respiratory tract infection
SKIN: Diaphoresis, erythema multiforme, pruritus, rash, Stevens-Johnson syndrome, urticaria
Other: Anaphylaxis, angioedema, hyponatremia, weight loss

Nursing Considerations

• Avoid giving duloxetine to patients with severe renal impairment or end-stage renal disease that requires hemodialysis because blood drug levels increase significantly in these patients. Also avoid duloxetine in patients with hepatic insufficiency because drug is metabolized by the liver.
• Use duloxetine cautiously in patients with delayed gastric emptying because drug has an enteric coating that resists dissolution until it reaches an area where pH exceeds 5.5.
• Give duloxetine cautiously to patients with a history of mania, which it may activate.

Also give cautiously to patients with a seizure disorder because drug effects aren't known in these patients.
• Obtain patient's baseline blood pressure before duloxetine therapy starts, and assess it periodically thereafter for changes. If orthostatic hypotension occurs during duloxetine therapy, notify prescriber and anticipate that drug may need to be discontinued.
• Monitor patient's serum sodium level, especially if patient is elderly, taking a diuretic, or experiencing volume depletion, because drug may lower serum sodium level.
• Monitor patient's hepatic function, as ordered, because drug may increase the risk of hepatotoxicity.
• If patient takes duloxetine for depression (especially if he's a child or an adolescent), watch closely for evidence of suicidal thinking or behavior, especially when therapy starts or dosage changes.
• Avoid stopping duloxetine therapy abruptly, if possible, because withdrawal symptoms such as dizziness, nausea, headacle, fatigue, paresthesia, vomiting, irritability, nightmares, insomnia, diarrhea, anxiety, hyperhidrosis, and vertigo may occur. Taper dosage gradually, as ordered.

PATIENT TEACHING
• Tell patient to take capsule whole and not to chew it, crush it, or sprinkle contents on food or liquids because doing so alters enteric coating and may affect drug absorption.
• Inform patient that full effect of duloxetine may take weeks to occur; stress the importance of continuing to take the drug as directed.
• Caution patient against excessive alcohol consumption while taking duloxetine because it may increase risk of hepatic dysfunction.
• Advise patient not to stop duloxetine abruptly because adverse reactions may occur. Explain that drug will be stopped gradually.
• Instruct patient to notify prescriber if any serious or troublesome adverse effects develop.
• Advise patient to avoid potentially hazardous activities until drug's CNS effects are known.
• Instruct patient to rise from a lying or sitting position slowly to minimize drug's effect on lowering blood pressure.

D

•If patient takes duloxetine for depression, urge caregivers to watch closely for evidence of suicidal tendencies, especially if patient is a child or an adolescent and especially when therapy starts or dosage changes.

•Instruct female patients of childbearing potential to notify prescriber if they are, could be, or wish to become pregnant; duloxetine therapy may cause adverse reactions in neonates exposed to it during the third trimester.

dutasteride

Avodart

Class and Category
Chemical class: Synthetic 4-azasteroid compound

Therapeutic class: Benign prostatic hyperplasia agent

Pregnancy category: X

Indications and Dosages
➤ *To treat symptomatic benign prostatic hyperplasia (BPH); as adjunct with tamsulosin therapy to treat symptomatic BPH*

CAPSULES

Adult males. 0.5 mg daily.

Contraindications
Children; women; hypersensitivity to dutasteride, its components, or other 5-alpha reductase inhibitors

Interactions
DRUGS

cimetidine, ciprofloxacin, diltiazem, keto-

Mechanism of Action
Dutasteride reduces prostate gland enlargement by inhibiting the conversion of the male hormone testosterone to its active metabolite, 5-alpha dihydrotestosterone (DHT). DHT is the principal hormone that stimulates prostate cells to grow. As men age, they may become more sensitive to the effects of DHT, resulting in an excessive growth of prostatic cells and enlargement of the prostate. This condition, known as benign prostatic hyperplasia, may cause such signs and symptoms as urinary hesitancy, urinary urgency, and nocturia.

The intracellular enzyme 5-alpha-reductase (5α-R), which is present in the liver, prostate, and skin, converts testosterone to DHT, as shown below left. The two forms of 5α-R are type 1 and type 2. Dutasteride, a dual 5α-R inhibitor, deactivates both forms. When 5α-R is inhibited by dutasteride, the production of DHT is suppressed, as shown below right. With less circulating DHT, the prostate gland becomes smaller and the patient experiences an improvement in his symptoms.

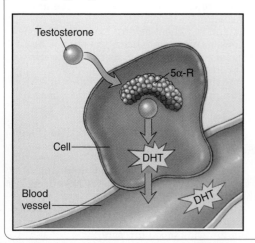

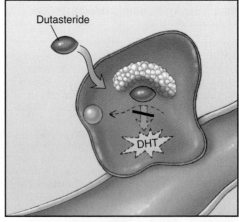

conazole, ritonavir, verapamil, and other CYP3A4 inhibitors: Risk of decreased metabolism and enhanced effects of dutasteride

Adverse Reactions

CNS: Dizziness
ENDO: Gynecomastia, increased serum testosterone and thyroid-stimulating hormone levels
GU: Decreased ejaculatory volume, decreased libido, impotence
SKIN: Localized edema, pruritus, rash, serious skin reactions, urticaria
ENDO: Angioedema

Nursing Considerations

•WARNING Be aware that dutasteride is absorbed through the skin. If you are female and pregnant or of childbearing age, do *not* handle the dutasteride capsule when administering it to a patient.
•Patient should be evaluated for other urologic conditions, including prostate cancer, before dutasteride therapy starts.
•Expect patient to undergo a digital rectal examination of the prostate before and periodically during dutasteride therapy.
•Anticipate the need to obtain a new baseline prostate-specific antigen (PSA) value after 3 to 6 months of dutasteride treatment because the drug can decrease PSA concentration by 40% to 50%.

PATIENT TEACHING

•WARNING Urge patient and female partners to use reliable contraceptive method during dutasteride therapy because semen of men who take drug can harm male fetuses. Caution women and children against handling capsules.
•Advise patient to inform prescriber if he has liver disease.
•Explain how to take drug properly, and advise patient to follow instructions that accompany drug. Instruct him to swallow capsule whole and to notify pharmacist if capsules are cracked or leaking.
•Inform patient that drug may decrease ejaculatory volume and libido and may cause impotence.
•Instruct patient to postpone blood donations for 6 months after final dose to avoid transmitting dutasteride to a pregnant woman during a blood transfusion.

•Urge patient to have periodic follow-up appointments.

dyphylline

Dilor, Lufyllin

Class and Category

Chemical class: Xanthine derivative
Therapeutic class: Bronchodilator
Pregnancy category: C

Indications and Dosages

➤ *To prevent or relieve bronchospasm from acute and chronic bronchial asthma, chronic bronchitis, and emphysema*

ELIXIR, TABLETS

Adults. Up to 15 mg/kg every 6 hr.

I.M. INJECTION

Adults. *Initial:* 500 mg. *Maintenance:* 250 to 500 mg every 2 to 6 hr, as needed.

Mechanism of Action

May cause bronchodilation by inhibiting phosphodiesterase enzymes. These enzymes normally inactivate cyclic adenosine monophosphate (cAMP) and cyclic guanosine monophosphate (cGMP), which are responsible for bronchial smooth-muscle relaxation. The drug may also foster calcium translocation, prostaglandin antagonism, catecholamine stimulation, and adenosine-receptor antagonism.

Contraindications

Hypersensitivity to dyphylline, xanthines, or their components; peptic ulcer disease; seizure disorder (unless controlled by anticonvulsant therapy)

Interactions

DRUGS

beta blockers: Possibly inhibited bronchodilation by dyphylline
ephedrine: Possibly increased frequency of insomnia, nausea, and nervousness
hydrocarbon inhalation anesthetics: Possibly increased risk of ventricular arrhythmias
probenecid: Possibly decreased renal excretion of dyphylline

sucralfate: Possibly adsorption of dyphylline if drugs given within 2 hours of each other

Adverse Reactions
CNS: Headache, insomnia, irritability, nervousness, seizures, tremor
CV: Arrhythmias, hypotension, tachycardia
GI: Diarrhea, gastroesophageal reflux, nausea, vomiting
GU: Increased diuresis

Nursing Considerations
•Inspect I.M. form of dyphylline for precipitate. If precipitate is present, discard drug and obtain a new ampule.
•Give oral drug at least 1 hour after meals for best absorption. However, if drug causes GI distress, give it with food if prescribed.
•Don't give parenteral drug by I.V. route.
•Evaluate for therapeutic response: decreased respiratory rate and effort.
•Assess for signs of dyphylline toxicity, including seizures and ventricular tachycardia.
PATIENT TEACHING
•Instruct patient to take oral dyphylline with a full glass of water and on an empty stomach to promote absorption.
•Advise patient to consult prescriber about taking drug with food if she experiences GI distress.

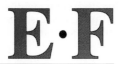

eflornithine hydrochloride

(alpha-difluoromethyl-ornithine, DFMO)

Ornidyl

Class and Category

Chemical class: Difluoromethylornithine
Therapeutic class: Antiprotozoal
Pregnancy category: C

Indications and Dosages

➤ *To treat the meningoencephalitic stage of* Trypanosoma brucei gambiense *infection (sleeping sickness)*

I.V. INFUSION
Adults. 100 mg/kg given over at least 45 min every 6 hr for 14 days.

Route	Onset	Peak	Duration
I.V.	Unknown	4 to 6 hr	Unknown

Mechanism of Action

Inhibits the enzyme ornithine decarboxylase, which is needed for decarboxylation of ornithine. This process is the first step in polyamine synthesis, which is needed for protozoal cell division and differentiation.

Incompatibilities

Don't give eflornithine with any other drug.

Contraindications

Hypersensitivity to eflornithine or its components

Adverse Reactions

CNS: Asthenia, dizziness, headache, seizures
EENT: Hearing loss
GI: Abdominal pain, anorexia, diarrhea, vomiting
HEME: Anemia, eosinophilia, leukopenia, myelosuppression, thrombocytopenia

Other: Alopecia, facial edema

Nursing Considerations

• Plan to reduce eflornithine dosage as prescribed, based on renal function. Monitor creatinine clearance in patients with renal dysfunction.
• Before infusion, dilute eflornithine concentrate with sterile water for injection. Using strict aseptic technique, withdraw the contents of a 100-ml vial and inject 25 ml into each of four I.V. diluent bags that contain 100 ml of sterile water. The resulting solution contains 40 mg/ml of eflornithine (5,000 mg of eflornithine in 125 ml total volume).
• Store bags of diluted eflornithine at 4° C (39° F) to reduce the risk of contamination. Use diluted drug within 24 hours.
• Expect to monitor the patient's CBC, including platelet count, before eflornithine treatment, twice weekly during treatment, and weekly after treatment stops until the patient's hematologic values return to baseline.
• Take infection-control and bleeding precautions because drug may cause myelosuppression. Adjust dosage or stop therapy as prescribed, based on severity.
• Take seizure precautions during eflornithine therapy.
• Consult prescriber about the need for serial audiography, if appropriate.
• Store undiluted vials of eflornithine at room temperature, and protect from freezing and light.

PATIENT TEACHING
• Stress the importance of follow-up visits because the risk of relapse lasts 24 months after treatment.
• Teach patient how to follow infection-control and bleeding precautions if myelosuppression occurs.
• Warn patient about risk of seizures; advise against performing potentially hazardous activities during therapy.

eletriptan hydrobromide

Relpax

Class and Category

Chemical class: Serotonin 5-HT$_{1D}$–receptor agonist

Therapeutic class: Antimigraine agent
Pregnancy category: C

Indications and Dosages

➤ *To relieve acute migraine attacks with or without aura*

TABLETS

Adults. *Initial:* 20 or 40 mg as a single dose. Repeated in 2 hr, as needed and ordered. *Maximum:* 40 mg as single dose, 80 mg daily.

Mechanism of Action

May stimulate 5-HT$_1$ receptors, causing selective vasoconstriction of inflamed and dilated cranial blood vessels in carotid circulation, which decreases carotid arterial blood flow and relieves acute migraines.

Contraindications

Bibasilar or hemiplegic migraine, cardiovascular disease (significant), cerebrovascular syndromes (stroke, transient ischemic attack), hepatic impairment (severe), hypersensitivity to eletriptan or components, ischemic bowel disease, ischemic or vasospastic coronary artery disease (CAD), peripheral vascular disease, uncontrolled hypertension, use within 24 hours of another serotonin 5-HT$_1$–receptor agonist or ergot-type drug, use within 72 hours of a potent CYP3A4 inhibitor

Interactions

DRUGS

clarithromycin, ketoconazole, itraconazole, nefazodone, nelfinavir, ritonavir, troleandomycin and other potent CYP3A4 inhibitors: Increased metabolism of eletriptan and decreased blood eletriptan level
ergot-containing drugs, 5-HT$_1$-receptor agonists: Possibly additive or prolonged vasoconstrictive effects
fluoxetine, fluvoxamine, paroxetine, sertraline: Increased risk of weakness, hyperreflexia, and incoordination

Adverse Reactions

CNS: Asthenia, dizziness, headache, paresthesia, somnolence, tiredness, weakness
CV: Chest tightness, pain, or pressure; coronary artery vasospasm; hypertension, MI or myocardial ischemia (transient); ventricular fibrillation or tachycardia
EENT: Dry mouth, throat tightness
GI: Abdominal pain, cramps, discomfort, or pressure; dysphagia; indigestion; nausea
SKIN: Flushing
Other: Feeling of warmth, pain, or pressure

Nursing Considerations

• Ensure that patients who are at risk for CAD undergo a satisfactory CV evaluation before you administer the first dose of eletriptan and that they have a periodic reevaluation of their cardiac status during intermittent long-term therapy.
• Obtain an ECG immediately after first dose of drug in patients who have CV risk factors but who have had a satisfactory CV evaluation because of the drug's potential to cause coronary vasospasm.
• Evaluate patient for CV signs and symptoms after administration of eletriptan and notify prescriber if they occur. Expect drug to be withheld, as ordered, while patient undergoes an extensive CV workup, and discontinued if abnormalities are detected.
• Monitor patient's blood pressure during therapy because of drug's potential to increase blood pressure.

PATIENT TEACHING

• Advise patient to take eletriptan as soon as possible after onset of migraine symptoms.
• Urge patient to contact prescriber and avoid taking drug if headache symptoms aren't typical.
• Advise against exceeding prescribed dose.
• Instruct patient to seek emergency care for chest, jaw, or neck tightness after taking drug because these may indicate adverse CV reactions; subsequent doses may require ECG monitoring.
• Urge patient to report palpitations.
• Advise patient to avoid hazardous activities until drug's CNS effects are known.
• Advise yearly ophthalmic examinations during prolonged eletriptan therapy.
• Instruct patient to inform prescriber of all drugs he's taking, including OTC products and herbal remedies.

eltrombopag olamine

Promacta

Class and Category

Chemical class: Biphenyl hydrazone

Therapeutic class: Platelet formation inducer
Pregnancy category: C

Indications and Dosages

➤ *To treat thrombocytopenia in patients with chronic immune (idiopathic) thrombocytopenic purpura who have had an insufficient response to corticosteroids, immunoglobulins, or splenectomy*

TABLETS

Adults. *Initial:* 50 mg daily, increased as needed to maintain a platelet count of 50 x 10⁹/L. Platelet counts usually increase in 1 to 2 wk. *Maximum:* 75 mg daily.

DOSAGE ADJUSTMENT For patients of East Asian ancestry or patients with moderate to severe hepatic impairment, starting dose of 25 mg daily.

Route	Onset	Peak	Duration
P.O.	Unknown	2 to 6 hr	Unknown

Mechanism of Action

Interacts with the transmembrane domain of the thrombopoietin receptor to signal cascades that induce proliferation and differentiation of megakaryocytes from bone marrow progenitor cells. This action increases platelet production, which is abnormally low in patients with thrombocytopenic purpura.

Contraindications

Hypersensitivity to eltrombopag or its components

Interactions

DRUGS

acetaminophen, atorvastatin, benzylpenicillin, fluvastatin, methotrexate, nateglinide, NSAIDs, opioids, pravastatin, repaglinide, rifampin, rosuvastatin: Possibly increased risk of adverse reactions related to excessive exposure to these drugs
antacids and mineral supplements containing aluminum, calcium, iron, magnesium, selenium, or zinc: Decreased eltrombopag absorption
ciprofloxacin, fluvoxamine, gemfibrozil, omeprazole, rifampin, trimethoprim: Increased risk of eltrombopag-induced adverse reactions

ACTIVITIES

smoking: Increased risk of eltrombopag-induced adverse reactions and possibly decreased eltrombopag efficacy

FOODS

all foods, especially diary: Decreased absorption of eltrombopag

Adverse Reactions

CNS: Headache, paresthesia
EENT: Cataract, conjunctival hemorrhage
GI: Abdominal pain, dyspepsia, elevated liver enzymes, hepatotoxicity, nausea, vomiting
GU: Menorrhagia
HEME: Hemorrhage, thrombocytopenia
MS: Fatigue, myalgia
SKIN: Ecchymosis

Nursing Considerations

•Eltrombopag should be used only to treat chronic immune (idiopathic) thrombocytopenia purpura and not any other kind of thrombocytopenia because of the risk of hematologic malignances.
•Eltrombopag can be used only through a restricted distribution program called, PROMACTA CARES. Patient, pharmacy, and prescriber must all be enrolled before therapy begins.
•Use cautiously in patients with hepatic impairment because drug may cause hepatotoxicity.
•Monitor liver enzymes and bilirubin level, as ordered, before starting eltrombopag therapy, every 2 weeks during dosage adjustment, and monthly once dose is stable. If abnormalities occur, repeat testing within 3 to 5 days and then weekly until liver enzymes return to baseline. Expect to discontinue drug if alanine aminothransferase level increases to three or more times the upper normal limit, progresses or persists for 4 or more weeks, or is accompanied by an increase in direct bilirubin or clinical symptoms of liver injury.
•Obtain baseline CBC, including platelet count and peripheral blood smears, before starting eltrombopag therapy, weekly until stable, and monthly thereafter, as ordered, because thrombopoietin receptor agonists (the same class as eltrombopag) have caused bone marrow fibrosis.
•Have patient undergo a baseline eye examination, as ordered, before starting eltrom-

E
F

bopag therapy and periodically throughout therapy, because drug may cause cataracts.
•Dosage adjustments are based on platelet count response and are not used to normalize platelet counts in order to prevent or minimize thrombotic complications.
•Give eltrombopag 1 hour before or 2 hours after the patient has eaten. Separate doses of other drugs by at least 4 hours to prevent drug interactions.
•Do not administer more than one dose of eltrombopag within any 24-hour period.
•Expect to discontinue drug if improvement doesn't occur within 4 weeks at maximum dose of 75 mg daily.
•Monitor patient for hematologic malignancies because eltrombopag stimulates thrombopoietin receptor on the surface of hematopoietic cells, which increases risk of malignancies.
•Monitor patient for increased bleeding after stopping eltrombopag because thrombocytopenia may worsen, increasing bleeding risk, especially if patient is on anticoagulants or antiplatelet therapy. If bleeding occurs, obtain weekly CBC, including platelet count, for at least 4 weeks after therapy stops, and provide supportive care, as indicated and ordered.

PATIENT TEACHING
•Inform patient that, before eltrombopag therapy can begin, he must be enrolled in the PROMACTA CARES program, which provides comprehensive education about the drug.
•Urge patient to tell prescriber about all health conditions and all prescribed drugs, OTC drugs, and herbs and supplements taken.
•Instruct patient to take eltrombopag on an empty stomach with a full glass of water 1 hour before or 2 hours after a meal and to separate use of other drugs by at least 4 hours because food and certain drugs (such as antacids and iron and vitamin supplements) may interfere with eltrombopag absorption.
•Instruct patient to take drug at the same time every day because no more than one dose should be taken within any 24-hour period.
•Urge patient to report any adverse reactions to prescriber and to keep all appointments for blood work and follow-up.

enalapril maleate

Vasotec

enalaprilat

Vasotec I.V.

Class and Category

Chemical class: Dicarbocyl-containing ACE inhibitor
Therapeutic class: Antihypertensive
Pregnancy category: C (first trimester), D (later trimesters)

Indications and Dosages

➤ *To control hypertension*

TABLETS
Adults. *Initial:* 5 mg daily, increased after 1 to 2 wk, as needed. *Maintenance:* 10 to 40 mg once daily or in divided doses b.i.d.
Children. 0.08 mg/kg daily, titrated according to blood pressure response up to 5 mg daily. *Maximum:* 0.58 mg/kg/dose or 40 mg/dose.

I.V. INJECTION
Adults. 1.25 mg every 6 hr.
DOSAGE ADJUSTMENT Initial dose 2.5 mg P.O. or 0.625 mg I.V. for patients who have sodium and water depletion from diuretic therapy, are receiving diuretics, or have a creatinine clearance below 30 ml/min/1.73 m^2. If response to I.V. dose is inadequate after 1 hr, I.V. dose of 0.625 mg is repeated and therapy continued at 1.25 mg every 6 hr.

➤ *To treat heart failure*

TABLETS
Adults. *Initial:* 2.5 mg once or twice daily, increased after 1 to 2 wk, as needed. *Maintenance:* 5 to 40 mg once daily or in divided doses b.i.d.

➤ *To treat asymptomatic left ventricular dysfunction*

TABLETS
Adults. *Initial:* 2.5 mg b.i.d., increased to 20 mg daily in divided doses.
DOSAGE ADJUSTMENT Initial dosage reduced to 2.5 mg daily and, if possible, diuretic dosage reduced in patients who have a serum sodium level below 130 mEq/L or a serum creatinine level above 1.6 mg/dl.

Route	Onset	Peak	Duration
P.O.	1 hr	4 to 6 hr	About 24 hr
I.V.	15 min	1 to 4 hr	About 6 hr

Mechanism of Action

May reduce blood pressure by affecting the renin-angiotensin-aldosterone system. By inhibiting angiotensin-convering enzyme (ACE), enalapril:

• prevents conversion of angiotensin I to angiotensin II, a potent vasoconstrictor that also stimulates the adrenal cortex to secrete aldosterone

• may inhibit renal and vascular production of angiotensin II

• decreases the serum angiotensin II level and increases serum renin activity, which decreases aldosterone secretion and slightly increases serum potassium level and fluid loss

• decreases vascular tone and blood pressure

• inhibits aldosterone release, which reduces sodium and water reabsorption and increases their excretion, further reducing blood pressure.

Contraindications

History of angioedema from previous ACE inhibitor; hypersensitivity to enalapril, enalaprilat, or their components

Interactions

DRUGS

allopurinol, bone marrow depressants (such as amphotericin B and methotrexate), procainamide, systemic corticosteroids: Possibly increased risk of fatal neutropenia or agranulocytosis

cyclosporine, potassium-sparing diuretics, potassium supplements: Increased risk of hyperkalemia

diuretics, other antihypertensives: Additive hypotensive effects

lithium: Increased blood lithium level and lithium toxicity

NSAIDs: Possibly reduced antihypertensive effects of enalapril and enalaprilat

sodium aurothiomalate: Increased risk of nitritoid reactions, such as facial flushing, nausea, vomiting, and hypotension

sympathomimetics: Possibly reduced therapeutic effects of enalapril and enalaprilat

FOODS

potassium-containing salt substitutes: Increased risk of hyperkalemia

ACTIVITIES

alcohol use: Possibly additive hypotensive effect

Adverse Reactions

CNS: Ataxia, confusion, depression, dizziness, dream disturbances, fatigue, headache, insomnia, nervousness, peripheral neuropathy, somnolence, stroke, syncope, vertigo, weakness

CV: Angina, arrhythmias, cardiac arrest, hypotension, MI, orthostatic hypotension, palpitations, pulmonary embolism and infarction, Raynaud's phenomenon

EENT: Blurred vision, conjunctivitis, dry eyes and mouth, glossitis, hoarseness, lacrimation, loss of smell, pharyngitis, rhinorrhea, stomatitis, taste perversion, tinnitus

ENDO: Gynecomastia

GI: Abdominal pain, anorexia, constipation, diarrhea, hepatic failure, hepatitis, ileus, indigestion, melena, nausea, pancreatitis, vomiting

GU: Flank pain, impotence, oliguria, renal failure, UTI

MS: Muscle spasms

RESP: Asthma, bronchitis, bronchospasm, cough, dyspnea, pneumonia, pulmonary edema, pulmonary infiltrates, upper respiratory tract infection

SKIN: Alopecia, diaphoresis, erythema multiforme, exfoliative dermatitis, flushing, pemphigus, photosensitivity, pruritus, rash, Stevens-Johnson syndrome, toxic epidermal necrolysis, urticaria

Other: Anaphylaxis, angioedema, herpes zoster, hyperkalemia

Nursing Considerations

•Use enalapril and enalaprilat cautiously in patients with impaired renal function. Avoid giving drug to children with a GFR less than 30 ml/min/1.73 m^2.

•For children who can't swallow tablets, consult with prescriber and pharmacist about preparation of an oral suspension from tablets as directed by manufacturer.

•Administer each I.V. dose over at least 5 minutes.

•Measure blood pressure immediately after first dose and frequently for at least 2 hours thereafter. If hypotension requires a dosage reduction, monitor blood pressure frequently for 2 hours after reduced dosage is administered and for another hour after blood pres-

E
F

sure has stabilized.
•Monitor blood pressure regularly during therapy. If hypotension develops, place patient in a supine position and expect to give I.V. normal saline solution or other volume expander as prescribed.
•Monitor patient's heart rate and rhythm. Expect to obtain repeated 12-lead ECG tracings.
•Monitor laboratory test results to check hepatic and renal function, leukocyte count, and serum potassium level.
•Monitor patient closely for angioedema of the face, lips, tongue, glottis, larynx, and limbs. For angioedema of the face and lips, stop drug and give an antihistamine, as prescribed. If tongue, glottis, or larynx is involved, assess patient for airway obstruction and prepare to give epinephrine 1:1,000 (0.3 to 0.5 ml) subcutaneously and maintain a patent airway.

PATIENT TEACHING
•Advise patient to take enalapril or enalaprilat at the same time each day.
•Instruct patient not to split, crush, or chew tablets.
•Inform patient that light-headedness and fainting may occur, especially during first few days of therapy. Advise him to change position slowly and avoid hazardous activities until drug's CNS effects are known.
•Inform patient that diarrhea, excessive sweating, vomiting, and other conditions may cause dehydration, which can lead to dizziness, fainting, and very low blood pressure during therapy. Urge sufficient fluid intake to prevent dehydration and related adverse reactions. If diarrhea or vomiting is severe or prolonged, instruct patient to notify prescriber.
•Urge patient to immediately notify prescriber if angioedema and other adverse reactions, including persistent dry cough, occur.
•Advise patient to consult prescriber before using salt substitutes, potassium supplements, or other drugs (including OTC drugs) while taking drug.
•WARNING Caution women of childbearing age that they should use a reliable form of contraception and should notify prescriber immediately if pregnancy is suspected because enalapril may cause fetal harm and should be discontinued.

enoxacin
Penetrex

Class and Category
Chemical class: Fluoroquinolone
Therapeutic class: Antibiotic
Pregnancy category: C

Indications and Dosages
➤ *To treat gonorrhea*
TABLETS
Adults. 400 mg as a single dose.
➤ *To treat uncomplicated UTI*
TABLETS
Adults. 200 mg every 12 hr for 7 days.
➤ *To treat complicated UTI*
TABLETS
Adults. 400 mg every 12 hr for 14 days.
DOSAGE ADJUSTMENT Dosage reduced to one-half in patients with creatinine clearance of 30 ml/min/1.73 m² or less.

Contraindications
History of tendinitis or tendon rupture, hypersensitivity to enoxacin or any quinolone antibiotic

Interactions
DRUGS
aluminum-, calcium-, or magnesium-containing antacids; didanosine (chewable or buffered tablets); ferrous sulfate; magnesium-containing laxatives; sucralfate; zinc: Interference with enoxacin absorption, decreased blood enoxacin level
bismuth: Decreased enoxacin bioavailability (by about 25% if given with or up to 60 minutes after enoxacin)
cyclosporine: Possibly increased blood cyclosporine level
digoxin: Increased serum digoxin level and risk of digitalis toxicity
NSAIDs: Possibly increased risk of CNS stimulation and seizures
theophylline: Interference with theophylline metabolism, increased risk of theophylline toxicity
warfarin: Possibly increased anticoagulant effect of warfarin and increased risk of bleeding
FOODS
caffeine: Decreased caffeine clearance, increased adverse effects of caffeine, increased blood enoxacin level

Mechanism of Action

Normally, the enzyme DNA gyrase is responsible for unwinding and supercoiling bacterial DNA before it replicates, as shown below left. Enoxacin inhibits this enzyme, as shown below right, interfering with bacterial cell replication and causing cell death.

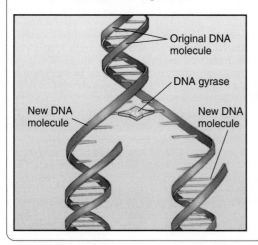
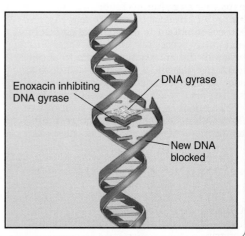

Adverse Reactions

CNS: Dizziness, drowsiness, hallucinations, headache, insomnia, nervousness, seizures, vertigo
EENT: Taste perversion
GI: Abdominal pain, diarrhea, indigestion, nausea, pseudomembranous colitis, vomiting
GU: Vaginitis
MS: Tendinitis, tendon rupture
SKIN: Photosensitivity, pruritus, rash
Other: Anaphylaxis

Nursing Considerations

•Be aware that enoxacin shouldn't be given to a patient under age 18 because it may cause arthropathy.
•Use drug cautiously in patients with a history of or susceptibility to seizures.
•Obtain a specimen for culture and sensitivity tests, as ordered, but expect to begin therapy before results are available.
•Monitor patient closely for signs and symptoms of anaphylaxis after first dose: shock, dyspnea, facial or laryngeal edema, loss of consciousness, paresthesia, pruritus, and urticaria. If they occur, stop enoxacin immediately, notify prescriber, and prepare to treat symptoms.
•Ask if patient has a history of seizures.

Take seizure and safety precautions because drug may induce seizures and other adverse CNS reactions after a single dose.
•Report severe or prolonged diarrhea, which may indicate pseudomembranous colitis.
•Watch for pain, inflammation, and tendon rupture, especially in shoulders, hands, and ankles.
•If patient has gonorrhea, expect to obtain a serologic test for syphilis at diagnosis and 3 months after enoxacin therapy ends.

PATIENT TEACHING
•Stress the importance of taking the full course of enoxacin exactly as prescribed, even if patient feels better before it's finished.
•Instruct patient to take drug at the same times each day—1 hour before or 2 hours after meals—with 8 oz of water.
•Urge patient to avoid potentially hazardous activities until CNS effects of enoxacin are known.
•Advise patient to notify prescriber if symptoms don't improve within a few days.
•Urge patient to drink plenty of fluids but to avoid caffeine during therapy.
•Caution patient not to take aluminum-, calcium-, or magnesium-containing antacids; bismuth; didanosine (chewable or buffered

tablets), if prescribed; or products that contain iron or zinc for 8 hours before or 2 hours after taking enoxacin.
•Tell patient to avoid direct sunlight and to use sunscreen and wear protective clothing outdoors. Urge him to report photosensitivity.
•Instruct patient to stop taking enoxacin and notify prescriber immediately if a rash or other allergic reaction develops.
•Instruct patient to take a missed dose as soon as he remembers, unless it's nearly time for the next. Warn against doubling the dose.
•Tell patient to report tendon pain or inflammation, stop enoxacin, and rest until tendinitis or tendon rupture is ruled out.

enoxaparin sodium

Lovenox

Class and Category

Chemical class: Low-molecular-weight heparin
Therapeutic class: Antithrombotic
Pregnancy category: B

Indications and Dosages

➤ *To prevent deep vein thrombosis (DVT) after hip or knee replacement and for continued prophylaxis after hospitalization for hip replacement*

SUBCUTANEOUS INJECTION

Adults. 30 mg every 12 hr, starting 12 to 24 hr after surgery for up to 14 days. Or, 40 mg daily, starting 9 to 15 hr after hip replacement surgery. *Prophylaxis:* 40 mg daily for 3 wk.

➤ *To prevent DVT after abdominal surgery for patients with thromboembolic risk factors (over age 40, obesity, general anesthesia lasting longer than 30 minutes, cancer, or a history of DVT or pulmonary embolism)*

SUBCUTANEOUS INJECTION

Adults. 40 mg daily, starting 2 hr before surgery and lasting 7 to 10 days.

➤ *To prevent ischemic complications of unstable angina and non–Q-wave MI*

SUBCUTANEOUS INJECTION

Adults. 1 mg/kg every 12 hr with 100 to 325 mg of aspirin daily for 2 to 8 days or until condition is stable.

DOSAGE ADJUSTMENT Dosage reduced to

30 mg daily if creatinine clearance is less than 30 ml/min/1.73 m^2 and patient is receiving drug as prophylaxis in abdominal, hip, or knee replacement surgery or is acutely ill. Reduced to 1 mg/kg daily if creatinine clearance is less than 30 ml/min/ 1.73 m^2 and drug is given with aspirin to prevent ischemic complications of unstable angina and non–Q-wave MI, with warfarin as inpatient treatment for acute DVT with or without pulmonary embolism, or with warfarin as outpatient treatment of acute DVT without pulmonary embolism.

➤ *To treat acute ST-segment–elevation MI (STEMI)*

I.V. INJECTION, THEN SUBCUTANEOUS INJECTION

Adults. 30 mg I.V. as a single dose, followed by 1 mg/kg subcutaneously (maximum, 100 mg for first two doses). Then, 1 mg/kg subcutaneously every 12 hr.

DOSAGE ADJUSTMENT If patient also receives a thrombolytic, enoxaparin should be given 15 to 30 min before and 30 min after fibrinolytic therapy starts. If patient has percutaneous coronary intervention, give 0.3-mg/kg I.V. bolus if last enoxaparin dose was given more than 8 hr before balloon inflation.

Route	Onset	Peak	Duration
SubQ	Unknown	3 to 5 hr	Up to 24 hr

Mechanism of Action

Potentiates the action of antithrombin III, a coagulation inhibitor. By binding with antithrombin III, enoxaparin rapidly binds with and inactivates clotting factors (primarily thrombin and factor Xa). Without thrombin, fibrinogen can't convert to fibrin and clots can't form.

Incompatibilities

Don't mix enoxaparin with other I.V. fluids or drugs.

Contraindications

Active major bleeding; hypersensitivity to benzyl alcohol (if only the multidose vial is available), enoxaparin, heparin (including low-molecular-weight heparins), or pork products; thrombocytopenia and positive antiplatelet antibody test while taking low-molecular-weight heparins

Interactions
DRUGS
cefamandole, cefoperazone, cefotetan, plica-mycin, valproic acid: Possibly increased risk of hemorrhage
NSAIDs; oral anticoagulants; platelet aggre-gation inhibitors, such as aspirin, dipyri-damole, sulfinpyrazone, and ticlopidine; thrombolytics, such as alteplase, anistreplase, streptokinase, and urokinase: Possibly in-creased risk of bleeding

Adverse Reactions
CNS: Confusion, epidural or spinal hema-toma, fever, paralysis, stroke
CV: Atrial fibrillation, congestive heart fail-ure, hyperlipidemia, peripheral edema
EENT: Epistaxis
GI: Bloody stools, diarrhea, elevated liver function test results, hematemesis, melena, nausea, vomiting
GU: Hematuria, menstrual irregularities
HEME: Anemia, hemorrhage, thrombocytopenia
RESP: Dyspnea, pneumonia, pulmonary edema or embolism
SKIN: Cutaneous vasculitis, ecchymosis, per-sistent bleeding or oozing from mucous membranes or surgical wounds, pruritus, skin necrosis at injection site or distant from injection site, urticaria, vesiculobullous rash
Other: Anaphylaxis; hyperkalemia; injection site erythema, hematoma, irritation, and pain

Nursing Considerations
• Use enoxaparin with extreme caution in patients with a history of heparin-induced thrombocytopenia or increased risk of hem-orrhage. Use cautiously in those with bleed-ing diathesis, diabetic retinopathy, hepatic or renal impairment, recent GI ulceration or hemorrhage, or uncontrolled hypertension. Expect delayed elimination in elderly pa-tients and those with renal insufficiency.
• Drug isn't recommended for patients with prosthetic heart valves, especially pregnant women, because of risk of prosthetic valve thrombosis. If enoxaparin is needed, monitor patient's peak and trough anti-factor Xa lev-els often and adjust dosage as needed.
• Use multidose vials cautiously in pregnant women because benzyl alcohol may cross the placenta and cause fetal harm.
• Don't give drug by I.M. injection.
• Expect to give drug with aspirin to patient with unstable angina, STEMI, and non–Q-wave MI. To minimize risk of bleeding after vascular procedures, be careful to give enoxaparin at recommended intervals.
• After percutaneous revascularization proce-dure, it is important to achieve hemostasis at the puncture site. A closure device may be removed right away; however, if a manual compression method is used, the sheath should be removed 6 hours after last enoxa-parin dose. If enoxaparin therapy will con-tinue, give next scheduled dose no sooner than 6 to 8 hours after sheath removal.
• Watch closely for bleeding. Notify pre-scriber immediately if platelet count falls below 100,000/mm³. Expect to stop drug and start treatment if patient has a thromboem-bolic event, such as a stroke.
• Test stool for occult blood, as ordered.
• Keep protamine sulfate nearby in case of accidental overdose.
• Check serum potassium level for elevation, especially in patients with renal impairment or concurrent use of potassium-sparing di-uretics.

PATIENT TEACHING
• Advise patient to notify prescriber about adverse reactions, especially bleeding.
• Instruct patient to seek immediate help for evidence of thromboembolism, such as neu-rologic changes and severe shortness of breath.
• Stress the importance of complying with follow-up visits with prescriber.
• Teach patient or family member how to give enoxaparin at home, if needed. Show patient how to give by deep subcutaneous injection while lying down. Instruct him not to expel air bubble from a prefilled syringe to avoid losing some of the drug. Tell him to insert the entire needle into a skin fold held between the thumb and forefinger. Remind him to alternate injection sites between the left and right anterolateral abdominal wall.
• To minimize bruising, caution patient not to rub the site after giving the injection.
• Review safe handling and disposal of sy-ringes and needles.

entacapone

Comtan

Class and Category
Chemical class: COMT inhibitor

Therapeutic class: Antidyskinetic
Pregnancy category: C

Indications and Dosages

➤ *As adjunct to manage symptoms of Parkinson's disease*

TABLETS

Adults. 200 mg with each dose of carbidopa and levodopa. *Maximum:* 1,600 mg daily.

Mechanism of Action

Inhibits peripheral catechol-*O*-methyltransferase (COMT), the major metabolizing enzyme for levodopa. During levodopa metabolism, COMT causes the formation of a levodopa metabolite that reduces the effectiveness of levodopa. By inhibiting COMT, entacapone leads to higher sustained blood levels of levodopa and its increased availability for diffusion into the CNS, where it is converted to dopamine. By replenishing dopamine stores, entacapone increases dopaminergic stimulation in the brain and reduces the symptoms of Parkinson's disease. Carbidopa is given with levodopa because it inhibits the peripheral distribution of levodopa, making more levodopa available for transport to the brain.

Contraindications

Hypersensitivity to entacapone or its components, use within 14 days of nonselective MAO inhibitor therapy

Interactions

DRUGS

ampicillin, chloramphenicol, cholestyramine, erythromycin, probenecid, rifampin: Decreased biliary excretion of entacapone
apomorphine, bitolterol, dobutamine, dopamine, epinephrine, isoetharine, isoproterenol, methyldopa, norepinephrine: Possibly increased heart rate, arrhythmias, and excessive changes in blood pressure
MAO inhibitors (nonselective): Possibly inhibited entacapone metabolism

Adverse Reactions

CNS: Agitation, anxiety, asthenia, dizziness, dyskinesia, fatigue, hallucinations, hyperkinesia, hypokinesia, somnolence
EENT: Dry mouth

GI: Abdominal pain, constipation, diarrhea, indigestion, gastritis, nausea
GU: Brown-orange urine
MS: Back pain
RESP: Dyspnea
SKIN: Diaphoresis, purpura

Nursing Considerations

•**WARNING** Be aware that entacapone should not be discontinued abruptly because doing so may precipitate signs and symptoms resembling those of neuroleptic malignant syndrome, such as fever, muscle rigidity, altered level of consciousness, confusion, and elevated creatine kinase level. Patients may also experience a rapid reemergence of parkinsonian symptoms.
•Monitor patient for drug-induced diarrhea during first 4 to 12 weeks of therapy.
•Help patient with activities as needed because drug may increase risk of orthostatic hypotension or syncope.
•Watch for worsening dyskinesia because entacapone potentiates dopaminergic adverse effects of levodopa.
•Be aware that drug may be taken with selective MAO inhibitors, such as selegiline.

PATIENT TEACHING

•Instruct patient to always take entacapone with carbidopa and levodopa because drug has no antidyskinetic effect of its own.
•Inform patient that dizziness and sleepiness are more common at beginning of treatment, especially in those with hypotension.
•Advise patient not to participate in potentially hazardous activities until drug's CNS effects are known, especially if he's also taking CNS depressants.
•If patient is scheduled for surgery, instruct him to inform surgeon and anesthesiologist about entacapone use before the prcedure because COMT inhibitors such as entacapone may interact with some drugs used in surgical procedures.
•Caution patient that entacapone may increase adverse effects of carbidopa and levodopa, such as nausea and uncontrolled movements. If these adverse effects do increase, advise him to contact prescriber immediately because carbidopa and levodopa dosage may need to be lowered.
•Inform patient that urine may turn brown-orange while he's taking entacapone but that this is a harmless effect.

epinephrine
(adrenaline)
Adrenalin, Adrenalin Chloride Solution, Ana-Guard, Bronkaid Mist, Bronkaid Mistometer (CAN), EpiPen (CAN), EpiPen Auto-Injector, EpiPen Jr. (CAN), EpiPen Jr. Auto-Injector, Primatene Mist

epinephrine bitartrate
Asthmahaler Mist, Bronkaid Suspension Mist

racepinephrine
AsthmaNefrin, MicroNefrin, Nephron, Vaponefrin

Class and Category
Chemical class: Catecholamine
Therapeutic class: Antianaphylactic, bronchodilator, cardiac stimulant, vasopressor
Pregnancy category: C

Indications and Dosages
➤ *To treat bronchospasm*
INHALED SOLUTION (EPINEPHRINE)
Adults and children age 4 and over. 1 to 3 inhalations (10 drops) by hand-bulb nebulizer no more than every 3 hr.
INHALED SOLUTION (RACEPINEPHRINE)
Adults and children age 4 and over. 3 inhalations of 0.5 ml (10 drops) by hand-bulb nebulizer, or 0.2 to 0.5 ml (4 to 10 drops) of diluted solution given over 15 min by jet nebulizer; repeated after 3 to 4 hr, if needed.
ORAL INHALED AEROSOL (EPINEPHRINE BITARTRATE)
Adults and children age 4 and over. 1 inhalation (160 mcg) repeated after 1 min, if needed; then repeated after at least 3 hr.
ORAL INHALER (EPINEPHRINE)
Adults and children age 4 and over. 1 inhalation (200 to 275 mcg) repeated after at least 1 min, if needed; then repeated after at least 3 hr.
➤ *To treat croup*
INHALED SOLUTION (RACEPINEPHRINE)
Children. 0.05 ml/kg diluted to 3 ml in normal saline solution and given over 15 min every 2 hr, as needed. *Maximum:* 0.5 ml/dose.
➤ *To treat anaphylaxis*
I.V. INFUSION
Adults and adolescents. 100 to 250 mcg given slowly.
I.M. OR SUBCUTANEOUS INJECTION

Adults and adolescents. 100 to 500 mcg repeated every 10 to 15 min, as needed. *Maximum:* 1 mg/dose; three doses.
Children. 10 mcg/kg repeated every 15 min for three doses. *Maximum:* 300 mcg/dose.
➤ *To treat severe anaphylactic shock*
I.V. INFUSION
Adults. 1 mcg/min titrated to 2 to 10 mcg/min for desired hemodynamic response.
➤ *To treat cardiac arrest*
I.V. INJECTION
Adults. 0.5 to 1 mg every 3 to 5 min during resuscitation.
Children. 10 mcg/kg followed by 100 mcg/kg every 3 to 5 min, if needed. If two doses produce no response, subsequent doses are increased to 200 mcg/kg every 5 min.
Neonates. 10 to 30 mcg/kg every 3 to 5 min.

Route	Onset	Peak	Duration
I.V., I.M.	Rapid	Unknown	1 to 2 min
SubQ	5 to 10 min	In 20 min	Short
Oral inhalation	1 to 5 min	In 5 to 15 min	Up to 3 hr

Mechanism of Action
Acts on alpha and beta receptors. This nonselective adrenergic agonist stimulates:
• alpha$_1$ receptors, which constricts arteries and may decrease bronchial secretions
• presynaptic alpha$_2$ receptors, which inhibits norepinephrine release by way of negative feedback
• postsynaptic alpha$_2$ receptors, which constricts arteries
• beta$_1$ receptors, which induces positive chronotropic and inotropic responses
• beta$_2$ receptors, which dilates arteries, relaxes bronchial smooth muscles, increases glycogenolysis, and prevents mast cells from secreting histamine and other substances, thus reversing bronchoconstriction and edema.

Incompatibilities
Don't mix epinephrine with alkalies or oxidizing agents, including bromine, chlorine, chromates, iodine, metal salts (as from iron), nitrites, oxygen, and permanganates, because these substances can destroy epinephrine.

Contraindications

Cerebral arteriosclerosis, coronary insufficiency, counteraction of phenothiazine-induced hypotension, dilated cardiomyopathy, general anesthesia with halogenated hydrocarbons or cyclopropane, hypersensitivity to epinephrine or its components, labor, angle-closure glaucoma, organic brain damage, shock (nonanaphylactic)

Interactions

DRUGS

alpha-adrenergic blockers, drugs with alpha-adrenergic action, rapid-acting vasodilators: Blockage of epinephrine's alpha-adrenergic effect, possibly causing severe hypotension and tachycardia

amyl nitrite, nitrates: Decreased antianginal effects

antihypertensives, diuretics used to treat hypertension: Decreased antihypertensive effects

beta blockers: Mutual inhibition of therapeutic effects, possibly severe hypertension and cerebral hemorrhage

chlorpheniramine, diphenhydramine, levothyroxine, MAO inhibitors, tricyclic antidepressants, tripelennamine: Possibly increased effects of epinepherine

digoxin, diuretics, quinidine: Increased risk of arrhythmias

dihydroergotamine, ergoloid mesylates, ergonovine, ergotamine, methylergonovine, methysergide, oxytocin: Increased risk of vasoconstriction, causing gangrene, peripheral vascular ischemia, or severe hypertension

ergot alkaloids: Possibly reversed pressor effects of epinephrine

hydrocarbon inhalation anesthetics: Increased risk of severe atrial and ventricular arrhythmias

insulin, oral antidiabetic drugs: Decreased effects of these drugs

MAO inhibitors: Possibly increased vasopressor effect of epinephrine and hypertensive crisis

maprotiline, tricyclic antidepressants: Potentiated cardiovascular effects of epinephrine, possibly causing arrhythmias, hyperpyrexia, severe hypertension, or tachycardia

sympathomimetics: Additive CNS stimulation, increased cardiovascular effects of either drug

thyroid hormones: Increased effects of either drug

xanthines: CNS stimulation and toxic effects

Adverse Reactions

CNS: Anxiety, apprehensiveness, chills, fever, dizziness, drowsiness, hallucinations, headache, insomnia, light-headedness, nervousness, restlessness, seizures, stroke, temporary worsening of Parkinson's disease, tremor, weakness

CV: Arrhythmias, including ventricular fibrillation; chest discomfort or pain; fast, irregular, or slow heartbeat; palpitations; severe hypertension; tachycardia

EENT: Blurred vision, dry mouth or throat, miosis

ENDO: Hyperglycemia in diabetics

GI: Anorexia, heartburn, nausea, vomiting

GU: Dysuria

MS: Muscle twitching, severe muscle spasms

RESP: Dyspnea

SKIN: Cold skin, diaphoresis, ecchymosis, flushed or red face or skin, pallor, tissue necrosis

Other: Hyperkalemia; hypokalemia; injection site coldness, hypoaesthesia, pain, pallor, and stinging

Nursing Considerations

• Use epinephrine with extreme caution in patients with angina, arrhythmias, asthma, degenerative heart disease, or emphysema. Epinephrine's inotropic effect equals that of dopamine and dobutamine; its chronotropic effect exceeds that of both.

• Use drug cautiously in elderly patients and those with cardiovascular disease (other than listed above), diabetes mellitus, hypertension, hyperthyroidism, prostatic hypertrophy, and psychoneurologic disorders.

• Be aware that some preparations contain sulfites, which may cause allergic-type reactions. However, the presence of sulfites in epinephrine should not deter its use in a patient with anaphylaxis, even if patient is sensitive to sulfites. Monitor patient closely for adverse effects.

• Dilute the 1:1,000 (1-mg/ml) solution of parenteral epinephrine before I.V. use.

• Shake suspension thoroughly before withdrawing dose; refrigerate it between uses.

• Inspect epinephrine solution or suspension before use. If it's pink or brown, air has entered a multidose vial. If it's discolored or contains particles, discard it. Also discard unused portions of parenteral epinephrine.

• When injecting drug, rotate sites because

repeated injections in the same site may cause vasoconstriction and localized necrosis.
•Be aware that drug shouldn't be given by intra-arterial injection because marked vaso-constriction may cause gangrene.
•Avoid giving injection into buttocks bec ause drug may be less effective when given there, especially for treating anaphylaxis.
•Monitor patient for potassium imbalances. Initially, hyperkalemia occurs when hepato-cytes release potassium. Hypokalemia may quickly follow as skeletal muscles take up potassium.
•To minimize insomnia, give last dose a few hours before bedtime.
•**WARNING** To treat cardiac arrest, at least twice the peripheral I.V. dose of epinephrine may be given by endotracheal instillation. Two dilutions are needed for this regimen; use great caution to avoid making medica-tion errors.

PATIENT TEACHING
•Warn patient not to exceed recommended dosage or to shorten interval because of the risk of adverse reactions and tolerance.
•Advise patient to notify prescriber if symp-toms don't improve or if they improve but then worsen.
•Instruct patient to take the day's last dose a few hours before bedtime to avoid in-somnia.
•Caution patient not to use inhalation solution that is pink or brown or that contains particles.
•Teach patient how to use oral inhaler or inhalation solution, as needed.
•If patient also uses an oral corticosteroid inhaler, instruct him to use epinephrine in-haler first, wait 5 minutes, and then use cor-ticosteroid inhaler to increase effectiveness.
•Teach patient and family how to adminis-ter epinephrine subcutaneously in an emer-gency. Tell them to inject drug into antero-lateral aspect of the thigh, through the clothing if necessary. Explain that solution is light sensitive and should be stored in the carrying case and at room temperature. Tell them not to refrigerate drug and to replace solution if it discolors.
•Caution patient to avoid accidental inject-ing drug into his fingers, hands, toes, or feet because epinephrine is a strong vasocon-strictor and could cause loss of blood flow to the area, resulting in gangrene. If acci-dental injection occurs in any of these areas,

instruct patient to go immediately to nearest emergency room.
•Advise patient to notify prescriber immedi-ately if he has blurred vision, chest pain, trouble breathing, a fast or irregular heart-beat, or increased sweating.
•Inform patient with diabetes that epineph-rine may cause hyperglycemia. Inform pa-tient with Parkinson's disease that symptoms my temporarily worsen but this should not deter use of drug.

eplerenone

Inspra

Class and Category
Chemical class: Methyl ester
Therapeutic class: Antihypertensive
Pregnancy category: B

Indications and Dosages
➤ *To improve survival of stable patients with left ventricular systolic dysfunction and congestive heart failure after an acute MI*
TABLETS
Adults. *Initial:* 25 mg daily, increased to 50 mg daily within 4 wk, if needed.
➤ *To treat hypertension alone or with other antihypertensive drugs*
TABLETS
Adults. *Initial:* 50 mg daily, increased to 50 mg b.i.d. after 4 wk, if needed.
DOSAGE ADJUSTMENT For patients taking weak CYP450 3A4 inhibitors, such as erythro-mycin, saquinavir, verapamil, and fluconazole, initial dosage reduced to 25 mg daily.

Mechanism of Action
Blocks the binding of aldosterone at its mineralocorticoid receptor sites located in the kidneys, heart, blood vessels, and brain. This action decreases blood pres-sure by preventing aldosterone from in-ducing sodium reabsorption and possibly other mechanisms that contribute to rais-ing blood pressure.

Contraindications
Hyperkalemia (serum potassium level greater than 5.5. mEq/L); hypersensitivity to eplere-

none or its components; renal insufficiency (serum creatinine level greater than 2.0 mg/dl in men or 1.8 mg/dl in women or creatinine clearance less than 50 ml/min/1.73 m^2); type 2 diabetes mellitus complicated by microalbuminuria; use of potassium supplements, potassium-sparing diuretics, or strong CYP3A4 inhibitors, such as ketoconazole or itraconazole

Interactions
DRUGS
ACE inhibitors, angiotensin II receptor antagonists: Increased risk of hyperkalemia
CYP450 3A4 inhibitors: Increased blood level and effect of eplerenone
lithium: Possibly lithium toxicity
NSAIDs: Possibly reduced antihypertensive effect of eplerenone
FOODS
grapefruit: Possibly increased blood level and effect of eplerenone

Adverse Reactions
CNS: Dizziness, fatigue, headache
CV: Angina pectoris, hypercholesterolemia, hypertriglyceridemia, MI
ENDO: Gynecomastia, mastodynia
GI: Abdominal pain, diarrhea, increased liver enzyme levels
GU: Albuminuria, elevated BUN and serum creatinine levels, vaginal bleeding
RESP: Cough
Other: Flulike symptoms, hyperkalemia, hyponatremia, increased uric acid level

Nursing Considerations
• Monitor patient's blood pressure regularly to evaluate the effectiveness of eplerenone therapy.
• Monitor patient's serum potassium level every 2 weeks for the first month or two of therapy and then monthly thereafter, as ordered.
• Be aware that patients who take an ACE inhibitor or an angiotensin II receptor antagonist during eplerenone therapy have an increased risk of hyperkalemia.
PATIENT TEACHING
• Caution patient not to use potassium-containing supplements or salt substitutes because increased potassium levels can lead to serious adverse reactions to eplerenone.
• Urge patient to tell all prescribers about eplerenone because of possible interactions.

epoetin alfa
(EPO, erythropoietin alfa, recombinant erythropoietin, r-HuEPO)
Epogen, Eprex (CAN), Procrit

Class and Category
Chemical class: 165–amino acid glycoprotein identical to human erythropoietin
Therapeutic class: Antianemic
Pregnancy category: C

Indications and Dosages
➤ *To treat anemia from renal failure*
I.V. OR SUBCUTANEOUS INJECTION
Adults and adolescents. *Initial:* 50 to 100 units/kg 3 times/wk, increased by 25 units/kg after 8 wk if hematocrit hasn't risen by 5 or 6 points or is below desired range (30% to 36%). *Maintenance:* Dosage gradually decreased by 25 units/kg at 4-wk intervals or longer to lowest dose that keeps hematocrit at 30% to 36%. *Maximum:* 300 units/kg 3 times/wk.
Children on dialysis. 50 units/kg 3 times/wk; increased after 8 wk if hematocrit hasn't risen by 5 or 6 points and is still below desired range of 30% to 36%. *Maintenance:* Dosage gradually decreased to lowest dose that keeps hematocrit at 30% to 36%.

➤ *To treat anemia in HIV-infected patients who take zidovudine*
I.V. OR SUBCUTANEOUS INJECTION
Adults with serum erythropoietin level of 500 mU/ml or less who receive 4,200 mg or less of zidovudine/wk. *Initial:* 100 units/kg 3 times/wk, increased by 50 to 100 units/kg every 4 to 8 wk after 8 wk of therapy. *Maintenance:* Dosage gradually titrated to maintain desired response, based on such factors as variations in zidovudine dosage and occurrence of infection or inflammation. *Maximum:* 300 units/kg 3 times/wk.

➤ *To treat anemia from chemotherapy*
SUBCUTANEOUS INJECTION
Adults. *Initial:* 150 units/kg 3 times/wk. Dosage decreased by 25% if hemoglobin level approaches 12 g/dl or increases more than 1 g/dl in any 2-wk period. Dose withheld if hemoglobin exceeds 13 g/dl and resumed at 25% less than previous dose after hemoglobin has fallen to 12 g/dl. Dosage increased to 300 units/kg 3 times/wk after 8 wk if re-

sponse is inadequate. *Maximum:* 300 units/ kg 3 times/wk. Alternatively, 40,000 units weekly. Dosage decreased by 25% if hemoglobin level approaches 12 g/dl or increases more than 1 g/dl in any 2-wk period. Dose withheld if hemoglobin level exceeds 13 g/dl and resumed at 25% less than previous dose after hemoglobin has fallen to 12 g/dl. Dosage increased to 60,000 units weekly after 8 wk if hemoglobin level has not increased at least 1 g/dl without RBC transfusion.

➤ *To reduce the need for blood transfusion in anemic patients having surgery*
SUBCUTANEOUS INJECTION
Adults. 300 units/kg daily for 10 days before surgery, on day of surgery, and 4 days after surgery; or 600 units/kg/wk starting 3 wk before surgery for a total of 3 doses. Dose of 300 units/kg repeated on day of surgery.
DOSAGE ADJUSTMENT For patients with anemia from renal failure, dosage temporarily reduced or drug discontinued if hematocrit reaches or exceeds 36%; drug is resumed at a lower dose when hematocrit returns to desired range. For patients with anemia from zidovudine use, therapy temporarily discontinued if hematocrit reaches or exceeds 40% and is resumed at a 25% lower dose when hematocrit returns to desired range.

Route	Onset	Peak	Duration
I.V., SubQ	In 2 to 6 wk	In 2 mo	About 2 wk

Mechanism of Action
Stimulates the release of reticulocytes from the bone marrow into the bloodstream, where they develop into mature RBCs.

Incompatibilities
Don't mix epoetin alfa with any other drug.

Contraindications
Hypersensitivity to human albumin or products made from mammal cells, uncontrolled hypertension

Interactions
DRUGS
antihypertensives: Increased blood pressure (to hypertensive level), especially when hematocrit rises rapidly
heparin: Increased heparin requirement in hemodialysis patients

iron supplements: Increased iron requirement and need for increased dose

Adverse Reactions
CNS: Anxiety, asthenia, dizziness, fatigue, fever, headache, insomnia, paresthesia, seizures, stroke
CV: Chest pain, deep vein thrombosis, edema, hypertension, MI, tachycardia
GI: Constipation, diarrhea, indigestion, nausea, vomiting
GU: UTI
HEME: Polycythemia
MS: Arthralgia, bone pain, muscle weakness
RESP: Cough, dyspnea, pulmonary congestion, upper respiratory tract infection
SKIN: Rash, pruritus, urticaria
Other: Flulike symptoms, hyperkalemia, injection site reaction, trunk pain

Nursing Considerations
• Use epoetin alfa cautiously in patients who have conditions that could decrease or delay response to drug, such as aluminum intoxication, folic acid deficiency, hemolysis, infection, inflammation, iron deficiency, malignant neoplasm, osteitis (fibrosa cystica), or vitamin B_{12} deficiency.
• Also use drug cautiously in patients with cardiovascular disorders caused by hypertension, a history of porphyria or seizures, vascular disease, or a hematologic disorder, such as hypercoagulation, myelodysplastic syndrome, or sickle cell disease.
• **WARNING** Be aware that the multidose vial of epoetin contains benzyl alcohol, which can cause a fatal toxic syndrome in neonates and immature infants characterized by CNS, respiratory, circulatory, and renal impairment and metabolic acidosis.
• Use lowest possible dose in cancer patients because drug has shortened survival rate and increased tumor progression in patients with certain types of cancers, such as breast, non-small cell lung, head and neck, and lymphoid cancers. Drug should only be used to treat anemia caused by myelosuppressive chemotherapy in cancer patients.
• Don't shake vial during preparation to avoid denaturing glycoprotein, inactivating drug.
• Discard unused portion of single-dose vial because it contains no preservatives. Discard unused portion of multidose vial after 21 days.
• Baseline hemoglobin level should be above 10 but below 13 g/dl if drug is given to pa-

tient scheduled for surgery. Watch closely throughout surgical period for deep vein thrombosis, especially in patients not receiving prophylactic anticoagulation, because risk of deep venous thromboses increases.

•**WARNING** Be aware that target hemoglobin shouldn't exceed 12 g/dl when treating anemia in patients with chronic renal failure. Exceeding 12 g/dl increases the risk of life-threatening adverse cardiovascular effects.

•Expect to increase heparin dose if patient receives hemodialysis because epoetin alfa can increase the RBC volume, which could cause clots to form in the dialyzer, hemodialysis vascular access, or both.

•Expect to give an iron supplement (I.V. iron dextran, if needed) because iron requirements rise when erythropoiesis consumes existing iron stores.

•Monitor drug effectiveness by checking hematocrit, typically twice weekly until it stabilizes at 30% to 36%. After that, monitoring can be less frequent.

•Take seizure precautions.

•Check hemoglobin and hematocrit levels, as ordered, with twice-weekly measurements recommended for chronic renal failure patients and weekly measurements recommended for zidovudine-treated HIV-infected and cancer patients.

•Be aware that the risk of hypertensive or thrombotic complications increases if the hematocrit rises more than 4 points in 2 weeks.

PATIENT TEACHING

•Before epoetin alfa therapy starts, explain its serious adverse effects.

•Teach patient how to administer drug and how to dispose of needles properly. Caution him against reusing needles.

•Advise patient that the risk of seizures is highest during the first 90 days of epoetin alfa therapy. Urge him not to engage in hazardous activities during this time.

•Stress the importance of complying with the dosage regimen and keeping follow-up medical appointments and appointments for laboratory tests.

•Encourage patient to eat iron-rich foods.

•Review possible adverse reactions, and urge patient to notify prescriber if he experiences chest pain, headache, hives, rapid heartbeat, rash, seizures, shortness of breath, or swelling.

•Advise women of childbearing age to use effective contraception throughout therapy if pregnancy isn't desired because menses may resume after epoetin alfa therapy.

epoprostenol sodium
(PGI$_2$, PGX, prostacyclin)
Flolan

Class and Category
Chemical class: Natural prostaglandin
Therapeutic class: Antihypertensive, vasodilator
Pregnancy category: B

Indications and Dosages
➤ *To provide long-term treatment of primary pulmonary hypertension*

I.V. INFUSION

Adults. *Initial:* 2 nanograms/kg/min, increased by 2 nanograms/kg/min every 15 min or longer until dose-limiting effects occur (abdominal, chest, or musculoskeletal pain; anxiety; bradycardia; dizziness; dyspnea; flushing; headache; hypotension; nausea; tachycardia; vomiting; or other adverse reactions). *Maintenance:* Dosage reduced by at least 4 nanograms/kg/min by continuous infusion.

DOSAGE ADJUSTMENT Infusion rate adjusted based on persistence, recurrence, or worsening of primary pulmonary hypertension and dose-related adverse reactions.

Mechanism of Action
Directly relaxes vascular smooth muscles through its action as a natural prostaglandin. This results in arterial dilation and inhibition of platelet aggregation. These actions decrease pulmonary vascular resistance, increase cardiac index and oxygen delivery, and limit thrombus formation.

Incompatibilities
Don't mix epoprostenol with other parenteral solutions or drugs.

Contraindications
Hypersensitivity to epoprostenol or its components; long-term use in patients with heart failure caused by severe left ventricular systolic dysfunction; pulmonary edema that developed while establishing epoprostenol dosage

Interactions

DRUGS

anticoagulants, antiplatelet drugs, NSAIDs: Increased risk of bleeding

antihypertensives, diuretics, vasodilators: Decreased blood pressure

Adverse Reactions

CNS: Anxiety, chills, confusion, dizziness, fever, headache, nervousness, paresthesia, syncope, weakness

CV: Bradycardia, chest pain, hypotension, tachycardia

GI: Abdominal pain, diarrhea, nausea, vomiting

HEME: Bleeding events, thrombocytopenia

MS: Arthralgia, jaw pain, myalgia

RESP: Dyspnea, hypoxia

SKIN: Flushing

Other: Flulike symptoms, injection site infection and pain, sepsis, weight loss or gain

Nursing Considerations

•Use epoprostenol cautiously in elderly patients because they may have decreased hepatic, renal, or cardiac function, or other diseases or may receive other drugs that can interact with epoprostenol.

•Reconstitute drug only with sterile diluent that comes with package. Don't dilute reconstituted epoprostenol.

•To make 100 ml of reconstituted solution at 3,000 nanograms/ml, dissolve contents of 0.5-mg vial with 5 ml of diluent; withdraw 3 ml and add diluent to make 100 ml. To make 100 ml of solution at 5,000 nanograms/ml, dissolve contents of 0.5-mg vial with 5 ml of diluent; withdraw contents and add diluent to make 100 ml. To make 100 ml of solution at 10,000 nanograms/ml, dissolve contents of two 0.5-mg vials each with 5 ml of diluent; withdraw contents and add diluent to make 100 ml. To make 100 ml of solution at 15,000 nanograms/ml, dissolve contents of 1.5-mg vial with 5 ml of diluent; withdraw contents and add diluent to make 100 ml.

•Give continuous infusion through a central venous catheter. Use peripheral I.V. infusion only until central access is established.

•Use a small, lightweight, ambulatory infusion pump able to deliver 2 nanograms/kg/min. It should have alarms for occlusion, end of infusion, and low battery. Use a polyvinyl chloride, polypropylene, or glass reservoir. Keep a backup pump and infusion set nearby to minimize disruptions in delivery.

•At room temperature, administer a single container of reconstituted solution over 8 hours. For extended use at temperatures above 77° F (25° C), use a cold pouch with frozen gel packs to keep drug at 36° to 46° F (2° to 8° C) for 12 hours.

•After a new infusion rate has been established, monitor patient closely for adverse reactions. Measure each blood pressure with patient standing and supine. Also, monitor heart rate for several hours after dosage adjustment.

•During prolonged infusion, monitor patient for dose-related adverse reactions. If they develop, expect to decrease infusion by 2 nanograms/kg/min every 15 minutes, as prescribed, until reactions resolve.

•Avoid abrupt withdrawal or a sudden large reduction in infusion rate, which could cause rebound pulmonary hypertension (asthenia, dizziness, and dyspnea) or death.

•Protect reconstituted drug from light, and refrigerate for no more than 48 hours. Discard solution that has been frozen or that has been refrigerated for more than 48 hours.

•Watch for evidence of bleeding, especially if patient has other risk factors for bleeding, because epoprostenol is a potent inhibitor of platelet aggregation.

PATIENT TEACHING

•Explain that epoprostenol is infused continuously through permanent indwelling central venous catheter by small infusion pump.

•Stress that patient must commit to long-term therapy, possibly for years.

•Teach patient or caregiver how to reconstitute drug, administer it, and care for the permanent central venous catheter.

•Urge patient to maintain prescribed infusion rate and to consult prescriber before altering it.

•Caution patient that even brief interruptions in drug delivery may cause rapid worsening of symptoms.

•Instruct patient to notify prescriber if adverse reactions occur.

•Make sure patient or caregiver has ready access to emergency phone numbers.

eprosartan mesylate

Teveten

Class and Category

Chemical class: Monomethanesulfonate, non-

biphenyl nontetrazole angiotensin II receptor antagonist
Therapeutic class: Antihypertensive
Pregnancy category: Not rated

Indications and Dosages

➤ *To control blood pressure in patients with essential hypertension*

TABLETS

Adults. *Initial:* 600 mg daily. *Maximum:* 800 mg once daily or in divided doses b.i.d.

Mechanism of Action

Blocks the effects of angiotensin II (a potent vasoconstrictor that's part of the renin-angiotensin-aldosterone system) by blocking its binding to angiotensin I receptors in vascular smooth muscles, adrenal glands, and other tissues. This action halts angiotensin II's negative feedback on renin secretion. Thus, circulating renin and angiotensin II levels rise and vascular resistance declines.

Contraindications

Hypersensitivity to eprosartan or components

Adverse Reactions

CNS: Depression, dizziness, drowsiness, fatigue
CV: Angina pectoris, atrial fibrillation, bradycardia, extrasystole, hypertriglyceridemia, hypotension, palpitations, tachycardia
EENT: Pharyngitis, rhinitis
GI: Abdominal pain
GU: Oliguria, UTI
MS: Myalgia, rhabdomyolysis
RESP: Cough, upper respiratory tract infection

Nursing Considerations

• Monitor for excessive hypotension if patient receives other cardiac drugs.
• Expect maximum blood pressure response after about 3 weeks.
• Be aware that, unlike ACE inhibitors, eprosartan doesn't affect bradykinin breakdown and cause the characteristic ACE cough.

PATIENT TEACHING

• Inform patient that maximum blood pressure response may not occur for 3 to 4 weeks.
• Explain that drug may cause dizziness, drowsiness, or very low blood pressure. Tell patient to rise slowly to upright positions.

eptifibatide

Integrilin

Class and Category

Chemical class: Cyclic heptapeptide
Therapeutic class: Platelet aggregation inhibitor
Pregnancy category: B

Indications and Dosages

➤ *To treat unstable angina and non–Q-wave MI*

I.V. INFUSION

Adults. *Initial:* 180 mcg/kg over 1 to 2 min as soon as possible after diagnosis. *Maintenance:* 2 mcg/kg/min by continuous infusion beginning immediately after initial dose and continuing until discharge or coronary artery bypass grafting, up to 72 hr.

DOSAGE ADJUSTMENT For patients with serum creatinine level of 2 to 4 mg/dl, initial dosage reduced to 135 mcg/kg over 1 to 2 min and maintenance dosage to 0.5 mcg/kg/min by continuous infusion. Dosage discontinued before coronary artery bypass graft surgery or if platelet count is less than 100,000/mm^3.

➤ *To prevent thrombosis related to percutaneous transluminal coronary angioplasty (PTCA)*

I.V. INFUSION

Adults. *Initial:* 135 mcg/kg over 1 to 2 min immediately before procedure. *Maintenance:* 0.5 mcg/kg/min by continuous infusion beginning just after initial dose and continuing for 20 to 24 hr. *Maximum:* 96 hr of therapy.

Route	Onset	Peak	Duration
I.V.	Immediate	In 15 min	4 to 8 hr

Mechanism of Action

Reversibly inhibits platelet aggregation by preventing fibrinogen, von Willebrand factor, and other adhesive ligands from binding to glycoprotein IIb/IIIa receptors on activated platelets. As a result, eptifibatide disrupts final cross-linking stage of platelet aggregation—and thrombus formation.

Incompatibilities

Don't administer eptifibatide through the same I.V. line as furosemide.

Contraindications

Active bleeding or stroke during prior 30 days, bleeding diathesis, dependency on dialysis, history of hemorrhagic stroke, hypersensitivity to eptifibatide, major surgery during previous 4 weeks, serum creatinine level of 2 mg/dl or higher for 180-mcg/kg dose or 2-mcg/kg/min infusion, serum creatinine level of 4 mg/dl or higher for 135-mcg/kg dose or 0.5-mcg/kg/min infusion, severe uncontrolled hypertension (systolic pressure above 200 mm Hg, diastolic pressure above 110 mm Hg), thrombocytopenia (platelet count below 100,000/mm³)

Interactions
DRUGS

anticoagulants, clopidogrel, dipyridamole, NSAIDs, thrombolytics, ticlopidine: Additive pharmacologic effects, increased risk of bleeding
other platelet aggregation inhibitors (especially inhibitors of platelet receptor glycoprotein IIb/IIIa, such as abciximab): Increased risk of additive pharmacologic effects

Adverse Reactions

CNS: Intracranial hemorrhage
CV: Hypotension
GI: Hematemesis
GU: Hematuria
HEME: Bleeding, decreased hemoglobin level, thrombocytopenia
Other: Anaphylaxis

Nursing Considerations

• Expect to obtain APTT and PT as a baseline and hematocrit, platelet count, and hemoglobin and serum creatinine levels before therapy.
• Withdraw bolus dose of eptifibatide from a 10-ml (2 mg/ml) vial into a syringe.
• Using a vented I.V. infusion set, administer a continuous infusion directly from the 100-ml (0.75 mg/ml) vial. Be sure to center the spike in the circle on top of vial stopper.
• Expect to keep APTT between 50 and 70 seconds or according to facility protocol during therapy unless patient undergoes PTCA.
• If patient undergoes PTCA, expect to maintain activated clotting time between 200 and 250 seconds during the procedure.
• During therapy, avoid arterial and venous punctures, I.M. injections, urinary catheter use, nasotracheal or nasogastric intubation, and use of noncompressible I.V. sites, such as subclavian and jugular veins.
• Expect to discontinue eptifibatide and heparin and monitor patient closely if platelet count falls below 100,000/mm³.
• Plan to discontinue drug, as prescribed, if patient undergoes coronary artery bypass surgery.

PATIENT TEACHING
• Instruct patient to immediately report bleeding during eptifibatide therapy.
• Reassure patient that he'll be monitored closely throughout therapy.
• Advise patient to avoid activities that may lead to bruising and bleeding.

ergoloid mesylates
(dihydrogenated ergot alkaloids)
Gerimal, Hydergine, Hydergine LC

Class and Category
Chemical class: Dihydrogenated ergot alkaloid derivative
Therapeutic class: Antidementia adjunct, cerebral metabolic enhancer
Pregnancy category: Not rated

Indications and Dosages

➤ *To treat age-related decline in mental capacity*

CAPSULES, ORAL SOLUTION, S.L. TABLETS, TABLETS
Adults. 1 to 2 mg t.i.d.

Route	Onset	Peak	Duration
P.O.	3 wk or more	Unknown	Unknown

Mechanism of Action
May increase cerebral metabolism, blood flow, and oxygen uptake. These actions may increase neurotransmitter levels.

Contraindications
Acute or chronic psychosis, hypersensitivity to ergoloid mesylates or their components

Interactions
DRUGS
delavirdine, efavirenz, indinavir, nelfinavir, saquinavir: Increased risk of ergotism

E
F

(blurred vision, dizziness, and headache)
dopamine: Increased risk of gangrene

Adverse Reactions

CNS: Dizziness, headache, light-headedness, syncope
CV: Bradycardia, orthostatic hypotension
EENT: Blurred vision, nasal congestion, tongue soreness (with S.L. tablets)
GI: Abdominal cramps, anorexia, nausea, vomiting
SKIN: Flushing, rash

Nursing Considerations

•Expect ergoloid mesylates to be prescribed only after a pathophysiologic cause for mental decline has been ruled out.
•Measure blood pressure and pulse rate and rhythm before therapy begins and monitor them frequently during therapy.
•If bradycardia or hypotension develops, expect to discontinue drug permanently.

PATIENT TEACHING
•Stress the importance of adhering to prescribed dosage and schedule.
•Teach caregiver to place S.L. tablet under patient's tongue and withhold food, fluids, and cigarettes until tablet dissolves.
•Instruct patient not to swallow S.L. tablets.
•Advise caregiver to skip a missed dose and resume the regular dosing schedule. Warn against doubling the dose, and urge caregiver to notify prescriber if patient misses two or more doses in a row.
•Instruct caregiver to store drug in a tightly closed, light-resistant container.
•Inform caregiver and family that drug may take 3 to 4 weeks to produce its effects.
•Stress the importance of follow-up care.

ergotamine tartrate

Ergomar (CAN), Ergostat, Gynergen (CAN), Medihaler Ergotamine (CAN)

Class and Category

Chemical class: Ergot alkaloid
Therapeutic class: Vascular headache suppressant
Pregnancy category: X

Indications and Dosages

➤ *To relieve vascular headaches, such as migraine, migraine variants, and cluster headaches*

S.L. TABLETS
Adults. *Initial:* 2 mg at first sign of attack and repeated every 30 min, p.r.n. *Maximum:* 6 mg/day and no more than twice/wk at least 5 days apart.

TABLETS
Adults. *Initial:* 1 to 2 mg at first sign of attack, repeated every 30 min, p.r.n. Increased to 3 mg for subsequent attacks if needed and if lower dose was well tolerated. *Maximum:* 6 mg daily.

ORAL INHALATION AEROSOL
Adults: 1 (360-mcg) inhalation at first sign of attack and repeated every 5 min, p.r.n. *Maximum:* 2.16 mg daily and no more than twice/wk at least 5 days apart.

Route	Onset	Peak	Duration
P.O., S.L.	Unknown	1 to 5 hr	Unknown

Mechanism of Action

Directly stimulates vascular smooth muscles, constricting arteries and veins and depressing vasomotor centers in the brain.

Contraindications

Coronary artery disease, hypersensitivity to ergot alkaloids, hypertension, impaired hepatic or renal function, malnutrition, peripheral vascular disease (Raynaud's disease, severe arteriosclerosis, syphilitic arteritis, thromboangiitis obliterans, thrombophlebitis), pregnancy or risk of pregnancy, sepsis, severe pruritus

Interactions

DRUGS
beta blockers: Increased risk of vasoconstriction and, possibly, peripheral gangrene
erythromycin, troleandomycin: Possibly increased risk of peripheral vasospasm and ischemia
nitrates: Increased ergotamine effects, decreased antianginal effects of nitrates, increased risk of hypertension
sumatriptan: Possibly additive vasoconstriction
vasoconstrictors: Increased risk of dangerous hypertension

ACTIVITIES
smoking: Possibly increased risk of peripheral vasoconstriction and ischemia

Adverse Reactions

CNS: Anxiety, confusion, dizziness, drowsiness, paresthesia, severe headache
CV: Chest pain, fast or slow heart rate, heart valve fibrosis, increased or decreased blood pressure, MI, weak pulse
EENT: Dry mouth, miosis, vision changes
GI: Nausea, vomiting
MS: Arm, back, or leg pain; muscle weakness in legs
SKIN: Cold, cyanotic, or pale feet or hands; pruritus
Other: Edema of face, feet, fingers, or lower legs; physical dependence

Nursing Considerations

• Use ergotamine cautiously in elderly patients.
• If patient receives long-term therapy, monitor pain control; he may need increasingly higher doses to obtain relief.
• Notify prescriber at the first sign of vasospasm and expect to discontinue drug.

PATIENT TEACHING

• Teach patient to take a tablet at the first sign of headache and to lie down in a quiet, dark room.
• Instruct patient not to swallow S.L. tablet but to let it dissolve under his tongue. Advise him not to drink, eat, or smoke until tablet has dissolved.
• Stress the importance of adhering to prescribed dosage and schedule because of drug's potential for dependence.
• Warn patient not to smoke while taking ergotamine (especially heavy smokers) because the combination of drug and nicotine, which also constricts vessels, may increase the risk of peripheral vascular ischemia.
• Advise patient to notify prescriber if usual doses fail to relieve headaches or if headache frequency or severity increases.
• Urge patient to avoid alcohol because it worsens headaches. Also suggest that patient avoid excessive cold, which may increase peripheral vasoconstriction.
• Instruct patient to notify prescriber if an infection develops because severe infection may increase sensitivity to drug.
• Advise patient to notify prescriber if he experiences chest pain; numbness, pain, or tingling in fingers or toes; pulse rate changes; swelling of face, feet, fingers, or lower legs; or vision changes.

ertapenem sodium

Invanz

Class and Category

Chemical class: Synthetic 1-β methyl-carbapenem
Therapeutic class: Antibiotic
Pregnancy category: B

Indications and Dosages

➤ *To treat moderate to severe infections, such as complicated intra-abdominal infections due to* Escherichia coli, Clostridium clostridioforme, Eubacterium lentum, Peptostreptococcus *species,* Bacteroides fragilis, B. distasonis, B. ovatus, B. thetaiotaomicron, *or* B. uniformis; *complicated skin and skin-structure infections due to* Staphylococcus aureus *(methicillin-susceptible strains only),* Streptococcus pyogenes, E. coli, *or* Peptostreptococcus *species; community-acquired pneumonia due to* Streptococcus pneumoniae *(penicillin-susceptible strains only, including cases with concurrent bacteremia),* Haemophilus influenzae *(beta-lactamase–negative strains only), or* Moraxella catarrhalis; *complicated UTI (including pyelo-nephritis) due to* E. coli *(including cases with concurrent bacteremia) or* Klebsiella pneumoniae; *and acute pelvic infections (including postpartum endo-myometritis, septic abortion, and post-surgical gynecologic infections) due to* Streptococcus agalactiae, E. coli, B. fragilis, Porphyromonas asaccharolytica, Peptostreptococcus *species, or* Prevotella bivia

I.V. INFUSION

Adults and adolescents. 1 g daily, infused over 30 min, for up to 14 days.
Children ages 3 months to 13 years. 15 mg/kg b.i.d., infused over 30 min, for up to 14 days. *Maximum:* 1 g daily.

I.M. INJECTION

Adults and adolescents. 1 g daily for up to 7 days.
Children ages 3 months to 13 years. 15 mg/kg b.i.d. for up to 7 days. *Maximum:* 1 g daily.
DOSAGE ADJUSTMENT Dosage decreased to 500 mg daily for patients with advanced

renal insufficiency (creatinine clearance less than or equal to 30 ml/min/1.73 m^2) or end-stage renal insufficiency (creatinine clearance less than or equal to 10 ml/min/1.73 m^2). For patients on hemodialysis who have received 500 mg of ertapenem within 6 hr of hemodialysis, supplemental dose of 150 mg given after hemodialysis.

Mechanism of Action
Inhibits bacterial cell wall synthesis by binding to specific penicillin-binding proteins inside the cell wall. Penicillin-binding proteins are responsible for various steps in bacterial cell wall synthesis. By binding to these proteins, ertapenem leads to bacterial cell wall lysis.

Incompatibilities
Don't mix ertapenem with other drugs. Don't dilute it with solutions containing dextrose.

Contraindications
Hypersensitivity to ertapenem, its components, or other drugs in the same class; hypersensitivity to local anesthetics (I.M. form only, because lidocaine hydrochloride 1% is used as a diluent); patients who have experienced anaphylactic reactions to beta-lactam drugs

Interactions
DRUGS
probenecid: Increased ertapenem half-life, increased and prolonged blood ertapenem level
valproic acid: Possibly decreased serum valproic acid level

Adverse Reactions
CNS: Agitation, anxiety, asthenia, confusion, disorientation, dizziness, fatigue, fever, hallucinations, headache, hypothermia, insomnia, mental changes, seizures, somnolence, stupor
CV: Chest pain, edema, hypertension, hypotension, tachycardia, thrombophlebitis
EENT: Nasopharyngitis, oral candidiasis, viral pharyngitis
ENDO: Hyperglycemia
GI: Abdominal pain, acid regurgitation, *Clostridium difficile* colitis, constipation, diarrhea, elevated liver function test results, indigestion, nausea, small-intestine obstruction, vomiting

GU: Dysuria, elevated serum creatinine level, proteinuria, RBCs and WBCs in urine, UTI, vaginitis
HEME: Anemia, decreased hematocrit, decreased WBC count, eosinophilia, increased WBC count, neutropenia, prolonged PT, thrombocytopenia, thrombocytosis
MS: Leg pain
RESP: Atelectasis, cough, crackles, dyspnea, pneumonia, respiratory distress, upper respiratory tract infection, wheezing
SKIN: Cellulitis, dermatitis, erythema, extravasation, pruritus, rash
Other: Anaphylaxis; death; hyperkalemia; hypokalemia; infusion site induration, pain, phlebitis, redness, swelling, or warmth

Nursing Considerations
• Obtain sputum, urine, or other specimens for culture and sensitivity testing, as ordered, before giving ertapenem. Expect to begin therapy before results are available.
• When preparing drug for I.V. use, reconstitute 1 g with 10 ml of sterile water for injection, 0.9% sodium chloride injection, or bacteriostatic water for injection. Don't use solutions that contain dextrose. Shake well to dissolve. Immediately transfer reconstituted drug to 50 ml normal saline solution. Use within 6 hours if stored at room temperature, 24 hours if refrigerated at 5° C (41° F). Don't freeze. Give I.V. infusion over 30 minutes.
• Inspect drug for particles and discoloration after reconstitution.
• For I.M. injection, reconstitute 1 g of drug with 3.2 ml of 1% lidocaine hydrochloride injection (*without* epinephrine). Shake thoroughly to form solution. Use within 1 hour after preparation. Withdraw contents of vial and inject deep into a large muscle mass such as the gluteal muscle.
• **WARNING** Don't give reconstituted I.M. solution by I.V. route because of risk of adverse reactions to the lidocaine hydrochloride injection used to reconstitute drug.
• Monitor patient closely for a life-threatening anaphylactic reaction. Patients with a history of hypersensitivity to penicillin, cephalosporins, other beta-lactams, or other allergens are at increased risk.
• **WARNING** If ertapenem triggers an anaphylactic reaction, stop drug, notify prescriber immediately, and provide appropriate therapy. Anaphylaxis requires immediate treatment with epinephrine as well as airway

management and administration of oxygen and I.V. corticosteroids, as needed.

•Be aware that patients with a history of seizures, other CNS disorders that predispose them to seizures (such as brain lesions), or compromised renal function may be at increased risk for seizures. Administer anticonvulsant, as ordered.

•Monitor patient for diarrhea during and for at least 2 months after drug therapy; diarrhea may signal pseudomembranous colitis caused by *Clostridium difficile*. If diarrhea occurs, notify prescriber and expect to withhold ertapenem and treat with fluids, electrolytes, protein, and an antibiotic effective against *C. difficile*.

•Be aware that because ertapenem is excreted in breast milk, its use by nursing mothers is carefully evaluated.

PATIENT TEACHING

•Instruct patient receiving ertapenem to immediately report signs of anaphylaxis, such as rash, itching, or shortness of breath; or signs of superinfection, such as severe diarrhea or white patches on tongue or in mouth.

•Urge patient to tell prescriber about diarrhea that's severe or lasts longer than 3 days. Remind patient that watery or bloody stools can occur 2 or more months after antibiotic therapy and can be serious, requiring prompt treatment.

erythromycin

(contains 250, 333, or 500 mg of base per delayed-release capsule, delayed-release tablet, or tablet)

Apo-Erythro (CAN), E-Mycin, Erybid (CAN), ERYC, Ery-Tab, Ilotycin, Novo-Rythro Encap (CAN), PCE

erythromycin estolate

(contains 250 mg of base per capsule or tablet, or 125 or 250 mg of base per 5 ml of oral suspension)

Ilosone, Novo-Rythro (CAN)

erythromycin ethylsuccinate

(contains 1 g of base per 1.6 g of oral suspension or tablet)

Apo-Erythro-ES (CAN), E.E.S., EryPed, Erythro, Novo-Rythro (CAN)

erythromycin gluceptate

(contains 500 or 1,000 mg of base per vial)

Ilotycin

erythromycin lactobionate

(contains 500 or 1,000 mg of base per vial)

Erythrocin

erythromycin stearate

(contains 125 or 250 mg of base per 5 ml of oral suspension, or 250 or 500 mg of base per tablet)

Apo-Erythro-S (CAN), Erythrocin, Erythrocot, My-E, Novo-Rythro (CAN), Wintrocin

Class and Category

Chemical class: Macrolide
Therapeutic class: Antiacne agent, antibiotic
Pregnancy category: B

Indications and Dosages

➤ *To treat mild to moderate upper respiratory tract infections caused by* Haemophilus influenzae, Streptococcus pneumoniae, *or* Streptococcus pyogenes *(group A beta-hemolytic streptococcus)*

CAPSULES, CHEWABLE TABLETS, DELAYED-RELEASE CAPSULES, DELAYED-RELEASE TABLETS, ORAL SUSPENSION, TABLETS, I.V. INFUSION

Adults. 250 to 500 mg (base) every 6 hr for 10 days.

Children. 250 to 500 mg (base) q.i.d. or 20 to 50 mg (base)/kg daily in divided doses for 10 days. For *H. influenzae* infections, erythromycin ethylsuccinate is administered with 150 mg/kg daily of sulfisoxazole. *Maximum:* Adult dosage, or 6 g daily for erythromycin ethylsuccinate.

➤ *To treat lower respiratory tract infections caused by* S. pneumoniae *or* S. pyogenes *(group A beta-hemolytic streptococcus)*

CAPSULES, CHEWABLE TABLETS, DELAYED-RELEASE CAPSULES, DELAYED-RELEASE TABLETS, ORAL SUSPENSION, TABLETS, I.V. INFUSION

Adults. 250 to 500 mg (base) every 6 hr for 10 days.

Children. 250 to 500 mg (base) q.i.d. or 20 to 50 mg (base)/kg daily in divided doses for 10 days. *Maximum:* Adult dosage.

➤ *To treat respiratory tract infections caused by* Mycoplasma pneumoniae

CAPSULES, CHEWABLE TABLETS, DELAYED-RELEASE CAPSULES, DELAYED-RELEASE TABLETS, ORAL SUSPENSION, TABLETS, I.V. INFUSION

Adults. 500 mg (base) every 6 hr for 5 to 10 days or up to 3 wk for severe infections.

➤ *To treat mild to moderate skin and soft-tissue infections caused by* S. pyogenes *or* Staphylococcus aureus

CAPSULES, CHEWABLE TABLETS, DELAYED-RELEASE CAPSULES, DELAYED-RELEASE TABLETS, ORAL SUSPENSION, TABLETS, I.V. INFUSION

Adults. 250 mg (base) every 6 hr or 500 mg (base) every 12 hr for 10 days. *Maximum:* 4 g (base) daily.

Children. 250 to 500 mg (base) q.i.d. or 20 to 50 mg (base)/kg daily in divided doses for 10 days. *Maximum:* Adult dosage.

➤ *To treat acne vulgaris*

DELAYED-RELEASE CAPSULES, DELAYED-RELEASE TABLETS, TABLETS

Adults and adolescents. *Initial:* 250 mg (base) every 6 hr, 333 mg (base) every 8 hr, or 500 mg (base) every 12 hr for 4 wk. *Maintenance:* 333 to 500 mg (base) daily.

➤ *To treat pertussis (whooping cough) caused by* Bordetella pertussis

CAPSULES, CHEWABLE TABLETS, DELAYED-RELEASE CAPSULES, DELAYED-RELEASE TABLETS, ORAL SUSPENSION, TABLETS, I.V. INFUSION

Children. 500 mg (base) q.i.d. or 40 to 50 mg (base)/kg daily in divided doses for 5 to 14 days.

➤ *To treat diphtheria*

CAPSULES, CHEWABLE TABLETS, DELAYED-RELEASE CAPSULES, DELAYED-RELEASE TABLETS, ORAL SUSPENSION, TABLETS, I.V. INFUSION

Adults and children. 500 mg (base) every 6 hr for 10 days.

➤ *To treat erythrasma*

CAPSULES, CHEWABLE TABLETS, DELAYED-RELEASE CAPSULES, DELAYED-RELEASE TABLETS, ORAL SUSPENSION, TABLETS, I.V. INFUSION

Adults and children. 250 mg (base) t.i.d. for 21 days.

➤ *To treat intestinal amebiasis*

CAPSULES, CHEWABLE TABLETS, DELAYED-RELEASE CAPSULES, DELAYED-RELEASE TABLETS, ORAL SUSPENSION, TABLETS, I.V. INFUSION

Adults. 250 mg (base) every 6 hr for 10 to 14 days.

Children. 30 to 50 mg (base)/kg daily in divided doses for 10 to 14 days

➤ *To treat pelvic inflammatory disease caused by* Neisseria gonorrhoeae

CAPSULES, CHEWABLE TABLETS, DELAYED-RELEASE CAPSULES, DELAYED-RELEASE TABLETS, ORAL SUSPENSION, TABLETS, I.V. INFUSION

Adults. 500 mg (base) I.V. every 6 hr for 3 days and then 250 mg (base) P.O. or I.V. every 6 hr for 7 days.

➤ *To treat conjunctivitis in newborns*

I.V. INFUSION

Neonates. 50 mg (base)/kg daily in 4 divided doses for 14 days.

➤ *To treat pneumonia in neonates*

I.V. INFUSION

Neonates. 50 mg (base)/kg daily in divided doses for 21 days.

➤ *To treat urogenital infections caused by* Chlamydia trachomatis *during pregnancy*

CAPSULES, CHEWABLE TABLETS, DELAYED-RELEASE CAPSULES, DELAYED-RELEASE TABLETS, ORAL SUSPENSION, TABLETS

Adults. 500 mg (base) on an empty stomach every 6 hr for 7 days; or 250 mg (base) on an empty stomach every 6 hr for at least 14 days.

➤ *To treat nongonococcal urethritis or uncomplicated urethral, endocervical, or rectal infections caused by* C. trachomatis

CAPSULES, CHEWABLE TABLETS, DELAYED-RELEASE CAPSULES, DELAYED-RELEASE TABLETS, ORAL SUSPENSION, TABLETS

Adults. 500 mg (base) every 6 hr for 7 days. If patient can't tolerate high doses, 250 mg (base) every 6 hr for 14 days.

➤ *To treat primary syphilis*

CAPSULES, CHEWABLE TABLETS, DELAYED-RELEASE CAPSULES, DELAYED-RELEASE TABLETS, ORAL SUSPENSION, TABLETS

Adults. 20 to 40 g (base) in divided doses over 10 to 15 days.

➤ *To treat Legionnaire's disease*

CAPSULES, CHEWABLE TABLETS, DELAYED-RELEASE CAPSULES, DELAYED-RELEASE TABLETS, ORAL SUSPENSION, TABLETS, I.V. INFUSION

Adults. 1 to 4 g (base) daily in divided doses for 10 to 14 days.

➤ *To treat rheumatic fever*

CAPSULES, CHEWABLE TABLETS, DELAYED-RELEASE CAPSULES, DELAYED-RELEASE TABLETS, ORAL SUSPENSION, TABLETS, I.V. INFUSION

Adults. 250 mg (base) every 12 hr.

➤ *To prevent bacterial endocarditis in patients with penicillin allergy who plan dental or upper respiratory tract surgery*
CAPSULES, CHEWABLE TABLETS, DELAYED-RELEASE CAPSULES, DELAYED-RELEASE TABLETS, ORAL SUSPENSION, TABLETS, I.V. INFUSION
Adults. 1 g (base) given 1 to 2 hr before procedure and then 500 mg (base) 6 hr after initial dose.
Children. 20 mg (base)/kg given 2 hr before procedure and then 10 mg (base)/kg 6 hr after initial dose.

➤ *To treat listeriosis*
CAPSULES, CHEWABLE TABLETS, DELAYED-RELEASE CAPSULES, DELAYED-RELEASE TABLETS, ORAL SUSPENSION, TABLETS, I.V. INFUSION
Adults. 250 mg (base) every 6 hr or 500 mg (base) every 12 hr. *Maximum:* 4 g (base) daily.

Mechanism of Action
Binds with the 50S ribosomal subunit of the 70S ribosome in many types of aerobic, anaerobic, gram-positive, and gram-negative bacteria. This action inhibits RNA-dependent protein synthesis in bacterial cells, causing them to die.

Contraindications
Astemizole, cisapride, pimozide, or terfenadine therapy; hypersensitivity to erythromycin, macrolide antibiotics, or their components; hepatic disease (erythromycin estolate)

Interactions
DRUGS
alfentanil: Decreased alfentanil clearance, prolonged alfentanil action
astemizole, cisapride, terfenadine: Increased risk of cardiotoxicity, torsades de pointes, ventricular tachycardia, and death
atorvastatin, lovastatin, pravastatin, simvastatin: Increased risk of rhabdomyolysis
carbamazepine, valproic acid: Possibly inhibited metabolism of these drugs, increasing their blood levels and risk of toxicity
chloramphenicol, lincomycins: Antagonized effects of these drugs
cyclosporine: Increased risk of nephrotoxicity
digoxin: Increased serum digoxin level and risk of digitalis toxicity
diltiazem, verapamil: Increased risk of life-threatening cardiac events

ergotamine: Decreased ergotamine metabolism, increased risk of vasospasm from ergotamine use
hepatotoxic drugs: Increased risk of hepatotoxicity
midazolam, triazolam: Increased pharmacologic effects of these drugs
oral contraceptives: Failed contraception, hepatotoxicity
ototoxic drugs: Increased risk of ototoxicity if patient with impaired renal function receives high doses of erythromycin
penicillins: Interference with bactericidal effects of penicillins
sildenafil: Increased effects of sildenafil
warfarin: Prolonged PT and risk of hemorrhage, especially in elderly patients
xanthines (except dyphylline): Increased serum theophylline level and risk of theophylline toxicity
ACTIVITIES
alcohol use: Increased alcohol level (by 40%) with I.V. erythromycin

Adverse Reactions
CNS: Fatigue, fever, malaise, weakness
CV: Prolonged QT interval, torsades de pointes, ventricular arrhythmias
EENT: Hearing loss, oral candidiasis
GI: Abdominal cramps and pain, diarrhea, hepatotoxicity, nausea, pseudomembranous colitis, vomiting
GU: Vaginal candidiasis
MS: New or aggravated myasthenia gravis syndrome
SKIN: Erythema, jaundice, pruritus, rash
Other: Fluid overload (from I.V. infusion), injection site inflammation and phlebitis

Nursing Considerations
•Use erythromycin cautiously in patients with impaired hepatic function because drug is metabolized by the liver.
•Use erythromycin cautiously elderly patients, especially those with renal or hepatic dysfunction, because they're at increased risk of hearing loss and torsades de pointes. They're also at increased risk of bleeding if taking an oral anticoagulant.
•Before administering the first erythromycin dose, expect to obtain body fluid or tissue sample for culture and sensitivity testing.
•Reconstitute parenteral form before administration. Add at least 10 ml of preservative-free sterile water for injection to each 500-mg vial

E
F

or at least 20 ml of diluent to each 1-g vial.
•For prolonged infusion, expect to infuse a buffered solution up to 24 hours after dilution.
•For intermittent infusion, dilute dose in 100 to 250 ml normal saline solution or D_5W if needed; give slowly over 20 to 60 minutes.
•When giving I.V. erythromycin gluceptate, dilute the solution if needed to 1 g/L in normal saline solution or D_5W injection for slow, continuous infusion. Diluted solution remains potent for 7 days if refrigerated.
•When giving I.V. erythromycin lactobionate, dilute the solution if needed to 1 to 5 mg/ml in normal saline solution, lactated Ringer's solution, or other electrolyte solution for slow, continuous infusion. Diluted solution remains potent for 14 days if refrigerated and for 24 hours at room temperature.
•Be aware that infusions prepared in piggyback infusion bottles stay potent for 30 days if frozen, 24 hours if refrigerated, or 8 hours at room temperature. Don't store infusions prepared in the ADD-vantage system.
•Don't use diluent with benzyl alcohol if parenteral erythromycin is for a neonate. It may cause a fatal toxic syndrome of CNS depression, hypotension, metabolic acidosis, renal failure, respiratory problems, and, possibly, seizures and intracranial hemorrhage.
•Periodically monitor liver function test results to detect hepatotoxicity, which is most common with erythromycin estolate. Signs typically appear within 2 weeks after continuous therapy starts and resolve when it stops.
•Assess hearing regularly, especially in elderly patients and those who receive 4 g or more daily or have hepatic or renal disease. Hearing impairment begins 36 hours to 8 days after treatment starts and usually begins to improve 1 to 14 days after it stops.
•During I.V. therapy, watch for signs of fluid overload, such as acute dyspnea and crackles.
•Monitor infants for vomiting or irritability with feeding because infantile hypertrophic pyloric stenosis has been reported.
•Assess myasthenia gravis patients for weakness because drug may aggravate it. Keep in mind that myasthenic syndrome may arise in patients previously undiagnosed with myasthenia gravis.
•Watch closely for signs and symptoms of superinfection. If they occur, notify prescriber and expect to stop drug and provide appropriate therapy.

•Monitor patient for diarrhea during and for at least 2 months after drug therapy; diarrhea may signal pseudomembranous colitis caused by *Clostridium difficile*. If diarrhea occurs, notify prescriber and expect to withhold drug and treat with fluids, electrolytes, protein, and an antibiotic effective against *C. difficile*.
•If patient receives an order for urine catecholamine analysis, notify prescriber; erythromycin interferes with fluorometric measurement of urine catecholamines.

PATIENT TEACHING
•Urge patient to complete prescribed therapy, even if he feels better before it's finished.
•Tell patient to notify prescriber if symptoms worsen or don't improve after a few days.
•Teach patient how to administer prescribed drug form. Instruct him to swallow capsules or tablets whole. For an oral suspension, teach him to use the measuring device provided to ensure accurate doses. Remind him to shake the suspension before measuring a dose.
•Advise patient to take oral form with a full glass of water on an empty stomach (except erythromycin ethylsuccinate, which is better absorbed with food).
•If GI distress occurs, instruct patient to take oral form with food.
•Instruct patient to promptly notify prescriber about allergic reactions, hearing changes, or signs of hepatic dysfunction.
•Urge patient to tell prescriber about diarrhea that's severe or lasts longer than 3 days. Remind patient that watery or bloody stools can occur 2 or more months after antibiotic therapy and can be serious, requiring prompt treatment.

escitalopram oxalate

Lexapro

Class and Category

Chemical class: Pure S+ enantiomer of racemic bicyclic phthalane derivative citalopram
Therapeutic class: Antidepressant
Pregnancy category: C

Indications and Dosages

➤ *To treat generalized anxiety disorder or major depression*
ORAL SOLUTION, TABLETS

Adults. *Initial:* 10 mg daily in morning or evening, increased to 20 mg daily after 1 or more wk, as needed.
DOSAGE ADJUSTMENT Dosage shouldn't exceed 10 mg daily for elderly patients and those with hepatic impairment.

Mechanism of Action

Inhibits reuptake of the neurotransmitter serotonin by CNS neurons, thereby increasing the amount of serotonin available in nerve synapses. An elevated serotonin level may result in elevated mood and reduced depression.

Contraindications

Hypersensitivity to escitalopram, citalopram or its components; use within 14 days of MAO inhibitor therapy

Interactions

DRUGS

aspirin, NSAIDs, warfarin: Possibly increased risk of bleeding
carbamazepine: Possibly increased clearance of escitalopram
cimetidine: Possibly increased plasma escitalopram level
CNS drugs: Additive CNS effects
lithium: Possible enhancement of the serotonergic effects of escitalopram
MAO inhibitors: Possibly hyperpyretic episodes, hypertensive crisis, serotonin syndrome, and severe seizures
metoprolol: Increased plasma metoprolol levels with decreased cardioselectivity of metoprolol
naratriptan, sumatriptan, zolmitriptan: Possibly weakness, hyperreflexia, and incoordination
St. John's wort: Increased risk of serotonin syndrome
sibutramine: Increased risk of serotonin syndrome

ACTIVITIES

alcohol use: Possibly increased cognitive and motor effects of alcohol

Adverse Reactions

CNS: Abnormal gait, acute psychosis, aggression, akathisia, delirium, dizziness, dyskinesia, dystonia, extrapyramidal effects, fatigue, headache, hypomania, insomnia, lethargy, mania, myoclonus, neuroleptic malignant syndrome, paresthesia, seizures, serotonin syndrome, somnolence, suicidal ideation
CV: Atrial fibrillation, cardiac failure, deep vein or phlebitis thrombosis, hypotension, MI, prolonged QT interval, thrombosis, torsades de pointes, ventricular arrhythmias
EENT: Diplopia, dry mouth, glaucoma, nystagmus, rhinitis, sinusitis, toothache, visual hallucinations
ENDO: Diabetes mellitus, hyperprolactinemia, syndrome of inappropriate ADH secretion
GI: Abdominal pain, constipation, decreased appetite, diarrhea, flatulence, GI bleeding or hemorrhage, hepatic necrosis, hepatitis, indigestion, nausea, pancreatitis, rectal hemorrhage, vomiting
GU: Acute renal failure, anorgasmia, decreased libido, ejaculation disorders, impotence, priapism
HEME: Bleeding, decreased prothrombin time, hemolytic anemia, leukopenia, thrombocytopenia
MS: Neck or shoulder pain, rhabdomyolysis
RESP: Pulmonary embolism
SKIN: Ecchymosis, erythema multiforme, increased sweating, photosensitivity, Stevens-Johnson syndrome, toxic epidermal necrolysis, urticaria
Other: Anaphylaxis, angioedema, flulike symptoms, hyponatremia

Nursing Considerations

•Use escitalopram cautiously in patients with history of mania or seizures, patients with severe renal impairment, and those with diseases or conditions that produce altered metabolism or hemodynamic responses.
•Monitor patient—especially elderly patient—for hypoosmolarity of serum and urine and for hyponatremia (headache, trouble contentrating, impaired memory, weakness, unsteadiness) because they may may indicate escitalopram-induced syndrome of inappropriate ADH secretion.
•Watch for signs of misuse or abuse, such as development of tolerance, increasing dosage without approval, and drug-seeking behavior; drug's potential for physical and psychological dependence is unknown.
•Monitor patient for bleeding, especially if patient is also taking aspirin, an NSAID, or

an anticoagulant. Bleeding can range from ecchymoses, hemtomas, epitaxis and petechiae to life-threatening hemorrhages.

•Expect prescriber to reassess patient periodically to determine the continued need for therapy and confirm the appropriate dosage.

•If patient (particularly a child or an adolescent) takes escitalopram for depression, watch closely for suicidal tendencies, especially when therapy starts or dosage changes, because depression may worsen temporarily.

•If drug will be stopped, expect to taper dosage to avoid serious adverse reactions.

PATIENT TEACHING

•Inform patient that alcohol use isn't recommended during escitalopram therapy because it may decrease his ability to think clearly and perform motor skills.

•Advise patient to avoid hazardous activities until drug's CNS effects are known.

•Instruct patient that drug shouldn't be taken with citalopram hydrobromide because of potentially additive effects.

•Tell patient that improvement may not be noticed for 1 to 4 weeks after therapy begins. Emphasize the importance of continuing therapy as prescribed.

•If patient (particularly a child or an adolescent) takes drug for depression, urge caregivers to watch closely for suicidal tendencies, especially when therapy starts or dosage changes.

•Warn patient not to stop taking drug abruptly. Explain that gradual tapering helps to avoid withdrawal symptoms.

•Urge patient to inform prescriber of any OTC drugs he takes because of potential for interactions.

•Review signs and symptoms of hyponatremia, and instruct patient to report them to prescriber.

•Warn patient that escitalopram increases bleeding risk if taken with aspirin, an NSAID, or an anticoagulants and that bleeding events could range from mild to severe. Tell patient to seek emergency care for serious or prolonged bleeding.

esmolol hydrochloride

Brevibloc

Class and Category

Chemical class: Beta blocker

Therapeutic class: Antiarrhythmic, antihypertensive

Pregnancy category: C

Indications and Dosages

➤ *To treat supraventricular tachycardia*

I.V. INFUSION

Adults. *Loading:* 500 mcg/kg over 1 min. *Maintenance:* If response to loading dose is adequate after 5 min, 50 mcg/kg/min infused for 4 min. If response is inadequate after 5 min, another 500 mcg/kg may be given over 1 min followed by 100 mcg/kg/min for 4 min. Sequence repeated, as needed, until adequate response occurs, increasing maintenance dosage by 50 mcg/kg/min at each step. *Maximum:* 200 mcg/kg/min for 48 hr.

Children. 50 mcg/kg/min titrated every 10 min up to 300 mcg/kg/min.

➤ *To treat intraoperative and postoperative tachycardia and hypertension*

I.V. INFUSION

Adults. *Initial:* 250 to 500 mcg/kg over 1 min. *Maintenance:* 50 mcg/kg/min infused over 4 min. If response is inadequate after 5 min, another 250 to 500 mcg/kg may be given over 1 min followed by 100 mcg/kg/ min for 4 min. Sequence repeated, as needed, up to 4 times, increasing by 50 mcg/kg/min each time. *Maximum:* 200 mcg/kg/min for 48 hr.

DOSAGE ADJUSTMENT Loading doses omitted, increments decreased to 25 mcg/kg/min, and titration intervals increased to 10 min as heart rate approaches desired level or if blood pressure decreases too much.

Route	Onset	Peak	Duration
I.V.	Immediate	Unknown	10 to 20 min

Mechanism of Action

Inhibits stimulation of beta$_1$ receptors primarily in the heart, which decreases cardiac excitability, cardiac output, and myocardial oxygen demand. Esmolol also decreases renin release from the kidneys, which helps reduce blood pressure.

Incompatibilities

Don't mix esmolol with 5% sodium bicarbonate injection.

Contraindications

Cardiogenic shock, hypersensitivity to beta

blockers, overt heart failure, second- or third-degree heart block, sinus bradycardia

Interactions

DRUGS

antihypertensives: Possibly hypotension
insulin, oral antidiabetic drugs: Possibly masking of signs and symptoms of hypoglycemia caused by these drugs
MAO inhibitors: Possibly severe hypertension if esmolol is administered within 14 days of discontinuing MAO inhibitor therapy
neuromuscular blockers: Possibly potentiated and prolonged action of these drugs
phenytoin: Possibly increased cardiac depression
reserpine: Possibly bradycardia and hypotension
sympathomimetics, xanthine derivatives: Possibly inhibited therapeutic effects of both drugs

Adverse Reactions

CNS: Anxiety, confusion, depression, dizziness, fatigue, fever, headache, syncope
CV: Bradycardia, chest pain, decreased peripheral circulation, heart block, hypotension
GI: Nausea, vomiting
RESP: Dyspnea, wheezing
SKIN: Diaphoresis, flushing, pallor
Other: Infusion site pain, redness, and swelling

Nursing Considerations

• Use esmolol cautiously if patient has supraventricular arrhythmias with decreased cardiac output, hypotension, or other hemodynamic compromise or is taking drugs that decrease peripheral resistance or myocardial filling, contractility, or impulse generation.
• Also use drug cautiously in patients with impaired renal function because drug is excreted by the kidneys. Patients with end-stage renal disease have an increased risk of adverse reactions.
• Avoid giving esmolol for intraoperative or postoperative hypertension caused by hypothermia-induced vasoconstriction.
• Expect to give lowest possible dose to patients with allergies, asthma, bronchitis, or emphysema. If patient develops bronchospasm, expect to discontinue infusion immediately and give a beta₂-stimulating drug, as ordered.
• Don't give 250 mg/ml (2,500 mg/10 ml) dosage strength by direct I.V. push. Dilute it to a 10-mg/ml infusion by first removing 20 ml from 500 ml of a compatible I.V. solution,

such as D_5W or dextrose 5% in normal saline solution, and then adding 5 g of esmolol to the solution.
• Use diluted solution within 24 hours if stored at room temperature.
• Use 100-mg vial (prediluted to 10 mg/ml) for loading dose. For 70-kg (154-lb) patient, loading dose for 500 mcg/kg/min is 3.5 ml.
• Monitor blood pressure and heart rate often during therapy. Hypotension can occur at any dose but usually is dose related. It typically reverses within 30 minutes after dose is decreased or infusion is stopped.
• Inspect site often for thrombophlebitis (pain, redness, swelling at site). Infusion of 20 mg/ml is more likely to cause serious vein irritation than 10 mg/ml. Extravasation of 20 mg/ml may cause a serious local reaction and skin necrosis. Don't give more than 10 mg/ml into a small vein or using a butterfly catheter.

PATIENT TEACHING

• Urge patient to report adverse reactions immediately.
• Reassure patient that his blood pressure, heart rate, and response to therapy will be monitored throughout esmolol therapy.

esomeprazole magnesium

Nexium, Nexium I.V.

Class and Category

Chemical class: Substituted benzimidazole
Therapeutic class: Antiulcerative
Pregnancy category: B

Indications and Dosages

➤ *To treat gastroesophageal reflux disease (GERD)*

DELAYED-RELEASE CAPSULES

Adults. 20 to 40 mg daily for 4 to 8 wk; may be repeated for another 4 to 8 wk if ulcer hasn't healed. *Maintenance:* 20 mg daily for up to 6 mo.
Adolescents ages 12 to 17. 20 or 40 mg once daily for up to 8 wk.
Children ages 1 to 11. 10 mg once daily for up to 8 wk.
DOSAGE ADJUSTMENT For children weighing 20 kg (44 lb) or more and being treated for healing of erosive esophagitis in GERD, dosage may be increased to 20 mg once daily for 8 wk, if needed.

➤ *To treat GERD in a patient with a history of erosive esophagitis who can't take the drug by mouth*

I.V. INFUSION, I.V. INJECTION
Adults. 20 to 40 mg daily infused for no less than 3 min (I.V. injection) or 10 to 30 min (I.V. infusion).

➤ *As adjunct to treat duodenal or gastric ulcer associated with* Helicobacter pylori

DELAYED-RELEASE CAPSULES
Adults. 40 mg daily with amoxicillin 1,000 mg b.i.d. and clarithromycin 500 mg b.i.d. for 10 days.

➤ *To reduce the risk of gastric ulcer formation in patients who are receiving continuous NSAID therapy and who either are over age 60 or have a history of gastric ulcer*

DELAYED-RELEASE CAPSULES
Adults. 20 to 40 mg daily for up to 6 mo.

➤ *To treat pathological hypersecretory conditions, including Zollinger-Ellison syndrome*

DELAYED-RELEASE CAPSULES
Adults. 40 mg b.i.d.
DOSAGE ADJUSTMENT Maximum, 20 mg daily for patients with severe hepatic insufficiency.

Mechanism of Action

Interferes with gastric acid secretion by inhibiting the hydrogen-potassium-adenosine triphosphatase (H^+-K^+-ATPase) enzyme system, or proton pump, in gastric parietal cells. Normally, the proton pump uses energy from hydrolysis of ATPase to drive H^+ and chloride (Cl^-) out of parietal cells and into the stomach lumen in exchange for potassium (K^+), which leaves the stomach lumen and enters parietal cells. After this exchange, H^+ and Cl^- combine in the stomach to form hydrochloric acid (HCl). Esomeprazole irreversibly inhibits the final step in gastric acid production by blocking exchange of intracellular H^+ and extracellular K^+, thus preventing H^+ from entering the stomach and additional HCl from forming.

Incompatibilities
Don't give esomeprazole with any other drug through the same I.V. site or tubing.

Contraindications
Hypersensitivity to esomeprazole or its components

Interactions
DRUGS
antimicrobials: Increased blood esomeprazole levels
atazanavir: Decreased blood atazanavir level
diazepam: Possibly increased diazepam level
digoxin, iron salts, ketoconazole: Possibly decreased absorption of these drugs
voriconazole: Increased esomeprazole exposure and risk of adverse effects
warfarin: Possibly increased INR and PT, leading to abnormal bleeding

FOODS
all foods: Decreased bioavailability of esomeprazole

Adverse Reactions
CNS: Agitation, aggression, depression, dizziness, headache, hallucinations, hepatic encephalopathy
EENT: Blurred vision, dry mouth, mucosal discoloration, sinusitis, stomatitis, taste disturbance
ENDO: Gynecomastia
GI: Abdominal pain; Barrett's esophagus; benign polyps or nodules; candidiasis; constipation; diarrhea; duodenitis; dyspepsia; esophagitis; esophageal stricture, ulceration, or varices; flatulence; gastric ulcer; gastritis; hepatic failure; hepatitis; jaundice; nausea; pancreatitis
GU: Interstitial nephritis
HEME: Agranulocytosis, pancytopenia
MS: Muscle weakness, myalgia
RESP: Bronchospasm, respiratory tract infection
SKIN: Alopecia, diaphoresis, erythema multiforme, photosensitivity, pruritus, Stevens-Johnson syndrome, toxic epidermal necrolysis
Other: Anaphylaxis, infusion site redness or pruritus

Nursing Considerations
•Give oral esomeprazole at least 1 hour before meals because food decreases bioavailability.
•WARNING If patient takes drug with amoxicillin or clarithromycin for *H. pylori*–related ulcer, severe diarrhea may indicate pseudomembranous colitis. Obtain stool cultures, as ordered.

•Always flush I.V. line with normal saline solution injection, lactated Ringer's injection, or 5% dextrose injection before and after giving esomeprazole intravenously.

•For I.V. injection, reconstitute powder with 5 ml of normal saline solution injection and give as a bolus dose over 3 or more minutes. Once reconstituted, drug may be stored at room temperature for up to 12 hours.

•For I.V. infusion, reconstitute powder with 5 ml of normal saline solution injection, lactated Ringer's injection, or 5% dextrose injection. Further dilute reconstituted solution to make a final volume of 50 ml, and infuse over 10 to 30 minutes. Reconstituted drug may be stored at room temperature up to 6 hours if mixed with 5% dextrose injection or up to 12 hours if mixed with normal saline solution or lactated Ringer's injection.

•Be aware that patient receiving I.V. esomeprazole should be switched to oral form as soon as possible.

PATIENT TEACHING

•If patient has trouble swallowing esomeprazole capsules, tell him to open capsule and sprinkle pellets into a tablespoon of cool applesauce. Tell him not to chew pellets and to discard any unused pellets.

•Urge patient to tell prescriber if he takes antacids.

estazolam

Class, Category, and Schedule
Chemical class: Benzodiazepine
Therapeutic class: Sedative-hypnotic
Pregnancy category: X
Controlled substance schedule: IV

Indications and Dosages
➤ *To treat insomnia*
TABLETS
Adults. 1 to 2 mg at bedtime.
DOSAGE ADJUSTMENT Starting dose 0.5 mg for small or debilitated elderly patients.

Route	Onset	Peak	Duration
P.O.	Unknown	Unknown	6 to 8 hr

Contraindications
Acute angle-closure glaucoma; hypersensitivity to estazolam, other benzodiazepines, or their components; pregnancy; psychosis

Mechanism of Action
May potentiate the effects of gamma-aminobutyric acid (GABA) and other inhibitory neurotransmitters by binding to specific benzodiazepine receptors in the limbic and cortical areas of the CNS. By binding to these receptors, estazolam increases GABA's inhibitory effects and blocks cortical and limbic arousal.

Interactions
DRUGS
barbiturates, carbamazepine, phenytoin, rifampin: Possibly decreased estazolam levels
carbamazepine: Possibly increased blood carbamazepine level
cimetidine, diltiazem, disulfiram, erythromycin, fluoxetine, fluvoxamine, isoniazid, itraconazole, ketoconazole, nefazodone, oral contraceptives, propoxyphene, ranitidine, verapamil: Possibly increased blood level and impaired hepatic metabolism of estazolam
clozapine: Possibly cardiac arrest or respiratory depression
CNS depressants: Possibly potentiated CNS depression
levodopa: Possibly decreased therapeutic effects of levodopa
FOODS
grapefruit juice: Possibly increased blood level and impaired hepatic metabolism of drug
ACTIVITIES
alcohol use: Possibly potentiated CNS depression

Adverse Reactions
CNS: Amnesia, anxiety, ataxia, confusion, delusions, depression, dizziness, drowsiness, euphoria, headache, hypokinesia, irritability, malaise, nervousness, slurred speech, tremor
CV: Chest pain, palpitations, tachycardia
EENT: Blurred vision, dry mouth, increased salivation, photophobia
GI: Abdominal pain, constipation, diarrhea, nausea, thirst, vomiting
GU: Libido changes
RESP: Respiratory depression
SKIN: Diaphoresis
Other: Physical or psychological dependence

Nursing Considerations
•Use estazolam with extreme caution in patients with a history of drug or alcohol abuse because of the risk of addiction. Expect to

E
F

give drug for no more than 12 weeks.
•Use cautiously in elderly or debilitated patients and those with depression or impaired hepatic, renal, or respiratory function.
•Expect to stop estazolam gradually to prevent withdrawal symptoms. Avoid stopping abruptly if patient has a history of seizures.
•Monitor respiratory status, especially in patients with respiratory compromise, who are at increased risk for respiratory depression.
•If patient takes estazolam for depression, watch for suicidal tendencies, especially when therapy starts or dosage changes.

PATIENT TEACHING
•Warn patient not to exceed prescribed amount of time because of risk of addiction.
•Because estazolam can reduce alertness, advise patient to avoid hazardous activities until CNS effects of the drug are known.
•Advise patient not to drink alcohol or take other CNS depressants during therapy because of the risk of additive effects.
•Warn elderly and debilitated patients and those with impaired hepatic or renal function about the risk of excessive sedation or mental impairment and need to report them.
•If patient takes 2-mg dosage for a long time, warn against stopping drug abruptly.

estradiol

Estrace, Estrasorb, Estring, Estrogel, Evamist

estradiol acetate

Femring, Femtrace

estradiol cypionate

depGynogen, Depo-Estradiol, Depogen, Dura-Estrin, E-Cypionate, Estragyn LA 5, Estro-Cyp, Estrofem, Estro-L.A.

estradiol transdermal system

Alora, Climara, Esclim, Estraderm, Estrasorb, Estrogel, FemPatch, Menostar, Vivelle, Vivelle-Dot

estradiol valerate

Clinagen LA 40, Delestrogen, Dioval 40, Dioval XX, Duragen-20, Estra-L 40, Estro-Span, Femogex (CAN), Gynogen L.A. 20, Gynogen L.A. 40, Menaval-20, Valergen 10, Valergen 20, Valergen 40

ethinyl estradiol

Estinyl

Class and Category

Chemical class: Estrogen derivative, steroid hormone
Therapeutic class: Antineoplastic, antiosteoporotic agent, ovarian hormone replacement
Pregnancy category: X

Indications and Dosages

➤ *To treat menopausal symptoms*
TABLETS (ESTRADIOL)
Adult menopausal and postmenopausal women. Starting on day 5 of a cycle, 0.5 to 2 mg daily in cycles of 3 wk on, 1 wk off.
Adult postmenopausal women with intact uterus receiving progestin. 0.5 to 2 mg daily with daily progestin. Alternatively, 0.5 to 2,mg daily on days 1 through 25 of a 28-day cycle, with progestin starting day 12 or 16 and continuing through day 25 of the cycle; then no drugs on days 26 through 28, as prescribed.
VAGINAL RING (ESTRADIOL ACETATE [FEMRING])
Adult women. One ring (0.05 mg or 0.1 mg of estradiol/24 hr) inserted into upper third of vaginal vault and replaced every 3 mo.
TABLETS (ESTRADIOL ACETATE [FEMTRACE])
Adult menopausal and postmenopausal women. *Initial:* 0.45 mg daily. May be increased to 0.9 mg daily and then 1.8 mg daily as needed.
TABLETS (ETHINYL ESTRADIOL)
Adult menopausal and postmenopausal women. 0.02 to 0.05 mg daily in cycles of 3 wk on, 1 wk off.
Adult postmenopausal women with intact uterus receiving progestin. 0.02 to 0.05 mg daily with daily progestin; or 0.02 to 0.05 mg daily on days 1 through 25 of a 28-day cycle, with progestin starting day 12 or 16 and continuing through day 25; then no drugs on days 26 through 28, as prescribed.
DOSAGE ADJUSTMENT Dosage may be reduced to less than 1 mg daily (estradiol) or 0.05 mg daily (ethinyl estradiol) for patients with only vaginal or vulvar symptoms.
I.M. INJECTION (ESTRADIOL CYPIONATE IN OIL)
Adult women. 1 to 5 mg as a single dose every 3 to 4 wk as needed.
I.M. INJECTION (ESTRADIOL VALERATE IN OIL)
Adult women. 10 to 20 mg every 4 wk as needed.

TRANSDERMAL (ALORA, ESTRADERM, VIVELLE, VIVELLE-DOT)

Adult menopausal and postmenopausal women. *Initial:* 0.025 to 0.05 mg daily in cycles of 3 wk on, 1 wk off. One patch applied to trunk or buttocks and replaced twice/wk (every 3 to 4 days). Adjust dosage to control symptoms, as prescribed.

TRANSDERMAL (CLIMARA)

Adult women. *Initial:* 0.025 mg daily. One patch applied to trunk or buttocks and replaced every wk. Titrate dosage to control symptoms, as prescribed. Schedule will be cyclic unless patient has had a hysterectomy.

TRANSDERMAL (ESCLIM)

Adult women. *Initial:* 0.025 mg daily. One patch applied to upper arm, upper thigh, or buttocks and replaced twice/wk (every 3 to 4 days). Adjust dosage to control symptoms, as prescribed. Use a cyclic schedule, as prescribed, unless patient has had a hysterectomy.

TRANSDERMAL (ESTRASORB)

Adult women. 3.48 g daily in morning. Half of dose (1 pouchful) applied to one thigh and rubbed over entire thigh and calf for 3 min, and then repeated on other thigh and calf.

TRANSDERMAL (ESTROGEL)

Adult women. 1.25 g daily applied in thin layer from wrist to shoulder on inside and outside of one arm.

TRANSDERMAL (FEMPATCH)

Adult women. *Initial:* 0.025 mg daily. One patch applied to buttocks and replaced every wk. If symptoms aren't relieved after 4 to 6 wk, increased to two patches every wk, as prescribed. Follow a cyclic schedule, as prescribed, unless patient has had a hysterectomy.

TRANSDERMAL MIST (EVAMIST)

Adult women. *Initial:* 1.53 mg (1 spray) once daily in the morning. Dosage may be increased to 3.06 mg (2 sprays) once daily in the morning and then to 4.59 mg (3 sprays) once daily in the morning as needed.

➤ *To treat menopausal symptoms as combination therapy in patients with an intact uterus*

TRANSDERMAL estradiol (ALORA, ESTRADERM, VIVELLE, VIVELLE-DOT) IN COMBINATION WITH ESTRADIOL AND NORETHINDRONE ACETATE (COMBIPATCH)

Adult women. 0.05 mg daily estradiol-only transdermal system applied for first 14 days of a 28-day cycle and replaced twice/wk, according to product directions. Estradiol and norethindrone acetate transdermal system applied for remaining 14 days of 28-day cycle and replaced twice/wk during this period.

➤ *To treat postmenopausal vaginal and urogenital symptoms*

VAGINAL CREAM (ESTRACE)

Adult women. *Initial:* 2 to 4 g (200 to 400 mcg) daily for 1 to 2 wk. Then, dosage gradually reduced to one-half of initial dose, as prescribed, for 1 to 2 wk. *Maintenance:* 1 g (100 mcg) daily 1 to 3 times/wk for 3 wk, followed by 1 wk of no drugs. Repeat cyclically as needed.

VAGINAL RING (ESTRING)

Adult women. One ring (7.5 mcg of estradiol/24 hr) inserted into upper third of vaginal vault and replaced every 3 mo.

VAGINAL RING (FEMRING)

Adult women. One ring (0.05 or 0.1 mg of estradiol/24 hr) inserted into upper third of vaginal vault and replaced every 3 mo.

➤ *To prevent osteoporosis secondary to estrogen deficiency due to either natural or surgical menopause*

TABLETS (ESTRADIOL)

Adult women. At least 0.5 mg daily cyclically or continuously, adjusted as needed to control concurrent menopausal symptoms, as prescribed.

TABLETS (ETHINYL ESTRADIOL)

Adult females. At least 0.02 mg daily cyclically or continuously, as prescribed.

TRANSDERMAL (ALORA, VIVELLE-DOT)

Adult women. *Initial:* 0.025 mg daily continuously. One patch applied to lower abdomen or buttocks and replaced twice/wk. Adjust dosage to control symptoms and maintain bone density, as prescribed.

TRANSDERMAL (CLIMARA)

Adult women. *Initial:* 0.025 mg daily. One patch applied to trunk or buttocks and replaced every wk. Adjust dosage to control symptoms, as prescribed. Follow a cyclic schedule, as prescribed, unless patient has had a hysterectomy.

TRANSDERMAL (ESTRADERM)

Adult women. *Initial:* 0.05 mg daily. One patch applied to trunk or buttocks and replaced twice/wk. Adjust dosage to control symptoms, as prescribed. Follow a cyclic schedule, as prescribed, unless patient has had a hysterectomy.

TRANSDERMAL (MENOSTAR)

Adult women. *Initial:* 0.014 mg daily. One patch applied to lower abdomen and replaced every wk. Follow a cyclic schedule, as prescribed, unless patient has had a hysterectomy.

➤ *To treat estrogen deficiency due to oophorectomy, primary ovarian failure, or female hypogonadism*

TABLETS (ESTRADIOL)
Adult women. 0.5 to 2 mg daily continuously or in cycles of 3 wk on, 1 wk off.

TABLETS (ETHINYL ESTRADIOL)
Adult women. For primary ovarian failure or oophorectomy, 0.05 mg t.i.d. initially, then 0.05 mg daily after a few weeks, cyclically or continuously. For female hypogonadism, 0.05 mg once daily to t.i.d. for first 2 wk of a theoretical menstrual cycle. A progestin may be added, as prescribed, during last half of cycle to help induce menses.

I.M. INJECTION (ESTRADIOL CYPIONATE IN OIL)
Adult women. 1.5 to 2 mg every mo (for female hypogonadism only).

I.M. INJECTION (ESTRADIOL VALERATE IN OIL)
Adult women. 10 to 20 mg every mo as needed.

TRANSDERMAL (ALORA, ESTRADERM, VIVELLE)
Adult women. *Initial:* 0.05 mg daily. One patch applied to trunk or buttocks and replaced twice/wk. Titrate dosage to control symptoms, as prescribed. Follow a cyclic schedule, as prescribed, unless patient has had a hysterectomy.

TRANSDERMAL (CLIMARA)
Adult women. *Initial:* 0.05 mg daily. One patch applied to trunk or buttocks and replaced every wk. Adjust dosage to control symptoms, as prescribed. Follow a cyclic schedule, as prescribed, unless patient has had a hysterectomy.

TRANSDERMAL (ESCLIM)
Adult women. *Initial:* 0.025 mg daily. One patch applied to upper arm, upper thigh, or buttocks and replaced twice/wk (every 3 to 4 days). Adjust dosage to control symptoms, as prescribed. Follow a cyclic schedule, as prescribed, unless patient has had a hysterectomy.

TRANSDERMAL (FEMPATCH)
Adult women. *Initial:* 0.025 mg. One patch applied to buttocks and replaced every wk. If symptoms aren't relieved after 4 to 6 wk, increased to two patches every wk, as prescribed. Follow a cyclic schedule, as prescribed, unless patient has had a hysterectomy.

➤ *To treat dysfunctional uterine bleeding caused by hormonal imbalance in patients with a hypoplastic or atrophic endometrium and without uterine disease*

TRANSDERMAL (CLIMARA)
Adult women. *Initial:* 0.05 mg daily. One patch applied to trunk or buttocks and replaced every wk. Adjust dosage to control symptoms, as prescribed. Follow a cyclic schedule, as prescribed.

TRANSDERMAL (FEMPATCH)
Adult women. *Initial:* 0.025 mg daily. One patch applied to buttocks and replaced every wk. If symptoms aren't relieved after 4 to 6 wk, increased to two patches every wk, as prescribed. Follow a cyclic schedule, as prescribed.

➤ *To provide palliative treatment for inoperable, progressive breast cancer in selected men and postmenopausal women*

TABLETS (ESTRADIOL)
Adults. 10 mg t.i.d. for at least 3 mo.

TABLETS (ETHINYL ESTRADIOL)
Adults. 1 mg t.i.d. for at least 3 mo.

➤ *To treat advancing, inoperable prostate cancer*

TABLETS (ESTRADIOL)
Adult men. 1 to 2 mg b.i.d. or t.i.d., adjusted or continued, as prescribed, according to patient response.

TABLETS (ETHINYL ESTRADIOL)
Adult men. 0.15 to 3 mg daily, adjusted or continued, as prescribed, according to patient response.

I.M. INJECTION (ESTRADIOL VALERATE)
Adult men. 30 mg every 1 to 2 wk, adjusted or continued, as prescribed, according to patient response.

Contraindications

Active deep vein thrombosis, pulmonary embolism, or history of these conditions; active or recent (within past year) arterial thromboembolic disease, such as stroke or MI; hepatic dysfunction or disease; hypersensitivity to estradiol, ethinyl estradiol, or their components; hypersensitivity to tartrazine dye (contained in 0.02-mg estradiol and ethinyl estradiol tablets); known or suspected breast cancer or history of breast cancer except in appropriately selected patients being treated for metastatic disease; known or suspected estrogen-dependent cancer; pregnancy; undiagnosed abnormal genital bleeding

Mechanism of Action

Increases the rate of DNA and RNA synthesis in cells of female reproductive organs, pituitary gland, hypothalamus, and other target organs. In the hypothalamus, estrogens reduce release of gonadotropin-releasing hormone, which decreases pituitary release of follicle-stimulating hormone and luteinizing hormone. In women, these hormones are required for normal genitourinary and other essential body functions.

At the cellular level, estrogens increase cervical secretions, cause endometrial cell proliferation, and improve uterine tone. Estrogen replacement helps maintain genitourinary function and reduces vasomotor symptoms when estrogen production declines as a result of menopause, surgical removal of ovaries, or other estrogen deficiency states. Estrogen replacement also helps prevent osteoporosis by inhibiting bone resorption.

In men, estrogens inhibit pituitary secretion of luteinizing hormone and decrease testicular secretion of testosterone. These actions may decrease prostate tumor growth and lower the level of prostate-specific antigen (PSA).

Interactions

DRUGS

aminocaproic acid: Possibly increased hypercoagulability caused by aminocaproic acid
barbiturates, carbamazepine, hydantoins, rifabutin, rifampin: Possibly reduced activity of estradiol
bromocriptine: Possibly decreased therapeutic effects of bromocriptine
calcium: Possibly increased calcium absorption
corticosteroids: Increased therapeutic and toxic effects of corticosteroids
cyclosporine: Increased risk of hepatotoxicity and nephrotoxicity
didanosine, lamivudine, zalcitabine: Possibly pancreatitis
hepatotoxic drugs, such as isoniazid: Increased risk of hepatitis and hepatotoxicity
oral antidiabetic drugs: Decreased therapeutic effects of these drugs
somatrem, somatropin: Possibly accelerated epiphyseal maturation
tamoxifen: Possibly decreased therapeutic effects of tamoxifen
thyroid hormone replacement: Decreased effectiveness
vitamin C: Decreased metabolism and possibly increased adverse effects of estradiol
warfarin: Decreased anticoagulant effect

FOODS

grapefruit juice: Decreased metabolism and possibly increased adverse effects of estradiol

ACTIVITIES

smoking: Increased risk of stroke, pulmonary embolism, thrombophlebitis, and transient ischemic attack

Adverse Reactions

CNS: Dementia, depression, dizziness, headache, migraine headache, stoke
CV: Hypertension, MI, peripheral edema, pulmonary embolism, thromboembolism, thrombophlebitis
EENT: Intolerance of contact lenses, retinal vascular thrombosis, vision changes
ENDO: Breast enlargement, pain, tenderness, or tumors; gynecomastia; hyperglycemia
GI: Abdominal cramps or pain, anorexia, bowel obstruction (vaginal ring), constipation, diarrhea, elevated liver function test results, enlargement of hepatic hemangiomas, gallbladder disease or obstruction, hepatitis, increased appetite, nausea, pancreatitis, vomiting
GU: Amenorrhea, breakthrough bleeding, cervical erosion, clear vaginal discharge, decreased libido (males), dysmenorrhea, endometrial cancer, impotence, increased libido (females), ovarian cancer, pelvic pain, prolonged or heavy menstrual bleeding, ring adherence, testicular atrophy, vaginal candidiasis, worsening of endometriosis
MS: Arthralgia
SKIN: Acne, alopecia, hirsutism, jaundice, melasma, oily skin, purpura, rash, seborrhea, urticaria
Other: Angioedema, folic acid deficiency, hypercalcemia (in metastatic bone disease), toxic shock syndrome (vaginal ring), weight gain

Nursing Considerations

•WARNING Be aware that estradiol (Estrace)

and ethinyl estradiol (Estinyl) are distinct and separate products and that their dosing isn't equivalent.

• Use estradiol cautiously in patients with asthma, chorea, diabetes mellitus, epilepsy, migraine headaches, porphyria, systemic lupus erythematosus, or hepatic hemangiomas because estradiol may worsen these disorders.

• Administer oral preparations with or immediately after food to decrease nausea.

• For I.M. injection of estradiol cypionate or estradiol valerate, roll vial and syringe between palms to evenly disperse drug. Use at least a 21-gauge needle because of viscosity of oil-based solution. Use a dry, sterile syringe. Inject deep into upper outer quadrant of gluteal muscle. Aspirate before injection to avoid injection into a blood vessel.

• Be aware that, in patients who are converting from oral estrogen to transdermal system, oral estrogen should be stopped 1 week before skin patches are applied.

• Expect to begin prophylaxis treatment against osteoporosis at the start of menopause.

• Be aware that estrogen therapy should be given cyclically or combined with a progestin for 10 to 14 days per month in women with an intact uterus to minimize the risk of endometrial hyperplasia.

• **WARNING** Be aware that severe hypercalcemia may occur in patients with bone metastasis due to breast cancer because estrogens influence the metabolism of calcium and phosphorus. Monitor for toxic effects of increased calcium absorption in patients who are predisposed to hypercalcemia or nephrolithiasis.

• **WARNING** Assess patient for possible contact lens intolerance or changes in vision or visual acuity because estrogens can cause keratoconus, leading to increased curvature of the cornea. Be prepared to discontinue drug immediately, as prescribed, if patient experiences sudden partial or complete loss of vision or sudden onset of diplopia, migraine, or proptosis.

• Monitor PT test results of patients receiving warfarin for loss of anticoagulant effect because estrogens increase production of clotting factors VII, VIII, IX, and X and promote platelet aggregation.

• Watch for elevated liver function test results because estrogens may worsen such

conditions as acute intermittent or variegate hepatic porphyria.

• Closely monitor patient's blood pressure. A few patients may experience a substantial increase in blood pressure as an indiosyncratic reaction to estrogen. Monitor patients who already have hypertension for increases in blood pressure because estrogens may cause fluid retention. Also monitor patients with asthma, heart disease, migraines, renal disease, or seizure disorder for exacerbation of these conditions.

• Watch for peripheral edema or mild weight gain because estrogens can cause sodium and fluid retention.

• Frequently monitor serum glucose level in patients who have diabetes mellitus because estrogens may decrease insulin sensitivity and alter glucose tolerance.

• **WARNING** Expect to stop estrogen therapy in any woman who develops signs or symptoms of cancer; cardiovascular disease, such as stroke, MI, pulmonary embolism, or venous thrombosis; or dementia.

• Be aware that exogenous estradiol and progestins may worsen mood disorders, including depression. Monitor patient for anxiety, depression, dizziness, fatigue, insomnia, or mood changes.

• Assess skin for melasma (tan or brown patches), which may develop on forehead, cheeks, temples, and upper lip. These patches may persist after drug is stopped.

• Check patient's triglyceride level routinely because, in patients with hypertriglyceridemia, estrogen therapy may increase serum triglyceride level enough to cause pancreatitis and other complications.

• Monitor serum PSA level in patients with inoperable prostate cancer to determine if patient is responding to hormone therapy. If patient responds (usually within 3 months), expect therapy to continue until disease is significantly advanced.

• Monitor thyroid function test results in patients with hypothyroidism because longterm use of ethinyl estradiol may decrease effectiveness of thyroid therapy.

• Expect to stop estrogen therapy several weeks before patient undergoes major surgery, as prescribed, because certain procedures are associated with prolonged immobilization and therefore pose a risk of thromboembolism.

•If patient takes thyroid hormone replacement therapy, monitor her for increased signs and symptoms of hypothyroidism because estradiol may increase thyroid binding globulin levels, which may make the patient's current dose of thyroid hormone insufficient.

PATIENT TEACHING

•Before therapy starts, inform patient of risks involved in estrogen therapy, such as increased risk of breast, endometrial, or ovarian cancer; cardiovascular disease; dementia (if age 65 or over); gallbladder disease; and vision abnormalities.

•Advise patient to remain recumbent for at least 30 minutes after applying estradiol vaginal cream. Inform her that she may use a sanitary napkin (but not a tampon) to protect clothing after application.

•Teach patient proper application and use of transdermal patch. Instruct her not to apply patch to breasts, waistline, or other areas where it may not adhere properly. Advise her to rotate application sites at least weekly and to remove old patch before applying new one. If patch falls off, instruct her to reapply it to another area or to apply a new patch and continue the original treatment schedule. Caution her not to expose patch to sun for long periods. Explain that she may bathe while wearing the patch.

•Teach patient to apply Estrogel to clean, dry skin of one arm, using applicator. Stress importance of transferring all of the gel from applicator to arm. Tell patient to spread gel as thinly as possible over entire inside and outside of arm from wrist to shoulder. Advise her to wash her hands with soap and water afterward and to avoid fire and smoking until gel has dried because it's flammable. Tell patient never to apply gel to breasts. Warn that gel is alcohol-based and that patient should avoid fire, flame, or smoking until gel has dried.

•Inform patient that each pouch of Estrasorb contains half of daily dose. Instruct her to apply emulsion to clean, dry skin on top of thigh and to rub it into entire thigh and calf for 3 minutes. Tell her to rub any excess emulsion onto her buttocks. Then, advise her to repeat procedure on her other thigh and calf using the second pouch. Tell her to wash her hands with soap and water after the application and to dress only after affected areas are dry.

•Teach patient proper use of estradiol vaginal ring. Instruct her to insert ring in upper third of vagina, to keep it there for 90 days, and then to remove it and insert a new ring. Or she may remove it during the 90-day dosage period, rinse it with lukewarm (not hot or boiling) water, and reinsert it as needed for personal hygiene. Remind patient that she shouldn't be able to feel the ring when it's in place. If she does, she should use a finger to push the ring farther into her vagina. If vaginal wall ulceration or erosion occurs, suggest that patient leave ring out and not replace it until healing is complete to keep ring from adhering to healing tissue.

•Instruct patient prescribed transdermal Evamist to prime the pump of a new device before the first dose by holding the container upright with the cover in place and spraying 3 sprays. Then, to deliver a dose, she should spray the mist on the inner aspect of her forearm starting near the elbow. Instruct her to let the mist dry for 2 minutes and to not wash the area for at least 30 minutes.

•Inform patient receiving estradiol treatment that she should have an annual pelvic examination to screen for cervical dysplasia.

•Tell patient who has an intact uterus and is prescribed transdermal Menostar that she will need to receive progestin for 14 days every 6 to 12 months and have an endometrial biopsy yearly.

estrogens (conjugated)

C.E.S. (CAN), Congest (CAN), Premarin, Premarin Vaginal Cream, Synthetic Conjugated Estrogens A (SCE-A) Vaginal Cream

estrogens (conjugated) and medroxyprogesterone

Premphase, Prempro

synthetic estrogens, A (conjugated)

Cenestin

synthetic estrogens, B (conjugated)

Enjuvia

Class and Category

Chemical class: Estrogen derivative, steroid hormone
Therapeutic class: Antiosteoporotic agent, ovarian hormone replacement
Pregnancy category: X

Indications and Dosages

➤ *To treat moderate to severe vasomotor menopausal symptoms*

TABLETS (CENESTIN, PREMARIN)

Adults. 0.3 to 1.25 mg daily (Cenestin, Premarin) or cyclicly 25 days on, 5 days off (Premarin only). Dosage increased as needed to control symptoms.

TABLETS (ENJUVIA)

Adults. 0.625 mg daily. Dosage increased as needed to control symptoms.

TABLETS (PREMPRO)

Adults. 0.3 mg of conjugated estrogens and 1.5 mg of medroxyprogesterone daily. Increased up to 0.625 mg of conjugated estrogens and 5 mg of medroxyprogesterone daily as needed.

TABLETS (PREMPHASE)

Adults. 0.625 mg of conjugated estrogens daily on days 1 through 14 and combination product (0.625 mg of conjugated estrogens and 5 mg of medroxyprogesterone) on days 15 through 28.

➤ *To treat vaginal and vulvar atrophy*

TABLETS (CENESTIN, PREMARIN)

Adults. 0.3 to 1.25 mg daily (Cenestin, Premarin) or cyclicly 25 days on, 5 days off (Premarin only). Dosage increased as needed to control symptoms.

TABLETS (PREMPRO)

Adults. 0.3 mg of conjugated estrogens and 1.5 mg of medroxyprogesterone daily. Increased up to 0.625 mg of conjugated estrogens and 5 mg of medroxyprogesterone daily as needed.

TABLETS (PREMPHASE)

Adults. 0.625 mg of conjugated estrogens daily on days 1 through 14 and combination product (0.625 mg of conjugated estrogens and 5 mg of medroxyprogesterone) on days 15 through 28.

➤ *To treat atrophic vaginitis and vaginal and vulvar atrophy*

VAGINAL CREAM (PREMARIN)

Adults. 0.5 to 2 g daily in cycles of 3 wk on, 1 wk off.

➤ *To treat moderate to severe vaginal dryness and pain with intercourse and symptoms of vulvar and vaginal atrophy in menopause*

TABLETS (ENJUVIA)

Adults. 0.3 mg daily.

VAGINAL CREAM (PREMARIN)

Adults. 0.5 gram twice/wk. Or, 0.5 gram daily for 21 days followed by 7 days off, with cycle repeated every 28 days.

VAGINAL CREAM (SCE-A)

Adults. 1 gram daily for 1 wk, followed by 1 gram twice/wk.

➤ *To prevent postmenopausal osteoporosis*

TABLETS (CENESTIN, PREMARIN)

Adults. 0.625 mg daily continuously or in cycles of 25 days on, 5 days off.

TABLETS (PREMPRO)

Adults. 0.3 mg of conjugated estrogens and 1.5 mg of medroxyprogesterone daily. Increased to 0.625 mg conjugated estrogens and 5 mg medroxyprogesterone daily as needed.

TABLETS (PREMPHASE)

Adults. 0.625 mg of conjugated estrogens daily on days 1 through 14 and combination product (0.625 mg of conjugated estrogens and 5 mg of medroxyprogesterone) on days 15 through 28.

➤ *To provide palliative treatment for advanced androgen-dependent prostate cancer*

TABLETS (PREMARIN)

Adults. 1.25 to 2.5 mg t.i.d.

➤ *To provide palliative treatment for metastatic breast cancer*

TABLETS (PREMARIN)

Adults. 10 mg t.i.d. for 3 mo or longer.

➤ *To treat dysfunctional uterine bleeding*

I.V. INFUSION, I.M. INJECTION (PREMARIN)

Adults. 25 mg, repeated in 6 to 12 hr if needed.

➤ *To treat estrogen deficiency from oophorectomy or primary ovarian failure*

TABLETS (PREMARIN)

Adults. 1.25 mg daily in cycles of 3 wk on, 1 wk off.

➤ *To treat female hypogonadism*

TABLETS (PREMARIN)

Adults. 0.3 to 0.625 mg daily in cycles of 3 wk on, 1 wk off. Increased as needed every 6 to 12 mo.

Mechanism of Action

Increase the rate of DNA and RNA synthesis in the cells of female reproductive organs, hypothalamus, pituitary glands, and other target organs. In the hypothalamus, estrogens reduce the release of gonadotropin-releasing hormone, which decreases pituitary release of follicle-stimulating hormone and luteinizing hormone. In women, these hormones are required for normal genitourinary and other essential body functions. At the cellular level, estrogens increase cervical secretions, cause endometrial cell proliferation, and increase uterine tone. Estrogen replacement helps maintain genitourinary function and reduce vasomotor symptoms when estrogen production declines from menopause, surgical removal of ovaries, or other estrogen deficiency. Estrogen also helps prevent osteoporosis by keeping bone resorption from exceeding bone formation.

In men, estrogens inhibit pituitary secretion of luteinizing hormone and decrease testicular secretion of testosterone. These actions may decrease prostate tumor growth and lower the level of prostate-specific antigen.

Contraindications

Active deep vein thrombosis, pulmonary embolism, or history of these conditions; active or recent (within past year) arterial thromboembolic disease such as stroke or MI; hepatic dysfunction or disease; hypersensitivity to estrogens or their components; known or suspected breast cancer or history of breast cancer; known or suspected estrogen-dependent cancer; pregnancy; undiagnosed abnormal genital bleeding

Incompatibilities

Don't combine I.V. estrogens with acid solutions, ascorbic acid, and protein hydrolysate because they're incompatible.

Interactions

DRUGS

aminocaproic acid: Possibly increased level of hypercoagulability caused by aminocaproic acid
barbiturates, carbamazepine, hydantoins, rifabutin, rifampin: Possibly reduced activity of estrogen and medroxyprogesterone
bromocriptine: Possibly interference with bromocriptine's therapeutic effects
calcium: Possibly increased calcium absorption
corticosteroids: Increased therapeutic and toxic effects of corticosteroids
cyclosporine: Increased risk of hepatotoxicity and nephrotoxicity
didanosine, lamivudine, zalcitabine: Possibly pancreatitis
hepatotoxic drugs (such as isoniazid): Increased risk of hepatitis and hepatotoxicity
oral antidiabetic drugs: Decreased therapeutic effects of these drugs
somatrem, somatropin: Possibly accelerated epiphyseal maturation
tamoxifen: Possibly interference with tamoxifen's therapeutic effects
thyroid hormone replacement: Decreased effectiveness
warfarin: Decreased anticoagulant effect

ACTIVITIES

smoking: Increased risk of stroke, pulmonary embolism, thrombophlebitis, and transient ischemic attack

Adverse Reactions

CNS: Asthenia, dementia, depression, dizziness, growth benign meningioma, headache, insomnia, migraine headache, mood disturbance, nervousness, paresthesia, stroke
CV: Hypertension, MI, peripheral edema, thromboembolism, thrombophlebitis, vasodilation
EENT: Intolerance of contact lenses, pharyngitis, retinal vascular thrombosis, rhinitis, sinusitis
ENDO: Breast enlargement, pain, tenderness, or tumors; gynecomastia (men); hot flashes; hyperglycemia
GI: Abdominal cramps or pain, anorexia, cholestatic jaundice, constipation, diarrhea, flatulence, gallbladder disease or obstruction, hepatic hemangioma enlargement, hepatitis, increased appetite, ischemic colitis, nausea, pancreatitis, vomiting
GU: Amenorrhea, breakthrough bleeding, cervical erosion, clear vaginal discharge, decreased libido (men), dysmenorrhea, endometrial cancer or hyperplasia, impotence, increased libido (women), leukorrhea, ovarian cancer, prolonged or heavy menstrual bleeding, testicular atrophy, uterine leiomyomata

E
F

enlargement, vaginal candidiasis, vaginitis, vaginal site reactions (vaginal administration only) such as burning, irritation, and genital pruritus
MS: Arthralgias, back pain
RESP: Bronchitis, increased cough, pulmonary embolism
SKIN: Acne, alopecia, chloasma, erythema multiforme, erythema nodosum, hemorrhagic eruption, hirsutism, melasma, oily skin, pruritus, purpura, rash, seborrhea, urticaria
Other: Anaphylaxis, angioedema, flu syndrome, folic acid deficiency, hypercalcemia (in metastatic bone disease), weight gain

Nursing Considerations
•Use conjugated estrogens cautiously in patients with severe hypocalcemia because a sudden increase in serum calcium level may cause adverse reactions.
•Reconstitute conjugated estrogens with normal saline solution, dextrose, or invert sugar solution and use within a few hours. Discard solution that contains precipitate.
•**WARNING** Monitor serum calcium level to detect severe hypercalcemia in patients with bone metastasis from breast cancer.
•Watch for elevated liver function test results because estrogen and progestins may worsen such conditions as acute intermittent or variegate hepatic porphyria.
•Assess hypertensive patients for increases in blood pressure because estrogens may cause fluid retention.
•Monitor patients with asthma, diabetes mellitus, endometriosis, heart disease, lupus erythematosus, migraine headaches, renal disease, or seizure disorder for worsening of these conditions.
•If patient takes warfarin, assess PT for loss of anticoagulant effects because estrogens increase production of clotting factors and promote platelet aggregation.
•Expect to stop drug during periods of immobilization, 4 weeks before elective surgery, and if jaundice develops.
•**WARNING** Expect to stop estrogen combination therapy in any woman who develops signs or symptoms of cancer; cardiovascular disease, such as MI, pulmonary embolism, venous thrombosis, or stroke; or dementia.
•Check patient's triglyceride level routinely because, in hypertriglyceridemia, estrogen therapy may increase triglycerides enough to cause pancreatitis and other complications.

•If patient takes thyroid hormone replacement therapy, monitor her for increased signs and symptoms of hypothyroidism because estrogen may increase thyroid binding globulin level, which may make the patient's current dose of thyroid hormone insufficient.
•Estrogen may worsen mood disorders, including depression. Monitor patient for depression, fatigue, insomnia, or mood changes.

PATIENT TEACHING
•Explain the risks of estrogen therapy, including increased risk of breast, endometrial, or ovarian cancer; cardiovascular disease; dementia; and gallbladder disease.
•Instruct patient how to use vaginal cream and to cleanse plunger by removing it from barrel and washing it with mild soap and warm water after each use.
•Urge patient to immediately report breakthrough bleeding to prescriber.
•Instruct patient to perform a monthly breast self-examination and to comply with all prescribed follow-up examinations.
•Warn female patient that long-term use may increase risk of dementia, heart disease, stroke, gallbladder disease, and breast or endometrial cancer.
•Inform patient that estrogen vaginal cream may alter effectiveness of condoms, diaphragms, or cervical caps made of latex or rubber.

eszopiclone

Lunesta

Class, Category, and Schedule
Chemical class: Pyrrolopyrazine derivative of cyclopyrrolone class
Therapeutic class: Sedative-hypnotic
Pregnancy category: C
Controlled substance schedule: IV

Indications and Dosages
➤ *To treat insomnia*
TABLETS
Adults. *Initial:* 2 mg immediately at bedtime. May be increased to 3 mg at bedtime, as needed. *Maintenance:* 3 mg at bedtime.
DOSAGE ADJUSTMENT For elderly patients who have trouble falling asleep or patients with severe hepatic impairment, dosage decreased to 1 mg at bedtime. For elderly patients who have trouble staying asleep, dosage may be increased to 2 mg at bedtime.

Route	Onset	Peak	Duration
P.O.	Unknown	1 hr	Unknown

Mechanism of Action

May potentiate the effects of the inhibitory neurotransmitter gamma-aminobutyric acid (GABA) by binding close to or with benzodiazepine receptors in limbic and cortical areas of the CNS. By binding to these receptor sites and areas, eszopiclone increases GABA's inhibitory effects and blocks cortical and limbic arousal, thereby inducing and maintaining sleep.

Contraindications

Hypersensitivity to eszopiclone or its components

Interactions

DRUGS

clarithromycin, itraconazole, ketoconazole, nefazodone, nelfinavir, ritonavir, troleandomycin: Increased blood level of eszopiclone
rifampin: Decreased blood level of eszopiclone

ACTIVITIES

alcohol use: Additive effect on psychomotor performance

Adverse Reactions

CNS: Agitation, anxiety, bizarre behavior such as sleep driving, confusion, depersonalization, depression, dizziness, hallucinations, headache (including migraine), nervousness, neuralgia, somnolence, unusual dreams
CV: Chest pain, peripheral edema
EENT: Dry mouth, taste perversion
ENDO: Gynecomastia
GI: Diarrhea, hepatitis, indigestion, nausea, vomiting
GU: Decreased libido, dysmenorrhea, UTI
RESP: Asthma, respiratory tract infection
SKIN: Pruritus, rash
Other: Generalized pain, heat stroke, viral infection

Nursing Considerations

• Use eszopiclone cautiously in patients with severe mental depression or reduced respiratory function; drug may intensify depression and lead to respiratory depression.

PATIENT TEACHING

• Instruct patient not to exceed prescribed dosage and not to stop drug abruptly because withdrawal symptoms may occur.
• Because eszopiclone can reduce alertness, advise patient to take drug immediately before bedtime and to avoid potentially hazardous activities until drug's CNS effects are known.
• Urge patient to avoid alcohol and CNS depressants because of additive effects.
• Advise female patient of childbearing age to notify prescriber if she becomes or intends to become pregnant during therapy.
• Inform patient that sleep may be disturbed for the first few nights after therapy.
• Warn patient and caregiver that some patients have performed bizarre activities after taking drug, such as driving the car, preparing and eating food, making phone calls, or having sex while not fully awake and often with no memory of the event. These episodes usually occur in patients who have taken the drug with alcohol or other CNS depressant or who have exceeded the recommended dose. If such an episode occurs, the prescriber should be notified and eszopiclone therapy discontinued immediately.

etanercept

Enbrel

Class and Category

Chemical class: Dimeric recombinant human p75 tumor necrosis factor receptor (TNFR)
Therapeutic class: Disease-modifying antirheumatoid drug
Pregnancy category: B

Indications and Dosages

➤ *To reduce signs and symptoms of rheumatoid or psoriatic arthritis, slow structural damage in active arthritis, and improve physical function in patients with psoriatic arthritis, alone or in combination with methotrexate*

SUBCUTANEOUS INJECTION

Adults. 50 mg once weekly on the same day each week.

➤ *To reduce signs and symptoms of active ankylosing spondylitis*

SUBCUTANEOUS INJECTION

Adults. 50 mg once weekly on the same day each week.

E
F

➤ *To reduce signs and symptoms of juvenile rheumatoid arthritis*

SUBCUTANEOUS INJECTION
Children ages 4 to 17. 0.4 mg/kg twice/wk 3 to 4 days apart for 3 to 7 mo; or 0.8 mg/kg once weekly on the same day each week for 3 to 7 mo. *Maximum:* 25 mg twice/wk or 50 mg weekly.

➤ *To treat chronic moderate-to-severe plaque psoriasis in candidates for systemic therapy or phototherapy*

SUBCUTANEOUS INJECTION
Adults. *Initial:* 50 mg twice/wk 3 to 4 days apart for 3 mo; then reduced to 50 mg/wk.

➤ *To reduce signs and symptoms of moderately to severely active polyarticular juvenile idiopathic arthritis*

SUBCUTANEOUS INJECTION
Children ages 2 to17. 0.8 mg/kg/wk. *Maximum:* 50 mg/wk.

Incompatibilities
Don't combine etanercept with other drugs.

Contraindications
Hypersensitivity to etanercept, hamster protein, or their components, sepsis or risk of it

Interactions
DRUGS
cyclophosphamide: Possibly increased risk of malignancy
sulfasalazine: Possibly decreased neutrophil count

Adverse Reactions
CNS: Asthenia, chills, dizziness, fever, headache, multiple sclerosis, seizures
CV: Congestive heart failure, hypertension, hypotension, peripheral edema
EENT: Optic neuritis, pharyngitis, rhinitis, sinusitis
GI: Abdominal abscess, abdominal pain, autoimmune hepatitis, cholecystitis, diarrhea, gastroenteritis, indigestion, nausea, noninfectious hepatitis, vomiting
GU: Pyelonephritis
HEME: Aplastic anemia, neutropenia, pancytopenia
MS: Osteomyelitis, septic arthritis, transverse myelitis
RESP: Bronchitis, cough, pneumonia, upper respiratory tract infection
SKIN: Cellulitis, foot abscess, leg ulceration, pruritus, rash, urticaria
Other: Angioedema; injection site edema, erythema, itching, and pain; lymphoma; sepsis; varicella infection

Nursing Considerations
•Screen patient for latent tuberculosis with a tuberculin skin test before starting etanercept therapy. If test is positive, expect to give treatment, as ordered, before starting etanercept. Also screen patient for hepatitis B. If present, expect etanercept therapy to be withdrawn because antirheumatic therapies like etanercept may reactivate hepatitis B.
•Use cautiously in patients with a history of recurrent infection, underlying conditions that may predispose them to infections, or an existing chronic, latent, or localized infection because etanercept increases their risk of infection.
•Use cautiously in patients with COPD, and monitor respiratory status closely because etanercept therapy may increase patient's risk of adverse respiratory reactions.
•Use cautiously in patients with preexisting or recent onset CNS demyelinating disorders because drug may worsen these conditions. Also use cautiously in patients with heart failure because drug may worsen it.
•Tumor necrosis factor antagonists shouldn't be given with etanercept because doing so increases the risk of serious infection.
•**WARNING** Don't use the diluent provided with etanercept (bacteriostatic water for injection, USP, with 0.9% benzyl alcohol) for patients who have benzyl alcohol hypersensitivity. Instead, use sterile water for injection for these patients.
•**WARNING** If you have a latex allergy, don't handle needle cover of diluent syringe because it contains dry natural rubber (latex).
•When giving etanercept to children, don't use the 25-mg prefilled syringe if the child weighs less than 31 kg (68 lb). The 50-mg prefilled syringe or SureClick autoinjector may be used for children who weigh 63 kg (138 lb) or more.
•**WARNING** Expect to stop etanercept if patient develops sepsis.
•Avoid giving live-virus vaccines to patients who are taking etanercept because the drug decreases immune response and increases the risk of secondary transmission of vaccine virus.
•Monitor patients with immunosuppression

Mechanism of Action

Etanercept reduces joint inflammation from rheumatoid arthritis by binding with tumor necrosis factor (TNF), a cytokine, or protein, that plays an important role in normal inflammatory and immune responses.

In rheumatoid arthritis, the immune and inflammatory process triggers release of TNF, mainly from macrophages. TNF then binds to TNF receptors on cell membranes, as shown below left. This action renders TNF biologically active and triggers a cas-

cade of inflammatory events that results in increased inflammation of the synovial membrane, release of destructive lysosomal enzymes, and further joint destruction.

Etanercept binds specifically to TNF and prevents it from binding with TNF receptors on the cell membranes, as shown below right. This action renders the bound TNF biologically inactive, prevents TNF-mediated cellular responses, and results in significant reduction in inflammatory activity.

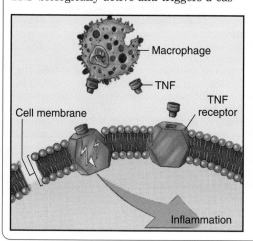

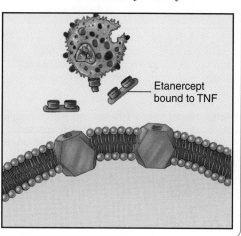

for evidence of acute or chronic infection, including chills, fever, and tachycardia, because etanercept decreases defenses against infection. This drug also increases the patient's risk of developing malignant tumors.
•Continue giving corticosteroids, NSAIDs, and other analgesics, as prescribed, during etanercept therapy.

PATIENT TEACHING
•Inform patient that etanercept is given by a small injection under the skin, and teach him proper injection technique if needed.
•If patient will be taking a 50-mg dose, explain that a prefilled syringe is available to eliminate the need to mix or draw up drug.
•If patient will be taking less than a 50-mg dose or prefers not to use prefilled syringe, advise him to use drug as soon as possible after dissolving powder. Dissolved powder may be kept in refrigerator for up to 6 hours after mixing and then should be discarded.

•Instruct patient to rotate injection sites among the thigh, stomach, and upper arms and to avoid areas that are tender, red, bruised, or hard. Advise him to keep each site at least 1″ away from a previous site.
•Urge patient to use needles and syringes once and discard in puncture-proof container.
•Caution patient that the risk of lymphoma may be higher in those who take etanercept; tell him to seek medical attention promptly for any suspicious signs and symptoms.
•Urge patient to consult prescriber immediately if he develops an infection because drug may decrease infection-fighting ability.
•Caution patient who hasn't had chickenpox to contact prescriber right away if he's exposed because he may develop a more serious infection.
•Urge patient to seek immediate emergency care if he develops a persistent fever, bruising, bleeding, or pallor while taking drug.

ethacrynic acid

Edecrin

ethacrynate sodium

Edecrin

Class and Category

Chemical class: Ketone derivative of anyloxyacetic acid
Therapeutic class: Diuretic
Pregnancy category: B

Indications and Dosages

➤ *To promote diuresis in heart failure; hepatic cirrhosis; renal disease; ascites of short duration caused by cancer, idiopathic edema, or lymphedema; and edema in children (excluding infants with congenital heart disease or nephrotic syndrome)*

ORAL SOLUTION, TABLETS

Adults. *Initial:* 50 to 100 mg daily as a single dose or in divided doses. Dosage increased by 25 to 50 mg daily, if needed. *Maintenance:* 50 to 200 mg daily. *Maximum:* 400 mg daily.
Children (except infants). *Initial:* 25 mg daily. Dosage increased in 25-mg increments daily, if needed.

I.V. INFUSION

Adults. *Initial:* 50 mg or 0.5 to 1 mg/kg. Dose repeated in 2 to 4 hr, if needed, then every 4 to 6 hr based on patient response. In an emergency, dose repeated every 1 hr, if needed. *Maximum:* 100 mg as a single dose.

Route	Onset	Peak	Duration
P.O.	30 min	2 hr	6 to 8 hr
I.V.	5 min	15 to 30 min	2 hr

Mechanism of Action

Probably inhibits the sulfhydryl-catalyzed enzyme systems that cause sodium and chloride resorption in the proximal and distal tubules and the ascending limb of the loop of Henle. These inhibitory effects increase urinary excretion of sodium, chloride, and water, causing profound diuresis. The drug also increases the excretion of potassium, hydrogen, calcium, magnesium, bicarbonate, ammonium, and phosphate.

Contraindications

Anuria; hypersensitivity to ethacrynic acid, ethacrynate sodium, sulfonylureas, or their components; infancy; severe diarrhea

Interactions

DRUGS

ACE inhibitors, antihypertensives: Possibly hypotension
aminoglycosides: Increased risk of ototoxicity
amiodarone: Increased risk of arrhythmias
amphotericin B: Increased risk of electrolyte imbalances, nephrotoxicity, and ototoxicity
anticoagulants, thrombolytics: Possibly potentiated anticoagulation and risk of hemorrhage
corticosteroids: Increased risk of gastric hemorrhage
digoxin: Increased risk of digitalis toxicity
insulin, oral antidiabetic drugs: Possibly increased serum glucose level and decreased therapeutic effects of these drugs
lithium: Increased risk of lithium toxicity
neuromuscular blockers: Possibly increased neuromuscular blockade
NSAIDs: Possibly decreased effects of ethacrynic acid
sympathomimetics: Possibly interference with hypotensive effects of ethacrynic acid and ethacrynate sodium

ACTIVITIES

alcohol use: Possibly potentiated hypotensive and diuretic effects of ethacrynic acid and ethacrynate sodium

Adverse Reactions

CNS: Confusion, fatigue, headache, malaise, nervousness
CV: Orthostatic hypotension
EENT: Blurred vision, hearing loss, ototoxicity (ringing or buzzing in ears), sensation of fullness in ears, yellow vision
ENDO: Hyperglycemia, hypoglycemia
GI: Abdominal pain, anorexia, diarrhea, dysphagia, GI bleeding (I.V. form), nausea, vomiting
GU: Hematuria (I.V. form), interstitial nephritis, polyuria
HEME: Agranulocytosis, severe neutropenia, thrombocytopenia
SKIN: Rash
Other: Hyperuricemia, hypochloremic alkalosis, hypokalemia, hypomagnesemia, hyponatremia, hypovolemia, infusion site irritation and pain

Nursing Considerations

•**WARNING** Administer ethacrynic acid and ethacrynate sodium cautiously in patients with advanced hepatic cirrhosis, especially those who also have a history of electrolyte imbalance or hepatic encephalopathy; both forms of drug may lead to lethal hepatic coma.

•Dilute ethacrynate sodium with D_5W or normal saline solution for I.V. infusion. Discard unused portion after 24 hours.

•Don't use diluted ethacrynate sodium that's cloudy or opalescent.

•Infuse I.V. ethacrynate sodium slowly over 30 minutes.

•Weigh patient daily and assess for signs of electrolyte imbalances and dehydration.

•Monitor blood pressure and fluid intake and output, and check laboratory test results.

•Report significant changes. Prescriber may reduce dosage or temporarily stop drug.

•If hypokalemia develops, administer replacement potassium, as ordered.

•Monitor serum glucose level frequently, especially if patient has diabetes mellitus; both forms of drug may cause hyperglycemia or hypoglycemia.

•Notify prescriber if patient experiences hearing loss, vertigo, or ringing, buzzing, or sense of fullness in his ears. Drug may need to be discontinued.

Patient Teaching

•Instruct patient to take the last dose of ethacrynic acid several hours before bedtime to avoid sleep interruption from diuresis. If patient receives once-daily dosing, advise him to take the dose in the morning to avoid sleep disturbance caused by nocturia.

•Suggest that patient take ethacrynic acid with food or milk to reduce the likelihood of GI distress.

•Advise patient to change position slowly to minimize effects of orthostatic hypotension, especially if he also takes an antihypertensive.

•Unless contraindicated, urge patient to eat more high-potassium foods and to take a potassium supplement, if prescribed, to prevent hypokalemia.

•Caution patient not to drink alcohol, stand for prolonged periods, or exercise during hot weather because these activities may exacerbate orthostatic hypotension.

•Instruct patient to notify prescriber if he has diarrhea; buzzing, fullness, or ringing in his ears; hearing loss; severe nausea; vertigo; or vomiting. Drug may need to be discontinued.

•Remind diabetic patients to check their serum glucose levels often for changes.

ethambutol hydrochloride

Etibi (CAN), Myambutol

Class and Category

Chemical class: Diisopropylethylene diamide derivative
Therapeutic class: Antitubercular
Pregnancy category: C

Indications and Dosages

➤ *As adjunct to treat tuberculosis and atypical mycobacterial infections caused by* Mycobacterium tuberculosis

Tablets

Adults and adolescents who haven't received previous antituberculotic therapy. 15 mg/kg daily.

Adults and adolescents who have received antituberculotic therapy. 25 mg/kg daily; after 60 days, decreased to 15 mg/kg daily.

Mechanism of Action

May suppress bacterial multiplication by interfering with RNA synthesis in susceptible bacteria that are actively dividing.

Contraindications

Hypersensitivity to ethambutol or its components, inability to report changes in vision, optic neuritis

Interactions

Drugs

antacids that contain aluminum hydroxide: Decreased absorption of ethambutol
other neurotoxic drugs: Increased risk of neurotoxicity, such as optic and peripheral neuritis

Adverse Reactions

CNS: Burning sensation or weakness in arms and legs, confusion, disorientation, dizziness, fever, headache, malaise, paresthesia, peripheral neuritis
EENT: Blurred vision, decreased visual acuity, eye pain, optic neuritis, red-green color

E
F

blindness
GI: Abdominal pain, anorexia, hepatic dysfunction, nausea, vomiting
HEME: Leukopenia, neutropenia, thrombocytopenia
MS: Arthralgia, gouty arthritis, joint pain
RESP: Pulmonary infiltrates
SKIN: Dermatitis, erythema multiforme, pruritus, rash
Other: Anaphylaxis, hypersensitivity syndrome (rash or exfoliative dermatitis, eosinophilia, and one of the following: hepatitis, pneumonitis, nephritis, myocarditis, pericarditis), lymphadenopathy

Nursing Considerations
•Expect prescriber to refer patient for an ophthalmologic examination that includes tests for visual fields, acuity, and red-green color blindness before taking ethambutol and monthly thereafter. This is especially likely if therapy is prolonged or dosage exceeds 15 mg/kg daily.
•WARNING Notify prescriber immediately if the patient develops vision changes; expect ethambutol therapy to be discontinued if they occur.
•Expect to give the patient at least one other antituberculotic with ethambutol, as prescribed, because bacteria may become resistant quickly to a single drug.
•Monitor laboratory test results for changes in liver function or for increased serum uric acid level if patient has gouty arthritis or impaired renal function. Notify prescriber of any abnormalities.
•Obtain a monthly sputum specimen, as ordered, to check bacteriologic response in sputum-positive patient.
•Knowthat successful ethambutol therapy typically takes 6 to 12 months but may take years.
PATIENT TEACHING
•Teach patient to recognize possible adverse reactions to ethambutol.
•Advise patient to take drug with food if he experiences adverse GI reactions.
•Instruct patient to take a missed dose as soon as he remembers, unless it's nearly time for the next dose, but not to double-dose.
•Inform patient that therapy may last months or years and that compliance is essential.
•Advise patient to notify prescriber if no improvement occurs within 3 weeks of taking

drug; if bothersome or severe adverse reactions occur; if his vision changes; or if a rash, fever, or joint pain (signs of hypersensitivity) develops.

ethchlorvynol
Placidyl

Class, Category, and Schedule
Chemical class: Chlorinated tertiary acetylenic carbinol
Therapeutic class: Sedative-hypnotic
Pregnancy category: C
Controlled substance schedule: IV

Indications and Dosages
➤ *To provide short-term relief from insomnia*
CAPSULES
Adults. 0.5 to 1 g at bedtime for no longer than 1 wk.

Route	Onset	Peak	Duration
P.O.	15 to 60 min	Unknown	5 hr

Mechanism of Action
Exerts sedative-hypnotic, muscle relaxant, and anticonvulsant effects possibly by depressing the reticular activating system.

Contraindications
Hypersensitivity to ethchlorvynol or its components, porphyria

Interactions
DRUGS
CNS depressants, tricyclic antidepressants: Increased CNS depression
oral anticoagulants: Decreased anticoagulant effects
ACTIVITIES
alcohol use: Increased CNS depression

Adverse Reactions
CNS: Ataxia, dizziness, facial numbness, fatigue, light-headedness, syncope, unsteadiness, weakness
CV: Hypotension
EENT: Blurred vision, unpleasant aftertaste
GI: Epigastric pain, indigestion, nausea, vomiting
HEME: Thrombocytopenia

SKIN: Jaundice, rash, urticaria
Other: Physical and psychological dependence

Nursing Considerations
•If patient awakens too early after taking 0.5 or 0.75 g of ethchlorvynol at bedtime, ask prescriber if he may take a single supplemental dose of 200 mg.
•Assess for signs of addiction if patient has taken drug for 2 weeks or longer.
•Be aware that ethchlorvynol shouldn't be given for longer than 1 week. If patient has received prolonged therapy, expect to discontinue drug gradually to prevent withdrawal symptoms. Notify prescriber if you detect evidence of withdrawal, such as diaphoresis, hallucinations, irritability, muscle twitching, nausea, nervousness, restlessness, seizures, sleep disturbance, tremor, vomiting, and weakness.
PATIENT TEACHING
•Caution patient not to exceed prescribed dosage or dosing frequency because of ethchlorvynol's habit-forming potential. Instruct him not to use drug for more than 1 week.
•Advise patient to take ethchlorvynol with food or milk to minimize adverse GI reactions.
•If patient has taken long-term ethchlorvynol therapy, warn against stopping drug abruptly; advise him to contact prescriber for guidelines to reduce dosage.
•Direct patient to avoid alcohol and other CNS depressants during ethchlorvynol therapy because they increase the risk of adverse reactions.
•Advise patient to avoid potentially hazardous activities until drug's CNS effects are known.

ethionamide

Trecator-SC

Class and Category
Chemical class: Thiamide analogue of isonicotinic acid
Therapeutic class: Antituberculotic
Pregnancy category: Not rated

Indications and Dosages
➤ *As adjunct to treat tuberculosis*
TABLETS
Adults. 0.5 to 1 g daily in divided doses every 8 to 12 hr, together with other antituberculotics. *Maximum:* 1 g daily.
Children. 15 to 20 mg/kg daily in divided doses every 8 to 12 hr, together with other antituberculotics. *Maximum:* 750 mg daily.

Mechanism of Action
May inhibit peptide synthesis, resulting in bacteriostatic action against *Mycobacterium tuberculosis.*

Contraindications
Hypersensitivity to ethionamide or its components, severe hepatic damage

Interactions
DRUGS
cycloserine: Increased risk of adverse CNS effects, especially seizures
other neurotoxic drugs: Increased risk of neurotoxicity, such as optic and peripheral neuritis

Adverse Reactions
CNS: Burning or pain in arms and legs, clumsiness, confusion, depression, mental or mood changes, paresthesia, unsteadiness
CV: Orthostatic hypotension
EENT: Blurred vision, eye pain, increased salivation, metallic taste, optic neuritis, stomatitis, vision loss
ENDO: Goiter, hypoglycemia, hypothyroidism
GI: Anorexia, hepatitis, nausea, vomiting
SKIN: Jaundice, rash

Nursing Considerations
•Use ethionamide cautiously in patients with a history of hypersensitivity to isoniazid, niacin, pyrazinamide, or chemically related drugs; these ptients also may be hypersensitive to ethionamide.
•Expect to give another antituberculotic with ethionamide to decrease the risk of development of bacterial resistance.
•Also plan to give pyridoxine to prevent or minimize peripheral neuritis (burning, numbness, pain, or tingling in hands and feet), especially if patient has already had isoniazid-induced peripheral neuritis.
•Monitor liver function test results, and assess for signs of impaired function, such as hepatitis and jaundice.
•Question patient regularly about vision

changes. Notify prescriber about blurred vision, eye pain, or loss of vision or acuity.
•Monitor compliance; treatment may need to continue for 1 to 2 years or indefinitely.

PATIENT TEACHING
•Advise patient to take ethionamide with food if adverse GI reactions occur.
•Instruct patient to take a missed dose as soon as he remembers unless it's nearly time for the next dose. Caution him not to double the dose.
•Encourage patient to notify prescriber if no improvement occurs within 3 weeks; if bothersome or severe adverse reactions occur; if his vision changes; or if he has burning, numbness, pain, or tingling in his hands and feet.
•Inform patient that therapy may have to continue for months or years and that compliance is essential.

ethosuximide

Zarontin

Class and Category

Chemical class: Succinimide derivative
Therapeutic class: Anticonvulsant
Pregnancy category: Not rated

Indications and Dosages

➤ *To manage absence seizures in a patient who also has generalized tonic-clonic seizures*

CAPSULES, SYRUP
Adults and children age 6 and over. *Initial:* 500 mg daily. *Maintenance:* Increased by 250 mg every 4 to 7 days until control is achieved with minimal adverse reactions.
Children ages 3 to 6. *Initial:* 250 mg daily. *Maintenance:* Increased by 250 mg every 4 to 7 days until control is achieved with minimal adverse reactions.

Contraindications

Hypersensitivity to ethosuximide, succinimides, or their components

Mechanism of Action

Elevates the seizure threshold and reduces the frequency of attacks by depressing the motor cortex and elevating the threshold of CNS response to convulsive stimuli.

Interactions

DRUGS
carbamazepine, phenobarbital, phenytoin, primidone: Possibly decreased blood ethosuximide level
CNS depressants: Possibly increased CNS depression
haloperidol: Possibly decreased blood haloperidol level
loxapine, MAO inhibitors, maprotiline, molindone, phenothiazines, pimozide, tricyclic antidepressants: Possibly lowered seizure threshold and reduced therapeutic effect of ethosuximide
valproic acid: Increased or decreased blood ethosuximide level

ACTIVITIES
alcohol use: Possibly increased CNS depression

Adverse Reactions

CNS: Aggressiveness, ataxia, decreased concentration, dizziness, drowsiness, euphoria, fatigue, headache, hyperactivity, irritability, lethargy, nightmares, sleep disturbance
EENT: Gingival hypertrophy, myopia, tongue swelling
GI: Abdominal and epigastric pain, abdominal cramps, anorexia, diarrhea, hiccups, indigestion, nausea, vomiting
GU: Increased libido, microscopic hematuria, vaginal bleeding
HEME: Agranulocytosis, aplastic anemia, eosinophilia, leukopenia, pancytopenia
SKIN: Erythematous and pruritic rash, hirsutism, Stevens-Johnson syndrome, systemic lupus erythematosus, urticaria
Other: Hypersensitivity reaction, weight loss

Nursing Considerations

•Use ethosuximide with extreme caution in patients with hepatic or renal disease.
•Give other anticonvulsants concurrently, as prescribed, to control generalized tonic-clonic seizures.
•Monitor CBC and platelet count and assess for signs of infection, such as cough, fever, and pharyngitis. Also routinely evaluate liver and renal function test results.
•Take safety precautions because drug may cause adverse CNS reactions, such as dizziness and drowsiness.

PATIENT TEACHING
•Stress the importance of complying with

ethosuximide regimen.
• Advise patient to take a missed dose as soon as he remembers unless it's nearly time for the next dose. Warn him not to double the dose.
• Instruct patient not to engage in potentially hazardous activities until drug's CNS effects are known.
• Caution patient not to stop taking drug abruptly; doing so increases the risk of absence seizures.

ethotoin

Peganone

Class and Category
Chemical class: Hydantoin derivative
Therapeutic class: Anticonvulsant
Pregnancy category: D

Indications and Dosages
➤ *To treat tonic-clonic and simple or complex partial seizures as initial or adjunct therapy, or when other drugs are ineffective*

TABLETS

Adults and adolescents. *Initial:* 0.5 to 1 g on the first day in four to six divided doses, increased over several days until desired response is reached. *Maintenance:* 2 to 3 g daily in four to six divided doses. *Maximum:* 3 g daily.
Children. *Initial:* Up to 750 mg daily, based on weight and age, in 4 to 6 divided doses, adjusted as needed and tolerated. *Maintenance:* 0.5 to 1 g daily in 4 to 6 divided doses. *Maximum:* 3 g daily.
DOSAGE ADJUSTMENT For debilitated patients, initial dosage lowered to reduce the risk of adverse reactions.

Contraindications
Hematologic disorders; hepatic dysfunction; hypersensitivity to ethotoin, phenytoin, other hydantoins, or their components

Interactions
DRUGS

acetaminophen: Increased risk of hepatotoxicity with long-term acetaminophen use
amiodarone: Possibly increased blood ethotoin level and risk of toxicity
antacids: Possibly decreased ethotoin effectiveness

bupropion, clozapine, loxapine, MAO inhibitors, maprotiline, phenothiazines, pimozide, thioxanthenes: Possibly lowered seizure threshold and decreased therapeutic effects of ethotoin; possibly intensified CNS depressant effects of these drugs
chloramphenicol, cimetidine, disulfiram, fluconazole, isoniazid, methylphenidate, metronidazole, omeprazole, phenylbutazone, ranitidine, salicylates, sulfonamides, trimethoprim: Possibly impaired metabolism of these drugs and increased risk of ethotoin toxicity
corticosteroids, cyclosporine, digoxin, disopyramide, doxycycline, furosemide, levodopa, mexiletine, quinidine: Decreased therapeutic effects of these drugs
diazoxide: Possibly decreased therapeutic effects of both drugs
estrogens, progestins: Decreased therapeutic effects of these drugs, increased blood ethotoin level
folic acid, leucovorin: Increased ethotoin metabolism, decreased seizure control
haloperidol: Possibly lowered seizure threshold and decreased therapeutic effects of ethotoin; possibly decreased blood haloperidol level
insulin, oral antidiabetic drugs: Possibly increased blood glucose level and decreased therapeutic effects of these drugs
lidocaine: Increased lidocaine metabolism, leading to reduced concentration
methadone: Possibly increased methadone metabolism, leading to withdrawal symptoms
molindone: Possibly lowered seizure threshold and impaired absorption and decreased therapeutic effects of ethotoin
oral anticoagulants: Possibly impaired metabolism of these drugs and increased risk of ethotoin toxicity; possibly increased anticoagulant effect initially, but decreased effect with prolonged therapy
oral contraceptives that contain estrogen and progestin: Possibly breakthrough bleeding and decreased contraceptive effectiveness
rifampin: Possibly decreased therapeutic effects of ethotoin
streptozocin: Possibly decreased therapeutic effects of streptozocin
sucralfate: Possibly decreased ethotoin absorption
tricyclic antidepressants: Possibly lowered seizure threshold and decreased therapeutic

E
F

effects of ethotoin; possibly decreased blood level of tricyclic antidepressants
valproic acid: Possibly decreased blood ethotoin level, increased blood valproic acid level
vitamin D analogues: Decreased vitamin D analogue activity; risk of anticonvulsant-induced rickets and osteomalacia
xanthines: Possibly inhibited ethotoin absorption and increased clearance of xanthines
ACTIVITIES
alcohol use: Possibly decreased ethotoin effectiveness, enhanced CNS depressant effects

Mechanism of Action
Limits the spread of seizure activity and the start of new seizures by:
• regulating voltage-dependent sodium and calcium channels in neurons
• inhibiting calcium movement across neuronal membranes
• enhancing sodium-potassium adenosine triphosphatase activity in neurons and glial cells.
   These actions may result from ethotoin's ability to slow the recovery rate of inactivated sodium channels.

Adverse Reactions
CNS: Clumsiness, confusion, drowsiness, excitement, peripheral neuropathy, sedation, slurred speech, stuttering, tremor
EENT: Nystagmus
GI: Constipation, diarrhea, nausea, vomiting
HEME: Agranulocytosis, leukopenia, thrombocytopenia
SKIN: Rash, Stevens-Johnson syndrome, toxic epidermal necrolysis
Other: Lymphadenopathy, systemic lupus erythematosus

Nursing Considerations
•Obtain CBC and differential before treatment and at monthly intervals for the first few months of ethotoin therapy, as ordered.
•WARNING Be aware that ethotoin shouldn't be discontinued abruptly because of a risk of causing status epilepticus. Plan to reduce dosage gradually or substitute another drug, as prescribed.
•Monitor patient for signs and symptoms of infection or unusual bleeding because ethotoin may cause hematologic toxicity.
•Because of ethotoin's potential for hepato-

toxicity, monitor liver function test results and expect drug to be discontinued if test results are abnormal.
•Notify prescriber immediately and expect ethotoin to be stopped and replaced with another drug if patient develops decreased blood counts, enlarged lymph nodes, or rash.
•Be aware that ethotoin may be substituted for phenytoin without loss of seizure control if patient develops severe gingival hyperplasia or other adverse reactions. Expect ethotoin dosage to be 4 to 6 times greater than phenytoin dosage.
•Institute and maintain seizure precautions according to facility protocol.
PATIENT TEACHING
•Instruct patient to take ethotoin exactly as prescribed and not to discontinue drug abruptly.
•Advise patient to take drug with food to enhance absorption and reduce adverse GI effects.
•Advise patient to report easy bruising, epistaxis, fever, malaise, petechiae, or sore throat to prescriber immediately.
•Instruct patient to keep medical appointments to monitor drug effectiveness and check for adverse reactions. Explain the need for periodic laboratory tests.
•Urge patient to avoid alcohol during therapy.
•Caution patient to avoid hazardous activities until drug's adverse effects are known.
•Encourage patient to wear or carry medical identification indicating his diagnosis and drug therapy.

etidronate disodium

Didronel

Class and Category
Chemical class: Bisphosphonate
Therapeutic class: Antihypercalcemic agent, bone resorption inhibitor
Pregnancy category: B (oral), C (parenteral)

Indications and Dosages
➤ *To treat Paget's disease of bone (osteitis deformans)*
TABLETS
Adults. 5 to 10 mg/kg daily for up to 6 mo, or 11 to 20 mg/kg daily for up to 3 mo.

➤ *To prevent and treat heterotopic ossification after total hip replacement*

TABLETS

Adults. 20 mg/kg daily for 1 mo before surgery and then 20 mg/kg daily for 3 mo after surgery for a total of 4 mo of treatment.

➤ *To prevent and treat heterotopic ossification after spinal cord injury*

TABLETS

Adults. 20 mg/kg daily for 2 wk and then 10 mg/kg daily for 10 wk for a total of 12 wk of treatment.

➤ *To treat moderate to severe hypercalcemia caused by cancer*

I.V. INFUSION

Adults. *Initial:* 7.5 mg/kg daily infused over at least 2 hr for 3 to 7 successive days. Oral etidronate may begin at 20 mg/kg/day for 30 days on the day after last infusion.

DOSAGE ADJUSTMENT Dosage reduced if patient has renal impairment. Drug not given if serum creatinine level exceeds 5 mg/dl.

Mechanism of Action

Inhibits normal and abnormal bone resorption by reducing bone turnover and slowing the remodeling of pagetic or heterotopic bone. Etidronate also decreases the elevated cardiac output that's seen in Paget's disease of bone and reduces local increases in skin temperature. It also inhibits the abnormal bone resorption that may occur with cancer and reduces the amount of calcium that enters the blood from resorbed bone.

Contraindications

Hypersensitivity to etidronate, bisphosphonates, or their components; severe renal impairment

Interactions

DRUGS

antacids that contain aluminum, calcium, or magnesium; vitamin and mineral supplements that contain aluminum, calcium, iron, or magnesium: Decreased etidronate absorption

FOODS

high-calcium food (such as milk and other dairy products): Decreased etidronate absorption

Adverse Reactions

EENT: Altered taste, metallic taste

GI: Diarrhea, elevated liver function test results, nausea

GU: Nephrotoxicity

MS: Bone fractures, bone pain

Other: Hypocalcemia

Nursing Considerations

•Anticipate starting etidronate as soon as possible after spinal cord injury, preferably before signs of heterotopic ossification.

•Expect etidronate not to inhibit healing of spinal fractures, affect prosthesis, or disrupt trochanter attachment when used after total hip replacement.

•Give oral form 2 hours before meals to prevent decreased absorption.

•Dilute parenteral form in at least 250 ml of normal saline solution.

•Give parenteral form slowly over at least 2 hours.

•Store diluted parenteral solution at room temperature for up to 48 hours.

•**WARNING** Watch for hypocalcemia if patient receives parenteral form for more than 3 days.

•When treating hypercalcemia, expect to continue giving drug for up to 90 days if serum calcium level remains within acceptable range.

PATIENT TEACHING

•Instruct patient to take etidronate tablets on an empty stomach—2 hours before meals, antacids, or calcium supplements. Urge him to drink a full glass of water with tablets and to avoid taking drug with milk or other high-calcium foods.

•Tell patient to take a missed dose as soon as he remembers as long as 2 hours have elapsed since his last meal. Instruct him not to eat for another 2 hours. Warn against doubling the dose.

•Inform patient with Paget's disease that his response to etidronate may be slow and may continue for months after treatment.

etodolac

Lodine, Lodine XL

Class and Category

Chemical class: Pyranoindoleacetic acid derivative

Therapeutic class: Analgesic, anti-inflammatory

Pregnancy category: C

Indications and Dosages

➤ *To manage osteoarthritis*
CAPSULES, TABLETS
Adults. *Initial:* 800 to 1,200 mg daily in divided doses. *Maintenance:* 600 to 1,200 mg daily in divided doses. *Maximum:* 1,200 mg daily for patients weighing 60 kg (132 lb) or more; 20 mg/kg daily for those less than 60 kg.
E.R. TABLETS
Adults. 400 to 1,000 mg daily.

➤ *To relieve mild to moderate pain*
CAPSULES, TABLETS
Adults. *Initial:* 400 mg and then 200 to 400 mg every 6 to 8 hr. *Maximum:* 1,200 mg daily for patients weighing 60 kg or more; 20 mg/kg/day for patients weighing less than 60 kg.

Route	Onset	Peak	Duration
P.O.	30 min	1 to 2 hr	4 to 12 hr

Mechanism of Action

Blocks the activity of cyclooxygenase, the enzyme needed for prostaglandin synthesis. Prostaglandins, important mediators of the inflammatory response, cause local vasodilation with swelling and pain. By inhibiting cyclooxygenase and prostaglandins, this NSAID causes inflammatory symptoms and pain to subside.

Contraindications

Angioedema, asthma, bronchospasm, nasal polyps, rhinitis, or urticaria induced by aspirin, iodides, or NSAIDs; coronary artery bypass graft surgery; hypersensitivity to etodolac or its components

Interactions

DRUGS
ACE inhibitors: Possibly decreased hypotensive effects of these drugs
acetaminophen (long-term use): Increased risk of adverse renal effects
antacids: Decreased blood etodolac level
antiplatelets, oral anticoagulants, thrombolytics: Prolonged PT (with warfarin), increased risk of bleeding
cidofovir: Possibly nephrotoxicity
corticosteroids: Increased risk of adverse GI effects

cyclosporine: Increased nephrotoxic effects, increased blood cyclosporine level
digoxin: Increased blood digoxin level and risk of digitalis toxicity
insulin, oral antidiabetic drugs: Increased risk of hypoglycemia
lithium: Increased blood lithium level and, possibly, toxicity
loop diuretics: Possibly decreased effects of loop diuretics
methotrexate: Increased risk of methotrexate toxicity
phenylbutazone: Possibly altered etodolac clearance
salicylates: Decreased blood etodolac level, increased risk of adverse GI effects
warfarin: Synergistic bleeding effects
ACTIVITIES
alcohol use, smoking: Increased risk of adverse GI effects

Adverse Reactions

CNS: Asthenia, chills, depression, dizziness, drowsiness, fatigue, fever, insomnia, irritability, malaise, nervousness, seizures, somnolence, syncope, stroke
CV: Edema, heart failure, hypertension, MI, palpitations, tachycardia, vasculitis
EENT: Blurred vision, deafness, loss of taste, photophobia, tinnitus
ENDO: Hyperglycemia in diabetics
GI: Abdominal pain or distention, anorexia, constipation, diarrhea, diverticulitis, dyspepsia, dysphagia, elevated liver function test results, esophagitis, flatulence, gastritis, gastroenteritis, gastroesophageal reflux disease, GI bleeding and ulceration, GI perforation, hemorrhoids, hepatic failure, hepatitis, hiatal hernia, indigestion, melena, nausea, pancreatitis, peptic ulcer, perforation of stomach or intestines, stomatitis, vomiting
GU: Dysuria, elevated serum creatinine level, hematuria, renal failure or insufficiency, renal papillary necrosis, urinary frequency
HEME: Agranulocytosis, aplastic anemia, easy bruising, hemolytic anemia, leukopenia, neutropenia, pancytopenia, thrombocytopenia
MS: Arthralgia, muscle pain
RESP: Asthma, bronchospasm, pulmonary infiltrate with eosinophilia, respiratory depression
SKIN: Erythema multiforme, exfoliative dermatitis, flushing, leukocytoclastic vasculitis,

pruritus, Stevens-Johnson syndrome, toxic epidermal necrolysis, urticaria, vesiculobullous or other rash

Other: Anaphylaxis, angioedema, lymphadenopathy, sepsis

Nursing Considerations

•Assess patient's hydration status and rehydrate, if needed and as ordered, before starting etodolac therapy.

•Use etodolac with extreme caution in patients with a history of ulcer disease or GI bleeding because NSAIDs such as etodolac increase the risk of GI bleeding and ulceration. Expect to use etodolac for the shortest time possible in these patients. Also use with extreme caution in patients with advanced renal disease because etodolac is eliminated mainly by the kidneys.

•Be aware that serious GI tract ulceration, bleeding, and perforation may occur without warning symptoms. Elderly patents are at greater risk. To minimize risk, give drug with food. If GI distress occurs, withhold drug and notify prescriber immediately.

•Use etodolac cautiously in patients with hypertension, and monitor blood pressure closely throughout therapy. Drug may cause hypertension or worsen it.

•**WARNING** Monitor patient closely for thrombotic events, including stroke and MI, because NSAIDs increase the risk.

•Especially if patient is elderly or taking etodolac long-term, watch for less common but serious adverse GI reactions, including anorexia, constipation, diverticulitis, dysphagia, esophagitis, gastritis, gastroenteritis, gastroesophageal reflux disease, hemorrhoids, hiatal hernia, melena, stomatitis, and vomiting.

•Monitor liver function test results because, in rare cases, elevated levels may progress to severe hepatic reactions, including fatal hepatitis, hepatic necrosis, and hepatic failure.

•Monitor BUN and serum creatinine levels in patients with heart failure, hepatic dysfunction, or impaired renal function; those taking diuretics or ACE inhibitors; and elderly patients because drug may cause renal failure.

•Monitor CBC for decreased hemoglobin level and hematocrit because drug may worsen anemia.

•**WARNING** If patient has bone marrow suppression or is receiving antineoplastic drug therapy, monitor laboratory results (including WBC count), and watch for evidence of infection because anti-inflammatory and antipyretic actions of etodolac may mask it, such as fever and pain.

•Assess patient's skin routinely for rash or other signs of hypersensitivity reaction because etodolac and other NSAIDs may cause serious skin reactions without warning, even in patients with no history of NSAID hypersensitivity Stop drug at first sign of reaction and notify prescriber.

•If patient also takes acetaminophen, monitor fluid intake and output and BUN and serum creatinine levels for signs of adverse renal reactions.

PATIENT TEACHING

•Tell patient to take etodolac with food or after meals if adverse GI reactions occur.

•Caution him to avoid aspirin or aspirin-containing products while taking drug.

•Advise patient not to smoke or drink alcohol during therapy because these activities increase the risk of adverse GI reactions.

•Inform patient that he may experience dizziness or drowsiness.

•Instruct him to notify prescriber immediately if he experiences blood in urine, easy bruising, itching, rash, swelling, or yellow eyes or skin.

•Caution pregnant patient not to take etodolac or other NSAIDs during the third trimester because drug may cause premature closure of the ductus arteriosus.

•Explain that etodolac may increase the risk of serious adverse cardiovascular reactions; urge patient to seek immediate medical attention for possible reactions, chest pain, shortness of breath, weakness, and slurring of speech.

•Tell patient that etodolac therapy also may increase the risk of serious adverse GI reactions; stress the importance of seeking immediate medical attention for such signs and symptoms as epigastric or abdominal pain, indigestion, black or tarry stools, or vomiting blood or material that looks like coffee grounds.

•Explain the possibility of rare but serious skin reactions. Urge patient to seek immediate medical attention for rash, blisters, itching, fever, or other indications of hypersensitivity.

E

F

exenatide

Byetta

Class and Category

Chemical class: Amino acid peptide amide
Therapeutic class: Antidiabetic drug
Pregnancy category: C

Indications and Dosages

➤ *Adjunct treatment to improve blood glucose levels in patients with type 2 diabetes mellitus who are taking metformin, a sulfonylurea, a thiazolidinedione, or a combination of metformin and a sulfonylurea or metformin and a thiazolidinedione but have not achieved adequate glucose control*

SUBCUTANEOUS INJECTION

Adults. *Initial:* 5 mcg b.i.d. within 60 min before morning and evening meals. After 1 mo, increased as needed to 10 mcg b.i.d. within 60 min before morning and evening meals.

Route	Onset	Peak	Duration
SubQ	Immediate	2.1 hr	Unknown

Contraindications

Hypersensitivity to exenatide or its components, ketoacidosis, type 1 diabetes mellitus

Interactions

DRUGS

oral antidiabetics: Increased risk of hypoglycemia
oral drugs: May decrease rate and extent of absorption of these drugs
warfarin: Possibly increased INR with increased risk of bleeding

Adverse Reactions

CNS: Asthenia, dizziness, headache, jitteriness, somnolence
CV: Chest pain
EENT: Decreased taste
ENDO: Hypoglycemia
GI: Abdominal distention or pain, anorexia, constipation, diarrhea, dyspepsia, flatulence, gastroesophageal reflux, indigestion, nausea,

Mechanism of Action

Normally, when serum glucose level rises, insulin is secreted within 10 minutes. This first-phase insulin response is absent in patients with type 2 diabetes.

Exenatide, an incretin mimetic, restores the first-phase insulin response and improves the second-phase response that immediately follows. It does so by promoting incretins that spur insulin synthesis and release from beta cells by binding and activating human GLP-1 receptors to reduce fasting and postprandial serum glucose levels.

The drug also suppresses inappropriately elevated glucagon secretion. Lower serum glucagon level leads to decreased hepatic glucose output and decreased insulin demand. It also slows gastric emptying and thus the rise of serum glucose level.

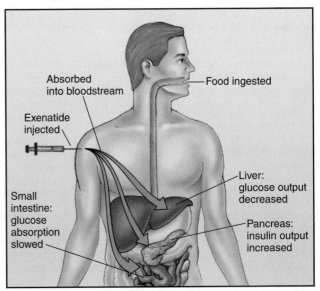

Food ingested

Absorbed into bloodstream

Exenatide injected

Liver: glucose output decreased

Pancreas: insulin output increased

Small intestine: glucose absorption slowed

pancreatitis, vomiting
RESP: Chronic hypersensitivity pneumonitis
SKIN: Diaphoresis, pruritus, rash, urticaria
Other: Anaphylaxis, angioedema, anti-exenatide antibodies, dehydration, elevated anti-exenatide antibody level, injection site reactions, weight loss

Nursing Considerations
•Know that exenatide is not recommended for patients with severe GI disease, patients with creatinine clearance less than 30 ml/min/1.73 m^3, or patients undergoing dialysis because of drug's adverse GI effects.
•Be aware that if patient also takes a sulfonylurea, the sulfonylurea dosage may need to be decreased to reduce the risk of hypoglycemia. Usually, no dosage adjustment is needed for a patient taking metformin.
•If patient also takes a sulfonylurea, monitor him for hypoglycemia and provide treatment as needed.
•Administer drug into the patient's thigh, abdomen, or upper arm.
•Monitor patient's blood glucose level. If control decreases despite the patient's best efforts, drug may need to be discontinued because of the possibility that anti-exenatide antibodies have formed.
•Monitor patient for evidence of acute pancreatitis, such as persistent, severe abdominal pain accompanied by vomiting. Notify prescriber, and expect exenatide therapy to be discontinued.
PATIENT TEACHING
•Teach patient how to give a subcutaneous injection and how to use the pen injection device.
•Inform patient that exenatide may be administered in the thigh, abdomen, or upper arm. Stress the need to rotate injection sites.
•Stress the need to use drug within 60 minutes before morning and evening meals or the two main meals of the day, about 6 hours or more apart, never after a meal.
•If patient misses a dose, tell him to resume treatment with the next scheduled dose.
•Advise patient that drug should look clear and colorless. Caution against using any prefilled pen device in which the solution looks cloudy or colored or contains particles.
•Instruct patient to check expiration date on the vial and not to use drug if date has passed.

•Advise patient to refrigerate drug before first use and protect it from light. After first use, drug may be stored at room temperature if it does not exceed 77° F (25° C).
•Tell patient to discard pen injector 30 days after initial use, even if some drug is left.
•Alert patient that pen doesn't come with needles and that he'll need to buy them.
•Warn patient that nausea may occur at the beginning of therapy.
•Inform patient taking a sulfonylurea to be alert for hypoglycemic reactions because risk increases with both drugs. Review ways to treat such reactions, and tell patient to alert prescriber if they occur often or are severe.
•Instruct female patient of childbearing potential to tell her prescriber if she is, could be, or is planning to become pregnant.
•Tell patient to seek emergency care for persistent, severe abdominal pain and vomiting.

ezetimibe
Zetia

Class and Category
Chemical class: Azetidinone
Therapeutic class: Antihypercholesterolemic
Pregnancy category: C

Indications and Dosages
➤ *To treat heterozygous familial and nonfamilial hypercholesterolemia or homozygous sitosterolemia; as adjunct with HMG-CoA reductase inhibitors to treat heterozygous familial and nonfamilial hypercholesterolemia; with fenofibrate to treat mixed hyperlipidemia and with atorvastatin or simvastatin to treat patients with homozygous familial hypercholesterolemia*
TABLETS
Adults. 10 mg daily.

Contraindications
Active hepatic dysfunction, hypersensitivity to ezetimibe or its components

Interactions
DRUGS
cholestyramine: Reduced effects of ezetimibe
cyclosporine: Increased blood cyclosporine and ezetimibe levels
fenofibrate, gemfibrozil: Increased blood ezetimibe level

Mechanism of Action

Reduces blood cholesterol by inhibiting its absorption through the small intestine. Normally, in the intestinal lumen, lipids break down to cholesterol and other substances that create smaller droplets called micelles, as shown below left. The micelles enter intestinal epithelial cells called enterocytes, where they combine with triglycerides, cholesterol, and other substances to form chylomicrons. Chylomicrons then pass through to the lymphatic system to be carried to the blood.

Ezetimibe blocks cholesterol absorption into enterocytes and keeps cholesterol from moving through the intestinal wall, as shown below right. Reduced cholesterol absorption from the intestine decreases chylomicron and LDL cholesterol content.

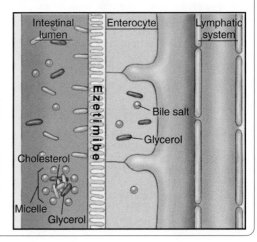

Adverse Reactions

CNS: Depression, dizziness, fatigue, headache, paresthesia
CV: Chest pain
EENT: Pharyngitis, sinusitis
GI: Abdominal pain, cholelithiasis, cholecystitis, diarrhea, elevated liver function test results, hepatitis, nausea, pancreatitis
HEME: Thrombocytopenia
MS: Arthralgia, back or limb pain, elevated CK level, myalgia, myopathy, rhabdomyolysis
RESP: Cough, upper respiratory tract infection
SKIN: Rash, urticaria
Other: Anaphylaxis, angioedema, influenza, viral infection

Nursing Considerations

•Monitor liver function test results before and during ezetimibe therapy, as ordered.
•Know that you should give ezetimibe 2 hours before or 4 hours after giving bile acid sequestrant, cholestyramine, or colestipol.

PATIENT TEACHING
•Direct patient to follow a low-cholesterol diet as an adjunct to ezetimibe therapy. Recommend weight loss and exercise programs, as appropriate.
•If patient also takes a bile acid sequestrant, tell him to take ezetimibe either 2 hours before or at least 4 hours after it to prevent drug interactions.
•Advise patient to report unexplained muscle pain, tenderness, or weakness.

famotidine

Act (CAN), Apo-Famotidine (CAN), Dyspep HB (CAN), Gen-Famotidine (CAN), Mylanta-AR, Novo-Famotidine (CAN), Nu-Famotidine (CAN), Pepcid, Pepcid AC, Pepcid RPD

Class and Category

Chemical class: Thiazole derivative
Therapeutic class: Antiulcer agent, gastric acid secretion inhibitor
Pregnancy category: B

Indications and Dosages

➤ *To provide short-term treatment of active duodenal ulcer*

ORAL SUSPENSION, TABLETS (CHEWABLE, ORAL DISINTEGRATING, AND REGULAR)

Adults and adolescents. 40 mg daily at bedtime or 20 mg b.i.d.

Children. 0.5 mg/kg daily as a single dose at bedtime or in divided doses b.i.d.

I.V. INFUSION OR INJECTION

Adults and adolescents over age 16. 20 mg every 12 hr, infused over 15 to 30 min or injected over at least 2 min.

Children ages 1 to 16. *Initial:* 0.25 mg/kg every 12 hr, infused over 15 to 30 min or injected over at least 2 min. *Maximum:* 40 mg daily.

➤ *To prevent recurrence of duodenal ulcer*

ORAL SUSPENSION, TABLETS (CHEWABLE, ORAL DISINTEGRATING, AND REGULAR)

Adults and adolescents. 20 mg daily at bedtime.

➤ *To provide short-term treatment for active, benign gastric ulcer*

ORAL SUSPENSION, TABLETS (CHEWABLE, ORAL DISINTEGRATING, AND REGULAR)

Adults and adolescents. 40 mg daily at bedtime.

Children. 0.5 mg/kg daily as a single dose at bedtime or in divided doses b.i.d.

I.V. INFUSION OR INJECTION

Adults and adolescents over age 16. 20 mg every 12 hr.

Children ages 1 to 16. *Initial:* 0.25 mg/kg every 12 hr. *Maximum:* 40 mg daily.

➤ *To treat gastroesophageal reflux disease (GERD)*

ORAL SUSPENSION, TABLETS (CHEWABLE, ORAL DISINTEGRATING, AND REGULAR)

Adults and adolescents. 20 mg b.i.d. for up to 6 wk.

Children weighing more than 10 kg (22 lb). 1 to 2 mg/kg daily in divided doses b.i.d.

Children weighing less than 10 kg. 1 to 2 mg/kg daily in divided doses t.i.d.

ORAL SUSPENSION

Infants age 4 months to 1 year. 0.5 mg/kg daily in divided doses b.i.d. for up to 8 wk.

Infants age 3 months or less. 0.5 mg/kg daily for up to 8 wk.

I.V. INFUSION OR INJECTION

Children ages 1 to 16. *Initial:* 0.25 mg/kg every 12 hr. *Maximum:* 40 mg daily.

➤ *To treat esophagitis caused by gastroesophageal reflux*

ORAL SUSPENSION, TABLETS (CHEWABLE, ORAL DISINTEGRATING, AND REGULAR)

Adults and adolescents. 20 to 40 mg b.i.d. for up to 12 wk.

➤ *To treat gastric hypersecretory conditions, such as Zollinger-Ellison syndrome*

ORAL SUSPENSION, TABLETS (CHEWABLE, ORAL DISINTEGRATING, AND REGULAR)

Adults and adolescents. *Initial:* 20 mg every 6 hr. Dosage adjusted, if needed, based on patient response.

I.V. INFUSION OR INJECTION

Adults and adolescents. 20 mg every 12 hr.

➤ *To prevent heartburn and indigestion*

TABLETS (CHEWABLE, ORAL DISINTEGRATING, AND REGULAR)

Adults and adolescents. 10 mg 1 hr before eating. *Maximum:* 20 mg every 24 hr.

➤ *To treat heartburn and indigestion*

TABLETS (CHEWABLE, ORAL DISINTEGRATING, AND REGULAR)

Adults and adolescents. 10 mg at onset of symptoms. *Maximum:* 20 mg every 24 hr for up to 2 wk unless prescribed otherwise.

DOSAGE ADJUSTMENT Oral or parenteral dosage reduced or dosing interval increased (to 36 to 48 hr), if needed, in patients with renal insufficiency and creatinine clearance of 49 ml/min/1.73 m^2 or less.

Route	Onset	Peak	Duration
P.O.	1 hr	1 to 4 hr	10 to 12 hr
I.V.	In 30 min	0.5 to 3 hr	10 to 12 hr

Contraindications

Hypersensitivity to famotidine, other H$_2$-receptor antagonists, or their components

Interactions

DRUGS

antacids, sucralfate: Possibly decreased absorption of famotidine

bone marrow depressants: Increased risk of blood dyscrasias

itraconazole, ketoconazole: Possibly decreased absorption of these drugs

ACTIVITIES

alcohol use: Possibly increased blood alcohol level

E
F

Mechanism of Action

In normal digestion, parietal cells in the gastric epithelium secrete hydrogen (H⁺) ions, which combine with chloride ions (Cl⁻) to form hydrochloric acid (HCl), as shown below left. However, HCl can inflame, ulcerate, and perforate the gastric and intestinal mucosa that's normally protected by mucus. Famotidine, an H_2-receptor antagonist, reduces HCl formation by preventing histamine from binding with H_2 receptors on the surface of parietal cells, as shown below right. By doing so, the drug helps prevent peptic ulcers from forming and helps heal existing ones.

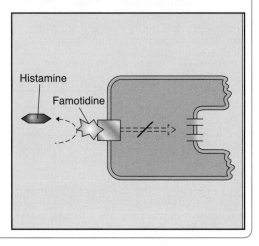

Adverse Reactions

CNS: Agitation (infants), anxiety, asthenia, confusion, depression, dizziness, fatigue, fever, hallucinations, headache, insomnia, mental or mood changes, paresthesia, seizures, somnolence
CV: Arrhythmias, AV block, palpitations
EENT: Dry mouth, laryngeal edema, taste alteration, tinnitus
GI: Abdominal pain, anorexia, cholestatic jaundice, constipation, diarrhea, elevated liver enzymes, hepatitis, nausea, vomiting
GU: Decreased libido
HEME: Agranulocytosis, aplastic anemia, leukopenia, neutropenia, pancytopenia, thrombocytopenia
MS: Arthralgia, muscle cramps
RESP: Bronchospasm, dyspnea, interstitial pneumonia, wheezing
SKIN: Acne, alopecia, dry skin, erythema multiforme, exfoliative dermatitis, flushing, jaundice, pruritus, rash, Stevens-Johnson syndrome, toxic epidermal necrolysis, urticaria
Other: Anaphylaxis, angioedema, facial edema, hyperuricemia

Nursing Considerations

•Shake famotidine oral suspension vigorously for 5 to 10 seconds before administration.
•Dilute injection form (2 ml) with normal saline solution or other solution to 5 to 10 ml; give I.V. injection over at least 2 minutes. Or dilute in 100 ml of D_5W and infuse over 15 to 30 minutes. Or infuse premixed injection (20 mg/50 ml normal saline solution) over 15 to 30 minutes.
•**WARNING** Be aware that Pepcid AC chewable tablets contain aspartame, which can be dangerous for patients who have phenylketonuria.

PATIENT TEACHING
•Instruct patient to store famotidine oral suspension at room temperature (below 86° F [30° C]) and to protect it from freezing. Tell her to shake the bottle vigorously for 5 to 10 seconds after adding water and right before use.
•Advise patient who uses Pepcid RPD to store drug in unopened package. For each dose, instruct her to open blister pack with

dry hands, place a tablet on her tongue, let it dissolve, and swallow it with saliva.
•If patient uses chewable tablets, instruct her to chew them thoroughly before swallowing.
•If patient also takes antacids, instruct her to wait 30 to 60 minutes after taking famotidine, if possible, before taking antacid.
•Caution patient to avoid alcohol and smoking during famotidine therapy because they irritate the stomach and can delay ulcer healing.
•Advise patient to notify prescriber if she develops pain or has trouble swallowing or if she has bloody vomit or black stools.
•Caution patient not to take famotidine with other acid-reducing products.

febuxostat

Uloric

Class and Category

Chemical class: Xanthine oxidase inhibitor
Therapeutic class: Antigout
Pregnancy category: C

Indications and Dosages

➤ *To treat chronic hyperuricemia in patients with gout*

TABLETS

Adults. *Initial:* 40 mg once daily, increased to 80 mg in 2 wk if serum uric acid level remains above 6 mg/dl. When therapy starts, given with gout flare prophylaxis drug, such as an NSAID or colchicine.

Route	Onset	Peak	Duration
P.O.	Unknown	1 to 1.5 hr	Unknown

Mechanism of Action

Inhibits the action of the enzyme xanthine oxidase. This enzyme is involved in purine metabolism to produce uric acid. Blocking its action causes uric acid production to decrease, thereby alleviating signs and symptoms of hyperuricemia found in gout.

Contraindications

Concurrent use of azathioprine, mercaptopurine, or theophylline; hypersensitivity to febuxotat or its components

Interactions

DRUGS

azathioprine, mercaptopurine, theophylline: Possibly increased serum levels of these drugs, leading to toxicity

Adverse Reactions

CNS: Dizziness, stroke
CV: MI, thrombosis
GI: Elevated liver enzymes, hepatic dysfunction, nausea
MS: Arthralgia
SKIN: Rash
Other: Gout flare

Nursing Considerations

•Febuxostat isn't recommended for patients with secondary hyperuricemia or patients in whom the rate of urate formation is greatly increased, such as in malignant disease.
•Use febuxostat cautiously in patients with severe renal or hepatic impairment.
•Monitor patient for gout flares after therapy starts because change in serum uric acid level mobilizes urate from tissue. To prevent gout flare-ups, expect to give an NSAID or colchicine for up to 6 months of febuxostat therapy.
•Monitor patient's serum uric acid level regularly starting as early as 2 weeks after febuxostat therapy starts. Drug is effective if serum uric acid level drops below 6 mg/dl.
•Monitor patient closely for thromboembolic events such as a MI or stroke. If cardiovascular or neurological abnormalities occur suggestive of an MI or strooke, notify prescriber immediately, discontinue drug, and provide supportive care, as ordered.
•Check patient's liver enzymes at 2 months, then 4 months, then periodically thereafter, as ordered, because febuxostat may adversely affect liver function.

PATIENT TEACHING

•Inform patient that gout flare-ups may occur with febuxostat therapy and that he may be prescribed an NSAID or colchicine to take with febuxostat for up to 6 months to prevent such flare-ups.
•Advise patient that periodic blood tests will be needed to monitor effectiveness of drug and detect liver abnormalities.
•Tell patient to notify prescriber immediately if he develops a rash, chest pain, shortness of breath, or neurological abnormalities.

E
F

felbamate

Felbatol

Class and Category

Chemical class: Dicarbamate
Therapeutic class: Anticonvulsant
Pregnancy category: C

Indications and Dosages

➤ *To treat partial seizures in patients who don't respond to other drugs*

ORAL SUSPENSION, TABLETS

Adults and adolescents over age 14. *Initial:* 1,200 mg daily in divided doses t.i.d. or q.i.d. Dosage increased over several weeks based on patient response. *Maximum:* 3,600 mg daily.

Children ages 2 to 14. *Initial:* 15 mg/kg daily in divided doses t.i.d. or q.i.d. Dosage increased over several weeks based on patient response. *Maximum:* 3,600 mg daily or 45 mg/kg daily.

➤ *As adjunct to treat generalized or partial seizures associated with Lennox-Gastaut syndrome in children*

ORAL SUSPENSION, TABLETS

Children ages 2 to 14. *Initial:* 15 mg/kg daily in divided doses t.i.d. or q.i.d. while decreasing other anticonvulsant drugs by 20% to control their blood levels. Felbamate dosage increased by 15 mg/kg daily every wk. *Maximum:* 3,600 mg daily or 45 mg/kg daily.

DOSAGE ADJUSTMENT Dosage reduced by 50% in patients with renal impairment.

Mechanism of Action

May exert its anticonvulsant effects by antagonizing the effects of the amino acid glycine. When glycine binds to *N*-methyl-D-aspartate (NMDA) receptors in the CNS, the frequency at which receptor-gated calcium ion channels open is increased—an important factor in initiating seizures. Felbamate may raise the seizure threshold by blocking NMDA receptors so that glycine can't bind to them.

Contraindications

Hepatic dysfunction; history of blood dyscrasias; hypersensitivity to felbamate, other carbamates, or their components

Interactions

DRUGS

carbamazepine: Decreased blood carbamazepine level and increased felbamate clearance, resulting in decreased blood felbamate level

fosphenytoin, phenytoin: Increased blood phenytoin level and increased felbamate clearance, resulting in decreased blood felbamate level

methsuximide: Increased adverse effects of methsuximide

oral contraceptives: Possibly decreased effectiveness of oral contraceptives

phenobarbital: Decreased blood felbamate level, increased blood phenobarbital level and risk of adverse effects

valproic acid: Increased blood valproic acid level and increased risk of adverse effects

Adverse Reactions

CNS: Abnormal gait, aggressiveness, agitation, anxiety, dizziness, drowsiness, fever, headache, insomnia, mood changes, tremor
EENT: Altered taste, diplopia, rhinitis
GI: Abdominal pain, anorexia, constipation, diarrhea, elevated liver function test results, hepatic failure, indigestion, nausea, vomiting
HEME: Aplastic anemia, leukopenia, pancytopenia, thrombocytopenia
RESP: Upper respiratory tract infection
SKIN: Photosensitivity, purpura, rash
Other: Anaphylaxis, lymphadenopathy, weight loss

Nursing Considerations

• Check liver function test results before starting felbamate therapy, and expect to monitor test results every 1 to 2 weeks during treatment. Notify prescriber immediately and expect to stop drug if test results become abnormal.

• Plan to taper dosage by one-third every 4 to 5 days as prescribed. If patient receives adequate amounts of other anticonvulsant drugs, felbamate may be stopped without tapering, if needed.

• **WARNING** Assess for signs of aplastic anemia and bone marrow depression, which may occur with felbamate use. Signs may not appear until several months after therapy begins. Expect to stop felbamate therapy if bone marrow depression develops.

• If patient receives adjunctive therapy, expect adverse reactions to resolve as other anticonvulsant dosages decrease.

PATIENT TEACHING
•Direct patient to shake suspension before using and to use a calibrated spoon or container to measure each dose.
•Instruct patient to store felbamate oral suspension and tablets at room temperature.
•Because drug may cause photosensitivity, urge patient to protect her skin from sun and to avoid sunlamps and tanning booths.
•Inform patient that dizziness and drowsiness may occur. Advise her to avoid hazardous activities until drug's CNS effects are known.
•Warn patient not to stop drug abruptly.
•Advise patient to return for ordered liver function tests and to report yellow skin or eyes and dark urine to prescriber.
•Instruct patient to tell prescriber if she experiences bleeding, infection, or fatigue.
•Advise patient to carry medical identification that indicates her condition and therapy.
•Because felbamate decreases oral contraceptive effectiveness, discuss alternate contraceptive methods.

felodipine

Plendil, Renedil (CAN)

Class and Category
Chemical class: Dihydropyridine derivative
Therapeutic class: Antihypertensive
Pregnancy category: C

Indications and Dosages
➤ *To manage essential hypertension alone or with other antihypertensives*

E.R. TABLETS
Adults. *Initial:* 5 mg daily. Dosage adjusted every 2 wk to 2.5 to 10 mg daily based on patient response.
DOSAGE ADJUSTMENT Initial or maintenance dosage reduced, if needed, in patients who are over age 65 or have impaired hepatic function.

Route	Onset	Peak	Duration
P.O.	2 to 5 hr	Unknown	16 to 24 hr

Contraindications
Hypersensitivity to felodipine or its components

Mechanism of Action
May slow the movement of extracellular calcium into myocardial and vascular smooth-muscle cells by deforming calcium channels in cell membranes, inhibiting ion-controlled gating mechanisms, and interfering with calcium release from the sarcoplasmic reticulum. The effect of these actions is a decrease in intracellular calcium ions, which inhibits contraction of smooth-muscle cells and dilates coronary and systemic arteries. As with other calcium channel blockers, felodipine's actions result in increased oxygen to the myocardium and reduced peripheral resistance, blood pressure, and afterload.

Interactions
DRUGS
anesthetics (hydrocarbon inhalation): Possibly hypotension
antihypertensives, prazocin: Increased risk of hypotension
beta blockers: Increased adverse effects of beta blockers
cimetidine: Increased felodipine bioavailability
digoxin: Transiently increased blood digoxin level and risk of digitalis toxicity
estrogens: Possibly increased fluid retention and decreased felodipine effects
lithium: Increased risk of neurotoxicity
NSAIDs, sympathomimetics: Possibly decreased therapeutic effect of felodipine
procainamide, quinidine: Increased risk of prolonged Q-T interval
tacrolimus: Possibly increased blood tacrolimus level and risk of adverse effects
FOODS
grapefruit juice: Doubled felodipine bioavailability

Adverse Reactions
CNS: Asthenia, dizziness, drowsiness, fatigue, headache, paresthesia, syncope, weakness
CV: Chest pain, hypotension, palpitations, peripheral edema, tachycardia
EENT: Gingival hyperplasia, pharyngitis, rhinitis
GI: Abdominal cramps, constipation, diarrhea, indigestion, nausea
HEME: Agranulocytosis
MS: Back pain
RESP: Cough

SKIN: Flushing, rash

Nursing Considerations
•Use felodipine cautiously in patients with heart failure or reduced ventricular function.
•Monitor blood pressure during dosage titration and throughout felodipine therapy, especially in elderly patients.
•Felodipine bioavailability increases up to twofold when taken with grapefruit juice.
•**WARNING** Be aware that felodipine may cause severe hypotension with syncope, which may lead to reflex tachycardia. This can precipitate angina in patients with coronary artery disease or a history of angina.
•Monitor for signs of overdose, such as excessive peripheral vasodilation, marked hypotension and, possibly, bradycardia. If they appear, place patient in supine position with legs elevated and give I.V. fluids, as ordered. Expect to give I.V. atropine for bradycardia.

PATIENT TEACHING
•Instruct patient to swallow tablets whole and not to crush or chew them.
•Caution patient not to alter her intake of grapefruit juice during therapy.
•Advise patient to store felodipine at room temperature and to protect it from light.
•Instruct patient to monitor her pulse rate and blood pressure.
•Teach patient how to minimize gingival hyperplasia.
•Advise patient to notify prescriber immediately if she has palpitations, pronounced dizziness, or swelling of hands or feet.

fenofibrate
Tricor

fenofibric acid
Trilipix

Class and Category
Chemical class: Aryloxisobutyric acid derivative
Therapeutic class: Antihyperlipidemic
Pregnancy category: C

Indications and Dosages
➤ *To treat primary hypercholesterolemia or mixed hyperlipidemia*
CAPSULES
Adults. 200 mg daily.

TABLETS
Adults. 145 mg daily.

➤ *To treat hypertriglyceridemia (Fredrickson types IV and V hyperlipidemia)*
CAPSULES
Adults. *Initial:* 67 mg daily with food, increased as needed every 4 to 8 wk. *Maximum:* 201 mg daily with meals.
TABLETS
Adults. 48 to 145 mg daily, increased as needed at 4- to 8-wk intervals. *Maximum:* 145 mg daily.
DOSAGE ADJUSTMENT For patients with mild to moderate renal impairment, initial dosage limited to 48 mg daily (tablets) or 67 mg daily (capsules), with dosage increase only after drug's therapeutic and renal effects are known. For elderly patients, dosage limited to 48 mg daily (tablets) or 67 mg daily (capsules).

➤ *As adjunct to diet to treat severe hypertriglyceridemia*
DELAYED-RELEASE CAPSULES
Adults. *Initial:* 45 mg once daily, increased, as needed every 4- to 8-wk intervals. *Maximum:* 135 mg daily.

➤ *As adjunct to diet to treat primary hyperlipidemia or mixed dyslipidemia; as adjunct to diet and a HMG-CoA reducatse inhibitor to treat mixed dyslipidemia*
DELAYED-RELEASE CAPSULES
Adults. 135 mg daily.
DOSAGE ADJUSTMENT For patients with mild to moderate renal impairment or elderly patients, initial dosage limited to 45 mg once daily, with dosage increase only after drug's therapeutic and renal effects are known.

Route	Onset	Peak	Duration
P.O.	6 to 8 wk	Unknown	Unknown

Contraindications
Breast-feeding; gallbladder disease; hypersensitivity to fenofibrate, fenofibric acid, choline fenofibrate, or their components; hepatic or severe renal impairment

Interactions
DRUGS
bile acid sequestrants: Decreased fenofibrate absorption

cyclosporine: Increased risk of nephrotoxicity

HMG-CoA reductase inhibitors (atorvastatin, cerivastatin, fluvastatin, lovastatin, pravastatin, simvastatin): Increased risk of myopathy, rhabdomyolysis, and acute renal failure

oral anticoagulants: Increased risk of bleeding

FOODS

all foods: Increased fenofibrate bioavailability when given in capsule form

Mechanism of Action

May increase the lipolysis of triglyceride-rich lipoproteins and decrease the synthesis of fatty acids and triglycerides by enhancing the activation of lipoprotein lipase and acyl-coenzyme A synthetase. Fenofibrate also may:
• increase hepatic elimination of cholesterol as bile salts
• promote the catabolism of larger, less dense LDLs with a high-binding affinity for cellular LDL receptors.

Adverse Reactions

CNS: Asthenia, fatigue, headache
CV: Deep vein thrombosis
EENT: Rhinitis
GI: Abdominal pain, cholelithiasis, cirrhosis, constipation, diarrhea, elevated liver function test results, hepatitis, nausea, pancreatitis
GU: Increased serum creatinine level, renal failure
HEME: Agranulocytosis, anemia, decreased hematocrit and hemoglobin levels, thrombocytopenia
MS: Arthralgia, back pain, muscle spasms, myopathy. myositis, rhabdomyolysis
RESP: Pulmonary embolus
SKIN: Rash, Stevens-Johnson syndrome, toxic epidermal necrolysis, urticaria
Other: Flulike symptoms

Nursing Considerations

• As ordered, stop drugs that increase serum triglycerides, such as beta blockers, estrogens, and thiazides, and obtain baseline lipid levels before starting fenofibrate.
• Give capsule form with a full glass of water with meals.
• Administer drug 1 hour before or 4 hours after bile acid sequestrants.

• Monitor results of liver and renal function tests. If liver enzyme levels rise to more than three times the upper limit of normal and persist, or if the patient develops gallstones, expect to stop drug.
• Monitor serum triglyceride and cholesterol levels at 4- to 8-week intervals. If levels don't decrease after 2 months at maximum dosage, expect to stop therapy.
• **WARNING** Monitor patient closely for acute hypersensitivity reactions, including severe rash, and notify prescriber if they occur. Patient may need inpatient corticosteroids.
• Assess blood counts periodically, as ordered, during the first 12 months of therapy to detect adverse hematologic effects.

PATIENT TEACHING

• Stress that drug will be effective only if patient carefully follows prescriber's instructions about diet and exercise.
• Instruct patient to take capsule form with a full glass of water and with food.
• Instruct patient prescribed tablet form to store the tablets in their original, desiccant-containing bottle and to avoid taking any chipped or broken tablets.
• Advise patient to have laboratory tests, as directed, to determine drug's effectiveness. They typically include liver function tests after 3 to 6 months, hematocrit and hemoglobin levels, and WBC counts periodically during first year.
• Urge patient to notify prescriber immediately about chills, fever, or sore throat. Also urge her to tell prescriber about unexplained muscle pain, tenderness, or weakness, especially if accompanied by fatigue or fever.

fenoldopam mesylate

Corlopam

Class and Category

Chemical class: Dopamine agonist
Therapeutic class: Antihypertensive
Pregnancy category: B

Indications and Dosages

➤ *To treat severe hypertension when rapid, but quickly reversible, emergency reduction of blood pressure is clinically indicated, including malignant hypertension with deteriorating end-organ function*

E
F

I.V. INFUSION
Adults. *Initial:* 0.025 to 0.3 mcg/kg/min, individualized according to patient weight and desired effect. *Usual:* 0.01 to 1.6 mcg/kg/min. *Maximum:* 1.6 mcg/kg/min for up to 48 hr.

Route	Onset	Peak	Duration
I.V.	Rapid	Unknown	Unknown

Mechanism of Action
Stimulates dopamine-1 postsynaptic receptors, which mediate renal and mesenteric vasodilation. Vasodilation lowers blood pressure and total peripheral resistance while increasing renal blood flow.

Contraindications
Hypersensitivity to fenoldopam or its components

Interactions
DRUGS
antihypertensives: Additive hypotensive effect
beta blockers: Increased risk of hypotension
dopamine antagonists, metoclopramide: Possibly decreased effects of fenoldopam

Adverse Reactions
CNS: Anxiety, headache, light-headedness
CV: Hypotension, ST- and T-wave changes, tachycardia
EENT: Increased intraocular pressure
GI: Abdominal pain, nausea
SKIN: Diaphoresis, flushing
Other: Hypokalemia, injection site pain

Nursing Considerations
•Reconstitute by adding 40 mg fenoldopam (4 ml of concentrate) to 1,000 ml normal saline solution or D₅W, or 20 mg fenoldopam (2 ml of concentrate) to 500 ml normal saline solution or D₅W, or 10 mg fenoldopam (1 ml of concentrate) to 250 ml normal saline solution or D₅W to produce a final fenoldopam concentration of 40 mcg/ml.
•Infuse through a mechanical infusion pump for proper control of infusion rate.
•Expect to titrate fenoldopam dosage in increments of 0.05 to 0.1 mcg/kg/min, as prescribed.
•Expect to monitor heart rate and blood pressure every 15 minutes during therapy because most effect on blood pressure occurs within 15 minutes of any dosage change.

•Be aware that patient may be started on oral antihypertensive therapy, as prescribed, any time after blood pressure is stable during fenoldopam infusion.
•Discard any reconstituted solution not used within 24 hours.
•**WARNING** Assess patient for signs of increased myocardial oxygen demand, especially if patient has heart failure or a history of angina, because fenoldopam may produce a rapid decline in blood pressure, resulting in symptomatic hypotension and a dose-dependent increase in heart rate.
•Monitor serum potassium level because fenoldopam decreases serum potassium concentrations, which may result in hypokalemia, exacerbate arrhythmias, or precipitate conduction abnormalities, especially in patients with cardiac disease.
•Monitor patients with glaucoma or increased intraocular pressure for changes in vision because drug may cause a dose-dependent increase in intraocular pressure.
•Be alert for possible allergic- or anaphylactic-type reaction to sodium metabisulfite, a component of fenoldopam injection, especially in patients with asthma.

PATIENT TEACHING
•Inform patient that she'll be switched to an oral antihypertensive once her blood pressure is controlled.
•Instruct patient to expect frequent monitoring of vital signs.

fenoprofen calcium

Nalfon

Class and Category
Chemical class: Propionic acid derivative
Therapeutic class: Analgesic, anti-inflammatory, antirheumatic
Pregnancy category: Not rated

Indications and Dosages
➤ *To manage mild to moderate pain*
CAPSULES, TABLETS
Adults. 200 mg every 4 to 6 hr, as needed.

➤ *To relieve pain, stiffness, and swelling from rheumatoid arthritis or osteoarthritis*
CAPSULES, TABLETS
Adults. 300 to 600 mg t.i.d. or q.i.d. *Maximum:* 3,200 mg daily.

Route	Onset	Peak	Duration
P.O.	15 to 30 min*	Unknown†	4 to 6 hr‡

Mechanism of Action

Blocks the activity of cyclooxygenase, the enzyme needed for prostaglandin synthesis. Prostaglandins, important mediators of the inflammatory response, cause local vasodilation with swelling and pain. When cyclooxygenase is blocked and prostaglandins inhibited, inflammatory symptoms subside. Prostaglandin inhibition also relieves pain because prostaglandins play a role in pain transmission from the periphery to the spinal cord.

Contraindications

Angioedema, asthma, bronchospasm, nasal polyps, rhinitis, or urticaria induced by aspirin, iodides, or NSAIDs; hypersensitivity to fenoprofen or its components; renal impairment; severe hepatic impairment

Interactions

DRUGS

acetaminophen: Increased risk of renal impairment with concurrent long-term use
antacids: Decreased fenoprofen effectiveness
anticoagulants, cefamandole, cefoperazone, cefotetan, heparin, plicamycin, thrombolytics, valproic acid: Increased risk of bleeding
antineoplastics: Increased adverse hematologic effects
cyclosporine: Increased risk of nephrotoxicity
diuretics, triamterene: Decreased effectiveness of these drugs
glucocorticoids, NSAIDs, potassium supplements: Increased adverse GI effects
insulin, oral antidiabetic drugs: Increased risk of hypoglycemia
lithium: Increased risk of lithium toxicity
methotrexate: Increased risk of methotrexate toxicity
phenobarbital: Possibly decreased elimination half-life of fenoprofen

---

* For analgesia; 2 days for antirheumatic effects.
† For analgesia; 2 to 3 wk for antirheumatic effects.
‡ For analgesia; unknown for antirheumatic effects.

salicylates: Increased risk of GI bleeding

ACTIVITIES

alcohol use, smoking: Increased risk of GI bleeding

Adverse Reactions

CNS: Agitation, confusion, dizziness, drowsiness, headache, seizures, sleep disturbance, stroke, tremor, weakness
CV: Hypertension, MI, palpitations, peripheral edema, tachycardia, vasodilation
EENT: Blurred vision, dry or sore mouth, hearing loss, tinnitus
GI: Abdominal cramps, distention, and pain; anorexia; constipation; diarrhea; diverticulitis; dysphagia; esophagitis; flatulence; gastritis; gastroenteritis; gastroesophageal reflux disease; GI bleeding or ulceration; hemorrhoids; hepatitis; hiatal hernia; indigestion; jaundice; liver failure; melena; nausea; perforation of stomach or intestines; vomiting
GU: Acute renal failure, dysuria, interstitial nephritis
HEME: Agranulocytosis, anemia, hemolytic anemia, leukopenia, neutropenia, pancytopenia
MS: Muscle spasms and twitching, myalgia
RESP: Dyspnea
SKIN: Diaphoresis, erythema, erythema multiforme, exfoliative dermatitis, pruritus, Stevens-Johnson syndrome, toxic epidermal necrolysis, urticaria
Other: Anaphylaxis, angioedema

Nursing Considerations

•Use fenoprofen with extreme caution in patients with a history of ulcer disease or GI bleeding because NSAIDs such as fenoprofen increase the risk of GI bleeding and ulceration. Expect to use fenoprofen for the shortest time possible in these patients.
•Be aware that serious GI tract ulceration, bleeding, and perforation may occur without warning symptoms. Elderly patients are at greater risk. To minimize risk, give drug with food. If GI distress occurs, withhold drug and notify prescriber immediately.
•Use fenoprofen cautiously in patients with hypertension, and monitor blood pressure closely throughout therapy. Drug may cause hypertension or worsen it.
•Give drug with food, milk, or antacids to decrease adverse GI reactions.
•WARNING If patient receives long-term therapy, watch for signs of toxicity, such as agi-

E
F

tation; blurred vision; coma; confusion; drowsiness; elevated BUN and serum creatinine levels; indigestion; nausea; rash; seizures; severe headache; slow, labored breathing; tinnitus; and vomiting.

•**WARNING** Monitor patient closely for thrombotic events, including MI and stroke, because NSAIDs increase the risk.

•**WARNING** If patient has bone marrow suppression or is receiving antineoplastic drug therapy, monitor laboratory results (including WBC count), and watch for evidence of infection because anti-inflammatory and antipyretic actions of fenoprofen may mask signs and symptoms of infection, such as fever and pain.

•Monitor patient—especially if she's elderly or receiving long-term fenoprofen therapy—for less common but serious adverse GI reactions, including anorexia, constipation, diverticulitis, dysphagia, esophagitis, gastritis, gastroenteritis, gastroesophageal reflux disease, hemorrhoids, hiatal hernia, melena, stomatitis, and vomiting.

•Monitor patient's liver function test results because, in rare cases, elevations may progress to severe hepatic reactions, including fatal hepatitis, liver necrosis, and hepatic failure.

•Monitor BUN and serum creatinine levels in elderly patients, patients taking diuretics or ACE inhibitors, and patients with heart failure, impaired renal function, or hepatic dysfunction because drug may cause renal failure.

•Monitor CBC for decreased hemoglobin and hematocrit because drug may worsen anemia.

•Assess patient's skin regularly for signs of rash or other hypersensitivity reaction because fenoprofen is an NSAID and may cause serious skin reactions without warning, even in patients with no history of NSAID sensitivity. At first sign of reaction, stop drug and notify prescriber.

PATIENT TEACHING

•Advise patient to take fenoprofen with food, milk, or antacids to minimize GI distress. Also instruct her to take drug with a full glass of water and to stay upright for 30 minutes afterward to decrease the risk of drug lodging in the esophagus and causing irritation.

•Instruct patient to swallow drug whole and not to crush, break, chew, or open capsules.

•Caution patient to avoid alcohol, aspirin, and other NSAIDs, unless prescribed, while taking fenoprofen.

•If patient takes an anticoagulant, urge her to immediately report bleeding, including bloody or tarry stools and bloody vomitus.

•Caution patient to avoid potentially hazardous activities until drug's CNS effects are known.

•Explain that NSAIDs may increase the risk of serious adverse cardiovascular reactions; urge patient to seek immediate medical attention if signs or symptoms arise, such as chest pain, shortness of breath, weakness, and slurring of speech.

•Explain that fenoprofen also may increase the risk of serious adverse GI reactions; stress the importance of seeking immediate medical attention for such signs and symptoms as epigastric or abdominal pain, indigestion, black or tarry stools, or vomiting blood or material that looks like coffee grounds.

•Alert patient to the possibility of rare but serious skin reactions. Urge her to seek immediate medical attention for rash, blisters, itching, fever, or other indications of hypersensitivity.

fentanyl citrate
Actiq, Sublimaze

fentanyl transdermal system
Duragesic

fentanyl iontophoretic transdermal
Ionsys

Class, Category, and Schedule
Chemical class: Opioid, phenylpiperidine derivative
Therapeutic class: Analgesic, anesthesia adjunct
Pregnancy category: C
Controlled substance schedule: II

Indications and Dosages
➤ *To provide surgical premedication*
I.M. INJECTION

Adults. 0.05 to 0.1 mg 30 to 60 min before surgery.

➤ *As adjunct to regional anesthesia*
I.V. OR I.M. INJECTION
Adults. 0.05 to 0.1 mg I.M. or slow I.V. over 1 to 2 min.

➤ *To manage postoperative pain in post-anesthesia care unit*
I.M. INJECTION
Adults. 0.05 to 0.1 mg. Repeated in 1 to 2 hr, if needed.

➤ *To manage acute postoperative pain in hospitalized patients requiring opioid analgesia*
IONTOPHORETIC TRANSDERMAL
Adults. 40 mg on-demand, released over 10 min. *Maximum:* Six 40-mcg doses/hour and eighty 40-mcg doses/24 hours for maximum of 72 hours.

➤ *To treat breakthrough pain in cancer patients who are receiving opioid therapy and have developed tolerance to it*
TRANSMUCOSAL LOZENGE
Adults. *Initial:* 200 mcg placed between cheek and gum for up to 15 min followed by second dose 15 min after first dose ends, if needed. Dosage increased according to patient's needs.

➤ *To relieve persistent moderate to severe chronic pain that doesn't respond to less potent drugs and requires around-the-clock opioid administration for an extended time*
TRANSDERMAL SYSTEM
Adults and children age 2 and over. *Initial:* One 25-mcg/hr patch, replaced every 72 hr (or 48 hr, if needed). Dosage increased by 12.5 mcg/hr, as needed, after first 72 hr and then every 6 days. For more than 100 mcg/hr, more than one patch is used.

DOSAGE ADJUSTMENT For elderly, cachectic, or debilitated patients, initial dosage should not exceed 25 mcg/hr unless patient is already receiving more than 135 mg of oral morphine daily or an equivalent dose of another opioid. For patients receiving long-term opioid therapy, dosage adjusted based on previous day's drug requirement. For cancer patients who need more than 800 mcg/day for breakthrough pain, dosage altered or another long-acting opioid given, as prescribed.

Route	Onset	Peak	Duration
I.V.	1 to 2 min	3 to 5 min	30 to 60 min
I.M.	7 to 15 min	20 to 30 min	1 to 2 hr
Trans-dermal	12 to 24 hr	Unknown	Over 72 hr

Mechanism of Action
Binds to opioid receptor sites in the CNS, altering perception of and emotional response to pain by inhibiting ascending pain pathways. Fentanyl may alter neurotransmitter release from afferent nerves responsive to painful stimuli, and it causes respiratory depression by acting directly on respiratory centers in the brain stem.

Contraindications
I.V. or I.M. form: Under age 2, asthma, myasthenia gravis, opioid hypersensitivity or intolerance, significant respiratory depression, upper airway obstruction; *transmucosal form:* acute or chronic pain, body weight less than 10 kg (22 lb), doses above 5 mcg/kg in adults or 15 mcg/kg in children; *transdermal form:* acute or postoperative pain, under age 12 (under age 18 if weight is less than 50 kg [110 lb]), dosage that exceeds 25 mcg/hr at the start of therapy, hypersensitivity to fentanyl (or alfentanil, sufentanil, or adhesives), intermittent pain, treatment of mild to moderate pain responsive to nonopioid drugs

Interactions
DRUGS
amiodarone, amprenavir, aprepitant, clarithromycin, diltiazem, erythromycin, fluconazole, fosamprenavir, itraconazole, ketoconazole, nefazodone, nelfinavir, ritonavir, troleandomycin, verapamil: Possibly increased opioid effect, leading to increased or prolonged adverse effects, including severe respiratory depression
anticholinergics, antidiarrheals (such as loperamide and paregoric): Increased risk of severe constipation
antihypertensives, diuretics: Possibly potentiated hypotension
benzodiazepines: Possibly reduced fentanyl dose required for anesthesia induction
buprenorphine: Possibly decreased therapeu-

tic effects of buprenorphine
CNS depressants: Possibly increased CNS and respiratory depression and hypotension
cytochrome P-450 inducers (such as rifampin, carbamazepine, and phenytoin): Possibly induced metabolism and increased clearance of fentanyl
hydroxyzine: Possibly increased analgesic effect of fentanyl and increased CNS depression and hypotension
MAO inhibitors: Possibly unpredictable, even fatal, effects if taken within 14 days of fentanyl
metoclopramide: Possibly antagonized effect of metoclopramide on gastric motility
nalbuphine, pentazocine: Possibly antagonized analgesic, respiratory depressant, and CNS depressant effects of fentanyl; possibly additive hypotensive and CNS and respiratory depressant effects of both drugs
naloxone: Antagonized analgesic, hypotensive, CNS, and respiratory depressant effects of fentanyl
naltrexone: Possibly blocked therapeutic effects of fentanyl
neuromuscular blockers: Possibly prevention or reversal of muscle rigidity by fentanyl

ACTIVITIES
alcohol use: Increased CNS and respiratory depression and hypotension

FOODS
grapefruit juice: Increased blood fentanyl level

Adverse Reactions

CNS: Agitation, amnesia, anxiety, asthenia, ataxia, confusion, delusions, depression, dizziness, drowsiness, euphoria, fever, hallucinations, headache, lack of coordination, light-headedness, nervousness, paranoia, sedation, seizures, sleep disturbance, slurred speech, syncope, tremor, weakness, yawning
CV: Asystole, bradycardia, chest pain, edema, hypotension, orthostatic hypotension, tachycardia
EENT: Blurred vision, dental caries, dry mouth, gum line erosion, laryngospasm, rhinitis, sneezing, tooth loss
GI: Anorexia, constipation, ileus, indigestion, nausea, vomiting
GU: Anorgasmia, decreased libido, ejaculatory difficulty, urinary hesitancy, urine retention
RESP: Apnea, depressed cough reflex, dyspnea, hypoventilation, respiratory depression
SKIN: Diaphoresis, exfoliative dermatitis, localized skin redness and swelling (with transdermal form), pruritus, rash
Other: Anaphylaxis, drug tolerance, physical or psychological dependence with long-term use, weight loss

Nursing Considerations

•**WARNING** Fentanyl transdermal system should be used only in patients already receiving opioid therapy and with demonstrated opioid tolerance (taking for a week or longer at least 60 mg of morphine daily, 30 mg of oral oxycodone daily, 8 mg of oral hydromorphone daily, or an equianalgesic dose of another opioid), and require at least a fentanyl dosage of 25 mcg per hour to manage their pain.
•Use caution when titrating fentanyl dosage in elderly patients, especially when using the intravenous route, because these patients are more sensitive to the drug's effects.
•Use cautiously in patients at increased risk for opioid abuse, such as those with a mental illness or a personal or family history of substance abuse. Monitor patient throughout therapy for fentanyl abuse or addiction.
•To reduce skin irritation, spray the allergy inhaler triamcinolone on the patient's skin, as prescribed, before applying a fentanyl patch.
•Expect the blood fentanyl level to be prolonged if patient chews or swallows the transmucosal form because drug is absorbed slowly from GI tract.
•**WARNING** Never apply a transdermal patch if the seal has been broken or patch has been cut, damaged, or changed in any way because excessive exposure could occur, resulting in a fentanyl overdose that could be fatal.
•Be aware that 100 mcg of fentanyl is equivalent in potency to 10 mg of morphine.
•To achieve optimum pain control with the lowest possible fentanyl dose, also plan to give a nonopioid analgesic, such as acetaminophen, as prescribed.
•**WARNING** Monitor patient's respiratory status closely, especially during the first 24 to 72 hours after therapy starts or dosage increases, because severe hypoventilation may occur without warning at any time during therapy.
•To prevent withdrawal symptoms after long-term use, expect to taper drug dosage

gradually, as prescribed.

•Assess patient for withdrawal symptoms after dosage reduction or conversion to another opioid analgesic.

•For patient with bradycardia, implement cardiac monitoring, as ordered, and assess heart rate and rhythm frequently during fentanyl therapy because drug may further slow heart rate.

•**WARNING** Expect respiratory depressant effects to last longer than analgesic effects. Also be prepared for residual drug to potentiate the effects of subsequent doses. Residual drug can be detected for at least 6 hours after I.V. dose and 17 hours after dose of other forms. Monitor patient closely for at least 24 hours after therapy ends.

•**WARNING** Assess patient for signs of overdose, such as cardiopulmonary arrest, hypoventilation, pupil constriction, respiratory and CNS depression, seizures, and shock. Give naloxone (possibly in repeated doses), as prescribed. Be prepared to assist with endotracheal intubation and mechanical ventilation and to provide fluids.

•Monitor the blood glucose level of diabetic patients who are receiving transdermal fentanyl because each unit contains about 2 g of sugar.

PATIENT TEACHING

•Instruct patient to avoid alcohol and other CNS depressants during fentanyl therapy unless prescribed.

•Advise patient not to stop taking drug unless directed by prescriber because withdrawal symptoms may occur. Warn against increasing dose or frequency without consulting prescriber because drug can cause dependency.

•For transdermal form, instruct patient to choose a site with intact (not irritated or irradiated) skin on a flat surface, such as the chest, back, flank, or upper arm, and, if appropriate, to clip, not shave, hair from the site and clean it with water (no soaps, lotions, oils, or alcohol). After site preparation, instruct patient to press patch firmly in place with palm for 30 seconds, making sure edges are sealed. If patch loosens, tell her to tape edges down but not cover the entire patch. If more than one patch is needed, the edges shouldn't touch or overlap. Instruct patient to remove patch after 72 hours, fold it in half with adhesive sides together, and flush it down the toilet. Remind her not to reuse a site for at least 3 days.

•Warn patient never to apply a fentanyl transdermal patch if the seal has been broken or the patch has been cut, damaged, or changed in any way because drug may be released too rapidly. Also warn patient not to expose the application site and surrounding area to direct external heat sources, such as heating pads or electric blankets, heat or tanning lamps, saunas, hot tubs, and heated water beds, while wearing the patch. She should also avoid hot baths or sunbathing because increased body temperature may increase fentanyl release, resulting in a possible overdose. If she develops a fever or becomes overheated from strenuous exercise while wearing a patch, she should contact the prescriber immediately.

•For iontophoretic transdermal form, instruct patient to press button twice firmly within 3 seconds to release a dose. An audible tone will sound when a dose is activated, and a red light will stay on throughout the 10-minute administration. Explain that no more than six doses can be given per hour and no more than 80 doses per 24 hours. Tell the patient that the patch may be replaced once 80 doses are released or 24 hours pass, but that 72 hours is the maximum time the drug can be delivered in this way.

•For transmucosal form, instruct patient to open the package just before use and to save plastic cap for discarding the unused part of the lozenge. Tell her to place lozenge between her cheek and gum and to suck, not chew, it for 15 minutes. Show her how to move lozenge from one side of her mouth to the other using the handle provided separately.

•For transmucosal form, urge patient to see a dentist regularly, to brush teeth and floss after each meal, and to avoid frequent consumption of products high in sugar because of an increased risk of dental caries.

•For transmucosal form, inform diabetic patient that each unit contains 2 g of sugar. Instruct her to monitor her blood glucose levels closely.

•Remind patient to keep used and unused dosage units out of reach of children and to dispose of drug properly. For buccal tablet form, patient should flush remaining drug down the toilet when no longer needed.

E
F

•Caution patient that accidentally exposing others to transdermal fentanyl could cause serious adverse reactions. If accidental exposure occurs, the person should remove the patch, wash the area well with water, and seek medical attention.
•Caution patient to avoid potentially hazardous activities until drug's CNS effects are known.
•Tell patient to increase fiber and fluid intake, unless contraindicated, because drug may cause severe constipation. If it persists or becomes severe, urge patient to notify prescriber.

ferrous salts

ferrous fumarate

(contains 100 mg of elemental iron per capsule or per 5 ml of oral suspension, 33 mg of elemental iron per chewable tablet or per 5 ml of oral suspension, 106 mg of elemental iron per E.R. capsule, 15 mg of elemental iron per 0.6 ml of oral solution, and 20 to 115 mg of elemental iron per tablet)

Femiron, Feostat, Feostat Drops, Ferretts, Fumasorb, Fumerin, Hemocyte, Ircon, Neo-Fer (CAN), Nephro-Fer, Novofumar (CAN), Palafer (CAN), Span-FF

ferrous gluconate

(contains 10 mg of elemental iron per capsule, 34 mg of elemental iron per 5 ml of elixir, 37 mg of elemental iron per E.R. tablet, 35 mg of elemental iron per 5 ml of syrup, and 34 to 38 mg of elemental iron per tablet)

Apo-Ferrous Gluconate (CAN), Fergon, Ferralet, Ferralet Slow Release, Fertinic (CAN), Novoferrogluc (CAN), Simron

ferrous sulfate

(contains 50 mg of elemental iron per capsule, 60 mg of elemental iron per dried capsule, 30 to 50 mg of elemental iron per dried E.R. capsule, 50 mg of elemental iron per dried E.R. tablet, 65 mg of elemental iron per dried tablet, 44 mg of elemental iron per 5 ml of elixir, 60 to 65 mg of elemental iron per enteric-coated tablet, 65 to 105 mg of elemental iron per E.R. tablet, 15 mg of elemental iron per 0.6 ml of oral solution, 18 mg of elemental iron per 0.5 ml of oral solution,

25 mg of elemental iron per ml of oral solution, 30 or 60 mg of elemental iron per 5 ml of oral solution, and 39 to 65 mg of elemental iron per tablet)

Apo-Ferrous Sulfate (CAN), Feosol, Feratab, Fer-gen-sol, Fer-In-Sol Capsules, Fer-In-Sol Drops, Fer-In-Sol Syrup, Fer-Iron Drops, Fero-Grad (CAN), Fero-Gradumet, Ferospace, Ferralyn Lanacaps, Ferra-TD, Mol-Iron, Novoferrosulfa (CAN), PMS-Ferrous Sulfate (CAN), Slow-Fe

iron, carbonyl

(contains 50 mg of elemental iron per caplet)

Feosol

Class and Category

Chemical class: Trace element, mineral
Therapeutic class: Antianemic, nutritional supplement
Pregnancy category: Not rated

Indications and Dosages

➤ *To prevent iron deficiency based on U.S. and Canadian recommended daily allowances*

CAPLETS, CAPSULES, CHEWABLE TABLETS, DRIED CAPSULES, DRIED E.R. CAPSULES, DRIED E.R. TABLETS, DRIED TABLETS, ELIXIR, ENTERIC-COATED TABLETS, E.R. CAPSULES, E.R. TABLETS, ORAL SOLUTION, ORAL SUSPENSION, SYRUP, TABLETS

Male adults and children age 11 and over. 10 mg (8 to 10 mg Canadian) elemental iron daily.
Female adults and children age 11 and over. 10 to 15 mg (8 to 13 mg Canadian) elemental iron daily.
Pregnant females. 30 mg (17 to 22 mg Canadian) elemental iron daily.
Breast-feeding females. 15 mg (8 to 13 mg Canadian) elemental iron daily.
Children ages 7 to 10. 10 mg (8 to 10 mg Canadian) elemental iron daily.
Children ages 4 to 6. 10 mg (8 mg Canadian) elemental iron daily.
Children from birth to age 3. 6 to 10 mg (0.3 to 6 mg Canadian) elemental iron daily.

➤ *To replace iron in deficiency states*
CAPLETS, CAPSULES, CHEWABLE TABLETS, DRIED CAPSULES, DRIED E.R. CAPSULES, DRIED E.R. TABLETS, DRIED TABLETS, ELIXIR, ENTERIC-COATED TABLETS, E.R. CAPSULES, E.R. TABLETS, ORAL SOLUTION, ORAL

SUSPENSION, SYRUP, TABLETS
Adults and adolescents. 100 to 200 mg elemental iron t.i.d. for 4 to 6 mo.
Children ages 2 to 12 weighing 30 to 50 kg (66 to 110 lb). 50 to 100 mg elemental iron daily in divided doses t.i.d. or q.i.d. for 4 to 6 mo.
Children ages 6 months to 2 years. Up to 6 mg/kg elemental iron daily in divided doses t.i.d. or q.i.d. for 4 to 6 mo.
Infants under age 6 months. 10 to 25 mg elemental iron daily in divided doses t.i.d. or q.i.d. for 4 to 6 mo.

➤ *To provide iron supplementation during pregnancy*
CAPLETS, CAPSULES, CHEWABLE TABLETS, DRIED CAPSULES, DRIED E.R. CAPSULES, DRIED E.R. TABLETS, DRIED TABLETS, ELIXIR, ENTERIC-COATED TABLETS, E.R. CAPSULES, E.R. TABLETS, ORAL SOLUTION, ORAL SUSPENSION, SYRUP, TABLETS
Pregnant females. 15 to 30 mg elemental iron daily during second and third trimesters.
DOSAGE ADJUSTMENT Dosage increased if needed for elderly patients, who may not absorb iron as easily as younger adults do.

Mechanism of Action
Acts to normalize RBC production by binding with hemoglobin or by being oxidized and stored as hemosiderin or aggregated ferritin in reticuloendothelial cells of the liver, spleen, and bone marrow. Iron is an essential component of hemoglobin, myoglobin, and several enzymes, including cytochromes, catalase, and peroxidase. Iron is needed for catecholamine metabolism and normal neutrophil function.

Contraindications
Hemochromatosis, hemolytic anemias, hemosiderosis, hypersensitivity to iron salts or their components, other anemic conditions unless accompanied by iron deficiency

Interactions
DRUGS
acetohydroxamic acid: Reduced absorption of both drugs
antacids, calcium supplements: Decreased iron absorption and effectiveness
ascorbic acid (with doses of 200 mg or more): Increased iron absorption

cholestyramine, cimetidine: Decreased iron absorption
ciprofloxacin, enoxacin, etidronate, lomefloxacin, norfloxacin, ofloxacin, oral tetracyclines: Decreased effectiveness of these drugs
dimercaprol: Possibly combination with iron in body to form a harmful chemical
levodopa: Possibly chelation with iron, decreasing levodopa absorption and blood level
levothyroxine: Decreased levothyroxine effectiveness and, possibly, hypothyroidism
methyldopa: Decreased methyldopa absorption and efficacy
penicillamine: Decreased penicillamine absorption because penicillamine chelates heavy metals
vitamin E: Decreased vitamin E absorption
FOODS
coffee; eggs; foods that contain bicarbonates, carbonates, oxalates, or phosphates; milk and milk products; tea that contains tannic acid; whole-grain breads and cereals and other high-fiber foods: Decreased iron absorption and effectiveness
ACTIVITIES
alcohol abuse (acute or chronic): Increased serum iron level

Adverse Reactions
CNS: Dizziness, fever, headache, paresthesia, syncope
CV: Chest pain, tachycardia
EENT: Metallic taste, tooth discoloration
GI: Abdominal cramps, constipation, epigastric pain, nausea, stool discoloration, vomiting
HEME: Hemochromatosis, hemolysis, hemosiderosis
RESP: Dyspnea
SKIN: Diaphoresis, flushing, rash, urticaria

Nursing Considerations
•Give iron tablets and capsules with a full glass of water or juice. Don't crush enteric-coated tablets or open capsules.
•Because iron solutions may stain teeth, dilute and administer with a straw or place drops in back of patient's throat. Mix the elixir form in water. Fer-In-Sol Drops or Syrup may be mixed with water or juice.
•To maximize absorption, give iron salts 1 hour before or 2 hours after meals. If GI irritation occurs, give with or just after meals.

E
F

•Protect liquid form from freezing.

•Be aware that at usual dosages, serum hemoglobin level usually normalizes in about 2 months unless blood loss continues. Treatment lasts for 3 to 6 months to help replenish iron stores.

•**WARNING** Monitor patient for signs of iron overdose, which may include abdominal pain, diarrhea (possibly bloody), nausea, severe vomiting, and sharp abdominal cramps. In case of iron toxicity or accidental iron overdose (a leading cause of fatal poisoning in children under age 6), give deferoxamine, as prescribed. As few as 3 adult iron tablets can cause serious poisoning in young children.

•Don't give antacids, coffee, tea, dairy products, eggs, or whole-grain cereals or breads within 1 hour before or 2 hours after iron.

•Remember that unabsorbed iron turns stool green or black and can mask blood in stool. Check stool for occult blood, as ordered.

PATIENT TEACHING

•Instruct patient not to chew any solid dosage form of iron except for chewable tablets.

•Inform patient that iron deficiency may cause decreased stamina, learning problems, shortness of breath, and tiredness.

•To improve iron absorption, encourage patient to eat lean red meat, chicken, turkey, and fish as well as foods rich in vitamin C (such as citrus fruits and fresh vegetables).

•Urge patient to avoid foods that impair iron absorption, including dairy products, eggs, spinach, and high-fiber foods, such as whole-grain breads and cereals and bran. Also advise her to avoid drinking coffee or tea within 1 hour of iron intake.

•Caution patient not to take antacids or calcium supplements within 1 hour before and 2 hours after taking iron supplement.

•Inform patient that her stool should become dark green or black during therapy. Advise her to notify prescriber if it doesn't.

•To minimize tooth stains from liquid iron, instruct patient to mix each dose with water, fruit juice, or tomato juice and to drink it with a straw. When patient must take liquid iron by dropper, direct her to place drops well back on the tongue and to follow with water or juice. Inform patient that iron stains can be removed by brushing with baking soda (sodium bicarbonate) or medicinal peroxide (hydrogen peroxide 3%).

•Advise patient to consult prescriber before taking large amounts of iron for longer than 6 months.

•Warn patient about the high risk of accidental poisoning, and urge her to keep iron preparations out of the reach of children.

fesoterodine fumarate

Toviaz

Class and Category

Chemical class: Muscarinic receptor antagonist

Therapeutic class: Antispasmodic

Pregnancy category: C

Indications and Dosages

➤ *To treat overactive bladder with symptoms of urinary incontinence, urgency, and frequency*

E.R. TABLETS

Adults. *Initial:* 4 mg daily, increased to 8 mg, as needed. *Maximum:* 8 mg daily.

DOSAGE ADJUSTMENT For patients with severe renal insufficiency or who are taking potent CYP3A4 inhibitors (such as clarithromycin, itraconazole, and ketoconazole), dosage shouldn't exceed 4 mg daily.

Route	Onset	Peak	Duration
P.O.	Unknown	5 hr	Unknown

Mechanism of Action

Exerts antimuscarinic (atropine-like) and potent direct antispasmodic (papaverine-like) actions on smooth muscle in the bladder. The result is increased bladder capacity and a decreased urge to void. Fesoterodine has an active metabolite that inhibits bladder contraction and decreases detrussor pressure.

Contraindications

Gastric retention, GI obstruction, hypersensitivity to fesoterodine or its components, ileus, pyloric stenosis, uncontrolled narrow-angle glaucoma, urine retention

Interactions

DRUGS

antimuscarinic agents: Possibly increased anticholinergic effects; possibly altered absorption of oral drugs taken concurrently potent CYP3A4 inhibitors, such as clar-ithromycin, itraconazole, ketoconazole: Possibly increased serum fesoterodine level and increased risk of adverse effects

FOODS

caffeine: May aggravate bladder symptoms

ACTIVITIES

alcohol use: Increased drowsiness

Adverse Reactions

CNS: Drowsiness, insomnia
CV: Angina, chest pain, peripheral edema, QT-interval prolongation
EENT: Blurred vision; dry eyes, mouth, or throat
GI: Constipation, diverticulitis, dyspepsia, elevated liver enzymes, gastroenteritis, irritable bowel syndrome, nausea, upper abdominal pain
GU: Dysuria, urine retention, UTI
MS: Back pain
RESP: Cough, upper respiratory tract infection
SKIN: Decreased sweating, rash

Nursing Considerations

• Use cautiously in patients with significant bladder outlet obstruction because fesoterodine can cause urine retention.
• Use cautiously in patients with myasthenia gravis, decreased GI motility, and controlled narrow-angle glaucoma because fesoterodine can make these conditions worse.
• Use cautiously in patients taking other drugs with anticholinergic effects, such as antihistamines.

PATIENT TEACHING

• Instruct patient to take drug exactly as prescribed.
• Tell patient to take drug with a full glass of water and not to cut, crush, or chew the tablets.
• Alert patient that drug can cause adverse effects such as constipation and urine retention. If adverse effects occur and are severe or prolonged, patient should notify prescriber.
• Advise patient to avoid alcohol consumption during fesoterodine therapy.
• Tell patient to avoid hazardous activities until drug's CNS effects are known.
• Caution patient to avoid strenuous exercise and excessive sun exposure because of increased risk of heatstroke.
• Advise patient to limit caffeine consump-

tion during drug therapy.
• Explain that full benefits of fesoterodine therapy may take 2 to 3 months.
• Inform patient that chewing sugarless gum or sucking hard candy (especially lemon drops) may help ease dry mouth.

filgrastim

(granulocyte colony-stimulating factor, rG-CSF)

Neupogen

Class and Category

Chemical class: Granulocyte colony-stimulating factor
Therapeutic class: Antineutropenic, hematopoietic stimulator
Pregnancy category: C

Indications and Dosages

➤ To prevent infection after myelosuppressive chemotherapy

I.V. INFUSION

Adults. 5 mcg/kg daily over 15 to 30 min. Increased, if needed, by 5 mcg/kg with each chemotherapy cycle.

SUBCUTANEOUS INJECTION

Adults. 5 mcg/kg daily for up to 2 wk. Increased, if needed, by 5 mcg/kg with each chemotherapy cycle.

➤ To reduce the duration of neutropenia after bone marrow transplantation

I.V. INFUSION

Adults. 10 mcg/kg daily over 4 hr or as a continuous infusion over 24 hr.

SUBCUTANEOUS INFUSION

Adults. 10 mcg/kg as a continuous infusion over 24 hr.

➤ To enhance peripheral blood progenitor cell collection in autologous hematopoietic stem cell transplantation

SUBCUTANEOUS INFUSION OR INJECTION

Adults. 10 mcg/kg as continuous infusion over 24 hr or a single injection, beginning 4 days before first leukapheresis and continuing until last day of leukapheresis.

➤ To reduce the occurrence and duration of neutropenia in congenital neutropenia

SUBCUTANEOUS INJECTION

Adults. 6 mcg/kg b.i.d.

E
F

➤ *To reduce the occurrence and duration of neutropenia in idiopathic or cyclic neutropenia*

SUBCUTANEOUS INJECTION

Adults. 5 mcg/kg daily.

DOSAGE ADJUSTMENT Dosage reduced for patients whose absolute neutrophil count remains above 10,000/mm^3.

Route	Onset	Peak	Duration
I.V.	In 5 min	Unknown	Unknown

Mechanism of Action

Is pharmacologically identical to human granulocyte colony-stimulating factor, an endogenous hormone synthesized by monocytes, endothelial cells, and fibroblasts. Filgrastim induces the formation of neutrophil progenitor cells by binding directly to receptors on the surface of granulocytes, which then divide and differentiate. It also potentiates the effects of mature neutrophils, which reduces fever and the risk of infection raised by severe neutropenia.

Incompatibilities

Don't mix filgrastim in vial or syringe with normal saline solution because precipitate will form.

Contraindications

Hypersensitivity to filgrastim, its components, or proteins derived from *Escherichia coli*

Interactions

DRUGS

growth hormone: Increased bone marrow hematopoetic activity
lithium: Increased neutrophil production

Adverse Reactions

CNS: Fever, headache
CV: Transient supraventricular tachycardia
GI: Splenic rupture, splenomegaly
HEME: Leukocytosis
MS: Arthralgia; myalgia; pain in arms, legs, lower back, or pelvis
SKIN: Pruritus, rash, Sweet's syndrome (acute febrile neutrophilic dermatosis)
Other: Anaphylaxis, injection site pain and redness

Nursing Considerations

• Warm filgrastim to room temperature before injection. Discard drug if stored longer than 6 hours at room temperature or 24 hours in refrigerator.
• Withdraw only one dose from a vial; don't repuncture the vial.
• Don't shake the solution.
• For continuous infusion, dilute in D$_5$W (not normal saline solution) to produce less than 15 mcg/ml.
• For subcutaneous dose larger than 1 ml, give by divided doses in more than one site.
• After chemotherapy, give filgrastim over 15 to 30 minutes. Don't give within 24 hours before or after cytotoxic chemotherapy.
• Be aware that the needle cover on the single-use prefilled syringe contains dry natural rubber and may cause sensitivity reaction. It shouldn't be handled by susceptible people.
• Monitor CBC, hematocrit, and platelet count two or three times weekly, as appropriate.
• Inform prescriber and expect to stop drug if leukocytosis develops or absolute neutrophil count consistently exceeds 10,000/mm^3.
• Anticipate decreased response to drug if patient has received extensive radiation therapy or long-term chemotherapy.

PATIENT TEACHING

• Teach patient how to prepare, administer, and store filgrastim. Caution her not to reuse needle, syringe, or vial.
• Advise patient prescribed the single-use prefilled syringe to notify prescriber if she has an allergy to dry natural rubber because the needle cover may cause a sensitivity reaction.
• Provide patient with puncture-resistant container for needle and syringe disposal.
• Advise patient to promptly report left-upper-quadrant abdominal pain or shoulder-tip pain.
• Stress the importance of returning for follow-up laboratory tests.

finasteride

Propecia, Proscar

Class and Category

Chemical class: 4-Azasteroid compound
Therapeutic class: Benign prostatic hyperpla-

sia agent, hair growth stimulant
Pregnancy category: X

Indications and Dosages
➤ *To treat symptomatic benign prostatic hyperplasia; to reduce the risk of symptomatic progression of benign prostatic hyperplasia when given with doxazocin*

TABLETS
Adults. 5 mg daily.
➤ *To treat male-pattern baldness*

TABLETS
Adults. 1 mg daily.

Route	Onset	Peak	Duration
P.O.*	Unknown	8 hr	24 hr†
P.O.‡	In 3 mo	Unknown	Unknown

Mechanism of Action
Inhibits 5-alpha reductase, an intracellular enzyme that converts testosterone to its metabolite (5-alpha dihydrotestosterone) in the liver, prostate, and skin. This metabolite is a potent androgen that's partially responsible for benign prostatic hyperplasia and hair loss.

Contraindications
Age (childhood), hypersensitivity to finasteride, sex (female)

Interactions
DRUGS
theophylline: Decreased blood theophylline level

Adverse Reactions
CNS: Asthenia, dizziness, headache
CV: Hypotension, peripheral edema
EENT: Lip swelling, rhinitis
ENDO: Gynecomastia
GI: Abdominal pain, diarrhea
GU: Decreased ejaculatory volume, decreased libido, impotence, testicular pain
MS: Back pain
RESP: Dyspnea

---

* For benign prostatic hyperplasia.
† With single-dose therapy; 2 wk with multiple-dose therapy.
‡ For male-pattern baldness.

SKIN: Pruritus, rash, urticaria
Other: Angioedema

Nursing Considerations
•Expect patient to have a digital rectal examination of the prostate before and periodically during finasteride therapy.
PATIENT TEACHING
•WARNING Urge patient and female partners to use reliable contraception during therapy because semen of men who take drug can harm male fetuses. Caution women and children not to handle broken tablets.
•Explain how to take drug, and urge patient to follow instructions that accompany drug.
•Inform patient that drug may cause decreased ejaculatory volume, decreased libido, and impotence.
•Urge patient to have periodic follow-up appointments to determine drug effectiveness.

flavoxate hydrochloride
Urispas

Class and Category
Chemical class: Flavone derivative
Therapeutic class: Urinary tract antispasmodic
Pregnancy category: B

Indications and Dosages
➤ *To relieve dysuria, nocturia, suprapubic pain, urinary frequency and urgency, and urinary incontinence caused by cystitis, prostatitis, urethrocystitis, or urethrotrigonitis*

TABLETS
Adults and adolescents. 100 to 200 mg t.i.d. or q.i.d.

Route	Onset	Peak	Duration
P.O.	55 min	112 min	Unknown

Mechanism of Action
Relaxes muscles by cholinergic blockade and counteracts smooth-muscle spasms in the urinary tract.

Contraindications
Achalasia; GI hemorrhage; hypersensitivity to flavoxate or its components; obstruction of the duodenum, ileum, or pylorus; ob-

E
F

structive uropathies of the lower urinary tract

Interactions
DRUGS
bethanechol, metoclopramide: Possibly antagonized GI motility effects of these drugs

Adverse Reactions
CNS: Confusion, decreased concentration, dizziness, drowsiness, fever, headache, nervousness, vertigo
CV: Palpitations, tachycardia
EENT: Accommodation disturbances, blurred vision, dry mouth, eye pain, photophobia, worsening of glaucoma
GI: Constipation, nausea, vomiting
GU: Dysuria
HEME: Eosinophilia, leukopenia
SKIN: Decreased sweating, dermatoses, urticaria

Nursing Considerations
•Monitor for eye pain if patient has glaucoma because flavoxate's anticholinergic effects may worsen glaucoma.
PATIENT TEACHING
•Caution patient about possible dry mouth and photophobia. Advise her to wear sunglasses outdoors, and suggest sugarless candy or gum, ice chips, sips of water, or saliva substitute for dry mouth.
•Advise patient to avoid potentially hazardous activities until CNS effects of flavoxate are known.
•Caution patient not to become overheated or to take hot baths or saunas because drug reduces sweating, which can lead to dizziness, fainting, or heatstroke.
•Instruct patient to notify prescriber immediately if she experiences confusion, drowsiness, dysuria, headache, high fever, hives, nausea, nervousness, palpitations, rash, tachycardia, vertigo, vision problems, vomiting, or worsening dry mouth.

flecainide acetate

Tambocor

Class and Category
Chemical class: Benzamide derivative
Therapeutic class: Class IC antiarrhythmic
Pregnancy category: C

Indications and Dosages
➤ *To prevent and suppress recurrent life-threatening ventricular tachycardia*
TABLETS
Adults. *Initial:* 100 mg every 12 hr (every 8 hr for some patients). Increased by 50 mg b.i.d. every 4 days, if needed, until response occurs. *Maintenance:* Up to 150 mg every 12 hr. *Maximum:* 400 mg daily.
DOSAGE ADJUSTMENT Initial dose reduced to 100 mg daily or 50 mg every 12 hr for patients with creatinine clearance of less than 35 ml/min/1.73 m².

➤ *To prevent paroxysmal atrial fibrillation or flutter or paroxysmal supraventricular tachycardia*
TABLETS
Adults. *Initial:* 50 mg every 12 hr (every 8 hr for some patients). Increased by 50 mg b.i.d. every 4 days, if needed, until response occurs. *Maintenance:* Up to 150 mg every 12 hr. *Maximum:* 300 mg daily.

Mechanism of Action
Achieves antiarrhythmic effect by inhibiting fast sodium channels of myocardial cell membranes, which increase myocardial recovery after repolarization, and by depressing the upstroke of the action potential. Flecainide also produces its antiarrhythmic effect by:
• slowing intracardiac conduction, which slightly increases the duration of the action potential in atrial and ventricular muscle, thus prolonging the PR interval, QRS complex, and QT interval
• shortening the action potential of Purkinje fibers without affecting surrounding myocardial tissue
• inhibiting extracellular calcium influx (at high doses)
• stopping paroxysmal reentrant supraventricular tachycardias by acting on antegrade pathways of dysfunctional AV conduction
• decreasing conduction in accessory pathways in those with Wolff-Parkinson-White syndrome.

Contraindications
Cardiogenic shock, hypersensitivity to flecainide or its components, recent MI, right

bundle-branch block associated with left hemiblock or second- or third-degree AV block unless pacemaker is present

Interactions
DRUGS
amiodarone: Increased blood flecainide level
beta blockers, disopyramide, verapamil: Possibly myocardial depression and increased blood levels of both drugs
calcium channel blockers: Increased risk of arrhythmias
digoxin: Possibly increased blood digoxin level
urinary acidifiers: Possibly increased flecainide elimination and decreased therapeutic effects
urinary alkalinizers: Possibly decreased flecainide elimination and increased therapeutic effects
FOODS
acidic juices, foods that decrease urine pH below 5.0: Increased flecainide elimination and decreased therapeutic effects
foods that increase urine pH above 7.0, strict vegetarian diet: Decreased flecainide elimination and increased therapeutic effects
ACTIVITIES
smoking: Increased flecainide clearance

Adverse Reactions
CNS: Anxiety, depression, dizziness, drowsiness, fatigue, headache, light-headedness, tremor, weakness
CV: Arrhythmias, chest pain, heart failure, hypotension
EENT: Blurred vision
GI: Abdominal pain, anorexia, constipation, hepatic dysfunction, nausea, vomiting
RESP: Dyspnea
SKIN: Rash

Nursing Considerations
•Monitor urine pH at the start of flecainide therapy.
•Check blood pressure, fluid intake and output, and weight regularly during therapy.
•Monitor blood trough level of flecainide, as needed; therapeutic level is 0.2 to 1 mcg/ml.
•Expect drug to cause mild to moderate negative inotropic effects, minimal cardiovascular effects, and no effect on blood pressure, heart rate, and left ventricular function.
•**WARNING** Because hypokalemia or hyperkalemia may interfere with flecainide's therapeutic effects, monitor serum potassium level before and during therapy and notify prescriber immediately if potassium imbalance develops. Also monitor for and notify prescriber about prolonged PR interval, QRS complex, or QT interval; chest pain; hypotension; and signs of heart failure. Keep in mind that drug can cause fatal proarrhythmias, which is why it isn't considered a first-line antiarrhythmic.
•Expect prolonged flecainide therapy to raise blood alkaline phosphatase level.
PATIENT TEACHING
•Instruct patient to take flecainide at regular intervals to keep a constant blood level.
•Advise patient to take a missed dose as soon as she remembers if it's within 6 hours of the scheduled time.
•Teach patient how to take her pulse, and instruct her to record it daily, along with her weight. Advise her to bring record to follow-up visits.
•Encourage family members to obtain instruction in basic cardiac life support.
•Advise patient to notify prescriber immediately about chest pain, difficulty breathing, and dizziness.
•Caution patient not to stop taking drug suddenly but to taper dosage gradually according to prescriber's instructions.

fluconazole

Diflucan

Class and Category
Chemical class: Triazole derivative
Therapeutic class: Antifungal
Pregnancy category: C

Indications and Dosages
➤ *To treat oral and esophageal candidiasis*
ORAL SUSPENSION, TABLETS, I.V. INJECTION
Adults and adolescents. 200 mg on day 1 followed by 100 mg daily for at least 2 (oral) or 3 (esophageal) wk after symptoms resolve.
Children. 3 mg/kg daily for at least 2 (oral) or 3 (esophageal) wk and then for 2 wk after esophageal symptoms resolve.
➤ *To treat systemic candidiasis*
ORAL SUSPENSION, TABLETS, I.V. INJECTION
Adults and adolescents. 400 mg on day 1, followed by 200 mg daily for at least 4 wk and then for additional 2 wk after symptoms resolve.

E
F

➤ *To treat cryptococcal meningitis*

ORAL SUSPENSION, TABLETS, I.V. INJECTION

Adults and adolescents. 400 mg daily until patient responds to treatment, then 200 to 400 mg daily for 10 to 12 wk after CSF culture is negative. *Maintenance:* 200 mg daily to suppress relapse.

Children. 6 to 12 mg/kg daily for 10 to 12 wk after CSF culture is negative.

➤ *To prevent candidiasis after bone marrow transplantation*

ORAL SUSPENSION, TABLETS, I.V. INJECTION

Adults and adolescents. 400 mg daily starting several days before procedure if severe neutropenia is expected and continued for 7 days after absolute neutrophil count exceeds 1,000/mm³.

➤ *To treat vaginal candidiasis*

CAPSULES, ORAL SUSPENSION, TABLETS

Adults. 150 mg as a single dose.

DOSAGE ADJUSTMENT Dosage reduced for patients with hepatic or renal impairment. Dosage reduced by 50% for patients with creatinine clearance of 11 to 50 ml/min/1.73 m².

Mechanism of Action

Damages fungal cells by interfering with a cytochrome P-450 enzyme needed to convert lanosterol to ergosterol, an essential part of the fungal cell membrane. Decreased ergosterol synthesis causes increased cell permeability, which allows cell contents to leak. Fluconazole also may inhibit endogenous respiration, interact with membrane phospholipids, inhibit transformation of yeasts to mycelial forms, inhibit purine uptake, and impair biosynthesis of triglycerides and phospholipids.

Incompatibilities

Don't add fluconazole to I.V. bag that contains any other drug.

Contraindications

Hypersensitivity to fluconazole or its components

Interactions

DRUGS

astemizole, terfenadine: Increased blood levels of these drugs

benzodiazepines (short-acting): Possibly increased blood benzodiazepine level and psychomotor effects

cimetidine: Decreased blood fluconazole level

cisapride: Possibly increased QT interval, leading to torsades de pointes

cyclosporine: Increased blood cyclosporine level

glipizide, glyburide, tolbutamide: Increased risk of hypoglycemia

hydrochlorothiazide: Increased blood fluconazole level from decreased excretion

isoniazid, rifampin: Decreased fluconazole effects

nonsedating antihistamines: Increased blood antihistamine level, increased risk of cardiotoxicity

oral anticoagulants: Increased anticoagulant effects

phenytoin: Increased blood phenytoin level

rifabutin: Increased blood rifabutin level

theophylline: Increased blood theophylline level

zidovudine: Increased blood zidovudine level

Adverse Reactions

CNS: Chills, dizziness, drowsiness, fever, headache, seizures

CV: Prolonged QT interval, torsades de pointes

GI: Abdominal pain, anorexia, constipation, diarrhea, hepatic failure, nausea, vomiting

HEME: Agranulocytosis, leukopenia, thrombocytopenia

SKIN: Exfoliative dermatitis, photosensitivity, pruritus, rash

Other: Anaphylaxis, angioedema

Nursing Considerations

• Use fluconazole cautiously in patients with potentially proarrhythmic conditions because drug may prolong the QT interval, which can lead to life-threatening torsades de pointes.

• Expect to obtain BUN and serum creatinine levels and culture and sensitivity and liver function test results before therapy starts.

• Refrigerate, but don't freeze, fluconazole oral suspension. Shake well before administering.

• Discard I.V. solution that's cloudy or contains precipitate. Don't infuse more than 200 mg/hr or add supplemental drugs to infusion.

• Monitor hepatic and renal function periodically during therapy, and notify prescriber if

you detect signs of dysfunction.
• Assess for rash every 8 hours during therapy, and notify prescriber if rash occurs.
• If patient receives an oral anticoagulant, monitor coagulation test results and assess patient for bleeding.
• Monitor patient for symptoms of overdose, such as hallucinations and paranoia. If they occur, provide supportive treatment, gastric lavage, and, possibly, hemodialysis, which can reduce blood fluconazole level by half after about 3 hours.

PATIENT TEACHING
• Instruct patient to take fluconazole tablets or oral suspension 30 minutes before or 2 hours after meals. Inform her that tablets may be crushed for easier swallowing if needed.
• Advise patient to complete entire course of therapy, even if she feels better.
• If patient takes an oral antidiabetic, urge her to monitor blood glucose level often because of increased risk of hypoglycemia.
• Alert patient that fluconazole may change the taste of food.
• Encourage patient to notify prescriber immediately about diarrhea, headache, nausea, rash, right-upper-quadrant abdominal pain, yellow skin or whites of eyes, or vomiting.
• Suggest that breast-feeding patient consult prescriber because breast-feeding may need to be stopped during therapy.

fludrocortisone acetate

Florinef

Class and Category
Chemical class: Glucocorticoid
Therapeutic class: Mineralocorticoid replacement
Pregnancy category: C

Indications and Dosages
➤ *To treat primary and secondary chronic adrenocortical insufficiency*

TABLETS
Adults and adolescents. *Usual:* 100 mcg daily. Dosage may range from 100 mcg three times/wk to 200 mcg daily.
Children. 50 to 100 mcg daily.

➤ *To treat salt-losing adrenogenital syndrome*

TABLETS
Adults. 100 to 200 mcg daily.
Children. 50 to 100 mcg daily.
DOSAGE ADJUSTMENT Dosage reduced to 50 mcg daily if transient hypertension develops during therapy.

Route	Onset	Peak	Duration
P.O.	Unknown	Unknown	1 to 2 days

Mechanism of Action
Enhances sodium reabsorption, hydrogen and potassium excretion, and water retention by the distal renal tubules, much like aldosterone, an endogenous mineralocorticoid. In large doses, fludrocortisone can inhibit endogenous adrenocortical secretion, thymic activity, and pituitary corticotropin excretion. It also can promote glycogen deposits in the liver and induce a negative nitrogen balance when protein intake is deficient.

Contraindications
Hypersensitivity to fludrocortisone, adrenocorticoids, or their components; systemic fungal infections

Interactions
DRUGS
digoxin: Increased risk of digitalis toxicity and arrhythmias from hypokalemia
phenytoin, rifampin: Decreased fludrocortisone effects
potassium-wasting drugs, such as loop diuretics and amphotericin B: Increased risk of severe hypokalemia

Adverse Reactions
CNS: Dizziness, headache, mental changes, seizures
CV: Arrhythmias, heart failure, hypertension, peripheral edema
EENT: Cataracts (with long-term use), increased intraocular pressure
ENDO: Adrenal insufficiency, growth suppression in children, hyperglycemia
GI: Anorexia, nausea, vomiting
GU: Menstrual irregularities
HEME: Easy bruising
MS: Arthralgia, muscle weakness, myalgia,

osteoporosis (with long-term use), tendon contractures
SKIN: Acne, diaphoresis, rash, urticaria
Other: Hypokalemia, hypokalemic alkalosis, impaired wound healing, weight gain

Nursing Considerations
•Monitor blood pressure, fluid status, and serum electrolyte levels periodically during fludrocortisone therapy. Watch for signs of heart failure, including adventitious breath sounds, peripheral edema, and weight gain.
•Monitor for signs and symptoms of overdose, such as cardiomegaly, edema, excessive weight gain, hypertension, and hypokalemia. These effects usually subside a few days after therapy stops. Potassium supplementation may be needed.
•Notify prescriber if patient experiences dizziness, headache, hypertension, hypokalemia, signs of infection, or weight gain.

PATIENT TEACHING
•Instruct patient to take a missed dose of fludrocortisone as soon as she remembers if it's within 12 hours of scheduled time. Warn against double-dosing. Advise her to notify prescriber if she misses more than one dose or if nausea or vomiting prevents her from taking drug.
•Instruct patient to reduce dietary sodium and to eat more potassium-rich foods during therapy.
•Direct patient to weigh herself each morning before breakfast in clothes of similar weight and to notify prescriber if she gains more than 2 lb (0.9 kg) per day or 5 lb (2.3 kg) per week. Instruct her to monitor how tightly her rings and shoes fit.
•Advise patient to notify prescriber about stressful events—such as dental extractions, emotional upset, illness, surgery, and trauma—because a dosage increase may be required.
•Instruct patient to notify prescriber about dizziness, fever, fluid retention, headache, joint pain, irregular heart rate, muscle weakness, or palpitations.
•Inform patient that drug may delay wound healing.
•Caution patient not to stop taking drug abruptly but to taper dosage gradually, as prescribed.
•Urge patient to wear or carry medical identification that documents corticosteroid use.

flumazenil
Anexate (CAN), Romazicon

Class and Category
Chemical class: Imidazobenzodiazepine derivative
Therapeutic class: Benzodiazepine antidote
Pregnancy category: C

Indications and Dosages
➤ *To reverse sedation from benzodiazepine therapy*
I.V. INJECTION
Adults. 0.2 mg, repeated after 45 to 60 sec if response is inadequate and then repeated every 1 min, if needed. If sedation recurs, regimen is repeated every 20 min or more. *Maximum:* 1 mg over 5 min or 3 mg over 1 hr.

➤ *To reverse benzodiazepine toxicity or suspected overdose*
I.V. INJECTION
Adults. 0.2 mg followed by 0.3 mg 30 to 60 sec later if response is inadequate and then 0.5 mg repeated every 1 min. If sedation recurs, regimen is repeated every 20 min. *Maximum:* 3 mg in 1-hr period.

Route	Onset	Peak	Duration
I.V.	1 to 2 min	6 to 10 min	Variable

Mechanism of Action
Antagonizes CNS effects of benzodiazepines by competing for their binding sites.

Contraindications
Evidence of tricyclic antidepressant overdose; hypersensitivity to flumazenil, benzodiazepines, or their components; use of benzodiazepine to control intracranial pressure, status epilepticus, or a potentially life-threatening condition

Interactions
DRUGS
benzodiazepines: Benzodiazepine withdrawal symptoms, including seizures
nonbenzodiazepine agonists: Loss of effectiveness of these drugs
tetracyclic or tricyclic antidepressant overdose: High risk of seizures

FOODS

all foods: Increased flumazenil clearance (by half) with food ingestion during I.V. injection

Adverse Reactions

CNS: Agitation, anxiety, ataxia, confusion, dizziness, drowsiness, emotional lability, fatigue, headache, hypoesthesia, insomnia, paresthesia, resedation, seizures, tremor, vertigo
CV: Hot flashes, hypertension, palpitations
EENT: Blurred vision, diplopia, dry mouth
GI: Nausea, vomiting
RESP: Dyspnea, hyperventilation, hypoventilation
SKIN: Diaphoresis, flushing, rash
Other: Injection site pain and thrombophlebitis

Nursing Considerations

• Use flumazenil cautiously in patients with cardiac disease. Assess for increased stress or anxiety from benzodiazepine withdrawal because patient's blood pressure may rise.
• Give flumazenil undiluted or diluted in a syringe with D₅W, normal saline solution, or lactated Ringer's solution. Administer over 15 to 30 seconds directly into tubing of a free-flowing compatible I.V. solution. Use a large vein, if possible, to minimize pain at site. Avoid extravasation because drug may irritate tissue.
• Be aware that drug may cause signs of benzodiazepine withdrawal in drug-dependent patient. Also, abrupt awakening from benzodiazepine overdose can cause agitation, dysphoria, and increased adverse reactions.
• Be aware that benzodiazepine reversal may cause an anxiety or a panic attack for patient with a history of these episodes. Expect to adjust dosage carefully.
• Monitor for signs of resedation and hypoventilation for at least 2 hours after giving flumazenil because drug has a short half-life. Be aware that patient shouldn't be discharged until the risk of resedation has resolved.

PATIENT TEACHING

• Caution patient to avoid alcohol and OTC drugs for 10 to 24 hours after taking drug.
• Advise patient to avoid hazardous activities for 18 to 24 hours after discharge.
• Inform patient and family that agitation, emotional lability, fear, and panic attack (if patient has a history of them) may occur. Tell them to seek medical care if patient has depression, trouble breathing, flushing, hyperventilation, insomnia, palpitations, or tremor.
• Because drug doesn't always reverse postprocedure amnesia, provide written instructions or instructions to caregiver even if patient is alert.

flunisolide

AeroBid, AeroBid-M, Bronalide (CAN), Nasalide, Nasarel, Rhinalar (CAN)

Class and Category

Chemical class: Corticosteroid
Therapeutic class: Antiasthmatic, anti-inflammatory
Pregnancy category: C

Indications and Dosages

➤ *To provide maintenance treatment of asthma, alone or with oral corticosteroids*

INHALATION AEROSOL

Adults and adolescents age 15 and over.
500 mcg (2 inhalations) b.i.d. morning and evening. *Maximum:* 2,000 mcg daily (4 inhalations b.i.d.).
Children ages 6 to 15. 500 mcg (2 inhalations) b.i.d. *Maximum:* 1,000 mcg daily.

➤ *To relieve symptoms of seasonal or perennial rhinitis*

NASAL SOLUTION

Adults. 50 mcg (2 sprays) b.i.d. in each nostril. *Maximum:* 400 mcg daily (16 sprays).
Children. 25 mcg (1 spray) t.i.d. in each nostril. *Maximum:* 200 mcg daily (8 sprays).

Route	Onset	Peak	Duration
Inhalation	In 4 wk	Unknown	Unknown
Nasal	3 to 7 days	Unknown	4 to 6 hr

Mechanism of Action

Inhibits cells involved in inflammatory response, such as mast cells, eosinophils, basophils, lymphocytes, macrophages, and neutrophils. Also inhibits production of chemical mediators, such as histamine, eicosanoids, leukotrienes, and cytokines.

Contraindications

Hypersensitivity to flunisolide or its components, primary treatment of status asthmaticus or other asthma episodes that require emer-

E
F

gency care, recent nasal surgery (nasal form), untreated localized infection of nasal mucosa (nasal form)

Adverse Reactions
CNS: Anxiety, chills, depression, dizziness, headache, hyperactivity, insomnia, irritability, lethargy, mood changes, nervousness, tremor, vertigo
CV: Hypertension
EENT: Candidiasis (oral and throat), dry mouth and throat, earache, eye infection, hoarseness, loss of smell or taste, mouth irritation, pharyngitis, rhinitis, sinusitis, sneezing
GI: Abdominal pain, anorexia, constipation, diarrhea, flatulence, heartburn, increased appetite, indigestion, nausea, vomiting
GU: Menstrual irregularities
HEME: Eosinophilia
RESP: Bronchitis, dyspnea, pleurisy, pneumonia
SKIN: Acne, eczema, pruritus, rash, urticaria
Other: Growth suppression (children), lymphadenopathy

Nursing Considerations
• Use flunisolide cautiously in patients with ocular herpes simplex, pulmonary tuberculosis, or untreated systemic bacterial, fungal, parasitic, or viral infection.
• If patient receives an oral corticosteroid, expect to taper it slowly 1 week after changing to flunisolide. For patient who receives prednisone, expect to reduce it by no more than 2.5 mg daily at weekly intervals, beginning at least 1 week after flunisolide therapy starts.
• **WARNING** Assess patient switched from systemic corticosteroid to flunisolide for adrenal insufficiency (fatigue, hypotension, lassitude, nausea, vomiting, weakness) during initial treatment and during stress, trauma, surgery, infection, or other electrolyte-depleting conditions. Notify prescriber immediately if signs or symptoms arise.
• Monitor growth in children; corticosteroids may increase risk of growth suppression.
PATIENT TEACHING
• Teach patient how to use inhaler. When starting a new canister, advise spraying once into the air (avoiding her eyes) to check for mist.
• Instruct patient to gargle or rinse after each use to help prevent mouth and throat dryness, relieve throat irritation, and prevent oropharyngeal infection.

• Urge patient to contact prescriber if symptoms haven't improved after 3 weeks.
• **WARNING** Caution patient not to use flunisolide to relieve acute bronchospasm.
• If patient switches from an oral corticosteroid to flunisolide, advise her to carry medical identification indicating the need for supplemental systemic corticosteroids during stress or severe asthma attack. Advise her to ask prescriber how to respond to these problems.
• Caution patient to avoid exposure to chickenpox and measles and to contact prescriber immediately if exposure occurs.

fluoxetine hydrochloride

Prozac, Prozac Weekly, Sarafem

Class and Category
Chemical class: Phenylpropylamine derivative
Therapeutic class: Antibulimic, antidepressant, antiobsessive-compulsive
Pregnancy category: C

Indications and Dosages
➤ *To treat depression*
CAPSULES, ORAL SOLUTION, TABLETS (PROZAC)
Adults. *Initial:* 20 mg daily in the morning. Dosage increased every 4 to 8 wk as needed. Dosage greater than 20 mg daily given b.i.d. morning and noon. *Maximum:* 80 mg daily.
Children and adolescents. *Initial:* 10 mg daily. Increased after 1 wk to 20 mg daily.
DOSAGE ADJUSTMENT For lower-weight children, dosage increased to 20 mg daily only if improvement insufficient after several wk.
DELAYED-RELEASE CAPSULES (PROZAC WEEKLY)
Adults. 90 mg/wk, beginning 7 days after last 20-mg daily dose.

➤ *To treat obsessive-compulsive disorder*
CAPSULES, ORAL SOLUTION, TABLETS (PROZAC)
Adults. *Initial:* 20 mg daily in the morning. Dosage increased every 4 to 8 wk as needed. Dosage greater than 20 mg daily given b.i.d. morning and noon. *Maximum:* 80 mg daily.
Children and adolescents. *Initial:* 10 mg daily. Dosage increased after 2 wk to 20 mg daily. Subsequent dosage increased, as needed, at intervals of at least several wk. *Maintenance:* 20 to 60 mg daily.
DOSAGE ADJUSTMENT For lower-weight children, dosage should be increased above 10 mg daily only if clinical improvement re-

mains insufficient after several wk. Maintenance dosage for such patients should not exceed 30 mg daily.

➤ *To treat moderate to severe bulimia nervosa*

CAPSULES, ORAL SOLUTION, TABLETS (PROZAC)
Adults. 60 mg daily in the morning. Some patients may be prescribed a lower dose, which is titrated to 60 mg daily as tolerated.

➤ *To treat panic disorder with or without agoraphobia*

CAPSULES, ORAL SOLUTION, TABLETS (PROZAC)
Adults. *Initial:* 10 mg daily. Dosage increased in 1 wk to 20 mg daily, as needed. *Maximum:* 60 mg daily.

➤ *To treat premenstrual dysmorphic disorder*

CAPSULES (SARAFEM)
Adults. 20 mg daily. Dosage increased as needed. *Maximum:* 80 mg daily.

DOSAGE ADJUSTMENT Dose or frequency reduced for patients with hepatic impairment or concurrent illness, those who take multiple medications, and for elderly patients.

Route	Onset	Peak	Duration
P.O.*	1 to 6 wk†	Unknown	Unknown

Mechanism of Action

Selectively inhibits reuptake of the neurotransmitter serotonin by CNS neurons and increases the amount of serotonin that's available in nerve synapses. An elevated serotonin level may result in elevated mood and, consequently, reduced depression.

Contraindications

Hypersensitivity to selective serotonin reuptake inhibitors or their components, use within 14 days of MAO inhibitor therapy

Interactions

DRUGS
alprazolam, diazepam: Possibly prolonged half-life of these drugs
aspirin, NSAIDs, warfarin: Increased anticoagulant activity and risk of bleeding

---

* Capsules, oral solution, and tablets.
† For depression and bulimia; 5 wk for obsessive-compulsive disorder.

astemizole: Increased risk of serious arrhythmias
buspirone: Decreased buspirone effects
clozapine, fluphenazine, haloperidol, maprotiline, trazodone: Increased risk of adverse effects
CYP2D6-metabolized drugs, such as antiarrhythmics (especially flecainide, propafenone), selected antidepressants (tricyclics), antipyschotics (phenothiazines and most atypicals), thioridazine, and vinblastine: Increased plasma levels of these drugs and increased risk of serious adverse reactions
linezolid, lithium, serotonergics (such as amphetamines and other psychostimulants, antidepressants, and dopamine agonists), St. John's wort, tramadol, triptans: Increased risk of serotonin syndrome
MAO inhibitors: Possibly severe and life-threatening adverse effects
phenytoin: Increased blood phenytoin level and risk of toxicity
pimozide: Possibly bradycardia
sumatriptan: Increased risk of weakness, hyperreflexia, and difficulty with coordination
tryptophan: Increased risk of central and peripheral toxicity

Adverse Reactions

CNS: Anxiety, chills, dream disturbances, drowsiness, fatigue, fever, headache, hypomania, insomnia, mania, nervousness, restlessness, seizures, somnolence, suicidal ideation, tremor, vertigo, weakness, yawning
CV: Hypotension, palpitations
EENT: Abnormal vision, dry mouth, pharyngitis, sinusitis
ENDO: Galactorrhea, gynecomastia, hypoglycemia, syndrome of inappropriate antidiuretic hormone secretion (SIADH)
GI: Anorexia, diarrhea, indigestion, nausea
GU: Decreased libido, ejaculation disorders, impotence
HEME: Altered platelet function, unusual bleeding
MS: Arthralgia, myalgia
RESP: Dyspnea
SKIN: Diaphoresis, pruritus, rash, urticaria
Other: Flulike symptoms, hyponatremia, weight loss

Nursing Considerations

•Use fluoxetine cautiously in patients with a history of seizures.
•**WARNING** Avoid giving fluoxetine within

14 days of an MAO inhibitor or starting MAO inhibitor therapy within 5 weeks of discontinuing fluoxetine.

• In patients taking fluoxetine for depression (especially children, adolescents, and young adults), watch closely for suicidal tendencies, particularly when therapy starts and dosage changes, because depression may worsen temporarily during those times.

• Monitor patient closely for evidence of GI bleeding, especially if patient takes another drug known to increase the risk, such as aspirin, an NSAID, or warfarin.

• Monitor patient—especially an elderly patient—for hypoosmolarity of serum and urine and for hyponatremia (headache, difficulty concentrating, memory impairment, weakness, unsteadiness), which may indicate fluoxetine-induced SIADH.

• To discontinue, expect to taper drug, as ordered, to minimnize adverse reactions.

• WARNING If patient receives another drug that raises serotonin level (such as dopamine agonists, MAO inhibitors and other antidepressants, tryptophan, and amphetamines and other psychostimulants), watch for serotonin syndrome, a rare but serious adverse effect of selective serotonin reuptake inhibitors. Signs and symptoms include agitation, confusion, diaphoresis, diarrhea, fever, hyperactive reflexes, poor coordination, restlessness, shaking, talking or acting with uncontrolled excitement, tremor, and twitching.

• Monitor patient with diabetes mellitus for altered blood glucose level because drug may cause hypoglycemia during therapy and hyperglycemia when it stops. Expect to adjust dosage of antidiabetic drug, as prescribed.

• Expect patient to be reevaluated periodically to determine continued need for therapy.

• When stopping therapy, expect to taper drug to minimize adverse reactions.

PATIENT TEACHING

• WARNING Tell patient that drug increases the risk of serotonin syndrome, a rare but serious complication, when taken with certain other drugs. Teach patient to recognize its signs and symptoms, and advise her to notify prescriber immediately if they occur.

• Urge family or caregiver to watch patient closely for suicidal tendencies, especially when therapy starts or dosage changes and particularly if patient is a child, teenager, or young adult.

• Caution patient to avoid hazardous activities until CNS effects of drug are known.

• Caution against stopping drug abruptly because serious adverse effects may result.

• Advise patient to consult prescriber before taking OTC or prescription drugs, if a rash or hives develop, or if she becomes or intends to become pregnant during therapy.

• Inform patient that drug may take several weeks to achieve full effects.

fluphenazine decanoate

Modecate (CAN), Modecate Concentrate (CAN), Prolixin Decanoate

fluphenazine enanthate

Moditen Enanthate (CAN), Prolixin Enanthate

fluphenazine hydrochloride

Apo-Fluphenazine (CAN), Moditen HCl (CAN), Permitil, Permitil Concentrate, PMS Fluphenazine (CAN), Prolixin, Prolixin Concentrate

Class and Category

Chemical class: Phenothiazine, propylpiperazine derivative
Therapeutic class: Antipsychotic
Pregnancy category: Not rated

Indications and Dosages

➤ *To control psychotic disorders*

ELIXIR, ORAL SOLUTION, TABLETS (FLUPHENAZINE HYDROCHLORIDE)

Adults and adolescents. *Initial:* 2.5 to 10 mg/day in divided doses every 6 to 8 hr. When symptoms are controlled, dosage reduced to 1 to 5 mg daily. *Maximum:* 20 mg/dose with caution.

Children. 250 to 750 mcg once daily to q.i.d.

I.M. INJECTION (FLUPHENAZINE HYDROCHLORIDE)

Adults and adolescents. *Initial:* 1.25 mg, increased as clinical condition tolerates up to 2.5 to 10 mg daily in divided doses every 6 to 8 hr. *Maximum:* 10 mg daily.

DOSAGE ADJUSTMENT For elderly or debilitated patients, dosage reduced to 1 to 2.5 mg daily in divided doses every 6 to 8 hr.

I.M. OR SUBCUTANEOUS INJECTION (FLUPHENAZINE DECANOATE OR ENANTHATE)

Adults. *Initial:* 12.5 to 25 mg every 1 to

4 wk, as needed (decanoate). For doses over 50 mg, next dose increased cautiously by 12.5 mg. Or 25 mg every 2 wk, with dose and dosing interval adjusted based on patient response (enanthate). *Maximum:* 100 mg/dose.
Adolescents and children age 12. *Initial:* 6.25 to 18.75 mg/wk (decanoate), increased to 12.5 to 25 mg every 1 to 3 wk, according to condition.
Children ages 5 to 12. 3.125 to 12.5 mg every 1 to 3 wk (decanoate), according to condition.

Incompatibilities
Don't mix fluphenazine hydrochloride oral solution with beverages that contain caffeine, such as coffee and cola; tannins, such as tea; or pectins, such as apple juice. They're physically incompatible.

Contraindications
Blood dyscrasias, bone marrow depression, cerebral arteriosclerosis, coma, concomitant use of large amounts of another CNS depressant, coronary artery disease, hepatic dysfunction, hypersensitivity to phenothiazines, myeloproliferative disorders, severe CNS depression, severe hypertension or hypotension, subcortical brain damage

Route	Onset	Peak	Duration
P.O.	In 1 hr	Variable	6 to 8 hr
I.M.*	In 1 hr	Variable	6 to 8 hr
I.M., SubQ†	In 24 to 72 hr	Variable	1 to 6 wk‡

Mechanism of Action
May block postsynaptic dopamine receptor sites in the CNS. This action may depress areas of the brain that control activity and aggression, including the cerebral cortex, hypothalamus, and limbic system.

Interactions
DRUGS
adsorbent antidiarrheals, aluminum- or magnesium-containing antacids: Possibly inhibited absorption of fluphenazine

---

* For hydrochloride.
† For decanoate and enanthate.
‡ For decanoate; 2 wk for enanthate.

amantadine, anticholinergics: Possibly intensified adverse effects of both drugs
amphetamines: Possibly decreased therapeutic effects of both drugs
antihypertensives: Possibly severe hypotension
antithyroid drugs: Increased risk of agranulocytosis
beta blockers: Possibly increased blood levels and risk of adverse effects of both drugs
bromocriptine: Decreased bromocriptine effects
CNS depressants: Possibly prolonged and intensified CNS depression
erythromycin: Possibly inhibited fluphenazine metabolism
guanethidine: Decreased hypotensive effect of guanethidine
levodopa: Possibly decreased antidyskinetic effect of levodopa
lithium: Possibly neurotoxicity (disorientation, extrapyramidal reactions, unconsciousness)
meperidine: Excessive sedation and hypotension
metrizamide: Increased risk of seizures when injected in subarachnoid area during fluphenazine therapy
oral anticoagulants: Possibly decreased anticoagulant effects
pimozide, other drugs that prolong QT interval: Prolonged QT interval and risk of arrhythmias
thiazide diuretics: Increased risk of hyponatremia, hypotension, and water intoxication
tricyclic antidepressants: Possibly prolonged and intensified sedation
ACTIVITIES
alcohol use: Possibly increased CNS depression and increased risk of heatstroke

Adverse Reactions
CNS: Ataxia, cerebral edema, dizziness, drowsiness, headache, insomnia, light-headedness, nervousness, seizures, slurred speech, syncope, worsening psychotic symptoms
CV: AV conduction disorders, bradycardia, cardiac arrest, hypercholesterolemia, hypertension, orthostatic hypotension, QT prolongation, shock, ST-segment depression, tachycardia
EENT: Blurred vision, dry mouth, glaucoma, increased salivation, laryngeal edema, laryngospasm, miosis, mydriasis, nasal congestion, papillary hypertrophy of the tongue, parotid gland enlargement, photophobia, pigmentary retinopathy, ptosis

ENDO: Breast engorgement (females), galactorrhea, hyperglycemia, hypoglycemia, mastalgia, syndrome of inappropriate ADH secretion
GI: Anorexia, constipation, diarrhea, fecal impaction, ileus, increased appetite, nausea, vomiting
GU: Amenorrhea, bladder paralysis, decreased libido, enuresis, menstrual irregularities, polyuria, urinary frequency, urinary incontinence, urine retention
HEME: Anemia, aplastic anemia, eosinophilia, leukopenia, thrombocytopenia, thrombocytopenic or nonthrombocytopenic purpura
RESP: Bronchospasm, dyspnea, increased respiratory depth
SKIN: Contact dermatitis, dry skin, eczema, erythema, jaundice, photosensitivity, pruritus, seborrhea
Other: Heatstroke, hyponatremia, lupuslike symptoms, weight gain

Nursing Considerations
• Fluphenazine shouldn't be used to treat dementia-related psychosis in the elderly because of an increased mortality risk.
• Use fluphenazine cautiously in patients with a history of glaucoma or renal impairment.
• For I.M. and subcutaneous injection, use at least a 21G needle.
• Monitor temperature; a significant, unexplained rise can indicate intolerance and a need to discontinue drug. Notify prescriber immediately if this occurs.
• Watch for signs of hepatic failure, such as jaundice.
• Notify prescriber about worsening psychotic symptoms: agitation, catatonic state, confusion, depression, hallucinations, lethargy, paranoid reactions.

PATIENT TEACHING
• If patient takes elixir form of fluphenazine, instruct her to keep it in an amber or opaque bottle because drug is sensitive to light.
• Advise patient not to mix oral solution with beverages that contain caffeine (coffee, cola), tannins (tea), or pectins (apple juice).
• Caution patient about possible dizziness or light-headedness.
• Teach patient how to prevent heatstroke, orthostatic hypotension, and photosensitivity reactions.
• Warn against stopping drug abruptly.

flurazepam hydrochloride

Apo-Flurazepam (CAN), Dalmane, Novo-Flupam (CAN), Somnol (CAN)

Class, Category, and Schedule
Chemical class: Benzodiazepine
Therapeutic class: Sedative-hypnotic
Pregnancy category: Not rated
Controlled substance schedule: IV

Indications and Dosages
➤ *To treat insomnia characterized by difficulty falling asleep, frequent nocturnal awakenings, or early-morning awakening*

CAPSULES
Adults. 15 to 30 mg at bedtime.
DOSAGE ADJUSTMENT Initial dose reduced to 15 mg for elderly or debilitated patients until individual response is known.

Route	Onset	Peak	Duration
P.O.	15 to 45 min	Unknown	7 to 8 hr

Mechanism of Action
May potentiate the effects of gamma-aminobutyric acid (GABA) and other inhibitory neurotransmitters by binding to specific benzodiazepine receptor sites in the limbic and cortical areas of the CNS. As a result, flurazepam increases GABA's inhibitory effects and blocks cortical and limbic arousal.

Contraindications
Acute angle-closure glaucoma, breastfeeding, hypersensitivity to other benzodiazepines, itraconazole or ketoconazole therapy, psychosis

Interactions
DRUGS
cimetidine, diltiazem, disulfiram, erythromycin, fluoxetine, fluvoxamine, itraconazole, nefazodone, estrogen-containing oral contraceptives, propoxyphene, ranitidine, verapamil: Possibly increased blood level and impaired hepatic metabolism of flurazepam
clozapine: Possibly cardiac arrest or respiratory depression

CNS depressants: Possibly potentiated CNS depression
levodopa: Possibly decreased therapeutic effects of levodopa

FOODS
grapefruit juice: Possibly increased blood level and impaired hepatic metabolism of flurazepam

ACTIVITIES
alcohol use: Possibly potentiated CNS and respiratory depression

Adverse Reactions

CNS: Amnesia, anxiety, ataxia, bizarre behavior (such as sleep driving), confusion, delusions, depression, dizziness, drowsiness, euphoria, headache, hypokinesia, irritability, malaise, nervousness, slurred speech, tremor
CV: Chest pain, palpitations, tachycardia
EENT: Blurred vision, dry mouth, increased salivation, photophobia
GI: Abdominal pain, constipation, diarrhea, nausea, thirst, vomiting
GU: Libido changes
SKIN: Diaphoresis
Other: Anaphylaxis, angioedema, physical or psychological dependence

Nursing Considerations

• Use flurazepam cautiously in patients with severe mental depression or reduced respiratory function; drug may intensify depression and lead to respiratory depression.
• Expect to use lowest effective dose in elderly or debilitated patients to minimize the risk of ataxia, confusion, dizziness, and oversedation.
• Monitor liver function test results, as appropriate.

PATIENT TEACHING
• Instruct patient not to exceed prescribed dosage and not to stop flurazepam abruptly.
• WARNING Warn patient that, although rare, drug may cause swelling of the oral cavity or throat, which could cause airway obstruction. If swelling occurs, patient should seek emergency care immediately and never take flurazepam again.
• Caution patient about possible morning dizziness or drowsiness.
• Because flurazepam can reduce alertness, advise patient to avoid potentially hazardous activities until drug's CNS effects are known.
• Caution patient to avoid alcohol and CNS depressants during therapy.

• Advise patient to notify prescriber if she becomes or intends to become pregnant during therapy.
• Inform patient that sleep may be disturbed for the first few nights after stopping drug.
• Warn patient and caregiver that some patients have performed bizarre activities after taking drug, such as driving their car, preparing and eating food, making phone calls, or having sex while not fully awake and often with no memory of the event. These episodes usually occur in patients who have taken the drug with alcohol or other CNS depressant or who have exceeded the recommended dose. If such an episode occurs, the prescriber should be notified and flurazepam therapy discontinued immediately.

flurbiprofen

Ansaid, Froben (CAN), Froben SR (CAN), Novo-Flurprofen (CAN)

Class and Category

Chemical class: Propionic acid derivative
Therapeutic class: Antiarthritis, anti-inflammatory
Pregnancy category: B (first trimester), Not rated (later trimesters)

Indications and Dosages

➤ *To treat acute or chronic rheumatoid arthritis and osteoarthritis*

E.R. CAPSULES
Adults. 200 mg daily in the evening.

TABLETS
Adults. *Initial:* 200 to 300 mg daily in divided doses b.i.d. to q.i.d. *Maximum:* 300 mg daily (100 mg/dose).

Mechanism of Action

Blocks the activity of cyclooxygenase, the enzyme necessary for prostaglandin synthesis. Prostaglandins, important mediators in the inflammatory response, cause local vasodilation with swelling and pain. They also play a role in pain transmission from the periphery to the spinal cord. By blocking cyclooxygenase and inhibiting prostaglandins, this NSAID causes inflammatory symptoms and pain to subside.

Contraindications

Angioedema, asthma, bronchospasm, nasal polyps, rhinitis, or urticaria induced by aspirin, iodides, or NSAIDs; hypersensitivity to NSAIDs

Interactions

Drugs

acetaminophen: Increased risk of renal impairment with long-term use of both drugs
antacids: Decreased flurbiprofen effectiveness
anticoagulants, cefamandole, cefoperazone, cefotetan, heparin, plicamycin, thrombolytics, valproic acid: Increased risk of bleeding
antineoplastics: Increased adverse hematologic effects
cyclosporine: Increased risk of nephrotoxicity
diuretics, triamterene: Decreased effectiveness of these drugs
glucocorticoids, other NSAIDs, potassium supplements: Increased adverse GI effects
insulin, oral antidiabetic drugs: Increased risk of hypoglycemia
lithium: Increased risk of lithium toxicity
methotrexate: Increased risk of methotrexate toxicity
salicylates: Increased risk of GI bleeding

Activities

alcohol use, smoking: Increased risk of GI bleeding

Adverse Reactions

CNS: Anxiety, cerebral hemorrhage, depression, dizziness, drowsiness, forgetfulness, headache, insomnia, malaise, nervousness, stroke, tremor, weakness
CV: Arrhythmias, heart failure, hypertension, hypotension, palpitations, peripheral edema, tachycardia
EENT: Amblyopia, blurred vision, rhinitis, stomatitis, tinnitus, vision changes
GI: Abdominal cramps or distress, anorexia, constipation, diarrhea, diverticulitis, dysphagia, esophagitis, flatulence, gastritis, gastroenteritis, gastroesophageal reflux disease, GI bleeding or ulceration, hemorrhoids, hiatal hernia, hepatitis, increased appetite, indigestion, jaundice, liver failure, melena, nausea, perforation of stomach or intestines, stomatitis, vomiting
GU: Hematuria, interstitial nephritis, renal failure, UTI
HEME: Agranulocytosis, aplastic anemia, eosinophilia, leukopenia, neutropenia, pancytopenia, thrombocytopenia
SKIN: Erythema multiforme, exfoliative dermatitis, flushing, rash, Stevens-Johnson syndrome, toxic epidermal necrolysis
Other: Anaphylaxis, angioedema, hyponatremia

Nursing Considerations

• Use flurbiprofen with extreme caution in patients who have a history of ulcer disease or GI bleeding because NSAIDs such as flurbiprofen increase the risk of GI bleeding and ulceration. Expect to use flurbiprofen for the shortest time possible in these patients.

• Be aware that serious GI tract ulceration, bleeding, and perforation may occur without warning signs or symptoms. Elderly patients are at greater risk. To minimize the risk, give flurbiprofen with food. If GI distress occurs, withhold drug and notify prescriber immediately.

• Use flurbiprofen cautiously in patients with hypertension, and monitor blood pressure closely throughout therapy. Drug may cause hypertension or worsen it.

• **WARNING** Monitor patient closely for thrombotic events, including MI and stroke, because NSAIDs increase the risk.

• Monitor patient—especially if she's elderly or receiving long-term flurbiprofen therapy—for less common but serious adverse GI reactions, including anorexia, constipation, diverticulitis, dysphagia, esophagitis, gastritis, gastroenteritis, gastroesophageal reflux disease, hemorrhoids, hiatal hernia, melena, stomatitis, and vomiting.

• Monitor liver function test results because, in rare cases, elevations may progress to severe hepatic reactions, including fatal hepatitis, liver necrosis, and hepatic failure.

• Monitor BUN and serum creatinine levels in elderly patients, patients taking diuretics or ACE inhibitors, and patients with heart failure, impaired renal function, or hepatic dysfunction; flurbiprofen may cause renal failure.

• Monitor CBC for decreased hemoglobin and hematocrit because drug may worsen anemia.

• **WARNING** If patient has bone marrow suppression or is receiving an antineoplastic drug, monitor laboratory results (including WBC count), and watch for evidence of infection because anti-inflammatory and antipyretic actions of flurbiprofen may mask

signs and symptoms, such as fever and pain.
•Assess patient's skin regularly for signs of rash or other hypersensitivity reaction because flurbiprofen is an NSAID and may cause serious skin reactions without warning, even in patients with no history of NSAID sensitivity. At first sign of reaction, stop drug and notify prescriber.

PATIENT TEACHING
•Encourage patient to take flurbiprofen with food or milk to avoid GI distress.
•Caution patient about possible blurred vision, dizziness, and drowsiness.
•Advise patient to avoid aspirin, alcohol, and smoking during flurbiprofen therapy.
•Urge patient to notify prescriber immediately if she has blood in urine, easy bruising, itching, rash, swelling, or yellow eyes or skin.
•Caution pregnant patient not to take NSAIDs such as flurbiprofen during the last trimester because they may cause premature closure of the ductus arteriosus.
•Explain that flurbiprofen may increase the risk of serious adverse cardiovascular reactions; urge patient to seek immediate medical attention if signs or symptoms arise, such as chest pain, shortness of breath, weakness, and slurring of speech.
•Explain that flurbiprofen may increase the risk of serious adverse GI reactions; stress the importance of seeking immediate medical attention for such signs and symptoms as epigastric or abdominal pain, indigestion, black or tarry stools, or vomiting blood or material that looks like coffee grounds.
•Alert patient to rare but serious skin reactions. Urge her to seek immediate medical attention for rash, blisters, itching, fever, or other indications of hypersensitivity.

fluticasone propionate

Flonase, Flovent

fluticasone furoate

Veramyst

Class and Category

Chemical class: Trifluorinated corticosteroid
Therapeutic class: Antiasthmatic, anti-inflammatory
Pregnancy category: C

Indications and Dosages

➤ *To prevent asthma attacks, alone or with oral corticosteroids*

INHALATION AEROSOL
Adults and children age 12 and over using bronchodilator therapy. *Initial:* 88 mcg inhaled b.i.d. *Maximum:* 440 mcg inhaled b.i.d.
Adults and children age 12 and over switching from another inhaled corticosteroid. *Initial:* 88 to 220 mcg inhaled b.i.d. *Maximum:* 440 mcg inhaled b.i.d.
Adults and children age 12 and over using oral corticosteroid therapy. *Initial and maximum:* 880 mcg inhaled b.i.d.
Children ages 4 to 11 regardless of previous therapy. 88 mcg b.i.d. *Maximum:* 88 mcg b.i.d.

➤ *To prevent seasonal or perennial allergic rhinitis*

NASAL SUSPENSION (FLONASE)
Adults and children age 12 and over. *Initial:* 100 mcg (2 sprays) in each nostril daily or 50 mcg (1 spray) in each nostril b.i.d, as needed. *Maintenance:* 50 mcg (1 spray) in each nostril daily, as tolerated and needed. *Maximum:* 200 mcg daily (4 sprays).
Children ages 4 to 11. 50 or 100 mcg (1 or 2 sprays) in each nostril daily in the morning, as needed. *Maximum:* 200 mcg daily (4 sprays).

➤ *To treat seasonal or perennial allergic rhinitis*

NASAL SUSPENSION (FLONASE)
Adults and children age 12 and over. *Initial:* 100 mcg (2 sprays) in each nostril daily or 50 mcg (1 spray) in each nostril b.i.d, as needed. *Maintenance:* 50 mcg (1 spray) in each nostril daily, as tolerated and needed. *Maximum:* 200 mcg daily (4 sprays).
Children ages 4 to 11. 50 or 100 mcg (1 or 2 sprays) in each nostril daily in the morning, as needed. *Maximum:* 200 mcg daily (4 sprays).

NASAL SUSPENSION (VERAMYST)
Adults and children age 12 and over. *Initial:* 110 mcg (2 sprays) in each nostril once daily, decreasedto 55 mcg (1 spray) in each nostril once daily when symptoms are controlled. *Maintenance:* 55 mcg (1 spray) in each nostril once daily.
Children ages 2 to 11. *Initial:* 55 mcg (1 spray) in each nostril once daily, increased to 110 mcg (2 sprays) in each nostril once

E
F

daily, as needed. *Maintenance:* 55 mcg (1 spray) in each nostril once daily.

Route	Onset	Peak	Duration
Inhalation	In 24 hr	1 to 2 wk	Several days
Nasal	12 hr to 3 days	4 to 7 days	1 to 2 wk

Mechanism of Action

Inhibits cells involved in the inflammatory response of asthma, such as mast cells, eosinophils, basophils, lymphocytes, macrophages, and neutrophils. Fluticasone also inhibits production or secretion of chemical mediators, such as histamine, eicosanoids, leukotrienes, and cytokines.

Contraindications

Hypersensitivity to fluticasone or its components, primary treatment of status asthmaticus or other acute asthma episodes that require intensive measures, untreated nasal mucosal infection (nasal suspension)

Interactions

DRUGS

ketoconazole, ritonavir and other strong cytochrome P-450 3A4 inhibitors (long-term use): Possibly increased fluticasone level and increased risk of reduced serum cortisol level

Adverse Reactions

CNS: Aggressiveness, agitation, depression, difficulty speaking, dizziness, fatigue, fever, headache, insomnia, malaise, restlessness
EENT: Allergic rhinitis, cataracts, conjunctivitis, dry mouth and throat, eye irritation, glaucoma, hoarseness, laryngitis, loss of voice, nasal congestion or discharge, nasal sinus pain, oropharyngeal candidiasis, otitis media, pharyngitis, sinusitis, throat irritation, tonsillitis
ENDO: Adrenal insufficiency, cushingoid symptoms, hyperglycemia, slower growth in children
GI: Abdominal pain, diarrhea, indigestion, nausea, vomiting
GU: Dysmenorrhea
HEME: Churg-Strauss syndrome, easy bruising, eosinophilia
MS: Arthralgia, myalgia, osteoporosis

RESP: Asthma exacerbation, bronchitis, bronchospasm, chest congestion and tightness, cough, dyspnea, pneumonia, upper respiratory tract infection, wheezing
SKIN: Dermatitis, ecchymosis, pruritus, rash, urticaria
Other: Anaphylaxis, angioedema, flulike symptoms, weight gain

Nursing Considerations

- Use fluticasone cautiously in patients with ocular herpes simplex, pulmonary tuberculosis, or untreated systemic bacterial, fungal, parasitic, or viral infection.
- Although anaphylaxis is rare, monitor patient closely at start of therapy, especially if patient has severe allergy to milk.
- If patient takes a systemic corticosteroid, expect to taper dosage by no more than 2.5 mg daily at weekly intervals, starting 1 week after fluticasone therapy begins.
- **WARNING** If patient is switched from systemic corticosteroid to fluticasone, assess for adrenal insufficiency (fatigue, hypotension, lassitude, nausea, vomiting, weakness) early in therapy and when patient has infection, stress, trauma, surgery, or other electrolyte-depleting conditions or procedures. Notify prescriber immediately if signs or symptoms develop.
- As prescribed, administer a fast-acting inhaled bronchodilator if bronchospasm occurs immediately after fluticasone use. Expect to stop fluticasone and start another drug therapy.
- Expect to titrate fluticasone to lowest effective dosage after asthma has stabilized.

PATIENT TEACHING

- Urge patient to use fluticasone regularly, as prescribed, but not for acute bronchospasm.
- Teach patient how to administer drug according to the form prescribed (nasal spray or oral inhaler).
- Instruct patient to shake canister and to use inhaler according to package insert instructions. On first use, advise her to spray 4 times into the air (away from her eyes and shaking inhaler between each test spray) and look for a fine mist. If inhaler hasn't been used for more than 7 days or it's dropped, it will need to be primed again by shaking well and then releasing 1 test spray into the air (away from her face).

•If 2 inhalations are prescribed, direct patient to wait at least 1 minute between them.

•Instruct patient to gargle and rinse her mouth after each dose to help prevent dry mouth and throat, relieve throat irritation, and prevent oropharyngeal yeast infection.

•If patient uses more than 1 inhaler, instruct her to use fluticasone last, at least 5 minutes after previous inhaler.

•Instruct patient to clean inhaler according to manufacturer guidelines at least once a week after her evening dose.

•Inform patient that, when counter reads 020, she should obtain a refill, if needed. When counter reaches 000, she should discard the inhaler.

•Instruct patient using nasal spray to shake container well before each use.

•Explain that symptoms may improve within 2 days but that full improvement may not occur for 1 to 2 weeks or longer.

•Caution patient not to increase dosage but to contact prescriber after 1 week if symptoms continue or worsen.

•Instruct patient to notify prescriber immediately if asthma attacks don't respond to bronchodilators during fluticasone therapy.

•If patient is switching from an oral corticosteroid to fluticasone, urge her to carry medical identification indicating the need for supplemental systemic corticosteroids during stress or severe asthma attack.

•Caution patient to avoid contact with people who have infections because fluticasone suppresses the immune system, increasing the risk of infection. Instruct patient to notify prescriber about exposure to chickenpox, measles, or other infections because additional treatment may be needed.

fluvastatin sodium

Lescol, Lescol XL

Class and Category

Chemical class: Heptenoic acid derivative
Therapeutic class: Antihyperlipidemic
Pregnancy category: X

Indications and Dosages

➤ *As adjunct to lower cholesterol level in primary hypercholesterolemia, to decrease progression of coronary atherosclerosis, to reduce risk in patients with coronary artery disease undergoing coronary revascularization*

CAPSULES

Adults. 20 to 40 mg daily in the evening or 40 mg b.i.d. *Maximum:* 40 mg b.i.d.

E.R. TABLETS

Adults. 80 mg in the evening. *Maximum:* 80 mg daily.

➤ *As adjunct to lower cholesterol level in children with heterozygous familial hypercholesterolemia*

CAPSULES

Girls ages 10 to 16 who are at least 1 year past menarche. *Initial:* 20 mg once daily, increased every 6 wk, as needed. *Maximum:* 40 mg b.i.d.

DOSAGE ADJUSTMENT For pediatric patients, if maximum dose of 40 mg b.i.d. is reached with immediate-release capsules, child may be switched to extended-release tablets, 80 mg once daily.

Route	Onset	Peak	Duration
P.O.	In 1 to 2 wk	In 4 to 6 wk	Unknown
P.O. (E.R.)	In 2 wk	In 4 wk	Unknown

Mechanism of Action

Interferes with the hepatic enzyme hydroxymethylglutaryl-coenzyme A reductase, reducing formation of mevalonic acid (a cholesterol precursor) and interrupting the pathway by which cholesterol is synthesized. When cholesterol level declines in hepatic cells, LDLs are consumed, which reduces circulating total cholesterol and serum triglycerides.

Contraindications

Acute hepatic disease, breast-feeding, hypersensitivity to fluvastatin or its components, pregnancy, unexplained persistently elevated liver enzyme levels

Interactions

DRUGS

bile acid sequestrants: Possibly decreased fluvastatin bioavailability

cimetidine, omeprazole, ranitidine: Significantly increased blood fluvastatin level

colchicine, cyclosporine, erythromycin, gem-

fibrozil, niacin: Increased risk of severe myopathy and rhabdomyolysis

cyclosporine, erythromycin, gemfibrozil, niacin: Increased risk of acute renal failure

fluconazole: Increased serum fluconazole level

itraconazole, ketoconazole: Increased risk of myopathy

oral contraceptives: Increased risk of bleeding

rifampin: Significantly decreased blood fluvastatin level, increased plasma clearance

ACTIVITIES

alcohol use: Increased bioavailability and blood level of fluvastatin

Adverse Reactions

CNS: Dizziness, fatigue, headache, insomnia, weakness

EENT: Pharyngitis, rhinitis, sinusitis

GI: Abdominal cramps and pain, constipation, diarrhea, flatulence, indigestion, nausea, vomiting

GU: UTI

MS: Arthritis, back pain, myalgia, myositis, rhabdomyolysis

RESP: Bronchitis, cough, upper respiratory tract infection

SKIN: Pruritus, rash

Nursing Considerations

•**WARNING** Expect to stop drug if serum CK level rises sharply or myopathy is suspected.

PATIENT TEACHING

•Urge patient to comply with monthly laboratory tests early in treatment.

•Tell patient to follow prescribed low-fat diet.

•Encourage patient to notify prescriber promptly about muscle pain or unexplained weakness.

fluvoxamine maleate

Luvox, Luvox CR

Class and Category

Chemical class: Aralkylketone derivative
Therapeutic class: Antiobsessional
Pregnancy category: C

Indications and Dosages

➤ *To treat obsessive-compulsive disorder*

TABLETS

Adults. *Initial:* 50 mg at bedtime, increased by 50 mg every 4 to 7 days, if needed. *Maximum:* 300 mg daily.

Children ages 8 to 17. *Initial:* 25 mg at bedtime, increased by 25 mg every 4 to 7 days, if needed. *Maximum:* 200 mg daily.

DOSAGE ADJUSTMENT Doses divided for adults taking more than 100 mg daily and for children taking more than 50 mg daily; given in 2 equal doses b.i.d. or in 2 unequal doses with the larger dose at bedtime.

CAPSULES

Adults. *Initial:* 100 mg at bedtime, increased by 50 mg weekly, if needed. *Maximum:* 300 mg daily.

DOSAGE ADJUSTMENT For elderly patients or those with hepatic impairment, dosage increases with extended-release form are made more slowly.

➤ *To treat social anxiety disorder*

CAPSULES

Adults. *Initial:* 100 mg at bedtime, increased by 50 mg weekly, if needed. *Maximum:* 300 mg daily.

DOSAGE ADJUSTMENT For elderly patients or those with hepatic impairment, dosage increases with extended-release form are made more slowly.

Route	Onset	Peak	Duration
P.O.	3 to 10 wk	Unknown	Unknown

Mechanism of Action

May potentiate serotonin's action by blocking its reuptake at neuronal membranes. An elevated serotonin level may elevate mood and decrease depression and anxiety, which often accompany obsessive-compulsive disorder.

Contraindications

Alosetron, astemizole, cisapride, pimozide, terfenadine, thioridazine, or tizanidine therapy, hypersensitivity to fluvoxamine maleate or its components, use within 14 days of MAO inhibitor

Interactions

DRUGS

alosetron: Increased plasma alosetron level

alprazolam: Increased plasma alprazolam level

antihistamines: Increased risk of impaired

mental and motor skills

aspirin, NSAIDs, warfarin: Risk of bleeding
astemizole, cisapride, pimozide, terfenadine: Possibly fatal QT prolongation
benzodiazepines: Decreased benzodiazepine clearance, possibly impaired memory and motor skills
buspirone: Decreased buspirone effects, increased blood fluvoxamine level, and paradoxical worsening of obsessive-compulsive disorder
carbamazepine: Increased risk of carbamazepine toxicity
clozapine: Increased blood clozapine level
diltiazem: Increased risk of bradycardia
haloperidol: Increased blood haloperidol level, possibly delayed recall and reduced memory and attention span
lithium: Possibly increased serotonin reuptake action of fluvoxamine
MAO inhibitors: Possibly serious or fatal reactions (such as agitation, autonomic instability, coma, delirium, fluctuating vital signs, hyperthermia, myoclonus, and rigidity)
methadone: Possibly significantly increased blood methadone level, increased risk of methadone toxicity
metoprolol, propranolol: Increased blood levels of these drugs, possibly reduced diastolic blood pressure and heart rate induced by these drugs
serotonergics (such as amphetamines and other psychostimulants, antidepressants, and dopamine agonists): Increased risk of serotonin syndrome
sympathomimetics: Possibly increased effects of sympathomimetics and increased risk of serotonin syndrome
tacrine: Increased blood level and therapeutic and adverse effects of tacrine
theophylline: Decreased theophylline clearance, increased risk of theophylline toxicity
tizanidine: Increased risk of serious adverse effects, such as hypotension and profound sedation
tricyclic antidepressants: Increased blood levels of antidepressants
warfarin: Increased blood warfarin level, prolonged PT

FOODS

caffeine: Possibly decreased hepatic clearance of caffeine

ACTIVITIES

smoking: Increased fluvoxamine metabolism

Adverse Reactions

CNS: Agitation, anxiety, apathy, chills, confusion, depression, dizziness, drowsiness, fatigue, headache, hypomania, insomnia, malaise, mania, nervousness, sedation, suicidal ideation, tremor, vertigo, yawning
CV: Palpitations, tachycardia
EENT: Altered taste, blurred vision, dry mouth
GI: Anorexia, constipation, diarrhea, flatulence, indigestion, nausea, upper GI bleeding, vomiting
GU: Decreased libido, ejaculation disorders, impotence, urinary frequency, urine retention
HEME: Bleeding events
MS: Muscle twitching
RESP: Dyspnea, upper respiratory tract infection
SKIN: Diaphoresis, rash
Other: Flulike symptoms, weight gain

Nursing Considerations

• Use fluvoxamine cautiously in patients with cardiovascular disease, impaired hepatic or renal function, mania, seizures, or suicidal tendencies.
• **WARNING** Fluvoxamine shouldn't be given within 14 days of an MAO inhibitor.
• **WARNING** If patient receives another drug that raises the serotonin level by a different mechanism, assess for serotonin syndrome, a rare but serious complication of certain selective serotonin reuptake inhibitors. Signs and symptoms include agitation, confusion, diaphoresis, diarrhea, fever, hyperactive reflexes, lack of coordination, muscle twitching, restlessness, shivering, talking or acting with uncontrolled excitement, and tremor. Drugs that raise the serotonin level include MAO inhibitors, tryptophan, amphetamines and other psychostimulants, antidepressants (buspirone, lithium), and dopamine agonists.
• Watch patient closely (especially children, adolescents, and young adults), for suicidal tendencies, particularly when therapy starts and dosage changes, because depression may worsen temporarily during these times and lead to suicidal ideation.
• Monitor patient for bleeding, especially if patient also takes aspirin, an NSAID, or an anticoagulant. Bleeding can range from ecchymoses, hemtomas, epitaxis, and petechiae to life-threatening hemorrhage.

E
F

• Discontinue fluvoxamine therapy gradually, as ordered, to prevent unpleasant adverse reactions.

PATIENT TEACHING

• Caution patient not to drink alcohol during fluvoxamine therapy.

• Urge patient to avoid potentially hazardous activities until drug's CNS effects are known.

• **WARNING** Inform patient that fluvoxamine increases the risk of a rare but serious problem: serotonin syndrome. Encourage her to notify prescriber immediately if symptoms develop.

• Caution patient not to stop taking drug abruptly. Explain that gradual tapering helps avoid withdrawal symptoms.

• Urge family or caregiver to watch patient closely for suicidal tendencies, especially when therapy starts or dosage changes and particularly if patient is a child, teenager, or young adult.

• Warn patient that fluvoxamine increases bleeding risk if taken with aspirin, an NSAID, or an anticoagulant and that bleeding events could range from mild to severe. Tell patient to seek emergency care for serious or prlonged bleeding.

• Advise pregnant patient to consult with prescriber before her third trimester about ongoing fluvoxamine therapy because of an increased risk to her unborn child during the third trimester.

folic acid

(vitamin B₉)

Apo-Folic (CAN), Folvite, Novo-Folacid (CAN)

Class and Category

Chemical class: Water-soluble B-complex vitamin
Therapeutic class: Nutritional supplement
Pregnancy category: A

Indications and Dosages

➤ *To prevent deficiency based on U.S. and Canadian recommended daily allowances*

TABLETS

Male adults and children age 11 and over. 150 to 400 mcg (150 to 220 mcg Canadian) daily.

Female adults and children age 11 and over. 150 to 400 mcg (145 to 190 mcg Canadian) daily.

Pregnant females. 400 to 800 mcg (445 to 475 mcg Canadian) daily.

Breast-feeding females. 260 to 800 mcg (245 to 275 mcg Canadian) daily.

Children ages 7 to 10. 100 to 400 mcg (125 to 180 mcg Canadian) daily.

Children ages 4 to 6. 75 to 400 mcg (90 mcg Canadian) daily.

Children from birth to age 3. 25 mcg (50 to 80 mcg Canadian) daily.

I.V INFUSION

Adults and children age 11 and over. Dosage individualized based on patient need and given as part of total parenteral nutrition solution.

➤ *To treat folic acid deficiency*

TABLETS

Adults and children age 11 and over. Dosage individualized based on severity of deficiency, as prescribed.

I.V. INFUSION, I.M. OR SUBCUTANEOUS INJECTION

Adults and children age 11 and over. 0.25 to 1 mg daily until hematologic response occurs.

Mechanism of Action

Acts as a catalyst for normal production of red blood cells, helping to prevent megaloblastic anemia, and helps maintain normal homocysteine levels. After being converted to tetrahydrofolic acid in the intestines, folic acid promotes synthesis of several enzymes, including purine and thymidylates; metabolism of amino acids, including glycine and methionine; and metabolism of histidine, all of which are essential for normal cell structure and growth.

Contraindications

Hypersensitivity to folic acid or its components

Interactions

DRUGS

analgesics, carbamazepine, estrogens (including oral contraceptives), phenobarbital, primidone: Possibly increased folic acid requirements

antacids (aluminum- or magnesium-containing), cholestyramine, sulfasalazine: Possibly decreased folic acid absorption

hydantoin anticonvulsants: Possibly decreased effectiveness of these drugs, possibly

increased folic acid requirements
methotrexate, pyrimethamine, triamterene, trimethoprim: Possibly decreased effectiveness of folic acid

Adverse Reactions
Other: Allergic reaction (bronchospasm, erythema, fever, malaise, rash, pruritus)

Nursing Considerations
•**WARNING** Don't give injection form containing benzyl alcohol to neonates or immature infants because a fatal toxic syndrome may occur with CNS, respiratory, circulatory, and renal impairment and metabolic acidosis.
•To prevent decreased absorption, give folic acid supplements at least 1 hour before or 4 hours after cholestyramine or sulfasalazine and don't give antacids within 1 hour before or 2 hours after giving folic acid.
•Know that folic acid will correct hematologic disorders in pernicious anemia, but neurologic problems will progressively worsen.

PATIENT TEACHING
•Advise against taking folic acid supplements as a substitute for proper dietary intake. Explain that good sources of folic acid include green vegetables, potatoes, cereals, and organ meats. Recommend eating raw green vegetables because heat used during cooking destroys up to 90% of folic acid found in food.
•Explain to patients with pernicious anemia that folic acid won't affect the neurologic symptoms associated with the disease.

fondaparinux sodium

Arixtra

Class and Category
Chemical class: Synthetic pentasaccharide factor Xa inhibitor
Therapeutic class: Antithrombolytic
Pregnancy category: B

Indications and Dosages
➤ *To provide prophylaxis against deep vein thrombosis, which may lead to pulmonary embolism in patients undergoing hip fracture surgery, hip replacement surgery, knee replacement surgery, or abdominal surgery in patients at risk for thromboembolic complications*

SUBCUTANEOUS INJECTION
Adults. *Initial:* After hemostasis has been established, 2.5 mg subcutaneously 6 to 8 hr after surgery, followed by 2.5 mg subcutaneously daily for 5 to 9 days. *Maximum:* 2.5 mg subcutaneously daily for 11 days for hip or knee replacement and abdominal surgery and 24 days for hip fracture surgery.

➤ *To treat acute deep vein thrombosis (with warfarin); to treat acute pulmonary embolism (with warfarin) in a hospital setting*

SUBCUTANEOUS INJECTION
Adults. *Initial:* 5 mg if body weight is less than 50 kg (110 lb), 7.5 mg if body weight is 50 to 100 kg (110 to 220 lb), and 10 mg if body weight exceeds 100 kg daily for at least 5 days and until INR is between 2.0 and 3.0 (usually in 5 to 9 days)

Mechanism of Action
Selectively binds to antithrombin III, which enhances the inactivation of clotting factor Xa by antithrombin III. Inactivation of factor Xa interrupts the blood coagulation pathway, which then inhibits thrombin formation. Without thrombin, fibrinogen can't convert to fibrin and clots can't form.

Incompatibilities
Don't mix fondaparinux sodium with other injections or infusions.

Contraindications
Active major bleeding; bacterial endocarditis; body weight less than 50 kg (110 lb) if patient is having hip repair or replacement or knee replacement surgery; fondaparinux-induced thrombocytopenia associated with a positive in vitro test for antiplatelet antibodies; hypersensitivity to fondaparinux; prophylactic fondaparinux therapy in patients weighing less than 50 kg (110 lb) undergoing hip repair or replacement, knee replacement, or abdominal surgery; severe renal impairment (creatinine clearance less than 30 ml/min/1.73 m^2)

Interactions
DRUGS
abciximab, thrombolytics, other drugs that

enhance risk of bleeding: Increased risk of hemorrhage

Adverse Reactions

CNS: Confusion, dizziness, fever, headache, insomnia
CV: Edema, elevated serum aminotransferase level, hypotension
GI: Constipation, diarrhea, elevated liver function test results, indigestion, nausea, vomiting
GU: Urine retention, UTI
HEME: Anemia, bleeding, elevated APTT, hematoma, postoperative hemorrhage, thrombocytopenia, thrombocytopenia with thrombosis
SKIN: Bullous eruption, increased wound drainage, rash, purpura
Other: Generalized pain; hypokalemia; injection site bleeding, pruritus, and rash

Nursing Considerations

• Use fondaparinux cautiously in elderly patients, especially those weighing less than 50 kg (110 lb) and are receiving the drug for pulmomary embolism or deep vein thrombosis, because the risk of drug-induced bleeding increases with age.
• Inspect fondaparinux for particles or discoloration before administration. Be aware that needle guard on prefilled syringe contains dry natural latex rubber and shouldnm't be handled by those sensitive to latex.
• Alternate injection sites during treatment using the left and right anterolateral or left and right posterolateral abdominal wall. Don't expel air bubble from prefilled syringe before injection to prevent expelling drug from syringe. Don't give drug by I.M. injection.
• **WARNING** Closely monitor patients who have had epidural or spinal anesthesia or a spinal puncture for signs of neurologic impairment. They're at risk for epidural or spinal hematoma, which can put them at risk for paralysis.
• Closely monitor patient for bleeding (such as ecchymosis, epistaxis, hematemesis, hematuria, and melena), especially those at risk for decreased drug elimination (such as elderly patients and patients with mild to moderate renal impairment) and those at increased risk for bleeding (such as patients with congenital or acquired bleeding disorders; active ulcerative GI disease; hemor-

rhagic stroke; recent brain, spinal, or ophthalmologic surgery; diabetic retinopathy; or a history of heparin-induced thrombocytopenia; and those being treated concomitantly with platelet inhibitors).
• Perform periodic CBC, including platelet count, as ordered. Expect prescriber to discontinue drug if platelet count falls below 100,000/mm^3. Be aware that routine coagulation tests, such as PT and INR, are not used to monitor fondaparinux therapy; an anti-Xa assay may be used instead. Also, test stools for occult blood, as ordered.
• Monitor patient with thrombocytopenia for evidence of thrombosis that may appear similar to heparin-induced thrombocytopenia even when no exposure to heparin has taken place. If patient's platelet count falls below 100,000/mm^3, fondaparinux should be discontinued.
• Monitor renal function test results, as ordered. Expect to discontinue drug if severe renal impairment or labile renal function occurs during fondaparinux therapy because the risk of hemorrhage increases as renal function decreases.
• Store drug at a controlled room temperature.

PATIENT TEACHING

• Inform patient that fondaparinux can't be taken orally.
• Instruct patient to seek immediate help if she experiences signs of thromboembolism, such as neurologic changes and severe shortness of breath.
• Inform patient about the increased risk of bleeding. Instruct her or family member to watch for and report abdominal or lower back pain, black stools, bleeding gums, bloody urine, or severe headaches.
• Teach patient or family member how to administer fondaparinux by subcutaneous injection at home, if needed. Instruct her not to expel air bubble from a prefilled syringe to avoid expelling some of the drug. Tell her to insert the entire needle into a skinfold held between thumb and forefinger, and remind her to alternate administration sites.
• To minimize bruising, caution the patient not to rub the injection site after giving the drug.
• Review safe handling and disposal of syringes and needles.
• Advise patient to have follow-up appointments and prescribed laboratory tests.

formoterol fumarate dihydrate

Foradil Aerolizer, Oxeze Turbuhaler (CAN), Perforomist

Class and Category

Chemical class: Racemic acid salt
Therapeutic class: Bronchodilator
Pregnancy category: C

Indications and Dosages

➤ *To prevent asthma-induced broncho-spasm*

POWDER FOR ORAL INHALATION

Adults and children age 5 and over. 12 mcg every 12 hr through inhaler device. *Maximum:* 24 mcg daily.

➤ *To prevent exercise-induced broncho-spasm*

POWDER FOR ORAL INHALATION

Adults and adolescents age 12 and over. 12 mcg at least 15 min before exercise every 12 hr p.r.n. *Maximum:* 24 mcg daily.

➤ *To provide long-term treatment of bronchospasm in patients with chronic bronchitis and emphysema*

POWDER FOR ORAL INHALATION

Adults. 12 mcg every 12 hr through inhaler device. *Maximum:* 24 mcg daily.

SOLUTION FOR ORAL INHALATION

Adults. 20 mcg b.i.d. by nebulization. *Maximum:* 40 mcg daily.

Route	Onset	Peak	Duration
Oral inhalation	1 to 3 min	Unknown	12 hr

Mechanism of Action

Selectively attaches to beta$_2$ receptors on bronchial membranes, stimulating the intracellular enzyme adenyl cyclase to convert adenosine triphosphate to cAMP. The resulting increase in the intracellular cAMP level relaxes bronchial smooth-muscle cells, stabilizes mast cells, and inhibits histamine release.

Contraindications

Acute asthma, hypersensitivity to formoterol fumarate or its components

Interactions

DRUGS

adrenergics: Possibly increased sympathetic effects of formoterol
beta blockers: Decreased effects of formoterol, possibly severe bronchospasm
corticosteroids, non–potassium-sparing diuretics, xanthine derivatives: Possibly increased hypokalemic effect of formoterol
disopyramide, MAO inhibitors, phenothiazines,
procainamide, quinidine, tricyclic antidepressants: Possibly prolonged QTc interval, increasing risk of ventricular arrhythmias

Adverse Reactions

CNS: Anxiety, dizziness, fatigue, fever, headache, insomnia, malaise, tremor
CV: Angina, arrhythmias, chest pain, hypertension, hypotension, palpitations, tachycardia
EENT: Dry mouth; laryngeal spasm, irritation, or swelling; hoarseness; pharyngitis; rhinitis and tonsillitis (in children); sinusitis
ENDO: Hyperglycemia
GI: Abdominal pain, gastroenteritis, indigestion (in children); nausea
MS: Back pain, leg cramps, muscle spasms
RESP: Asthma exacerbation, bronchitis, bronchospasm (paradoxical or hypersensitivity-induced), cough, dyspnea, increased sputum production, upper respiratory tract infection
SKIN: Dermatitis, pruritus, rash
Other: Anaphylaxis, angioedema, hypokalemia, metabolic acidosis, viral infection (in children)

Nursing Considerations

• Administer formoterol capsules or solution only by oral inhalation.
• Store capsules and solution in their original packaging, and open immediately before use.
• To use delivery system for powder form, place capsule in well of inhaler device. Press and release buttons on side of device to pierce capsule. Have patient inhale rapidly and deeply through mouthpiece; drug is dispersed into airways as patient inhales.
• Give inhalation solution only by standard jet nebulizer connected to an air compressor.
• **WARNING** Monitor patient for worsening or deteriorating asthma because drug isn't rapid-acting and shouldn't be used as a sub-

E
F

stitute for corticosteroid therapy.
•Watch closely for paradoxical bronchospasm; if this occurs, discontinue formoterol immediately and notify prescriber.
•Monitor patients with a history of cardiovascular disorders, especially coronary insufficiency, arrhythmias, or hypertension. Notify prescriber of any significant increases in pulse rate or blood pressure or exacerbation of chronic conditions because formoterol may produce cardiovascular reactions, including angina, arrhythmias, hypertension or hypotension, palpitations, and tachycardia. Drug may need to be discontinued if such reactions occur.

PATIENT TEACHING
•Advise patient, especially if she has significant cardiac history, to inform prescriber of any other drugs she takes before beginning formoterol therapy to prevent harmful drug interactions.
•Instruct patient to use manufacturer's plastic device for inhaling powder form of formoterol, to always use new inhaler that comes with each refill, and not to use a spacer. Tell her never to swallow capsules.
•Teach patient how to properly store powdered drug and inhaler. Instruct her to avoid exposing capsules to moisture and to always handle them with dry hands because powder inside capsules must be dry to be inhaled. Also advise her to keep inhaler in a dry place and *not* to wash it.
•Teach patient proper use of powdered formoterol delivery system. Instruct her to remove capsule from blister pack just before use, to place capsule in well of inhaler device, to press and release buttons on side of device to pierce capsule, and then to inhale rapidly and deeply through mouthpiece. Emphasize that she should only inhale, *not exhale*, into device.
•For solution form of formoterol, teach patient how to use, clean, and store nebulizer equipment. Tell her to leave the vial in its original foil pack until just before use.
•Instruct patient who currently uses oral or inhaled corticosteroids to continue using them, as prescribed, even if she feels better after starting formoterol.
•Caution patient not to increase formoterol dosage or frequency without consulting prescriber because she may need a rapid-acting bronchodilator.

•Urge patient to notify prescriber if her symptoms worsen, if formoterol becomes less effective, or if she needs more inhalations of short-acting beta₂-agonist than usual. This may indicate that her asthma is worsening.
•Instruct patient to notify prescriber immediately if she experiences palpitations, chest pain, rapid heart rate, tremor, or nervousness while taking formoterol because dosage may need to be adjusted.

fosfomycin tromethamine

Monurol

Class and Category
Chemical class: Phosphonic acid derivative
Therapeutic class: Antibiotic
Pregnancy category: B

Indications and Dosages
➤ *To treat uncomplicated UTI (acute cystitis) caused by* Enterococcus faecalis *or* Escherichia coli
GRANULES FOR ORAL SOLUTION
Women age 18 and over. 3 g as a single dose mixed with water.

Route	Onset	Peak	Duration
P.O.	2 to 3 days	48 hr	Unknown

Mechanism of Action
Disrupts the formation of bacterial cell walls by blocking cell wall precursors. Specifically, fosfomycin inactivates enolpyruvyl transferase, which irreversibly blocks the condensation of uridine diphosphate-*N*-acetylglucosamine with phosphoenolpyruvate, a preliminary step in bacterial cell wall synthesis. Fosfomycin also decreases adherence of bacteria to epithelial cells of the urinary tract.

Contraindications
Hypersensitivity to fosfomycin or its components

Interactions
DRUGS
metoclopramide: Decreased blood level and urinary excretion of fosfomycin

Adverse Reactions

CNS: Asthenia, dizziness, fever, headache, insomnia, nervousness, paresthesia, somnolence
EENT: Dry mouth, pharyngitis, rhinitis
GI: Abdominal pain, anorexia, constipation, diarrhea, flatulence, indigestion, nausea, pseudomembranous colitis, vomiting
GU: Dysmenorrhea, dysuria, hematuria, menstrual irregularities, vaginitis
MS: Back pain
SKIN: Pruritus, rash
Other: Flulike symptoms, lymphadenopathy

Nursing Considerations

• Use fosfomycin cautiously in patients with impaired renal function because drug clearance may be decreased.
• Expect to obtain urine specimens for culture and sensitivity tests before and after fosfomycin therapy.
• To reconstitute granules, pour contents of single-dose packet into 90 to 120 ml (3 to 4 oz) of water (not hot water) and stir. Administer immediately after dissolving.
•WARNING Expect adverse reactions to increase if more than one dose is used to treat a single episode of acute cystitis.
• Monitor patient for diarrhea during and for at least 2 months after drug therapy; diarrhea may signal pseudomembranous colitis caused by *Clostridium difficile*. If diarrhea occurs, notify prescriber and expect to withhold fosfomycin and treat with fluids, electrolytes, protein, and an antibiotic effective against *C. difficile*.

PATIENT TEACHING

• Explain how to reconstitute fosfomycin, and instruct patient to take drug immediately after it dissolves. Tell her not to take dry granules or mix them with hot water.
• To treat each episode of acute cystitis, advise patient to use only a single dose, as prescribed, to avoid increasing the risk of adverse reactions.
• Urge patient to notify prescriber if symptoms don't improve in 2 to 3 days.
• Instruct patient to return to prescriber for further urine testing after taking fosfomycin.
• Urge patient to tell prescriber about diarrhea that's severe or lasts longer than 3 days. Explain that watery or bloody stools can occur 2 or more months after therapy and can be serious, requiring prompt treatment.

fosinopril sodium

Monopril

Class and Category

Chemical class: Phosphinic acid derivative
Therapeutic class: Antihypertensive, vasodilator
Pregnancy category: C (first trimester), D (later trimesters)

Indications and Dosages

➤ *To manage blood pressure, alone or with other antihypertensives*

TABLETS

Adults. *Initial:* 10 mg daily. *Maintenance:* 20 to 40 mg daily. *Maximum:* 80 mg daily.

➤ *To treat heart failure*

TABLETS

Adults. 10 mg daily.
DOSAGE ADJUSTMENT Initial dosage reduced to 5 mg daily, if needed, for patients with acute heart failure, moderate to severe renal failure, or recent aggressive diuresis. Dosage may be increased over several weeks to maximum of 40 mg daily.

Route	Onset	Peak	Duration
P.O.	1 hr	2 to 6 hr	24 hr

E
F

Mechanism of Action

May reduce blood pressure by affecting renin-angiotensin-aldosterone system. By inhibiting angiotensin-converting enzyme, fosinopril:
• prevents conversion of angiotensin I to angiotensin II, a potent vasoconstrictor that also stimulates the adrenal cortex to secrete aldosterone
• may inhibit renal and vascular production of angiotensin II
• decreases serum angiotensin II level and increases serum renin activity, which decreases aldosterone secretion, slightly increasing the serum potassium level and fluid loss
• decreases vascular tone and blood pressure
• inhibits aldosterone release, which reduces sodium and water reabsorption and increases their excretion, further reducing blood pressure.

Contraindications

Hypersensitivity to fosinopril, other ACE inhibitors, or their components

Interactions

DRUGS

allopurinol, bone marrow depressants, procainamide, systemic corticosteroids: Increased risk of potentially fatal neutropenia or agranulocytosis

antacids: Impaired fosinopril absorption

cyclosporine, potassium-sparing diuretics, potassium supplements: Increased risk of hyperkalemia

diuretics, other antihypertensives: Possibly additive hypotension

lithium: Increased blood lithium level and risk of lithium toxicity

NSAIDs: Possibly decreased antihypertensive effect of fosinopril

FOODS

salt substitutes: Increased risk of hyperkalemia

ACTIVITIES

alcohol use: Possibly additive hypotension

Adverse Reactions

CNS: Confusion, depression, dizziness, drowsiness, fatigue, fever, headache, insomnia, mood changes, sleep disturbance, syncope, tremor, vertigo, weakness

CV: Angina, arrhythmias (including AV conduction disorders, bradycardia, and tachycardia), claudication, hypotension, MI, orthostatic hypotension, palpitations

EENT: Dry mouth, epistaxis, eye irritation, hoarseness, rhinitis, sinus problems, taste perversion, tinnitus, vision changes

GI: Abdominal distention and pain, anorexia, constipation, diarrhea, flatulence, hepatic failure, hepatitis, hepatomegaly, nausea, pancreatitis, vomiting

GU: Decreased libido, flank pain, renal insufficiency, sexual dysfunction, urinary frequency

MS: Arthralgia, gout, myalgia

RESP: Asthma; bronchitis; bronchospasm; dry, persistent, tickling cough; dyspnea; tracheobronchitis; upper respiratory tract infection

SKIN: Diaphoresis, jaundice, photosensitivity, pruritus, rash, urticaria

Other: Anaphylaxis, angioedema, hyperkalemia, weight gain

Nursing Considerations

• Monitor serum potassium level before and during fosinopril therapy, as appropriate.

• Observe patient being treated for heart failure for at least 2 hours after giving drug to detect hypotension or orthostatic hypotension. If either develops, notify prescriber and monitor patient until blood pressure stabilizes. Keep in mind that orthostatic hypotension is unlikely to develop in patients with a systolic blood pressure over 100 mm Hg who receive a 10-mg dose.

• If patient also receives an antacid, separate administration times by at least 2 hours.

• If patient also receives a diuretic or another antihypertensive, expect to reduce its dosage over 2 to 3 days before starting fosinopril. If blood pressure isn't controlled with fosinopril alone, other antihypertensive therapy may resume, as prescribed. If so, observe for excessive hypotension.

• **WARNING** If angioedema affects the face, glottis, larynx, limbs, lips, mucous membranes, or tongue, notify prescriber immediately. Expect to discontinue fosinopril and start appropriate therapy at once. If airway obstruction threatens, promptly give 0.3 to 0.5 ml of epinephrine solution 1:1,000 subcutaneously, as prescribed.

PATIENT TEACHING

• Instruct patient to take fosinopril at the same time each day to improve compliance and maintain drug's therapeutic effect.

• Emphasize the importance of taking fosinopril as prescribed, even if patient feels well. Caution her not to stop taking drug without consulting prescriber.

• Explain that drug helps control—but doesn't cure—hypertension and that patient may need lifelong therapy.

• **WARNING** Urge patient to seek immediate medical attention for difficulty breathing or swallowing, hoarseness, or swelling of the face, lips, tongue, or throat.

• Instruct patient to notify prescriber about persistent, severe nausea, vomiting, and diarrhea; resulting dehydration may lead to hypotension.

• Advise patient not to take other drugs or use salt substitutes without consulting prescriber.

• Encourage patient to keep scheduled appointments with prescriber to monitor blood

pressure, blood test results, and effects of therapy.
•Caution patient about possible dizziness.
•To minimize effects of orthostatic hypotension, advise patient to rise slowly from a lying or sitting position and to dangle legs over bed for several minutes before standing.
•Reinforce prescriber's recommendations for lifestyle changes, such as smoking cessation, stress reduction, dietary improvements, alcohol avoidance, and regular exercise.
•If patient is a woman of childbearing age, urge her to use contraception during therapy because drug may harm fetus.
•Advise patient to use caution during exercise and hot weather because of the increased risk of dehydration from excessive sweating.

fosphenytoin sodium

Cerebyx

Class and Category

Chemical class: Hydantoin derivative
Therapeutic class: Anticonvulsant
Pregnancy category: D

Indications and Dosages

➤ *To treat status epilepticus*
I.V. INFUSION, I.M. INJECTION
Adults and adolescents. *Initial:* 15 to 20 mg of phenytoin equivalent (PE)/kg I.V. at 100 to 150 PE/min. *Maintenance:* 4 to 6 mg PE/kg daily I.V. or I.M. in divided doses b.i.d. to q.i.d.
Maximum: 30 mg PE/kg as total loading dose.
Children. *Initial:* 15 to 20 mg PE/kg I.V. given at up to 3 mg PE/kg/min. *Maintenance:* 4 to 6 mg PE/kg daily I.V. or I.M. in divided doses b.i.d. to q.i.d.

➤ *To prevent or treat seizures during and after neurosurgery*
I.V. INFUSION, I.M. INJECTION
Adults and adolescents. *Initial:* 10 to 20 mg PE/kg I.V., not to exceed 150 mg PE/min. *Maintenance:* 4 to 6 mg PE/kg daily I.V. or I.M. in divided doses b.i.d. to q.i.d. *Maximum:* 30 mg PE/kg as total loading dose.

Contraindications

Hypersensitivity to fosphenytoin, phenytoin, other hydantoins, or their components

Mechanism of Action

Is converted from fosphenytoin (a prodrug) to phenytoin, which limits the spread of seizure activity and the start of new seizures. Phenytoin does so by regulating voltage-dependent sodium and calcium channels in neurons, inhibiting calcium movement across neuronal membranes, and enhancing the sodium-potassium-adenosine triphosphatase activity in neurons and glial cells. These actions may stem from phenytoin's ability to slow the recovery rate of inactivated sodium channels.

Interactions

DRUGS

acetaminophen (long-term use): Increased risk of hepatotoxicity
acyclovir: Decreased blood phenytoin level, loss of seizure control
alfentanil: Increased clearance and decreased effectiveness of alfentanil
amiodarone, fluoxetine: Possibly increased blood phenytoin level and risk of toxicity
antacids: Possibly decreased phenytoin effectiveness
antineoplastics: Increased phenytoin metabolism
beta blockers: Increased myocardial depression
bupropion, clozapine, loxapine, MAO inhibitors, maprotiline, phenothiazines, pimozide, thioxanthenes: Possibly lowered seizure threshold and decreased therapeutic effects of phenytoin, possibly intensified CNS depressant effects of these drugs
calcium: Possibly impaired phenytoin absorption
calcium channel blockers: Possibly increased blood phenytoin level
carbamazepine: Decreased blood carbamazepine level, possibly increased blood phenytoin level and risk of toxicity
chloramphenicol, cimetidine, disulfiram, isoniazid, methylphenidate, metronidazole, phenylbutazone, ranitidine, salicylates, sulfonamides, trimethoprim: Possibly impaired metabolism of these drugs, increased risk of phenytoin toxicity
CNS depressants: Possibly increased CNS depression

E
F

corticosteroids, cyclosporine, digoxin, diso-pyramide, doxycycline, furosemide, levodopa, mexiletine, quinidine: Decreased therapeutic effects of these drugs

diazoxide: Possibly decreased therapeutic effects of both drugs

dopamine: Possibly sudden hypotension or cardiac arrest after I.V. fosphenytoin administration

estrogen- and progestin-containing contraceptives: Possibly breakthrough bleeding and decreased contraceptive effectiveness

estrogens, progestins: Decreased therapeutic effects, increased blood phenytoin level

felbamate: Possibly impaired metabolism and increased blood level of phenytoin

fluconazole, itraconazole, ketoconazole, miconazole: Increased blood phenytoin level

folic acid: Increased phenytoin metabolism, decreased seizure control

haloperidol: Possibly lowered seizure threshold and decreased therapeutic effects of phenytoin; possibly decreased blood haloperidol level

insulin, oral antidiabetic drugs: Possibly increased blood glucose level and decreased therapeutic effects of these drugs

lamotrigine: Possibly decreased therapeutic effects of lamotrigine

lidocaine: Possibly decreased blood lidocaine level, increased myocardial depression

lithium: Increased risk of lithium toxicity

methadone: Possibly increased methadone metabolism, leading to withdrawal symptoms

molindone: Possibly lowered seizure threshold, impaired absorption, and decreased therapeutic effects of phenytoin

omeprazole: Possibly increased blood phenytoin level

oral anticoagulants: Possibly impaired metabolism of these drugs and increased risk of phenytoin toxicity; possibly increased anticoagulant effects initially and then decreased effects with prolonged therapy

rifampin: Possibly decreased therapeutic effects of phenytoin

streptozocin: Possibly decreased therapeutic effects of streptozocin

sucralfate: Possibly decreased phenytoin absorption

tricyclic antidepressants: Possibly lowered seizure threshold and decreased therapeutic effects of phenytoin; possibly decreased

blood antidepressant level

valproic acid: Decreased blood phenytoin level, increased blood valproic acid level

vitamin D analogues: Decreased vitamin D analogue activity

xanthines: Possibly inhibited phenytoin absorp-tion and increased clearance of xanthines

zaleplon: Increased clearance and decreased effectiveness of zaleplon

ACTIVITIES

alcohol use: Possibly decreased phenytoin effectiveness

Adverse Reactions

CNS: Agitation, amnesia, asthenia, ataxia, cerebral edema, chills, coma, confusion, delusions, depression, dizziness, emotional lability, encephalitis, encephalopathy, extrapyramidal reactions, fever, headache, hemiplegia, hostility, hypoesthesia, lack of coordination, malaise, meningitis, nervousness, neurosis, paralysis, personality disorder, positive Babinski's sign, seizures, somnolence, speech disorders, stroke, stupor, subdural hematoma, syncope, transient paresthesia, tremor, vertigo

CV: Atrial flutter, bradycardia, bundle-branch block, cardiac arrest, cardiomegaly, edema, heart failure, hypertension, hypotension, orthostatic hypotension, palpitations, PVCs, shock, tachycardia, thrombophlebitis

EENT: Amblyopia, conjunctivitis, diplopia, dry mouth, earache, epistaxis, eye pain, gingival hyperplasia, hearing loss, hyperacusis, increased salivation, loss of taste, mydriasis, nystagmus, pharyngitis, photophobia, rhinitis, sinusitis, taste perversion, tinnitus, tongue swelling, visual field defects

ENDO: Diabetes insipidus, hyperglycemia, ketosis

GI: Anorexia, constipation, diarrhea, dysphagia, elevated liver function test results, flatulence, gastritis, GI bleeding, hepatic necrosis, hepatitis, ileus, indigestion, nausea, vomiting

GU: Albuminuria, dysuria, incontinence, oliguria, polyuria, renal failure, urine retention, vaginal candidiasis

HEME: Anemia, easy bruising, leukopenia, thrombocytopenia

MS: Arthralgia, back pain, leg cramps, muscle twitching, myalgia, myasthenia, myoclonus, myopathy

RESP: Apnea, asthma, atelectasis, bronchitis, dyspnea, hemoptysis, hyperventilation, hypoxia, increased cough, increased sputum production, pneumonia, pneumothorax
SKIN: Contact dermatitis, diaphoresis, maculopapular or pustular rash, photosensitivity, skin discoloration, skin nodule, Stevens-Johnson syndrome, transient pruritus, urticaria
Other: Cachexia, cryptococcosis, dehydration, facial edema, flulike symptoms, hyperkalemia, hypokalemia, hypophosphatemia, infection, injection site reaction, lymphadenopathy, sepsis

Nursing Considerations
• Express the dosage, concentration, and infusion rate of fosphenytoin in PE units. Misreading an order or a label could result in massive overdose.
• Refrigerate unopened fosphenytoin at 2° to 8° C (36° to 46° F), but don't freeze.
• Dilute drug in D_5W or normal saline solution to 1.5 to 25 mg PE/ml.
• Inspect parenteral solution before administration. Discard solution that contains particles or is discolored.
• Be aware that drug shouldn't be given I.M. for status epilepticus because I.V. route allows faster onset and peak.
• Keep in mind that I.V. fosphenytoin administration doesn't require use of a filter, as with phenytoin administration.
• Don't give fosphenytoin solution faster than 150 mg PE/minute because of the risk of hypotension. For a 50-kg (110-lb) patient, infusion typically takes 5 to 7 minutes. Fosphenytoin can be given more rapidly than I.V. phenytoin.
• Follow loading dose with maintenance dosage of oral or parenteral phenytoin or parenteral fosphenytoin, as prescribed.
• As prescribed, give I.V. benzodiazepine (such as lorazepam or diazepam) with fosphenytoin; otherwise, drug's full antiepileptic effect won't be immediate.
• Monitor ECG, blood pressure, and respiratory function for 10 to 20 minutes after infusion ends.
• Expect to obtain blood fosphenytoin (phenytoin) level 2 hours after I.V. infusion or 4 hours after I.M. injection. Therapeutic level generally ranges from 10 to 20 mcg/ml; steady-state may take several days to several

weeks to reach.
• Be aware that I.V. or I.M. fosphenytoin may be substituted for oral phenytoin sodium at same total daily dose and frequency. If prescribed, give daily amount in two or more divided doses to maintain seizure control.
• When switching between phenytoin and fosphenytoin, remember that small differences in phenytoin bioavailability can lead to significant changes in blood phenytoin level and an increased risk of toxicity.
• If drug causes transient, infusion-related paresthesia and pruritus, decrease or discontinue infusion, as ordered.
• Monitor CBC for thrombocytopenia or leukopenia—signs of hematologic toxicity. Also monitor serum albumin level and results of renal and liver function tests.
• Anticipate increased frequency and severity of adverse reactions after I.V. administration in patients with hepatic or renal impairment or hypoalbuminemia.
• Discontinue drug, as ordered, if signs of hypersensitivity develop: acute hepatotoxicity (hepatic necrosis and hepatitis), fever, lymphadenopathy, and skin reactions during first 2 months of therapy.
• Monitor blood phenytoin level to detect early signs of toxicity, such as diplopia, nausea, severe confusion, slurred speech, and vomiting. Expect to reduce or stop drug.
• **WARNING** Monitor patient for seizures; at toxic levels, phenytoin is excitatory.
• **WARNING** If patient has bradycardia or heart block rhythm, notify prescriber and expect to withhold drug; severe cardiovascular reactions and death have occurred.
• Expect to provide vitamin D supplement if patient has inadequate dietary intake and is receiving long-term anticonvulsant treatment.
• Document type, onset, and characteristics of seizures as well as response to treatment.

PATIENT TEACHING
• Inform patient that fosphenytoin typically is used for short-term treatment.
• Instruct patient to notify prescriber immediately about bothersome symptoms, especially rash and swollen glands.
• Because gingival hyperplasia may develop during long-term therapy, emphasize need for good oral hygiene and gum massage.
• Urge patient to consume adequate amounts of vitamin D.

E
F

frovatriptan succinate

Frova

Class and Category

Chemical class: Selective 5-hydroxytryptamine$_1$ (5-HT$_1$) receptor agonist, triptan
Therapeutic class: Antimigraine agent
Pregnancy category: C

Indications and Dosages

➤ *To treat acute migraine with or without aura*

TABLETS

Adults. 2.5 mg, repeated in 2 hr if needed. *Maximum:* 7.5 mg daily.

Mechanism of Action

Binds to 5-HT$_{1B}$ and 5-HT$_{1D}$ receptors on extracerebral and intracranial arteries to inhibit excessive dilation of these vessels. This action may decrease carotid arterial blood flow, thus relieving acute migraines. Frovatriptan may also relieve pain by inhibiting the release of proinflammatory neuropeptides and reducing transmission of trigeminal nerve impulses from sensory nerve endings during a migraine attack.

Contraindications

Hypersensitivity to frovatriptan or its components, basilar or hemiplegic migraines, cerebrovascular or peripheral vascular disease, ischemic or vasospastic coronary artery disease (CAD), uncontrolled hypertension, use within 24 hours of other serotonin-receptor agonists or ergotamine-containing or ergot-type drugs

Interactions

DRUGS

dihydroergotamine mesylate, other ergotamine-containing drugs: Possibly prolonged vasospastic reaction
fluoxetine, other selective serotonin-reuptake inhibitors: Possibly weakness, hyperreflexia, and incoordination
oral contraceptives, propranolol: Possibly increased blood frovatriptan level

Adverse Reactions

CNS: Anxiety, dizziness, dysesthesia, fatigue, headache, hypoesthesia, insomnia, paresthesia

CV: Arrhythmias (such as bradycardia and tachycardia), chest pain, coronary artery vasospasm, ECG changes, MI, myocardial ischemia (transient), palpitations, ventricular fibrillation, ventricular tachycardia
EENT: Abnormal vision, dry mouth, indigestion, rhinitis, sinusitis, tinnitus
GI: Abdominal pain, diarrhea, indigestion, vomiting
MS: Skeletal pain
SKIN: Diaphoresis, flushing
Other: Generalized pain

Nursing Considerations

•Use frovatriptan cautiously in patients with peripheral vascular disease because drug may cause vasospastic reactions, leading to vascular and colonic ischemia with abdominal pain and bloody diarrhea. Assess patient's peripheral circulation and bowel sounds during frovatriptan therapy.
•Don't administer frovatriptan within 24 hours of another 5-HT$_1$ receptor agonist, such as sumatriptan or rizatriptan, or of an ergotamine-containing or ergot-type drug, such as dihydroergotamine or methysergide.
•Administer tablet with fluids.
•Assess patient for headache before administering second dose. Don't administer more than three 2.5-mg tablets a day.
•**WARNING** Be aware that some patients have had serious adverse cardiac reactions—including fatal ones—after using 5-HT$_1$ receptor agonists. However, these reactions are extremely rare; most were reported in patients with risk factors for CAD.
•Assess patient's cardiovascular status and institute continuous ECG monitoring, as ordered, immediately after drug administration in patients with cardiovascular risk factors because they're at risk for asymptomatic cardiac ischemia.
•Assess patient for arrhythmias, chest pain, and other signs of heart disease in patients with risk factors for CAD. Expect to periodically assess cardiovascular status of patients on long-term therapy.
•Be aware that the safety of treating more than four migraine attacks in 30 days (on average) has not been established.
•Regularly monitor blood pressure of hypertensive patients during therapy because frovatriptan may produce a transient increase in blood pressure.

•Instruct patient to read and follow manufacturer's instructions for using frovatriptan to ensure maximum therapeutic results.
•Remind patient not to exceed prescribed daily dosage.
•Encourage patient to lie down in a dark, quiet room after taking drug to help relieve migraine.
•Instruct patient to seek emergency care for chest, jaw, or neck tightness after drug use because drug may cause coronary artery vasospasm.
•Urge patient to report palpitations.
•Caution patient about possible adverse CNS effects, and advise her to avoid hazardous activities until drug's CNS effects are known.

furazolidone

Furoxone

Class and Category

Chemical class: MAO inhibitor, nitrofuran derivative
Therapeutic class: Antibiotic, antiprotozoal
Pregnancy category: C

Indications and Dosages

➤ *To treat bacterial diarrhea and cholera*
ORAL SUSPENSION, TABLETS
Adults and adolescents. 100 mg every 6 hr for 5 to 7 days.
Infants and children age 1 month and over. 1.25 mg/kg every 6 hr for 5 to 7 days. *Maximum:* 8.8 mg/kg daily.

➤ *To treat giardiasis*
ORAL SUSPENSION, TABLETS
Adults and adolescents. 100 mg every 6 hr for 7 to 10 days.
Infants and children age 1 month and over. 1.25 to 2 mg/kg every 6 hr for 7 to 10 days. *Maximum:* 8.8 mg/kg daily.

Mechanism of Action

May interfere with several bacterial enzyme systems through DNA strand damage. Furazolidone also prevents the inactivation of tyramine by GI and hepatic MAO because it is similar in structure and actions to MAO inhibitors.

Contraindications

Age less than 1 month; hypersensitivity to furazolidone, other nitrofurans, or their components

Interactions
DRUGS
levodopa: Increased therapeutic and adverse effects (particularly hypertension) of levodopa
meperidine: Possibly agitation, apnea, coma, diaphoresis, fever, and seizures
other MAO inhibitors, sedatives, sympathomimetics, tranquilizers, tricyclic antidepressants: Possibly sudden and severe hypertensive crisis
selective serotonin reuptake inhibitors: Increased risk of serotonin syndrome
FOODS
foods and beverages with high content of tyramine or other vasopressor amines: Possibly sudden and severe hypertensive crisis
ACTIVITIES
alcohol use: Possibly disulfiram-like reaction

Adverse Reactions
CNS: Headache, malaise
ENDO: Hypoglycemia
GI: Abdominal pain, diarrhea, nausea, vomiting
GU: Darkened urine
HEME: Hemolytic anemia, leukopenia
Other: Allergic reaction (arthralgia, dyspnea, fever, hypotension, urticaria, vesicular morbilliform rash)

Nursing Considerations
•Ask patient if she has a history of blood disorders—especially glucose-6-phosphate dehydrogenase (G6PD) deficiency—before giving furazolidone.
•As ordered, check G6PD level before giving furazolidone to whites of Mediterranean and Near Eastern origin, Asians, or blacks; G6PD deficiency may worsen drug's hemolytic effect.
•If no response occurs within 7 days, expect to discontinue drug because organism is resistant. Provide therapy with other antibiotics, as prescribed.
•If giardiasis symptoms persist, expect to obtain three stool specimens for analysis several days apart, starting 3 to 4 weeks after treatment ends.

E
F

PATIENT TEACHING

•Instruct patient to take drug at evenly spaced intervals around the clock.
•Advise patient to take drug with food if GI distress occurs.
•Direct patient to take a missed dose as soon as she remembers, unless it's nearly time for the next scheduled dose. Caution against double-dosing.
•Instruct patient to take furazolidone for the full time prescribed, even if she feels better before finishing the prescription, because stopping too soon could result in reinfection.
•Advise patient to store furazolidone between 59° and 86° F (15° and 30° C), protected from moisture and light.
•Inform patient that drug may cause dizziness and usually turns urine brown.
•Instruct patient to avoid alcohol during therapy and for 4 days afterward.
•Give patient a list of products to avoid during furazolidone therapy and for at least 2 weeks afterward, such as foods and beverages that contain tyramine and other vasopressor amines (for example, ripe cheese, beer, red and white wine, and smoked or pickled meat, poultry, or fish), OTC appetite suppressants, cough and cold medicines, and other drugs, unless prescribed.
•Instruct patient to notify prescriber if she experiences difficult breathing, fever, flushing, itching, muscle aches, or rash.

furosemide

Apo-Furosemide (CAN), Furoside (CAN), Lasix, Lasix Special (CAN), Myrosemide, Novosemide (CAN), Uritol (CAN)

Class and Category

Chemical class: Sulfonamide
Therapeutic class: Antihypertensive, diuretic
Pregnancy category: C

Indications and Dosages

➤ *To reduce edema caused by cirrhosis, heart failure, and renal disease, including nephrotic syndrome*

ORAL SOLUTION, TABLETS

Adults. 20 to 80 mg as a single dose, increased by 20 to 40 mg every 6 to 8 hr until desired response occurs. *Maximum:* 600 mg daily.

Children. 2 mg/kg as a single dose, increased by 1 to 2 mg/kg every 6 to 8 hr until desired response occurs. *Maximum:* 6 mg/kg/dose.

I.V. INFUSION, I.V. OR I.M. INJECTION

Adults. 20 to 40 mg as a single dose, increased by 20 mg every 2 hr until desired response occurs.

Children. 1 mg/kg as a single dose, increased by 1 mg/kg every 2 hr until desired response occurs. *Maximum:* 6 mg/kg/dose.

DOSAGE ADJUSTMENT Initial single dose limited to 20 mg for elderly patients.

➤ *To manage mild to moderate hypertension, as adjunct to treat acute pulmonary edema and hypertensive crisis*

ORAL SOLUTION, TABLETS

Adults. *Initial:* 40 mg b.i.d., adjusted until desired response occurs. *Maximum:* 600 mg daily.

I.V. INFUSION OR INJECTION

Adults with normal renal function. 40 to 80 mg as a single dose over several minutes.
Adults with acute renal failure or pulmonary edema. 100 to 200 mg as a single dose over several minutes.

DOSAGE ADJUSTMENT For patients with acute pulmonary edema without hypertensive crisis, dosage reduced to 40 mg followed by 80 mg 1 hr later if therapeutic response doesn't occur.

Route	Onset	Peak	Duration
P.O.	20 to 60 min	1 to 2 hr	6 to 8 hr
I.V.	5 min	In 30 min	2 hr
I.M.	30 min	Unknown	2 hr

Mechanism of Action

Inhibits sodium and water reabsorption in the loop of Henle and increases urine formation. As the body's plasma volume decreases, aldosterone production increases, which promotes sodium reabsorption and the loss of potassium and hydrogen ions. Furosemide also increases the excretion of calcium, magnesium, bicarbonate, ammonium, and phosphate. By reducing intracellular and extracellular fluid volume, the drug reduces blood pressure and decreases cardiac output. Over time, cardiac output returns to normal.

Incompatibilities
Don't mix furosemide (a milky, buffered alkaline solution) with highly acidic solutions.

Contraindications
Anuria unresponsive to furosemide; hypersensitivity to furosemide, sulfonamides, or their components

Interactions
DRUGS
ACE inhibitors: Possibly first-dose hypotension
aminoglycosides, cisplatin: Increased risk of ototoxicity
amiodarone: Increased risk of arrhythmias from hypokalemia
chloral hydrate: Possibly diaphoresis, hot flashes, and hypertension
digoxin: Increased risk of digitalis toxicity related to hypokalemia
insulin, oral antidiabetic drugs: Increased blood glucose level
lithium: Increased risk of lithium toxicity
NSAIDs: Possibly decreased diuresis
phenytoin, probenecid: Possibly decreased therapeutic effects of furosemide
propranolol: Possibly increased blood propranolol level
thiazide diuretics: Possibly profound diuresis and electrolyte imbalances

ACTIVITIES
alcohol use: Possibly increased hypotensive and diuretic effects of furosemide

Adverse Reactions
CNS: Dizziness, fever, headache, paresthesia, restlessness, vertigo, weakness
CV: Orthostatic hypotension, shock, thromboembolism, thrombophlebitis
EENT: Blurred vision, oral irritation, ototoxicity, stomatitis, tinnitus, transient hearing loss (rapid I.V. injection), yellow vision
ENDO: Hyperglycemia
GI: Abdominal cramps, anorexia, constipation, diarrhea, gastric irritation, hepatocellular insufficiency, indigestion, jaundice, nausea, pancreatitis, vomiting
GU: Bladder spasms, glycosuria
HEME: Agranulocytosis (rare), anemia, aplastic anemia (rare), azotemia, hemolytic anemia, leukopenia, thrombocytopenia
MS: Muscle spasms
SKIN: Bullous pemphigoid, erythema multiforme, exfoliative dermatitis, photosensitivity, pruritus, purpura, rash, urticaria
Other: Allergic reaction (interstitial nephritis, necrotizing vasculitis, systemic vasculitis), dehydration, hyperuricemia, hypochloremia, hypokalemia, hyponatremia, hypovolemia

Nursing Considerations
•**WARNING** Use furosemide cautiously in patients with advanced hepatic cirrhosis, especially those who also have a history of electrolyte imbalance or hepatic encephalopathy; drug may lead to lethal hepatic coma.
•Obtain patient's weight before and periodically during furosemide therapy to monitor fluid loss.
•For once-a-day dosing, give drug in the morning so patient's sleep won't be interrupted by increased need to urinate.
•Prepare drug for infusion with normal saline solution, lactated Ringer's solution, or D_5W.
•Administer drug slowly I.V. over 1 to 2 minutes to prevent ototoxicity.
•Expect patient to have periodic hearing tests during prolonged or high-dose I.V. therapy.
•Monitor blood pressure and hepatic and renal function as well as BUN, blood glucose, and serum creatinine, electrolyte, and uric acid levels, as appropriate.
•Be aware that elderly patients are more susceptible to hypotensive and electrolyte-altering effects and thus are at greater risk for shock and thromboembolism.
•If patient is at high risk for hypokalemia, give potassium supplements along with furosemide, as prescribed.
•Expect to discontinue furosemide at maximum dosage if oliguria persists for more than 24 hours.
•Be aware that furosemide may worsen left ventricular hypertrophy and adversely affect glucose tolerance and lipid metabolism.
•Notify prescriber if patient experiences hearing loss, vertigo, or ringing, buzzing, or sense of fullness in her ears. Drug may need to be discontinued.

PATIENT TEACHING
•Instruct patient to take furosemide at the same time each day to maintain therapeutic effects. Urge her to take it as prescribed, even if she feels well.
•Instruct patient to take the last dose of furosemide several hours before bedtime to

E
F

avoid sleep interruption from diuresis. If patient receives once-daily dosing, advise her to take the dose in the morning to avoid sleep disturbance caused by nocturia.

•Advise patient to change position slowly to minimize effects of orthostatic hypotension and to take furosemide with food or milk to reduce GI distress.

•Caution patient about drinking alcoholic beverages, standing for prolonged periods, and exercising in hot weather because these actions increase the hypotensive effect of furosemide.

•Emphasize the importance of weight and diet control, especially limiting sodium intake.

•Unless contraindicated, urge patient to eat more high-potassium foods and to take a potassium supplement, if prescribed, to prevent hypokalemia.

•Instruct patient to keep follow-up appointments with prescriber to monitor progress. Urge her to notify prescriber about persistent, severe nausea, vomiting, and diarrhea because they may cause dehydration.

•Inform diabetic patient that furosemide may increase blood glucose level, and advise her to check her blood glucose level frequently.

G·H·I

gabapentin

Neurontin

Class and Category

Chemical class: Cyclohexane-acetic acid derivative
Therapeutic class: Anticonvulsant
Pregnancy category: C

Indications and Dosages

➤ *To manage postherpetic neuralgia*

CAPSULES, ORAL SOLUTION, TABLETS

Adults. *Initial:* 300 mg on day 1, increased to 300 mg b.i.d. on day 2, increased to 300 mg t.i.d. on day 3, and increased gradually thereafter according to pain response, up to 600 mg t.i.d. *Maximum:* 1,800 mg daily.

➤ *As adjunct to treat partial seizures*

CAPSULES, ORAL SOLUTION, TABLETS

Adults and adolescents. *Initial:* 300 mg t.i.d., increased gradually according to clinical response. *Maintenance:* 900 to 1,800 mg daily. *Maximum:* 3,600 mg daily.

DOSAGE ADJUSTMENT If creatinine clearance is 30 to 60 ml/min/1.73 m², dosage reduced to 300 mg b.i.d.; if 15 to 29 ml/min/1.73 m², to 300 mg daily; and if less than 15 ml/min/1.73 m², to 300 mg every other day.

Mechanism of Action

Is structurally like gamma-aminobutyric acid (GABA), the main inhibitory neurotransmitter in the brain. Although gabapentin's exact mechanism of action is unknown, GABA inhibits the rapid firing of neurons associated with seizures.

Contraindications

Hypersensitivity to gabapentin or its components

Interactions

DRUGS

aluminum- and magnesium-containing antacids: Decreased gabapentin bioavail-ability

CNS depressants: Increased CNS depression

ACTIVITIES

alcohol use: Increased CNS depression

Adverse Reactions

CNS: Agitation, altered proprioception, amnesia, anxiety, apathy, aphasia, asthenia, ataxia, cerebellar dysfunction, chills, CNS tumors, decreased or absent reflexes, delusions, depersonalization, depression, disappearance of aura, dizziness, dream disturbances, dysesthesia, dystonia, emotional lability, euphoria, facial paralysis, fatigue, fever, hallucinations, headache, hemiplegia, hostility, hyperkinesia, hyperreflexia, hypoesthesia, hypotonia, intracranial hemorrhage, lack of coordination, malaise, migraine headache, nervousness, occipital neuralgia, paranoia, paresis, paresthesia, positive Babinski's sign, psychosis, sedation, seizures, somnolence, stupor, subdural hematoma, suicidal tendencies, syncope, tremor, vertigo

CV: Angina, hypertension, hypotension, murmur, palpitations, peripheral edema, peripheral vascular insufficiency, tachycardia, vasodilation

EENT: Abnormal vision, amblyopia, blepharospasm, cataracts, conjunctivitis, diplopia, dry eyes and mouth, earache, epistaxis, eye hemorrhage, eye pain, gingival bleeding, gingivitis, glossitis, hearing loss, hoarseness, increased salivation, inner ear infection, loss of taste, nystagmus, pharyngitis, photophobia, ptosis (bilateral or unilateral), rhinitis, sensation of fullness in ears, stomatitis, taste perversion, tinnitus, tooth discoloration, visual field defects

GI: Abdominal pain, anorexia, constipation, diarrhea, fecal incontinence, flatulence, gastroenteritis, hemorrhoids, hepatitis, hepatomegaly, increased appetite, indigestion, melena, nausea, thirst, vomiting

GU: Acute renal failure, decreased libido, impotence

HEME: Anemia, coagulation defect, decreased WBC count, leukopenia, thrombocytopenia

MS: Arthralgia, arthritis, back pain, bone fractures, dysarthria, joint stiffness or swelling, muscle twitching, myalgia, positive Romberg test, tendinitis

RESP: Apnea, cough, dyspnea, pneumonia, pseudocroup

SKIN: Abrasion, acne, alopecia, cyst, dia-

G
H
I

phoresis, dry skin, eczema, hirsutism, pruritus, purpura, rash, seborrhea, urticaria
Other: Dehydration, facial edema, lymphadenopathy, viral infection, weight gain or loss

Nursing Considerations
• As needed, open gabapentin capsules and mix contents with water, fruit juice, applesauce, or pudding before administration.
• Administer initial dose at bedtime to minimize adverse reactions, especially ataxia, dizziness, fatigue, and somnolence.
• Give drug at least 2 hours after giving an antacid.
• Don't exceed 12 hours between doses on a 3-times-a-day schedule.
• Be aware that routine monitoring of blood gabapentin level isn't necessary.
• WARNING To discontinue drug or switch to an alternate anticonvulsant, expect to change gradually over at least 1 week, as prescribed, to avoid loss of seizure control.
• Monitor renal function test results, and expect to adjust dosage, if necessary.

PATIENT TEACHING
• If patient has trouble swallowing gabapentin capsules, advise him to open them and sprinkle contents in juice or on soft food immediately before use.
• Instruct patient not to take drug within 2 hours after taking an antacid.
• Urge patient to take a missed dose as soon as he remembers. If the next dose is in less than 2 hours, tell him to wait 1 to 2 hours before taking it and then resume his regular schedule. Caution against doubling the dose.
• Caution patient not to stop drug abruptly.
• Inform patient about possible ataxia, dizziness, drowsiness, and nystagmus. Advise him to avoid potentially hazardous activities until drug's CNS effects are known.
• To prevent complications from adverse oral reactions (such as gingivitis), encourage patient to use good oral hygiene and to seek routine dental care.
• Explain that adverse effects usually are mild to moderate and decline with time.
• Urge patient to keep follow-up appointments with prescriber to check progress.

galantamine hydrobromide

Razadyne, Razadyne ER

Class and Category
Chemical class: Tertiary alkaloid
Therapeutic class: Antidementia agent
Pregnancy category: B

Indications and Dosages
➤ *To treat mild to moderate Alzheimer's-type dementia*

ORAL SOLUTION, TABLETS
Adults. *Initial:* 4 mg b.i.d. Dosage increased by 8 mg daily every 4 wk, if tolerated. *Maximum:* 12 mg b.i.d.
DOSAGE ADJUSTMENT For patients with moderately impaired hepatic or renal function, maximum dosage shouldn't exceed 16 mg daily.

E.R. CAPSULES
Adults. *Initial:* 8 mg daily. Dosage increased by 8 mg daily every 4 wk if tolerated. *Maximum:* 24 mg daily.

Route	Onset	Peak	Duration
P.O.	Unknown	About 1 hr	Unknown

Mechanism of Action
Reduces acetylcholine metabolism by competitively and reversibly inhibiting the brain enzyme acetylcholinesterase. Acetylcholine-producing neurons degenerate in the brains of patients with Alzheimer's disease. Inhibition of acetylcholinesterase increases the amount of acetylcholine, which is necessary for nerve impulse transmission.

Contraindications
Hypersensitivity to galantamine hydrobromide or its components, severe hepatic or renal impairment (creatinine clearance less than 9 ml/min/1.73 m^2)

Interactions
DRUGS
amitriptyline, fluoxetine, fluvoxamine, quinidine: Possibly decreased galantamine clearance
anticholinergics: Possibly interference with cholinesterase activity
cholinergic agonists, cholinesterase inhibitors, neuromuscular blockers: Possibly exaggerated effects of these drugs and galantamine
cimetidine: Possibly increased galantamine bioavailability
ketoconazole, paroxetine: Increased galantamine bioavailability

Adverse Reactions
CNS: Aggression, asthenia, depression, dizziness, fatigue, fever, headache, insomnia, malaise, somnolence, stroke, suicidal ideation, syncope, tremor
CV: AV block, bradycardia, chest pain, MI, myocardial ischemia
EENT: Rhinitis
GI: Abdominal pain, anorexia, diarrhea, flatulence, GI bleeding, indigestion, nausea, vomiting
GU: Hematuria, incontinence, renal failure or insufficiency, UTI
HEME: Anemia
Other: Dehydration, hypokalemia, weight loss

Nursing Considerations
• Administer galantamine twice daily with morning and evening meals, and ensure adequate fluid intake to prevent GI symptoms.
• If therapy is interrupted for several days, expect to restart drug at lowest dose because drug's benefits are lost when it is discontinued.
• Monitor patient's CV status closely because cholinesterase inhibitors like galantamine may have depressive effect on sinoatrial and AV nodes and may lead to bradycardia and AV block.
• Monitor patient for progressive deterioration of mental status because drug is less effective as Alzheimer's disease progresses and intact cholinergic neurons decrease.

PATIENT TEACHING
• Instruct patient to take or caregiver to give regular-strength drug with morning and evening meals. Extended-release capsules should be given once in the morning, preferably with food.
• Tell patient or caregiver to notify prescriber immediately if therapy is stopped for several days. Prescriber may restart at lowest dose.
• Instruct patient to maintain an adequate fluid intake throughout galantamine therapy.
• Advise patient not to drive or perform activities requiring high levels of alertness, especially during first weeks of treatment, because drug may cause dizziness and drowsiness.
• Inform patient and family members that drug isn't a cure for Alzheimer's disease.

gemfibrozil

Apo-Gemfibrozil (CAN), Gen-Fibro (CAN), Lopid, Novo-Gemfibrozil (CAN), Nu-Gemfibrozil (CAN)

Class and Category
Chemical class: Fibric acid derivative, phenoxypentanoic acid
Therapeutic class: Antihyperlipidemic
Pregnancy category: C

Indications and Dosages
➤ *As adjunct (with diet) to treat hyperlipidemia types IIb, IV, and V*
CAPSULES, TABLETS
Adults. 600 mg a.c. b.i.d.

Route	Onset	Peak	Duration
P.O.	2 to 5 days	4 wk	Unknown

Mechanism of Action
May decrease hepatic triglyceride production by reducing VLDL synthesis, inhibiting peripheral lipolysis, and decreasing hepatic extraction of free fatty acids. Gemfibrozil also may inhibit synthesis and increase clearance of apolipoprotein B, a carrier molecule for VLDL. In addition, it may accelerate turnover and removal of total cholesterol from the liver while increasing cholesterol excretion in the feces. As a result of these actions, triglyceride, total cholesterol, and VLDL levels decrease; the HDL level increases; and the LDL level is unaffected.

Contraindications
Gallbladder disease, hepatic or severe renal dysfunction, hypersensitivity to gemfibrozil or its components

Interactions
DRUGS
chenodiol, ursodiol: Decreased effectiveness of gemfibrozil
HMG-CoA reductase inhibitors: Increased risk of rhabdomyolysis and acute renal failure
oral anticoagulants: Increased anticoagulation
repaglinide: Increased serum repaglinide level

Adverse Reactions
CNS: Chills, fatigue, headache, hypoesthesia, paresthesia, seizures, somnolence, syncope, vertigo
CV: Vasculitis
EENT: Blurred vision, cataracts, hoarseness, retinal edema, taste perversion
GI: Abdominal or epigastric pain, cholelithi-

G
H
I

asis, colitis, diarrhea, flatulence, heartburn, hepatoma, nausea, pancreatitis, vomiting
GU: Decreased male fertility, dysuria, impotence
HEME: Anemia, bone marrow hypoplasia, eosinophilia, leukopenia, thrombocytopenia
MS: Arthralgia, back pain, myalgia, myasthenia, myopathy, myositis, rhabdomyolysis, synovitis
RESP: Cough
SKIN: Eczema, jaundice, pruritus, rash
Other: Anaphylaxis, angioedema, increased risk of bacterial and viral infections, lupus-like symptoms, weight loss

Nursing Considerations
•Monitor serum triglyceride and cholesterol levels, as appropriate.
•Periodically review CBC and liver function test results during therapy, as ordered.
•If serum triglyceride and cholesterol levels don't improve within 3 months, expect to switch to a different drug, as prescribed.
PATIENT TEACHING
•Instruct patient to take gemfibrozil 30 minutes before breakfast and 30 minutes before dinner.
•Advise patient to take a missed dose as soon as he remembers, unless it's nearly time for the next dose. Caution against doubling the dose.
•Stress the importance of a low-fat diet, regular exercise, alcohol avoidance, and smoking cessation, as appropriate.
•Caution patient to avoid hazardous activities until drug's CNS effects are known.
•Instruct patient to notify prescriber if he experiences chills; cough; fever; hoarseness; lower back, side, or muscle pain; painful or difficult urination; severe abdominal pain with nausea and vomiting; tiredness; or weakness.
•If patient also takes an oral anticoagulant, urge him to report unusual bleeding or bruising; anticoagulant dosage may need to be reduced.
•Advise patient to keep scheduled appointments with prescriber to check progress.

gemifloxacin mesylate
Factive

Class and Category
Chemical class: Fluoroquinolone

Therapeutic class: Antibiotic
Pregnancy category: C

Indications and Dosages
➤ *To treat acute bacterial exacerbation of chronic bronchitis caused by* Streptococcus pneumoniae, Haemophilus influenzae, H. parainfluenzae, *or* Moraxella catarrhalis
TABLETS
Adults. 320 mg daily for 5 days.
➤ *To treat mild to moderate community-acquired pneumonia caused by* S. pneumoniae, H. influenzae, M. catarrhalis, Mycoplasma pneumoniae, Chlamydia pneumoniae, *or* Klebsiella pneumoniae
TABLETS
Adults. 320 mg daily for 7 days.
DOSAGE ADJUSTMENT Dosage should be decreased to 160 mg daily in patients with creatinine clearance of 40 ml/min/1.73 m² or less.

Route	Onset	Peak	Duration
P.O.	0.5 to 2 hr	Unknown	Unknown

Mechanism of Action
Inhibits the actions of the enzymes DNA gyrase and topoisomerase IV, which are required for bacterial growth, and thereby causes bacterial cells to die.

Contraindications
Hypersensitivity to gemifloxacin, its components, or other fluroroquinolones

Interactions
DRUGS
aluminum and magnesium antacids, didanosine as chewable or buffered tablets or pediatric powder for oral solution, ferrous sulfate, sucralfate, zinc or other metal cations: Reduced blood gemifloxacin level
antipsychotics; class Ia antiarrhythmics, such as procainamide and quinidine; class III antiarrhythmics, such as amiodarone and sotalol; erythromycin; tricyclic antidepressants: Possibly prolonged QT interval
probenecid: Increased blood gemifloxacin level
warfarin: Possibly enhanced warfarin anticoagulant effects

Adverse Reactions

CNS: Dizziness, fever, headache, syncope, transient ischemic attack
CV: Peripheral edema, prolonged QT interval, supraventricular tachycardia, vasculitis
EENT: Taste perversion
GI: Abdominal pain, acute hepatic necrosis or failure, diarrhea, elevated liver function test results, hepatitis, jaundice, nausea, pseudomembranous colitis, vomiting
GU: Acute renal insufficiency or failure, interstitial nephritis
HEME: Agranulocytosis, aplastic or hemolytic anemia, elevated platelet count, elevated INR, hemorrhage, leukopenia, pancytopenia, thrombocytopenia
MS: Arthralgia, myalgia, tendinitis, tendon rupture
RESP: Allergic pneumonitis
SKIN: Erythema multiforme, exfoliation, facial swelling, photosensitivity, rash, Stevens-Johnson syndrome, toxic epidermal necrolysis, urticaria
OTHER: Anaphylaxis, angioedema, serum sickness

Nursing Considerations

• Review patient's medical history before administering gemifloxacin, which should not be used in a patient with a history of prolonged QT interval, in patients with uncorrected electrolyte disorders, or in patients receiving class IA or III antiarrhythmics because of a heightened risk for prolonged QT interval. Monitor elderly patients closely because they may be more susceptible to prolonged QT interval.
• Use cautiously in patients with CNS disorders, such as epilepsy, or in those prone to seizures because other fluroquinolones have caused seizures, increased intracranial pressure, and toxic psychosis. Monitor patient closely; if CNS alterations occur, notify prescriber immediately and expect drug to be discontinued.
• Monitor patient closely for a hypersensitivity reaction, which may occur as soon as the first dose. If signs of hypersensitivity, such as angioedema, bronchospasm, dyspnea, itching, rash, jaundice, shortness of breath, and urticaria, occur, notify prescriber immediately and expect drug to be discontinued.
• Monitor patients who are prone to tendinitis, such as the elderly, athletes, and those taking corticosteroids, for complaints of tendon pain, inflammation, or rupture. If present, notify prescriber; expect gemifloxacin to be discontinued, patient placed on bedrest with no exercise of the suspected limb, and diagnostic studies ordered to confirm rupture.
• Notify prescriber if severe or prolonged diarrhea develops; it may indicate pseudomembranous colitis caused by *Clostridium difficile*. If diarrhea occurs, notify prescriber and expect to withhold gemifloxacin and treat with fluids, electrolytes, protein, and an antibiotic effective against *C. difficile*.
• Monitor patients, especially women under age 40 and postmenopausal women who are receiving hormone replacement therapy, for rash. Rash may appear days after therapy is initiated and resolve in 7 days. Notify prescriber immediately if rash occurs because it can be severe in about 10% of patients.
• If patient takes warfarin, monitor coagulation status, as ordered, because adding gemifloxacin may increase the risk of bleeding.

Patient Teaching
• Tell patient to swallow tablet whole and take with a full glass of liquid.
• Warn patient not to increase dose because doing so may cause life-threatening cardiac arrhythmias.
• Instruct patient to complete entire course of therapy, even if symptoms decrease before prescription is finished.
• Caution patient to avoid sun exposure as much as possible while taking gemifloxacin. Patient who can't avoid sun exposure should apply sunscreen and wear a hat, sunglasses, and long sleeves to cover as much skin as possible.
• Instruct patient to maintain adequate hydration throughout therapy to keep urine from becoming too concentrated. Tell patient to increase fluid intake if urine darkens or amount voided decreases.
• Caution patient to avoid performing hazardous activities until the CNS effects of the drug are known.
• Instruct patient to seek medical attention and notify prescriber immediately if he experiences tendon pain, tenderness, or rupture; evidence of a hypersensitivity reaction, such as rash, urticaria, difficulty breathing, or facial swelling; or palpitations or fainting spells. The drug may need to be stopped.
• Urge patient to tell prescriber about diar-

G
H
I

rhea that's severe or lasts longer than 3 days. Explain that watery or bloody stools can occur 2 or more months after therapy and can be serious, requiring prompt treatment.
• Tell patient to consult prescriber before starting any new medications, including OTC products, because gemifloxacin may interact adversely.
• Inform patient that antacids containing magnesium and/or aluminum; products containing iron; multivitamin preparations containing zinc or other metal cations; and didanosine (Videx) chewable or buffered tablets and pediatric powder for oral solution (if prescribed) should not be taken within 3 hours before or 2 hours after taking gemifloxacin and that gemifloxacin should be taken at least 2 hours before sucralfate (if prescribed).
• Instruct patient to alert prescriber about severe diarrhea, even up to 2 months after gemifloxacin therapy has ended.

gentamicin sulfate

Cidomycin (CAN), Garamycin, G-Mycin, Jenamicin

Class and Category
Chemical class: Aminoglycoside derived from *Micromonospora purpurea*
Therapeutic class: Antibiotic
Pregnancy category: D

Indications and Dosages
➤ *To treat serious bacterial infections caused by aerobic gram-negative organisms and some gram-positive organisms, including* Citrobacter *species,* Enterobacter *species,* Escherichia coli, Klebsiella *species,* Proteus *species,* Pseudomonas aeruginosa, Serratia *species,* Staphylococcus aureus, *and many strains of* Streptococcus *species*

I.V. INFUSION, I.M. INJECTION
Adults and adolescents. 1 to 1.7 mg/kg every 8 hr for 7 to 10 days.
Children. 2 to 2.5 mg/kg every 8 hr for 7 to 10 days.
Infants. 2.5 mg/kg every 8 to 16 hr for 7 to 10 days.
Premature or full-term neonates up to age 1 week. 2.5 mg/kg every 12 to 24 hr for 7 to 10 days.

INTRATHECAL (INTRALUMBAR OR INTRAVENTRICULAR) INJECTION
Adults and adolescents. 4 to 8 mg daily.
Infants and children age 3 months and over. 1 to 2 mg daily.

➤ *To treat uncomplicated UTI*

I.V. INFUSION, I.M. INJECTION
Adults and adolescents weighing more than 60 kg (132 lb). 160 mg once daily or 80 mg every 12 hr.
Adults and adolescents weighing less than 60 kg. 3 mg/kg once daily or 1.5 mg/kg every 12 hr.
DOSAGE ADJUSTMENT Supplemental dose of 1 to 1.7 mg/kg (2 to 2.5 mg/kg for children) given by I.M. injection or I.V. infusion after hemodialysis, based on infection severity.

Mechanism of Action
Binds to negatively charged sites on the outer cell membrane of bacteria, thereby disrupting the membrane's integrity. Gentamicin also binds to bacterial ribosomal subunits and inhibits protein synthesis. Both actions lead to cell death.

Incompatibilities
Don't administer gentamicin through same I.V. line as other drugs, especially beta-lactam antibiotics (penicillins and cephalosporins), because substantial mutual inactivation may occur. Give drugs through separate sites.

Contraindications
Hypersensitivity or serious toxic reaction to other aminoglycosides, hypersensitivity to gentamicin or its components

Interactions
DRUGS
aminoglycosides (concurrent use of two or more): Decreased bacterial uptake of each drug, increased risk of ototoxicity and nephrotoxicity
cephalosporins, enflurane, methoxyflurane, vancomycin: Increased risk of nephrotoxicity
loop diuretics: Increased risk of ototoxicity and nephrotoxicity
neuromuscular blockers: Prolonged respiratory depression, increased neuromuscular blockade
penicillins: Inactivation of gentamicin by certain penicillins, increased risk of nephrotoxicity

Adverse Reactions

CNS: Acute organic mental syndrome, confusion, depression, fever, headache, increased protein in cerebrospinal fluid, lethargy, myasthenia gravis–like syndrome, neurotoxicity (dizziness, hearing loss, tinnitus, vertigo), peripheral neuropathy or encephalopathy (muscle twitching, numbness, seizures, skin tingling), pseudotumor cerebri
CV: Hypertension, hypotension, palpitations
EENT: Blurred vision, increased salivation, laryngeal edema, ototoxicity, stomatitis, vision changes
GI: Anorexia, nausea, splenomegaly, transient hepatomegaly, vomiting
GU: Nephrotoxicity
HEME: Anemia, eosinophilia, granulocytopenia, increased or decreased reticulocyte count, leukopenia, thrombocytopenia
MS: Arthralgia, leg cramps
RESP: Pulmonary fibrosis, respiratory depression
SKIN: Alopecia, generalized burning sensation, pruritus, purpura, rash, urticaria
Other: Anaphylaxis, injection site pain, superinfection, weight loss

Nursing Considerations

• Before gentamicin therapy begins, expect to obtain a body fluid or tissue specimen for culture and sensitivity testing, as ordered, or check test results, if available.
• Be aware that drug is best absorbed when administered by I.V. route. The blood level is unpredictable after I.M. administration.
• For I.V. use, dilute each dose with 50 to 200 ml of normal saline solution or D5W to yield no more than 1 mg/ml. Administer slowly over 30 to 60 minutes.
• Don't administer gentamicin through same I.V. line as other drugs without first consulting pharmacist.
• Expect to adjust dosage based on peak and trough blood drug levels drawn after third maintenance dose, as prescribed.
• Don't give gentamicin by subcutaneous route because it may be painful.
• When assisting with intrathecal injection, use only 2 mg/ml of preservative-free preparation. Drug may be injected directly or delivered by implanted reservoir.
• Don't give gentamicin to pregnant patient because drug can cause hearing loss in fetus.
• **WARNING** When giving pediatric injectable

form of drug, be alert for allergic reactions—including anaphylaxis and, possibly, life-threatening asthmatic episodes—because drug contains sodium bisulfite.
• Assess for signs of other infections because gentamicin may cause overgrowth of nonsusceptible organisms.
• Be aware that premature infants, neonates, and elderly patients have an increased risk of nephrotoxicity.
PATIENT TEACHING
• Stress the importance of completing the full course of gentamicin therapy.
• Instruct patient to immediately report adverse reactions, such as hearing loss, to avoid permanent effects.

glimepiride

Amaryl

Class and Category

Chemical class: Sulfonylurea
Therapeutic class: Antidiabetic
Pregnancy category: C

Indications and Dosages

➤ *To control blood glucose level in type 2 diabetes mellitus*
TABLETS
Adults. 1 to 2 mg daily with first meal of the day. *Maintenance:* 1 to 4 mg daily, increased by 1 to 2 mg every 1 to 2 wk as needed for blood glucose control. *Maximum:* 8 mg daily.
DOSAGE ADJUSTMENT Initial dosage reduced to 1 mg daily if needed for patients with renal impairment.

➤ *As adjunct (with insulin) to control blood glucose level*
TABLETS
Adults. 8 mg daily with low-dose insulin.

Route	Onset	Peak	Duration
P.O.	2 to 3 hr	Unknown	Over 24 hr

Mechanism of Action

Stimulates insulin release from beta cells in the pancreas. The drug also increases peripheral tissue sensitivity to insulin, either by enhancing insulin binding to cellular receptors or by increasing the number of insulin receptors.

Contraindications

Diabetes complicated by pregnancy; diabetic coma; hypersensitivity to glimepiride, sulfonylureas, or their components; ketoacidosis; sole therapy for type 1 diabetes mellitus

Interactions

DRUGS

ACE inhibitors, anabolic steroids, androgens, azole antifungals, bromocriptine, chloramphenicol, disopyramide, fibric acid derivatives, guanethidine, H₂-receptor antagonists, insulin, magnesium salts, MAO inhibitors, methyldopa, octreotide, oral anticoagulants, oxyphenbutazone, phenylbutazone, probenecid, quinidine, salicylates, sulfonamides, tetracycline, theophylline, tricyclic antidepressants, urinary acidifiers: Increased risk of hypoglycemia

asparaginase, calcium channel blockers, cholestyramine, clonidine, corticosteroids, danazol, diazoxide, estrogen, glucagon, hydantoins, isoniazid, lithium, morphine, nicotinic acid, oral contraceptives, phenothiazines, rifabutin, rifampin, sympathomimetics, thiazide diuretics, thyroid drugs, urinary alkalinizers: Increased risk of hyperglycemia

beta blockers: Possibly hyperglycemia or masking of hypoglycemia signs
digoxin: Increased risk of digitalis toxicity
pentamidine: Initially hypoglycemia and then hyperglycemia if beta cell damage occurs

ACTIVITIES

alcohol use: Altered blood glucose control (usually hypoglycemia)

Adverse Reactions

CNS: Abnormal gait, anxiety, asthenia, chills, depression, dizziness, fatigue, headache, hypertonia, hypoesthesia, insomnia, malaise, migraine headache, nervousness, paresthesia, somnolence, syncope, tremor, vertigo
CV: Arrhythmias, edema, hypertension, vasculitis
EENT: Blurred vision, conjunctivitis, eye pain, pharyngitis, retinal hemorrhage, rhinitis, taste perversion, tinnitus
ENDO: Hypoglycemia
GI: Anorexia, constipation, diarrhea, elevated liver function test results, epigastric discomfort or fullness, flatulence, heartburn, hunger, nausea, proctocolitis, trace blood in stool, vomiting
GU: Darkened urine, decreased libido, dysuria, polyuria
HEME: Agranulocytosis, aplastic anemia, eosinophilia, hemolytic anemia, hepatic porphyria, leukopenia, pancytopenia
MS: Arthralgia, leg cramps, myalgia
RESP: Dyspnea
SKIN: Allergic skin reactions, diaphoresis, eczema, erythema multiforme, exfoliative dermatitis, flushing, jaundice, lichenoid reactions, maculopapular or morbilliform rash, photosensitivity, urticaria
Other: Disulfiram-like reaction

Nursing Considerations

•Monitor fasting blood glucose level to determine response to glimepiride. Expect to check glycosylated hemoglobin level every 3 to 6 months to evaluate long-term blood glucose control.
•Arrange for dietary consultation and diabetic teaching, if appropriate. Ask dietitian to discuss the amount of alcohol patient can consume without risking hypoglycemia.
•Expect to switch patient to insulin therapy, as prescribed, during physical stress, such as infection, surgery, and trauma.
•WARNING Expect a higher risk of hypoglycemia when giving glimepiride to a malnourished or debilitated patient or one with renal, hepatic, pituitary, or adrenal insufficiency.

PATIENT TEACHING

•Instruct patient to take glimepiride just before the first meal of the day. Caution him not to skip the meal after taking drug.
•Urge patient not to skip doses or increase dosage without consulting prescriber.
•Urge patient to report signs of hypoglycemia, such as anxiety, confusion, dizziness, excessive sweating, headache, and nausea.
•Encourage patient to carry candy or other simple sugars to treat mild hypoglycemia.
•Advise patient to consult prescriber before taking any OTC drug.
•Urge patient to carry identification indicating that he has diabetes.
•Teach patient how to monitor his blood glucose level.
•Teach patient about exercise, diet, signs of hyperglycemia and hypoglycemia, hygiene, foot care, and ways to avoid infection.
•Instruct patient to notify prescriber about darkened urine, difficulty controlling his blood glucose level, easy bruising, fever, rash, sore throat, or unusual bleeding.

•If photosensitivity is a problem, instruct patient to avoid direct sunlight and to wear sunscreen.

glipizide

Glucotrol, Glucotrol XL

Class and Category
Chemical class: Sulfonylurea
Therapeutic class: Antidiabetic
Pregnancy category: C

Indications and Dosages
➤ *To control blood glucose level in type 2 diabetes mellitus*

E.R. TABLETS
Adults. *Initial:* 5 mg daily with breakfast. Dosage increased by 5 mg daily every 3 mo, if needed. *Maintenance:* 5 to 10 mg daily. *Maximum:* 20 mg daily.

TABLETS
Adults. *Initial:* 5 mg 30 min before first meal of the day. Dosage adjusted by 2.5 to 5 mg every 2 to 3 days. For daily dose of 15 mg or less, give as a single dose. For dose above 15 mg daily, give in 2 divided doses. *Maximum:* 40 mg daily.

➤ *As adjunct to or replacement for insulin therapy in type 2 diabetes mellitus*

CAPSULES, TABLETS
Adults who need more than 20 units insulin daily. 5 mg daily, while decreasing insulin dosage by one-half. Further insulin reductions are based on clinical response.

DOSAGE ADJUSTMENT Initial dosage reduced to 2.5 mg daily if needed for patients over age 65 and those with hepatic disease.

Route	Onset	Peak	Duration
P.O.	10 to 30 min	30 min to 2 hr	12 to 24 hr
P.O. (E.R.)	Unknown	Unknown	18 to 24 hr

Mechanism of Action
Stimulates insulin release from beta cells in the pancreas. Glipizide also increases peripheral tissue sensitivity to insulin, either by enhancing insulin binding to cellular receptors or by increasing the number of insulin receptors.

Contraindications
Diabetes complicated by pregnancy; diabetic coma; hypersensitivity to glipizide, sulfonylureas, or their components; ketoacidosis; sole therapy for type 1 diabetes mellitus

Interactions
DRUGS
ACE inhibitors, anabolic steroids, androgens, azole antifungals, bromocriptine, chloramphenicol, disopyramide, fibric acid derivatives, guanethidine, H_2-receptor antagonists, insulin, magnesium salts, MAO inhibitors, methyldopa, octreotide, oral anticoagulants, oxyphenbutazone, phenylbutazone, probenecid, quinidine, salicylates, sulfonamides, tetracycline, theophylline, tricyclic antidepressants, urinary acidifiers: Increased risk of hypoglycemia
asparaginase, calcium channel blockers, cholestyramine, clonidine, corticosteroids, danazol, diazoxide, estrogen, glucagon, hydantoins, isoniazid, lithium, morphine, nicotinic acid, oral contraceptives, phenothiazines, rifabutin, rifampin, sympathomimetics, thiazide diuretics, thyroid drugs, urinary alkalinizers: Increased risk of hyperglycemia
beta blockers: Possibly hyperglycemia or masking of hypoglycemia signs
digitalis glycosides: Increased risk of digitalis toxicity
pentamidine: Initially hypoglycemia and then hyperglycemia if beta cell damage occurs

FOODS
all foods: Possibly delayed drug absorption of tablets if taken within 30 minutes of meal

ACTIVITIES
alcohol use: Altered blood glucose control (usually hypoglycemia)

Adverse Reactions
CNS: Abnormal gait, anxiety, asthenia, chills, depression, dizziness, fatigue, headache, hypertonia, hypoesthesia, insomnia, malaise, migraine headache, nervousness, paresthesia, somnolence, syncope, tremor, vertigo
CV: Arrhythmias, edema, hypertension, vasculitis
EENT: Blurred vision, conjunctivitis, eye pain, pharyngitis, retinal hemorrhage, rhinitis, taste perversion, tinnitus
ENDO: Hypoglycemia
GI: Abdominal pain, anorexia, constipation,

G
H
I

diarrhea, elevated liver function test results, epigastric discomfort or fullness, flatulence, heartburn, hunger, nausea, proctocolitis, trace blood in stool, vomiting
GU: Darkened urine, decreased libido, dysuria, polyuria
HEME: Agranulocytosis, aplastic anemia, eosinophilia, hemolytic anemia, hepatic porphyria, leukopenia, pancytopenia
MS: Arthralgia, leg cramps, myalgia
RESP: Dyspnea
SKIN: Allergic skin reactions, diaphoresis, eczema, erythema multiforme, exfoliative dermatitis, flushing, jaundice, lichenoid reactions, maculopapular or morbilliform rash, photosensitivity, urticaria
Other: Disulfiram-like reaction

Nursing Considerations
•To improve blood glucose control, give glipizide in divided doses instead of once a day.
•Check blood glucose level at least 3 times daily for a patient switching from insulin to glipizide. Patients who take more than 40 units of insulin daily may need hospitalization during transition.
•If patient gradually loses responsiveness to glipizide, expect to give a second antidiabetic to maintain blood glucose control.
•Monitor fasting blood glucose level to determine response to drug. Expect to check glycosylated hemoglobin level every 3 to 6 months or as ordered to evaluate long-term blood glucose control.
•Expect to switch patient to insulin therapy, as prescribed, during physical stress, such as infection, surgery, or trauma.
•WARNING Risk of hypoglycemia is higher when giving glipizide to a malnourished or debilitated patient or one with renal, hepatic, pituitary, or adrenal insufficiency.

PATIENT TEACHING
•Tell patient to take glipizide 30 minutes before the first meal of the day. Caution him not to skip the meal after taking the drug.
•Advise patient not to skip doses or increase the dosage without consulting prescriber.
•Urge patient to report evidence of hypoglycemia, such as anxiety, confusion, dizziness, excessive sweating, headache, and nausea.
•Encourage patient to carry candy or other simple sugars to treat mild hypoglycemia.
•Caution patient to consult prescriber before taking any OTC drugs.

•Urge patient to carry identification indicating that he has diabetes.
•Teach patient how to monitor his blood glucose level.
•Teach patient about exercise, diet, signs of hyperglycemia and hypoglycemia, hygiene, foot care, and ways to avoid infection.
•Instruct patient to notify prescriber if he experiences darkened urine, easy bruising, fever, hypoglycemia or hyperglycemia, rash, sore throat, and unusual bleeding.
•If photosensitivity is a problem, instruct patient to avoid direct sunlight and to wear sunscreen.

glucagon
GlucaGen, Glucagon Diagnostic Kit, Glucagon Emergency Kit

Class and Category
Chemical class: Synthetic hormone
Therapeutic class: Antihypoglycemic, diagnostic aid adjunct
Pregnancy category: B

Indications and Dosages
➤ *To provide emergency treatment of severe hypoglycemia*
I.V., I.M., OR SUBCUTANEOUS INJECTION
Adults and children weighing more than 20 kg (44 lb) or, with GlucaGen, more than 25 kg (55 lb). 1 mg, repeated in 15 min if needed.
Children weighing 20 kg or less or, when using GlucaGen, 25 kg or less. 0.5 mg, or 0.02 to 0.03 mg/kg, repeated in 15 min, if needed.
➤ *To provide diagnostic assistance by inhibiting bowel peristalsis in radiologic examination of GI tract*
I.V. INJECTION
Adults. 0.25 to 2 mg before procedure. Dose, route, and timing vary with segment of GI tract examined and length of procedure.

Incompatibilities
Don't mix glucagon with sodium chloride or solutions that have a pH of 3.0 to 9.5; use with dextrose solutions instead.

Contraindications
Hypersensitivity to glucagon or its components, pheochromocytoma

Route	Onset	Peak	Duration
I.V.	5 to 20 min*†	Unknown	90 min*‡
I.M.	15 to 26 min*§	Unknown	90 min*‖
SubQ	30 to 45 min*	Unknown	90 min*

Mechanism of Action

Increases production of adenylate cyclase, which catalyzes the conversion of adenosine triphosphate to cAMP, a process that in turn activates phosphorylase. Phosphorylase promotes the breakdown of glycogen to glucose (glycogenolysis) in the liver. As a result, the blood glucose level increases and GI smooth muscles relax.

Interactions

DRUGS

oral anticoagulants: Possibly increased anticoagulant effects

Adverse Reactions

CV: Hypertension, hypotension (with hypersensitivity reaction), tachycardia
GI: Nausea, vomiting
RESP: Bronchospasm, respiratory distress
SKIN: Urticaria

Nursing Considerations

• Rouse patient as quickly as possible because prolonged hypoglycemia can cause cerebral damage.
• For I.V. use, reconstitute a 1-mg vial of glucagon with 1 ml of diluent or a 10-mg vial with 10 ml of diluent. Don't give more than 1 mg/ml. For large doses, dilute with sterile water for injection.
• Before injecting glucagon, place unconscious patient on his side to prevent aspiration of vomitus when he regains consciousness.
• Administer by slow I.V. injection to decrease the risk of adverse reactions, such as tachycardia and vomiting.
• If patient doesn't respond to glucagon, expect to administer I.V. dextrose.

---

* For antihypoglycemic action.
† 45 sec to 1 min for smooth-muscle relaxation.
‡ 9 to 25 min for smooth-muscle relaxation.
§ 4 to 10 min for smooth-muscle relaxation.
‖ 12 to 32 min for smooth-muscle relaxation.

• When patient has regained consciousness or diagnostic procedure is completed, give oral carbohydrates to restore hepatic glycogen stores and prevent secondary hypoglycemia.
• Keep in mind that glucagon isn't effective in patients with depleted hepatic glycogen stores caused by such conditions as adrenal insufficiency, chronic hypoglycemia, and starvation.

PATIENT TEACHING

• Instruct patient to monitor blood glucose level, especially with signs of hypoglycemia.
• Teach patient and family members how to recognize signs of hypoglycemia and when to notify prescriber.
• Advise patient to carry candy or other simple sugars to treat early hypoglycemia.
• Emphasize the importance of a consistent diet, regular exercise, and proper use of insulin or an oral antidiabetic drug.
• Make sure unstable diabetic patients and family members know how to give glucagon subcutaneously in case of hypoglycemia. Instruct family members to keep patient on his side and give him a carbohydrate when he awakens. Advise against giving fluids by mouth until patient is fully conscious.
• Instruct patient and family members to call for emergency medical assistance after glucagon treatment, especially if patient can't ingest oral glucose or if he's taking the sulfonylurea chlorpropamide, in case secondary hypoglycemia occurs.

glyburide
(glibenclamide)

Albert Glyburide (CAN), Apo-Glyburide (CAN), DiaBeta, Euglucon (CAN), Gen-Glybe (CAN), Glynase PresTab, Medi-Glybe (CAN), Micronase, Novo-Glyburide (CAN), Nu-Glyburide (CAN)

Class and Category

Chemical class: Sulfonylurea
Therapeutic class: Antidiabetic
Pregnancy category: C (B for Glynase PresTab and Micronase)

Indications and Dosages

➤ *To control blood glucose level in type 2 diabetes mellitus*

MICRONIZED TABLETS

Adults. *Initial:* 1.5 to 3 mg daily with first

G
H
I

meal of the day, increased by up to 1.5 mg at weekly intervals, if needed. *Maintenance:* 0.75 to 12 mg as a single dose or in divided doses with meals.

NONMICRONIZED TABLETS

Adults. *Initial:* 2.5 to 5 mg daily with first meal of the day, increased by up to 2.5 mg at weekly intervals, if needed. *Maintenance:* 1.25 to 20 mg daily as a single dose or in divided doses with meals.

DOSAGE ADJUSTMENT For conversion from insulin to glyburide for adults who use more than 40 units of insulin daily, initial dosage adjusted to 5 mg nonmicronized or 3 mg micronized glyburide as a single dose with 50% of usual insulin dose; glyburide dosage increased gradually, as needed. For adults who use less than 40 units insulin daily, usual glyburide dosage is used when insulin is discontinued.

For elderly patients, initial dosage possibly reduced to 1.25 mg nonmicronized glyburide daily, gradually increased by 2.5 mg/wk, as needed; or 0.75 to 3 mg micronized daily, gradually increased by 1.5 mg/wk, as needed.

Route	Onset	Peak	Duration
P.O.*	1 hr	2.3 to 3.5 hr	12 to 24 hr
P.O.†	15 to 60 min	1 to 3 hr	24 hr

Mechanism of Action

Stimulates insulin release from beta cells in the pancreas. Glyburide also increases peripheral tissue sensitivity to insulin either by enhancing insulin binding to cellular receptors or by increasing the number of insulin receptors.

Contraindications

Diabetes complicated by pregnancy; diabetic coma; hypersensitivity to glyburide, sulfonylureas, or their components; ketoacidosis; sole therapy for type 1 diabetes mellitus

Interactions

DRUGS

ACE inhibitors, anabolic steroids, androgens, azole antifungals, bromocriptine, chloram-

* Micronized.
† Nonmicronized.

phenicol, disopyramide, fibric acid derivatives, guanethidine, H$_2$-receptor antagonists, insulin, magnesium salts, MAO inhibitors, methyldopa, octreotide, oral anticoagulants, oxyphenbutazone, phenylbutazone, probenecid, quinidine, salicylates, sulfonamides, tetracycline, theophylline, tricyclic antidepressants, urinary acidifiers: Increased risk of hypoglycemia

asparaginase, calcium channel blockers, cholestyramine, clonidine, corticosteroids, danazol, diazoxide, estrogen, glucagon, hydantoins, isoniazid, lithium, morphine, nicotinic acid, oral contraceptives, phenothiazines, rifabutin, rifampin, sympathomimetics, thiazide diuretics, thyroid drugs, urinary alkalinizers: Increased risk of hyperglycemia

beta blockers: Possibly hyperglycemia or masking of hypoglycemia signs

digitalis glycosides: Increased risk of digitalis toxicity

pentamidine: Initial hypoglycemia and then hyperglycemia if beta cell damage occurs

FOODS

high-fat foods: Reduced bioavailability of nonmicronized glyburide

ACTIVITIES

alcohol use: Altered blood glucose control (usually hypoglycemia)

Adverse Reactions

CNS: Abnormal gait, anxiety, asthenia, chills, depression, dizziness, fatigue, headache, hypertonia, hypoesthesia, insomnia, malaise, migraine headache, nervousness, paresthesia, somnolence, syncope, tremor, vertigo

CV: Arrhythmias, edema, hypertension, vasculitis

EENT: Blurred vision, conjunctivitis, eye pain, pharyngitis, retinal hemorrhage, rhinitis, taste perversion, tinnitus

ENDO: Hypoglycemia

GI: Anorexia, constipation, diarrhea, elevated liver function test results, epigastric discomfort or fullness, flatulence, heartburn, hunger, nausea, proctocolitis, trace blood in stool, vomiting

GU: Decreased libido, dysuria, polyuria

HEME: Agranulocytosis, aplastic anemia, eosinophilia, hemolytic anemia, hepatic porphyria, leukopenia, pancytopenia

MS: Arthralgia, leg cramps, myalgia

RESP: Dyspnea

SKIN: Allergic skin reactions, diaphoresis, eczema, erythema multiforme, exfoliative dermatitis, flushing, jaundice, lichenoid reactions, maculopapular or morbilliform rash, photosensitivity, urticaria
Other: Disulfiram-like reaction

Nursing Considerations

•Give glyburide as a single dose before the first meal of the day. If patient takes more than 10 mg daily or if severe GI distress occurs, give in 2 divided doses before meals.
•Monitor fasting blood glucose level to determine patient's response to glyburide. Expect to check glycosylated hemoglobin level every 3 to 6 months or as ordered to evaluate long-term blood glucose control.
•When patient switches from insulin to glyburide, check blood glucose level 3 times daily before meals.
•Be aware that micronized tablets aren't equal to nonmicronized tablets; they contain smaller particles, which affects drug bioavailability.
•WARNING Expect a higher risk of hypoglycemia when giving drug to a malnourished or debilitated patient or one with renal, hepatic, pituitary, or adrenal insufficiency.
•Administer insulin as needed and prescribed during periods of increased stress, such as infection, surgery, and trauma.
•Arrange for diabetic teaching and consultation between patient and dietitian, if appropriate.

PATIENT TEACHING

•Instruct patient to take glyburide just before the day's first meal. Caution him not to skip the meal after taking drug.
•Advise patient not to take nonmicronized glyburide with a high-fat meal because doing so can reduce glyburide bioavailability.
•Caution patient to avoid skipping doses, discontinuing glyburide, or taking OTC drugs without first consulting prescriber.
•Teach patient how to monitor his blood glucose level and when to notify prescriber about changes.
•Urge patient to report signs of hypoglycemia, such as anxiety, confusion, dizziness, excessive sweating, headache, and nausea.
•Suggest that patient carry candy or other simple sugars to treat mild hypoglycemia.
•Urge patient to avoid alcohol because it increases the risk of hypoglycemia.

•Advise patient to carry identification indicating that he has diabetes.
•Teach patient about exercise, diet, signs of hyperglycemia and hypoglycemia, hygiene, foot care, and ways to avoid infection.
•Instruct patient to notify prescriber if he experiences easy bruising, fever, hypoglycemia or hyperglycemia, rash, sore throat, and unusual bleeding.
•If photosensitivity is a problem, instruct patient to avoid direct sunlight and to wear sunscreen.

glycopyrrolate

Robinul, Robinul Forte

Class and Category

Chemical class: Quaternary ammonium compound
Therapeutic class: Antiarrhythmic, anticholinergic, cholinergic adjunct
Pregnancy category: B

Indications and Dosages

➤ *To treat peptic ulcer disease*
TABLETS
Adults and adolescents. 1 to 2 mg b.i.d. or t.i.d. *Maximum:* 8 mg daily.
I.V. OR I.M. INJECTION
Adults and adolescents. 0.1 to 0.2 mg every 4 hr, p.r.n. *Maximum:* 4 doses daily.

➤ *To reduce gastric acid and respiratory secretions before anesthesia*
I.M. INJECTION
Adults and adolescents. 0.0044 mg/kg 30 to 60 min before anesthesia or when preanesthesia sedative or narcotic is given.
Children over age 2. 0.0044 to 0.0088 mg/kg 30 to 60 min before anesthesia or when preanesthesia sedative or narcotic is given.

➤ *To counteract intraoperative and anesthesia-induced arrhythmias*
I.V. INJECTION
Adults and adolescents. 0.1 mg, repeated every 2 to 3 min, if needed.
Children over age 2. 0.0044 mg/kg. Dose repeated every 2 to 3 min, if needed. *Maximum:* 0.1 mg as a single dose.

➤ *As cholinergic adjunct in curariform block*
I.V. INJECTION
Adults and children over age 2. 0.2 mg gly-

G
H
I

copyrrolate for each 1 mg neostigmine or 5 mg pyridostigmine when given together.

Route	Onset	Peak	Duration
P.O.	60 min	Unknown	8 to 12 hr
I.V.	1 min	Unknown	2 to 3 hr*
I.M., SubQ.	15 to 30 min	30 to 45 min	2 to 3 hr*

Mechanism of Action
Inhibits acetylcholine's action on postganglionic muscarinic receptors throughout the body. Depending on the receptors' location, glycopyrrolate produces various effects, such as:
• reducing the volume and acidity of gastric secretions
• controlling excessive bronchial, pharyngeal, and tracheal secretions and dilating the bronchi
• inhibiting vagal stimulation of the heart
• relaxing smooth muscle in the GI and GU tracts.

Incompatibilities
Don't mix glycopyrrolate with alkaline drugs or solutions that have a pH over 6.0 because drug stability may be affected. A pH over 6.0 may occur if glycopyrrolate is mixed with dexamethasone sodium phosphate or LR solution. Gas or precipitate may form if glycopyrrolate is mixed in same syringe as chloramphenicol, diazepam, dimenhydrinate, methohexital sodium, pentobarbital sodium, secobarbital sodium, sodium bicarbonate, or thiopental sodium.

Contraindications
Angle-closure glaucoma, asthma, hemorrhage with unstable cardiovascular status, hepatic disease, hypersensitivity to anticholinergics, ileus, intestinal atony, myasthenia gravis, obstructive GI or urinary disorders, severe ulcerative colitis, toxic megacolon

Interactions
DRUGS
anticholinergics, antiparkinsonian drugs, phenothiazines, tricyclic antidepressants:

---

* For vagal blocking effect; up to 7 hr for reduction of saliva.

Possibly increased anticholinergic effects
antidiarrheals (adsorbent): Decreased glycopyrrolate absorption, leading to decreased therapeutic effectiveness
antimyasthenics: Possibly reduced intestinal motility
atenolol: Possibly potentiated atenolol effects
calcium- or magnesium-containing antacids, carbonic anhydrase inhibitors, citrates, sodium bicarbonate: Possibly reduced excretion of glycopyrrolate and increased therapeutic and adverse effects
cyclopropane: Possibly ventricular arrhythmias
digoxin: Possibly potentiated digoxin effects
haloperidol, phenothiazines: Possibly decreased effectiveness of these drugs
ketoconazole: Possibly decreased ketoconazole absorption
metoclopramide: Possibly antagonized effects of metoclopramide
opioids: Possibly severe constipation and urine retention, risk of ileus
potassium chloride: Possibly increased severity of potassium chloride–induced gastric lesions

Adverse Reactions
CNS: Confusion, dizziness, drowsiness, headache, insomnia, nervousness, weakness
CV: Bradycardia (low doses), heart block, palpitations, prolonged QT interval, tachycardia (high doses)
EENT: Blurred vision, cycloplegia, dilated pupils, dry mouth, increased intraocular pressure, loss of taste, mydriasis, nasal congestion, photophobia, taste perversion
GI: Abdominal distention, constipation, dysphagia, nausea, vomiting
GU: Impotence, urinary hesitancy, urine retention
RESP: Dyspnea
SKIN: Decreased sweating (heat exhaustion), dry skin, flushing, pruritus, urticaria
Other: Anaphylaxis

Nursing Considerations
• Use glycopyrrolate cautiously in patients with autonomic neuropathy, hepatic disease, mild to moderate ulcerative colitis, prostatic hypertrophy, or hiatal hernia because drug's anticholinergic effect can worsen these conditions; gastric ulcer because drug may delay gastric emptying; and renal disease because drug excretion may be altered.
• Give tablets 30 to 60 minutes before meals.
• As needed and prescribed, give 2-mg dose

at bedtime to ensure overnight control of symptoms.
•For I.V. use, administer by direct injection without diluting. Or inject into tubing of a flowing I.V. solution unless it contains an alkaline drug or sodium bicarbonate.
•Closure system contains dry natural rubber that may cause hypersensitivity reaction if handled by or used to inject someone with latex sensitivity.
•Use continuous cardiac monitoring, as ordered, to assess patient for arrhythmias during drug administration.
•**WARNING** Check all doses carefully because even a slight overdose can lead to toxicity.
•To prevent overheating caused by decreased sweating, adjust the room temperature and make sure patient is well hydrated.

PATIENT TEACHING
•Advise patient to take glycopyrrolate tablets 30 to 60 minutes before meals.
•Instruct patient to consult prescriber before taking any OTC drugs.
•Caution patient about possible drowsiness and dizziness and need to avoid hazardous activities until drug's effects are known.
•Suggest that he use sugarless hard candy, ice, or saliva substitute to relieve dry mouth.
•Instruct patient to avoid exertion and hot environments because he's prone to heat exhaustion while taking glycopyrrolate.
•Urge patient to drink at least 8 glasses of water daily, unless contraindicated.
•Tell patient to notify prescriber about abdominal distention, trouble breathing or urinating, eye pain, irregular heartbeat, sensitivity to light, or severe constipation.
•Advise patient to wear sunglasses in bright light.
•Inform male patient that reversible impotence may occur during therapy.
•If urinary hesitancy occurs, advise patient to void before taking each dose.

granisetron hydrochloride

Kytril, Sancuso

Class and Category
Chemical class: Carbazole
Therapeutic class: Antiemetic
Pregnancy category: B

Indications and Dosages
➤ *To prevent nausea and vomiting caused by chemotherapy*
ORAL SOLUTION, TABLETS
Adults and adolescents. 1 mg up to 1 hr before chemotherapy and repeated 12 hr later; or 2 mg up to 1 hr before chemotherapy.
I.V. INFUSION
Adults and adolescents. 10 mcg/kg diluted and infused over 5 min, starting 30 min before chemotherapy; or 10 mcg/kg undiluted and infused over 30 sec, starting 30 min before chemotherapy.
TRANSDERMAL
Adults. 3.1 mg/24 hr patch applied to upper outer arm 24 to 48 hr before chemotherapy and worn up to 7 days. Patch removed no sooner than 24 hr after chemotherapy is completed.
➤ *To prevent nausea and vomiting caused by radiation therapy*
ORAL SOLUTION, TABLETS
Adults and adolescents. 2 mg daily given 1 hr before radiation therapy.
➤ *To prevent or treat postoperative nausea and vomiting*
I.V. INJECTION
Adults and adolescents. 1 mg administered over 30 sec before induction of anesthesia or immediately before reversal anesthesia for prevention. 1 mg administered over 30 sec after surgery for treatment.

Mechanism of Action
Has a high affinity for serotonin receptors along vagal nerve endings in the intestines. Because of this affinity, granisetron prevents the nausea and vomiting that usually result when serotonin is released by damaged enterochromaffin cells.

Incompatibilities
Don't mix granisetron in same solution as other drugs.

Contraindications
Hypersensitivity to granisetron or its components

Adverse Reactions
CNS: Asthenia, chills, CNS stimulation, drowsiness, fever, headache, insomnia, somnolence
CV: Hypertension

G
H
I

EENT: Taste perversion
GI: Abdominal pain, anorexia, constipation, diarrhea, elevated liver function test results, nausea, vomiting
HEME: Anemia, leukopenia, thrombocytopenia
SKIN: Alopecia, reactions at patch application site (pruritus, rash, redness)

Nursing Considerations
•For use with chemotherapy, dilute I.V. preparation of granisetron with normal saline solution or D_5W to a total volume of 20 to 50 ml. Mixture may be stored for up to 24 hours. Use only on days when chemotherapy is given.
•Apply transdermal patch to patient's upper outer arm 24 to 48 hours before chemotherapy, and don't remove it until at least 24 hours after chemotherapy is completed.

PATIENT TEACHING
•Inform patient that granisetron is given orally or I.V. before chemotherapy to help prevent nausea.
•Instruct patient to take granisetron tablet without food to avoid reducing drug bioavailability.
•Advise patient to report constipation, fever, severe diarrhea, or severe headache to prescriber. Also caution him about possible drowsiness.
•Advise patient wearing granisetron patch to cover it with clothing if there's a risk of exposure to sunlight. Tell patient to continue covering the application site with clothing for 10 days after removal of patch.

guaifenesin

Anti-Tuss, Balminil Expectorant (CAN), Benylin-E (CAN), Breonesin, Calmylin Expectorant (CAN), Gee-Gee, Genatuss, GG-CEN, Glycotuss, Glytuss, Guaituss, Halotussin, Hytuss, Hytuss 2X, Mucinex, Organidin NR, Resyl (CAN), Robitussin, Scot-tussin Expectorant, Uni-tussin

Class and Category
Chemical class: Glyceryl guaiacolate
Therapeutic class: Expectorant
Pregnancy category: C

Indications and Dosages
➤ *To relieve cough, especially when secretions are thick*

CAPSULES, ORAL SOLUTION, SYRUP, TABLETS
Adults and adolescents. 200 to 400 mg every 4 hr. *Maximum:* 2,400 mg daily.
CAPSULES, ORAL SOLUTION, SYRUP
Children ages 6 to 12. 100 to 200 mg every 4 hr. *Maximum:* 1,200 mg daily.
➤ *To promote productive cough*
E.R. TABLETS (MUCINEX)
Adults and adolescents. 600 to 1,200 mg every 12 hr. *Maximum:* 2,400 mg daily.

Route	Onset	Peak	Duration
P.O.	30 min	Unknown	4 to 6 hr

Mechanism of Action
Increases fluid and mucus removal from the upper respiratory tract by increasing the volume of secretions and reducing their adhesiveness and surface tension.

Contraindications
Hypersensitivity to guaifenesin

Adverse Reactions
CNS: Dizziness, headache
GI: Nausea and vomiting (with large doses)
SKIN: Rash, urticaria

Nursing Considerations
•As prescribed and as appropriate, give liquid forms of guaifenesin to children.
•Watch for signs of more serious condition, such as cough that lasts longer than 1 week, fever, persistent headache, and rash.

PATIENT TEACHING
•Instruct patient to take each dose with a full glass of water.
•Advise patient not to break, crush, or chew E.R. tablets but to swallow them whole.
•Instruct patient to increase fluid intake (unless contraindicated) to help thin secretions.
•Advise patient not to take drug longer than 1 week and to notify prescriber about fever, persistent headache, or rash.

guanadrel sulfate

Hylorel

Class and Category
Chemical class: Guanidine derivative
Therapeutic class: Antihypertensive

Pregnancy category: B

Indications and Dosages
➤ *To manage hypertension*
TABLETS
Adults. 5 mg b.i.d., increased to 20 to 75 mg daily in divided doses t.i.d. or q.i.d., if needed.
DOSAGE ADJUSTMENT Initial dosage reduced to 5 mg daily if needed for patients with renal impairment or creatinine clearance of 30 to 60 ml/min/1.73 m². Then dosage adjusted after at least 7 days. Initial dosage reduced to 5 mg every other day if needed for patients with creatinine clearance of less than 30 ml/min/1.73 m². Then dosage adjusted after at least 2 wk.

Route	Onset	Peak	Duration
P.O.	30 min to 2 hr	4 to 6 hr	4 to 14 hr

Mechanism of Action
Exerts its antihypertensive effect at peripheral sympathetic nerve endings. Through an uptake mechanism, guanadrel is stored in adrenergic neurons, where it displaces norepinephrine from its storage sites. This action blocks the normal release of norepinephrine in response to nerve impulses, which depletes norepinephrine stores in the synapses and relaxes vessel walls, thus reducing peripheral resistance and blood pressure.

Contraindications
Heart failure not caused by hypertension, hypersensitivity to guanadrel or its components, MAO inhibitor use within 1 week of guanadrel use, pheochromocytoma

Interactions
DRUGS
alpha blockers, beta blockers, rauwolfia alkaloids: Possibly orthostatic hypotension or bradycardia
amphetamines, appetite suppressants, cyclobenzaprine, haloperidol, loxapine, maprotiline, methylphenidate, phenothiazines, thioxanthenes, tricyclic antidepressants: Decreased antihypertensive effect of guanadrel
anticholinergics: Possibly decreased inhibition of gastric acid secretion
barbiturates, opioids: Increased hypotensive effect
MAO inhibitors: Possibly severe blood pressure increase
NSAIDs: Possibly sodium and water retention and decreased antihypertensive effect of guanadrel
sympathomimetics: Possibly reduced antihypertensive effect of guanadrel, leading to hypertension; possibly potentiated effects of sympathomimetics
vasodilators: Increased orthostatic hypotension
ACTIVITIES
alcohol use: Increased hypotensive effect

Adverse Reactions
CNS: Confusion, drowsiness, fatigue, headache, light-headedness, paresthesia, sleep disturbance
CV: Chest pain, orthostatic hypotension, palpitations, peripheral edema
EENT: Blurred vision, dry mouth and throat, glossitis
GI: Abdominal cramps or pain, anorexia, constipation, diarrhea, indigestion, nausea, vomiting
GU: Difficult ejaculation, hematuria, impotence, nocturia, urinary frequency or urgency
MS: Arthralgia, back or neck pain, joint inflammation, leg cramps, muscle weakness, myalgia
RESP: Cough, dyspnea
Other: Excessive weight gain or loss

Nursing Considerations
• Use guanadrel cautiously in patients with asthma because drug may aggravate this condition. Monitor patient for acute dyspnea, wheezing, and other evidence of asthma attack. Notify prescriber immediately if they develop.
• **WARNING** Assess patient for evidence of overdose, such as blurred vision, dizziness, and syncope.
• Be aware that elderly patients have a greater risk of dizziness and syncope.
• Assess for signs of fluid retention and heart failure, including crackles, a new S₃ heart sound, and sudden weight gain.
PATIENT TEACHING
• Inform patient that guanadrel won't cure high blood pressure but will help control it.
• Instruct patient to take drug at the same time each day to improve compliance and

G
H
I

blood pressure control.
•Caution patient about possible dizziness, light-headedness, and fainting, especially when getting up from a lying or sitting position. Advise him to rise slowly, especially in the morning, and to sit with his feet dangling for 1 to 2 minutes before standing up.
•Instruct patient to sit or lie down immediately if he feels dizzy.
•To prevent fainting, advise patient to avoid alcohol, standing for long periods, pursuing excessive exercise, and being overly exposed to hot weather.
•Instruct patient to check with prescriber before taking OTC drugs during therapy.
•Advise patient to follow a low-sodium diet to help reduce blood pressure and prevent fluid retention.

guanethidine monosulfate

Apo-Guanethidine (CAN), Ismelin

Class and Category
Chemical class: Guanidine derivative
Therapeutic class: Antihypertensive
Pregnancy category: C

Indications and Dosages
➤ *To manage moderate to severe hypertension and renal hypertension*

TABLETS
Adults. *Initial:* 10 to 12.5 mg daily, increased as needed by 10 to 12.5 mg every wk. *Maintenance:* 25 to 50 mg daily. Some patients may need up to 300 mg daily.
Children. 0.2 mg/kg daily, increased p.r.n. by 0.2 mg/kg every 7 to 10 days. *Maximum:* 3 mg/kg every 24 hr.
DOSAGE ADJUSTMENT Initial dosage increased to 25 to 50 mg daily for adult hospitalized patients because they can be monitored more closely. Then dosage increased by 25 to 50 mg every other day, p.r.n.

Route	Onset	Peak	Duration
P.O.	Unknown	8 hr	Unknown

Contraindications
Heart failure not caused by hypertension, hypersensitivity to guanethidine or its components, MAO inhibitor use within 1 week of guanethidine use, pheochromocytoma

Mechanism of Action
Exerts antihypertensive effect at peripheral sympathetic nerve endings. Through an uptake mechanism, guanethidine is stored in adrenergic neurons, where it displaces norepinephrine from its storage sites. This action blocks the normal release of norepinephrine in response to nerve impulses, which depletes norepinephrine stores in the synapses and relaxes vessel walls, thus reducing peripheral resistance and blood pressure.

Interactions
DRUGS
alpha blockers, beta blockers, rauwolfia alkaloids: Possibly orthostatic hypotension or bradycardia
amphetamines, appetite suppressants, cyclobenzaprine, haloperidol, loxapine, maprotiline, methylphenidate, phenothiazines, thioxanthenes, tricyclic antidepressants: Decreased antihypertensive effect of guanethidine
anticholinergics: Possibly decreased inhibition of gastric acid secretion
barbiturates, opioids: Increased hypotensive effect
insulin, oral antidiabetic drugs: Possibly increased antidiabetic effect of these drugs
MAO inhibitors: Possibly severe blood pressure increase
NSAIDs: Possibly sodium and water retention and decreased antihypertensive effect of guanethidine
sympathomimetics: Possibly reduced antihypertensive effect of guanethidine, leading to hypertension; possibly potentiated effects of sympathomimetics
vasodilators: Increased orthostatic hypotension
ACTIVITIES
alcohol use: Increased hypotensive effect

Adverse Reactions
CNS: Depression, dizziness, fatigue, headache, lassitude, paresthesia, syncope
CV: Angina, bradycardia, orthostatic hypotension, palpitations, peripheral edema
EENT: Blurred vision, dry mouth, glossitis, nasal congestion, parotid gland tenderness, ptosis

GI: Anorexia, constipation, diarrhea (severe), indigestion, nausea, vomiting
GU: Ejaculation disorders, elevated BUN level, impotence, nocturia, priapism, urinary frequency
HEME: Anemia, leukopenia, thrombocytopenia
MS: Leg cramps, muscle twitching, myalgia
RESP: Asthma exacerbation, dyspnea
SKIN: Alopecia, dermatitis
Other: Weight gain

Nursing Considerations
• As prescribed, discontinue MAO inhibitor therapy at least 1 week before starting guanethidine.
• Because guanethidine has cumulative effects, give a small initial dose and increase gradually, as prescribed. When blood pressure is controlled, expect to reduce dosage to lowest effective level.
• Monitor for orthostatic hypotension, which occurs most often when arising in the morning and is exacerbated by hot weather, exercise, and alcohol. Assess supine and standing blood pressures, especially after dosage adjustments.
• Measure daily weight to help detect fluid retention. Also observe for edema and other signs of heart failure. A thiazide diuretic may be prescribed to decrease sodium and fluid retention.
• Notify prescriber if severe diarrhea occurs. Drug may need to be discontinued.
• Monitor febrile patient for increased hypotension and adverse reactions because fever decreases drug requirements.
• As ordered, stop giving guanethidine 2 weeks before surgery to reduce the risk of cardiac arrest during anesthesia.

PATIENT TEACHING
• Teach patient how to recognize signs of orthostatic hypotension, and advise changing position slowly. Inform patient that symptoms are worse in the morning and exacerbated by exercise, hot weather, alcohol, and hot showers.
• Instruct patient to report fainting, frequent dizziness, and severe diarrhea.
• Caution patient to avoid alcohol because it may increase the risk of orthostatic hypotension.
• Instruct patient to weigh himself daily at the same time, on the same scale, and wearing the same amount of clothing. Advise him to report signs of fluid retention, such as reduced urine volume, sudden weight increase, and limb swelling.
• Urge patient to consult prescriber before taking OTC drugs during guanethidine therapy.
• If a diabetic patient takes insulin or a sulfonylurea, instruct him to monitor his blood glucose level more frequently to check for hypoglycemia.
• Advise patient to follow a low-sodium diet to help reduce blood pressure and prevent fluid retention.

guanfacine hydrochloride

Tenex

Class and Category
Chemical class: Dichlorobenzine derivative
Therapeutic class: Antihypertensive
Pregnancy category: B

Indications and Dosages
➤ *To manage hypertension, alone or with other antihypertensives*
TABLETS
Adults. 1 mg daily at bedtime, increased if needed to 2 mg after 3 to 4 wk. Then increased to 3 mg if needed after another 3 to 4 wk. *Maintenance:* 2 or 3 mg daily.
DOSAGE ADJUSTMENT Twice-daily administration used if blood pressure tends to rise at the end of 24-hr period.

Mechanism of Action
Decreases sympathetic nerve impulse outflow from the vasomotor center of the brain to the heart and blood vessels by stimulating central alpha$_2$-adrenergic receptors. This action reduces peripheral vascular resistance, renovascular resistance, heart rate, and blood pressure. Prolonged use of guanfacine may reduce total peripheral vascular resistance, slightly reducing the heart rate. Guanfacine also stimulates growth hormone secretion, reduces circulating levels of plasma catecholamines, and reduces left ventricular hypertrophy.

G
H
I

Route	Onset	Peak	Duration
P.O.	Unknown*	8 to 12 hr†	24 hr

Contraindications

Hypersensitivity to guanfacine

Interactions

DRUGS

CNS depressants: Possibly increased CNS depression
NSAIDs, sympathomimetics, tricyclic antidepressants: Possibly decreased antihypertensive effect of guanfacine
other antihypertensives: Possibly increased antihypertensive effect, resulting in hypotension

ACTIVITIES

alcohol use: Possibly increased CNS depression

Adverse Reactions

CNS: Anxiety, confusion, depression, dizziness, drowsiness, headache, nervousness, weakness
CV: Bradycardia, orthostatic hypotension
EENT: Conjunctivitis, dry mouth
GI: Constipation, nausea
GU: Decreased libido, impotence
SKIN: Dermatitis, diaphoresis, pruritus, purpura, rash

Nursing Considerations

•Use guanfacine cautiously in patients with cerebrovascular disease, chronic renal or hepatic failure, recent MI, or severe coronary insufficiency.
•Give drug at bedtime to minimize daytime sedation.
•**WARNING** Expect to discontinue drug by decreasing dosage gradually over 2 to 4 days. Typically, if patient hasn't taken the drug for 2 or more days, he may experience withdrawal symptoms, including abdominal cramps, anxiety, chest pain, diaphoresis, headache, increased salivation, insomnia, irregular heart rate and rhythm, nausea, nervousness, restlessness, tremor, and vomiting.
•If you suspect that patient has drug-related depression, notify prescriber immediately and expect to discontinue drug.

---

* For single dose; in 1 wk for multiple doses.
† For single dose; 1 to 3 mo for multiple doses.

PATIENT TEACHING

•Instruct patient to take guanfacine at bedtime to reduce daytime drowsiness.
•Caution patient about possible drowsiness, and advise him to avoid potentially hazardous activities until drug's CNS effects are known.
•Urge patient to avoid consuming alcohol and other CNS depressants while taking guanfacine.
•Advise patient to report rash.
•Inform male patient that guanfacine may cause impotence. Suggest that he discuss impotence with prescriber, if it occurs.
•Caution patient not to stop taking drug abruptly because doing so can cause a dangerous rise in blood pressure along with anxiety and nervousness.

halazepam

Paxipam

Class, Category, and Schedule

Chemical class: Benzodiazepine
Therapeutic class: Antianxiety
Pregnancy category: D
Controlled substance schedule: IV

Indications and Dosages

➤ *To manage anxiety*
TABLETS
Adults. 20 to 40 mg t.i.d. or q.i.d. *Optimal:* 80 to 160 mg daily.
DOSAGE ADJUSTMENT Dosage reduced to 20 mg once or twice daily if needed for debilitated patients.

Route	Onset	Peak	Duration
P.O.	Slow	Unknown	6 to 8 hr

Mechanism of Action

May potentiate the effects of gamma-aminobutyric acid (GABA) and other inhibitory neurotransmitters by binding to specific benzodiazepine receptor sites in the limbic and cortical areas of the CNS. By binding to these receptor sites, halazepam increases the inhibitory effects of GABA and blocks cortical and limbic arousal.

Contraindications
Acute angle-closure glaucoma, hypersensitivity to halazepam or its components, itraconazole or ketoconazole therapy, psychosis

Interactions
DRUGS
antacids: Possibly altered rate of halazepam absorption
barbiturates, CNS depressants, narcotics: Increased CNS depression, possibly sedation and impaired motor function
cimetidine, diltiazem, disulfiram, erythromycin, fluoxetine, fluvoxamine, isoniazid, itraconazole, ketoconazole, metoprolol, nefazodone, oral contraceptives, propoxyphene, propranolol, ranitidine, valproic acid, verapamil: Decreased clearance, increased blood level, and increased risk of adverse effects of halazepam
clozapine: Possibly respiratory depression
digoxin: Increased blood digoxin level and risk of digitalis toxicity
levodopa: Decreased antidyskinetic effect
neuromuscular blockers: Increased or blocked neuromuscular blockade
theophyllines: Decreased sedative effect of halazepam
ACTIVITIES
alcohol use: Increased CNS depression, possibly sedation and impaired motor function
smoking: Decreased halazepam effectiveness

Adverse Reactions
CNS: Agitation, anxiety, ataxia, confusion, depression, dizziness, drowsiness, euphoria, headache, irritability, nervousness, slurred speech, tremor, weakness
CV: Angina, palpitations, sinus tachycardia
EENT: Diplopia, dry mouth, tinnitus
GI: Abdominal cramps or pain, constipation, diarrhea, increased salivation, nausea, vomiting
GU: Decreased libido, dysuria
MS: Arthralgia
SKIN: Pruritus, rash

Nursing Considerations
•Use halazepam cautiously in patients with impaired hepatic or renal function, seizure disorders, or suicidal tendencies.
•Be aware that risk of halazepam addiction and abuse is relatively high.
•Monitor renal and liver function test results, as appropriate, during long-term treatment.

•Expect to withdraw drug gradually over 2 weeks to avoid withdrawal symptoms, which include anxiety, confusion, insomnia, psychosis, and seizures.
PATIENT TEACHING
•Instruct patient to take halazepam exactly as prescribed and not to stop abruptly because withdrawal symptoms may occur.
•Caution patient to avoid alcohol and other CNS depressants during therapy. Advise patient to avoid OTC drugs, such as cough and cold remedies, because they may contain CNS depressants.
•Advise patient to avoid hazardous activities until drug's CNS effects are known.
•Instruct patient to report depression, difficulty voiding, double vision, persistent drowsiness, and rash.
•Explain that drug's full effects may not occur for 6 weeks.

haloperidol
Apo-Haloperidol (CAN), Haldol, Novo-Peridol (CAN), Peridol (CAN)

haloperidol decanoate
Haldol Decanoate, Haldol LA (CAN)

haloperidol lactate
Haldol Concentrate

Class and Category
Chemical class: Butyrophenone derivative
Therapeutic class: Antidyskinetic, antipsychotic
Pregnancy category: C (haloperidol decanoate), not rated (haloperidol, haloperidol lactate)

Indications and Dosages
➤ *To treat psychotic disorders*
ORAL SOLUTION, TABLETS
Adults and adolescents. 0.5 to 5 mg b.i.d. or t.i.d. *Maximum:* Usually 100 mg daily.
Children ages 3 to 12. 0.05 mg/kg daily in divided doses b.i.d. or t.i.d. Increased by 0.5 mg every 5 to 7 days, if needed. *Maximum:* 0.15 mg/kg daily.

➤ *To treat nonpsychotic behavior disorders and Tourette's syndrome*
ORAL SOLUTION, TABLETS
Adults and adolescents. 0.5 to 5 mg b.i.d. or

t.i.d. *Maximum:* Usually 100 mg daily.
Children ages 3 to 12. 0.05 to 0.075 mg/kg
daily in divided doses b.i.d. or t.i.d. Increased
by 0.5 mg every 5 to 7 days, if needed. *Maxi-mum:* 0.075 mg/kg daily.

DOSAGE ADJUSTMENT Initial dosage reduced
to 0.5 to 2 mg b.i.d. or t.i.d. if needed for elderly or debilitated patients.

➤ *To treat acute psychotic episodes*
I.M. INJECTION
Adults and adolescents. *Initial:* 2 to 5 mg
followed by subsequent doses as frequently
as every 60 min. Alternatively, if symptoms
are controlled, dose may be repeated every
4 to 8 hr. *Maximum:* Usually 100 mg daily.
First oral dose may be given 12 to 24 hr
after last parenteral dose.

➤ *To provide long-term antipsychotic therapy for patients who require parenteral
therapy*
LONG-ACTING I.M. (DECANOATE) INJECTION
Adults. *Initial:* 10 to 15 times the daily oral
dose up to 100 mg. Repeated every 4 wk, if
needed. *Maximum:* 300 mg/mo.

Route	Onset	Peak	Duration
I.M.*	Unknown	3 to 4 days†	Unknown

Mechanism of Action
May block postsynaptic dopamine receptors in the limbic system and increase
brain turnover of dopamine, producing an
antipsychotic effect.

Contraindications
Blood dyscrasias, bone marrow depression,
cerebral arteriosclerosis, coma, concurrent use
of large amounts of other CNS depressants,
coronary artery disease, epilepsy, hepatic
dysfunction, hypersensitivity to haloperidol
or its components, Parkinson's disease, severe hypertension or hypotension, severe
CNS depression, subcortical brain damage

Interactions
DRUGS
amphetamines: Possibly decreased stimulant

---

* For haloperidol decanoate and lactate.
† For haloperidol decanoate only; 30 to
  45 min for haloperidol lactate.

effects of amphetamines and decreased antipsychotic effect of haloperidol
*anticholinergics, antidyskinetics, antihista-
mines:* Increased anticholinergic effect and
risk of decreased antipsychotic effect of
haloperidol
anticonvulsants: Possibly decreased effectiveness of anticonvulsants and decreased blood
haloperidol level
bromocriptine: Possibly decreased effectiveness of bromocriptine
bupropion: Lowered seizure threshold, increased risk of major motor seizure
CNS depressants: Increased CNS depression
and risk of respiratory depression and hypotension
diazoxide: Possibly hypoglycemia
dopamine (high-dose therapy): Possibly decreased vasoconstriction
ephedrine: Possibly decreased vasopressor
effect of ephedrine
epinephrine: Possibly severe hypotension and
tachycardia
fluoxetine: Increased risk of severe and frequent extrapyramidal effects
guanadrel, guanethidine: Decreased hypotensive effects of these drugs
levodopa, pergolide: Possibly decreased therapeutic effects of these drugs
lithium: Increased risk of neurotoxicity
*MAO inhibitors, maprotiline, tricyclic anti-
depressants:* Increased sedative and anticholinergic effects of these drugs
metaraminol: Possibly decreased vasopressor
effect of metaraminol
methoxamine: Decreased vasopressor effect,
shortened duration of action of methoxamine
methyldopa: Possibly disorientation, slowed
or difficult thought processes
phenylephrine: Decreased vasopressor response to phenylephrine
ACTIVITIES
alcohol use: Increased CNS depression and
risk of respiratory depression and hypotension

Adverse Reactions
CNS: Agitation, anxiety, confusion, drowsiness, dystonia, euphoria, extrapyramidal reactions that may be irreversible (akathisia,
pseudoparkinsonism, tardive dyskinesia),
hallucinations, headache, insomnia, neuroleptic malignant syndrome, restlessness,
slurred speech, tremor, vertigo

CV: Cardiac arrest, hypertension, orthostatic hypotension, QT prolongation, ventricular arrymias, tachycardia, torsades de pointes
EENT: Blurred vision, dry mouth, increased salivation (all drug forms); stomatitis (oral solution)
ENDO: Breast engorgement, galactorrhea
GI: Constipation, nausea, vomiting
GU: Decreased libido, difficult ejaculation, impotence, menstrual irregularities, urine retention
HEME: Anemia, leukocytosis, leukopenia
SKIN: Diaphoresis, photosensitivity, rash
Other: Heatstroke, weight gain

Nursing Considerations
• Haloperidol shouldn't be used to treat dementia-related psychosis in the elderly because of an increased mortality risk.
• Use haloperidol cautiously in patients with a history of prolonged QT interval, patients with uncorrected electrolyte disturbances, and patients receiving Class IA or III antiarrhythmics because of an increased risk of prolonged QT interval. Monitor elderly patients closely because they may have an increased risk of prolonged QT interval.
• Dilute oral solution with a beverage, such as cola or orange, apple, or tomato juice.
• Administer haloperidol decanoate (long-acting form prepared in sesame oil to produce slow, sustained release) by deep I.M. injection into gluteal muscle using Z-track technique and 21G needle. Don't give more than 3 ml at one site. Expect to reach a stable plasma level after third or fourth dose.
• If injection solution has a slight yellow discoloration, be aware that this change doesn't affect potency.
• Monitor for tardive dyskinesia (potentially irreversible involuntary movements) in patients receiving long-term therapy, especially elderly women who take large doses.
• If extrapyramidal reactions occur during the first few days of treatment, reduce dosage, as prescribed. If symptoms persist, drug may have to be discontinued. Dystonia also may occur during first few days of treatment, especially in patients receiving higher doses and in males and younger age groups. Notify prescriber.
• Avoid stopping haloperidol abruptly unless severe adverse reactions occur.
• Monitor for signs of neuroleptic malignant

syndrome, a rare but possibly fatal disorder linked to antipsychotic drugs. Signs include altered mental status, arrhythmias, fever, and muscle rigidity.
• **WARNING** Sudden death, QT-interval prolongation, and torsades de pointes, although uncommon, may occur in patients receiving haloperidol despite the lack of such predisposing factors as electrolyte imbalance, concurrent therapy with drugs known to prolong QT interval, underlying cardiac abnormalities, hypothyroidism, and familial long-QT syndrome.

PATIENT TEACHING
• Advise patient to take haloperidol exactly as prescribed and not to stop taking it abruptly because withdrawal symptoms may occur.
• To prevent oral mucosal irritation, instruct patient to dilute liquid form with juice or cola before taking it.
• Caution patient to avoid skin contact with oral solution because it may cause a rash.
• Advise patient to take tablets with food or a full glass of milk or water to reduce GI distress.
• Instruct patient to consume adequate fluids and to take precautions against heatstroke.
• Urge patient not to drink alcohol during therapy.
• If sedation occurs, caution patient to avoid driving and other hazardous activities.
• Instruct patient to report repetitive movements, tremor, and vision changes.

heparin calcium
Calcilean (CAN), Calciparine
heparin sodium
Hepalean (CAN), Heparin Leo (CAN), Heparin Lock Flush, Liquaemin

Class and Category
Chemical class: Glycosaminoglycan
Therapeutic class: Anticoagulant
Pregnancy category: C

Indications and Dosages
➤ *To prevent and treat deep vein thrombosis and pulmonary embolism, to treat peripheral arterial embolism, and to prevent thromboembolism before and after cardioversion of chronic atrial fibrillation*

I.V. INFUSION OR INJECTION
Adults. *Loading:* 35 to 70 units/kg or 5,000 units by injection. Then 20,000 to 40,000 units infused over 24 hr.
Children. *Loading:* 50 units/kg by injection. Then 100 units/kg infused every 4 hr or 20,000 units/m² infused over 24 hr.
I.V. INJECTION
Adults. *Initial:* 10,000 units. *Maintenance:* 5,000 to 10,000 units every 4 to 6 hr.
Children. *Initial:* 50 units/kg. *Maintenance:* 100 units/kg/dose every 4 hr.
I.V. OR SUBCUTANEOUS INJECTION
Adults. *Loading:* 5,000 units I.V., then 10,000 to 20,000 units subcutaneously. *Maintenance:* 8,000 to 10,000 units subcutaneously every 8 hr or 15,000 to 20,000 units subcutaneously every 12 hr.

➤ *To diagnose and treat disseminated intravascular coagulation (DIC)*
I.V. INFUSION OR INJECTION
Adults. 50 to 100 units/kg every 4 hr. Drug may be discontinued if no improvement occurs in 4 to 8 hr.
Children. 25 to 50 units/kg every 4 hr. Drug may be discontinued if no improvement occurs in 4 to 8 hr.

➤ *To prevent postoperative thromboembolism*
SUBCUTANEOUS INJECTION
Adults. 5,000 units 2 hr before surgery and then 5,000 units every 8 to 12 hr for 7 days or until patient is fully ambulatory.

➤ *To prevent clots in patients undergoing open-heart and vascular surgery*
I.V. INFUSION OR INJECTION
Adults. 300 units/kg for procedures that last less than 60 min; 400 units/kg for procedures that last longer than 60 min. *Minimum:* 150 units/kg.
Children. 300 units/kg for procedures that last less than 60 min. Then dosage based on coagulation test results. *Minimum:* 150 units/ kg.

➤ *To maintain heparin lock patency*
I.V. INJECTION
Adults. 10 to 100 units/ml heparin flush solution (enough to fill device) after each use of device.

Incompatibilities
Don't mix heparin with any other drug unless you have an order to do so and have

checked with pharmacist. Heparin is incompatible with many drugs and solutions, especially ones that contain a phosphate buffer, sodium bicarbonate, or sodium oxalate.

Route	Onset	Peak	Duration
I.V.	Immediate	Minutes	Unknown
SubQ	In 20 to 60 min	Unknown	Unknown

Mechanism of Action
Binds with antithrombin III, enhancing antithrombin III's inactivation of the coagulation enzymes thrombin (factor IIa) and factors Xa and XIa. At low doses, heparin inhibits factor Xa and prevents the conversion of prothrombin to thrombin. Thrombin is necessary for the conversion of fibrinogen to fibrin; without fibrin, clots can't form. At high doses, heparin inactivates thrombin, preventing fibrin formation and existing clot extension.

Contraindications
Hypersensitivity to heparin or its components; severe thrombocytopenia; uncontrolled bleeding, except in DIC

Interactions
DRUGS
antihistamines, digoxin, nicotine, tetracyclines: Decreased anticoagulant effect of heparin
aspirin, NSAIDs, platelet aggregation inhibitors, sulfinpyrazone: Increased platelet inhibition and risk of bleeding
cefamandole, cefoperazone, cefotetan, methimazole, plicamycin, propylthiouracil, valproic acid: Possibly hypoprothrombinemia and increased risk of bleeding
chloroquine, hydroxychloroquine: Possibly thrombocytopenia and increased risk of hemorrhage
ethacrynic acid, glucocorticoids, salicylates: Increased risk of bleeding and GI ulceration and hemorrhage
nitroglycerin (I.V.): Possibly decreased anticoagulant effect of heparin
probenecid: Possibly increased anticoagulant effect of heparin
thrombolytics: Increased risk of hemorrhage

ACTIVITIES

smoking: Decreased anticoagulant effect of heparin

Adverse Reactions

CNS: Chills, dizziness, fever, headache, peripheral neuropathy
CV: Chest pain, thrombosis
EENT: Epistaxis, gingival bleeding, rhinitis
GI: Abdominal distention and pain, hematemesis, melena, nausea, vomiting
GU: Hematuria, hypermenorrhea
HEME: Easy bruising, excessive bleeding from wounds, thrombocytopenia
MS: Back pain, myalgia, osteoporosis
RESP: Dyspnea, wheezing
SKIN: Alopecia, cyanosis, petechiae, pruritus, urticaria
Other: Anaphylaxis; injection site hematoma, irritation, pain, redness, and ulceration

Nursing Considerations

• Use heparin cautiously in alcoholics; menstruating women; patients over age 60, especially women; and patients with mild hepatic or renal disease or a history of allergies, asthma, or GI ulcer.
• **WARNING** Give heparin only by subcutaneous or I.V. route; I.M. use causes hematoma, irritation, and pain.
• Avoid injecting any drugs by I.M. route during heparin therapy to decrease the risk of bleeding and hematoma.
• **WARNING** Don't use heparin sodium injection as a catheter lock flush because fatal medication errors have occurred in children when 1-ml heparin sodium injection vials were confused with 1-ml catheter lock flush vials. Always examine vial labels closely to ensure correct product is being used.
• Administer subcutaneous heparin into the anterior abdominal wall, above the iliac crest, and 5 cm (2″) or more away from the umbilicus. To minimize subcutaneous tissue trauma, lift adipose tissue away from deep tissues; don't aspirate for blood before injecting drug; don't move needle while injecting drug; and don't massage the injection site before or after injection. Keep in mind that you can apply gentle pressure to the site after you withdraw the needle.
• Alternate injection sites, and observe for signs of bleeding and hematoma formation.
• To prepare heparin for continuous infusion, invert container at least six times to prevent drug from pooling. Anticipate slight discoloration of prepared solution; this doesn't indicate a change in potency.
• During continuous I.V. therapy, expect to obtain APTT after 8 hours of therapy. Use the arm opposite the infusion site.
• For intermittent I.V. therapy, expect to adjust dose based on coagulation test results performed 30 minutes earlier. Therapeutic range is typically 1.5 to 2.5 times the control.
• Bleeding is the major adverse effect of heparin therapy. Take safety precautions to prevent bleeding, such as having patient use a soft-bristled toothbrush and an electric razor. Bleeding may occur at any site and also may indicate an underlying problem, such as GI or urinary tract bleeding. Other sites of bleeding that could be fatal and require immediate attention includes adrenal, ovarian, and retroperitoneal hemorrhage.
• Monitor blood test results and observe for signs of bleeding, such as ecchymosis, epistaxis, hematemesis, hematuria, melena, and petechiae. If platelet count drops below $1,000,000/mm^3$ or recurrent thrombosis develops, notify prescriber and expect heparin to be discontinued.
• Make sure all health care providers know that patient is receiving heparin.
• Keep protamine sulfate on hand to use as an antidote for heparin. Be aware that each milligram of protamine sulfate neutralizes 100 units of heparin.
• Be aware that prescriber may order oral anticoagulants before discontinuing heparin to avoid increased coagulation caused by heparin withdrawal. Heparin may be discontinued when full therapeutic effect of oral anticoagulant is achieved.
• Know that women over age 60 have the highest risk of hemorrhage during therapy.
• Watch closely if patient is receiving heparin therapy and nitroglycerin I.V. because PTT may decrease and then rebound after nitroglycerin is discontinued. Monitor PTT closely, and be prepared to adjust heparin dose, as prescribed.
• **WARNING** Be aware that delayed-onset, heparin-induced thrombocytopenia may occur several weeks after heparin is discontinued and may progress to venous and arterial thromboses.
• Various heparin products contain the preservative benzyl alcohol, which isn't recom-

mended for children under age 1 month because it may cause gasping syndrome, which may be fatal.

PATIENT TEACHING
•Explain that heparin can't be taken orally.
•Inform patient about the increased risk of bleeding; urge her to avoid injuries and to use a soft-bristled toothbrush and an electric razor.
•Urge patient to report any abnormal sign or symptom to prescriber, even weeks after heparin has been discontinued, because of the potential for delayed adverse reactions.
•Advise patient to avoid drugs that interact with heparin, such as aspirin and ibuprofen.
•Instruct patient and family to watch for and report abdominal or lower back pain, black stools, bleeding gums, bloody urine, excessive menstrual bleeding, nosebleeds, and severe headaches.
•Explain that temporary hair loss may occur.
•Advise patient to wear or carry appropriate medical identification.

hyaluronan (high-molecular-weight)

Euflexxa, Orthovisc

Class and Category
Chemical class: Natural complex glycosaminoglycan sugar
Therapeutic class: Analgesic
Pregnancy category: Not rated

Indications and Dosages
➤ *To relieve osteoarthritic knee pain in patients who respond inadequately to conservative nonpharmacologic therapy and to simple analgesics*
INTRA-ARTICULAR INJECTION (ORTHOVISC)
Adults. 30 mg/wk for 3 to 4 wk.
INTRA-ARTICULAR INJECTION (EUFLEXXA)
Adults. 20 mg/wk for 3 wk.

Mechanism of Action
Instilling hyaluronan, a viscoelastic substance normally found in joint tissues and in the fluid that fills joints, directly into the joint relieves pain associated with osteoarthritis by lubricating the joint and absorbing shock when the joint moves.

Contraindications
Hypersensitivity to hyaluronan avian, avian-derived products (such as eggs, feathers, or poultry) or any of their components; knee infections; skin diseases affecting the knee area

Adverse Reactions
CNS: Headache
MS: Acute arthritis, arthralgia, back pain, bursitis
Other: Injection site bruising, edema, erythema, pain, pruritus, or rash

Nursing Considerations
•Prepare the patient for removal of joint effusion, if present, before hyaluronan injection.
•Assist the trained health care professional who gives the intra-articular injections, as needed, making sure that strict aseptic technique is followed throughout the procedure.
•Be aware that the prefilled syringe is for single use and that contents of the syringe should be used immediately after opening.

PATIENT TEACHING
•Inform patient that transient knee pain, swelling, or other localized reactions, such as itchiness or bruising, may occur after hyaluronan injection.
•Instruct patient to avoid strenuous or weight-bearing activities lasting longer than 1 hour for 48 hours after the injection.
•Inform patient that she may feel achy after the injection but that this discomfort is typically mild and brief.
•Advise patient that pain may not be relieved until after third injection.

hydralazine hydrochloride

Apo-Hydralazine (CAN), Apresoline (CAN), Novo-Hylazin (CAN)

Class and Category
Chemical class: Phthalazine derivative
Therapeutic class: Antihypertensive, vasodilator
Pregnancy category: C

Indications and Dosages
➤ *To manage essential hypertension, alone or with other antihypertensives*
TABLETS
Adults. *Initial:* 40 mg daily in divided doses

b.i.d. or q.i.d. for first 2 to 4 days and then increased to 100 mg daily in divided doses b.i.d. or q.i.d. for remainder of first wk. *Maximum:* Usually 200 mg daily, but sometimes 300 to 400 mg daily.

Children. 0.75 mg/kg daily in divided doses b.i.d. or q.i.d. Increased gradually over 3 to 4 wk. *Maximum:* 7.5 mg/kg or 200 mg daily.

➤ *To manage severe essential hypertension when drug can't be taken orally or when the need to reduce blood pressure is urgent*

I.V. OR I.M. INJECTION

Adults. 5 to 40 mg, repeated as needed.

Children. 1.7 to 3.5 mg/kg daily in divided doses every 4 to 6 hr, as needed.

Incompatibilities

Don't mix hydralazine in I.V. infusion solutions.

Route	Onset	Peak	Duration
P.O.	20 to 30 min	1 to 2 hr	2 to 4 hr
I.V.	5 to 20 min	10 to 80 min	2 to 6 hr
I.M.	10 to 30 min	1 hr	2 to 6 hr

Mechanism of Action

May act in a manner that resembles organic nitrates and sodium nitroprusside, except that hydralazine is selective for arteries. It:

• exerts a direct vasodilating effect on vascular smooth muscle

• interferes with calcium movement in vascular smooth muscle by altering cellular calcium metabolism

• dilates arteries rather than veins, which minimizes orthostatic hypotension and increases cardiac output and cerebral blood flow

• causes a reflex autonomic response that increases the heart rate, cardiac output, and left ventricular ejection fraction

• has a positive inotropic effect on the heart.

Contraindications

Coronary artery disease, hypersensitivity to hydralazine or its components, mitral valve disease

Interactions

DRUGS

beta blockers: Increased effects of both drugs

diazoxide, MAO inhibitors, other antihypertensives: Risk of severe hypotension

epinephrine: Possibly decreased vasopressor effect of epinephrine

NSAIDs: Decreased hydralazine effects

sympathomimetics: Possibly decreased antihypertensive effect of hydralazine

FOODS

all foods: Possibly increased bioavailability of hydralazine

Adverse Reactions

CNS: Chills, fever, headache, peripheral neuritis

CV: Angina, edema, orthostatic hypotension, palpitations, tachycardia

EENT: Lacrimation, nasal congestion

GI: Anorexia, constipation, diarrhea, nausea, vomiting

RESP: Dyspnea

SKIN: Blisters, flushing, pruritus, rash, urticaria

Other: Lupus-like symptoms, especially with high doses; lymphadenopathy

Nursing Considerations

• Monitor CBC, lupus erythematosus cell preparation, and ANA titer before therapy and periodically as appropriate during long-term treatment.

• Anticipate that drug may change color in solution. Consult pharmacist if color change occurs.

• Be aware that hydralazine may undergo color changes when exposed to a metal filter.

• Give tablets with food to increase bioavailability.

• Monitor blood pressure and pulse rate regularly and weigh patient daily during therapy.

• Check blood pressure with patient in lying, sitting, and standing positions, and watch for signs of orthostatic hypotension. Expect orthostatic hypotension to be most common in the morning, during hot weather, and with exercise.

• **WARNING** Expect to discontinue drug immediately if patient experiences lupus-like symptoms, such as arthralgia, fever, myalgia, pharyngitis, and splenomegaly.

G
H
I

•Expect prescriber to withdraw hydralazine gradually to avoid a rapid increase in blood pressure.

•Expect to treat peripheral neuritis with pyridoxine.

PATIENT TEACHING

•Instruct patient to take hydralazine tablets with food.

•Advise patient to change position slowly, especially in the morning. Caution her that hot showers may increase hypotension.

•Instruct patient to immediately notify prescriber about fever, muscle and joint aches, and sore throat.

•Urge patient to report numbness and tingling in her limbs, which may require treatment with another drug.

•Caution patient against stopping drug abruptly because doing so may cause severe hypertension.

hydrochlorothiazide

Esidrix, Hydro-chlor, Hydro-D, Hydro-DIURIL, Microzide, Neo-Codema (CAN), Novo-Hydrazide (CAN), Oretic, Urozide (CAN)

Class and Category

Chemical class: Benzothiadiazide
Therapeutic class: Antihypertensive, diuretic
Pregnancy category: B

Indications and Dosages

➤ *To manage hypertension*

CAPSULES

Adults. 12.5 mg daily.

ORAL SOLUTION, TABLETS

Adults. 25 to 100 mg daily as a single dose or in divided doses b.i.d.

Children age 6 months and over. 1 to 2 mg/kg daily as a single dose or in divided doses b.i.d.

Infants under age 6 months. Up to 3 mg/kg daily.

➤ *As adjunct to treat edema caused by cirrhosis, corticosteroids, estrogen, heart failure, or renal disorders*

ORAL SOLUTION, TABLETS

Adults. 25 to 100 mg b.i.d., once daily, or every other day for 3 to 5 days/wk.

Children age 6 months and over. 1 to 2 mg/kg daily as a single dose or in divided doses b.i.d.

Infants under age 6 months. Up to 3 mg/kg daily.

Route	Onset	Peak	Duration
P.O.	2 hr	4 hr	6 to 12 hr

Contraindications

Anuria; hypersensitivity to hydrochlorothiazide, other thiazides, sulfonamide derivatives, or their components; renal failure

Interactions

DRUGS

ACTH, amphotericin B, corticosteroids: Increased electrolyte depletion, especially potassium

amantadine: Possibly increased blood level and risk of toxicity of amantadine

amiodarone: Increased risk of arrhythmias from hypokalemia

antihypertensives: Increased antihypertensive effects

barbiturates, opioids: Possibly orthostatic hypotension

calcium: Possibly increased serum calcium level

cholestyramine, colestipol: Reduced GI absorption of hydrochlorothiazide

diazoxide: Increased antihypertensive and hyperglycemic effects of hydrochlorothiazide

diflunisal: Possibly increased blood hydrochlorothiazide level

digoxin: Increased risk of digitalis toxicity from hypokalemia

dopamine: Possibly increased diuretic effects of both drugs

insulin, oral antidiabetic drugs: Possibly increased blood glucose level

lithium: Decreased lithium clearance, increased risk of lithium toxicity

neuromuscular blockers: Possibly enhanced neuromuscular blockade from hypokalemia

nondeplarizing skeletal muscle relaxants: Possibly increased response to muscle relaxants

NSAIDs: Decreased diuretic effect of hydrochlorothiazide, increased risk of renal failure

oral anticoagulants: Possibly decreased anticoagulant effects

sympathomimetics: Possibly decreased antihypertensive effect of hydrochlorothiazide

Mechanism of Action

A thiazide diuretic, hydrochlorothiazide promotes the movement of sodium (Na^+), chloride (Cl^-), and water (H_2O) from blood in the peritubular capillaries into the nephron's distal convoluted tubule, as shown at right. Initially, hydrochlorothiazide may decrease extracellular fluid volume, plasma volume, and cardiac output, which helps explain blood pressure reduction. It also may reduce blood pressure by causing direct dilation of arteries. After several weeks, extracellular fluid volume, plasma volume, and cardiac output return to normal, and peripheral vascular resistance remains decreased.

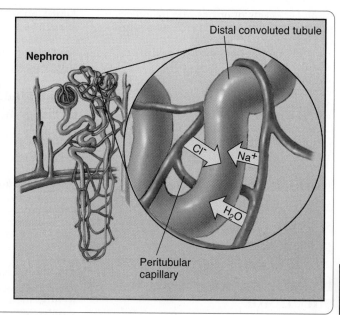

Distal convoluted tubule

Nephron

Cl^- Na^+

H_2O

Peritubular capillary

vitamin D: Increased risk of hypercalcemia

ACTIVITIES

alcohol use: Possibly orthostatic hypotension

Adverse Reactions

CNS: Dizziness, fever, headache, insomnia, paresthesia, vertigo, weakness
CV: Hypotension, orthostatic hypotension, vasculitis
EENT: Blurred vision, dry mouth
ENDO: Hyperglycemia
GI: Abdominal cramps, anorexia, constipation, diarrhea, indigestion, jaundice, nausea, pancreatitis, vomiting
GU: Decreased libido, impotence, interstitial nephritis, nocturia, polyuria, renal failure
HEME: Agranulocytosis, aplastic anemia, hemolytic anemia, leukopenia, neutropenia, thrombocytopenia
MS: Muscle spasms and weakness
SKIN: Alopecia, cutaneous vasculitis, erythema multiforme, exfoliative dermatitis, photosensitivity, purpura, rash, Stevens-Johnson syndrome, toxic epidermal necrolysis, urticaria
Other: Anaphylaxis, dehydration, hypercalcemia, hyperuricemia, hypochloremia, hypokalemia, hyponatremia, hypovolemia, metabolic alkalosis, weight loss

Nursing Considerations

• Give hydrochlorothiazide in the morning and early in the evening to avoid nocturia.
• Monitor fluid intake and output, daily weight, blood pressure, and serum levels of electrolytes, especially potassium.
• Assess for signs of hypokalemia, such as muscle spasms and weakness.
• Monitor BUN and serum creatinine levels.
• Frequently monitor blood glucose level as ordered in diabetic patients, and expect to increase antidiabetic drug dosage, as needed.
• If patient has gouty arthritis, expect an increased risk of gout attacks during therapy.

PATIENT TEACHING

• Advise patient to take hydrochlorothiazide in the morning and early in the evening to avoid awakening during the night to urinate.
• Instruct patient to take drug with food or milk if adverse GI reactions occur.
• Tell patient to weigh herself at the same time each day wearing the same amount of clothing and to notify prescriber if she gains more than 2 lb (0.9 kg) per day or 5 lb (2.3 kg) per week.
• Instruct patient to eat a diet high in potassium-rich food, including citrus fruits, bananas, tomatoes, and dates.
• Advise patient to change position slowly to

G
H
I

minimize effects of orthostatic hypotension.
•Urge patient to notify prescriber about decreased urination, muscle cramps and weakness, and unusual bleeding or bruising.

hydrocortisone
(cortisol)
Cortef, Cortenema, Hydrocortone

hydrocortisone acetate
Cortifoam, Hydrocortone Acetate

hydrocortisone cypionate
Cortef

hydrocortisone sodium phosphate
Hydrocortone Phosphate

hydrocortisone sodium succinate
A-hydroCort, Solu-Cortef

Class and Category
Chemical class: Glucocorticoid
Therapeutic class: Adrenocorticoid replacement, anti-inflammatory
Pregnancy category: Not rated; C (Cortifoam)

Indications and Dosages
➤ *To treat severe inflammation or acute adrenal insufficiency*
ORAL SUSPENSION, TABLETS (HYDROCORTISONE, HYDROCORTISONE CYPIONATE)
Adults. 20 to 240 mg daily as a single dose or in divided doses.
I.V. INFUSION OR I.V., I.M., OR SUBCUTANEOUS INJECTION (HYDROCORTISONE SODIUM PHOSPHATE); I.M. INJECTION (HYDROCORTISONE)
Adults. 15 to 240 mg daily as a single dose or in divided doses. *Usual:* ½ to ⅓ the oral dose.
DOSAGE ADJUSTMENT Dosage increased to more than 240 mg daily if needed to treat acute disease.
I.V. INFUSION; I.V. OR I.M. INJECTION (HYDROCORTISONE SODIUM SUCCINATE)
Adults. 100 to 500 mg every 2, 4, or 6 hr.
➤ *To treat joint and tissue inflammation*
INTRA-ARTICULAR INJECTION (HYDROCORTISONE ACETATE)

Adults. 25 to 37.5 mg injected into large joints or bursae as a single dose, or 10 to 25 mg into small joints as a single dose.
INTRALESIONAL INJECTION (HYDROCORTISONE ACETATE)
Adults. 5 to 12.5 mg injected into tendon sheaths as a single dose, or 12.5 to 25 mg injected into ganglia as a single dose.
SOFT-TISSUE INJECTION (HYDROCORTISONE ACETATE)
Adults. 25 to 50 mg as a single dose. Sometimes a dose of up to 75 mg is needed.
➤ *As adjunct to treat ulcerative proctitis of the distal portion of the rectum in patients who can't retain hydrocortisone or other corticosteroid enemas*
RECTAL AEROSOL (HYDROCORTISONE ACETATE)
Adult males. *Initial:* 1 applicatorful once or twice daily for 2 to 3 wk; then every other day thereafter. *Maintenance:* Highly individualized.
➤ *To treat ulcerative colitis*
ENEMA (HYDROCORTISONE)
Adults. 100 mg every night for 2 to 3 wk or until condition improves.

Contraindications
Hypersensitivity to hydrocortisone or its components, idiopathic thrombocytopenic purpura (I.M.), intestinal conditions prohibiting intrarectal steroids (P.R.), recent live-virus vaccination, systemic fungal infection

Route	Onset	Peak	Duration
P.O. (hydrocortisone)	Unknown	1 hr	1.25 to 1.5 days
P.O. (cypionate)	Unknown	1 to 2 hr	Unknown
I.V. (phosphate, succinate)	Rapid	Unknown	Unknown
I.M. (hydrocortisone)	Unknown	4 to 8 hr	Unknown
I.M. (phosphate)	Rapid	1 hr	Unknown
I.M. (succinate)	Rapid	1 hr	Variable
Other* (acetate)	Unknown	24 to 48 hr	3 days to 4 wk

* Intra-articular, intralesional, and soft-tissue injection.

Mechanism of Action

Binds to intracellular glucocorticoid receptors and suppresses the inflammatory and immune responses by:

- inhibiting neutrophil and monocyte accumulation at the inflammation site and suppressing their phagocytic and bactericidal activity
- stabilizing lysosomal membranes
- suppressing the antigen response of macrophages and helper T cells
- inhibiting the synthesis of cellular mediators of the inflammatory response, such as cytokines, interleukins, and prostaglandins.

Interactions

DRUGS

acetaminophen: Increased risk of hepatotoxicity
amphotericin B, carbonic anhydrase inhibitors: Possibly severe hypokalemia
anabolic steroids, androgens: Increased risk of edema and severe acne
anticholinergics: Possibly increased intraocular pressure
anticoagulants, thrombolytics: Increased risk of GI ulceration and hemorrhage, possibly decreased therapeutic effects of these drugs
asparaginase: Increased risk of hyperglycemia and toxicity
aspirin, NSAIDs: Increased risk of GI distress and bleeding
cholestyramine: Possibly increased hydrocortisone clearance
cyclosporine: Possibly increased action of both drugs; increased risk of seizures
digoxin: Possibly hypokalemia-induced arrhythmias and digitalis toxicity
ephedrine, phenobarbital, phenytoin, rifampin: Decreased blood hydrocortisone level
estrogens, oral contraceptives: Increased therapeutic and toxic effects of hydrocortisone
insulin, oral antidiabetic drugs: Possibly increased blood glucose level
isoniazid: Possibly decreased therapeutic effects of isoniazid
macrolide antibiotics: Possibly decreased hydrocortisone clearance
mexiletine: Decreased blood mexiletine level
neuromuscular blockers: Possibly increased neuromuscular blockade, causing respiratory depression or apnea
potassium-depleting drugs, such as thiazide diuretics: Possibly severe hypokalemia
potassium supplements: Possibly decreased effects of these supplements
somatrem, somatropin: Possibly decreased therapeutic effects of these drugs
streptozocin: Increased risk of hyperglycemia
vaccines: Decreased antibody response and increased risk of neurologic complications

ACTIVITIES

alcohol use: Increased risk of GI distress and bleeding

Adverse Reactions

CNS: Ataxia, behavioral changes, depression, dizziness, euphoria, fatigue, headache, increased intracranial pressure with papilledema, insomnia, malaise, mood changes, paresthesia, seizures, steroid psychosis, syncope, vertigo
CV: Arrhythmias (from hypokalemia), fat embolism, heart failure, hypertension, hypotension, thromboembolism, thrombophlebitis
EENT: Exophthalmos, glaucoma, increased intraocular pressure, nystagmus, posterior subcapsular cataracts
ENDO: Adrenal insufficiency during stress, cushingoid symptoms (buffalo hump, central obesity, moon face, supraclavicular fat pad enlargement), diabetes mellitus, growth suppression in children, hyperglycemia, negative nitrogen balance from protein catabolism
GI: Abdominal distention; hiccups; increased appetite; nausea; pancreatitis; peptic ulcer; rectal abnormalities, such as bleeding, blistering, burning, itching, or pain (rectal form); ulcerative esophagitis; vomiting
GU: Amenorrhea, glycosuria, menstrual irregularities, perineal burning or tingling
HEME: Easy bruising, leukocytosis
MS: Arthralgia; aseptic necrosis of femoral and humeral heads; compression fractures; muscle atrophy, twitching, or weakness; myalgia; osteoporosis; spontaneous fractures; steroid myopathy; tendon rupture
SKIN: Acne; altered skin pigmentation; diaphoresis; erythema; hirsutism; necrotizing vasculitis; petechiae; purpura; rash; scarring; sterile abscess; striae; subcutaneous fat atrophy; thin, fragile skin; urticaria
Other: Anaphylaxis, hypocalcemia, hypokalemia, hypokalemic alkalosis, impaired wound healing, masking of signs of infection,

G
H
I

metabolic alkalosis, suppressed skin test reaction, weight gain

Nursing Considerations

• Be aware that systemic hydrocortisone shouldn't be given to immunocompromised patients, such as those with fungal and other infections, including amebiasis, hepatitis B, tuberculosis, vaccinia, and varicella.
• Give daily dose of hydrocortisone in the morning to mimic the normal peak in adrenocortical secretion of corticosteroids.
• When possible, give oral dose with food or milk to avoid GI distress.
• Don't give acetate injectable suspension by I.V.
• Give hydrocortisone sodium succinate as a direct I.V. injection over 30 seconds to several minutes, or as an intermittent or a continuous infusion. For infusion, dilute to 1 mg/ml or less with D_5W, normal saline solution, or dextrose 5% in normal saline solution.
• Inject I.M. form deep into gluteal muscle, and rotate injection sites to prevent muscle atrophy. Subcutaneous injection may cause atrophy and sterile abscess.
• Shake foam container vigorously for 5 to 10 seconds before each use. Gently withdraw applicator plunger past the fill-line on the applicator barrel while container is upright on a level surface. Administer rectal foam only with provided applicator. After each use, wash applicator, container cap, and underlying tip with warm water.
• Be aware that high-dose therapy shouldn't be given for longer than 48 hours. Be alert for depression and psychotic episodes.
• Regularly monitor weight, blood pressure, and serum electrolyte levels during therapy.
• Expect hydrocortisone to exacerbate infections or mask their signs and symptoms.
• Monitor blood glucose level in diabetic patients, and increase insulin or oral antidiabetic drug dosage, as prescribed.
• Know that elderly patients are at high risk for osteoporosis during long-term therapy.
• Anticipate the possibility of acute adrenal insufficiency with stress, such as emotional upset, fever, surgery, and trauma. Increase hydrocortisone dosage, as prescribed.
• **WARNING** Avoid withdrawing drug suddenly after long-term therapy because adrenal crisis can result. Expect to reduce dosage gradually as prescribed and monitor response.

PATIENT TEACHING
• Advise patient to take daily dose of hydrocortisone at 9 a.m.
• Instruct patient to take tablets or oral suspension with milk or food.
• Teach patient how to use foam or enema form, if prescribed.
• Caution patient not to stop taking drug abruptly without first consulting prescriber.
• Instruct patient to report early signs of adrenal insufficiency: anorexia, difficulty breathing, dizziness, fainting, fatigue, joint pain, muscle weakness, and nausea.
• Inform patient that he may bruise easily.
• Advise patient on long-term therapy to have periodic eye examinations.
• If patient receives long-term therapy, urge her to carry or wear medical identification.
• Caution patient to avoid people with infections because drug can suppress immune system, increasing risk of infection. If patient comes into contact with chickenpox or measles, instruct him to call prescriber because he may need prophylactic care.

hydromorphone hydrochloride
(dihydromorphinone)

Dilaudid, Dilaudid-5, Dilaudid-HP, Hydrostat IR, Palladone, PMS-Hydromorphone (CAN), PMS-Hydromorphone Syrup (CAN)

Class, Category, and Schedule

Chemical class: Phenanthrene derivative, semisynthetic opioid derivative
Therapeutic class: Analgesic
Pregnancy category: C
Controlled substance schedule: II

Indications and Dosages

➤ *To relieve moderate to severe pain*
ORAL SOLUTION
Adults. 2.5 to 10 mg every 3 to 6 hr, p.r.n.
TABLETS
Adults. 2 mg every 3 to 6 hr, p.r.n. Increased to 4 mg or more every 4 to 6 hr, if indicated.
E.R. CAPSULES
Adults. Highly individualized and dependent on patient's previous total daily 24-hour opioid use. Once dosage is determined, drug is given daily.

I.V. INJECTION

Adults. 1 mg every 3 hr, p.r.n.

I.M. OR SUBCUTANEOUS INJECTION

Adults. 1 or 2 mg every 3 to 6 hr, p.r.n. Increased to 3 or 4 mg every 4 to 6 hr, if needed for severe pain.

SUPPOSITORIES

Adults. 3 mg every 4 to 8 hr, p.r.n.

Route	Onset	Peak	Duration
P.O.	30 min	1.5 to 2 hr	4 hr
I.V.	10 to 15 min	15 to 30 min	2 to 3 hr
I.M.	15 min	30 to 60 min	4 to 5 hr
SubQ	15 min	30 to 90 min	4 hr
P.R.	30 min	Unknown	4 hr

Mechanism of Action

May bind with opioid receptors in the spinal cord and higher levels in the CNS. In this way, hydromorphone is believed to stimulate mu and kappa receptors, thus altering the perception of and emotional response to pain.

Contraindications

Acute asthma; hypersensitivity to hydromorphone, other narcotics, or their components; increased intracranial pressure; severe respiratory depression; upper respiratory tract obstruction

Interactions

DRUGS

anticholinergics: Increased risk of ileus, severe constipation, or urine retention

antihypertensives, diuretics, guanadrel, guanethidine, mecamylamine: Increased risk of orthostatic hypotension

barbiturate anesthetics: Increased sedative effect of hydromorphone

belladonna alkaloids, difenoxin and atropine, diphenoxylate and atropine, kaolin pectin, loperamide, paregoric: Increased risk of CNS depression and severe constipation

buprenorphine, butorphanol, dezocine, nalbuphine, pentazocine: Possibly potentiated or suppressed symptoms of spontaneous narcotic withdrawal

CNS depressants, other opioid analgesics: Additive CNS depression and hypotension

hydroxyzine: Increased analgesia, CNS depression, and hypotension

metoclopramide: Decreased effect of metoclopramide on GI motility

naloxone: Possibly withdrawal symptoms in physically dependent patients

naltrexone: Possibly prolonged respiratory depression or cardiac arrest

neuromuscular blockers: Additive CNS depression

ACTIVITIES

alcohol use: Increased CNS depression

Adverse Reactions

CNS: Anxiety, confusion, dizziness, drowsiness, euphoria, hallucinations, headache, nervousness, restlessness, sedation, somnolence, tremor, weakness

CV: Hypertension, orthostatic hypotension, palpitations, tachycardia

EENT: Blurred vision, diplopia, dry mouth, laryngeal edema, laryngospasm, nystagmus, tinnitus

GI: Abdominal cramps, anorexia, biliary tract spasm, constipation, hepatotoxicity, nausea, vomiting

GU: Dysuria, urine retention

RESP: Dyspnea, respiratory depression, wheezing

SKIN: Diaphoresis, flushing

Other: Injection site pain, redness, and swelling; physical and psychological dependence

Nursing Considerations

• To improve analgesic action, give hydromorphone before pain becomes intense.

• Give I.V. form by direct injection over at least 2 minutes. For infusion, mix drug with D₅W, normal saline solution, or Ringer's solution.

• Monitor for respiratory depression when using I.V. route. Keep resuscitation equipment and naloxone nearby.

• Rotate I.M. and subcutaneous injection sites.

• Monitor effectiveness of hydromorphone in relieving pain; consult prescriber as needed.

• Assess patient for constipation.

• Monitor patient for signs of physical dependence or abuse.

• Anticipate that drug may mask or worsen gallbladder pain.

• Be aware that all other around-the-clock opioid analgesics should be stopped when

G
H
I

E.R. capsules are prescribed. Expect to give immediate-release nonopioid analgesics for exacerbations of pain and for preventing pain during certain activities.

PATIENT TEACHING
•Instruct patient to take hydromorphone exactly as prescribed and before pain is severe.
•Advise patient to take drug with food to avoid GI distress.
•Tell patient not to break open or chew E.R. capsules but to swallow them whole.
•Instruct patient to refrigerate suppositories.
•Caution patient to avoid alcohol and OTC drugs during therapy, unless prescriber approves.
•Instruct patient to report constipation, difficulty breathing, severe nausea, or vomiting.
•Inform patient that drug may cause drowsiness and sedation. Advise her to avoid potentially hazardous activities until drug's CNS effects are known.
•Tell patient to change position slowly to minimize effects of orthostatic hypotension.
•To avoid withdrawal, instruct physically dependent patient not to stop taking hydromorphone abruptly.

hydroxychloroquine sulfate

Plaquenil

Class and Category
Chemical class: 4-aminoquinoline compound
Therapeutic class: Antiprotozoal, antirheumatic, lupus erythematosus suppressant
Pregnancy category: C

Indications and Dosages
➤ *To prevent malaria*
TABLETS
Adults. 400 mg the same day of each week starting 2 wk before entering endemic area and continuing until departure from endemic area. If this isn't possible, initially 800 mg in two divided doses 6 hr apart, followed 1 wk later with 400 mg and then 400 mg on the same day of each week thereafter until departure from endemic area.
Infants and children. 5 mg/kg the same day of each week, starting 2 wk before entering endemic area and continuing until departure from endemic area. If this isn't possible, initially 10 mg/kg in two divided doses 6 hr

apart, followed 1 wk later with 5 mg/kg and then 5 mg/kg on the same day of each week thereafter until departure from endemic area. *Maximum:* Adult dosage.

➤ *To treat acute attacks of malaria caused by* Plasmodium vivax, P. malariae, P. ovale, *and susceptible strains of* P. falciparum
TABLETS
Adults. *Initial:* 800 mg, followed by 400 mg in 6 to 8 hr and 400 mg on next 2 consecutive days. Alternatively, 800 mg given as a single dose or an initial dose of 10 mg base/kg (maximum, 620 mg base [800 mg]), followed by 5 mg base/kg (maximum, 310 mg base [400 mg]) 6 hr after first dose, 5 mg base/kg 18 hr after second dose, and 5 mg base/kg 24 hr after third dose.
Infants and children. *Initial:* 10 mg base/kg (maximum, 620 mg base [800 mg]), followed by 5 mg base/kg (maximum, 310 mg base [400 mg]) 6 hr after first dose, 5 mg base/kg 18 hr after second dose, and 5 mg base/kg 24 hr after third dose.

➤ *To treat chronic discoid and systemic lupus erythematosus*
TABLETS
Adults. *Initial:* 400 mg once or twice daily for several weeks or months. *Maintenance:* 200 to 400 mg daily.

➤ *To treat acute or chronic rheumatoid arthritis*
TABLETS
Adults. *Initial:* 400 to 600 mg daily for 4 to 12 wk. *Maintenance:* 200 mg to 400 mg daily.
DOSAGE ADJUSTMENT For patients with rheumatoid arthritis who develop troublesome adverse reactions, initial dosage decreased for 5 to 10 days and then gradually increased to optimum response level.

Contraindications
Hypersensitivity to 4-aminoquinoline compounds (including hydroxychloroquine), long-term therapy in children, retinal or visual changes related to 4-aminoquinoline compounds

Interactions
DRUGS
aurothioglucose: Increased risk of blood dyscrasias
digoxin: Increased digoxin concentrations

Mechanism of Action

May mildly suppress the immune system, inhibiting production of rheumatoid factor and acute phase reactants. Hydroxychloroquine also accumulates in WBCs, stabilizing lysosomal membranes and inhibiting enzymes such as collagenase and the proteases that cause cartilage breakdown. These actions may decrease symptoms of rheumatoid arthritis and lupus erythematosus.

Hydroxychloroquine also binds to and alters the DNA of the malaria parasite to prevent it from reproducing. In addition, it may increase the pH of acid vesicles, which interferes with vesicle function and may inhibit parasitic phospholipid metabolism in erythrocytes, thereby halting plasmodial activity.

Adverse Reactions

CNS: Abnormal nerve conduction, ataxia, dizziness, emotional lability, headache, irritability, lassitude, nervousness, neuromuscular sensory abnormalities, nightmares, psychosis, seizures, vertigo
CV: Cardiomyopathy (with prolonged high doses)
EENT: Abnormal pigmentation (bull's eye appearance) or colored vision, blurred vision, central scotoma with decreased visual acuity, corneal deposits, decreased corneal sensitivity, diplopia, irreversible retinal damage (in lupus erythematosus or rheumatoid arthritis), halo vision, lassitude, macular edema or atrophy, nerve-related hearing loss, nystagmus, pericentral or paracentral scotoma, photophobia, retinal fundus changes, tinnitus, visual abnormalities
ENDO: Hypoglycemia
GI: Abdominal cramps, anorexia, diarrhea, elevated liver function test results, fulminant hepatic failure, nausea, vomiting
HEME: Agranulocytosis, aplastic anemia, hemolysis (in patients with glucose-6-phosphate dehydrogenase [G6PD] deficiency), leukopenia, thrombocytopenia
MS: Atrophy of proximal skeletal muscle groups, depressed tendon reflexes, muscle weakness
RESP: Bronchospasm
SKIN: Acute generalized exanthematous pustulosis, alopecia, altered mucosal and skin pigmentation, bleaching of hair, dermatitis (including exfoliative dermatitis), non–light-sensitive psoriasis, pruritus, psoriasis exacerbation, rash, Stevens-Johnson syndrome, urticaria
Other: Angioedema, porphyria, weight loss

Nursing Considerations

• Use hydroxychloroquine cautiously in patients with G6PD deficiency, patients with hepatic disease or alcoholism, and patients taking hepatotoxic drugs.
• Monitor children closely for adverse reactions because they are especially sensitive to 4-aminoquinoline compounds.
• Observe patients with psoriasis closely because hydroxychloroquine may lead to severe psoriasis attack. Also monitor patients with porphyria closely because hydroxychloroquine may worsen the condition. Expect to use hydroxychloroquine in patients with psoriasis or porphyria only after risks and benefits have been considered.
• During prolonged therapy, obtain periodic blood cell counts, as ordered, to detect adverse hematologic effects. Expect to stop drug if severe adverse effects occur.
• Monitor patient's vision when giving hydroxychloroquine for lupus erythematosus or rheumatoid arthritis because irreversible retinal damage may occur in some patients during long-term or high-dose therapy. Ask regularly about visual abnormalities, such as light flashes or streaks, that may indicate retinopathy. Expect patient to have an initial ophthalmologic examination, followed by examinations every 3 months. Report changes to prescriber immediately, and expect drug to be stopped. Retinal changes may progress even after therapy stops.
• Monitor patient on long-term therapy for muscle weakness and abnormal knee and ankle reflexes. If present, notify prescriber and expect drug to be stopped.
• Expect drug to be stopped if patient with rheumatoid arthritis shows no improvement, such as reduced joint swelling or increased mobility, in 6 months.
• If serious adverse reactions occur, notify prescriber immediately. Expect drug to be stopped. Also expect to give ammonium chloride (8 g daily in divided doses for adults) 3 or 4 days weekly for several

months because acidification of urine increases renal excretion of drug.

PATIENT TEACHING

• Instruct patient to take drug with meals or milk to minimize stomach upset.

• Tell patient to take hydroxychloroquine exactly as prescribed because taking too much may cause serious adverse reactions and taking too little or skipping doses decreases effectiveness.

• Caution patient to notify prescriber about troublesome adverse reactions. Hydroxychloroquine dosage may need to be adjusted or drug stopped.

• Caution patient who takes drug for rheumatoid arthritis or lupus erythematosus about possible visual reactions and the need for periodic eye examinations. Tell patient to notify prescriber about abnormal visual changes, including blurred vision, halos around lights, and light flashes or streaks; explain that drug will need to be stopped.

• Tell patient receiving prolonged therapy about the need for periodic blood tests to detect adverse effects.

• Advise patient to notify prescriber if muscle weakness develops.

hydroxyzine hydrochloride

Apo-Hydroxyzine (CAN), Atarax, Multipax (CAN), Novo-Hydroxyzin (CAN)

hydroxyzine pamoate

Vistaril

Class and Category

Chemical class: Piperazine derivative
Therapeutic class: Antianxiety, antiemetic, antihistamine, sedative-hypnotic
Pregnancy category: C

Indications and Dosages

➤ *To relieve anxiety and induce sedation and hypnosis*

CAPSULES, ORAL SUSPENSION, SYRUP, TABLETS

Adults and adolescents. 50 to 100 mg as a single dose.
Children. 600 mcg/kg as a single dose.

I.M. INJECTION

Adults and adolescents. 50 to 100 mg every 4 to 6 hr, p.r.n. (antianxiety); 50 mg as a single dose (sedative-hypnotic).

➤ *To treat pruritus*

CAPSULES, ORAL SUSPENSION, SYRUP, TABLETS

Adults and adolescents. 25 to 100 mg t.i.d. or q.i.d., p.r.n.
Children. 500 mcg/kg every 6 hr, p.r.n.

➤ *To provide antiemetic effects*

CAPSULES, ORAL SUSPENSION, SYRUP, TABLETS

Adults and adolescents. 25 to 100 mg t.i.d. or q.i.d., p.r.n.
Children. 500 mcg/kg every 6 hr, p.r.n.

I.M. INJECTION

Adults and adolescents. 25 to 100 mg, p.r.n.
Children. 1.1 mg/kg as a single dose.

➤ *As adjunct to permit reduction in preoperative and postoperative opioid dosage*

I.M. INJECTION

Adults and adolescents. 25 to 100 mg given with prescribed opioid.
Children. 1.1 mg/kg given with prescribed opioid.

DOSAGE ADJUSTMENT For elderly patients, treatment is started at lowest possible dosage.

Route	Onset	Peak	Duration
P.O.	15 to 60 min	Unknown	4 to 6 hr
I.M.	20 to 30 min	Unknown	4 to 6 hr

Mechanism of Action

Competes with histamine for histamine$_1$ receptor sites on the surfaces of effector cells. This suppresses the results of histaminic activity, including edema, flare, and pruritus. Hydroxyzine's antiemetic effect may stem from its central anticholinergic actions. Its sedative actions occur at the subcortical level of the CNS and are dose-related.

Contraindications

Breastfeeding; early pregnancy; hypersensitivity to cetirizine, hydroxyzine, or their components

Interactions

DRUGS

CNS depressants: Increased CNS depression

ACTIVITIES

alcohol use: Increased CNS depression

Adverse Reactions

CNS: Drowsiness, hallucinations, headache, involuntary motor activity, seizures, tremor

EENT: Dry mouth
SKIN: Pruritus, rash, urticaria
Other: Allergic reaction, injection site pain

Nursing Considerations
• Don't give hydroxyzine by subcutaneous or I.V. route because tissue necrosis may occur.
• Inject I.M. form deep into a large muscle, using the Z-track method.
• Observe for oversedation if patient takes another CNS depressant.

PATIENT TEACHING
• Urge patient to avoid alcohol.
• Caution patient about drowsiness; tell her to avoid potentially hazardous activities until drug's CNS effects are known.
• Instruct female patient to tell prescriber if she is or could be pregnant because drug is contraindicated in early pregnancy.

hyoscyamine sulfate

Anaspaz, A-Spas S/L, Cystospaz, Cystospaz-M, Donnamar, ED-SPAZ, Gastrosed, Levbid, Levsin, Levsin/SL, Levsinex Timecaps, Symax SL, Symax SR

Class and Category
Chemical class: Belladonna alkaloid, tertiary amine
Therapeutic class: Antimuscarinic, antispasmodic
Pregnancy category: C

Indications and Dosages
➤ *To treat peptic ulcers and GI tract disorders caused by spasm*
ELIXIR, ORAL SOLUTION
Adults and adolescents. 0.125 to 0.25 mg every 4 to 6 hr.
Children. Dosage individualized by weight.
E.R. CAPSULES
Adults and adolescents. 0.375 mg every 12 hr.
E.R. TABLETS
Adults and adolescents. 0.375 to 0.75 mg every 12 hr. *Maximum:* 1.5 mg daily.
TABLETS
Adults and adolescents. 0.125 to 0.5 mg t.i.d. or q.i.d.
Children. Dosage individualized by weight.
I.V., I.M., OR SUBCUTANEOUS INJECTION
Adults and adolescents. 0.25 to 0.5 mg every 4 to 6 hr.
Children. Dosage individualized by weight.

➤ *To control salivation and excessive secretions during surgical procedures*
I. V. INJECTION
Adults and adolescents. 0.5 mg 30 to 60 min before procedure.

Route	Onset	Peak	Duration
P.O.*	20 to 30 min	30 to 60 min	4 hr
P.O. (E.R.)†	20 to 30 min	40 to 90 min	12 hr
I.V., I.M., SubQ.	2 to 3 min	15 to 30 min	4 hr

Mechanism of Action
Competitively inhibits acetylcholine at autonomic postganglionic cholinergic receptors. Because the most sensitive receptors are in the salivary, bronchial, and sweat glands, hyoscyamine acts mainly to reduce salivary, bronchial, and sweat gland secretions. It also causes GI smooth muscle to contract and decreases gastric secretion and GI motility. In addition, hyoscyamine causes the bladder detrusor muscle to contract; reduces nasal and oropharyngeal secretions; and decreases airway resistance from relaxation of smooth muscle in the bronchi and bronchioles.

Contraindications
Acute hemorrhage and hemodynamic instability; angle-closure glaucoma; hepatic disease; hypersensitivity to hyoscyamine, other anticholinergics, or their components; ileus; intestinal atony; myasthenia gravis; myocardial ischemia; obstructive GI disease; obstructive uropathy; renal disease; severe ulcerative colitis; tachycardia; toxic megacolon

Interactions
DRUGS
anticholinergics: Possibly increased anticholinergic effects

---

* For tablets only; for elixir and oral solution, onset is 5 to 20 min, and peak and duration are unknown.
† For E.R. tablets only; for E.R. capsules, onset and peak are unknown, and duration is 12 hr.

antidiarrheals (adsorbent): Possibly decreased therapeutic effects of hyoscyamine
calcium- and magnesium-containing antacids, carbonic anhydrase inhibitors, citrates, sodium bicarbonate, urinary alkalinizers: Possibly potentiated therapeutic and adverse effects of hyoscyamine
haloperidol: Possibly decreased therapeutic effects of haloperidol
ketoconazole: Possibly reduced ketoconazole absorption
metoclopramide: Possibly antagonized therapeutic effects of metoclopramide
opioid analgesics: Increased risk of severe constipation and ileus

Adverse Reactions
CNS: Drowsiness, insomnia
EENT: Blurred vision; dry mouth, nose, and throat; photophobia
ENDO: Decreased lactation
GI: Constipation
GU: Impotence, urine retention
SKIN: Decreased sweating
Other: Heatstroke, injection site redness and urticaria

Nursing Considerations
•Use hyoscyamine cautiously in patients who have arrhythmias, autonomic neuropathy, coronary artery disease, heart failure, hiatal hernia with reflux esophagitis, hypertension, hyperthyroidism, renal failure, or tachycardia.
•Give drug 30 to 60 minutes before meals and at bedtime. Give bedtime dose at least 2 hours after the day's last meal.
•Anticipate that tablets may not disintegrate and may appear in stool.
•WARNING Anticipate an increased risk of drug-induced heatstroke in hot or humid weather because hyoscyamine decreases sweating.
•WARNING Be aware that lower doses may paradoxically decrease heart rate. Higher doses affect nicotinic receptors in autonomic ganglia, causing delirium, disorientation, hallucinations, and restlessness.
•Monitor urine output, and be alert for urine retention.

Patient Teaching
•Instruct patient to void before taking each dose and to notify prescriber if she has trouble urinating during hyoscyamine therapy.

•Advise patient to take drug 30 to 60 minutes before meals and at bedtime. Bedtime dose should be taken at least 2 hours after the day's last meal.
•Inform patient that drug may cause drowsiness. Advise her to avoid potentially hazardous activities until drug's CNS effects are known.
•If patient reports dry mouth, suggest using sugarless hard candy or gum.
•Inform male patient that drug may cause impotence. If it occurs, suggest that he discuss it with prescriber.
•Advise patient to avoid exposure to high temperatures and to increase fluid intake, unless contraindicated.

ibuprofen

Actiprofen Caplets (CAN), Advil, Apo-Ibuprofen (CAN), Bayer Select Ibuprofen Pain Relief Formula Caplets, Children's Advil, Children's Motrin, Dolgesic, Excedrin IB, Genpril, Haltran, Ibifon 600 Caplets, Ibuprin, Ibuprohm Caplets, Ibu-Tab, Medipren, Midol IB, Motrin, Motrin-IB, Novo-Profen (CAN), Nu-Ibuprofen (CAN), Nuprin, Pamprin-IB, Q-Profen, Rufen, Trendar

Class and Category
Chemical class: Propionic acid derivative
Therapeutic class: Analgesic, anti-inflammatory, antipyretic
Pregnancy category: Not rated

Indications and Dosages
➤ *To relieve pain in rheumatoid arthritis and osteoarthritis*
CAPSULES, CHEWABLE TABLETS, ORAL SUSPENSION, TABLETS
Adults. 300 mg q.i.d., or 400, 600, or 800 mg t.i.d. or q.i.d. *Range:* 1.2 to 3.2 g daily.
➤ *To relieve mild to moderate pain*
CAPSULES, CHEWABLE TABLETS, ORAL SUSPENSION, TABLETS
Adults. 400 mg every 4 to 6 hr, p.r.n.
➤ *To relieve acute migraine pain*
CAPSULES, CHEWABLE TABLETS, ORAL SUSPENSION, TABLETS
Adults. 200 to 400 mg at onset of migraine pain. *Maximum:* 400 mg daily.
➤ *To relieve pain in primary dysmenorrhea*

CAPSULES, CHEWABLE TABLETS, ORAL SUSPENSION, TABLETS
Adults. 400 mg every 4 hr, p.r.n.

➤ *To relieve pain in juvenile arthritis*
CAPSULES, CHEWABLE TABLETS, ORAL SUSPENSION, TABLETS
Children. 30 to 70 mg/kg daily in divided doses t.i.d. or q.i.d.; 20 mg/kg daily for mild disease.

➤ *To relieve minor aches, pains, and dysmenorrhea and to reduce fever*
CAPSULES, CHEWABLE TABLETS, ORAL SUSPENSION, TABLETS
Adults. 200 to 400 mg every 4 to 6 hr. *Maximum:* 1.2 g daily.

➤ *To reduce fever*
CAPSULES, CHEWABLE TABLETS, ORAL SUSPENSION, TABLETS
Children ages 6 months to 12 years. 5 to 10 mg/kg every 4 to 6 hr. *Maximum:* 40 mg/kg daily.

Route	Onset	Peak	Duration
P.O.*	30 min	Unknown	4 to 6 hr
P.O.†	Up to 7 days	1 to 2 wk	Unknown
P.O.‡	In 1 hr	2 to 4 hr	6 to 8 hr

Mechanism of Action
Blocks the activity of cyclooxygenase, the enzyme needed to synthesize prostaglandins, which mediate the inflammatory response and cause local vasodilation, swelling, and pain. By inhibiting prostaglandins, this NSAID reduces inflammatory symptoms and relieves pain. Ibuprofen's antipyretic action probably stems from its effect on the hypothalamus, which increases peripheral blood flow, causing vasodilation and encouraging heat dissipation.

Contraindications
Angioedema, asthma, bronchospasm, nasal polyps, rhinitis, or urticaria caused by hypersensitivity to aspirin, ibuprofen, iodides, or other NSAIDs

---

* For analgesic effects.
† For anti-inflammatory effects.
‡ For antipyretic effects.

Interactions
DRUGS
acetaminophen: Possibly increased renal effects with long-term use of both drugs
antihypertensives: Decreased effectiveness of these drugs
aspirin: Possibly decreased cardioprotective and stroke-preventive effects of aspirin
aspirin, other NSAIDs: Increased risk of bleeding and adverse GI effects
bone marrow depressants: Possibly increased leukopenic and thrombocytopenic effects of bone marrow depressants
cefamandole, cefoperazone, cefotetan: Increased risk of hypoprothrombinemia and bleeding
colchicine, platelet aggregation inhibitors: Increased risk of GI bleeding, hemorrhage, and ulcers
corticosteroids, potassium supplements: Increased risk of adverse GI effects
cyclosporine: Increased risk of nephrotoxicity from both drugs, increased blood cyclosporine level
digoxin: Increased blood digoxin level and risk of digitalis toxicity
diuretics (loop, potassium-sparing, and thiazide): Decreased diuretic and antihypertensive effects
gold compounds, nephrotoxic drugs: Increased risk of adverse renal effects
heparin, oral anticoagulants, thrombolytics: Increased anticoagulant effects, increased risk of hemorrhage
insulin, oral antidiabetic drugs: Possibly increased hypoglycemic effects of these drugs
lithium: Increased blood lithium level
methotrexate: Decreased methotrexate clearance, increased risk of methotrexate toxicity
plicamycin, valproic acid: Increased risk of hypoprothrombinemia and GI bleeding, hemorrhage, and ulcers
probenecid: Possibly increased blood level, effectiveness, and risk of toxicity of ibuprofen
ACTIVITIES
alcohol use: Increased risk of adverse GI effects

Adverse Reactions
CNS: Aseptic meningitis, dizziness, headache, nervousness, seizures, stroke
CV: Fluid retention, heart failure, hypertension, MI, peripheral edema, tachycardia
EENT: Amblyopia, epistaxis, stomatitis, tinnitus

GI: Abdominal cramps, distention, or pain; anorexia; constipation; diarrhea; diverticulitis; dyspepsia; dysphagia; elevated liver function test results; epigastric discomfort; esophagitis; flatulence; gastritis; gastroenteritis; gastroesophageal reflux disease; GI bleeding, hemorrhage, perforation, or ulceration; heartburn; hemorrhoids; hepatic failure; hepatitis; hiatal hernia; indigestion; melena; nausea; stomatitis; vomiting
GU: Cystitis, hematuria, renal failure (acute)
HEME: Agranulocytosis, anemia, aplastic anemia, eosinophilia, hemolytic anemia, leukopenia, neutropenia, pancytopenia, prolonged bleeding time, thrombocytopenia
RESP: Bronchospasm, dyspnea, wheezing
SKIN: Blisters, erythema multiforme, photosensitivity, pruritus, rash, Stevens-Johnson syndrome, toxic epidermal necrolysis, urticaria
Other: Anaphylaxis, angioedema, flulike symptoms, weight gain

Nursing Considerations

•Use ibuprofen with extreme caution in patients with a history of ulcer disease or GI bleeding because NSAIDs such as ibuprofen increase the risk of GI bleeding and ulceration. Expect to use ibuprofen for the shortest time possible in these patients.
•Be aware that serious GI tract ulceration, bleeding, and perforation may occur without warning symptoms. Elderly patients are at greater risk. To minimize risk, give drug with food. If GI distress occurs, withhold drug and notify prescriber immediately.
•Use ibuprofen cautiously in patients with hypertension, and monitor blood pressure closely throughout therapy. Drug may cause hypertension or worsen it.
•**WARNING** Monitor patient closely for thrombotic events, including MI and stroke, because NSAIDs increase the risk.
•Monitor patient—especially if he's elderly or receiving long-term ibuprofen therapy—for less common but serious adverse GI reactions, including anorexia, constipation, diverticulitis, dysphagia, esophagitis, gastritis, gastroenteritis, gastroesophageal reflux disease, hemorrhoids, hiatal hernia, melena, stomatitis, and vomiting.
•Monitor liver function test results because, in rare cases, elevations may progress to severe hepatic reactions, including fatal hepa-

titis, liver necrosis, and hepatic failure.
•Monitor BUN and serum creatinine levels in elderly patients, patients taking diuretics or ACE inhibitors, and patients with heart failure, impaired renal function, or hepatic dysfunction; drug may cause renal failure.
•Monitor CBC for decreased hemoglobin and hematocrit. Drug may worsen anemia.
•**WARNING** If patient has bone marrow suppression or is receiving an antineoplastic drug, monitor laboratory results (including WBC count), and watch for evidence of infection because anti-inflammatory and antipyretic actions of ibuprofen may mask signs and symptoms, such as fever and pain.
•Assess patient's skin regularly for signs of rash or other hypersensitivity reaction because ibuprofen is an NSAID and may cause serious skin reactions without warning, even in patients with no history of NSAID sensivitity. At first sign of reaction, stop drug and notify prescriber.
•Although drug's analgesic effect occurs at low doses, expect to give at least 400 mg four times daily for anti-inflammatory effect.
•Expect higher doses for rheumatoid arthritis than for osteoarthritis.
•Be aware that ibuprofen oral suspension may contain sucrose, which may affect blood glucose level in patients with diabetes.

PATIENT TEACHING
•Instruct patient to take tablets with a full glass of water, and caution him not to lie down for 15 to 30 minutes to prevent esophageal irritation.
•Advise patient to take drug with food or after meals to reduce GI distress.
•Urge patient not to take more than prescribed because stomach bleeding may occur.
•Instruct patient to consult prescriber if he needs to take drug for more than 3 days for fever or 10 days for pain; if stomach problems (heartburn, upset, pain) recur; if he has a history of ulcers, bleeding problems, hypertension, or heart or renal disease; if he takes a diuretic; or if he's over age 65.
•Inform patient with phenylketonuria that Motrin chewable tablets contain aspartame.
•Inform patient that full therapeutic effect for arthritis may take 2 weeks or longer.
•Advise patient to avoid taking two different NSAIDs at the same time, unless directed, and to alert prescriber before taking ibuprofen if he has ever had an allergic reaction to

any other analgesic or fever-reducing drug.
•Urge patient to avoid alcohol, aspirin, and
corticosteroids while taking ibuprofen, unless
prescribed. If patient takes aspirin as prevention against MI or stroke, explain that
ibuprofen may interfere with this effect.
•Suggest that patient wear sunscreen and
protective clothing when outdoors.
•Advise patient to report flulike symptoms,
rash, signs of GI bleeding, swelling, vision
changes, and weight gain.
•Urge parents to tell prescriber promptly if
child receiving drug develops a severe or
persistent sore throat, high fever, headache,
persistent diarrhea, nausea, or vomiting or
hasn't been drinking fluids.
•Advise parents to consult prescriber before
giving OTC ibuprofen to a child if the child
has ulcers, bleeding problems, high blood
pressure, heart or kidney disease, a need for
diuretic therapy, serious adverse effects from
previous use of fever reducers or pain reliev-
ers, or persistent stomach problems, such as
heartburn, upset stomach, or stomach pain.
•Caution pregnant patient not to take
NSAIDs such as ibuprofen during the last
trimester because they may cause premature
closure of the ductus arteriosus.
•Explain that ibuprofen may increase the
risk of serious adverse cardiovascular reactions; urge patient to seek immediate medical attention if signs or symptoms arise,
such as chest pain, shortness of breath,
weakness, and slurring of speech.
•Explain that ibuprofen may increase the
risk of serious adverse GI reactions; stress
the importance of seeking immediate medical
attention for such signs and symptoms as
epigastric or abdominal pain, indigestion,
black or tarry stools, or vomiting blood or
material that looks like coffee grounds.
•Alert patient to rare but serious skin reactions. Urge him to seek immediate medical
attention for rash, blisters, itching, fever, or
other indications of hypersensitivity.

ibutilide fumarate

Corvert

Class and Category
Chemical: Methanesulfonanilide derivative
Therapeutic: Class III antiarrhythmic
Pregnancy category: C

Indications and Dosages
➤ *To rapidly convert recent-onset atrial
flutter or fibrillation to sinus rhythm*
I.V. INFUSION
Adults weighing 60 kg (132 lb) or more. 1 mg
over 10 min. Dose repeated 10 min after first
dose is finished if arrhythmia persists.
Adults weighing less than 60 kg. 0.01 mg/kg
over 10 min. Dose is repeated 10 min after
first dose is completed if arrhythmia persists.
DOSAGE ADJUSTMENT Infusion stopped if arrhythmia is terminated or if sustained or
nonsustained ventricular tachycardia or prolonged QT or QTc interval develops.

Mechanism of Action
May promote sodium movement through
slow inward sodium channels in myocardial cell membranes. Ibutilide also may
inhibit potassium channels in myocardial
cell membranes involved in cardiac repolarization. These actions prolong the cardiac action potential by delaying repolarization and increasing atrial and ventricular refractoriness. As a result, the sinus
rate slows and AV conduction is delayed.

Contraindications
Hypersensitivity to ibutilide or components

Interactions
DRUGS
*amiodarone, astemizole, disopyramide, ma-
protiline, phenothiazines, procainamide,
quinidine, sotalol, tricyclic antidepressants:*
Possibly prolonged QT interval, leading to
increased risk of proarrhythmias

Adverse Reactions
CNS: Headache, syncope
CV: AV block, bradycardia, bundle-branch
block, heart failure, hypertension, hypotension, idioventricular rhythm, orthostatic hypotension, palpitations, prolonged QT interval, sinus and supraventricular tachycardia,
supraventricular arrhythmias, ventricular arrhythmias, ventricular tachycardia (sustained
and nonsustained)
GI: Nausea
GU: Renal failure

Nursing Considerations
•Before giving ibutilide, check serum elec-

trolyte levels and expect to correct abnormalities, as prescribed. Be especially alert for hypokalemia and hypomagnesemia, which can lead to arrhythmias.

• Give drug undiluted, or dilute it in 50 ml of normal saline solution or D_5W. Add contents of 10-ml vial (0.1 mg/ml) to 50 ml of solution to obtain 0.017 mg/ml. Use polyvinyl chloride plastic bags or polyolefin bags for admixtures. Give drug within 24 hours (48 hours if refrigerated).

• Infuse drug slowly over 10 minutes.

• As ordered, monitor patient's cardiac rhythm continuously during drug infusion and for at least 4 hours afterward—longer if arrhythmias appear or if patient has abnormal hepatic function. Observe patient for ventricular ectopy.

• Make sure that a defibrillator and drugs to treat sustained ventricular tachycardia are available during therapy and when monitoring patient after therapy.

PATIENT TEACHING

• Inform patient that ibutilide will be administered by I.V. infusion and that his heart rhythm will be monitored continuously during the infusion.

• Ask patient to report chest pain, faintness, numbness, tingling, palpitations, and shortness of breath.

• Advise patient to keep follow-up appointments to monitor heart rhythm.

iloprost

Ventavis

Class and Category

Chemical class: Synthetic analogue of prostacyclin PGI_2
Therapeutic class: Pulmonary arterial antihypertensive
Pregnancy category: C

Indications and Dosages

➤ *To improve symptoms and exercise tolerance and prevent further deterioration from pulmonary arterial hypertension in patients with New York Heart Association (NYHA) Class III or IV symptoms*

INHALATION SOLUTION

Adults. *Initial:* 2.5 mcg as one-time dose. If tolerated well for 2 hr, dosage increased to 5 mcg. *Maintenance:* 5 mcg six to nine times daily during waking hours with at least 2 hr between each dose. *Maximum:* 45 mcg daily.

Mechanism of Action

Dilates systemic and pulmonary arterial vascular beds, which lowers blood pressure in the pulmonary arterial system.

Contraindications

Hypersensitivity to iloprost or its components

Interactions

DRUGS

anticoagulants: Increased risk of bleeding
antihypertensives, vasodilators: Increased hypotensive effect

Adverse Reactions

CNS: Apathy, dizziness, headache, insomnia, restlessness, syncope
CV: Chest pain, congestive heart failure, hypotension, palpitations, peripheral edema, supraventricular tachycardia, thrombosis, vasodilation
EENT: Epistaxis, gingival bleeding, tongue pain
ENDO: Hyperglycemia
GI: Abdominal cramps, diarrhea, nausea, vomiting
GU: Renal failure
MS: Back pain, muscle cramps or spasms
RESP: Bronchospasm, dyspnea, hemoptysis, increased cough, pneumonia, wheezing
SKIN: Flushing
Other: Flulike symptoms, increased alkaline phosphatase level

Nursing Considerations

• Use iloprost cautiously in patients with hepatic or renal impairment.

• Give iloprost only with the Prodose AAD System, a pulmonary drug delivery device. Avoid contact between solution and skin or eyes.

• **WARNING** Don't give iloprost if patient's systolic blood pressure is less than 85 mm Hg.

• Notify prescriber if patient develops exertional syncope because dosage may need to be adjusted.

• **WARNING** Stop iloprost immediately if patient develops signs of pulmonary edema, such as shortness of breath, anxiety, restless-

ness, and abnormal breath sounds. Notify prescriber and provide supportive care, as prescribed.
•Monitor patient's vital signs while initiating iloprost therapy because drug may cause syncope.

PATIENT TEACHING
•Instruct patient to use iloprost inhalation therapy exactly as prescribed. Tell patient that at least 2 hours must elapse between doses but that the benefits of iloprost therapy may not last for 2 hours.
•Teach patient how to administer iloprost via the Prodose AAD System. Tell patient to have a backup system available in case of equipment malfunction.
•Advise patient to stand up slowly because drug may cause dizziness or faintness. If these symptoms persist or worsen, tell patient to notify prescriber because a dosage adjustment may be required.

imipramine hydrochloride

Apo-Imipramine (CAN), Impril (CAN), Norfranil, Novopramine (CAN), Tipramine, Tofranil

imipramine pamoate

Tofranil-PM

Class and Category
Chemical class: Dibenzazepine derivative
Therapeutic class: Antidepressant
Pregnancy category: Not rated

Indications and Dosages
➤ *To treat depression*
CAPSULES
Adults. *Initial:* 75 mg daily at bedtime, gradually increased as needed and tolerated. *Maximum:* 300 mg daily (hospitalized patients), 200 mg/day (outpatients).
TABLETS
Adults. *Initial:* 25 to 50 mg t.i.d. or q.i.d., gradually increased as needed and tolerated. *Maximum:* 300 mg daily (hospitalized patients), 200 mg daily (outpatients).
DOSAGE ADJUSTMENT Initial dosage reduced to 25 mg at bedtime for depressed elderly patients; then adjusted as needed and tolerated up to 100 mg daily in divided doses.
Adolescents. *Initial:* 25 to 50 mg daily in di-

vided doses, adjusted as needed and tolerated. *Maximum:* 100 mg daily.
Children ages 6 to 12. 10 to 30 mg daily in divided doses b.i.d.

➤ *As adjunct to treat childhood enuresis*
TABLETS
Children age 6 and over. 25 mg 1 hr before bedtime. Increased to 50 mg if no response occurs within 1 wk and child is under age 12; increased to 75 mg if child is age 12 or over. *Maximum:* 2.5 mg/kg daily.

Route	Onset	Peak	Duration
P.O.	2 to 3 wk*	Unknown	Unknown

Mechanism of Action
May interfere with reuptake of serotonin (and possibly other neurotransmitters) at presynaptic neurons, thus enhancing serotonin's effects at postsynaptic receptors. Mood elevation may result from restoration of normal levels of neurotransmitters at nerve synapses. This tricyclic antidepressant also blocks acetylcholine receptors, which may explain how it relieves enuresis.

Contraindications
Acute recovery period after MI; hypersensitivity to imipramine, other tricyclic antidepressants, or their components; use within 2 weeks of MAO inhibitor therapy

Interactions
DRUGS
amantadine, anticholinergics, antidyskinetics, antihistamines: Risk of increased anticholinergic effects, including confusion, hallucinations, and nightmares
anticonvulsants: Increased risk of CNS depression, increased risk of seizures, decreased effectiveness of imipramine
antithyroid drugs: Possibly agranulocytosis
barbiturates, carbamazepine: Possibly decreased blood level and effectiveness of imipramine
cimetidine, fluoxetine: Possibly increased blood imipramine level
clonidine, guanadrel, guanethidine: Possibly decreased antihypertensive effects of these drugs, increased CNS depression (clonidine)
CNS depressants: Increased CNS depression,

* For antidepressant effect.

respiratory depression, and hypotension
disulfiram, ethchlorvynol: Risk of delirium,
increased CNS depression (ethchlorvynol)
*estramustine, estrogen-containing oral con-
traceptives, estrogens:* Risk of increased bioavailability of imipramine, increased depression
MAO inhibitors: Increased risk of hypertensive crisis, severe seizures, and death
oral anticoagulants: Possibly increased anticoagulant activity
pimozide, probucol: Risk of arrhythmias
*sympathomimetics (including ophthalmic
epinephrine and vasoconstrictive local anesthetics):* Increased risk of arrhythmias, hyperpyrexia, hypertension, tachycardia
thyroid hormones: Risk of increased therapeutic and adverse effects of both drugs

ACTIVITIES
alcohol use: Increased CNS depression, increased alcohol effects
sun exposure: Increased risk of photosensitivity

Adverse Reactions

CNS: Anxiety, ataxia, chills, confusion, delirium, dizziness, drowsiness, excitation, extrapyramidal reactions, fever, hallucinations,
headache, insomnia, nervousness, nightmares, parkinsonism, seizures, stroke, suicidal ideation, tremor
CV: Arrhythmias, orthostatic hypotension,
palpitations
EENT: Blurred vision, dry mouth, increased
intraocular pressure, pharyngitis, taste perversion, tinnitus, tongue swelling
ENDO: Gynecomastia, syndrome of inappropriate ADH secretion
GI: Constipation, diarrhea, heartburn, ileus,
increased appetite, nausea, vomiting
GU: Impotence, libido changes, testicular
swelling, urine retention
HEME: Agranulocytosis, bone marrow depression
RESP: Wheezing
SKIN: Alopecia, diaphoresis, jaundice, photosensitivity, pruritus, rash, urticaria
Other: Allergic reaction, facial edema, weight
gain

Nursing Considerations

•Use imipramine cautiously in patients with
a history of urine retention or angle-closure
glaucoma because drug's anticholinergic effects may cause urine retention and in-

creased intraocular pressure.
•**WARNING** Don't give MAO inhibitors within
2 weeks of imipramine. Patient may experience hypertensive crisis, seizures, and death.
•Frequently assess for adverse reactions during first 2 hours of therapy.
•Check supine and standing blood pressure
for orthostatic hypotension before and during imipramine therapy and before dosage
increases.
•Anticipate an increased risk of arrhythmias
in patients with a history of cardiac disease.
•When drug is used for depression, expect
mood elevation to take 2 to 3 weeks. Watch
patient closely for suicidal tendencies, especially children and adolescents and especially when therapy starts or dosage changes,
because depression may worsen temporarily
at these times.
•Avoid abrupt withdrawal of drug in patients who receive long-term therapy. Such
withdrawal may cause headache, malaise,
nausea, sleep disturbance, and vomiting.
•Taper drug gradually, as ordered, a few
days before surgery to avoid the risk of hypertension during surgery.
•Obtain CBC, as ordered, if patient experiences signs and symptoms of infection, such
as fever or pharyngitis.
•Limit amount of drug given to potentially
suicidal patient.

PATIENT TEACHING
•Advise patient to take imipramine exactly
as prescribed. Warn him that stopping drug
abruptly may cause headache, malaise, nausea, trouble sleeping, and vomiting.
•Caution parents to monitor child or adolescent closely for suicidal tendencies, especially when therapy starts or dosage changes.
•Urge patient to report chills, trouble urinating, dizziness, excess sedation, fever, palpitations, signs of allergic reaction, and sore
throat.
•Caution patient to avoid hazardous activities until drug's CNS effects are known.
•Urge patient to avoid alcohol during imipramine therapy because it increases CNS depression and alcohol effects.
•Suggest that patient eat small, frequent
meals to help relieve nausea.
•Instruct patient to avoid prolonged exposure to sunlight because of the risk of photosensitivity.
•Inform male patient about possible impo-

tence and increased or decreased libido.
•If patient reports dry mouth, suggest sugar-less candy or gum to relieve it. Tell him to check with prescriber if dry mouth persists after 2 weeks.

immune globulin intramuscular (human)
(gamma globulin, IG)

BayGam, WinRho SDF

immune globulin intravenous (human)
(IGIV, immune serum globulin, ISG, IVIG)

Gamimune N 5% S/D, Gamimune N 10% S/D, Gammagard Liquid, Gammagard S/D, Gammagard S/D 0.5 g, Gammar-P IV, Gamunex 10%, Iveegam EN, Octagam 5%, Polygam S/D, Rhophylac, Sandoglobulin, Venoglobulin-I, Venoglobulin-S 5%, Venoglobulin-S 10%, WinRho SDF

Class and Category
Chemical class: Polyvalent antibody
Therapeutic class: Antibacterial, anti–Kawasaki disease agent, antipoly-neuropathy agent, antiviral, immunizing agent, platelet count stimulator
Pregnancy category: C

Indications and Dosages
➤ *To treat primary immunodeficiency*
I.M. INJECTION (BAYGAM)
Adults. 0.66 ml/kg (at least 200 mg/kg) every 3 to 4 wk; initial dose may be doubled.
I.V. INFUSION (GAMIMUNE N 5% S/D OR 10% S/D)
Adults. 100 to 200 mg/kg every mo. If response is inadequate, dose may be increased to as high as 400 mg/kg or dosing frequency may be increased.
I.V. INFUSION (GAMMAGARD S/D, POLYGAM S/D)
Adults. 200 to 400 mg/kg initially, then at least 100 mg/kg every mo thereafter. If response is inadequate, dose or frequency may be adjusted.
I.V. INFUSION (GAMMAR-P IV)
Adults. 200 to 400 mg/kg every 3 to 4 wk.
Adolescents and children. 200 mg/kg every 3 to 4 wk.

I.V. INFUSION (GAMUNEX 10%)
Adults. 300 to 600 mg/kg every 3 or 4 wk.
I.V. INFUSION (IVEEGAM EN)
Adults. 200 mg/kg every mo.
I.V. INFUSION (OCTAGAM 5%)
Adults. *Initial:* 30 mg/kg/hr for first 30 minutes; increased, if tolerated, to 60 mg/kg/hr for second 30 minutes and, if tolerated, to 120 mg/kg/hr for another 30 minutes; followed by maintenance infusion of up to 200 mg/kg/hr.
I.V. INFUSION (SANDOGLOBULIN)
Adults and children. 200 mg/kg every mo. If response is inadequate, dose may be increased to 300 mg/kg or dosing frequency may be increased.
I.V. INFUSION (VENOGLOBULIN-I)
Adults and children. 200 mg/kg every mo. If response is inadequate, dose may be increased to 300 to 400 mg/kg every mo or dosing frequency may be increased.
I.V. INFUSION (VENOGLOBULIN-S 5% OR 10%)
Adults and children. 200 mg/kg every mo. If response is inadequate, dose may be increased to as high as 400 mg/kg or dosing frequency may be increased.

➤ *To treat primary immunodeficiency disorders associated with defects in humoral immunity*
I.V. INFUSION (GAMMAGARD LIQUID)
Adults and children. 300 to 600 mg/kg daily every 3 to 4 wk.

➤ *To treat idiopathic thrombocytopenic purpura (ITP)*
I.V. INFUSION (GAMIMUNE N 5% S/D)
Adults and children. 400 mg/kg daily for 5 days. Or, 1,000 mg/kg for 1 or 2 days for patients not at risk for increased fluid volume.
I.V. INFUSION (GAMIMUNE N 10% S/D)
Adults and children. 1,000 mg/kg for 1 or 2 days for patients not at risk for increased fluid volume.
I.V. INFUSION (GAMUNEX 10%)
Adults. 1 g/kg daily for 2 consecutive days (second dose may be withheld if adequate increase in platelet count occurs 24 hours after first dose). Alternatively, 0.4 g/kg daily for 5 consecutive days.
DOSAGE ADJUSTMENT In acute ITP of childhood, I.V. Sandoglobulin therapy may be discontinued after second day of 5-day course if initial platelet count response is adequate

G
H
I

(30,000 to 50,000/mm³). In chronic ITP, an additional I.V. infusion of 400 mg/kg (of either Sandoglobulin or Gamimune) may be prescribed if platelet count falls below 30,000/mm³ or if patient develops significant bleeding. If response remains inadequate, an additional I.V. infusion of 800 to 1,000 mg/kg may be given.

I.V. INFUSION (GAMMAGARD S/D)

Adults. 1 g/kg. If response is inadequate, up to three separate doses may be administered on alternate days.

I.V. INFUSION (RHOPHYLAC)

Adults. 50 mcg/kg at 2 ml/15 to 60 seconds.

I.V. INFUSION (SANDOGLOBULIN)

Adults and adolescents. 400 mg/kg daily for 2 to 5 consecutive days.

I.V. INFUSION (VENOGLOBULIN-I)

Adults and children. *Induction:* Cumulative dose up to 2 g/kg over 2 to 7 consecutive days. *Maintenance (adults):* 2 g/kg as a single dose every 2 wk as needed to maintain platelet count above 30,000/mm³ or prevent bleeding episodes. *Maintenance (children):* 1 g/kg as a single dose every 2 wk as needed to maintain platelet count above 30,000/mm³ or prevent bleeding episodes.

I.V. INFUSION (VENOGLOBULIN-S 5% OR 10%)

Adults and children. Cumulative dose up to 2,000 mg/kg over 5 consecutive days.

DOSAGE ADJUSTMENT An additional I.V. infusion of 1,000 mg/kg may be administered to maintain a platelet count of 30,000/mm³ in children or 20,000/mm³ in adults or to prevent bleeding episodes.

➤ *To treat acute or chronic pediatric immune thrombocytopenia purpura; to treat chronic adult-onset immune thrombocytopenia purpura; to treat prediatric- and adult-onset immune thrombocytopenia purpura secondary to HIV infection*

I.V. INJECTION (WINRHO SDF)

Adults and children. *Initial:* 250 international units/kg given as a single injection over 3 to 5 min. Or 125 international units/kg given as a single injection over 3 to 5 min and repeated once on a separate day. *Maintenance:* Frequency and dosage highly individualized based on patient's hemoglobin and platelet levels.

DOSAGE ADJUSTMENT For patients with a hemoglobin level less than 10 g/dl, dose re-

duced to 125 to 200 international units/kg.

➤ *As adjunct to treat Kawasaki disease*

I.V. INFUSION (GAMMAGARD S/D)

Adults and adolescents. 1 g/kg as a single dose; alternatively, 400 mg/kg daily for 4 consecutive days.

I.V. INFUSION (IVEEGAM EN, VENOGLOBULIN-S 5% OR 10%)

Adults and adolescents. 2 g/kg as a single dose; alternatively, Iveegam EN may be given at 400 mg/kg daily for 4 days.

➤ *To decrease the risk of graft-versus-host disease, interstitial pneumonia, septicemia, and other infections during first 100 days after bone marrow transplantation*

I.V. INFUSION (GAMIMUNE N 5% S/D OR 10% S/D)

Adults over age 20. 500 mg/kg on 7th and 2nd days before transplant (or at time conditioning therapy for transplantation begins), and then weekly through 90th day after transplant.

➤ *As adjunct to treat bacterial infections secondary to B-cell chronic lymphocytic leukemia*

I.V. INFUSION (GAMMAGARD S/D, POLYGAM S/D)

Adults and adolescents. 400 mg/kg every 3 to 4 wk.

➤ *To prevent bacterial infection in children with HIV who are immunosuppressed*

I.V. INFUSION (GAMIMUNE N 5% S/D OR 10% S/D)

Children. 400 mg/kg daily every 28 days.

➤ *To prevent hepatitis A*

I.M. INJECTION (BAYGAM)

Adults with household or institutional contacts. 0.02 ml/kg (0.01 ml/lb).

Adults traveling to areas where hepatitis A is common. 0.02 ml/kg if staying less than 3 mo, 0.06 ml/kg (repeated every 4 to 6 mo) if staying 3 mo or longer.

➤ *To prevent or lessen severity of measles (rubeola) in susceptible persons*

I.M. INJECTION (BAYGAM)

Adults. 0.2 ml/kg (0.11 ml/lb) for persons exposed fewer than 6 days previously.

➤ *To provide passive immunization against varicella in immunosuppressed patients*

I.M. INJECTION (BAYGAM)

Adults. 0.6 to 1.2 ml/kg if varicella-zoster immune globulin (human) is unavailable.

➤ *To reduce the risk of infection and fetal*

damage in women who have been exposed to rubella in early pregnancy
I.M. INJECTION (BAYGAM)
Adults. 0.55 ml/kg.

➤ *To suppress Rh isoimmunization*
I.M. INJECTION, I.V. INFUSION (RHOPHYLAC)
Adult pregnant females. 1,500 international units as a single dose at 28 to 30 wk gestation followed by 1,500 international units within 72 hr after delivery of an Rh-positive newborn.
I.M. INJECTION (WINRHO SDF)
Adult pregnant females. 1,500 international units as a single dose at 28 wk gestation followed by 600 international units within 72 hr after delivery of an Rh-positive newborn.
I.V. INJECTION (WINRHO SDF)
Adult pregnant females. 1,500 international units as a single dose infused over 3 to 5 min at 28 wk gestation followed by 600 international units over 3 to 5 min within 72 hr after delivery of an Rh-positive newborn.
DOSAGE ADJUSTMENT For patients who are more than 34 wk gestation and are having an abortion, amniocentesis, or other manipulative procedure, 600 international units given within 72 hr but preferably immediately after procedure. For patients who are 34 wk gestation or less and are having amniocentesis or chorionic villus sampling, 1,500 international units given immediately after procedure and repeated every 12 wk for duration of pregnancy. For patients with a threatened abortion at any stage of pregnancy, 1,500 international units given immediately.

➤ *To treat incompatible blood transfusions*
I.M. INJECTION, I.V. INFUSION (RHOPHYLAC)
Adults exposed to Rh-positive RBCs. 100 international units/2 ml transfused blood or 1 ml erythrocyte concentrate within 72 hr of exposure.
I.M. INJECTION (WINRHO SDF)
Adults exposed to Rh-positive whole blood. 6,000 international units every 12 hr until total dose (60 international units/ml of blood) is given.
Adults exposed to Rh-positive RBCs. 6,000 international units every 12 hr until total dose (120 international units/ml of cells) is given.
I.V. INJECTION (WINRHO SDF)
Adults exposed to Rh-positive whole blood. 3,000 international units infused over 3 to

5 min every 8 hr until total dose (45 international units/ml of blood) is given.
Adults exposed to Rh-positive RBCs. 3,000 international units infused over 3 to 5 min every 8 hr until total dose (90 international units/ml of cells) is given.

➤ *To treat massive fetomaternal hemorrhage*
I.M. INJECTION, I.V. INFUSION (RHOPHYLAC)
Adults exposed to Rh-positive RBCs. 1,500 international units plus 100 international units for every 1 ml of fetal RBCs exceeding 15 ml if transplacental bleeding is quantified or an additional 1,500 international units if transplacental bleeding can't be quantified within 72 hours of hemorrhage.
I.M. INJECTION (WINRHO SDF)
Adults exposed to Rh-positive whole blood. 6,000 international units every 12 hr until total dose (60 international units/ml of blood) is given.
Adults exposed to Rh-positive RBCs. 6,000 international units every 12 hr until total dose (120 international units/ml of cells) is given.
I.V. INJECTION (WINRHO SDF)
Adults exposed to Rh-positive whole blood. 3,000 international units infused over 3 to 5 min every 8 hr until total dose (45 international units/ml of blood) is given.
Adults exposed to Rh-positive RBCs. 3,000 international units infused over 3 to 5 min every 8 hr until total dose (90 international units/ml of cells) is given.

Route	Onset	Peak	Duration
I.V.	Unknown	Unknown	21 to 28 days

Incompatibilities
Don't mix immune globulin with any other drugs, including other immune globulins, or with any I.V. solutions other than D_5W or manufacturer's supplied diluent because effects of doing so are unknown.

Contraindications
Hypersensitivity to immune globulin (human) or its components, IgA deficiency in patients with known antibody to IgA

Interactions
DRUGS
vaccines, live-virus: Possibly decreased response to vaccine

Mechanism of Action

Releases antibody-specific globulins to produce an antibody-antigen reaction that results in bacterial lysis and facilitates bacterial phagocytosis. In treatment of ITP, immune globulin blocks iron receptors on macrophages to increase immunoglobulin action. Immune globulin also increases cytokine production and improves B-cell immune function by regulating T-cell and macrophage activity. Newly formed antigen-antibody complexes produce split complement components that cause bacterial lysis.

In Kawasaki disease and bacterial infections with B-cell chronic lymphocytic leukemia, immune globulin neutralizes bacterial and viral toxins that harm immune and inflammatory responses.

Adverse Reactions

CNS: Headache, malaise
CV: Tachycardia
GI: Nausea, vomiting
MS: Arthralgia, back pain, myalgia
RESP: Dyspnea

Nursing Considerations

• Before administering immune globulin, monitor patient's fluid volume and BUN and serum creatinine levels, as ordered, to determine if he's at risk for acute renal failure. Those at increased risk include patients with renal insufficiency, diabetes mellitus, volume depletion, sepsis, or paraproteinemia; those taking nephrotoxic drugs; and those over age 65. Expect drug to be discontinued if renal function deteriorates.
• When preparing immune globulin, verify that appropriate form of immune globulin is being used—either immune globulin intramuscular for I.M. injection or immune globulin intravenous for I.V. infusion.
• To reconstitute drug (except Gammagard Liquid, which doesn't need reconstitution), follow manufacturer's guidelines and use only diluent recommended by manufacturer. Don't shake solution; excessive shaking causes foaming. If drug or diluent is cold, drug may take up to 20 minutes to dissolve.
• If drug is reconstituted outside of sterile laminar airflow conditions, administer it immediately and discard unused portions.
• Consult manufacturer's guidelines to determine appropriate flow rate for starting infusion. Expect to increase flow rate after 15 to 30 minutes, according to guidelines.
• When giving drug by I.M. injection, inject it only into deltoid muscle of the upper arm or anterolateral aspect of the upper thigh. If giving a dose larger than 5 ml, divide it and administer at separate sites.
• **WARNING** Watch for an acute inflammatory reaction in patients who have never received immune globulin therapy before, in those whose last treatment was more than 8 weeks before, and in those whose initial infusion rate exceeded 1 ml/minute. Within 30 minutes to 1 hour after beginning of infusion, assess for chills, fever, facial flushing, feeling of tightness in chest, dizziness, nausea and vomiting, diaphoresis, and hypotension. Notify prescriber immediately if such symptoms occur, and be prepared to stop infusion until symptoms have subsided.
• **WARNING** After immune globulin administration, monitor patient closely for aseptic meningitis. Notify prescriber if patient develops drowsiness, fever, nausea and vomiting, nuchal rigidity, photophobia, painful eye movements, or severe headache.
• Be aware that immune globulin intravenous is made from human plasma and therefore may contain infectious agents, such as viruses. However, the risk of transmitting a virus by infusion has been reduced by screening blood donors, testing donated blood, and inactivating or removing certain viruses from the product.
• For patient receiving WinRho SDF to treat immune thrombocytopenia purpura, assess clinical response by monitoring patient's platelet count, RBC count, hemoglobin level, and reticulocyte level.
• For patient receiving WinRho SDF for exposure to incompatible blood transfusions or massive fetal hemorrhage, give drug within 72 hours of incident.

Patient Teaching

• Instruct patient to immediately report any symptoms he experiences after receiving immune globulin.
• Inform patient to postpone live-virus vaccinations for up to 11 months after receiving immune globulin because drug may delay or inhibit his response to vaccine.

inamrinone
(amrinone)

Inocor

Class and Category
Chemical class: Bipyridine derivative
Therapeutic class: Cardiac inotrope
Pregnancy category: C

Indications and Dosages
➤ *To treat heart failure in patients who haven't responded sufficiently to digoxin, diuretics, or vasodilators*

I.V. INFUSION
Adults. *Initial:* 0.75 mg/kg by bolus over 2 to 3 min and repeated after 30 min, if needed. *Maintenance:* 5 to 10 mcg/ kg/min by infusion. *Maximum:* 10 mg/kg daily.

Route	Onset	Peak	Duration
I.V.	2 to 5 min	In 10 min	30 min to 2 hr

Incompatibilities
Don't administer inamrinone through same I.V. line as furosemide because doing so could result in precipitate formation. Don't dilute inamrinone in solution that contains dextrose because a chemical interaction occurs over 24 hours.

Contraindications
Hypersensitivity to inamrinone, bisulfites, or their components; severe aortic or pulmonary valvular disease

Interactions
DRUGS
disopyramide: Possibly severe hypotension

Adverse Reactions
CNS: Fever
CV: Chest pain, hypotension, pericarditis, supraventricular tachycardia, ventricular arrhythmias
GI: Abdominal pain, anorexia, elevated liver function test results, hepatotoxicity, nausea, vomiting
HEME: Elevated erythrocyte sedimentation rate, thrombocytopenia (especially with high-dose or prolonged treatment)
MS: Myositis
RESP: Hypoxemia, pleuritis
SKIN: Jaundice
Other: Infusion site burning

Mechanism of Action
Inhibits phosphodiesterase enzymes that normally degrade myocardial cAMP. This action increases intracellular levels of cAMP, which regulates intracellular and extracellular calcium balance. An increased intracellular cAMP level enhances the influx of calcium into the cell, thereby increasing the force of myocardial contractions. Inamrinone also acts directly on peripheral vascular smooth-muscle cells, causing relaxation and dilation. This action reduces preload and afterload.

Nursing Considerations
•**WARNING** Be aware that inamrinone may increase the risk of ventricular arrhythmias in patients with atrial flutter or fibrillation. To minimize this risk, expect to pretreat such patients with digoxin.
•Give drug undiluted or diluted in normal or half-normal (0.45) saline solution to a concentration of 1 to 3 mg/ml, as prescribed. Use diluted solution within 24 hours.
•**WARNING** Monitor vital signs regularly. If blood pressure falls significantly, slow or stop inamrinone infusion and notify prescriber.
•Monitor weight, cardiac index, central venous pressure, pulmonary artery wedge pressure, and fluid intake and output as appropriate to assess effectiveness of therapy.
•**WARNING** Assess frequently for signs of thrombocytopenia, such as bruising or bleeding and altered platelet count. If signs appear, expect to decrease inamrinone dose or discontinue drug.
PATIENT TEACHING
•Instruct patient to notify you or another nurse if he becomes dizzy, which may indicate hypotension.

indapamide

Apo-Indapamide (CAN), Gen-Indapamide (CAN), Lozide (CAN), Lozol, Novo-Indapamide (CAN), Nu-Indapamide (CAN)

Class and Category
Chemical class: Sulfonamide
Therapeutic class: Antihypertensive, diuretic
Pregnancy category: B

Indications and Dosages

➤ *To treat edema caused by heart failure*

TABLETS

Adults. 2.5 mg daily in the morning, increased to 5 mg daily after 1 wk, if indicated.

➤ *To manage hypertension*

TABLETS

Adults. 2.5 mg daily, increased to 5 mg after 4 wk, if needed.

Route	Onset	Peak	Duration
P.O.*	1 to 2 hr	Unknown	36 hr
P.O.†	1 to 2 wk	8 to 12 wk	Up to 8 wk

Mechanism of Action

Acts mainly on distal convoluted tubules, where it enhances excretion of sodium, chloride, and water by inhibiting sodium ion movement across renal tubules. The resulting decrease in plasma and extracellular fluid volume decreases peripheral vascular resistance and reduces blood pressure. This thiazide diuretic also may cause arterial vasodilation by blocking calcium channels in smooth-muscle cells.

Contraindications

Anuria; hypersensitivity to thiazide or related diuretics or to sulfonamide-derived drugs

Interactions

DRUGS

amiodarone: Increased risk of arrhythmias if hypokalemia develops

cholestyramine, colestipol: Decreased indapamide absorption

diazoxide: Increased risk of hyperglycemia

digoxin: Increased risk of digitalis toxicity if hypokalemia develops

hypotension-producing drugs: Increased antihypertensive or diuretic effects

lithium: Increased risk of lithium toxicity

neuromuscular blockers: Possibly increased neuromuscular blockade, risk of respiratory depression

oral anticoagulants: Possibly decreased anticoagulant effects

---

* For edema.
† For hypertension (with multiple doses).

Adverse Reactions

CNS: Anxiety, dizziness, drowsiness, fatigue, fever, headache, mood changes, nervousness, sleep disturbance, vertigo, weakness

CV: Arrhythmias, hypercholesterolemia, orthostatic hypotension, palpitations

EENT: Dry mouth

ENDO: Hyperglycemia, hypoglycemia

GI: Anorexia, constipation, diarrhea, hepatitis, nausea, pancreatitis, thirst, vomiting

GU: Impotence, nocturia

MS: Gout, muscle spasms

SKIN: Jaundice, necrotizing vasculitis, photosensitivity, pruritus, rash, urticaria

Other: Dilutional hypochloremia and hyponatremia, hypokalemia, metabolic alkalosis, weight loss

Nursing Considerations

• Administer indapamide with food or milk to reduce adverse GI reactions.

• Give drug early in the day to avoid nocturia.

• Weigh patient daily, and monitor fluid intake and output, blood pressure, and serum electrolyte levels.

• Monitor BUN and serum creatinine levels regularly, as appropriate.

• If muscle cramps and weakness develop from hypokalemia, expect prescriber to order a potassium supplement or potassium-sparing diuretic.

• When managing hypertension, expect therapeutic response to indapamide to take several weeks.

PATIENT TEACHING

• Advise patient to take indapamide early in the day to avoid nighttime urination and to take it with food or milk to minimize GI distress.

• Encourage patient to eat high-potassium foods, such as oranges and bananas.

• Caution patient to change position slowly to minimize effects of orthostatic hypotension.

• Instruct patient to weigh himself daily at the same time and wearing similar clothing. Direct him to report a weight gain of more than 2 lb (0.9 kg) per day or 5 lb (2.3 kg) per week.

• Inform patient about possible photosensitivity.

• If patient has a dry mouth, suggest sugarless gum or hard candy to relieve it.

indomethacin

Apo-Indomethacin (CAN), Indocid (CAN), Indocin, Indocin SR, Novo-Methacin (CAN), Nu-Indo (CAN)

indomethacin sodium trihydrate

Apo-Indomethacin (CAN), Indameth, Indocid (CAN), Indocid PDA (CAN), Indocin, Indocin I.V., Novomethacin (CAN)

Class and Category

Chemical class: Indoleacetic acid derivative
Therapeutic class: Antigout, anti-inflammatory, antirheumatic
Pregnancy category: Not rated

Indications and Dosages

➤ *To relieve symptoms of ankylosing spondylitis, osteoarthritis, and rheumatoid arthritis*

CAPSULES, ORAL SUSPENSION
Adults. 25 to 50 mg b.i.d. to q.i.d., increased by 25 or 50 mg daily every wk, if needed. *Maximum:* 200 mg daily. After adequate response, dosage reduced as low as possible.

E.R. CAPSULES (ANTIRHEUMATIC)
Adults. 75 mg daily, increased to 75 mg b.i.d, if needed.

SUPPOSITORIES
Adults. 50 mg up to q.i.d.

➤ *To relieve symptoms of acute gouty arthritis*

CAPSULES, ORAL SUSPENSION
Adults. *Initial:* 100 mg. Increased up to 50 mg t.i.d. *Maximum:* 200 mg daily. After pain is relieved, dosage tapered until drug is discontinued.

SUPPOSITORIES
Adults. 50 mg up to q.i.d. *Maximum:* 200 mg daily.

➤ *To treat inflammation and relieve acute shoulder pain from bursitis or tendinitis*

CAPSULES, ORAL SUSPENSION
Adults. 75 to 150 mg daily in divided doses t.i.d. or q.i.d. for 7 to 14 days.

SUPPOSITORIES
Adults. 50 mg up to q.i.d. *Maximum:* 200 mg daily.

DOSAGE ADJUSTMENT Dosage reduced for elderly patients.

➤ *To treat hemodynamically significant*

patent ductus arteriosus in premature infants weighing 500 to 1,750 g (1 to 3.9 lb)

I.V. INJECTION
Infants over age 7 days. *Initial:* 200 mcg/kg (0.2 mg/kg) over 5 to 10 sec; 1 or 2 additional doses of 250 mcg/kg (0.25 mg/kg) given at 12- to 24-hr intervals, if needed.
Neonates ages 2 to 7 days. *Initial:* 200 mcg/kg (0.2 mg/kg) over 5 to 10 sec; 1 or 2 additional doses of 200 mcg/kg (0.2 mg/kg) given at 12- to 24-hr intervals, if needed.
Neonates under age 48 hours. *Initial:* 200 mcg/kg (0.2 mg/kg) over 5 to 10 sec; 1 or 2 additional doses of 100 mcg/kg (0.1 mg/kg) given at 12- to 24-hr intervals, if needed.

Route	Onset	Peak	Duration
P.O.*	2 to 4 hr	2 to 5 days	Unknown
P.O.†	30 min	Unknown	4 to 6 hr
P.O.‡	In 7 days	1 to 2 wk	Unknown

Mechanism of Action

Blocks the activity of cyclooxygenase, the enzyme needed to synthesize prostaglandins, which mediate the inflammatory response and cause local vasodilation, swelling, and pain. By blocking cyclooxygenase and inhibiting prostaglandins, this NSAID reduces inflammatory symptoms and helps relieve pain.

Incompatibilities

Don't give indomethacin suspension with alkaline antacids or liquids. Don't mix reconstituted indomethacin sodium with I.V. infusion solutions.

Contraindications

Allergy or hypersensitivity to aspirin, indomethacin, iodides, other NSAIDs, or their components; history of proctitis or recent rectal bleeding (suppositories)

Interactions

DRUGS
Note: All effects listed are for oral forms and suppositories unless indicated.

---

* For antigout effects.
† For anti-inflammatory effects.
‡ For antirheumatic effects.

acetaminophen: Increased risk of adverse renal effects (with long-term use of both drugs)

aluminum- and magnesium-containing antacids: Possibly decreased blood indomethacin level

aminoglycosides: Increased risk of aminoglycoside toxicity

antihypertensives: Decreased effectiveness of these drugs

aspirin, other NSAIDs: Increased risk of adverse GI effects and non-GI bleeding

bone marrow depressants: Possibly increased leukopenic or thrombocytopenic effects of these drugs

cefamandole, cefoperazone, cefotetan: Increased risk of hypoprothrombinemia and bleeding

colchicine, platelet aggregation inhibitors: Increased risk of GI bleeding, hemorrhage, and ulcers

corticosteroids, potassium supplements: Increased risk of adverse GI effects

cyclosporine: Increased risk of nephrotoxicity from both drugs, increased blood cyclosporine level

diflunisal: Increased blood indomethacin level and risk of GI bleeding

digoxin: Increased blood digoxin level and risk of digitalis toxicity (all forms)

diuretics (thiazide, loop, and potassium-sparing): Decreased diuretic and antihypertensive effects

gold compounds, nephrotoxic drugs: Increased risk of adverse renal effects

heparin, oral anticoagulants, thrombolytics: Possibly increased anticoagulant effects and risk of hemorrhage

lithium: Increased blood lithium level and risk of toxicity

methotrexate: Increased risk of methotrexate toxicity

plicamycin, valproic acid: Increased risk of hypoprothrombinemia and GI bleeding, hemorrhage, and ulcers

probenecid: Increased blood level and effectiveness of indomethacin, increased risk of indomethacin toxicity

zidovudine: Increased blood zidovudine level and risk of toxicity, increased risk of indomethacin toxicity

ACTIVITIES

alcohol use: Increased risk of adverse GI effects

Adverse Reactions

Note: All reactions are for oral forms and suppositories unless indicated.

CNS: Confusion, depression, dizziness, drowsiness, fatigue, hallucinations, headache, intraventricular hemorrhage (I.V.), peripheral neuropathy, seizures, stroke, syncope, vertigo

CV: Arrhythmias, chest pain, edema, fluid retention (all forms), heart failure, hypertension, MI, pulmonary hypertension (I.V.), tachycardia

EENT: Blurred vision, corneal and retinal damage, epistaxis, hearing loss, tinnitus

ENDO: Hypoglycemia (I.V.)

GI: Abdominal cramps or pain, abdominal distention (I.V.), anorexia, constipation, diarrhea, diverticulitis, dyspepsia, dysphagia, epigastric discomfort, esophagitis, gastric perforation, gastritis, gastroenteritis, gastroesophageal reflux disease, GI bleeding and ulceration (all forms), hemorrhoids, hepatic dysfunction (I.V.), hepatic failure, hiatal hernia, ileus (I.V.), indigestion, melena, nausea, necrotizing enterocolitis (I.V.), pancreatitis, peptic ulcer, perforation of stomach or intestine, stomatitis, vomiting (all forms)

GU: Acute renal failure, hematuria, interstitial nephritis, nephrotic syndrome, oliguria (I.V.), proteinuria, renal dysfunction (I.V.), vaginal bleeding

HEME: Agranulocytosis, anemia, aplastic anemia, bone marrow depression, disseminated intravascular coagulation, hemolytic anemia, iron deficiency anemia, leukopenia, neutropenia, pancytopenia, thrombocytopenia, unusual bleeding or bruising (all forms)

RESP: Asthma, respiratory depression

SKIN: Ecchymosis, erythema multiforme, erythema nodosum, photosensitivity, pruritus, rash, Stevens-Johnson syndrome, toxic epidermal necrolysis, urticaria

Other: Anaphylaxis, angioedema, hyperkalemia (I.V.), hyponatremia (I.V.), injection site irritation

Nursing Considerations

•Use indomethacin with extreme caution in patients with a history of ulcer disease or GI bleeding because NSAIDs such as indomethacin increase the risk of GI bleeding and ulceration. Expect to use indomethacin for the shortest time possible in these patients.

•Be aware that serious GI tract ulceration,

bleeding, and perforation may occur without warning symptoms. Elderly patients are at greater risk. To minimize risk, give oral indomethacin with food, a full glass of water (not suspension), or an antacid to reduce GI distress.

• If GI distress occurs, withhold drug and notify prescriber immediately.

• Use indomethacin cautiously in patients with hypertension, and monitor blood pressure closely throughout therapy. Drug may cause hypertension or worsen it.

• Shake suspension well before giving it.

• Give up to 100 mg of daily dose (not E.R. capsules) at bedtime to reduce nighttime pain and morning stiffness in arthritis patients.

• Make sure suppository stays in rectum at least 1 hour to improve absorption.

• To reconstitute I.V. form, add 1 to 2 ml of preservative-free sodium chloride for injection or preservative-free sterile water to vial. Solution made with 1 ml of diluent contains 100 mcg (0.1 mg) of indomethacin/0.1 ml. Solution made with 2 ml of diluent contains 50 mcg (0.05 mg) of indomethacin/0.1 ml. Use solution immediately because it contains no preservatives. Discard unused portion.

• Be aware that scheduled I.V. doses may be withheld if infant or neonate has anuria or a significant decrease in urine output (less than 0.6 ml/kg/hr).

• When using I.V. form, avoid extravasation to protect surrounding tissue.

• Anticipate a second course (3 more doses) of I.V. indomethacin if patent ductus arteriosus fails to close or reopens. After 2 courses, surgery may be performed.

• WARNING Monitor patient closely for thrombotic events, including MI and stroke, because NSAIDs increase the risk.

• Monitor patient—especially if he's elderly or receiving long-term indomethacin therapy—for less common but serious adverse GI reactions, including anorexia, constipation, diverticulitis, dysphagia, esophagitis, gastritis, gastroenteritis, gastroesophageal reflux disease, hemorrhoids, hiatal hernia, melena, stomatitis, and vomiting.

• Monitor liver function test results because, in rare cases, elevations may progress to severe hepatic reactions, including fatal hepatitis, liver necrosis, and hepatic failure.

• Monitor BUN and serum creatinine levels in elderly patients, patients taking diuretics or ACE inhibitors, and patients with heart failure, impaired renal function, or hepatic dysfunction; drug may cause renal failure.

• Monitor CBC for decreased hemoglobin and hematocrit because drug may worsen anemia.

• WARNING If patient has bone marrow suppression or is receiving an antineoplastic drug, monitor laboratory results (including WBC count), and watch for evidence of infection because anti-inflammatory and antipyretic actions of indomethacin may mask signs and symptoms, such as fever and pain.

• Assess patient's skin regularly for signs of rash or other hypersensitivity reaction because indomethacin is an NSAID and may cause serious skin reactions without warning, even in patients with no history of NSAID sensivity. At first sign of reaction, stop drug and notify prescriber.

• Because indomethacin causes sodium retention, monitor weight and blood pressure, especially if patient has hypertension.

• When drug is used to treat gouty arthritis, expect its action to peak in 24 to 36 hours and significant swelling to gradually disappear over 3 to 5 days.

• Be aware that E.R. form shouldn't be used to treat gouty arthritis.

• Expect to use suppositories for patients who can't swallow oral form.

• To evaluate drug effectiveness, assess for reduced pain and inflammation and improved joint mobility.

• Expect patient to have intermittent checkups during long-term therapy and an ophthalmologic examination if vision changes develop.

PATIENT TEACHING

• Advise patient to take indomethacin capsules with a full glass of water and to avoid lying down for 15 to 30 minutes after taking drug. This helps prevent drug from lodging in esophagus and causing irritation. Caution him not to open or crush capsules.

• Instruct patient to take drug with food or an antacid to reduce GI distress.

• Instruct patient to make sure suppository stays in rectum at least 1 hour.

• Urge patient to avoid alcohol during therapy.

• Remind patient that improvement may not occur for 2 to 4 weeks after starting indomethacin and that he should continue taking drug, as prescribed.

•Inform breast-feeding patient that indomethacin appears in breast milk and may cause seizures in infants. Urge her to use another feeding method during indomethacin therapy.

•Caution against prolonged sun exposure during therapy.

•Urge patient to notify prescriber immediately about changes in vision or hearing, fever, itching, rash, sore throat, swelling in arms or legs, and weight gain.

•Stress the importance of undergoing ordered laboratory tests and eye examinations during long-term therapy.

•Caution pregnant patient not to take NSAIDs such as indomethacin during the last trimester because they may cause premature closure of the ductus arteriosus.

•Explain that indomethacin may increase the risk of serious adverse cardiovascular reactions; urge patient to seek immediate medical attention if signs or symptoms arise, such as chest pain, shortness of breath, weakness, and slurring of speech.

•Explain that indomethacin may increase the risk of serious adverse GI reactions; stress the need to seek immediate medical attention for such signs and symptoms as epigastric or abdominal pain, indigestion, black or tarry stools, or vomiting blood or material that looks like coffee grounds.

•Alert patient to rare but serious skin reactions. Urge him to seek immediate medical attention for rash, blisters, itching, fever, or other indications of hypersensitivity.

infliximab

Remicade

Class and Category

Chemical class: Monoclonal antibody
Therapeutic class: Anti-inflammatory
Pregnancy category: C

Indications and Dosages

➤ *To control moderate to severe Crohn's disease long-term*
I.V. INFUSION
Adults and children. *Induction:* 5 mg/kg over 2 hr, repeated 2 and 6 wk after first infusion.

Maintenance: 5 mg/kg over 2 hr every 8 wk.
DOSAGE ADJUSTMENT For adults who respond and then lose response, dosage may be increased to 10 mg/kg.

➤ *To reduce number of draining enterocutaneous and rectovaginal fistulas and to maintain fistula closure in fistulizing Crohn's disease*
I.V. INFUSION
Adults. *Induction:* 5 mg/kg over 2 hr, repeated 2 and 6 wk after first infusion. *Maintenance:* 5 mg/kg over 2 hr every 8 wk.
DOSAGE ADJUSTMENT For patients who respond and then lose response, dosage may be increased to 10 mg/kg.

➤ *To reduce signs and symptoms, to induce and maintain remission and mucosal healing, and to eliminate corticosteroid use in patients with moderately to severely active ulcerative colitis who have had an inadequate response to conventional therapy*
I.V. INFUSION
Adults. 5 mg/kg over 2 hr, repeated 2 and 6 wk after infusion. Maintenance: 5 mg/kg over 2 hr every 8 wk.

➤ *As adjunct to reduce signs and symptoms, inhibit progression of structural damage, and improve physical function in patients with moderate to severe active rheumatoid arthritis*
I.V. INFUSION
Adults. 3 mg/kg, with methotrexate, repeated 2 and 6 wk after first infusion and then every 8 wk thereafter.

➤ *To treat active ankylosing spondylitis*
I.V. INFUSION
Adults. 5 mg/kg, repeated 2 and 6 wk after first infusion and then every 6 wk thereafter.

➤ *To reduce signs and symptoms, inhibit progression of structural damage, and improve physical function in patients with psoriatic arthritis*
I.V. INFUSION
Adults. 5 mg/kg, with or without methotrexate, repeated 2 and 6 wk after first infusion and then every 8 wk thereafter.

➤ *To treat chronic severe plaque psoriasis in patients who are candidates for systemic therapy but those therapies are medically less appropriate*

I.V. INFUSION

Adults. 5 mg/kg, repeated 2 and 6 wk after first infusion and then every 8 wk thereafter.

Mechanism of Action

Binds with cytokine tumor necrosis factor-alpha (TNF-alpha), preventing it from binding with its receptors. As a result, TNF-alpha can't produce proinflammatory cytokines and endothelial permeability. Infiltration of inflammatory cells into inflamed intestine and joints declines.

Incompatibilities

Don't infuse infliximab in same I.V. line with other drugs or through plasticized polyvinyl chloride infusion equipment or devices.

Contraindications

Breastfeeding; hypersensitivity to infliximab, murine proteins, or their components; moderate or severe New York Heart Association (NYHA) Class III or IV heart failure

Interactions

DRUGS

anakinra, etanercept: Increased risk of neutropenia and serious infections

Adverse Reactions

CNS: Chills, dizziness, fatigue, fever, Guillain-Barre syndrome, headache, meningitis, neuritis, numbness, paresthesia, stroke, syncope, tingling

CV: Arrhythmias, chest pain, hypertension, hypotension, MI, myelitis, neuropathies, pericardial effusion, systemic and cutaneous vasculitis, thrombophlebitis

EENT: Oral candidiasis, pharyngitis, rhinitis, sinusitis, visual changes

GI: Abdominal hernia; abdominal pain; acute hepatic failure; cholecystitis; cholestasis; diarrhea; dyspepsia; elevated aminotranferases; GI hemorrhage; hepatitis; hepatotoxicity; ileus; intestinal obstruction, perforation, or stenosis; melena; pancreatitis; nausea; splenic infarction; splenomegaly; vomiting

GU: Kidney infection, renal failure, ureteral obstruction, UTI, vaginal candidiasis, vaginitis

HEME: Anemia, leukopenia, neutropenia, pancytopenia, thrombocytopenia

MS: Ankylosing spondylitis, arthralgia, back pain, extremity weakness, myalgia, psoriatic arthritis

RESP: Adult respiratory distress syndrome, bronchitis, cough, dyspnea, interstitial lung disease, pneumonia, tuberculosis, respiratory tract infection, wheezing

SKIN: Facial flushing, jaundice, pruritus, psoriasis, rash, urticaria

Other: Antibody formation to infliximab; bacterial, fungal, or viral infection; infusion reaction; lupuslike symptoms; lyphadenopathy; lymphoma; sepsis

Nursing Considerations

• Infliximab therapy shouldn't be started in a patient with an active infection, including serious localized infection.

• Use with extreme caution if patient has a history of chronic or recurrent infection, known exposure to tuberculosis, an underlying condition that predisposes to infection, or residence or travel to areas of endemic tuberculosis or mycoses, such as histoplasmosis, coccidioidomycosis, or blastomycosis.

• Use cautiously in elderly patients because they have a higher risk of infection.

• **WARNING** Because drug increases the risk of developing tuberculosis or reactivating latent tuberculosis, expect prescriber to evaluate patient's risk and start tuberculosis treatment, as needed, before starting infliximab.

• **WARNING** Be aware that infliximab increases the risk of serious or fatal opportunistic infections, including invasive fungal infections as well as bacterial and viral infections. The most common ones include aspergillosis, candidiasis, coccidioidomycosis, histoplasmosis, listeriosis, and pneumocytosis.

• **WARNING** Watch for infection, especially if patient receives immunosuppressant therapy or has a chronic infection. Upper respiratory tract infections and UTI are most common, but sepsis and fatal infections have occurred.

• To reconstitute infliximab, use a 21G (or smaller) needle to add 10 ml of sterile water for injection to each vial of drug. Swirl to mix; don't shake. Be aware that solution may foam and be clear or light yellow.

• Withdraw a volume equal to amount of reconstituted drug from a 250-ml glass bottle or polypropylene or polyolefin infusion bag of normal saline solution. Then add reconstituted infliximab to bottle to dilute to 250 ml. Use within 3 hours.

G
H
I

•Infuse over at least 2 hours using polyethyl-ene-lined infusion set and in-line, sterile, nonpyrogenic, low-protein-binding filter with pores of 1.2 microns or less. Don't reuse.

•Be prepared to stop infusion if a hypersensitivity or CNS reaction occurs. Keep acetaminophen, antihistamines, corticosteroids, and epinephrine on hand. A reaction may occur 2 hours to 12 days after infusion.

•**WARNING** Avoid giving infliximab to patients with New York Heart Association Class III or IV congestive heart failure (CHF) because it may worsen the condition or cause death. If patient does receive infliximab, expect to stop it if CHF worsens.

•Because severe hepatic reactions may occur, monitor liver function. Expect to stop drug if jaundice develops or liver enzymes are 5 times or more the upper limit of normal.

PATIENT TEACHING

•Inform patient that infliximab should take effect within 1 to 2 weeks.

•Urge patient to report signs of infection, such as painful urination, cough, and sore throat. Infusion reaction (chest pain, chills, dyspnea, facial flushing, fever, itching, headache, rash) may occur for up to 12 days.

•Explain that infliximab increases the risk of lymphoma; urge prompt medical attention for suspicious signs or symptoms.

ipecac syrup

Ipecac Syrup

Class and Category

Chemical class: Cephaelis acuminata or *Cephaelis ipecacuanha* derivative
Therapeutic class: Emetic
Pregnancy category: C

Indications and Dosages

➤ *To induce vomiting after drug overdose and certain types of poisoning*

SYRUP

Adults and children over age 12. 15 to 30 ml followed by 240 ml of water. Dose repeated if vomiting doesn't begin within 20 to 30 min.

Children ages 1 to 12. 15 ml preceded or followed by 120 to 240 ml of water. Dose repeated if vomiting doesn't begin within 20 to 30 min.

Infants ages 6 months to 1 year. 5 to 10 ml preceded or followed by 120 to 240 ml of water.

Route	Onset	Peak	Duration
P.O.	20 to 30 min	Unknown	20 to 25 min

Mechanism of Action

Induces vomiting by irritating the gastric mucosa and stimulating the medullary chemoreceptor trigger zone in the CNS.

Contraindications

Loss of gag reflex, poisoning with strychnine or corrosives (such as alkaloid substances, petroleum distillates, and strong acids), seizures, semiconsciousness or unconsciousness, severe inebriation, shock

Interactions

DRUGS

activated charcoal: Lack of emetic effect

Adverse Reactions

CNS: Depression, drowsiness
EENT: Aspiration of vomitus, coughing
GI: Diarrhea, indigestion

Nursing Considerations

•Give ipecac syrup only to conscious patients, and follow with adequate water. Give young or frightened children water before or after ipecac.

•Expect vomiting to start in 20 to 30 minutes.

•If vomiting doesn't start within 30 minutes of second dose, prepare for gastric lavage.

•Don't give ipecac after ingestion of petroleum distillates, such as gasoline, or caustic substances (to avoid further injury to esophagus).

•If activated charcoal also will be given, expect to do so after patient vomits or 30 minutes after second dose because activated charcoal adsorbs ipecac and inhibits its action.

•Arrhythmias, atrial fibrillation, bradycardia, fatal myocarditis, hypotension, myalgia, or muscle stiffness or weakness may develop if patient takes too much or doesn't vomit.

PATIENT TEACHING

•Inform patient of ipecac's effects.

•Tell adult patient to drink 8 oz (240 ml) of water after taking drug and child to drink

4 to 8 oz (120 to 240 ml) before or after taking drug.
•Inform patient or parents of child that diarrhea may occur after taking drug.
•Urge parents to keep ipecac syrup and phone number of a poison control center.
•**WARNING** Advise parents to replace their ipecac extract or tincture with ipecac syrup. Explain that ipecac fluid extract is 14 times more concentrated than ipecac syrup and can cause serious, possibly toxic, effects if given incorrectly.

ipratropium bromide

Apo-Ipravent (CAN), Atrovent, Kendral-Ipratropium (CAN)

Class and Category
Chemical class: Quaternary *N*-methyl isopropyl derivative of noratropine
Therapeutic class: Anticholinergic, bronchodilator
Pregnancy category: B

Indications and Dosages
➤ *To treat bronchitis and COPD*
INHALATION AEROSOL
Adults and adolescents. 2 to 4 inhalations (36 to 72 mcg) t.i.d. or q.i.d. *Maximum:* Up to 12 inhalations (216 mcg)/24 hr.
INHALATION SOLUTION FOR NEBULIZER
Adults and adolescents. 250 to 500 mcg dissolved in preservative-free sterile normal saline solution every 6 to 8 hr. For severe COPD exacerbations, 500 mcg every 4 to 8 hr.
➤ *To treat perennial and allergic rhinitis*
NASAL SPRAY
Adults and children age 6 and over. 2 sprays of 0.03% (21 mcg/spray) per nostril b.i.d. or t.i.d. *Maximum:* 12 sprays (252 mcg)/24 hr.
➤ *To treat rhinorrhea caused by the common cold*
NASAL SPRAY
Adults and children age 5 and over. 2 sprays of 0.06% (42 mcg/spray) per nostril t.i.d. or q.i.d. for up to 4 days. *Maximum:* 16 sprays (672 mcg)/24 hr.

Route	Onset	Peak	Duration
Inhalation	5 to 15 min	1 to 2 hr	3 to 8 hr
Nasal	5 min	1 to 4 hr	4 to 8 hr

Contraindications
Hypersensitivity to atropine, ipratropium

Mechanism of Action
After acetylcholine is released from cholinergic fibers, ipratropium prevents it from attaching to muscarinic receptors on membranes of smooth-muscle cells, as shown at right. By blocking acetycholine's effects in the bronchi and bronchioles, ipratropium relaxes smooth muscles and causes bronchodilation.

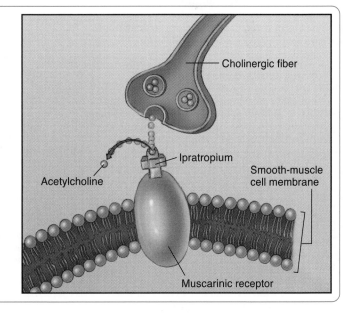

Cholinergic fiber

Ipratropium

Smooth-muscle cell membrane

Acetylcholine

Muscarinic receptor

bromide, or their components; hypersensitivity to peanuts, soya lecithin, soybeans, or related products (with aerosol inhaler)

Interactions
DRUGS
anticholinergics: Increased anticholinergic effects
tacrine: Decreased effects of both drugs

Adverse Reactions
CNS: Dizziness, insomnia
CV: Atrial fibrillation (oral inhalation), bradycardia (nasal spray), edema, hypertension, palpitations, supraventricular tachycardia (oral inhalation), tachycardia
EENT: Acute eye pain, dry mouth or pharyngeal area, laryngospasm, taste perversion (all drug forms); blurred vision, eye irritation and pain, glaucoma or worsening of existing glaucoma (if nasal spray comes in contact with eyes); epistaxis, mydriasis, nasal dryness and irritation, pharyngitis, rhinitis, sinusitis, tinnitus (with nasal spray)
GI: Bowel obstruction, constipation, diarrhea, ileus, nausea, vomiting
GU: Prostatitis, urine retention
MS: Arthritis
RESP: Bronchitis, bronchospasm, cough, dyspnea, increased sputum production, wheezing
SKIN: Dermatitis, pruritus, rash, urticaria
Other: Anaphylaxis, angioedema, flulike symptoms

Nursing Considerations
•Use ipratropium cautiously in patients with angle-closure glaucoma, benign prostatic hyperplasia, or bladder neck obstruction and in patients with hepatic or renal dysfunction.
•As prescribed, mix ipratropium inhalation solution with preservative-free albuterol, and preservative-free ipratropium inhalation solution with cromolyn inhalation solution. Use within 1 hour.
•When using a nebulizer, apply a mouthpiece to prevent drug from leaking out around mask and causing blurred vision or eye pain.
PATIENT TEACHING
•Caution patient not to use ipratropium to treat acute bronchospasm.
•Inform patient that although some people feel relief within 24 hours of drug use, maximum effect may take up to 2 weeks.

•Teach patient to use inhaler or nasal spray. Tell him to shake inhaler well with each use.
•Advise patient to keep spray out of his eyes because it may irritate them or blur his vision. If spray comes in contact with his eyes, instruct patient to flush them with cool tap water for several minutes and to contact prescriber.
•Instruct patient to rinse mouth after each nebulizer or inhaler treatment to help minimize throat dryness and irritation.
•If patient is using 0.06% nasal spray for a common cold, advise against use for longer than 4 days.
•Teach patient to track canister contents by counting and recording number of doses.
•Advise patient to report decreased response to ipratropium as well as difficulty voiding, eye pain, nasal dryness, nose bleeds, palpitations, and vision changes.

irbesartan

Avapro

Class and Category
Chemical class: Nonpeptide angiotensin II antagonist
Therapeutic class: Antihypertensive
Pregnancy category: D

Indications and Dosages
➤ *To manage hypertension, alone or with other antihypertensives*
TABLETS
Adults and adolescents. *Initial:* 150 mg daily. *Maximum:* 300 mg daily.
DOSAGE ADJUSTMENT Initial dosage reduced to 75 mg daily for patients with hypovolemia or hyponatremia from such causes as hemodialysis or vigorous diuretic therapy.
Children ages 6 to 12. *Initial:* 75 mg daily. *Maximum:* 150 mg daily.
➤ *To treat nephropathy in type 2 diabetes mellitus*
TABLETS
Adults. 300 mg daily.

Route	Onset	Peak	Duration
P.O.	Unknown	In 4 to 6 wk	Unknown

Contraindications
Hypersensitivity to irbesartan or its components

Mechanism of Action
Selectively blocks binding of the potent vasoconstrictor angiotensin (AT) II to AT_1 receptor sites in many tissues, including vascular smooth muscle and adrenal glands. This inhibits the vasoconstrictive and aldosterone-secreting effects of AT II, which reduces blood pressure.

Interactions
DRUGS
diuretics: Possibly additive hypotensive effects

Adverse Reactions
CNS: Anxiety, dizziness, fatigue, headache, nervousness
CV: Chest pain, hypotension, peripheral edema, tachycardia
EENT: Pharyngitis, rhinitis
GI: Abdominal pain, diarrhea, heartburn, hepatitis, indigestion, nausea, vomiting
GU: UTI
MS: Musculoskeletal pain
RESP: Upper respiratory tract infection
SKIN: Rash

Nursing Considerations
•If patient has known or suspected hypovolemia, provide treatment, such as I.V. normal saline solution, as prescribed, to correct this condition before beginning irbesartan therapy. Or expect to begin therapy with a lower dosage.
•Check blood pressure often to evaluate drug's effectiveness.
•If blood pressure isn't controlled with irbesartan alone, expect to also give a diuretic, such as hydrochlorothiazide, as prescribed.
•**WARNING** If patient receives a diuretic or another antihypertensive during irbesartan therapy, frequently monitor his blood pressure because he's at risk for developing hypotension.
•If patient experiences symptomatic hypotension, expect to stop drug temporarily. Immediately place patient in supine position and prepare to administer I.V. normal saline solution, as prescribed. Expect to resume drug therapy after blood pressure stabilizes.
•If patient receives a diuretic, provide adequate hydration, as appropriate, to help prevent hypovolemia. Also monitor patient for signs and symptoms of hypovolemia, such as hypotension, dizziness, and fainting.
•**WARNING** Monitor patient for increased BUN and serum creatinine levels if he has heart failure or impaired renal function because drug may cause acute renal failure. If increases are significant or persistent, notify prescriber immediately.

PATIENT TEACHING
•Advise patient to take drug at the same time each day to maintain its therapeutic effect.
•Explain the importance of regular exercise, proper diet, and other lifestyle changes in controlling hypertension.
•Caution patient to avoid hazardous activities until drug's CNS effects are known.
•Instruct patient to consult prescriber before taking any new drug.
•To reduce the risk of dehydration and hypotension, advise patient to drink adequate fluids during hot weather and exercise.
•Instruct patient to contact prescriber if severe nausea, vomiting, or diarrhea occurs and continues because of the risk of dehydration and hypotension.
•Advise female patient to notify prescriber immediately about known or suspected pregnancy. Explain that if she becomes pregnant, prescriber may replace irbesartan with another antihypertensive that's safe to use during pregnancy.
•Urge patient to keep follow-up appointments with prescriber to monitor progress.

iron dextran

(contains 50 mg of elemental iron per milliliter)
DexFerrum, DexIron (CAN), InFeD

Class and Category
Chemical class: Iron salt, mineral
Therapeutic class: Antianemic
Pregnancy category: C

Indications and Dosages
➤ *To treat iron deficiency anemia*
I.V. INFUSION
Adults and children weighing more than 15 kg (33 lb). Dose (ml) = 0.0442 (desired hemoglobin − observed hemoglobin) × lean body weight (in kg) + (0.26 × lean body weight). Alternatively, consult dosage table in package insert. *Maximum:* 2 ml (100 mg) daily.

Children over age 4 months weighing 5 to 15 kg (11 to 33 lb). Dose (ml) = 0.0442 (desired hemoglobin − observed hemoglobin) × weight (kg) + (0.26 × weight). Alternatively, consult dosage table in package insert. *Maximum:* 1 ml (50 mg) daily.

➤ *To replace iron lost in blood loss*
I.V. INFUSION
Adults. Replacement iron (mg) = ml of blood loss × hematocrit.

Mechanism of Action
Restores hemoglobin and replenishes iron stores. Iron, an essential component of hemoglobin, myoglobin, and several enzymes (including cytochromes, catalase, and peroxidase), is needed for catecholamine metabolism and normal neutrophil function.

In iron dextran therapy, iron binds to available protein parts after the drug has been split into iron and dextran by cells of the reticuloendothelial system. The bound iron forms hemosiderin or ferritin, physiologic forms of iron, and transferrin, which replenish hemoglobin and depleted iron stores. Dextran is metabolized or excreted.

Incompatibilities
Don't mix iron dextran with blood for transfusion, other drugs, or parenteral nutrition solutions for I.V. infusion.

Contraindications
Anemia other than iron deficiency, hypersensitivity to iron dextran or its components

Adverse Reactions
CNS: Chills, disorientation, dizziness, fever, headache, malaise, paresthesia, seizures, syncope, unconsciousness, weakness
CV: Arrhythmias, bradycardia, chest pain, hypertension, hypotension, shock, tachycardia
EENT: Altered taste
GI: Abdominal pain, diarrhea, nausea, vomiting
GU: Hematuria
HEME: Leukocytosis
MS: Arthralgia, arthritis, backache, myalgia, rhabdomyolysis
RESP: Bronchospasm, dyspnea, respiratory arrest, wheezing
SKIN: Cyanosis, diaphoresis, rash, pruritus, purpura, urticaria

Other: Anaphylaxis, infusion site phlebitis

Nursing Considerations
•Expect oral iron therapy to stop before iron dextran therapy starts. Iron dextran is given only when oral therapy isn't feasible; it also may be given by I.M. injection.
•Expect to monitor hemoglobin level, hematocrit, serum ferritin level, and transferrin saturation, as ordered, before, during, and after iron dextran therapy.
•**WARNING** Before starting iron dextran therapy, give a test dose of 0.5 ml of iron dextran gradually over 30 seconds, as prescribed, and monitor patient closely for an anaphylactic reaction.
•Wait 1 to 2 hours before administering the remainder of the dose. Infuse undiluted iron dextran slowly, at a rate not to exceed 1 ml/minute (50 mg/minute).
•**WARNING** Monitor patient closely for signs and symptoms of anaphylaxis (such as severe hypotension, loss of consciousness, collapse, dyspnea, and seizures) during and after infusion. Patients with a history of asthma or allergies are at increased risk for anaphylaxis and, possibly, death. Institute emergency resuscitation measures as needed, including epinephrine administration, as prescribed.
•**WARNING** Assess blood pressure frequently after iron dextran administration because hypotension is a common adverse effect that may be related to infusion rate; avoid rapid infusion.
•Be aware that patient may exhibit adverse reactions, including arthralgia, backache, chills, and vomiting, 1 to 2 days after drug therapy. Symptoms should resolve within 3 to 4 days.
•Assess patients with a history of rheumatoid arthritis for exacerbation of joint pain and swelling.
•If patient has cardiovascular disease, watch for worsening from drug's adverse effects.
•Assess patient for iron overload, characterized by sedation, decreased activity, pale eyes, and bleeding in GI tract and lungs.
•Store iron dextran at 15° to 30° C (59° to 86° F).
PATIENT TEACHING
•Instruct patient to immediately report signs of an adverse reaction, such as shortness of breath, wheezing, or rash, during iron dextran therapy.

•Advise patient not to take any oral iron preparations without first consulting prescriber.

•Inform patient that symptoms of iron deficiency may include decreased stamina, learning problems, shortness of breath, and fatigue. Encourage patient to plan periods of activity and rest in order to avoid excessive fatigue.

•Stress the need to follow dosage regimen and of keeping follow-up medical appointments and appointments for laboratory tests.

iron sucrose

(contains 100 mg of elemental iron per 5 ml)
Venofer

Class and Category
Chemical class: Iron salt, mineral
Therapeutic class: Antianemic
Pregnancy category: B

Indications and Dosages
➤ *To treat iron deficiency anemia in hemodialysis patients receiving erythropoietin*

I.V. INJECTION
Adults. *Initial:* 100 mg of elemental iron injected undiluted over 2 to 5 min during dialysis. *Usual:* 100 mg of elemental iron every wk to 3 times/wk to a total dose of 1,000 mg. Dosage repeated as needed to maintain target levels of hemoglobin and hematocrit and acceptable blood iron level. *Maximum:* 100 mg/dose.

I.V. INFUSION
Adults. *Initial:* 100 mg of elemental iron infused diluted over 15 min during dialysis. *Usual:* 100 mg of elemental iron every wk to 3 times/wk to a total dose of 1,000 mg. Dosage repeated as needed to maintain target levels of hemoglobin and hematocrit and acceptable blood iron level. *Maximum:* 100 mg/dose.

➤ *To treat iron deficiency anemia in peritoneal dialysis patients receiving erythropoietin*

I.V. INFUSION
Adults. *Initial:* 300 mg elemental iron infused diluted over 1.5 hr on days 1 and 14, followed by 400 mg of elemental iron infused over 2.5 hr on day 28. Dosage repeated as needed to maintain target levels of hemo-globin and hematocrit and acceptable blood iron level. *Maximum:* 1,000 mg/28 days.

➤ *To treat iron deficiency anemia in non-dialysis patients with chronic renal disease regardless of whether they're receiving erythropoietin*

I.V. INJECTION
Adults. *Initial:* 200 mg of elemental iron injected undiluted over 2 to 5 min and repeated 4 more times over a 14-day period for a total dose of 1,000 mg. Dosage repeated as needed to maintain target levels of hemoglobin and hematocrit and acceptable blood iron level. *Maximum:* 1,000 mg/14 days.

I.V. INFUSION
Adults. 500 mg of elemental iron infused diluted over 3.5 to 5 hr on days 1 and 14. Dosage repeated as needed to maintain target levels of hemoglobin and hematocrit and acceptable blood iron level. *Maximum:* 1,000 mg/14 days.

Mechanism of Action
Acts to replenish iron stores lost during dialysis because of increased erythropoiesis and insufficient absorption of iron from the GI tract. Iron is an essential component of hemoglobin, myoglobin, and several enzymes, including cytochromes, catalase, and peroxidase, and is needed for catecholamine metabolism and normal neutrophil function. Iron sucrose injection also normalizes RBC production by binding with hemoglobin or being stored as ferritin in reticuloendothelial cells of the liver, spleen, and bone marrow.

Incompatibilities
Don't mix with other drugs or parenteral nutrition solutions for I.V. infusion.

Contraindications
Anemia other than iron deficiency, hypersensitivity to iron salts or their components, iron overload

Interactions
DRUGS
chloramphenicol: Possibly decreased effectiveness of iron sucrose
oral iron preparations: Possibly reduced absorption of oral iron supplements

Adverse Reactions

CNS: Asthenia, dizziness, fatigue, fever, headache, hypoesthesia, malaise
CV: Chest pain, heart failure, hypertension, hypotension, peirpheral edema
EENT: Conjunctivitis, ear pain, nasal congestion, nasopharyngitis, rhinitis, sinusitis, taste perversion
ENDO: Hyperglycemia, hypoglycemia
GI: Abdominal pain, constipation, diarrhea, elevated liver function test results, nausea, occult-positive feces, peritoneal infection, vomiting
GU: UTI
MS: Arthralgia, arthritis, back pain, leg cramps, muscle pain or weakness, myalgia
RESP: Cough, dyspnea, pneumonia, upper respiratory tract infection
SKIN: Pruritus, rash
Other: Anaphylaxis; fluid overload; gout; hypervolemia; infusion or injection site burning, pain, or redness; sepsis

Nursing Considerations

• To reconstitute iron sucrose injection for infusion, dilute 100 mg of elemental iron in maximum of 100 ml of normal saline solution (for hemodialysis patients) or 250 ml (for peritoneal dialysis and nondialysis patients) immediately before infusion. Discard any unused diluted solution.
• Give drug directly into dialysis line by slow I.V. injection or by infusion.
• WARNING Monitor patient closely for evidence of anaphylaxis, such as severe hypotension, loss of consciousness, collapse, dyspnea, or seizures, during and after therapy. Institute emergency resuscitation measures as needed.
• WARNING Assess blood pressure frequently after drug administration because hypotension is a common adverse reaction that may be related to infusion rate (avoid rapid infusion) or total cumulative dose.
• Monitor hemoglobin, hematocrit, serum ferritin, and transferrin saturation, as ordered, before, during, and after iron sucrose therapy. Test serum iron level 48 hours after last dose. Notify prescriber and expect to stop therapy if blood iron levels are normal or elevated, to prevent iron toxicity.
• Watch for evidence of iron overload, such as sedation, decreased activity, pale eyes, and bleeding in GI tract and lungs.

• Advise patient not to take any oral iron preparations during iron sucrose therapy without first consulting prescriber.
• Inform patient that symptoms of iron deficiency may include decreased stamina, learning problems, shortness of breath, and fatigue.

isocarboxazid

Marplan

Class and Category

Chemical class: Hydrazine derivative
Therapeutic class: Antidepressant
Pregnancy category: C

Indications and Dosages

➤ *To treat major depression*
TABLETS
Adults and adolescents over age 16. *Initial:* 10 mg b.i.d., increased by 10 mg daily every 2 to 4 days, as needed and tolerated. *Maximum:* 60 mg daily.

Route	Onset	Peak	Duration
P.O.	7 to 10 days	Unknown	10 days

Mechanism of Action

Irreversibly binds to MAO, reducing its activity and increasing levels of neurotransmitters, including serotonin and the catecholamine neurotransmitters dopamine, epinephrine, and norepinephrine. This regulation of CNS neurotransmitters helps to ease depression. With long-term use, the drug results in down-regulation (desensitization) of alpha$_2$- or beta-adrenergic and serotonin receptors after 2 to 4 weeks, which also produces an antidepressant effect.

Contraindications

Cardiovascular disease; cerebrovascular disease; heart failure; hepatic disease; history of headaches; hypersensitivity to isocarboxazid or its components; hypertension; pheochromocytoma; severe renal impairment; use of anesthetics, antihypertensives, bupropion, buspirone, carbamazepine, CNS depressants, cyclobenzaprine, dextromethorphan, meperidine, selective serotonin reuptake inhibitors, sympathomimetics, or tricyclic antidepressants; use within 14 days of another MAO inhibitor

Interactions

DRUGS

anticholinergics, antidyskinetics, antihistamines: Increased anticholinergic effect, prolonged CNS depression (with antihistamines)
anticonvulsants: Increased CNS depression, possibly altered seizure pattern
antihypertensives, diuretics: Increased hypotensive effect
bromocriptine: Possibly interference with bromocriptine effects
bupropion: Increased risk of bupropion toxicity
buspirone, guanadrel, guanethidine: Increased risk of hypertension
caffeine-containing drugs: Increased risk of dangerous arrhythmias and severe hypertension
carbamazepine, cyclobenzaprine, maprotiline, other MAO inhibitors: Increased risk of hyperpyretic crisis, hypertensive crisis, severe seizures, and death; altered pattern of seizures (with carbamazepine)
CNS depressants: Increased CNS depression
dextromethorphan: Increased risk of excitation, hypertension, and hyperpyrexia
doxapram: Increased vasopressor effects of either drug
fluoxetine, paroxetine, sertraline, trazodone, tricyclic antidepressants: Increased risk of life-threatening serotonin syndrome
haloperidol, loxapine, molindone, phenothiazines, pimozide, thioxanthenes: Prolonged and intensified anticholinergic, hypotensive, and sedative effects
insulin, oral antidiabetic drugs: Increased hypoglycemic effects
levodopa: Increased risk of sudden, moderate to severe hypertension
local anesthetics (with epinephrine or levonordefrin): Possibly severe hypertension
meperidine, other opioid analgesics: Increased risk of coma, hyperpyrexia, hypotension, immediate excitation, rigidity, seizures, severe hypertension, severe respiratory depression, shock, sweating, and death
methyldopa: Increased risk of hallucinations, headache, hyperexcitability, and severe hypertension

methylphenidate: Increased CNS stimulant effects
metrizamide: Decreased seizure threshold and increased risk of seizures
oral anticoagulants: Increased anticoagulant activity
phenylephrine (nasal or ophthalmic): Potentiated vasopressor effect of phenylephrine
rauwolfia alkaloids: Increased risk of moderate to severe hypertension, CNS depression (when isocarboxazid is added to rauwolfia alkaloid therapy), CNS excitation and hypertension (when rauwolfia alkaloid is added to isocarboxazid therapy)
spinal anesthetics: Increased risk of hypotension
sympathomimetics: Prolonged and intensified cardiac stimulant and vasopressor effects
tryptophan: Increased risk of confusion, disorientation, hyperreflexia, hyperthermia, hyperventilation, mania or hypomania, and shivering

FOODS

aged cheese; avocados; bananas; fava or broad beans; cured meat or sausage; overripe fruit; pickled or smoked fish, meats or poultry; protein extract; soy sauce; yeast extract; and other foods high in tyramine or other pressor amines: Increased risk of dangerous arrhythmias and severe hypertensive crisis

ACTIVITIES

alcohol-containing products that also may contain tyramine, such as beer (including reduced-alcohol and alcohol-free beer), hard liquor, liqueurs, sherry, and wines (red and white): Increased risk of developing hypertensive crisis

Adverse Reactions

CNS: Agitation, dizziness, drowsiness, fever, headache, insomnia, intracranial bleeding, overstimulation, restlessness, sedation, suicidal ideation, tremor, weakness
CV: Bradycardia, chest pain, edema, hypertensive crisis, orthostatic hypotension, palpitations, tachycardia
EENT: Blurred vision, dry mouth, mydriasis, photophobia, yellowing of sclera
GI: Abdominal pain, anorexia, constipation, diarrhea, elevated liver function test results, increased appetite, nausea
GU: Darkened urine, oliguria, sexual dysfunction
HEME: Leukopenia

MS: Muscle spasms, myoclonus, neck stiffness
SKIN: Clammy skin, diaphoresis, jaundice, rash
Other: Unusual weight gain

Nursing Considerations
•Monitor patient's blood pressure during isocarboxazid therapy to detect hypertensive crisis and decrease the risk of orthostatic hypotension.
•WARNING Notify prescriber immediately if patient has signs and symptoms of hypertensive crisis (drug's most serious adverse effect), such as chest pain, headache, neck stiffness, and palpitations. Expect to stop drug immediately if these occur.
•Keep phentolamine readily available to treat hypertensive crisis. Give 5 mg by slow I.V. infusion, as prescribed, to reduce blood pressure without causing excessive hypotension. Use external cooling measures, as prescribed, to manage fever.
•To avoid hypertensive crisis, expect to wait 10 to 14 days, as prescribed, when switching patient from one MAO inhibitor to another or when switching from a dibenzazepine-related drug, such as amitriptyline or perphenazine.
•Monitor patient with a history of epilepsy for seizures because isocarboxazid may alter seizure threshold. Institute seizure precautions according to facility protocol.
•Monitor liver function test results and assess patient for abdominal pain, darkened urine, and jaundice because isocarboxazid may cause hepatic dysfunction.
•Expect to observe some therapeutic effect in 7 to 10 days, but keep in mind that full effect may not occur for 4 to 8 weeks.
•Be aware that, for maintenance therapy, the smallest dose possible should be used. Once clinical effect has been achieved, expect to decrease the dosage slowly over several weeks.
•Keep dietary restrictions in place for at least 2 weeks after stopping isocarboxazid because of the slow recovery from drug's enzyme-inhibiting effects.
•Ideally, expect to stop drug 10 days before elective surgery, as prescribed, to avoid hypotension.
•Anticipate that coadministration with a selective serotonin reuptake inhibitor may cause confusion, diaphoresis, diarrhea, seizures, and other less severe symptoms.
•Monitor depressed patient for suicidal tendencies, especially when therapy starts or dosage changes, because depression may worsen temporarily. If suicidal tendencies arise, institute suicide precautions, as appropriate and according to facility policy, and notify prescriber immediately.
•Monitor patient for sudden insomnia. If it develops, notify prescriber and be prepared to give drug early in the day.

PATIENT TEACHING
•Inform patient and family members that therapeutic effects of isocarboxazid may take several weeks to appear and that he should continue taking drug as prescribed.
•Caution parents to monitor pediatric patients, including adolescents, closely for suicidal tendencies, especially when therapy starts or dosage changes.
•Caution patient to rise slowly from a lying or sitting position to minimize effects of orthostatic hypotension.
•WARNING Instruct patient to avoid the following foods, beverages, and drugs during isocarboxazid therapy and for 2 weeks afterward: alcohol-free and reduced-alcohol beer and wine; appetite suppressants; beer; broad beans; cheese (except cottage and cream cheese); chocolate and caffeine in large quantities; dry sausage (including Genoa salami, hard salami, Lebanon bologna, and pepperoni); hay fever drugs; inhaled asthma drugs; liver; meat extract; OTC cold and cough medicines (including those containing dextromethorphan); nasal decongestants (tablets, drops, or spray); pickled herring; products that contain tyramine; protein-rich foods that may have undergone protein changes by aging, fermenting, pickling, or smoking; sauerkraut; sinus drugs; weight-loss preparations; yeast extracts (including brewer's yeast in large quantities); yogurt; and wine.
•Advise patient to notify prescriber immediately about chest pain, dizziness, headache, nausea, neck stiffness, palpitations, rapid heart rate, sweating, and vomiting.
•Advise patient to inform all health care providers (including dentists) that he takes an MAO inhibitor because certain drugs are contraindicated within 2 weeks of therapy.
•Urge patient to avoid potentially hazardous

activities until drug's adverse effects are known.

•Urge patient with diabetes mellitus who's taking insulin or an oral antidiabetic drug to monitor blood glucose level frequently during therapy because isocarboxazid may affect glucose control.

•Caution patient not to stop taking drug abruptly to avoid recurrence of original symptoms.

isoetharine hydrochloride

Arm-a-Med Isoetharine (0.062%, 0.125%, 0.167%, 0.2%, 0.25%), Beta-2 (1%), Bronkosol (1%), Dey-Lute Isoetharine (0.08%, 0.1%, 0.17%, 0.25%)

isoetharine mesylate

Bronkometer (0.61%)

Class and Category

Chemical class: Catecholamine
Therapeutic class: Bronchodilator
Pregnancy category: Not rated

Indications and Dosages

➤ *To prevent and treat reversible bronchospasm from chronic bronchitis or emphysema*

INHALATION AEROSOL

Adults and adolescents. 1 or 2 inhalations (340 or 680 mcg) every 4 hr.

INHALATION SOLUTION FOR HAND-BULB NEBULIZER

Adults. 3 to 7 inhalations of undiluted 0.5% or 1% solution every 4 hr.

INHALATION SOLUTION FOR NEBULIZER

Adults. 2.5 to 10 mg over 15 to 20 min. Repeated every 4 hr, p.r.n.

Route	Onset	Peak	Duration
Inhalation	5 min	5 to 15 min	2 to 3 hr

Mechanism of Action

Attaches to beta$_2$ receptors on bronchial cell membranes, which stimulates the intracellular enzyme adenylate cyclase to convert adenosine triphosphate to cyclic adenosine monophosphate (cAMP). Increased intracellular levels of cAMP help relax bronchial smooth-muscle cells, stabilize mast cells, and inhibit histamine release.

Contraindications

Hypersensitivity to isoetharine, sympathomimetic amines, or their components

Interactions

DRUGS

beta blockers: Decreased effects of both drugs
cyclopropane, halothane: Increased risk of arrhythmias
ephedrine: Increased cardiac stimulation
epinephrine: Increased effects of epinephrine
guanethidine: Decreased hypotensive effects
isoproterenol: Excessive cardiac stimulation
MAO inhibitors: Increased risk of hypertensive crisis, increased vascular effects of isoetharine
methyldopa: Increased vasopressor response
nitrates: Possibly decreased effects of both drugs
oxytocic drugs: Increased risk of hypotension
rauwolfia alkaloids: Increased risk of hypertension
tricyclic antidepressants: Increased risk of arrhythmias

Adverse Reactions

CNS: Anxiety, dizziness, headache, insomnia, tremor, vertigo, weakness
CV: Angina, arrhythmias, hypertension, palpitations, tachycardia
EENT: Choking sensation, eyelid or lip swelling, laryngospasm, taste perversion
GI: Nausea, vomiting
RESP: Bronchospasm, cough, paradoxical increased airway resistance (with excessive use), wheezing
SKIN: Dermatitis, flushing, pruritus, urticaria
Other: Angioedema, facial edema

Nursing Considerations

•Dilute 1% isoetharine inhalation solution with 1 to 4 ml of sterile normal saline solution; 0.062% to 0.25% solutions don't need to be diluted before use.

•Don't use a solution that's pink or darker than light yellow or one that contains precipitate.

•Wait 1 minute after initial inhaler dose to assess whether patient needs a second dose.

•Monitor blood pressure and pulse rate, and observe for arrhythmias during therapy.

PATIENT TEACHING

•Teach patient how to use isoetharine inhaler or nebulizer.

G
H
I

•Instruct patient to take drug exactly as directed and not to exceed dosage.
•Instruct patient not to take other drugs, even OTC drugs, unless prescribed.
•Teach patient how to determine when canister needs to be replaced by counting and recording number of doses.
•Instruct patient to report chest pain, difficulty breathing, failure to respond to usual isoetharine dose, irregular heartbeat, productive cough, or tremor.

isoniazid
(isonicotinic acid hydrazide, INH)

Isotamine (CAN), Laniazid, Nydrazid, PMS-Isoniazid (CAN)

Class and Category

Chemical class: Isonicotinic acid derivative
Therapeutic class: Antibiotic, antitubercular
Pregnancy category: C

Indications and Dosages

➤ *To prevent tuberculosis*
SYRUP, TABLETS, I.M. INJECTION
Adults and adolescents. 300 mg daily.
Children. 10 mg/kg daily (up to 300 mg).

➤ *As adjunct to treat active tuberculosis*
SYRUP, TABLETS
Adults and adolescents. 300 mg daily or 15 mg/kg (up to 900 mg) 2 or 3 times/wk, based on treatment regimen.
Children. 10 to 20 mg/kg (up to 300 mg) daily or 20 to 40 mg/kg (up to 900 mg) 2 or 3 times/wk, based on treatment regimen.
I.M. INJECTION
Adults and adolescents. 5 mg/kg (up to 300 mg) daily or 15 mg/kg (up to 900 mg) 2 or 3 times/wk, based on treatment regimen.
Children. 10 to 20 mg/kg (up to 300 mg) daily or 20 to 40 mg/kg (up to 900 mg) 2 or 3 times/wk, based on treatment regimen.

Mechanism of Action

Interferes with lipid and nucleic acid synthesis in actively growing tubercule bacilli cells. Isoniazid also disrupts bacterial cell wall synthesis and may interfere with mycolic acid synthesis in mycobacterial cells.

Contraindications

History of serious adverse reactions (such as hepatic injury) from isoniazid, hypersensitivity to isoniazid or its components

Interactions
DRUGS

acetaminophen: Increased risk of hepatotoxicity and, possibly, nephrotoxicity
alfentanil: Decreased alfentanil clearance and increased duration of effects
aluminum-containing antacids: Decreased isoniazid absorption
benzodiazepines: Decreased benzodiazepine clearance
carbamazepine: Increased blood carbamazepine level and toxicity, increased risk of isoniazid toxicity
corticosteroids: Decreased isoniazid effects
cycloserine: Increased risk of adverse CNS effects and CNS toxicity
disulfiram: Changes in behavior and coordination
enflurane: Increased risk of high-output renal failure
halothane: Increased risk of hepatotoxicity and hepatic encephalopathy
hepatotoxic drugs, rifampin: Increased risk of hepatotoxicity
ketoconazole: Possibly decreased blood ketoconazole level and resistance to antifungal treatment
meperidine: Risk of hypotensive episodes or CNS depression
nephrotoxic drugs: Increased risk of nephrotoxicity
oral anticoagulants: Increased anticoagulation
phenytoin: Increased blood phenytoin level, increased risk of phenytoin toxicity
theophylline: Increased theophylline level
FOODS

histamine-containing foods, such as tuna, skipjack, and other tropical fish: Inhibited action of the enzyme diamine oxidase in foods, possibly resulting in headache, sweating, palpitations, flushing, and hypotension.
tyramine-containing foods, such as cheese and fish: Increased responses to tyramine contained in foods, possibly resulting in chills; diaphoresis; headache; light-headedness; and red, itchy, clammy skin
ACTIVITIES

alcohol use: Increased risk of hepatotoxicity and increased isoniazid metabolism

Adverse Reactions

CNS: Clumsiness, confusion, dizziness, encephalopathy, fatigue, fever, hallucinations, neurotoxicity, paresthesia, peripheral neuritis, psychosis, seizures, weakness
CV: Vasculitis
EENT: Optic neuritis
ENDO: Gynecomastia, hyperglycemia
GI: Abdominal pain, anorexia, elevated liver function test results, epigastric distress, hepatitis, nausea, vomiting
GU: Glycosuria
HEME: Agranulocytosis, aplastic anemia, eosinophilia, hemolytic anemia, sideroblastic anemia, thrombocytopenia
MS: Arthralgia, joint stiffness
SKIN: Jaundice, pruritus, rash
Other: Hypocalcemia, hypophosphatemia, injection site irritation, lupus-like symptoms, lymphadenopathy

Nursing Considerations

• Administer isoniazid cautiously to diabetic, alcoholic, or malnourished patients and those at risk for peripheral neuritis.
• Give drug 1 hour before or 2 hours after meals to promote absorption. If GI distress occurs, give drug with a small amount of food or an antacid that doesn't contain aluminum 1 hour before or 2 hours after meal.
• Monitor liver enzyme studies, which may be ordered monthly, because isoniazid can cause severe (and possibly fatal) hepatitis.
• Be aware that about 50% of patients metabolize isoniazid more slowly, which may lead to increased toxic effects. Monitor for such adverse reactions as peripheral neuritis; if they occur, expect to decrease dosage.
• Give isoniazid with other antitubercular drugs, as prescribed, to prevent development of resistant organisms.
• Be aware that patients with advanced HIV infection may experience more severe adverse reactions in greater numbers.

PATIENT TEACHING

• Instruct patient to take isoniazid exactly as prescribed and not to stop taking it without first consulting prescriber. Explain that treatment may take months or years.
• Direct patient to take drug on an empty stomach 1 hour before or 2 hours after meals. If GI distress occurs, instruct him to take drug with food or an antacid that doesn't contain aluminum.

• Advise patient to report signs of hepatic dysfunction, including darkened urine, decreased appetite, fatigue, and jaundice.
• Caution patient not to drink alcohol while taking isoniazid because alcohol increases the risk of hepatotoxicity.
• Provide patient with a list of tyramine-containing foods to avoid when taking isoniazid, such as cheese, fish, salami, red wine, and yeast extracts. Inform him that consuming these foods during isoniazid therapy may cause unpleasant adverse reactions, such as chills, pounding heartbeat, and sweating.
• Tell patient to avoid histamine-containing foods such as tuna, skipjack, and other tropical fish during therapy to avoid such adverse reactions as headache, sweating, rapid heartbeat, flushing, and low blood pressure.
• Inform patient that he'll need periodic laboratory tests and physical examinations.
• Urge patient to report fever, nausea, numbness and tingling in arms and legs, rash, vision changes, vomiting, and yellowing skin.

isoproterenol
(isoprenaline)

Isuprel

isoproterenol hydrochloride

Isuprel, Isuprel Mistometer

isoproterenol sulfate

Medihaler-Iso

Class and Category

Chemical class: Catecholamine
Therapeutic class: Antiarrhythmic, bronchodilator
Pregnancy category: B (inhalation), C (I.V. infusion)

Indications and Dosages

➤ *To treat bronchospasm in asthma and to prevent and treat bronchospasm in COPD*

INHALATION AEROSOL (ISOPROTERENOL HYDROCHLORIDE)

Adults and adolescents. 1 oral inhalation (120 to 131 mcg), repeated in 2 to 5 min. Inhalations repeated every 3 to 4 hr, p.r.n.

INHALATION AEROSOL (ISOPROTERENOL SULFATE)

Adults and adolescents. 1 oral inhalation (80 mcg), repeated in 2 to 5 min. Inhalations repeated every 4 to 6 hr, p.r.n.

INHALATION SOLUTION FOR NEBULIZER (ISOPROTERENOL)

Adults and adolescents. 2.5 mg diluted and administered over 10 to 20 min. Repeated every 4 hr, p.r.n.

Children. 0.05 to 0.1 mg/kg (up to 1.25 mg) diluted and administered over 10 to 20 min. Repeated every 4 hr, p.r.n.

➤ *To manage bronchospasm during anesthesia*

I.V. INJECTION (ISOPROTERENOL HYDROCHLORIDE)

Adults. 0.01 to 0.02 mg, repeated p.r.n.

➤ *To treat bradycardia with significant hemodynamic change, such as third-degree heart block or prolonged QT intervals*

I.V. INFUSION (ISOPROTERENOL HYDROCHLORIDE)

Adults. *Initial:* 2 mcg/min. Titrated according to heart rate, as ordered. *Maximum:* 10 mcg/min.

Route	Onset	Peak	Duration
I.V.*	Unknown	Unknown	1 to 2 hr
I.V.†	In 5 min	Unknown	10 min
Inhalation	In 5 min	5 to 15 min	In 3 hr

Mechanism of Action

Stimulates beta$_1$ receptors in the myocardium and cardiac conduction system, resulting in positive inotropic and chronotropic effects. Isoproterenol also shortens the AV conduction time and refractory period in patients with AV block. This action increases the ventricular rate and halts bradycardia and associated syncope.

In addition, isoproterenol attaches to beta$_2$ receptors on bronchial cell membranes. This action stimulates the intracellular enzyme adenylate cyclase to convert adenosine triphosphate to cyclic adenosine monophosphate (cAMP). An increased intracellular level of cAMP relaxes bronchial smooth-muscle cells, stabilizes mast cells, and inhibits histamine release.

---

*For treatment of bronchospasm.
†For treatment of bradycardia.

Contraindications

Angina pectoris, heart block or tachycardia from digitalis toxicity, ventricular arrhythmias that require inotropic therapy (I.V. form); hypersensitivity to isoproterenol or its components, such as sulfite in some preparations (inhalation form); tachyarrhythmias (I.V. and inhalation forms)

Interactions

DRUGS

Note: All interactions listed are for I.V. form unless indicated.

alpha blockers, other drugs with this action: Possibly decreased peripheral vasoconstricting and hypertensive effects of isoproterenol

anesthetics (hydrocarbon inhalation): Increased risk of atrial and ventricular arrhythmias

astemizole, cisapride, drugs that prolong QTc interval, terfenadine: Possibly prolonged QTc interval

beta blockers (ophthalmic): Decreased effects of isoproterenol, increased risk of bronchospasm, wheezing, decreased pulmonary function, and respiratory failure

beta blockers (systemic): Increased risk of bronchospasm, decreased effects of both drugs (including inhaled isoproterenol)

digoxin: Increased risk of arrhythmias, hypokalemia, and digitalis toxicity

diuretics, other antihypertensives: Possibly decreased antihypertensive effects

ergot alkaloids: Increased vasoconstriction and vasopressor effects

MAO inhibitors: Intensified and extended cardiac stimulation and vasopressor effects

quinidine, other drugs that affect myocardial reaction to sympathomimetics: Increased risk of arrhythmias

theophylline: Increased risk of cardiotoxicity, decreased blood theophylline level

thyroid hormones: Increased effects of both drugs, increased risk of coronary insufficiency in patients with coronary artery disease

tricyclic antidepressants: Increased vasopressor response, increased risk of prolonged QTc interval and arrhythmias

Adverse Reactions

CNS: Dizziness, headache, insomnia, nervousness, syncope, tremor, weakness

CV: Angina, arrhythmias, bradycardia, hypertension, hypotension, palpitations, tachycardia, ventricular arrhythmias

EENT: Dry mouth, oropharyngeal edema,

taste perversion
ENDO: Hyperglycemia
GI: Heartburn, nausea, vomiting
MS: Muscle spasms and twitching
RESP: Bronchitis, bronchospasm, cough, dyspnea, increased sputum production, pulmonary edema, wheezing
SKIN: Dermatitis, diaphoresis, erythema multiforme, flushing, pallor, pruritus, rash, Stevens-Johnson syndrome, urticaria
Other: Angioedema, hypokalemia

Nursing Considerations
•Expect to give lowest possible dose for shortest possible time to minimize tolerance.
•Don't administer I.V. isoproterenol if it is pink or brown or contains precipitate.
•Administer infusion through large vein, and monitor for signs of extravasation.
•Monitor blood pressure, cardiac rhythm, central venous pressure, and urine output when giving I.V. drug. Adjust infusion rate to response, as ordered.
•Notify prescriber immediately if heart rate increases significantly or exceeds 110 beats/minute during I.V. infusion.
•Know that drug may increase pulse pressure and cause hypotension. Expect to reduce I.V. infusion slowly to decrease risk of hypotension.
•WARNING Be aware that drug markedly increases the risk of arrhythmias. If an arrhythmia develops, expect to give a cardioselective beta blocker, such as atenolol.
•Isoproterenol isn't used regularly to treat asthma, decreased cardiac output, hypotension, or shock because it increases the risk of arrhythmias, hypotension, and ischemia.
•WARNING If drug aggravates a ventilation-perfusion problem, expect blood oxygen level to fall even as breathing seems to improve.
PATIENT TEACHING
•Instruct patient not to use isoproterenol inhaler more often than prescribed because it may cause cardiac and respiratory problems.
•Teach patient to use the inhaler. Provide a spacer, as needed.
•Instruct patient to wait 2 to 5 minutes before taking second inhalation.
•Advise patient to rinse his mouth after inhalation to remove drug residue and minimize mouth dryness.
•Inform patient that saliva may appear pink after inhalation.
•If patient uses a corticosteroid inhaler, tell him to take isoproterenol first and wait at least 2 minutes before taking corticosteroid.
•Instruct patient to report chest pain, dizziness, hyperglycemic symptoms (such as abdominal cramps, lethargy, nausea, and vomiting), insomnia, irregular heartbeat, palpitations, tremor, and weakness.
•Advise patient to also report reduced drug effectiveness, increased use of inhaler, and increased symptoms after taking drug.

isosorbide dinitrate
Apo-ISDN (CAN), Cedocard-SR (CAN), Coradur (CAN), Coronex (CAN), Dilatrate-SR, Isordil Tembids, Isordil Titradose, Sorbitrate

isosorbide mononitrate
IMDUR, ISMO, Monoket

Class and Category
Chemical class: Organic nitrate
Therapeutic class: Antianginal, vasodilator
Pregnancy category: C

Indications and Dosages
➤ *To treat or prevent angina*
CHEWABLE TABLETS
Adults. 5 mg every 2 to 3 hr, p.r.n. (dinitrate).
E.R. CAPSULES
Adults. 40 to 80 mg every 8 to 12 hr (dinitrate).
E.R. TABLETS
Adults. 20 to 80 mg every 8 to 12 hr (dinitrate); 30 to 60 mg daily, increased gradually as tolerated to 120 mg daily (mononitrate).
S.L. TABLETS
Adults. 2.5 to 5 mg every 2 to 3 hr, p.r.n. (dinitrate).
TABLETS
Adults. 5 to 40 mg every 6 hr, adjusted as needed (dinitrate); 20 mg in 2 doses given 7 hr apart (mononitrate).

Route	Onset	Peak	Duration
P.O.*	1 hr†	Unknown	5 to 6 hr
P.O. (chewable)*	In 3 min	Unknown	30 min to 2 hr
P.O. (E.R.)*	30 min	Unknown	6 to 8 hr
P.O. (S.L.)*	In 3 min	Unknown	2 hr

*For dinitrate.
†For mononitrate, onset also is 1 hr; peak and duration are unknown.

Contraindications

Angle-closure glaucoma; cerebral hemorrhage; concurrent use of sildenafil; head trauma; hypersensitivity to isosorbide, other nitrates, or their components; orthostatic hypotension; severe anemia

Interactions

DRUGS

acetylcholine, norepinephrine: Possibly decreased effectiveness of these drugs
antihypertensives, calcium channel blockers, opioid analgesics, other vasodilators: Increased risk of orthostatic hypotension
aspirin: Increased blood level and pharmacologic action of isosorbide
sildenafil, tadalafil, vardenafil: Increased risk of hypotension and death
sympathomimetics: Increased risk of hypotension, possibly decreased therapeutic effects of isosorbide

ACTIVITIES

alcohol use: Increased risk of orthostatic hypotension

Adverse Reactions

CNS: Agitation, confusion, dizziness, headache, insomnia, restlessness, syncope, vertigo, weakness
CV: Arrhythmias, orthostatic hypotension, palpitations, peripheral edema, tachycardia
EENT: Blurred vision, diplopia (all drug forms); sublingual burning (S.L. form)
GI: Abdominal pain, diarrhea, indigestion, nausea, vomiting
GU: Dysuria, impotence, urinary frequency
HEME: Hemolytic anemia
MS: Arthralgia, muscle twitching
RESP: Bronchitis, pneumonia, upper respiratory tract infection
SKIN: Diaphoresis, flushing, rash

Nursing Considerations

•Use isosorbide cautiously in patients with hypovolemia or mild hypotension. Monitor for increased hypotension and reduced cardiac output.
•Give drug 1 hour before or 2 hours after meals. Give with meals if patient experiences severe headaches or adverse GI reactions.
•Know that patient may experience daily headaches from isosorbide's vasodilating effects. Give acetaminophen, as prescribed, to relieve pain.
•**WARNING** Be aware that abrupt drug discontinuation may cause angina and increase the risk of MI.

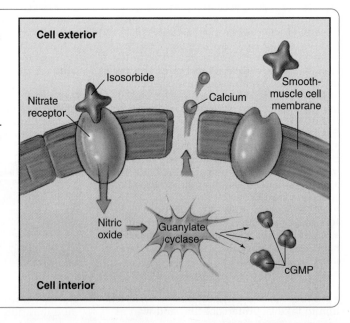

Mechanism of Action

Isosorbide may interact with nitrate receptors in vascular smooth-muscle cell membranes. By interacting with nitrate receptors' sulfhydryl groups, the drug is reduced to nitric oxide. Nitric oxide activates the enzyme guanylate cyclase, increasing intracellular formation of cyclic guanosine monophosphate (cGMP). An increased cGMP level may relax vascular smooth muscle by forcing calcium out of muscle cells, causing vasodilation. This improves cardiac output by reducing primarily preload but also afterload.

Cell exterior

Isosorbide

Nitrate receptor

Calcium

Smooth-muscle cell membrane

Nitric oxide

Guanylate cyclase

cGMP

Cell interior

• Monitor blood pressure frequently during isosorbide therapy, especially in the elderly; the drug may cause severe hypotension.
• Keep drug away from heat and light.

PATIENT TEACHING
• Teach patient and family to recognize signs and symptoms of angina, including chest pain, fullness, or pressure, which commonly is accompanied by sweating and nausea. Pain may radiate down the left arm or into the neck or jaw. Inform female patients and those with diabetes mellitus or hypertension that they may experience only fatigue and shortness of breath.
• Advise patient not to crush or chew isosorbide E.R. capsules or tablets or S.L. tablets unless specifically ordered to do so.
• Instruct patient to place S.L. tablet under tongue and not to swallow it, but to let it dissolve. Explain that moisture in mouth promotes drug absorption and that tingling or burning in the mouth indicates drug effectiveness.
• Advise patient to chew chewable tablets well and to keep them in his mouth for 1 to 2 minutes before swallowing to enhance drug absorption.
• Instruct patient to take drug before any situation or activity that might precipitate angina.
• Advise patient to carry isosorbide with him at all times.
• Caution patient that abrupt drug discontinuation may cause angina and increase the risk of MI.
• Instruct patient to report blurred vision, fainting, increased angina attacks, rash, and severe or persistent headaches.
• Teach patient to reduce the effects of orthostatic hypotension by changing position slowly. Advise him to lie down if he becomes dizzy.
• Inform patient that drug commonly causes headache, which typically resolves after a few days of continuous therapy. Suggest that patient take acetaminophen as needed and as prescribed.
• Advise patient to avoid potentially hazardous activities until drug's CNS effects are known.
• Urge patient to avoid alcohol consumption.
• Instruct patient to store drug in a tightly closed container away from light and heat.
• Advise male patients with erectile dysfunction to alert prescriber that he is taking isosorbide because sildenafil, tadalafil, and vardenafil can cause fatal reactions when taken with isosorbide.

isotretinoin

Accutane, Claravis

Class and Category
Chemical class: Retinoid
Therapeutic class: Acne inhibitor
Pregnancy category: X

Indications and Dosages
➤ *To treat severe recalcitrant nodular acne unresponsive to conventional therapy*

CAPSULES
Adults. *Initial:* 0.5 mg to 1 mg/kg daily in 2 divided doses, increased as needed up to 2 mg/kg daily given in 2 divided doses. *Maximum:* 2 mg/kg daily. Course of therapy given for 15 to 20 wk with second course given, as needed, after a period of 2 mo or more off therapy.

Mechanism of Action
Inhibits sebaceous gland function and keratinization, which results in diminished nodular formation associated with recalcitrant nodular acne.

Contraindications
Hypersensitivity to isotretinoin or any of its components, hypersensitivity to parabens, pregnancy

Interactions
DRUGS
corticosteroids (systemic): Possibly increased risk of osteoporosis
oral contraceptives including microdosed progesterone preparations, medroxyprogesterone injection, levonorgestrel implants: Possibly decreased effectiveness of contraceptive
phenytoin: Possibly increased risk of osteomalacia
tetracyclines: Increased risk of benign intracranial hypertension
vitamin A supplements: Increased risk of additive toxic effects

G
H
I

Adverse Reactions

CNS: Aggressive or violent behavior, depression, dizziness, drowsiness, emotional instability, fatigue, headache, insomnia, lethargy, malaise, nervousness, paresthesias, pseudotumor cerebri, psychosis, seizures, stroke, suicidal ideation, syncope, weakness

CV: Chest pain, decreased high-density lipoprotein level, edema, elevated creatinine phosphokinase level, hypercholesteremia, hypertriglyceridemia, palpitation, stroke, tachycardia, vascular thrombotic disease, vasculitis

ENDO: Abnormal menses, alterations in blood glucose levels

EENT: Bleeding and inflammation of gums, cataracts, color vision disorder, conjunctivitis, corneal opacities, decreased night vision, dry mouth or nose, dry eyes, epistaxis, eyelid inflammation, hearing impairment, keratitis, optic neuritis, photophobia, tinnitus, visual disturbances, voice alteration

GI: Colitis, hepatitis, ileitis, inflammatory bowel disease, liver enzyme elevation, nausea, pancreatitis

GU: Glomerulonephritis, hematuria, proteinuria, WBCs in urine

HEME: Anemia, agranulocytosis, neutropenia, platelet count elevation, sedimentation rate elevation, thrombocytopenia

MS: Arthralgia, arthritis, back pain (children), bone abnormalities, calcification of tendons and ligaments, premature epiphyseal closure, tendonitis

RESP: Bronchospasms, respiratory infection

SKIN: Alopecia, bruising, disseminated herpes simplex, dry lips or skin, eczema, eruptive xanthomas, facial erythema, flushing, fulminant acne, hair abnormalities, hirsutism, hyperpigmentation, hypopigmentation, increased sunburn susceptibility, infections, nail dystrophy, paronychia, peeling of palms and soles, photoallergic or photosensitizing reactions, pruritus, pyogenic granuloma, rash, seborrhea, skin fragility, sweating, urticaria

Other: Abnormal wound healing, alkaline phosphatase increase, allergic reactions, hyperuricemia, lymphadenopathy, weight loss

Nursing Considerations

•Ensure that women of childbearing age have had 2 negative urine or serum pregnancy tests with a sensitivity of at least 50 mIU/ml, joined the Accutane Survey, signed the consent form, and watched the videotape provided by manufacturer prior to beginning isotretinoin therapy.

•**WARNING** Notify prescriber if elevated serum triglyceride levels can't be controlled or if symptoms of pancreatitis occur (abdominal pain, nausea, vomiting). Drug may need to be discontinued because fatal hemorrhagic pancreatitis has occurred with drug use.

•Obtain serum lipid level before therapy and periodically thereafter, as ordered, to detect elevated lipid levels that result from isotretinoin therapy.

•Monitor liver enzyme levels periodically, as ordered, because drug can cause hepatitis.

•Assess patient frequently for adverse reactions and report to prescriber any that occur; drug may have serious adverse effects that require discontinuation.

PATIENT TEACHING

•Instruct patient to take isotretinoin with food or milk.

•Advise women of childbearing age that 2 forms of contraceptives must be used simultaneously (unless absolute abstinence is a chosen method) 1 month before therapy and for 1 month after therapy has stopped because of potential for fetal harm. Inform women who use oral contraceptives that drug may lessen effectiveness of oral contraceptives. Urge patient to notify prescriber immediately if pregnancy occurs.

•Stress importance of picking up isotretinoin prescription within 7 days of a pregnancy test or, for male patients or women not of childbearing potential, within 30 days of prescription.

•Urge patient to report headache, nausea, vomiting and visual disturbances immediately to prescriber because drug will need to be discontinued immediately and the patient referred to a neurologist.

•Caution patient and family that isotretinoin may cause aggressive or violent behavior, depression, psychosis, and suicidal ideation. Instruct patient to notify prescriber immediately if changes in mood occur.

•Tell patient to report hearing changes or tinnitus, visual difficulties, abdominal pain, rectal bleeding, or severe diarrhea to prescriber because drug may need to be discontinued.

•Advise patient to avoid hazardous activities

until drug's CNS effects are known. Caution her that changes in night vision may occur suddenly.

•Caution patient not to donate blood during therapy and for 1 month after therapy has stopped because blood might be given to a pregnant woman.

•Warn patient that transient exacerbation of acne may occur, especially during initial therapy and to notify prescriber if this occurs.

•Instruct patient to avoid wax epilation and skin resurfacing procedures during therapy and for at least 6 months thereafter because of scarring potential.

•Caution patient to avoid exposure to direct sunlight or UV light and to wear sunscreen when outdoors.

•Inform patient that contact lens tolerance may decrease during and after therapy.

•Alert patient to the potential for mild musculoskeletal adverse reactions, which usually clear rapidly after drug is discontinued. Urge patient to notify prescriber if symptoms become bothersome or serious because drug may need to be discontinued.

•Advise patient not to take vitamin A supplements while on drug therapy because of potential additive toxic effects.

•Instruct patient to notify all prescribers of isotretinoin use because of the risk of interactions.

•Inform patient of need for frequent laboratory tests and importance of complying with scheduled appointments.

isradipine

DynaCirc

Class and Category

Chemical class: Dihydropyridine derivative
Therapeutic class: Antihypertensive
Pregnancy category: C

Indications and Dosages

➤ *To manage essential hypertension*

CAPSULES

Adults. *Initial:* 2.5 mg b.i.d., increased by 5 mg every 2 to 4 wk, if needed. *Maximum:* 20 mg daily.

Route	Onset	Peak	Duration
P.O.	2 to 3 hr	2 to 4 wk	Unknown

Mechanism of Action

Inhibits calcium movement into coronary vascular smooth-muscle cells by blocking the slow calcium channels in their membranes. By decreasing the intracellular calcium level, isradipine inhibits smooth-muscle cell contractions. The result is relaxation of coronary and vascular smooth muscle, decreased peripheral vascular resistance, and reduced systolic and diastolic blood pressure, all of which decrease myocardial oxygen demand.

Contraindications

Hypersensitivity to isradipine or its components

Interactions

DRUGS

anesthetics (hydrocarbon inhalation), antihypertensives, hydrochlorothiazide, prazocin: Increased risk of hypotension
beta blockers: Increased adverse effects of beta blockers
cimetidine: Increased blood level and bioavailability of isradipine
digoxin: Transiently increased blood digoxin level and risk of digitalis toxicity
estrogens: Possibly increased fluid retention and decreased isradipine effects
lithium: Increased risk of neurotoxicity
NSAIDs, sympathomimetics: Possibly decreased therapeutic effects of isradipine
procainamide, quinidine: Increased risk of prolonged QT interval

FOODS

grapefruit juice: Doubled isradipine bioavailability
other foods: Prolonged time to achieve peak blood level

Adverse Reactions

CNS: Asthenia, dizziness, fatigue, headache, paresthesia, somnolence, stroke, syncope, transient ischemic attack, weakness
CV: Angina, atrial fibrillation, heart failure, hypotension, MI, orthostatic hypotension, palpitations, peripheral edema, tachycardia, ventricular fibrillation
EENT: Gingival hyperplasia, pharyngitis, rhinitis
GI: Abdominal cramps, constipation, diarrhea, elevated liver function test results, in-

digestion, nausea, vomiting
HEME: Leukopenia
MS: Back pain
RESP: Cough
SKIN: Flushing, photosensitivity, rash, urticaria
Other: Angioedema

Nursing Considerations
•Monitor blood pressure and heart rate frequently during isradipine therapy.
•Monitor patient with impaired hepatic or renal function for an increased blood isradipine level.
•Avoid giving isradipine with food because doing so increases time to peak effect by about 1 hour.
•Observe for mild peripheral edema caused by vasodilation of small blood vessels. Know that this type of edema doesn't result from fluid retention or heart failure.

PATIENT TEACHING
•Inform patient that isradipine therapy will be long-term and will require laboratory tests and follow-up visits to monitor drug effects.
•Instruct patient to take drug exactly as prescribed and to swallow capsules whole, not crush or chew them.
•Advise patient to take drug on an empty stomach 1 hour before or 2 hours after meals.
•Instruct patient to take a missed dose as soon as he remembers it unless it's nearly time for the next dose. In that case, advise him to wait and take the next scheduled dose, but not to double the dose. If more than one dose is missed, tell him to contact prescriber.
•WARNING Urge patient not to stop taking drug suddenly. Doing so may lead to life-threatening problems.
•Inform patient that fragments of capsules may be visible in stool.
•Caution patient not to drink grapefruit juice during isradipine therapy.
•Urge patient to avoid potentially hazardous activities until isradipine's CNS effects are known.
•Caution patient to change position slowly to minimize orthostatic hypotension.
•Urge patient to contact prescriber if he experiences chest pain, fainting, irregular heartbeat, rash, or swollen ankles while taking isradipine.
•Instruct patient to maintain good oral hygiene, perform gum massage, and see his dentist every 6 months to prevent gum bleeding and gum disorders.
•To help prevent photosensitivity reactions, caution patient to avoid direct sunlight and to wear protective clothing and apply sunscreen when outdoors.
•Instruct patient to store drug at room temperature in a dry place.

itraconazole

Sporanox

Class and Category
Chemical class: Triazole derivative
Therapeutic class: Antifungal
Pregnancy category: C

Indications and Dosages
➤ *To treat blastomycosis caused by* Blastomyces dermatitidis *and histoplasmosis caused by* Histoplasma capsulatum

CAPSULES
Adults and adolescents. *Initial:* 200 mg daily, increased by 100 mg daily, if needed. *Maximum:* 400 mg daily, with dosage greater than 200 mg given in divided doses b.i.d.

➤ *To treat aspergillosis unresponsive to amphotericin B*

CAPSULES
Adults and adolescents. 200 to 400 mg daily, with dosage greater than 200 mg daily given in divided doses b.i.d.

➤ *To treat oropharyngeal candidiasis*

ORAL SOLUTION
Adults and adolescents. 100 mg b.i.d. for 7 to 14 days.

➤ *To treat esophageal candidiasis*

ORAL SOLUTION
Adults and adolescents. 100 mg daily for at least 3 wk and continued for 2 wk after symptoms resolve.

➤ *To treat onychomycosis of toenails only or of toenails and fingernails*

CAPSULES
Adults and adolescents. 200 mg daily for 12 wk.

➤ *To treat onychomycosis of fingernails only*

CAPSULES

Adults and adolescents. 200 mg b.i.d. for 7 days; then repeated after 3 wk.

> ## Mechanism of Action
> Inhibits the synthesis of ergosterol, an essential component of fungal cell membranes, by binding with a cytochrome P-450 enzyme needed to convert lanosterol to ergosterol. The lack of ergosterol results in increased cellular permeability and leakage of cell contents. Itraconazole also may lead to fungal cell death by inhibiting fungal respiration under aerobic conditions.

Contraindications

Concurrent therapy with cisapride, dofetilide, ergot alkaloids, HMG-CoA inhibitors (lovastatin and simvastatin), levomethadyl, oral midazolam, pimozide, quinidine, or triazolam; evidence of ventricular dysfunction, as in congestive heart failure (CHF) or a history of it (onychomycosis treatment); hypersensitivity to itraconazole or its components; planning for pregnancy during onychomycosis treatment

Interactions

DRUGS

alfentanil, buspirone, busulfan, carbamazepine, cyclosporine, digoxin, docetaxel, dofetilide, indinavir, methylprednisolone, phenytoin, pimozide, quinidine, rifabutin, ritonavir, saquinavir, sirolimus, tacrolimus, trimetrexate, vinca alkaloids: Possibly increased blood levels of these drugs
alprazolam, diazepam, oral midazolam, triazolam: Elevated blood levels and possibly prolonged sedative effects of these drugs
antacids, anticholinergics, H₂-receptor antagonists, omeprazole, sucralfate: Possibly decreased itraconazole absorption
atorvastatin, lovastatin, simvastatin: Increased blood levels of these drugs; possibly rhabdomyolysis
calcium channel blockers: Possibly edema and increased blood levels of these drugs
carbamazepine, isoniazid, nevirapine, phenobarbital, phenytoin, rifabutin, rifampin: Possibly decreased blood itraconazole level
cisapride, pimozide, levomethadyl, quinidine: Possibly life-threatening cardiovascular com-

plications as well as sudden death
clarithromycin, erythromycin, indinavir, ritonavir: Possibly increased blood itraconazole level
didanosine: Possibly decreased therapeutic effects of itraconazole
oral antidiabetic drugs: Possibly increased blood levels of these drugs and risk of hypoglycemia
warfarin: Increased anticoagulant effect of warfarin

Adverse Reactions

CNS: Dizziness, drowsiness, fatigue, fever, headache, peripheral neuropathy, vertigo
CV: CHF, hypertriglyceridemia, hypertension, peripheral edema
GI: Abdominal pain, anorexia, constipation, diarrhea, elevated liver function test results, flatulence, hepatic failure, hepatitis, hepatotoxicity, hyperbilirubinemia, indigestion, nausea, vomiting
GU: Menstrual irregularities
HEME: Neutropenia
RESP: Cough, dyspnea, pulmonary edema
SKIN: Alopecia, diaphoresis, photosensitivity, pruritus, rash, Stevens-Johnson syndrome, urticaria
Other: Angioedema, anaphylaxis, hypokalemia

Nursing Considerations

•Because itraconazole has been linked to serious adverse cardiac and hepatic effects, expect to send appropriate nail specimens for laboratory testing to confirm onychomycosis before beginning therapy.
•WARNING Keep in mind that itraconazole is a potent inhibitor of the cytochrome P-450 3A4 (CYP3A4) isoenzyme system, which may increase blood levels of drugs metabolized by this system. Patients using such drugs as cisapride with itraconazole or other CYP3A4 inhibitors have experienced life-threatening cardiovascular complications, such as prolonged QT interval, torsades de pointes, and ventricular tachycardia, as well as sudden death.
•Administer itraconazole capsules (but not oral solution) with a meal to ensure maximal absorption.
•Keep in mind that a patient with AIDS may have hypochlorhydria, which reduces drug absorption. For such a patient, expect to administer higher doses of itraconazole.
•Monitor liver function test results in pa-

G
H
I

tients with impaired hepatic function and those who have experienced hepatotoxicity with other drugs.

•If patient develops signs and symptoms of peripheral neuropathy or CHF, such as fatigue, dyspnea, and peripheral edema, expect to discontinue drug.

•Assess patient for rash every 8 hours during therapy; notify prescriber if rash occurs.

•If patient also receives warfarin, monitor PT and assess patient for signs and symptoms of bleeding.

•If patient also receives digoxin, monitor blood digoxin level as appropriate to detect toxic level, and assess patient for signs and symptoms of digitalis toxicity, such as nausea and yellow vision.

PATIENT TEACHING

•Instruct patient to take itraconazole capsules with a meal, but oral solution without food.

•If patient also takes an oral antidiabetic drug, instruct him to monitor his blood glucose level frequently because of the increased risk of hypoglycemia.

•Advise patient to avoid taking antacids with oral itraconazole.

•Advise patient to notify prescriber immediately of changes in other drugs, such as new drugs and dosage changes.

•Advise patient to notify prescriber immediately about abdominal pain, diarrhea, headache, nausea, peripheral neuropathy, rash, or vomiting.

•Instruct patient to notify prescriber if he experiences signs of liver problems, such as abdominal pain, dark urine, fatigue, loss of appetite, pale stools, weakness, or yellow eyes or skin.

•Caution breastfeeding patient to consult prescriber about continuation of breastfeeding during itraconazole therapy.

J·K·L

kanamycin sulfate

Kantrex

Class and Category
Chemical class: Aminoglycoside
Therapeutic class: Antibiotic
Pregnancy category: D

Indications and Dosages
➤ *To treat infections caused by gram-negative organisms (including* Acinetobacter *species,* Enterobacter aerogenes, Escherichia coli, Haemophilus influenzae, Klebsiella pneumoniae, Neisseria *species,* Proteus *species,* Providencia *species,* Salmonella *species,* Serratia marcescens, Shigella *species, and* Yersinia *species) and gram-positive organisms (including* Staphylococcus aureus *and* Staphylococcus epidermidis)

I.M. INJECTION
Adults and children. 3.75 mg/kg every 6 hr, 5 mg/kg every 8 hr, or 7.5 mg/kg every 12 hr for 7 to 10 days. *Maximum:* 1.5 g daily.

I.V. INFUSION
Adults and children. 5 mg/kg every 8 hr or 7.5 mg/kg every 12 hr for 7 to 10 days. *Maximum:* 1.5 g daily.

➤ *As adjunct to suppress intestinal bacterial growth*

CAPSULES
Adults. 1 g/hr for 4 hr and then 1 g every 6 hr for 36 to 72 hr.

➤ *To treat hepatic coma*

CAPSULES
Adults. 8 to 12 g daily administered in divided doses.

➤ *To treat respiratory tract infection*

INHALATION NEBULIZER
Adults. 250 mg b.i.d. to q.i.d. *Maximum:* 1.5 g daily.

DOSAGE ADJUSTMENT For elderly patients and those with renal failure, dosage reduced and blood kanamycin level and renal function test results monitored.

Contraindications
Hypersensitivity to kanamycin, other aminoglycosides, or their components; intestinal obstruction (oral form)

Route	Onset	Peak	Duration
P.O.	Slow	Unknown	Unknown
I.V.	Rapid	Unknown	Unknown
I.M.	Unknown	1 to 2 hr	Unknown

Mechanism of Action
Binds to negatively charged sites on bacterial outer cell membranes, which disrupts cell membrane integrity. Kanamycin also binds to bacterial ribosomal subunits and inhibits protein synthesis; these actions lead to cell death.

Incompatibilities
Don't mix kanamycin in same syringe or administer through same I.V. line as other antibiotics.

Interactions
DRUGS
cephalosporins, vancomycin: Increased risk of nephrotoxicity
digoxin, loop diuretics: Increased ototoxic and nephrotoxic effects of kanamycin
general anesthetics, neuromuscular blockers: Increased risk of neuromuscular blockade
penicillins: Inactivation of kanamycin or synergistic effects

Adverse Reactions
CNS: Ataxia, dizziness, headache
EENT: Hearing loss
GI: Diarrhea
GU: Elevated BUN and serum creatinine levels, oliguria, proteinuria
MS: Muscle paralysis
RESP: Apnea
SKIN: Injection site irritation or pain

Nursing Considerations
• Obtain body fluid or tissue specimen for culture and sensitivity testing before kanamycin therapy begins, as indicated. Therapy may begin before test results are available.
• Administer I.M. injection deep into upper outer quadrant of gluteus maximus. Rotate

J
K
L

injection sites.

•Be aware that oral kanamycin is minimally absorbed from intact GI mucosa but may be more extensively absorbed from mechanically irrigated areas of the GI tract.

•For I.V. use, dilute 500-mg vial with 100 to 200 ml of normal saline solution or D_5W, or 1-g vial with 200 to 400 ml of normal saline solution or D_5W, and infuse over 30 to 60 min. Be aware that vial contents may darken during storage but potency isn't affected.

•Keep patient well hydrated before and during therapy.

•Monitor blood kanamycin level periodically during therapy, as appropriate.

•Be aware that prolonged treatment increases the risk of ototoxicity and nephrotoxicity. Monitor hearing and renal function if therapy lasts longer than 10 days.

PATIENT TEACHING

•Explain the need to take kanamycin at prescribed intervals around the clock until patient completes full course of therapy.

•Advise patient to report dizziness, hearing loss, and severe diarrhea or headache to prescriber.

ketoprofen

Actron, Apo-Keto (CAN), Orudis, Orudis KT, Orudis-SR (CAN), Oruvail, Rhodis

Class and Category

Chemical class: Propionic acid derivative
Therapeutic class: Analgesic, anti-inflammatory
Pregnancy category: B

Indications and Dosages

➤ *To treat symptoms of rheumatoid arthritis*

CAPSULES, TABLETS

Adults. *Initial:* 75 mg t.i.d. or 50 mg q.i.d. *Maximum:* 300 mg daily.

E.R. CAPSULES

Adults. *Maintenance:* 150 to 200 mg daily. *Maximum:* 300 mg daily.

➤ *To relieve pain in dysmenorrhea*

TABLETS

Adults. *Initial:* 25 to 50 mg every 6 to 8 hr p.r.n. *Maximum:* 300 mg daily.

DOSAGE ADJUSTMENT Dosage reduced by 33% to 50% for patients with renal impairment.

Mechanism of Action

Blocks the activity of cyclooxygenase, the enzyme needed for prostaglandin synthesis. Prostaglandins, important mediators of the inflammatory response, cause local vasodilation with swelling and pain. By blocking cyclooxygenase and inhibiting prostaglandins, this NSAID reduces inflammatory symptoms and relieves pain.

Contraindications

Angioedema; aspirin-, iodide-, or NSAID-induced asthma, bronchospasm, nasal polyps, rhinitis, or urticaria; hypersensitivity to ketoprofen or its components

Interactions

DRUGS

ACE inhibitors: Possibly decreased hypotensive effect of ACE inhibitors

acetaminophen: Possibly increased adverse renal effects with long-term acetaminophen use

aspirin, other NSAIDs: Increased risk of bleeding and adverse GI effects, increased and prolonged blood ketoprofen levels

cefamandole, cefoperazone, cefotetan: Increased risk of hypoprothrombinemia and bleeding

colchicine, platelet aggregation inhibitors: Increased risk of GI bleeding, hemorrhage, and ulcers

corticosteroids, potassium supplements: Increased risk of adverse GI effects

cyclosporine: Increased risk of nephrotoxicity from both drugs, increased blood cyclosporine level

diuretics (loop, potassium-sparing, and thiazide): Decreased diuretic and antihypertensive effects

gold compounds, nephrotoxic drugs: Increased risk of adverse renal effects

heparin, oral anticoagulants, thrombolytics: Increased anticoagulant effects, increased risk of hemorrhage

insulin, oral antidiabetic drugs: Possibly increased hypoglycemic effects of these drugs

lithium: Increased blood lithium level and possibly toxicity

methotrexate: Decreased methotrexate clearance, increased risk of methotrexate toxicity

plicamycin, valproic acid: Increased risk of hypoprothrombinemia and GI bleeding, hemorrhage, and ulcers

probenecid: Possibly increased blood level, effectiveness, and risk of toxicity of ketoprofen

ACTIVITIES

alcohol use: Increased risk of adverse GI effects

Adverse Reactions

CNS: Headache, irritability, nervousness, seizures, stroke

CV: Edema, fluid retention, hypertension, MI, tachycardia

EENT: Tinnitus, vision changes

GI: Abdominal pain, anorexia, constipation, diarrhea, diverticulitis, dyspepsia, dysphagia, flatulence, gastritis, gastroenteritis, gastroesophageal reflux disease, GI bleeding and ulceration, hepatic failure, hiatal hernia, indigestion, melena, nausea, perforation of stomach or intestines, stomatitis, vomiting

GU: Acute renal failure, decreased urine output

HEME: Agranulocytosis, anemia, easy bruising, hemolytic anemia, leukopenia, neutropenia, pancytopenia, thrombocytopenia

RESP: Asthma, respiratory depression

SKIN: Erythema multiforme, Stevens-Johnson syndrome, toxic epidermal necrolysis, rash

Other: Anaphylaxis, angioedema, rapid weight gain

Nursing Considerations

• Use ketoprofen with extreme caution in patients with a history of ulcer disease or GI bleeding because NSAIDs such as ketoprofen increase the risk of GI bleeding and ulceration. Expect to use ketoprofen for the shortest time possible in these patients.

• Be aware that serious GI tract ulceration, bleeding, and perforation may occur without warning symptoms. Elderly patients are at greater risk. To minimize risk, give drug with food. If GI distress occurs, withhold drug and notify prescriber immediately.

• Use ketoprofen cautiously in patients with hypertension, and monitor blood pressure closely throughout therapy. Drug may cause hypertension or worsen it.

• **WARNING** Monitor patient closely for thrombotic events, including MI and stroke, because NSAIDs increase the risk.

• Monitor patient—especially if he's elderly or receiving long-term ketoprofen therapy—

for less common but serious adverse GI reactions, including anorexia, constipation, diverticulitis, dysphagia, esophagitis, gastritis, gastroenteritis, gastroesophageal reflux disease, hemorrhoids, hiatal hernia, melena, stomatitis, and vomiting.

• Monitor liver function test results because, in rare cases, elevations may progress to severe hepatic reactions, including fatal hepatitis, liver necrosis, and hepatic failure.

• Monitor BUN and serum creatinine levels in elderly patients, patients taking diuretics or ACE inhibitors, and patients with heart failure, impaired renal function, or hepatic dysfunction; drug may cause renal failure.

• Monitor CBC for decreased hemoglobin level and hematocrit because drug may worsen anemia.

• **WARNING** If patient has bone marrow suppression or is receiving an antineoplastic drug, monitor laboratory results (including WBC count), and watch for evidence of infection because anti-inflammatory and antipyretic actions of ketoprofen may mask signs and symptoms, such as fever and pain.

• Assess patient's skin regularly for signs of rash or other hypersensitivity reaction because ketoprofen is an NSAID and may cause serious skin reactions without warning, even in patients with no history of NSAID sensitivity. At first sign of reaction, stop drug and notify prescriber.

• If patient takes acetaminophen, monitor fluid intake and output, BUN level, and serum creatinine level for evidence of adverse renal effects.

PATIENT TEACHING

• Instruct patient to take ketoprofen with food or after meals to prevent GI upset. Advise him to take drug with a full glass of water and to avoid lying down for 15 to 30 minutes afterward to prevent drug from lodging in esophagus and causing irritation.

• Advise patient to swallow drug whole and not to crush, break, chew, or open capsules.

• Instruct patient to avoid aspirin, aspirin-containing products, and alcohol while taking ketoprofen to decrease the risk of adverse GI effects.

• Tell patient not to take more drug than prescribed because stomach bleeding may occur.

• If patient takes an anticoagulant, tell him to watch for and immediately report bleeding problems, such as bloody or tarry stools

J
K
L

and bloody vomitus.
• If patient takes insulin or an oral antidiabetic, advise him to monitor his blood
glucose levels closely. Urge him to carry
candy or other simple sugars to treat mild
hypoglycemia. If he has frequent or severe
episodes, instruct him to consult with his
prescriber.
• Inform patient that he may be nervous and
irritable while taking ketoprofen.
• Instruct patient to notify prescriber immediately if he develops a rash, decreased urine
output, dark yellow or brown urine, or signs
of fluid retention, including swelling of extremities and unexplained rapid weight gain.
• Caution pregnant patient not to take
NSAIDs such as ketoprofen during the last
trimester because they may cause premature
closure of the ductus arteriosus.
• Explain that ketoprofen may increase the
risk of serious adverse cardiovascular reactions; urge patient to seek immediate medical attention if signs or symptoms arise,
such as chest pain, shortness of breath,
weakness, and slurring of speech.
• Explain that ketoprofen may increase the
risk of serious adverse GI reactions; stress
the importance of seeking immediate medical
attention for such signs and symptoms as
epigastric or abdominal pain, indigestion,
black or tarry stools, or vomiting blood or
material that looks like coffee grounds.
• Alert patient to rare but serious skin reactions. Urge him to seek immediate medical
attention for rash, blisters, itching, fever, or
other indications of hypersensitivity.

ketorolac tromethamine

Toradol

Class and Category

Chemical class: Acetic acid derivative
Therapeutic class: Analgesic, anti-
inflammatory
Pregnancy category: C

Indications and Dosages

➤ *To treat moderate to severe pain*
TABLETS
Adults ages 16 to 64. *Initial:* 20 mg as a single dose, followed by 10 mg every 4 to 6 hr
p.r.n., up to 4 times a day. *Maximum:* 40 mg
daily for no more than 5 days.

DOSAGE ADJUSTMENT For patients weighing
less than 50 kg, elderly patients, and patients
with impaired renal function, initial dose reduced to 10 mg.
I.M. INJECTION
Adults ages 16 to 64. *Initial:* 60 mg as a
single dose, followed by oral ketorolac if
needed; or 30 mg every 6 hr p.r.n. *Maximum:*
120 mg daily for no more than 5 days.
DOSAGE ADJUSTMENT For patients weighing
less than 50 kg, elderly patients, and patients
with impaired renal function, initial dose
reduced to 30 mg, followed by oral ketorolac
if needed; or 15 mg every 6 hr p.r.n., up to
maximum of 60 mg daily for no more than
5 days.
I.V. INJECTION
Adults ages 16 to 64. *Initial:* 30 mg as a single
dose, followed by oral ketorolac if needed; or
30 mg every 6 hr p.r.n. *Maximum:* 120 mg
daily for no more than 5 days.
DOSAGE ADJUSTMENT For patients weighing
less than 50 kg, elderly patients, and patients
with impaired renal function, initial dose
reduced to 15 mg, followed by oral ketorolac
if needed; or 15 mg every 6 hr p.r.n., up to
maximum of 60 mg daily for no more than
5 days.

Route	Onset	Peak	Duration
P.O.	30 to 60 min	2 to 3 hr	5 to 6 hr
I.M., I.V.	30 to 60 min	1 to 2 hr	4 to 6 hr

Mechanism of Action

Blocks cyclooxygenase, an enzyme needed
to synthesize prostaglandins. Prostaglandins mediate the inflammatory response
and cause local vasodilation, swelling,
and pain. They also promote pain transmission from the periphery to the spinal
cord. By blocking cyclooxygenase and inhibiting prostaglandins, this NSAID reduces inflammation and relieves pain.

Contraindications

Advanced renal impairment or risk of renal
impairment due to volume depletion; before
or during surgery if hemostasis is critical;
breastfeeding; cerebrovascular bleeding; concurrent use of aspirin or other salicylates,
other NSAIDs, or probenecid; hemorrhagic

diathesis; history of GI bleeding, GI perforation, or peptic ulcer disease; hemophilia or other bleeding problems, including coagulation or platelet function disorders; hypersensitivity to ketorolac tromethamine, aspirin, other NSAIDs, or their components; incomplete hemostasis; labor and delivery; treatment of perioperative pain during coronary artery bypass graft surgery

Interactions
DRUGS
ACE inhibitors, angiotensin II receptor antagonists: Increased risk of renal impairment; decreased effectiveness of these drugs
acetaminophen, gold compounds: Increased risk of adverse renal effects
amphotericin, penicillamine, and other nephrotoxic drugs: Increased risk or severity of adverse renal reactions
antihypertensives, diuretics: Possibly reduced effects of these drugs
aspirin and other salicylates, other NSAIDs: Additive toxicity
cefamandole, cefoperazone, cefotetan: Possibly hypoprothrombinemia
corticosteroids, potassium supplements: Increased risk of gastric ulcers or hemorrhage
furosemide: Decreased effects of furosemide
heparin, oral anticoagulants, platelet aggregation inhibitors, thrombolytics: Increased risk of GI bleeding and I.M. hematoma formation
lithium: Possibly increased blood lithium level and increased risk of lithium toxicity
methotrexate: Possibly methotrexate toxicity
nondepolarizing muscle relaxants: Increased risk of apnea
pentoxifylline, selective serotonin reuptake inhibitors: Increased risk of bleeding
plicamycin, valproic acid: Possibly hypoprothrombinemia and increased risk of bleeding
probenecid: Decreased elimination of ketorolac, increased risk of adverse effects
ACTIVITIES
alcohol use: Increased risk of adverse GI effects

Adverse Reactions
CNS: Aseptic meningitis, cerebral hemorrhage, coma, dizziness, drowsiness, headache, psychosis, seizures, stroke
CV: Edema, fluid retention, hypertension
EENT: Laryngeal edema, stomatitis
ENDO: Hyperglycemia

GI: Abdominal pain; acute pancreatitis; bloating; constipation; diarrhea; diverticulitis; flatulence; GI bleeding, perforation, or ulceration; hepatitis; hepatic failure; jaundice; indigestion; nausea; perforation of stomach or intestines; vomiting; worsening of inflammatory bowel disease
GU: Interstitial nephritis, renal failure, urine retention
HEME: Agranulocytosis, anemia, aplastic or hemolytic anemia, eosinophilia, leukopenia, lymphadenopathy, pancytopenia, thrombocytopenia
RESP: Bronchospasm, pneumonia, respiratory depression
SKIN: Diaphoresis, erythema multiforme, exfoliative dermatitis, photosensitivity, pruritus, rash, Stevens-Johnson syndrome, toxic epidermal necrolysis, urticaria
Other: Anaphylaxis, angioedema, hyperkalemia, hyponatremia, injection site pain, sepsis, unusual weight gain

Nursing Considerations
•Read ketorolac label carefully. Don't use I.M. form for I.V. route. Be aware that ketorolac isn't for intrathecal or epidural use.
•Inject I.M. ketorolac slowly, deep into a large muscle mass. Monitor site for bleeding, bruising, or hematoma.
•Administer I.V. injection over at least 15 seconds.
•Notify prescriber if pain relief is inadequate or if breakthrough pain occurs between doses because supplemental doses of an opioid analgesic may be required.
•**WARNING** Monitor liver function test results. If elevated levels persist or worsen, notify prescriber and expect to stop drug, as ordered, to prevent hepatic impairment.
•**WARNING** Monitor patients with a history of peripheral edema, heart failure, or hypertension for adequate fluid balance because drug can promote fluid retention and worsen these conditions. Assess patient for dyspnea, edema, unexplained rapid weight gain, and decreased activity tolerance. Notify prescriber if such symptoms develop.
•Use ketorolac with extreme caution in patients with a history of ulcer disease or prior gastrointestinal bleeding because NSAIDs like ketorolac increases risk of GI bleeding and ulceration. Be aware that use of ketorolac in these patients should be for the short-

J
K
L

est length of time possible.

•Be aware that serious GI tract ulceration and bleeding as well as perforation of stomach or intestines can occur without warning or symptoms. Elderly patients are at greater risk. To minimize this risk, give drug with food. If GI distress occurs, withhold drug and notify prescriber immediately.

•Monitor patient with a history of inflammatory bowel disease, such as ulcerative colitis or Crohn's disease, because ketorolac may worsen these conditions.

•Use ketorolac cautiously in patients with hypertension and monitor blood pressure closely throughout therapy because drug can lead to the onset of hypertension or worsen existing hypertension.

•WARNING Monitor patient closely for thrombotic events including MI and stroke because use of NSAIDs such as ketorolac increases patient's risk.

•Monitor patient—especially if he's elderly for less common but serious adverse GI reactions, including anorexia, constipation, diverticulitis, dysphagia, esophagitis, gastritis, gastroenteritis, gastroesophageal reflux disease, hemorrhoids, hiatal hernia, melena, stomatitis, and vomiting.

•Monitor liver function test results because in rare cases, elevations may progress to severe hepatic reactions, including fatal hepatitis, liver necrosis, and hepatic failure.

•Monitor BUN and serum creatinine levels in patients with heart failure, existing impaired renal function, or hepatic dysfunction; those who are taking diuretics or ACE inhibitors; and the elderly because drug may cause renal failure.

•Monitor CBC for decreased hemoglobin and hematocrit because drug may worsen anemia.

•WARNING In patient who has bone marrow suppression or is receiving antineoplastic drug therapy, monitor laboratory results (including WBC) and assess for signs and symptoms of infection because ketorolac has antiinflammatory and antipyretic actions that may mask signs and symptoms, such as fever and pain.

•Assess patient's skin routinely for evidence of rash or other hypersensitivity reactions because ketorolac is a NSAID and may cause serious skin reactions without warning even in patients with no history of NSAID hyper-

sensitivity. Discontinue drug at first sign of reaction, and notify prescriber.

PATIENT TEACHING

•Instruct patient to take ketorolac tablets with a meal, a snack, or an antacid to prevent stomach upset. Advise him to take ketorolac with a full glass of water and to stay upright for at least 15 minutes after taking it.

•Advise patient not to use aspirin, other salicylates, or other NSAIDs while taking ketorolac without consulting prescriber. Encourage patient to limit use of acetaminophen to only a few days during ketorolac therapy and to notify prescriber of use.

•Instruct him to notify prescriber immediately if he experiences blood in urine, easy bruising, itching, rash, swelling, or yellow eyes or skin.

•Caution pregnant patient that NSAIDs like ketolac should not be taken during her last trimester because drug may cause premature closure of the ductus arteriosus.

•Explain that ketorolac may increase the risk of serious adverse cardiovascular reactions; urge patient to seek immediate medical attention if signs or symptoms such as chest pain, shortness of breath, weakness, and slurring of speech arise.

•Tell patient that ketorolac may also increase the risk of serious adverse gastrointestinal reactions; stress importance of seeking immediate medical attention if signs or symptoms such as epigastric or abdominal pain, indigestion, black tarry stools, and vomiting blood or coffee ground material occurs.

•Alert patient to the possibility of serious skin reactions, although rare, occurring with ketorolac therapy. Urge patient to seek immediate medical attention if signs or symptoms such as a rash, blisters, fever, or other signs of hypersensitivity such as itching occurs.

•Caution patient to avoid hazardous activities until drug's CNS effects are known.

•Urge patient to avoid alcohol while taking drug.

•Encourage patient to have dental procedures performed before starting drug therapy because of increased risk of bleeding.

•Teach patient proper oral hygiene measures, and encourage him to use a soft-bristled toothbrush while taking ketorolac.

labetalol hydrochloride

Normodyne, Trandate

Class and Category

Chemical class: Benzamine derivative
Therapeutic class: Antihypertensive
Pregnancy category: C

Indications and Dosages

➤ *To manage hypertension*

TABLETS

Adults. *Initial:* 100 mg b.i.d., increased by 100 mg b.i.d. as needed and tolerated every 2 to 3 days. *Maintenance:* 200 to 400 mg b.i.d. For severe hypertension, 1.2 to 2.4 g daily in divided doses b.i.d. or t.i.d.

➤ *To manage severe hypertension and treat hypertensive emergencies*

I.V. INFUSION

Adults. 200 mg diluted in 160 ml of D_5W and infused at 2 mg/min until desired response occurs.

I.V. INJECTION

Adults. 20 mg given over 2 min; additional doses given in increments of 40 to 80 mg every 10 min as indicated until desired response occurs. *Maximum:* 300 mg.

Route	Onset	Peak	Duration
P.O.	20 min to 2 hr	1 to 4 hr	8 to 24 hr
I.V.	2 to 5 min	5 to 15 min	2 to 4 hr

Mechanism of Action

Selectively blocks alpha$_1$ and beta$_2$ receptors in vascular smooth muscle and beta$_1$ receptors in the heart to reduce peripheral vascular resistance and blood pressure. Potent beta blockade prevents reflex tachycardia, which commonly occurs when alpha blockers reduce resting heart rate, cardiac output, or stroke volume.

Incompatibilities

Don't dilute labetalol in sodium bicarbonate solution or administer through same I.V. line as alkaline drugs, such as furosemide; doing so may cause white precipitate to form.

Contraindications

Asthma, cardiogenic shock, heart failure, hypersensitivity to labetalol or its components, second- or third-degree heart block, severe bradycardia

Interactions

DRUGS

allergen immunotherapy, allergenic extracts for skin testing: Increased risk of serious systemic reaction or anaphylaxis
beta blockers, digoxin: Increased risk of bradycardia
calcium channel blockers, clonidine, diazoxide, guanabenz, reserpine: Possibly hypotension
cimetidine: Possibly increased labetalol effects
estrogens, NSAIDs: Possibly reduced antihypertensive effect of labetalol
general anesthetics: Increased risk of hypotension and myocardial depression
insulin, oral antidiabetic drugs: Increased risk of hyperglycemia
nitroglycerin: Possibly hypertension
phenoxybenzamine, phentolamine: Possibly additive alpha$_1$-blocking effects
sympathomimetics with alpha- and beta-adrenergic effects (such as pseudoephedrine): Possibly hypertension, excessive bradycardia, or heart block
xanthines (aminophylline and theophylline): Possibly decreased therapeutic effects of both drugs

FOODS

all food: Increased blood labetalol level

ACTIVITIES

alcohol use: Increased labetalol effects

Adverse Reactions

CNS: Anxiety, confusion, depression, dizziness, drowsiness, fatigue, paresthesia, syncope, vertigo, weakness, yawning
CV: Bradycardia, chest pain, edema, heart block, heart failure, hypotension, orthostatic hypotension, ventricular arrhythmias
EENT: Nasal congestion, taste perversion
GI: Elevated liver function test results, hepatic necrosis, hepatitis, indigestion, nausea, vomiting
GU: Ejaculation failure, impotence
RESP: Dyspnea, wheezing
SKIN: Jaundice, pruritus, rash, scalp tingling

Nursing Considerations

•During I.V. labetalol administration, moni-

J
K
L

tor blood pressure according to facility policy, usually every 5 minutes for 30 minutes, then every 30 minutes for 2 hours, and then every hour for 6 hours.
•Keep patient in supine position for 3 hours after I.V. administration.
•**WARNING** Be aware that labetalol masks common signs of shock.
•Monitor blood glucose level in diabetic patient because labetalol may conceal symptoms of hypoglycemia.
•Be aware that stopping labetalol tablets abruptly after long-term therapy could result in angina, MI, or ventricular arrhythmias. Expect to taper dosage over 2 weeks while monitoring response.

PATIENT TEACHING
•Advise patient to report confusion, difficulty breathing, rash, slow pulse, and swelling in arms or legs.
•Caution patient not to·discontinue drug abruptly because doing so could cause angina and rebound hypertension.
•Suggest that patient minimize the effects of orthostatic hypotension by rising slowly, avoiding sudden position changes, and taking labetalol at bedtime, if approved by prescriber.
•Instruct diabetic patient to monitor blood glucose level frequently and to be alert for signs of hypoglycemia.
•Inform patient that scalp tingling may occur during the early phase of treatment but is transient.
•Urge patient to avoid alcohol during labetalol therapy.

lacosamide

Vimpat

Class and Category

Chemical class: Functionalized amino acid
Therapeutic class: Anticonvulsant
Pregnancy category: C

Indications and Dosages

➤ *As adjunct to treat partial-onset seizures in patients with epilepsy*

TABLETS
Adults and adolescents age 17 and over. *Initial:* 50 mg b.i.d., increased by 100 mg/day at weekly intervals based on response and tolerance. *Maintenance:* 200 to 400 mg daily.

I.V. INFUSION
Adults and adolescents age 17 and over. *Initial:* 50 mg infused over 30 to 60 min b.i.d., increased by 100 mg/day at weekly intervals. *Maintenance:* 200 to 400 mg daily.
DOSAGE ADJUSTMENT For patients with creatinine clearance of 30 ml/min/1.73 m^2 or less, maximum is 300 mg daily.

Mechanism of Action
May selectively inactivate voltage-gated sodium channels, which prevents seizure activity by stabilizing hyperexcitable neuronal membranes and inhibiting repetitive neuronal firing in the brain.

Contraindications

Hypersensitivity to lacosamide and its components

Interactions

DRUGS
drugs that may prolong the QT interval: Possibly further QT-interval prolongation

Adverse Reactions

CNS: Asthenia, ataxia, attention deficit, cerebellar syndrome, confusion, depression, dizziness, feeling drunk, fever, headache, hypoaesthesia, impaired balance, irritability, memory impairment, mood alteration, paresthesia, somnolence, suicidal ideation, tremor, vertigo
CV: Palpitations, prolonged QT interval
EENT: Blurred vision, diplopia, dry mouth, nystagmus, oral hypoaesthesia, tinnitus
GI: Constipation, diarrhea, dyspepsia, nausea, vomiting
HEME: Anemia, neutropenia
MS: Dysarthria, muscle spasms
SKIN: Pruritus, rash
Other: Delayed multi-organ hypersensitivity reaction; injection site pain, irritation, and erythemia

Nursing Considerations

•Use cautiously in patients with conduction problems (such as AV block and sick sinus syndrome) and no pacemaker in place or in patients with severe cardiac disease (such as myocardial ischemia or heart failure) because lacosamide may affect conduction.
•Use cautiously in patients with diabetic

neuropathy or cardiovascular disease because drug may predispose them to atrial fibrillation or flutter.

•Watch patient closely for suicidal tendencies, particularly when therapy starts and dosage changes, because depression may worsen temporarily during these times and lead to suicidal ideation.

•Be aware that lacosamide therapy should be discontinued gradually over at least 1 week to minimize seizure frequency.

•Monitor patient closely for hypersensitivity reactions to lacosamide, such as rash, pruritus, and more than one organ abnormality, such as elevated liver enzymes and myocarditis or pancreatitis.

PATIENT TEACHING

•Urge family or caregiver to watch patient closely for suicidal tendencies, especially when therapy starts or dosage changes.

•Caution patient to avoid hazardous activities until drug's CNS effects are known.

•Encourage patient to carry medical identification that indicates her diagnosis and drug therapy.

lactulose

Acilac (CAN), Cephulac, Cholac, Chronulac, Constilac, Constulose, Duphalac, Enulose, Evalose, Heptalac, Lactulax (CAN), Laxilose (CAN), PMS-Lactulose (CAN), Portalac

Class and Category

Chemical: Synthetic disaccharide sugar
Therapeutic: Ammonia reducer, laxative
Pregnancy category: B

Indications and Dosages

➤ *To treat constipation*

POWDER, SYRUP

Adults. *Initial:* 10 to 20 g daily, increased p.r.n. *Maximum:* 40 g daily.

➤ *To prevent and treat hepatic encephalopathy*

POWDER, SYRUP

Adults. *Initial:* 20 to 30 g t.i.d. or q.i.d. until two or three soft stools occur daily. *Usual:* 60 to 100 g daily in divided doses. For acute episodes, 20 to 30 g every 2 hr initially to achieve rapid laxative effect and then reduced to usual dosage.

RETENTION ENEMA

Adults. 200 g (300 ml) diluted in 700 ml of water or normal saline solution and given every 4 to 6 hr, as needed.

Route	Onset	Peak	Duration
P.O.	24 to 48 hr	Unknown	Unknown

Mechanism of Action

Arrives unchanged in the colon, where it breaks down into lactic acid and small amounts of formic and acetic acids, acidifying fecal contents. Acidification leads to increased osmotic pressure in the colon, which, in turn, increases stool water content and softens stool.

Also, lactulose makes the intestinal contents more acidic than blood. This prevents ammonia diffusion from the intestines into the blood, as occurs in hepatic encephalopathy. The trapped ammonia is converted into ammonia ions and, by lactulose's cathartic effect, is expelled in the feces (with other nitrogenous wastes).

Contraindications

Hypersensitivity to lactulose or its components, low-galactose diet

Interactions

DRUGS

antacids, antibiotics (especially oral neomycin), other laxatives: Decreased effectiveness of lactulose

Adverse Reactions

GI: Abdominal cramps and distention, diarrhea, flatulence
ENDO: Hyperglycemia
Other: Hypernatremia, hypokalemia, hypovolemia

Nursing Considerations

•When giving lactulose by retention enema, use a rectal tube with a balloon to help patient retain enema for 30 to 60 minutes. If not retained for at least 30 minutes, repeat dose. Be sure to deflate balloon and remove rectal tube after completing administration.

•Expect to periodically check serum electrolyte levels of elderly or debilitated patient who uses oral drug longer than 6 months.

•Monitor blood ammonia level in patient

with hepatic encephalopathy. Also monitor for dehydration, hypernatremia, and hypokalemia when giving higher lactulose doses to treat this condition.
•Monitor diabetic patient for hyperglycemia because lactulose contains galactose and lactose.
•Plan to replace fluids if frequent bowel movements cause hypovolemia.

PATIENT TEACHING
•Advise patient to take lactulose with food or to dilute it with juice to minimize sweet taste.
•Direct patient not to use other laxatives while taking lactulose.
•Instruct patient to report abdominal distention or severe diarrhea.
•Advise diabetic patient to check blood glucose level often and to report hyperglycemia.
•Instruct patient to increase fluid intake if frequent bowel movements occur.
•Teach patient with chronic constipation the importance of exercising, increasing fiber in her diet, and increasing fluid intake.
•Inform patient that because oral lactulose must reach the colon to work, bowel movement may not occur for 24 to 48 hours after taking drug.

lamotrigine

Lamictal

Class and Category
Chemical class: Phenyltriazine
Therapeutic class: Anticonvulsant
Pregnancy category: C

Indications and Dosages
➤ *As adjunct to treat partial seizures; to treat generalized seizures of Lennox-Gastaut syndrome; to treat primary generalized tonic-clonic seizures*

CHEWABLE TABLETS, TABLETS
Adults and children age 12 and over taking valproate. 25 mg every other day for 2 wk, followed by 25 mg once daily for 2 wk. Increased by 25 to 50 mg every 1 to 2 wk, if needed. *Maintenance:* 100 to 400 mg daily.
Children ages 2 to 12 taking valproate. 0.15 mg/kg daily as a single dose or in divided doses b.i.d. for 2 wk and then 0.3 mg/kg daily as a single dose or in divided doses b.i.d. for next 2 wk. Increased by 0.3 mg/kg every 1 to 2 wk, if needed, to reach mainte-

nance dosage. *Maintenance:* 1 to 5 mg/kg daily as a single dose or in divided doses b.i.d. *Maximum:* 200 mg daily.
Adults and children age 12 and over taking an antiepileptic drug other than carbamazepine, phenytoin, phenobarbital, primidone, or valproate. 25 mg once daily for 2 wk, followed by 50 mg once daily for 2 wk. Increased by 50 mg every 1 to 2 wk, if needed. *Maintenance:* 225 to 375 mg daily in 2 divided doses b.i.d. *Maximum:* 400 mg daily.
Children ages 2 to 12 taking an an antiepileptic drug other than carbamazepine, phenytoin, phenobarbital, primidone, or valproate. 0.3 mg/kg daily in 1 or 2 divided doses for 2 wk; followed by 0.6 mg/kg daily in 2 divided doses for 2 wk. Increased by 0.6 mg/kg daily every 1 to 2 wk, if needed. *Maintenance:* 4.5 to 7.5 mg/kg daily in 2 divided doses. *Maximum:* 300 mg daily
Adults and children age 12 and over taking carbamazepine, phenytoin, phenobarbital, or primidone but not valproate. 50 mg once daily for 2 wk and then 100 mg daily in divided doses b.i.d. for 2 wk. Increased by 100 mg every 1 to 2 wk, if needed. *Maintenance:* 300 to 500 mg daily in divided doses b.i.d. *Maximum:* 700 mg daily in divided doses b.i.d.
Children ages 2 to 12 taking carbamazepine, phenytoin, phenobarbital, or primidone but not valproate. 0.6 mg/kg daily in divided doses b.i.d. for 2 wk and then 1.2 mg/kg daily in divided doses b.i.d. for 2 wk. Increased by 1.2 mg/kg every 1 to 2 wk, if needed to reach maintenance dosage. *Maintenance:* 5 to 15 mg/kg daily in divided doses b.i.d. *Maximum:* 400 mg daily.

➤ *To treat partial seizures after conversion from carbamazepine, phenytoin, phenobarbital, primidone, or valproate*

CHEWABLE TABLETS, TABLETS
Adults and adolescents age 16 and over converting from carbamazepine, phenytoin, phenobarbital, or primidone. 50 mg once daily for 2 wk, followed by 100 mg once daily for next 2 wk. Increased by 100 mg daily every 1 to 2 wk (while continuing to take carbamaze-pine, phenytoin, phenobarbital, or primidone), until usual maintenance dosage—500 mg daily in divided doses b.i.d.—is achieved. Then carbamazepine, phenytoin,

phenobarbital, or primidone dosage tapered in 20% increments weekly over 4 wk and then discontinued.

Adults and adolescents age 16 and over converting from valproate. 25 mg every other day for 2 wk followed by 25 mg once daily for 2 wk. Then increased by 25 to 50 mg daily every 1 to 2 wk until dosage of 200 mg daily is achieved. At this time valproate dosage decreased to 500 mg daily by decrements no greater than 500 mg daily every wk and then maintained at 500 mg daily for 1 wk. After completion of week, lamotrigine dosage increased to 300 mg daily and maintained for 1 wk while valproate dosage decreased to 250 mg daily and maintained for 1 wk. Then lamotrigine dosage increased by 100 mg daily every wk to achieve maintenance dose of 500 mg daily. Once achieved, valproate therapy is discontinued.

➤ As maintenance therapy for bipolar 1 disorder to delay occurrence of mood episodes (depression, mania, hypomania, mixed episodes)

CHEWABLE TABLETS, TABLETS
Adults not taking carbamazepine, phenytoin, phenobarbital, primidone, rifampin, or valproate. 25 mg once daily for 2 wk, followed by 50 mg once daily for 2 wk, followed by 100 mg once daily for 1 wk and then increased to 200 mg daily as maintenance dose. *Maximum:* 200 mg daily.

Adults taking valproate. 25 mg every other day for 2 wk, followed by 25 mg once daily for 2 wk, followed by 50 mg once daily for 1 wk, and then increased to 100 mg once daily as maintenance dose.

Adults taking carbamazepine, phenytoin, phenobarbital, primidone, or rifampin, but not valproate. 50 mg once daily for 2 wk followed by 100 mg once daily in divided doses for 2 wk, followed by 200 mg once daily in divided doses for 1 wk and then increased to 300 mg daily in divided doses for 1 wk and then increased to 400 mg daily in divided doses as maintenance dose.

DOSAGE ADJUSTMENT For patient starting or stopping estrogen-containing oral contraceptives, lamotrigine dosage may need to be adjusted on individual basis. For patient with moderate to severe liver impairment without ascites, dosage reduced by 25%. For patient with severe liver impairment with ascites, dosage reduced by 50%.

Route	Onset	Peak	Duration
P.O.	Days to wks	Unknown	Unknown

Mechanism of Action

May stabilize neuron membranes by blocking their sodium channels and inhibiting release of excitatory neurotransmitters, such as glutamate and aspartate, through these channels. By blocking the release of neurotransmitters, lamotrigine inhibits the spread of seizure activity in the brain and reduces seizure frequency.

Contraindications

Hypersensitivity to lamotrigine or its components

Interactions
DRUGS
acetaminophen (long-term use): Possibly decreased blood lamotrigine level
carbamazepine: Decreased blood lamotrigine level; possibly increased risk of dizziness, diplopia, ataxia, and blurred vision
folate inhibitors, such as co-trimoxazole and methotrexate: Increased blood lamotrigine level
oral contraceptives: Decreased blood lamotrigine level during 3 weeks of active hormonal therapy and increased blood lamotrigine level during 1 week of inactive hormonal therapy; possibly reduced effectiveness of oral contraceptives
oxcarbazepine: Possibly increased risk of headache, dizziness, nausea, and somnolence
phenobarbital, phenytoin, primidone: Decreased blood lamotrigine level, possibly increased CNS depression
topiramate: Increased blood topiramate level
valproic acid: Increased blood lamotrigine level, decreased lamotrigine clearance, decreased blood valproic acid level
ACTIVITIES
alcohol use: Possibly increased CNS depression

Adverse Reactions

CNS: Amnesia, anxiety, ataxia, confusion, depression, dizziness, drowsiness, emotional lability, fever, headache, increased seizure

J
K
L

activity, lack of coordination, suicidal thoughts

CV: Chest pain

EENT: Blurred vision, diplopia, dry mouth, nystagmus

GI: Abdominal pain, anorexia, constipation, diarrhea, hepatic failure, vomiting

HEME: Anemia, aplastic anemia, disseminated intravascular coagulation, eosinophilia, leukopenia, neutropenia, pancytopenia, pure red cell aplasia, thrombocytopenia

SKIN: Petechiae, photosensitivity, pruritus, rash, Stevens-Johnson syndrome, toxic epidermal necrolysis

Other: Acute multiorgan failure, angioedema, flulike symptoms, lymphadenopathy

Nursing Considerations

• Use cautiously in patients with illnesses that could affect metabolism or elimination of lamotrigine, such as renal, hepatic, or cardiac functional impairment.

• **WARNING** Lamotrigine may cause potentially life-threatening rash. Notify prescriber at first sign, and expect to discontinue drug. Be aware that lamotrigine therapy shouldn't be restarted after rash subsides.

• Monitor patient for adverse reactions, especially suicidal thoughts, at start of therapy and with each dosage increase.

• Monitor patient for seizure activity during lamotrigine therapy.

• Be aware that stopping lamotrigine abruptly may increase patient's seizure activity. Expect to taper dosage over at least 2 weeks, even for treatment of bipolar disorder.

PATIENT TEACHING

• Advise patient to take lamotrigine exactly as prescribed and not to stop drug abruptly because seizure activity may increase.

• Advise patient to notify prescriber immediately if rash occurs.

• Instruct patient to report increased seizure activity, vision changes, and vomiting.

• Caution patient to avoid potentially hazardous activities until drug's CNS effects are known.

• Advise patient to avoid direct sunlight and to wear protective clothing to minimize the risk of photosensitivity.

• Instruct patient to wear or carry medical identification stating that she takes an anticonvulsant.

• Caution patient or caregiver about possibility of suicidal thoughts, especially when therapy begins or dosage changes.

• Tell female patient to notify prescriber if she becomes pregnant, is considering pregnancy, or starts or stops an oral hormonal contraceptive or other female hormonal preparation.

lanreotide

Somatulin Depot

Class and Category

Chemical class: Somatostatin analog
Therapeutic class: Growth inhibitor
Pregnancy category: C

Indications and Dosages

➤ *To treat acromegaly in patients who have had an inadequate response to or cannot be treated with surgery or radiation*

SUBCUTANEOUS INJECTION

Adults. *Initial:* 90 mg every 4 wk for 3 mo; then dosage adjusted according to growth hormone (GH) level. If GH level is less than 1 nanogram/ml, dosage reduced to 60 mg every 4 wk. If GH level is 1 to 2.5 nanograms/ml, dosage is 90 mg every 4 wk. If GH level is above 2.5 nanograms/ml, dosage is increased to 120 mg every 4 wk.

DOSAGE ADJUSTMENT For patient with moderate to severe renal or hepatic failure, initial dose reduced to 60 mg every 4 wk for 3 mo; then adjusted according to GH level.

Mechanism of Action

Reduces growth hormone (GH) and insulin growth factor-1 levels, allowing for normalization of these hormones in patients with acromegaly. An octapeptide analog of natural somatostatin, lanreotide has a high affinity for human somatostatin receptors 2 and 5. Activity at these receptors may be responsible for GH inhibition.

Contraindications

Hypersensitivity to lanreotide or its components

Interactions
DRUGS
beta blockers, calcium channel blockers: Additive depressive effects on heart rate
bromocriptine: Possibly increased action of bromocriptine
cyclosporine: Possibly decreased cyclosporine effectiveness
drugs metabolized by the liver, quinidine, terfenadine: Possibly increased blood levels of these drugs
insulin, oral antidiabetic drugs: Possibly decreased effectiveness of these drugs
oral drugs: Possibly decreased absorption of these drugs

Adverse Reactions
CNS: Headache
CV: Bradycardia, hypertension
ENDO: Hyperglycemia, hypoglycemia
GI: Abdominal pain, cholelithiasis, constipation, diarrhea, flatulence, loose stools, nausea, vomiting
HEME: Anemia
MS: Arthralgia
SKIN: Erythema, pruritus
Other: Injection site reactions (induration, pain, pruritus, redness, swelling), weight loss

Nursing Considerations
• Check patient's blood glucose level before starting lanreotide therapy and whenever dosage changes because drug may cause hypoglycemia or hyperglycemia.
• Inject drug deep into subcutaneous tissue of upper, outer quadrant of buttock. Do not fold the skin. Insert needle perpendicular to the skin, rapidly and to its full length. Alternate between left and right buttocks.
• If patient has underlying cardiovascular disease, watch for changes in heart rate and blood pressure because drug may cause bradycardia or hypertension.
• Monitor GH and insulin growth factor-1 levels, as ordered, to assess drug effects.
PATIENT TEACHING
• Inform patient that lanreotide will be given as a subcutaneous injection every 4 weeks and that it may cause discomfort at the site.
• Tell patient that periodic blood tests will be needed to monitor lanreotide's effectiveness.
• Instruct diabetic patient to monitor blood glucose level closely.

lansoprazole
Prevacid, Prevacid I.V., Prevacid SoluTab

dexlansoprazole
Kapidex

Class and Category
Chemical class: Substituted benzimidazole
Therapeutic class: Antisecretory, antiulcer
Pregnancy category: B

Indications and Dosages
➤ *To treat duodenal ulcers and maintain healed duodenal ulcers*
DELAYED-RELEASE CAPSULES, DELAYED-RELEASE SUSPENSION, DELAYED-RELEASE ORALLY DISINTEGRATING TABLETS
Adults. 15 to 30 mg daily before morning meal for 4 wk. *Maximum:* 30 mg daily.

➤ *To treat gastric ulcers*
DELAYED-RELEASE CAPSULES, DELAYED-RELEASE SUSPENSION, DELAYED-RELEASE ORALLY DISINTEGRATING TABLETS
Adults. 15 to 30 mg daily before morning meal for up to 8 wk.

➤ *To treat gastroesophageal reflux disease*
DELAYED-RELEASE CAPSULES, DELAYED-RELEASE SUSPENSION, DELAYED-RELEASE ORALLY DISINTEGRATING TABLETS
Adults. 15 mg daily before morning meal for up to 8 wk.

➤ *To treat non-erosive gastroesophageal reflux disease*
CAPSULES (DEXLANSOPRAZOLE)
Adults. 30 mg once daily for 4 wk.

➤ *To heal all grades of erosive esophagitis*
CAPSULES (DEXLANSOPRAZOLE)
Adults. 60 mg once daily for up to 8 wk.

➤ *To maintain healed erosive esophagitis*
CAPSULES (DEXLANSOPRAZOLE)
Adults. 30 mg once daily.

➤ *To treat erosive esophagitis*
DELAYED-RELEASE CAPSULES, DELAYED-RELEASE SUSPENSION, DELAYED-RELEASE ORALLY DISINTEGRATING TABLETS
Adults. *Initial:* 30 mg daily before morning meal for up to 8 wk. Continued another 8 wk if indicated. *Maintenance:* 15 mg daily.

➤ *To treat erosive esophagitis short-term (up to 7 days) in patients unable to take oral medication*

J
K
L

I.V. INFUSION
Adults. 30 mg daily infused over 30 min for up to 7 days.

➤ *To treat pathological hypersecretory conditions, such as Zollinger-Ellison syndrome*
DELAYED-RELEASE CAPSULES, DELAYED-RELEASE SUSPENSION, DELAYED-RELEASE ORALLY DISINTEGRATING TABLETS
Adults. *Initial:* 60 mg daily before morning meal, increased as needed according to patient's condition. Doses exceeding 120 mg/day administered in divided doses. *Maximum:* 180 mg daily.

➤ *To eradicate* Helicobacter pylori *and reduce risk of duodenal ulcer recurrence*
DELAYED-RELEASE CAPSULES, DELAYED-RELEASE SUSPENSION, DELAYED-RELEASE ORALLY DISINTEGRATING TABLETS
Adults. 30 mg plus 1 g of amoxicillin and 500 mg of clarithromycin every 12 hr before meals for 10 to 14 days. Or, 30 mg plus 1 g of amoxicillin t.i.d. before meals for 14 days.

➤ *To treat symptomatic pediatric gastroesophageal reflux disease*
DELAYED-RELEASE CAPSULES, DELAYED-RELEASE SUSPENSION, DELAYED-RELEASE ORALLY DISINTEGRATING TABLETS
Children ages 12 to 17. 15 mg daily for up to 8 wk.
Children ages 1 to 11 weighing 30 kg (66 lb) or less. 15 mg daily for up to 12 wk.
Children ages 1 to 11 weighing more than 30 kg. 30 mg daily for up to 12 wk.

➤ *To treat symptomatic pediatric erosive esophagitis*
DELAYED-RELEASE CAPSULES, DELAYED-RELEASE SUSPENSION, DELAYED-RELEASE ORALLY DISINTEGRATING TABLETS
Children ages 12 to 17. 30 mg daily for up to 8 wk.
Children ages 1 to 11 weighing 30 kg (66 lb) or less. 15 mg daily for up to 12 wk.
Children ages 1 to 11 weighing more than 30 kg. 30 mg daily for up to 12 wk.

Route	Onset	Peak	Duration
P.O.	1 to 3 hr	Unknown	Over 24 hr

Incompatibilities

Don't give any other drugs with parenteral lansoprazole, and dilute only with solutions recommended by manufacturer (sterile water for initial reconstitution and normal saline solution, lactated Ringer's solution, or D_5W for further dilution).

Mechanism of Action

Binds to and inactivates the hydrogen-potassium adenosine triphosphate enzyme system (also called the proton pump) in gastric parietal cells. This action blocks the final step of gastric acid production.

Contraindications

Hypersensitivity to lansoprazole or its components

Interactions
DRUGS
ampicillin, digoxin, iron salts, ketoconazole, other drugs that depend on low gastric pH for bioavailability: Inhibited absorption of these drugs
atazanavir: Decreased blood level and possibly reduced effectiveness of atazanavir
sucralfate: Delayed absorption of lansoprazole
theophylline: Slightly decreased blood theophylline level
warfarin: Increased INR and PT with possibly increased risk of serious bleeding

Adverse Reactions
CNS: Dizziness, headache
GI: Abdominal pain, anorexia, diarrhea, elevated liver enzymes, hepatotoxicity, increased appetite, nausea, pancreatitis, pseudomembranous colitis, vomiting
GU: Interstitial nephritis, urine retention
HEME: Agranulocytosis, aplastic anemia, decreased hemoglobin, hemolytic anemia, leukopenia, neutropenia, pancytopenia, thrombocytopenia, thrombotic thrombocytopenic purpura
MS: Arthralgia, myositis
RESP: Upper respiratory tract infection
SKIN: Erythema multiforme, pruritus, rash, Stevens-Johnson syndrome, toxic epidermal necrolysis
Other: Anaphylaxis, hyperkalemia, injection site reaction

Nursing Considerations
• Give patient lansoprazole before meals. Antacids may be given as well, if needed.

•If patient is prescribed capsules and has trouble swallowing them, open capsule and sprinkle granules on applesauce, Ensure, pudding, cottage cheese, yogurt, or strained pears. Don't crush the granules, and have patient swallow the mixture immediately. Alternatively, empty granules into 2 ounces of apple, orange, or tomato juice; mix quickly, and have patient swallow immediately. Then add 2 or more ounces of juice to glass and have patient drink immediately to ensure a full dose.

•For patient prescribed delayed-release orally disintegrating tablets, place tablet on patient's tongue and let it dissolve, with or without water, until patient can swallow particles.

•For patient with nasogastric tube, don't use oral suspension. Instead use capsules or orally disintegrating tablets. For capsule form, open capsule, mix granules in 40 ml of apple juice only, and inject through tube. Then flush tube with apple juice only. For disintegrating tablets, place tablet in syringe and draw up 4 ml (for 15-mg tablet) or 8 ml (for 30-mg tablet) of water. Shake gently, and inject through tube within 15 minutes. Then refill syringe with 5 ml of water, shake gently, and inject through tube.

•For delayed-release oral suspension, empty packet contents into a container with 2 tablespoons of water (no other liquids or foods should be used), stir well, and have patient drink immediately. If any particles remain in container, add more water, stir, and have patient drink again immediately.

•Reconstitute parenteral form by injecting 5 ml of sterile water into 30-mg vial of drug. Mix gently until powder dissolves. Use within 1 hour. After reconstitution, dilute with 50 ml of normal saline solution, lactated Ringer's solution, or D_5W. Give within 12 hours if mixed with D_5W or 24 hours if mixed with normal saline solution or lactated Ringer's solution.

•Give parenteral drug with a filter following manufacturer's guidelines. Change filter every 24 hours. Give as an I.V. infusion over 30 minutes. Flush the line with normal saline solution, lactated Ringer's solution, or D_5W before and after giving lansoprazole.

•Expect to administer lansoprazole with antibiotics because decreased gastric acid secretion helps the antibiotics eradicate *H. pylori*.

•If lansoprazole is given with antibiotics, watch for diarrhea from possible pseudomembranous colitis caused by *Clostridium difficile*. If diarrhea occurs, notify prescriber and expect to withhold lansoprazole and treat with fluids, electrolytes, protein, and an antibiotic effective against *C. difficile*.

PATIENT TEACHING

•Urge patient to take lansoprazole exactly as prescribed, usually before a meal (preferably breakfast) to decrease gastric acid output.

•If patient has trouble swallowing dexlansoprazole capsules, tell her to open them and sprinkle granules on 1 tablespoon of applesauce and swallow immediately. If patient has trouble swallowing lansoprazole capsules, tell her to open them and sprinkle granules on applesauce, Ensure, pudding, cottage cheese, yogurt, or strained pears and to swallow immediately without chewing. Alternatively, she may empty granules into 2 ounces of apple, orange, or tomato juice, mix quickly, and swallow immediately. Tell her to refill glass with 2 or more ounces of juice and drink immediately to ensure a full dose.

•If patient was prescribed delayed-release orally disintegrating tablets, tell her to place the tablet on her tongue, let it dissolve, and then to swallow particles with or without water.

•If patient was prescribed delayed-release oral suspension, tell her to empty contents of packet into a container with 2 tablespoons of water (no other liquids or foods), stir well, and drink immediately. If particles remain in container, she should add water, stir, and drink immediately.

•Inform patient that she may take antacids with lansoprazole.

•Advise patient to report severe headache, or worsening of symptoms immediately to prescriber.

•Urge patient to tell prescriber about diarrhea that's severe or lasts longer than 3 days. Remind patient that watery or bloody stools can occur 2 or more months after antibiotic therapy and can be serious, requiring prompt treatment.

J
K
L

lanthanum carbonate

Fosrenol

Class and Category

Chemical class: Rare earth element
Therapeutic class: Phosphate binder
Pregnancy category: C

Indications and Dosages

➤ *To reduce serum phosphate levels in patients with end-stage renal disease*

TABLETS

Adults. *Initial:* 250 to 500 mg t.i.d. with meals; increased, as needed, by 750 mg daily every 2 to 3 wk until an acceptable serum phosphate level is reached.

Contraindications

Bowel obstruction, hypersensitivity to lanthanum carbonate or any of its components, hypophosphatemia

Adverse Reactions

CNS: Headache
CV: Hypotension
EENT: Rhinitis
ENDO: Hypercalcemia
GI: Abdominal pain, constipation, diarrhea, nausea, vomiting
GU: Dialysis graft occlusion
RESP: Bronchitis

Nursing Considerations

•Use lanthanum carbonate cautiously in patients with acute peptic ulcer, ulcerative colitis, Crohn's disease, or bowel obstruction because drug effects are unknown in these patients.
•Monitor the patient's serum phosphate levels, as ordered, especially during dosage adjustment, to determine effectiveness of lanthanum carbonate therapy. Serum phosphate levels should fall below 6.0 mg/dl.

PATIENT TEACHING

•Instruct patient to take lanthanum carbonate with or immediately after meals.
•Advise patient to chew each tablet thoroughly before swallowing. If patient has trouble chewing tablets, tell her she may crush them.

Mechanism of Action

During digestion, phosphate is released into the upper GI tract (below left) and absorbed into the bloodstream, increasing serum phosphate levels. In patients with end-stage renal disease, however, inefficient phosphate clearance from the blood leads to abnormally elevated levels.

Lanthanum dissociates in the upper GI tract, releasing ions that attach to unbound phosphate to form an insoluble complex (below right). Unabsorbed into the bloodstream, these altered phosphate molecules can't elevate the patient's serum phosphate level.

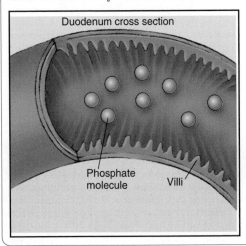

Duodenum cross section

Phosphate molecule   Villi

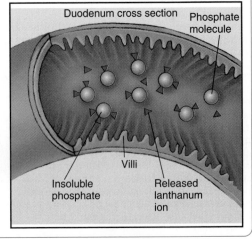

Duodenum cross section   Phosphate molecule

Villi

Insoluble phosphate   Released lanthanum ion

• Urge patient to take drug exactly as prescribed, and explain that it may take weeks to reach a desired serum phosphate level.

leflunomide

Arava

Class and Category

Chemical class: Malonitrilamide immuno-modulator
Therapeutic class: Antirheumatic
Pregnancy category: X

Indications and Dosages

➤ *To relieve symptoms of active rheumatoid arthritis, improve physical function and slow disease progression*

TABLETS

Adults. *Loading:* 100 mg daily for 3 days. *Maintenance:* 20 mg daily, reduced to 10 mg daily if poorly tolerated. *Maximum:* 20 mg/day.

Mechanism of Action

Inhibits dihydroorotate dehydrogenase, the enzyme in the autoimmune process that leads to rheumatoid arthritis. With this action, leflunomide relieves inflammation and prevents alteration of the autoimmune process.

Contraindications

Hypersensitivity to leflunomide or its components, pregnancy

Interactions

DRUGS

activated charcoal, cholestyramine: Decreased blood leflunomide level
methotrexate: Risk of hepatotoxicity
NSAIDs: Possibly impaired NSAID metabolism
rifampin, tolbutamide: Increased blood leflunomide level
vaccines (live-virus): Possibly adverse reactions to vaccines caused by leflunomide-induced immunosuppression

Adverse Reactions

CNS: Anxiety, dizziness, drowsiness, fatigue, fever, headache, paresthesia
CV: Chest pain, hypertension, palpitations, tachycardia

EENT: Blurred vision, conjunctivitis, dry mouth, epistaxis, mouth ulcers, pharyngitis, rhinitis, sinusitis
GI: Abdominal pain, cholestasis, constipation, diarrhea, elevated liver function test results, flatulence, gastritis, gastroenteritis, hepatic failure, hepatitis, nausea, vomiting
GU: UTI
HEME: Agranulocytosis, anemia, pancytopenia, thrombocytopenia
MS: Back pain, synovitis, tendinitis
RESP: Asthma, bronchitis, dyspnea, interstitial lung disease, respiratory tract infection
SKIN: Alopecia (transient), erythematous rash, jaundice, pruritus, urticaria
Other: Sepsis, weight loss

Nursing Considerations

• Leflunomide isn't recommended for patients with severe immunodeficiency, bone marrow dysplasia, or severe, uncontrolled infections because of its immunosuppressant effect.

• Assess liver enzyme (ALT and AST) levels at start of therapy, monthly during first 6 months, and if stable, every 6 to 8 weeks thereafter, as ordered. Expect to stop drug if hepatic dysfunction develops.

• Obtain platelet count, WBC count, and hemoglobin or hematocrit at start of therapy and every 4 to 8 weeks thereafter, as ordered.

• Notify prescriber if patient develops a serious infection because leflunomide may need to be interrupted and cholestyramine or charcoal given to eliminate drug rapidly.

• **WARNING** Monitor patient's respiratory function closely because drug may cause interstitial lung disease that could become life-threatening. If patient develops a cough and dyspnea, notify prescriber; drug may need to be stopped, and patient may need cholestyramine or charcoal to eliminate drug rapidly.

PATIENT TEACHING

• Advise patient that leflunomide doesn't cure arthritis but may relieve its symptoms and improve physical function.

• Inform patient that reversible hair loss may occur.

• Caution female patient of childbearing potential not to become pregnant while taking drug because of the high risk of birth defects.

• Instruct patient to report signs of hepatotoxicity, such as mouth ulcers, unusual bleeding or bruising, and yellow skin or eyes.

J
K
L

• Tell patient to report signs of respiratory dysfunction, such as cough and dyspnea.
• Advise patient to avoid live vaccines during leflunomide therapy.
• Instruct patient to notify prescriber if she develops an infection.

lepirudin

Refludan

Class and Category

Chemical class: Yeast-derived recombinant form of hirudin
Therapeutic class: Anticoagulant
Pregnancy category: B

Indications and Dosages

➤ *To prevent thromboembolic complications in patients with heparin-induced thrombocytopenia and associated thromboembolic disease*

I.V. INFUSION AND INJECTION
Adults. *Initial:* 0.4 mg/kg, but no more than 44 mg, given by bolus over 15 to 20 sec, followed by continuous infusion of 0.15 mg/kg/hr for 2 to 10 days or longer, as indicated. *Maximum:* 0.21 mg/kg/hr.
DOSAGE ADJUSTMENT For patients with renal insufficiency, bolus dose decreased to 0.2 mg/kg and infusion rate adjusted as follows: for creatinine clearance of 45 to 60 ml/min/1.73 m^2, 50% of standard infusion rate; for creatinine clearance of 30 to 44 ml/min/1.73 m^2, 30% of standard infusion rate; for creatinine clearance of 15 to 29 ml/min/1.73 m^2, 15% of standard infusion rate; for clearance of less than 15 ml/min/1.73 m^2, expect drug to be stopped.

Route	Onset	Peak	Duration
I.V.	Immediate	Unknown	Unknown

Incompatibilities

Don't mix lepirudin in same I.V. line with other drugs.

Contraindications

Hypersensitivity to lepirudin or other hirudins

Interactions

oral anticoagulants, platelet aggregation inhibitors, thrombolytics: Increased risk of bleeding complications and enhanced effects of lepirudin

Mechanism of Action

Forms a tight bond with thrombin, neutralizing this enzyme's actions, even when the enzyme is trapped within clots. One molecule of lepirudin binds with one molecule of thrombin. Thrombin causes fibrinogen to convert to fibrin, which is essential for clot formation.

Adverse Reactions

CNS: Chills, fever, intracranial hemorrhage
CV: Heart failure
EENT: Epistaxis
GI: GI or rectal bleeding, hepatic dysfunction
GU: Hematuria, vaginal bleeding
HEME: Anemia, easy bruising, hematoma
RESP: Hemoptysis, pneumonia
SKIN: Excessive bleeding from wounds, rash, pruritus, urticaria
Other: Anaphylaxis, injection site bleeding, sepsis

Nursing Considerations

• Be aware that patients with heparin-induced thrombocytopenia have low platelet counts, which can lead to severe bleeding and even death. Lepirudin works to prevent clotting without further reducing platelet count.
• To reconstitute, mix lepirudin with normal saline solution or sterile water for injection. Warm solution to room temperature before giving.
• For I.V. bolus delivery, reconstitute 50 mg of drug with 1 ml of sterile water for injection or sodium chloride for injection. Then further dilute by withdrawing reconstituted solution into a 10-ml syringe and adding enough sterile water for injection, sodium chloride for injection, or D$_5$W to produce a total volume of 10 ml, or 5 mg of lepirudin/ml. Administer prescribed dose over 15 to 20 seconds.
• For I.V. infusion, reconstitute 2 vials of drug and transfer to infusion bag that contains 250 or 500 ml of normal saline solution or D$_5$W. Concentration will be 0.4 or 0.2 mg/ml.
• Adjust infusion rate as prescribed, according to patient's APTT ratio, which is APTT divided by a control value. Target APTT ratio during treatment is 1.5 to 2.5.
• Expect to obtain first APTT 4 hours after

starting infusion and to obtain follow-up APTT daily (more often for patients with hepatic or renal impairment).

•Stop infusion for 2 hours, as ordered, if APTT is above target range. Expect to decrease infusion rate by one-half when restarting. If APTT is below target range, expect to increase rate in 20% increments and recheck APTT in 4 hours.

•Avoid I.M. injections or needle sticks during lepirudin therapy to minimize risk of hematoma.

•Observe I.M. injection sites, I.V. infusion sites, and wounds for bleeding.

•Monitor for ecchymoses on arms and legs, epistaxis, hematemesis, hematuria, melena, and vaginal bleeding.

•Be aware that when patient is scheduled to switch to an oral anticoagulant, lepirudin dosage may need to be tapered over a period of days, as ordered, until the patient's APTT is just above 1.5, before starting oral anticoagulant. In addition, INR and PT will need to be monitored closely, as ordered, to prevent bleeding adverse effects.

PATIENT TEACHING

•Tell patient to report unexpected bleeding, such as blood in urine, easy bruising, nosebleeds, tarry stools, and vaginal bleeding.

•Advise patient to avoid bumping arms and legs because of the risk of bruising.

•Instruct patient to use an electric razor and a soft toothbrush to reduce the risk of bleeding.

leuprolide acetate

Eligard 7.5 mg, Eligard 22.5 mg, Lupron, Lupron Depot, Lupron Depot-3 Month 11.25 mg, Lupron Depot-3 Month 22.5 mg, Lupron Depot-4 Month 30 mg, Lupron Depot-Ped, Lupron-3 Month SR Depot 22.5 mg

Class and Category

Chemical class: Synthetic peptide gonadotropin-releasing hormone analogue
Therapeutic class: Antianemic, antiendometrionic agent, antineoplastic, gonadotropin inhibitor
Pregnancy category: X

Indications and Dosages

➤ *To treat prostate cancer*
I.M. INJECTION (LEUPROLIDE ACETATE FOR INJECTION)

Adults. 7.5 mg/mo, 22.5 mg every 3 mo, or 45 mg every 4 mo.
SUBCUTANEOUS INJECTION (LEUPROLIDE ACETATE FOR INJECTABLE SUSPENSION)
Adults. 7.5 mg/mo.
SUBCUTANEOUS INJECTION (LEUPROLIDE ACETATE INJECTION)
Adults. 1 mg daily.

➤ *To provide palliative treatment of advanced prostate cancer*
SUBCUTANEOUS INJECTION (ELIGARD FOR INJECTABLE SUSPENSION)
Adults. 7.5 mg/mo. 22.5 mg every 3 mo, or 45 mg every 6 mo.

➤ *To treat precocious central puberty*
I.M. INJECTION (LEUPROLIDE ACETATE FOR INJECTION)
Children weighing more than 37.5 kg (83 lb). *Initial:* 15 mg every 4 wk. *Maintenance:* Dosage increased as needed in increments of 3.75 mg every 4 wk. *Maximum:* 15 mg every 4 wk.
Children weighing 25 to 37.5 kg (55 to 83 lb). *Initial:* 11.25 mg every 4 wk. *Maintenance:* Dosage increased as needed in increments of 3.75 mg every 4 wk. *Maximum:* 15 mg every 4 wk.
Children weighing less than 25 kg. *Initial:* 7.5 mg every 4 wk. *Maintenance:* Dosage increased as needed in increments of 3.75 mg every 4 wk. *Maximum:* 15 mg every 4 wk.
SUBCUTANEOUS INJECTION (LEUPROLIDE ACETATE INJECTION)
Children. 50 mcg/kg daily. Dosage increased in increments of 10 mcg/kg daily.

➤ *To treat endometriosis*
I.M. INJECTION (LEUPROLIDE ACETATE FOR INJECTION)
Adults. 3.75 mg every mo or 11.25 mg every 3 mo for up to 6 mo. *Maximum:* 33.75 mg total dose.

➤ *As adjunct to treat anemia due to uterine leiomyomas*
I.M. INJECTION (LEUPROLIDE ACETATE FOR INJECTION)
Adults. 3.75 mg every mo up to 3 mo or 11.25 mg single dose. *Maximum:* 11.25 mg total dose.

Contraindications

Women and children (leuprolide acetate injectable suspension); hypersensitivity to benzyl alcohol, gonadorelin, and gonadotropin-releasing hormone analogues, including leuprolide, and their components; pregnancy; undiagnosed abnormal vaginal bleeding

J K L

Route	Onset	Peak	Duration
I.M., SubQ*	1 wk	Unknown	4 to 12 wk after therapy
I.M., SubQ†	2 to 4 wk	After 1 to 2 mo	60 to 90 days after therapy

Mechanism of Action

After stimulating follicle-stimulating hormone (FSH) and luteinizing hormone (LH), continuous leuprolide therapy suppresses secretion of gonadotropin-releasing hormone, decreasing testosterone and estradiol levels. In children with central precocious puberty, this stops menses and reproductive organ development.

In adult males, continuous suppression decreases testosterone levels and causes pharmacologic castration, which slows the activity of prostatic neoplastic cells. In women with endometriosis or uterine leiomyomas, leuprolide suppresses ovarian function, inactivating endometrial tissues and resulting in amenorrhea.

Adverse Reactions

CNS: Depression, dizziness, fatigue, headache, insomnia, lethargy, malaise, memory loss, paresthesia, peripheral neuropathy, rigors, syncope, weakness; anxiety, mood changes, nervousness (adult women)
CV: Arrhythmias, edema, hypertension, hypotension, palpitations, vasodilation; angina, MI, thrombophlebitis (adult men)
EENT: Blurred vision
ENDO: Amenorrhea, androgenic effects in women. breast tenderness or swelling, decreased testicle size, gynecomastia, hot flashes, hyperglycemia, pituitary apoplexy
GI: Colitis, constipation in adult men, dyspepsia, gastroenteritis, hepatic dysfunction, nausea, vomiting
GU: Bladder spasm, decreased libido, decreased penis size, dysuria, endometriosis flareup, impotence, incontinence, nocturia, prostate cancer flareup, prostate pain, uterine bleeding, vaginal discharge in girls, vaginitis

*Gonadotropin inhibitor.
†Antiendometrionic, antineoplastic.

HEME: Leukopenia
MS: Arthralgia, body pain in children, bone density loss, bone or limb pain, myalgia, tenosynovitis
RESP: Asthma, dyspnea, pulmonary embolism
SKIN: Alopecia, clamminess, night sweats, photosensitivity, rash, urticaria
Other: Anaphylaxis; weight gain; injection site abscess, burning, edema, induration, itching, pain, or redness

Nursing Considerations

•Let drug come to room temperature before using. Reconstitute leuprolide acetate depot suspension with diluent provided by manufacturer. Add diluent to powder for suspension and thoroughly shake vials to disperse particles into a uniform milky suspension. Use within 30 minutes after mixing, and discard any unused portion. If using a prefilled dual-chamber syringe, follow manufacturer's instructions to release diluent into chamber containing powder. Shake gently after diluted to disperse particles evenly in solution. No dilution or reconstitution is needed for leuprolide acetate injection for subcutaneous administration. Rotate injection sites.
•WARNING Leuprolide acetate for injectable suspension (Eligard) is approved only for use in men for palliative treatment of prostate cancer. Use provided syringes and delivery system, and read and follow instructions carefully to ensure proper mixing of product; shaking alone is inadequate to mix it.
•WARNING Monitor patient for possible allergic reaction (erythema and induration) at injection site because leuprolide injections contain benzyl alcohol. Manufacturer recommends that injection be given by physician.
•During first weeks of leuprolide therapy, monitor patient being treated for prostate cancer for initial worsening of symptoms, such as increased bone pain, difficult urination, and paresthesia or paralysis (in patients with vertebral metastasis).
•During treatment for prostate cancer, monitor patient's serum testosterone and PSA levels periodically, as ordered, to determine response to leuprolide therapy.
•Expect to stop drug before age 11 in female patients and age 12 in male patients treated for precocious central puberty.
•Monitor bone density test results, as ordered, of women at risk for osteoporosis who

are receiving leuprolide because of potential for drug-induced estrogen loss, which may result in decreased bone density.
•Be aware that therapeutic doses of leuprolide suppress the pituitary-gonadal system and that normal function doesn't return until 4 to 12 weeks after drug is stopped.
•**WARNING** Monitor patient for evidence of pituitary apoplexy, such as sudden headache, vomiting, visual changes, ophthalmoplegia, altered mental status, and possibly cardiovascular collapse. Although rare, it may occur within 2 weeks of the first dose, sometimes within the first hour. Notify prescriber immediately and provide supportive care.

PATIENT TEACHING
•Instruct patient who is self-administering leuprolide injection to use syringe provided by manufacturer. If manufacturer's syringe is unavailable, advise her to use only a 0.5-ml disposable, low-dose, U-100 insulin syringe to ensure accurate dosage. Substitution of syringes is not recommended for leuprolide acetate for injectable suspension.
•Advise women to immediately report monthly menses or breakthrough bleeding to prescriber.
•Instruct female patient of childbearing age to use a nonhormonal form of contraception during leuprolide therapy. Advise her to stop taking drug and notify prescriber at once if she becomes pregnant.
•Inform patient with osteoporosis or at risk for developing it that drug may increase bone density loss.
•Inform parents of child being treated for central precocious puberty that they should expect normal gonadal-pituitary function to return 4 to 12 weeks after therapy ends.
•Advise patient to report symptoms of depression or memory problems.
•Caution patient being treated for prostate cancer that drug may initially worsen such symptoms as bone pain and that it may cause new signs or symptoms to occur during first few weeks of treatment. Reassure patient that this is transient.

levalbuterol hydrochloride

Xopenex, Xopenex HFA

Class and Category
Chemical class: Sympathomimetic amine

Therapeutic class: Bronchodilator
Pregnancy category: C

Indications and Dosages
➤ *To prevent or treat bronchospasm in reversible obstructive airway disease*

INHALATION AEROSOL
Adults and children age 4 and over. 45 or 90 mcg (1 or 2 inhalations) every 4 to 6 hr.
INHALATION SOLUTION
Adults and children age 12 and over. 0.63 to 1.25 mg t.i.d. every 6 to 8 hr. *Maximum:* 1.25 mg t.i.d.
Children ages 6 to 11. 0.31 to 0.63 mg t.i.d. *Maximum:* 0.63 mg t.i.d.
DOSAGE ADJUSTMENT For elderly patients, dosage limited to 0.63 mg t.i.d. every 6 to 8 hr.

Route	Onset	Peak	Duration
Inhalation	10 to 17 min	1.5 hr	5 to 6 hr

Mechanism of Action
Attaches to beta$_2$ receptors on bronchial cell membranes, which stimulates the intracellular enzyme adenyl cyclase to convert adenosine triphosphate to cAMP. An increased intracellular cAMP level relaxes bronchial smooth muscle and inhibits histamine release from mast cells.

Contraindications
Hypersensitivity to levalbuterol, other sympathomimetic amines, or their components

Interactions
DRUGS
beta blockers: Blocked effects of both drugs
digoxin: Decreased blood digoxin level
loop or thiazide diuretics: Increased risk of hypokalemia
MAO inhibitors, sympathomimetics, tricyclic antidepressants: Increased risk of adverse cardiovascular effects

Adverse Reactions
CNS: Anxiety, chills, dizziness, hypertonia, insomnia, migraine headache, nervousness, paresthesia, syncope, tremor
CV: Chest pain, hypertension, hypotension, tachycardia
EENT: Dry mouth and throat, rhinitis, sinusitis

J
K
L

GI: Diarrhea, indigestion, nausea, vomiting
MS: Leg cramps, myalgia
RESP: Asthma exacerbation, cough, dyspnea, paradoxical bronchospasm
Other: Flulike symptoms, lymphadeno-pathy

Nursing Considerations

•Use levalbuterol cautiously in patients with arrhythmias, diabetes mellitus, hypertension, hyperthyroidism, or a history of seizures.
•Give oral solution form only by nebulizer.
•Monitor the patient's pulse rate and blood pressure before and after nebulizer treatment.
•Because drug may provoke paradoxical bronchospasm, observe for dyspnea, wheezing, and increased coughing.

PATIENT TEACHING

•Teach patient how to use levalbuterol nebulizer and to measure correct dose.
•Intsruct patient to prime inhaler before using it for the first time or when it hasn't been used for more than 3 days by releasing 4 test sprays into the air, aiming it away from her face.
•Show patient how to clean nebulizer or inhaler, and explain the need to do so at least once weekly.
•Instruct patient to notify prescriber if drug fails to work or if she needs more frequent treatments because her asthma is worsening.
•Instruct patient not to increase the dosage or frequency unless advised to do so by prescriber.
•Urge patient to stop drug and contact prescriber if she develops paradoxical bronchospasm.
•Instruct patient to use inhalation solution within 2 weeks of opening the foil pouch and to protect drug from light and heat.
•Urge patient to consult prescriber before using OTC or other drugs.

levetiracetam

Keppra, Keppra XR

Class and Category

Chemical: Pyrrolidine derivative
Therapeutic: Anticonvulsant
Pregnancy category: C

Indications and Dosages

➤ *As adjunct to treat partial seizures*

ORAL SOLUTION, TABLETS

Adults and adolescents over age 16. *Initial:* 500 mg b.i.d., increased by 1,000 mg daily every 2 wk if needed. *Maximum:* 3,000 mg daily.

Children ages 4 to 16. *Initial:* 10 mg/kg b.i.d., increased by 20 mg/kg daily every 2 wk until recommended daily dose of 60 mg/kg is reached.

XR TABLETS

Adults and adolescents over age 16. 1,000 mg once daily, increased by 1,000 mg daily every 2 wk until recommended daily dose of 3,000 mg is reached.

I.V. INFUSION

Adults and adolescents over age 16. *Initial:* 500 mg infused over 15 minutes b.i.d., increased by 1,000 mg daily every 2 wk, if needed. *Maximum:* 3,000 mg daily.

➤ *As adjunct to treat myoclonic seizures in patients with juvenile myoclonic epilepsy*

ORAL SOLUTION, TABLETS

Adults and children age 12 and over. *Initial:* 500 mg b.i.d., increased by 1,000 mg daily every 2 wk, if needed. *Maximum:* 3,000 mg daily.

➤ *As adjunct to treat primary generalized tonic-clonic seizures in patients with idiopathic generalized epilepsy*

ORAL SOLUTION, TABLETS

Adults and children age 6 and over. *Initial:* 500 mg b.i.d., increased by 1,000 mg daily every 2 wk, as needed. *Maximum:* 3,000 mg daily.

DOSAGE ADJUSTMENT Maximum dosage reduced to 2,000 mg daily for patients with creatinine clearance of 50 to 80 ml/min/1.73 m^2; to 1,500 mg daily for creatinine clearance of 30 to 49 ml/min/1.73 m^2; and to 1,000 mg daily for creatinine clearance less than 30 ml/min/1.73 m^2. For patients with end-stage renal disease who are having dialysis, expect to give another 250 to 500 mg, as prescribed, after each dialysis session. For children who can't tolerate 60 mg/kg daily, dosage reduced to point of tolerance.

Contraindications

Hypersensitivity to levetiracetam or its components

Mechanism of Action
May protect against secondary generalized seizure activity by preventing coordination of epileptiform burst firing. Levetiracetam doesn't seem to involve inhibitory and excitatory neurotransmission.

Adverse Reactions
CNS: Abnormal gait, aggression, agitation, anger, anxiety, apathy, asthenia, ataxia, behavioral difficulties (children), confusion, coordination difficulties, depersonalization, depression, dizziness, emotional lability, fatigue, hallucinations, headache, hostility, increased reflexes, insomnia, irritability, mental or mood changes, nervousness, neurosis, paresthesia, personality disorder, psychosis, seizures, somnolence, suicidal thinking, vertigo
EENT: Amblyopia, conjunctivitis, diplopia, ear pain, nasopharyngitis, pharyngitis, rhinitis, sinusitis
GI: Anorexia, constipation, diarrhea, elevated liver enzyme levels, gastroenteritis, hepatic failure, hepatitis, pancreatitis, vomiting
GU: Albuminuria
HEME: Decreased hemtatocrit, hemoglobin, and total mean RBC count; leukopenia; neutropenia; pancytopenia; thrombocytopenia
MS: Neck pain
RESP: Asthma, cough
SKIN: Alopecia, ecchymosis, pruritus, skin discoloration, vesiculobullous rash
Other: Dehydration, facial edema, infection, influenza, weight loss

Nursing Considerations
• Know that children weighing 20 kg or less should be given only the oral solution form.
• For I.V. administration, dilute parenteral levetiracetam in 100 ml of a compatible diluent such as normal saline injection, lactated Ringer's injection, or dextrose 5% injection. Use within 24 hours.
• Assess compliance during first 4 weeks of therapy, when adverse reactions are most common.
• Monitor patient for seizure activity during levetiracetam therapy. As appropriate, implement seizure precautions according to facility policy.
• Stopping drug may increase seizure activity.

Expect to taper dosage gradually.
• Certain adverse effects, including somnolence, fatigue, coordination problems, and abnormal behaviors may be more likely in patieints taking levetiracetam for partial seizure disorders.

PATIENT TEACHING
• Caution patient that levetiracetam may cause dizziness and drowsiness, especially during first 4 weeks of therapy.
• Advise patient to avoid hazardous activities until drug's full CNS effects are known.
• Caution patient not to stop taking levetiracetam abruptly; inform her that drug dosage should be tapered under prescriber's direction to reduce the risk of breakthrough seizures.
• Explain that levetiracetam may cause mental and behavioral changes, such as aggression, depresison, irritability, and rarely psychotic symptoms or thoughts of suicide. Urge her to contact prescriber about any bothersome changes.
• Advise patient to keep taking other anticonvulsants, as ordered, while taking levetiracetam.
• Encourage patient to avoid alcohol during therapy because alcohol can increase incidence of drowsiness and dizziness.
• Instruct patient to see prescriber regularly so that her progress can be monitored.

levocetirizine
Xyzal

Class and Category
Chemical class: H_1-receptor antagonist
Therapeutic class: Antihistamine
Pregnancy category: B

Indications and Dosages
➤ *To treat chronic idiopathic urticaria; to treat allergic rhinitis*
TABLETS, ORAL SOLUTION
Adults and children age 12 and over. 2.5 to 5 mg once daily in evening. *Maximum:* 5 mg daily.
DOSAGE ADJUSTMENT For patient with mild renal impairment (creatinine clearance of 50 to 80 ml/min/1.73 m^2), dosage shouldn't exceed 2.5 mg daily. For patient with moderate renal impairment (creatinine clearance of 30 to 50 ml/min/1.73 m^2), dosage shouldn't

exceed 2.5 mg once every other day. For patient with severe renal impairment (creatinine clearance of 10 to 30 ml/min/1.73 m²), dosage shouldn't exceed 2.5 mg once every 3 to 4 days.
Children ages 6 to 11. 2.5 mg once daily in evening. *Maximum:* 2.5 mg daily.

Mechanism of Action
Binds to central and peripheral H_1 receptors, competing with histamine for these sites and preventing it from reaching its site of action. By blocking histamine, levocetirizine produces antihistamine effects, inhibiting respiratory, vascular, and GI smooth-muscle contraction; decreasing capillary permeability, which reduces wheals, flares, and itching; and decreasing salivary and lacrimal gland secretions to relieve chronic urticaria and signs and symptoms of allergic rhinitis.

Contraindications
Children ages 6 to 11 with impaired renal function; creatinine clearance less than 10 ml/min/1.73 m²; end-stage renal disease in adults and children age 12 and over; hypersensitivity to levocetirizine, cetirizine or their components; renal failure

Interactions
DRUGS
CNS depressants: Possibly increased CNS depression
MAO inhibitors: Possibly prolonged and intensified anticholinergic effects
ritonavir: Possibly increased risk of adverse effects of levocetirizine
theophylline: Possibly decreased clearance of levocetirizine
ACTIVITIES
alcohol use: Possibly increased CNS depression

Adverse Reactions
CNS: Aggression, agitation, asthenia, fatigue, fever, seizures, somnolence, syncope
CV: Palpitations
EENT: Dry mouth, epistaxis, nasopharyngitis, pharyngitis, visual disturbances
GI: Hepatitis, nausea
MS: Myalgia
RESP: Cough, dyspnea

SKIN: Pruritus, rash, urticaria
Other: Anaphylaxis, angioedema, weight gain

Nursing Considerations
•Expect to stop drug at least 72 hours before skin tests for allergies because drug may inhibit cutaneous histamine response, thus producing false-negative results.
PATIENT TEACHING
•Instruct patient to take drug exactly as prescribed. For oral solution, patient should use appropriate measuring device.
•Urge patient to avoid alcohol while taking levocetirizine
•Advise patient to avoid hazardous activities until drug's CNS effects are known.

levodopa

Dopar, Larodopa

Class and Category
Chemical class: Dihydroxyphenylalanine isomer, metabolic precursor of dopamine
Therapeutic class: Antidyskinetic
Pregnancy category: Not rated

Indications and Dosages
➤ *To manage symptoms of primary Parkinson's disease, postencephalitic parkinsonism, and parkinsonism caused by CNS injury from carbon monoxide or manganese intoxication*
CAPSULES, TABLETS
Adults and children age 12 and over. *Initial:* 250 mg daily in divided doses b.i.d. to q.i.d. Increased by 100 to 750 mg every 3 to 7 days, as indicated. *Maximum:* 8 g daily.

Route	Onset	Peak	Duration
P.O.	14 to 21 days*	Unknown	5 hr

Contraindications
Angle-closure glaucoma, history of melanoma, hypersensitivity to levodopa or its components, suspicious undiagnosed skin lesions, use within 14 days of MAO inhibitor therapy

Interactions
DRUGS
antacids: Increased blood levodopa level

---

* With multiple doses.

Mechanism of Action

By supplementing a low level of endogenous dopamine, levodopa helps control alterations in voluntary muscle movement (such as tremors and rigidity) associated with Parkinson's disease. Dopamine, a neurotransmitter that's synthesized and released by neurons leading from substantia nigra to basal ganglia, is essential for normal motor function. By stimulating peripheral and central dopaminergic$_2$ (D$_2$) receptors on postsynaptic cells, dopamine inhibits the firing of striatal neurons (such as cholinergic neurons). In Parkinson's disease, progressive degeneration of these neurons substantially reduces the supply of intrasynaptic dopamine. Levodopa, a dopamine precursor, increases the dopamine supply in neurons, making more available to stimulate dopaminergic receptors.

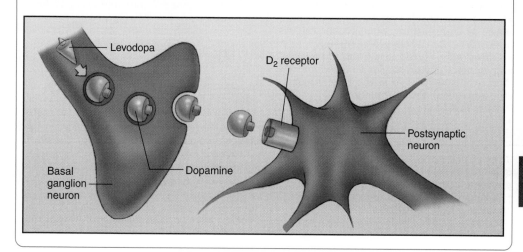

antihypertensives: Risk of orthostatic hypotension

benzodiazepines: Possibly decreased therapeutic effects of levodopa

bromocriptine: Possibly additive effects of levodopa

furazolidone, MAO inhibitors, procarbazine: Risk of severe hypertension

haloperidol, loxapine, molindone, papaverine, phenothiazines, phenytoin, rauwolfia alkaloids: Decreased effects of levodopa

inhaled anesthetics, sympathomimetics: Increased risk of arrhythmias

iron salts: Possibly decreased blood level and effectiveness of levodopa

methyldopa: Possibly toxic CNS effects

metoclopramide: Possibly worsening of Parkinson's disease and decreased therapeutic effects of metoclopramide

pyridoxine (vitamin B$_6$): Decreased antidyskinetic effect of levodopa

FOODS

high-protein food: Decreased levodopa absorption

ACTIVITIES

cocaine use: Increased risk of arrhythmias

Adverse Reactions

CNS: Aggressiveness, anxiety, ataxia, confusion, delusions, dizziness, dream disturbances, dyskinesia, dystonia, euphoria, hallucinations, headache, increased tremor, insomnia, malaise, mood changes, severe depression, suicidal tendencies, syncope, weakness

CV: Arrhythmias, hot flashes, orthostatic hypotension, palpitations

EENT: Bitter aftertaste, blurred vision, darkened saliva, diplopia, dry mouth, increased salivation, mydriasis, tooth clenching and grinding

GI: Abdominal pain, anorexia, constipation, diarrhea, flatulence, GI bleeding, hepato-

toxicity, hiccups, indigestion, nausea, vomiting
GU: Darkened urine, priapism, urine retention
SKIN: Darkened sweat, diaphoresis, rash

Nursing Considerations
•Expect to discontinue levodopa 6 to 8 hours before surgery to avoid interactions with anesthetics.
•Observe patient for mental or behavioral changes and suicidal tendencies. Notify prescriber immediately if they occur.
•Monitor for muscle twitching and blepharospasm (eyelid spasm), which are early signs of overdose. Report these signs immediately.
•Expect patient to be tested for acromegaly and diabetes during long-term levodopa therapy. Also expect to monitor hematopoietic, hepatic, and renal function.

PATIENT TEACHING
•Advise patient to take levodopa with meals if she experiences adverse GI reactions.
•Because protein impairs drug absorption, instruct patient to avoid high-protein meals during levodopa therapy and to distribute protein intake equally throughout the day.
•Caution patient to avoid excessive use of vitamins and fortified cereals that contain vitamin B_6 or iron, which can reduce levodopa's effects.
•Instruct patient to report fainting, increased muscle tremor, difficult urination, and severe or persistent nausea and vomiting.
•Urge patient to continue taking drug as prescribed even if results of therapy aren't evident immediately.
•Inform patient that saliva, sweat, and urine may darken but that this isn't harmful.
•Direct patient to protect drug from heat, light, and moisture and to discard darkened pills because they have lost their potency.
•Advise patient to change position slowly to minimize effects of orthostatic hypotension.
•Caution male patient about risk of priapism (persistent, painful erection), and urge him to seek medical help immediately if it occurs.

levofloxacin

Levaquin

Class and Category
Chemical class: Fluoroquinolone

Therapeutic class: Antibiotic
Pregnancy category: C

Indications and Dosages
➤ *To reduce incidence or progression of inhalation anthrax after exposure to aerosolized* Bacillus anthracis

TABLETS, I.V. INFUSION, ORAL SOLUTION
Adults and children weighing more than 50 kg (110 lb). 500 mg (over 60 min for I.V. infusion) daily for 60 days.
Children weighing less than 50 kg. 8 mg/kg (over 60 min for I.V. infusion) every 12 hr for 60 days. *Maximum:* 250 mg/dose.

➤ *To treat acute maxillary sinusitis caused by* Haemophilus influenzae, Moraxella catarrhalis, *or* Streptococcus pneumoniae

TABLETS, I.V. INFUSION, ORAL SOLUTION
Adults. 500 mg daily (over 60 to 90 min for I.V. infusion) for 10 to 14 days. Or 759 mg daily for 5 days.

➤ *To treat acute exacerbation of chronic bacterial bronchitis caused by* H. influenzae, H. parainfluenzae, M. catarrhalis, S. pneumoniae, *or* Staphylococcus aureus

TABLETS, I.V. INFUSION, ORAL SOLUTION
Adults. 500 mg daily (over 60 to 90 min for I.V. infusion) for 7 days.

➤ *To treat community-acquired pneumonia caused by* Chlamydia pneumoniae, H. influenzae, H. parainfluenzae, Klebsiella pneumoniae, Legionella pneumophila, M. catarrhalis, Mycoplasma pneumoniae, S. aureus, *or* S. pneumoniae

TABLETS, I.V. INFUSION, ORAL SOLUTION
Adults. 500 mg daily (over 60 to 90 min for I.V. infusion) for 7 to 14 days. Alternatively, for infection caused by *C. pneumoniae, H. influenzae, H. parainfluenzae, M. pneumoniae,* or *S. pneumoniae,* 750 mg daily (over 60 to 90 min for I.V. infusion) for 5 days.

➤ *To treat uncomplicated UTI caused by* Escherichia coli, K. pneumoniae, *or* Staphylococcus saprophyticus

TABLETS, I.V. INFUSION, ORAL SOLUTION
Adults. 250 mg daily (over 60 to 90 min for I.V. infusion) for 3 days.

➤ *To treat complicated UTI caused by* Enterococcus faecalis, E. cloacae, E. coli, K. pneumoniae, Proteus mirabilis, *or*

Pseudomonas aeruginosa *or acute pyelonephritis caused by* E. coli

TABLETS, I.V. INFUSION, ORAL SOLUTION
Adults. 250 mg daily (over 60 to 90 min for I.V. infusion) for 10 days.

➤ *To treat complicated UTI caused by* E. coli, K. pneumoniae, *or* P. mirabilis *or acute pyelonephritis caused by* E. coli

TABLETS, I.V. INFUSION, ORAL SOLUTION
Adults. 750 mg daily (over 90 min for I.V. infusion) for 5 days.

➤ *To treat mild to moderate skin and soft-tissue infections caused by* S. aureus *or* Streptococcus pyogenes

TABLETS, I.V. INFUSION, ORAL SOLUTION
Adults. 500 mg daily (over 60 to 90 min for I.V. infusion) for 7 to 10 days.

➤ *To treat complicated skin and soft-tissue infections caused by methicillin-sensitive* Enterococcus faecalis, Proteus mirabilis, S. aureus, *or* S. pyogenes; *to treat nosocomial pneumonia caused by* S. aureus, Pseudomonas aeruginosa, Serratia marcescens, E. coli, K. pneumoniae, H. influenzae, *or* S. pneumoniae

TABLETS, I.V. INFUSION, ORAL SOLUTION
Adults. 750 mg daily (over 60 to 90 min for I.V. infusion) for 7 to 14 days.

➤ *To treat chronic bacterial prostatitis caused by* E. coli, E. faecalis, *or* S. epidermidis

TABLETS, I.V. INFUSION, ORAL SOLUTION
Adults. 500 mg daily (over 60 to 90 min for I.V. infusion) for 28 days.

DOSAGE ADJUSTMENT For complicated UTI in patients with creatinine clearance of 10 to 19 ml/min/1.73 m^2, 250 mg initially and then maintenance dosage of 250 mg every 48 hr. For complicated skin and soft-tissue infections and nosocomial pneumonia when creatinine clearance is 19 ml/min/1.73 m^2 or less, 750 mg initially and then maintenance dosage of 500 mg every 48 hr; when creatinine clearance is 20 to 49 ml/min/1.73 m^2, 750 mg initially and then maintenance dosage of 750 mg every 48 hr. For all other indications, when creatinine clearance is 19 ml/min/1.73 m^2 or less, 500 mg initially and then maintenance of 250 mg every 48 hr; when creatinine clearance is 20 to 49 ml/min/1.73 m^2, 500 mg initially and then maintenance dosage of 250 mg every 24 hr.

Mechanism of Action
Interferes with bacterial cell replication by inhibiting the bacterial enzyme DNA gyrase, which is essential for replication and repair of bacterial DNA.

Contraindications
Hypersensitivity to levofloxacin, other fluoroquinolones, or their components

Interactions
DRUGS
aluminum-, calcium-, or magnesium-containing antacids; didanosine; iron; sucralfate; zinc: Reduced GI absorption of levofloxacin
antineoplastics: Decreased blood levofloxacin level
cimetidine: Increased blood levofloxacin level
cyclosporine: Increased risk of nephrotoxicity
NSAIDs: Possibly increased CNS stimulation and risk of seizures
oral anticoagulants: Increased anticoagulant effect and risk of bleeding
oral antidiabetic drugs: Possibly hyperglycemia or hypoglycemia
theophylline: Increased blood theophylline level and risk of toxicity
ACTIVITIES
sun exposure: Increased risk of photosensitivity

Adverse Reactions
CNS: Anxiety, CNS stimulation, dizziness, fever, headache, increased ICP, insomnia, light-headedness, nervousness, paranoia, peripheral neuropathy, psychosis, seizures, sleep disturbance, suicidal ideation
CV: Arrhythmias, leukocytoclastic vasculitis, prolonged QT interval, torsades de pointes, vasculitis, vasodilation
EENT: Blurred vision, decreased visual acuity, diplopia, dysphonia, scotoma, taste perversion, tinnitus
ENDO: Hyperglycemia, hypoglycemia
GI: Abdominal pain, acute hepatic necrosis or failure, anorexia, constipation, diarrhea, flatulence, hepatitis, hepatotoxicity, indigestion, jaundice, nausea, pseudomembranous colitis, vomiting
GU: Acute renal failure or insufficiency, crystalluria, interstitial nephritis, vaginal candidiasis
HEME: Agranulocytosis, aplastic anemia, eo-

sinophilia, hemolytic anemia, leukopenia, pancytopenia, thrombocytopenia
MS: Arthralgia, back pain, myalgia, rhabdomyolysis, tendon or muscle rupture
RESP: Allergic pneumonitis
SKIN: Photosensitivity, pruritus, rash, Stevens-Johnson syndrome, toxic epidermal necrolysis, urticaria
Other: Anaphylaxis, angioedema, multiorgan failure, serum sickness

Nursing Considerations

• Use levofloxacin cautiously in patients with renal insufficiency. Monitor renal function as appropriate during levofloxacin treatment.
• Use drug cautiously in patients with CNS disorders, such as epilepsy, that may lower the seizure threshold. Also use cautiously in patients taking corticosteroids, especially elderly patients, because of the increased risk of tendon rupture.
• Expect to obtain culture and sensitivity tests before levofloxacin treatment begins.
• Avoid giving drug within 2 hours of antacids.
• Give parenteral form over 60 to 90 minutes, depending on dosage, because bolus or rapid I.V. delivery may cause hypotension.
• **WARNING** Stop levofloxacin at the first sign of hypersensitivity, including rash and jaundice, because drug may lead to anaphylaxis. Reaction may occur after the first dose. Expect to give epinephrine, and provide supportive care.
• Monitor blood glucose level, especially in diabetic patient who takes an oral antidiabetic or uses insulin, because levofloxacin may alter blood glucose levels. If so, notify prescriber, stop drug immediately if patient has hypoglycemia, and provide prescribed treatment.
• Monitor QT interval if needed. If it lengthens, notify prescriber immediately and stop drug. Patients with hypokalemia, significant bradycardia, or cardiomyopathy and those receiving a class Ia or III antiarrhythmic shouldn't receive levofloxacin.
• Notify prescriber if patient has symptoms of peripheral neuropathy (pain, burning, tingling, numbness, weakness, or altered sensations of light touch, pain, temperature, position sense, or vibration sense), which could be permanent; or CNS abnormalities (seizures, psychosis, increased ICP or CNS stimulation), which may lead to more serious adverse reactions, such as suicidal thoughts. In each case, expect to discontinue levofloxacin.
• Watch for evidence of tendon rupture (inflammation, pain, swelling) during and up to several months after therapy is completed, especially in children, elderly patients, patients receiving corticosteroids, and patients with kidney, heart, and lung transplants. Notify prescriber about suspected tendon rupture, and have patient rest and refrain from exercise until tendon rupture has been ruled out. If present, expect to provide supportive care, as ordered.
• Monitor patient's bowel elimination. If diarrhea develops, obtain stool culture to check for pseudomembranous colitis. If confirmed, expect to stop drug and give fluid, electrolytes, and antibiotics effective against *Clostridium difficile.*

PATIENT TEACHING

• If patient will take oral solution form of levofloxacin, tell him to take it 1 hour before or 2 hours after eating.
• Advise patient to increase fluid intake during levofloxacin therapy to prevent crystalluria.
• Direct patient to take an antacid, didanosine, iron, sucralfate, or zinc at least 2 hours before or after levofloxacin.
• Tell patient to complete the drug as prescribed, even if symptoms subside.
• Urge patient to avoid excessive exposure to sunlight and to wear sunscreen because of increased risk of photosensitivity. Tell patient to notify prescriber at first sign.
• Caution patient to avoid hazardous activities until drug's CNS effects are known.
• Tell patient to stop drug and notify prescriber if he develops tendon pain or inflammation or abnormal changes in motor or sensory function.
• Urge patient to stop drug and tell prescriber about rash or other allergic reaction.
• Advise diabetic patient to monitor blood glucose level and tell prescriber of changes.
• Urge patient to tell prescriber about severe diarrhea, even for more than 2 months after drug therapy ends. Additional treatment may be needed.
• Advise patient to notify prescriber about heart palpitations or loss of consciousness. An ECG may be needed to detect adverse drug effects on the patient's heart.

levorphanol tartrate

Levo-Dromoran

Class, Category, and Schedule
Chemical class: Morphinan derivative
Therapeutic class: Analgesic, anesthesia adjunct
Pregnancy category: Not rated
Controlled substance schedule: II

Indications and Dosages
➤ *To relieve moderate to severe pain*
TABLETS
Adults. 2 mg every 6 to 8 hr, p.r.n. Increased to 3 mg every 6 to 8 hr, if indicated.
I.V. INJECTION
Adults. Up to 1 mg every 3 to 6 hr, p.r.n. *Maximum:* 8 mg daily for non–opioid-dependent patients.
I.M. OR SUBCUTANEOUS INJECTION
Adults. 1 to 2 mg every 6 to 8 hr, p.r.n. *Maximum:* 8 mg daily for non–opioid-dependent patients.

➤ *To provide preoperative sedation*
I.M. OR SUBCUTANEOUS INJECTION
Adults. 1 to 2 mg 60 to 90 min before procedure.

Route	Onset	Peak	Duration
P.O.	10 to 60 min	90 to 120 min	4 to 5 hr
I.V.	Unknown	In 20 min	4 to 5 hr
I.M.	Unknown	60 min	4 to 5 hr
SubQ	Unknown	60 to 90 min	4 to 5 hr

Mechanism of Action
Decreases intracellular level of cyclic adenosine monophosphate by inhibiting adenylate cyclase, which regulates release of pain neurotransmitters, such as substance P, gamma-aminobutyric acid, dopamine, acetylcholine, and noradrenaline. Levorphanol also stimulates mu and kappa opioid receptors, altering perception of and emotional response to pain.

Incompatibilities
Don't mix levorphanol tartrate with solutions that contain aminophylline, ammonium chloride, amobarbital sodium, chlorothiazide sodium, heparin sodium, methicillin sodium, nitrofurantoin sodium, novobiacin sodium, pentobarbital sodium, perphenazine, phenobarbital sodium, phenytoin, secobarbital sodium, sodium bicarbonate, sodium iodide, sulfadiazine sodium, sulfisoxazole diethanolamine, or thiopental sodium.

Contraindications
Acute alcoholism, acute or severe asthma, anoxia, hypersensitivity to levorphanol tartrate or its components, increased intracranial pressure, respiratory depression, upper airway obstruction

Interactions
DRUGS
alfentanil, CNS depressants, fentanyl, sufentanil: Possibly increased CNS and respiratory depression and hypotension
anticholinergics: Increased risk of severe constipation
antidiarrheals, such as difenoxin and atropine, kaolin, and loperamide: Increased risk of severe constipation and increased CNS depression
antihypertensives: Increased risk of hypotension
buprenorphine: Possibly decreased therapeutic effects of levorphanol and increased risk of respiratory depression
hydroxyzine: Increased risk of CNS depression and hypotension
metoclopramide: Possibly antagonized effects of metoclopramide
naloxone, naltrexone: Decreased therapeutic effects of levorphanol
neuromuscular blockers: Increased risk of prolonged CNS and respiratory depression
ACTIVITIES
alcohol use: Possibly increased CNS and respiratory depression and hypotension

Adverse Reactions
CNS: Amnesia, coma, confusion, delusions, depression, dizziness, drowsiness, dyskinesia, hypokinesia, insomnia, nervousness, personality disorder, seizures
CV: Bradycardia, cardiac arrest, hypotension, orthostatic hypotension, palpitations, shock, tachycardia
EENT: Abnormal vision, diplopia, dry mouth
GI: Abdominal pain, biliary tract spasm, constipation, hepatic failure, indigestion, nausea, vomiting
GU: Dysuria, urine retention
RESP: Apnea, hyperventilation

SKIN: Cyanosis, pruritus, rash, urticaria
Other: Injection site pain, redness, and swelling; physical and psychological dependence

Nursing Considerations

•**WARNING** Be aware that levorphanol may be habit-forming.
•Give drug with food if GI distress occurs.
•If respiratory depression occurs, expect to administer naloxone to reverse it.
•Monitor supine and standing blood pressure, and notify prescriber of orthostatic hypotension.
•Carefully assess for adverse reactions in elderly patients; they are especially sensitive to drug and are at increased risk for constipation.

PATIENT TEACHING

•Advise patient to avoid potentially hazardous activities until drug's CNS effects are known.
•Instruct patient to avoid alcoholic beverages while taking levorphanol.
•Direct patient to change position slowly to minimize effects of orthostatic hypotension.
•Advise patient to notify prescriber if constipation, nausea, or vomiting occurs.
•If patient reports dry mouth, suggest that she use sugarless candy or gum or ice chips.

levothyroxine sodium

(L-thyroxine sodium, T₄, thyroxine sodium)

Eltroxin (CAN), Levo-T, Levothroid, Levoxyl, PMS-Levothyroxine Sodium (CAN), Synthroid, Unithroid

Class and Category

Chemical class: Synthetic thyroxine (T_4)
Therapeutic class: Thyroid hormone replacement
Pregnancy category: A

Indications and Dosages

➤ *To treat mild hypothyroidism*
TABLETS
Adults. *Initial:* 50 mcg daily, increased by 25 to 50 mcg every 2 to 3 wk until desired response occurs or therapeutic blood level is reached. *Maintenance:* 75 to 125 mcg daily.
DOSAGE ADJUSTMENT For elderly patients and those with cardiovascular disease or chronic hypothyroidism, initial dosage usually reduced to 12.5 to 25 mcg daily and then increased by 12.5 to 25 mcg every 3 to 4 wk until desired response occurs. For elderly patients, maintenance dosage is limited to 75 mcg daily.
Children over age 10. 2 to 3 mcg/kg daily. *Usual:* 150 to 200 mcg daily.
Children ages 6 to 10. 4 to 5 mcg/kg daily. *Usual:* 100 to 150 mcg daily.
Children ages 1 to 5. 3 to 5 mcg/kg daily. *Usual:* 75 to 100 mcg daily.
Infants ages 6 to 12 months. 5 to 6 mcg/kg daily. *Usual:* 50 to 75 mcg daily.
Infants under age 6 months. 5 to 6 mcg/kg daily. *Usual:* 25 to 50 mcg daily.

➤ *To treat severe hypothyroidism*
TABLETS
Adults. *Initial:* 12.5 to 25 mcg daily. Increased by 25 mcg every 2 to 3 wk until desired response occurs or therapeutic blood level is reached. *Maintenance:* 75 to 125 mcg daily. *Maximum:* 200 mcg daily.
Children over age 10. 2 to 3 mcg/kg daily. *Usual:* 150 to 200 mcg daily.
Children ages 6 to 10. 4 to 5 mcg/kg daily. *Usual:* 100 to 150 mcg daily.
Children ages 1 to 5. 3 to 5 mcg/kg daily. *Usual:* 75 to 100 mcg daily.
Infants ages 6 to 12 months. 5 to 6 mcg/kg daily. *Usual:* 50 to 75 mcg daily.
Infants under age 6 months. 5 to 6 mcg/kg daily. *Usual:* 25 to 50 mcg daily.
I.V. OR I.M. INJECTION
Adults. 50 to 100 mcg daily until therapeutic blood level is reached.
Children. 75% of usual P.O. dose daily until therapeutic blood level is reached.

➤ *To treat myxedema coma*
I.V. INJECTION
Adults. 200 to 500 mcg on day 1. If no significant improvement, 100 to 300 mcg on day 2. Daily dose continued as prescribed until therapeutic blood level is reached and P.O. administration is tolerated.
Children. 75% of usual P.O. dose daily until therapeutic blood level is reached and P.O. administration is tolerated.

Route	Onset	Peak	Duration
P.O.	3 to 5 days	3 to 4 wk	1 to 3 wk
I.V.	6 to 8 hr	24 hr	Unknown
I.M.	Unknown	Unknown	1 to 3 wk

Contraindications

Acute MI (unless caused or complicated by

hyperthyroidism), hypersensitivity to levo-thyroxine or its components, uncorrected ad-renal insufficiency, untreated thyrotoxicosis

Mechanism of Action

Replaces endogenous thyroid hormone, which may exert its physiologic effects by controlling DNA transcription and protein synthesis. Levothyroxine exhibits all of the following actions of endogenous thyroid hormone. The drug:
• increases energy expenditure
• accelerates the rate of cellular oxidation, which stimulates body tissue growth, maturation, and metabolism
• regulates differentiation and prolifera-tion of stem cells
• aids in myelination of nerves and devel-opment of synaptic processes in the ner-vous system
• regulates growth
• decreases blood and hepatic cholesterol concentrations
• enhances carbohydrate and protein me-tabolism, increasing gluconeogenesis and protein synthesis.

Adverse Reactions

CNS: Fatigue, headache, insomnia, somno-lence
ENDO: Hyperthyroidism (with overdose)
GI: Dysphagia
MS: Muscle weakness, myalgia, slipped capi-tal femoral epiphysis
SKIN: Alopecia (transient), rash, urticaria
Other: Weight gain

Interactions

DRUGS
adrenocorticoids: Possibly adrenocorticoid dosage adjustments as thyroid status changes
aluminum- and magnesium-containing antacids, bile acid sequestrants, calcium car-bonate, cation exchange resins, cholestyra-mine, colestipol, ferrous sulfate, kayexalate, orlistat, sucralfate: Possibly reduced effects of levothyroxine
amiodarone, iodide: Possibly hyperthy-roidism
beta blockers: Possibly impaired action of beta blockers and decreased conversion of T_4 to triiodothyronine (T_3)

cholestyramine, colestipol: Delayed or inhib-ited levothyroxine absorption
digoxin: Reduced therapeutic effects of digoxin
estrogen, phenylbutazone, phenytoin: Re-duced binding of levothyroxine to protein, possibly requiring increased levothyroxine dosage
insulin, oral antidiabetic drugs: Possibly un-controlled diabetes mellitus, requiring in-creased dosage of insulin or oral antidiabetic drug
ketamine: Possibly hypertension and tachy-cardia
maprotiline: Increased risk of arrhythmias
oral anticoagulants: Altered anticoagulant activity, possibly need for anticoagulant dos-age adjustment
selective serotonin reuptake inhibitors, tri-cyclic and tetracyclic antidepressants: In-creased therapeutic and toxic effects of both drugs
sympathomimetics: Increased risk of coro-nary insufficiency in patients with coronary artery disease
theophylline: Decreased theophylline clear-ance
FOODS
dietary fiber, soybean flour (infant formula), walnuts: Possibly decreased absorption of levothyroxine from GI tract

Nursing Considerations

•Administer levothyroxine tablets as a single daily dose 30 to 60 minutes before breakfast. If patient has difficulty swallowing, crush tablet and suspend in a small amount of water or food.
•To prevent decreased drug absorption, ad-minister oral levothyroxine at least 4 hours before or after aluminum- or magnesium-containing antacids, bile acid sequestrants, calcium carbonate, cation exchange resins, cholestyramine, colestipol, ferrous sulfate, kayexalate, or sucralfate.
•Expect to give drug I.V. or I.M. if patient can't take tablets. Be aware that drug shouldn't be given subcutaneously.
•For I.V. use, reconstitute drug by adding 5 ml of normal saline solution.
•Monitor PT of patient who is receiving an-ticoagulants; she may require a dosage ad-justment.
•Monitor blood glucose level of diabetic pa-

tient. Prescriber may reduce antidiabetic drug dosage as thyroid hormone level enters therapeutic range.

• Expect patient to undergo thyroid function tests regularly during levothyroxine therapy.

PATIENT TEACHING

• Inform patient that levothyroxine replaces a hormone that is normally produced by the thyroid gland and that she'll probably need to take drug for life.

• Instruct patient to take drug at least 30 minutes before breakfast because drug absorption is increased on an empty stomach and evening doses may cause insomnia.

• Stress the need to take levothyroxine with a full glass of water to avoid choking, gagging, having tablet stick in throat, and developing heartburn afterward.

• Instruct patient to separate iron and calcium supplements and antacids by at least 4 hours from levothyroxine doses.

• Inform patient that drug may require a few weeks to take effect.

• Advise patient not to stop drug or change dosage unless instructed by prescriber.

• Instruct patient to report signs of hyperthyroidism, such as diarrhea, excessive sweating, heat intolerance, insomnia, palpitations, weight loss, chest pain, shortness of breath, leg cramps, headache, nervousness, irritability, tremors, changes in appetite, vomiting, fever, and changes in menstrual periods.

• Tell patient to notify prescriber if rash or hives develop during drug use.

• Inform patient that transient hair loss may occur during first few months of therapy.

• Instruct female patient of childbearing age to notify prescriber immediately if she becomes pregnant because levothyroxine dosage may need to be increased.

lidocaine hydrochloride
(lignocaine hydrochloride)

Alphacaine (CAN), Anestacon, DermaFlex, Dilocaine, L-Caine, Lidoderm, Xylocaine, Xylocard (CAN), Zingo

Class and Category

Chemical class: Aminoacetamide
Therapeutic class: Class IB antiarrhythmic, local anesthetic
Pregnancy category: B

Indications and Dosages

➤ *To treat ventricular tachycardia or ventricular fibrillation*

I.V. INFUSION AND INJECTION

Adults. *Loading:* 50 to 100 mg (or 1 to 1.5 mg/ kg), administered at 25 to 50 mg/min. If desired response isn't achieved after 5 to 10 min, second dose of 25 to 50 mg (or 0.5 to 0.75 mg/ kg) is given every 5 to 10 min until maximum loading dose (300 mg in 1 hr) has been given. *Maintenance:* 20 to 50 mcg/kg/min (1 to 4 mg/ min) by continuous infusion. Smaller bolus dose repeated 15 to 20 min after the start of infusion if needed to maintain therapeutic blood level. *Maximum:* 300 mg (or 3 mg/kg) over 1 hr.

Children. *Loading:* 1 mg/kg. *Maintenance:* 30 mcg/kg/min by continuous infusion. *Maximum:* 3 mg/kg.

DOSAGE ADJUSTMENT For elderly patients receiving I.V. lidocaine to treat arrhythmias and for patients with acute hepatitis or decompensated cirrhosis, loading dose and continuous infusion rate reduced by 50%.

I.M. INJECTION

Adults. 300 mg, repeated after 60 to 90 min, if needed.

➤ *To provide topical anesthesia for skin or mucous membranes*

FILM-FORMING GEL, JELLY, OR OINTMENT

Adults. Thin layer applied to skin or mucous membranes as needed before procedure.

TRANSDERMAL PATCH

Adults. 1 to 3 patches applied over most painful area only once for up to 12 hr within a 24-hr period.

➤ *To provide topical anesthesia before venous access procedures*

POWDER

Children ages 3 to 18. Compressed gas application of powder to selected skin site 1 to 3 minutes before procedure.

Route	Onset	Peak	Duration
I.V.	45 to 90 sec	Immediate	10 to 20 min
I.M.	5 to 15 min	Unknown	60 to 90 min
Topical	2 to 5 min	Unknown	0.5 to 1 hr

Contraindications

Adams-Stokes syndrome; hypersensitivity to lidocaine, amide anesthetics, or their components; severe heart block (without artificial pacemaker); Wolff-Parkinson-White syndrome

Mechanism of Action

Combines with fast sodium channels in myocardial cell membranes, which inhibits sodium influx into cells and decreases ventricular depolarization, automaticity, and excitability during diastole. Lidocaine also blocks nerve impulses by decreasing the permeability of neuronal membranes to sodium. This action produces local anesthesia.

Interactions
DRUGS

beta blockers, cimetidine: Increased blood lidocaine level and risk of toxicity
MAO inhibitors, tricyclic antidepressants: Risk of severe, prolonged hypertension
mexiletine, tocainide: Additive cardiac effects
neuromuscular blockers: Possibly increased neuromuscular blockade
phenytoin, procainamide: Increased cardiac depression

Adverse Reactions

CNS: Anxiety, confusion, difficulty speaking, dizziness, hallucinations, lethargy, paresthesia, seizures
CV: Bradycardia, cardiac arrest, hypotension, new or worsening arrhythmias
EENT: Blurred vision, diplopia, tinnitus
GI: Nausea
MS: Muscle weakness, myalgia
RESP: Respiratory arrest or depression
Other: Hypersensitivity; injection site burning, irritation, petechiae, redness, stinging, swelling, and tenderness; worsened pain

Nursing Considerations

• Observe for respiratory depression after bolus injection and during I.V. infusion of lidocaine.
• Keep life-support equipment and vasopressors nearby during I.V. use in case respiratory depression or other reactions occur.
• Carefully check prefilled syringes before using. Use only syringes labeled "for cardiac arrhythmias" for I.V. administration.
• As prescribed, titrate I.V. dose to minimum amount needed to prevent arrhythmias.

• During I.V. administration, place patient on cardiac monitor, as ordered, and closely observe her at all times. Monitor for worsening arrhythmias, widening QRS complex, and prolonged PR interval—possible signs of drug toxicity.
• Monitor blood lidocaine level, as ordered. Check for therapeutic level of 2 to 5 mcg/ml.
• If signs of toxicity, such as dizziness, occur, notify prescriber and expect to discontinue or slow infusion.
• Give I.M. injection in deltoid muscle only.
• Apply lidocaine jelly or ointment to gauze or bandage before applying to skin.
• Monitor vital signs as well as BUN and serum creatinine and electrolyte levels during and after therapy.

PATIENT TEACHING

• Inform patient who receives lidocaine as an anesthetic that she'll experience numbness.
• Advise patient to report difficulty speaking, dizziness, injection site pain, nausea, numbness or tingling, and vision changes.
• Caution patient to keep lidocaine topical preparations and patches out of reach of children and pets.
• Tell patient to wash hands thoroughly after handling lidocaine topical preparation or patch and to avoid getting drug in eyes.
• If patient uses patches, tell her to store them in their sealed envelopes until needed and to apply immediately after removing from the envelope. Tell patient to remove patch if irritation or burning occurs at the site and not to reapply until irritation is gone.
• Tell patient to fold used patches so that the adhesive side sticks to itself and discard where children or pets cannot get to them.

lincomycin hydrochloride

Lincocin

Class and Category

Chemical class: Lincosamide
Therapeutic class: Bacteriostatic or bactericidal antibiotic
Pregnancy category: C

Indications and Dosages

➤ *To treat serious respiratory, skin, and*

soft-tissue infections caused by suscepti-ble strains of streptococci, pneumococci, and staphylococci

CAPSULES

Adults and adolescents. 500 mg every 6 to 8 hr.

Children over age 1 month. 7.5 to 15 mg/kg every 6 hr; alternatively, 10 to 20 mg/kg every 8 hr.

I.V. INFUSION

Adults. 600 mg to 1 g every 8 to 12 hr. *Maxi-mum:* 8 g daily in divided doses for life-threatening infection.

Children over age 1 month. 10 to 20 mg/kg/day in divided doses every 8 to 12 hr, de-pending on severity of infection.

I.M. INJECTION

Adults and adolescents. 600 mg every 12 to 24 hr.

Children over age 1 month. 10 mg/kg every 12 to 24 hr.

DOSAGE ADJUSTMENT Dosage reduced by 25% to 30% for patients with severely impaired renal function.

Mechanism of Action

Inhibits protein synthesis in susceptible bacteria by binding to the 50S subunit of bacterial ribosomes and preventing pep-tide bond formation, thus causing bacter-ial cells to die.

Incompatibilities

Don't administer lincomycin with novobiocin or kanamycin.

Contraindications

Hypersensitivity to lincomycin, clindamycin, or their components

Interactions

DRUGS

antimyasthenic drugs: Possibly antagonized effects of these drugs

chloramphenicol, clindamycin, erythromycin: Possibly blocked access of lincomycin to its site of action

hydrocarbon inhalation anesthetics, neuro-muscular blockers: Increased neuromuscular blockade, possibly severe respiratory depres-sion

opioid analgesics: Increased risk of pro-longed or increased respiratory depression

Adverse Reactions

CNS: Fever, vertigo

CV: Cardiac arrest and hypotension (with rapid administration)

EENT: Glossitis, stomatitis, tinnitus

GI: Abdominal cramps, colitis, diarrhea, nausea, pseudomembranous colitis, rectal candidiasis, vomiting

GU: Vaginal candidiasis

HEME: Agranulocytosis, eosinophilia, leukopenia, neutropenia, thrombocytopenic purpura

SKIN: Erythema multiforme, rash, Stevens-Johnson syndrome, urticaria

Other: Anaphylaxis, angioedema, super-infection

Nursing Considerations

•Expect to obtain a specimen for culture and sensitivity testing before administering first dose of lincomycin.

•**WARNING** Be aware that some preparations of lincomycin contain benzyl alcohol, which can cause a fatal toxic syndrome in neonates or premature infants, characterized by CNS, respiratory, circulatory, and renal impairment and metabolic acidosis. Because drug enters breast milk, breastfeeding patient may need to stop drug or stop breastfeeding.

•Dilute 600-mg dose in at least 100 ml of D_5W, $D_{10}W$, normal saline solution, dextrose 5% in normal saline solution, or other com-patible diluent recommended by manufac-turer. Dilute higher doses in 100 ml of a compatible diluent for each gram being ad-ministered—for example, dilute a 3-g dose in at least 300 ml of diluent. Use diluted solu-tion within 24 hours if stored at room tem-perature.

•**WARNING** Give lincomycin over at least 1 hour for each gram being administered. For example, infuse 1 g over 1 hour and 3 g over 3 hours. Too-rapid infusion may result in cardiac arrest or hypotension.

•**WARNING** Monitor patient for hypersensitiv-ity reaction, such as rash, pruritus, wheez-ing, and dysphagia from laryngeal edema. If a reaction occurs, stop infusion and notify prescriber immediately. If anaphylaxis oc-curs, give epinephrine, antihistamines, oxy-gen, and corticosteroids, as prescribed. Be aware that patients with a history of asthma or significant allergies are at increased risk for a hypersensitivity reaction.

•Observe patient for evidence of superinfection, such as vaginal itching and sore mouth.
•Monitor patient for signs of pseudomembranous colitis, such as watery, loose stools. Patients with a history of GI disease, particularly colitis or regional enteritis, are at increased risk for colitis. In elderly patients, antibiotic-related diarrhea may be more severe and less well tolerated. Notify prescriber if severe or prolonged diarrhea develops; it may indicate pseudomembranous colitis caused by *Clostridium difficile*. Expect to withhold lincomycin and treat with fluids, electrolytes, protein, and an antibiotic effective against *C. difficile*.
•Monitor results of liver and renal function tests, CBC, and platelet counts periodically during lincomycin therapy.
•Before diluting drug, store it at a controlled room temperature of 20° to 25° C (68° to 77° F).

PATIENT TEACHING
•Advise patient to take lincomycin capsules with a full glass of water on an empty stomach 1 hour before or 2 hours after meals to maximize drug's effectiveness.
•Review with patient possibly serious adverse reactions associated with lincomycin use, such as difficulty breathing, rash, and chest tightness, and tell her to report any that occur.
•Inform patient that yogurt or buttermilk can help maintain intestinal flora and may decrease the risk of diarrhea.
•Urge patient to tell prescriber about diarrhea that's severe or lasts longer than 3 days. Remind patient that watery or bloody stools can occur 2 or more months after antibiotic therapy and can be serious, requiring prompt treatment.
•Stress the importance of following dosage regimen and keeping follow-up medical and laboratory appointments.

lindane

Bio-Well, GBH, G-well, Hexit (CAN), Kildane, Kwell, Kwellada (CAN), Kwildane, PMS-Lindane (CAN), Scabene, Thionex

Class and Category

Chemical class: Benzene derivative
Therapeutic class: Pediculicide, scabicide
Pregnancy category: B

Indications and Dosages

➤ *To treat scabies and pediculosis*
CREAM, LOTION
Adults and children. For scabies, thin layer applied once over entire skin surface. For pediculosis, thin layer applied once to affected skin and hair.
SHAMPOO
Adults and children. 30 ml (for short hair) or 45 ml (for long hair) applied to dry hair and worked into lather for 4 to 5 min.

Mechanism of Action

Penetrates parasite skeleton and inhibits neuronal membrane function, causing seizures and death. Lindane also kills parasite eggs.

Contraindications

Hypersensitivity to lindane or its components, prematurity (in neonates), seizure disorders

Interactions

ACTIVITIES
use of oil-based hair products: Possibly increased absorption of lindane

Adverse Reactions

CNS: Dizziness, irritability, nervousness, restlessness, seizures, unsteadiness
SKIN: Erythema, pruritus, rash, urticaria

Nursing Considerations

•Use lindane cautiously in patients at risk for CNS toxicity, such as infants and elderly patients, and in patients weighing less than 110 lb (50 kg).
•Wear gloves when applying drug. If another person will apply drug, supply gloves for use.
•For scabies, apply thin layer of preparation to dry skin and rub in thoroughly. Trim patient's nails, and apply under nails with toothbrush. Apply to body from neck down, including soles. Leave drug on for 8 to 12 hours (usually overnight), and then remove with bath or shower.
•Expect to reduce application time for infants and children to 6 to 8 hours, as prescribed, because of the risk of systemic absorption.
•Keep lindane away from mouth and eyes.

J
K
L

Don't use on open wounds, cuts, or sores.
•Expect to administer topical steroids or
oral antihistamines to reduce pruritus, which
may continue for several weeks with scabies.
•For hospitalized patients, use special linen-
handling precautions until treatment is completed.
•**WARNING** Be aware that lindane may cause
seizures or other adverse CNS reactions;
therefore, use it only after other treatments
have been tried.
•Monitor immunocompromised patients
closely because they're at increased risk for
adverse reactions.

PATIENT TEACHING
•Inform patient that lindane is for one-time
use but may be reapplied after 1 week if she
finds live lice or nits (eggs).
•Caution patient to avoid eyes, mucous
membranes, and open areas of skin when applying drug and not to inhale vapors.
•Instruct patient (or parents of a child) to
wear gloves when applying drug.
•For scabies, instruct patient to shake lotion
bottle well before using and to apply lotion
or cream in a thin layer all over body from
the neck down, avoiding face and scalp. Direct her to leave drug on for 8 to 12 hours
and then wash it off in the bath or shower.
Explain that itching may persist for several
weeks after treatment.
•For pubic lice, instruct patient to shake lotion bottle well before using and to apply a
thin layer of lotion to pubic hair and skin as
well as to groin, thighs, and lower stomach if
they're also affected. Direct her to leave lotion on for 12 hours and then thoroughly
wash it off in the bath or shower.
•For head lice, instruct patient to shake lotion bottle well before using and to apply lotion to affected areas of head and scalp as
well as nearby hairy areas and rub it in well.
Tell her to leave lotion on for 12 hours and
then thoroughly wash it off.
•For head or pubic lice, instruct patient to
wash and dry her hair before applying lindane shampoo, especially if she uses oil-
based hair products. Instruct her to shake
bottle well before using and then apply
shampoo to dry hair, working it in thoroughly and adding a small amount of water
if needed to form good lather. Direct her to
wait 4 minutes, rinse her hair well, and then
dry it with a clean towel. Instruct her to use
a fine-toothed comb or tweezers to remove
nits or nit shells. Direct patient not to use
shampoo again for 7 days and then only if
she finds live lice. Caution patient not to use
shampoo in the shower to avoid getting it in
her eyes and mouth.
•Advise patient to wash lindane off her skin
and to contact prescriber if irritation (severe
itching, hives, or redness) occurs.
•Explain that if lice come back, the problem
is probably reinfestation rather than treatment failure.
•Advise patient to notify family members
and sexual contacts about infestation.

linezolid

Zyvox

Class and Category

Chemical class: Oxazolidinone
Therapeutic class: Antibiotic
Pregnancy category: C

Indications and Dosages

➤ *To treat vancomycin-resistant* Enterococcus faecium *infections, including
bacteremia*

ORAL SUSPENSION, TABLETS, I.V. INFUSION

Adults and adolescents. 600 mg every 12 hr
for 14 to 28 days.
Infants and children. 10 mg/kg every 8 hr for
14 to 28 days.

➤ *To treat nosocomial pneumonia caused by*
Staphylococcus aureus *(methicillin-susceptible and -resistant strains) or* Streptococcus pneumoniae *(penicillin-susceptible
strains only) and community-acquired
pneumonia, including accompanying bacteremia, caused by* S. aureus *(methicillin-
susceptible strains only) or* S. pneumoniae *(penicillin-susceptible strains only);
to treat complicated skin and soft-tissue
infections, including diabetic foot infections without concomitant osteomyelitis,
caused by* S. aureus *(methicillin-susceptible and -resistant strains),* Streptococcus
pyogenes, *or* Streptococcus agalactiae

ORAL SUSPENSION, TABLETS, I.V. INFUSION

Adults and adolescents. 600 mg every 12 hr
for 10 to 14 days.
Infants and children. 10 mg/kg every 8 hr for
10 to 14 days.

➤ *To treat uncomplicated skin and soft-tissue infections caused by* S. aureus *(methicillin-susceptible strains only) or* S. pyogenes

ORAL SUSPENSION, TABLETS

Adults. 400 mg every 12 hr for 10 to 14 days.

Adolescents. 600 mg every 12 hr for 10 to 14 days.

Children age 5 to 11 years. 10 mg/kg every 12 hr for 10 to 14 days.

Infants and children to age 5 years. 10 mg/kg every 8 hr.

Incompatibilities

Don't add other drugs to linezolid solution. Don't infuse linezolid in the same I.V. line as amphotericin B, chlorpromazine hydrochloride, co-trimoxazole, diazepam, erythromycin lactobionate, pentamidine isethionate, or phenytoin sodium because these drugs are physically incompatible. Don't infuse linezolid with ceftriaxone sodium because these drugs are chemically incompatible.

Contraindications

Carcinoid syndrome; concurrent therapy with buspirone, dopaminergic agents, meperidine, sympathomimetic agents, serotonin 5-HT_1 receptor agonists, serotonin reuptake inhibitors, tricyclic antidepressants, or vasopressive agents without careful monitoring; hypersensitivity to linezolid or its components; phenylketonuria; thyrotoxicosis; un-

Mechanism of Action

Linezolid inhibits bacterial protein synthesis by interfering with translation of ribonucleic acid (RNA) to protein. In bacteria, protein synthesis begins with binding of a 30S ribosomal subunit and a 50S ribosomal subunit to a messenger RNA (mRNA) molecule to form a 70S initiation complex. The 50S ribosomal subunit consists of 23S ribosomal RNA (rRNA) and other ribosomal subunits. Then translation begins. Transfer RNA (tRNA) attaches to the 50S subunit and brings specific amino acids into place. As the tRNA and amino acids fall into place, they are joined together by peptide bonds and elongate to form a polypeptide chain, as shown below left. This chain eventually combines with other polypeptide chains to form a complete protein molecule. After translation is complete, the ribosomal subunits fall away and are ready to combine with more mRNA to start the translation process over again.

Linezolid binds to a site on the bacterial 23S rRNA of the 50S subunit. This action prevents formation of a functional 70S initiation complex, an essential component of the bacterial translation. Without proper protein production, as shown below right, susceptible bacteria can't multiply. Linezolid is bacteriostatic against staphylococci and enterococci and bactericidal against most streptococci.

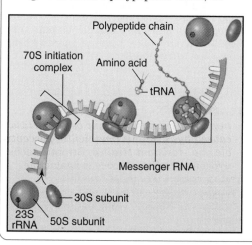

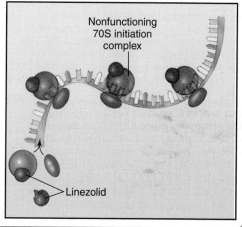

controlled hypertension; use within 14 days of an MAO inhibitor

Interactions

DRUGS

adrenergics, including pseudoephedrine and phenylpropanolamine: Possibly increased blood pressure

buspirone, meperidine, serotonergics, tricyclic antidepressants: Possibly serotonin syndrome

MAO inhibitors: Increased risk of life-threatening adverse effects

FOODS

tyramine-containing foods and beverages: Possibly hypertension

Adverse Reactions

CNS: Dizziness, fever, headache, insomnia, optic and peripheral neuropathy, serotonin syndrome

CV: Hypertension

EENT: Oral candidiasis, tongue discoloration

GI: Abdominal pain, constipation, diarrhea, indigestion, nausea, pseudomembranous colitis, vomiting

GU: Vaginal candidiasis

HEME: Anemia, leukopenia, pancytopenia, thrombocytopenia

SKIN: Pruritus, rash

Other: Lactic acidosis

Nursing Considerations

•Obtain body tissue and fluid specimens for culture and sensitivity tests, as ordered, before giving first dose of linezolid. Expect to begin drug before test results are known.

•Be aware that linezolid shouldn't be used to treat catheter-related bloodstream infections, catheter-site infections, or infections caused by gram-negative bacteria because the risk of death is higher in these infections.

•Infuse I.V. solution over 30 to 120 minutes with D_5W, normal saline solution, or lactated Ringer's solution.

•WARNING Monitor CBC weekly, as ordered, to detect or track worsening myelosuppression in patients who need more than 2 weeks of therapy, who have preexisting myelosuppression, or are receiving drugs that produce bone marrow suppression, or who have chronic infection and are receiving or have received antibiotic therapy.

•Notify prescriber if patient develops visual impairment that suggests optic neuropathy, such as changes in visual acuity or color vision, blurred vision, lost vision, or visual field defect. If optic or peripheral neuropathy develops, the drug may need to be stopped.

•If patient takes a dopaminergic agent, sympathomimetic agent, or vasopressive agent, monitor blood pressure closely; if monitoring isn't possible, linezolid shouldn't be prescribed.

•If patient takes buspirone, meperidine, a serotinergic, or a tricyclic antidepressant, watch closely for signs and symptoms of serotonin syndrome; if monitoring isn't possible, linezolid shouldn't be prescribed.

•Assess bowel pattern daily. Also assess patient for secondary infection, including oral candidiasis and profuse, watery diarrhea.

PATIENT TEACHING

•Caution patient with phenylketonuria that oral suspension contains phenylalanine.

•Advise patient not to take OTC cold remedies without consulting prescriber because medications that contain pseudoephedrine or propanolamine may cause or worsen hypertension.

•Instruct patient to avoid foods and beverages that contain large amounts of tyramine, including aged cheese, fermented or air-dried meats, sauerkraut, soy sauce, tap beers, red wines, and protein-rich foods that have been stored for long periods or poorly refrigerated.

•Instruct patient to notify prescriber immediately about severe diarrhea, even up to 2 months after linezolid therapy has ended, because additional treatment may be needed. Also tell patient to report vision changes and changes in limb sensation (such as pins and needles, numbness, or tingling) because drug may need to be stopped.

liothyronine sodium

(L-triiodothyronine, sodium L-triiodothyronine, T_3, thyronine sodium)

Cytomel, Triostat

Class and Category

Chemical class: Synthetic triiodothyronine (T_3)

Therapeutic class: Thyroid hormone replacement

Pregnancy category: A

Indications and Dosages

➤ *To treat mild hypothyroidism*
TABLETS
Adults. *Initial:* 25 mcg daily. Increased by
12.5 to 25 mcg every 1 to 2 wk until response
occurs. *Maintenance:* 25 to 50 mcg daily.
DOSAGE ADJUSTMENT For elderly patients
and those with cardiovascular disease, initial
dose reduced to 5 mcg daily and then increased by 5 mcg every 2 wk.

➤ *To treat congenital hypothyroidism*
TABLETS
Adults and children. *Initial:* 5 mcg daily. Increased by 5 mcg every 3 to 4 days until desired response occurs. *Maintenance:* Highly
individualized.

➤ *To treat simple nontoxic goiter*
TABLETS
Adults. *Initial:* 5 mcg daily. Increased by 5 to
10 mcg every 1 to 2 wk up to 25 mcg daily.
Then increased by 12.5 to 25 mcg/wk, as in-
dicated. *Maintenance:* 50 to 100 mcg daily.

➤ *To treat myxedema*
TABLETS
Adults. *Initial:* 2.5 to 5 mcg daily. Increased
5 to 10 mcg every 1 to 2 wk up to 25 mcg
daily. Then increased by 12.5 to 25 mcg every
1 to 2 wk, as indicated. *Maintenance:* 25 to
50 mcg daily.

➤ *To treat myxedema coma or premyx-*
edema coma (severe hypothyroidism)
I.V. INJECTION
Adults. *Initial:* 25 to 50 mcg. Repeated every
4 to 12 hr according to patient's response.
Then P.O. therapy is resumed as soon as possible.
DOSAGE ADJUSTMENT When treating myxedema coma in patients with known or suspected cardiovascular disease, initial dose
decreased to 10 to 20 mcg.

➤ *To differentiate hyperthyroidism from*
euthyroidism (T_3 suppression test)
TABLETS
Adults. 75 to 100 mcg daily for 7 days.

Route	Onset	Peak	Duration
P.O.	24 to 72 hr	48 to 72 hr	Up to 72 hr
I.V.	2 to 4 hr	2 days	Unknown

Contraindications
Acute MI (unless caused or complicated by
hypothyroidism), hypersensitivity to liothyronine or its components, uncorrected adrenal
insufficiency, untreated thyrotoxicosis

Mechanism of Action
Replaces endogenous thyroid hormone,
which may exert its physiologic effects by
controlling DNA transcription and protein
synthesis. Like endogenous thyroid hormone, liothyronine:
• increases energy expenditure
• accelerates the rate of cellular oxidation, which stimulates body tissue growth,
maturation, and metabolism
• regulates differentiation and proliferation of stem cells
• aids in myelination of nerves and development of synaptic processes in the nervous system
• regulates growth
• decreases blood and hepatic cholesterol
concentrations
• enhances carbohydrate and protein metabolism, increasing gluconeogenesis and
protein synthesis.

Interactions
DRUGS
adrenocorticoids: Possibly need for adrenocorticoid dosage adjustments as thyroid status changes
beta blockers: Possibly impaired action of
beta blockers
cholestyramine, colestipol: Decreased liothyronine absorption
digoxin: Reduced therapeutic effects of digoxin
estrogen, phenylbutazone, phenytoin: Reduced
binding of liothyronine to protein, possibly
requiring increased liothyronine dosage
insulin, oral antidiabetic drugs: Possibly uncontrolled diabetes mellitus, requiring increased dosage of insulin or oral antidiabetic
drug
ketamine: Possibly hypertension and tachycardia
maprotiline: Increased risk of arrhythmias
oral anticoagulants: Altered anticoagulant
activity, possibly need for anticoagulant dosage adjustment
sympathomimetics: Increased risk of coronary insufficiency in patients with coronary
artery disease

theophylline: Decreased theophylline clearance

tricyclic antidepressants: Increased therapeutic and toxic effects of both drugs

Adverse Reactions

CNS: Insomnia
ENDO: Hyperthyroidism (with overdose)
SKIN: Alopecia (transient), rash, urticaria

Nursing Considerations

• Be aware that liothyronine is used most often when rapid onset or rapidly reversible thyroid hormone replacement is needed.
• Administer tablet as a single daily dose before breakfast.
• Give I.V. injections more than 4 hours but less than 12 hours apart.
• Evaluate response to therapy by monitoring pulse rate and blood pressure.
• Expect patient to undergo regular tests of thyroid function during liothyronine therapy.
• Monitor PT of patient receiving anticoagulants because she may require a dosage adjustment.
• Frequently monitor blood glucose level of diabetic patient. Prescriber may reduce antidiabetic drug dosage as thyroid hormone level enters therapeutic range.
• Be aware that liothyronine is used in T_3 suppression test to differentiate hyperthyroidism from euthyroidism (normal thyroid function). For this test, ^{131}I uptake test is performed before and after liothyronine administration. Suppression of ^{131}I uptake by 50% indicates normal thyroid function.

PATIENT TEACHING
• Inform patient that liothyronine usually is taken for life. Caution her not to discontinue drug or change dosage unless instructed by prescriber.
• Instruct patient to take drug before breakfast; evening doses may cause insomnia.
• Advise patient to report signs of hyperthyroidism, such as chest pain, excessive sweating, heat intolerance, increased pulse rate, nervousness, and palpitations.
• Inform patient that transient hair loss may occur during first few months of therapy.
• Instruct diabetic patient to monitor blood glucose level frequently because antidiabetic drug dosage may need to be reduced.
• Inform patient of need for periodic blood tests to monitor drug effectiveness.

lisdexamfetamine dimesylate

Vyvanse

Class and Category

Chemical class: Sympathomimetic amine
Therapeutic class: CNS stimulant
Pregnancy category: C

Indications and Dosages

➤ *To treat attention deficit hyperactivity disorder (ADHD)*

CAPSULES
Adults and children ages 6 to 12. *Initial:* 30 mg once daily in the morning, increased as needed in increments of 10 or 20 mg daily every wk. *Maximum:* 70 mg daily.

Route	Onset	Peak	Duration
P.O.	Unknown	1 hr	Unknown

Mechanism of Action

Produces CNS stimulant effects, probably by facilitating release and blocking reuptake of norepinephrine at adrenergic nerve terminals and by stimulating alpha and beta receptors in the peripheral nervous system. The drug also releases and blocks reuptake of dopamine in the limbic regions of the brain. These actions cause decreased motor restlessness and increased alertness.

Contraindications

Advanced arteriosclerosis; agitation; glaucoma; history of drug abuse, hypersensitivity, or idiosyncratic reaction to lisdexamfetamine, other sympathomimetic amines, or their components; hyperthyroidism; MAO inhibitor therapy within 14 days; moderate to severe hypertension; symptomatic cardiovascular disease; history of seizures

Interactions

DRUGS
adrenergic blockers: Inhibited adrenergic blockade
acetazolamide, alkalinizers (such as sodium bicarbonate), some thiazides: Increased blood level and effects of lisdexamfetamine
antihistamines: Possibly reduced sedation from antihistamine

antihypertensives: Possibly decreased antihypertensive effects

chlorpromazine: Inhibited CNS stimulant effects of lisdexamfetamine

ethosuximide: Possibly delayed ethosuximide absorption

GI acidifiers (such as ascorbic acid), reserpine: Decreased amphetamine absorption

guanethine: Decreased antihypertensive effect and decreased lisdexamfetamine absorption

haloperidol: Decreased CNS stimulation

lithium carbonate: Possibly decreased anorectic and stimulant effects of lisdexamfetamine

MAO inhibitors: Potentiated effects of lisdexamfetamine, possibly hypertensive crisis

meperidine: Increased analgesia

methenamine: Increased urine excretion and decreased effects of lisdexamfetamine

norepinephrine: Possibly increased adrenergic effect of norepinephrine

phenobarbital, phenytoin: Synergistic anticonvulsant action

propoxyphene: Increased CNS stimulation, potentially fatal seizures

sympathomimetic drugs: Increased stimulant effect

tricyclic antidepressants: Possibly increased antidepressant effects and decreased lisdexamfetamine effects

urinary acidifiers (such as ammonium chloride and sodium acid phosphate): Increased amphetamine excretion and decreased amphetamine blood level and effects

veratrum alkaloids: Decreased hypotensive effect

Adverse Reactions

CNS: Affect lability, agitation, anxiety, dizziness, fever, headache, insomnia, irritability, jittery feeling, psychomotor hyperactivity, seizures, somnolence, tic, tremor
CV: Hypertension, tachycardia, ventricular hyperthrophy
EENT: Dry mouth
GI: Anorexia, diarrhea, nausea, vomiting, upper abdominal pain
RESP: Dyspnea
SKIN: Diaphoresis, rash, Stevens-Johnson syndrome, toxic epidermal necrolysis, urticaria
Other: Anaphylaxis, angioedema, physical or psychological dependence, weight loss

Nursing Considerations

•**WARNING** Patients with symptoms such as chest pain or fainting should contact their presciber immediately.

•**WARNING** Be aware that lisdexamfetamine shouldn't be given to patients with structural cardiac abnormalities, cardiomyopathy, or other serious heart problems or rhythm abnormalities because even usual CNS-stimulant dosages increase the risk of sudden death in patients with these conditions.

•Use lisdexamfetamine cautiously in patients with hypertension, heart failure, recent MI, or ventricular arrhythmia because the drug may increase blood pressure and worsen these conditions.

•Monitor patient's blood pressure closely; stimulant drugs such as lisdexamfetamine may increase it.

•Monitor patients with psychosis, bipolar illness, or a history of aggression or hostility; CNS stimulation may worsen symptoms.

•Assess growth pattern in pediatric patients because stimulants such as lisdexamfetamine may suppress growth. If this occurs, notify prescriber and expect therapy to be halted.

•If patient has a history of seizures or EEG abnormality, watch for seizure activity because stimulants may lower the seizure threshold. Rarely, lisamfetamine may cause seizures in a patient with no history of them. Take seizure precautions in all patients, and notify prescriber if a seizure occurs. Expect to discontinue lisdexamfetamine, as prescribed.

•Take safety precautions because stimulants may alter accommodation and cause blurred vision. Although these effects haven't been reported with lisdexamfetamine, the drug is a known stimulant.

•Be aware that therapy may be stopped temporarily to assess the continued need for it, as evidenced by a return of hyperactivity and attention deficit.

PATIENT TEACHING

•**WARNING** Patients with symptoms such as chest pain or fainting should contact their presciber immediately.

•Warn patient or caregiver that drug must be taken exactly as prescribed and dosage increased only at prescriber's instruction because drug can be abused or lead to dependence.

•Instruct patient or caregiver that capsule

may be opened and contents dissolved in a glass of water; it should be drunk immediately.

• Tell patient or caregiver that drug should only be taken in the morning because taking it later in the day may cause insomnia.

• Advise patient or caregiver to report any symptoms that suggest heart disease, such as such as exertional chest pain or unexplained syncope.

• Urge patient to avoid hazardous activities until drug effects are known.

• Tell female patient of childbearing age to notify prescriber if pregnancy is suspected.

lisinopril

Prinivil, Zestril

Class and Category

Chemical class: Lysine ester of enalaprilat
Therapeutic class: Antihypertensive, vasodilator
Pregnancy category: C (first trimester), D (later trimesters)

Indications and Dosages

➤ *To manage uncomplicated essential hypertension*

TABLETS

Adults. *Initial:* 10 mg daily. *Maintenance:* 20 to 40 mg daily. *Maximum:* 80 mg daily.

DOSAGE ADJUSTMENT For patients with renal failure, initial dosage reduced to 5 mg daily if creatinine clearance is 10 to 30 ml/min/ 1.73 m^2, and to 2.5 mg daily if creatinine clearance is less than 10 ml/min/1.73 m^2. For patients receiving a diuretic, initial dosage reduced to 5 mg daily.

Children age 6 and over with a GFR of at least 30 ml/min/1.73 m^2. *Initial:* 0.07 mg/kg daily, adjusted according to blood pressure response up to 5 mg daily. *Maximum:* 0.61 mg/kg or 40 mg daily.

➤ *To treat heart failure, along with digoxin and diuretics*

TABLETS

Adults. *Initial:* 5 mg daily. *Maintenance:* 5 to 20 mg daily. *Maximum:* 80 mg daily.

DOSAGE ADJUSTMENT For patients with hyponatremia or creatinine clearance of 30 ml/ min/1.73 m^2 or less, initial dosage reduced to 2.5 mg daily.

➤ *To improve survival in hemodynamically stable patient after acute MI*

TABLETS

Adults. 5 mg within 24 hr after onset of symptoms, followed by 5 mg after 24 hr and 10 mg after 48 hr. *Maintenance:* 10 mg daily for 6 wk. *Maximum:* 80 mg daily.

DOSAGE ADJUSTMENT For patients with baseline systolic blood pressure of 120 mm Hg or less, initial dosage decreased to 2.5 mg daily for first 3 days after MI. If systolic blood pressure falls to 100 mm Hg or less during therapy, maintenance dosage decreased to 2.5 to 5 mg as tolerated; if systolic blood pressure is 90 mm Hg or less for more than 1 hr, drug is discontinued.

Route	Onset	Peak	Duration
P.O.	1 hr	6 to 8 hr	24 hr

Mechanism of Action

May reduce blood pressure by inhibiting the conversion of angiotensin I to angiotensin II. Angiotensin II is a potent vasoconstrictor that also stimulates the adrenal cortex to secrete aldosterone. Lisinopril may also inhibit renal and vascular production of angiotensin II. Decreased release of aldosterone reduces sodium and water reabsorption and increases their excretion, thereby reducing blood pressure.

Contraindications

Hypersensitivity to lisinopril, other ACE inhibitors, or their components; history of angioedema related to previous treatment with an ACE inhibitor; hereditary or idiopathic angioedema

Interactions

DRUGS

allopurinol, bone marrow depressants (such as methotrexate), procainamide, systemic corticosteroids: Increased risk of potentially fatal neutropenia or agranulocytosis
cyclosporine, potassium-sparing diuretics, potassium supplements: Increased risk of hyperkalemia
diuretics, other antihypertensives: Increased hypotensive effect
insulin, oral antidiabetics: Increased risk of hypoglycemia

lithium: Increased blood lithium level and risk of lithium toxicity

NSAIDs: Possibly reduced antihypertensive effect, reduced renal function in patients with preexisting renal dysfunction

sympathomimetics: Possibly reduced antihypertensive effect

FOODS

high-potassium diet, potassium-containing salt substitutes: Increased risk of hyperkalemia

ACTIVITIES

alcohol use: Possibly increased hypotensive effect

Adverse Reactions

CNS: Ataxia, confusion, dizziness, fatigue, headache, stroke, syncope, transient ischemic attack, vertigo
CV: Arrhythmias, chest pain, hypotension, MI, orthostatic hypotension, palpitations, peripheral edema, vasculitis
ENDO: Hyperglycemia
GI: Abdominal pain, anorexia, cholestatic jaundice, diarrhea, elevated liver enzyme levels, fulminant hepatic necrosis, gastritis, hepatitis, indigestion, nausea, pancreatitis, vomiting
GU: Acute renal failure, decreased libido, impotence, pyelonephritis
HEME: Agranulocytosis, anemia, hemolytic anemia, neutropenia, thrombocytopenia
MS: Muscle spasms, myalgia
RESP: Bronchospasm, cough, dyspnea, paroxysmal nocturnal dyspnea, pulmonary embolism and infarction, upper respiratory tract infection
SKIN: Alopecia, cutaneous pseudolymphoma, diaphoresis, erythema, flushing, herpes zoster, infections, pemphigus, photosensitivity, pruritus, rash, Stevens-Johnson syndrome, toxic epidermal necrolysis, urticaria
Other: Anaphylaxis, angioedema

Nursing Considerations

•Use lisinopril cautiously in patients with fluid volume deficit, heart failure, impaired renal function, or sodium depletion.
•To prepare pediatric suspension, add 10 ml of purified water to a polyethylene terephthalate (PET) bottle containing ten 20-mg tablets and shake for at least 1 minute. Add 30 ml of Bicitra diluent and 160 ml of Ora-Sweet SF to the concentrate in the PET bot-

tle, and shake gently for several seconds. Store in refrigerator for up to 4 weeks. Shake the suspension before each use.
•Monitor blood pressure often, especially early in treatment. If excessive hypotension develops, expect to withhold drug for several days.
•**WARNING** If angioedema affects face, glottis, larynx, limbs, lips, mucous membranes, or tongue, notify prescriber immediately and expect to stop lisinopril and start appropriate therapy at once. If airway obstruction threatens, promptly give 0.3 to 0.5 ml of epinephrine 1:1,000 solution subcutaneously, as prescribed.
•Monitor patient for anaphylaxis, especially patient being dialyzed with high-flux membranes and treated concurrently with an ACE inhibitor such as lisinopril. If anaphylaxis occurs, stop dialysis immediately and treat aggressively (antihistamines are ineffective in this situation), as ordered. Anaphylaxis has also occurred with some patients undergoing low-density lipoprotein apheresis with dextran sulfate absorption.
•Notify prescriber if patient has persistent, nonproductive cough, a common adverse effect of ACE inhibitors such as lisinopril.
•Monitor for dehydration, which can lead to hypotension. Be aware that diarrhea and vomiting can cause dehydration.
•Monitor patient for hepatic dysfunction because lisinopril, an ACE inhibitor, may rarely cause a syndrome that starts with cholestatic jaundice or hepatitis and progresses to fulminant hepatic necrosis. If patient develops jaundice or a marked elevation in liver enzyme levels, withhold drug and notify prescriber.
•If patient takes insulin or an oral antidiabetic, monitor blood glucose level closely because risk of hypoglycemia increases, especially during the first month of therapy.

PATIENT TEACHING
•Explain to patient that lisinopril helps to control but doesn't cure hypertension and that she may need lifelong therapy.
•Advise patient to take lisinopril at the same time every day.
•Emphasize need to take drug as ordered, even if patient feels well; caution her not to stop drug without consulting prescriber.
•Instruct patient to report dizziness, especially during the first few days of therapy.

•Inform patient that a persistent, nonproductive cough may develop during lisinopril therapy. Urge her to notify prescriber immediately if cough becomes difficult to tolerate.
•Advise patient to drink adequate fluid and avoid excessive sweating, which can lead to dehydration and hypotension. Make sure she understands that diarrhea and vomiting also can cause hypotension.
•Caution patient not to use salt substitutes that contain potassium.
•Instruct patient to report signs of infection, such as fever and sore throat, which may indicate neutropenia.
•Advise patient to change position slowly to minimize the effects of orthostatic hypotension.
•If patient has diabetes and takes insulin or an oral antidiabetic, urge her to monitor her blood glucose level closely and watch for symptoms of hypoglycemia.
•Caution female patient to notify prescriber immediately if she is or could be pregnant.

lithium carbonate

Carbolith (CAN), Duralith (CAN), Eskalith, Eskalith CR, Lithane, Lithizine (CAN), Lithobid, Lithonate, Lithotabs

lithium citrate

Cibalith-S

Class and Category

Chemical class: Alkaline metal, monovalent cation
Therapeutic class: Antidepressant, antimanic
Pregnancy category: D

Indications and Dosages

➤ *To treat recurrent bipolar affective disorder, to prevent bipolar disorder depression*

CAPSULES, TABLETS

Adults and children age 12 and over. *Initial:* 300 to 600 mg t.i.d. *Maintenance:* 300 mg t.i.d. or q.i.d. *Maximum:* 2,400 g daily.
Children up to age 12. 15 to 20 mg/kg daily in divided doses b.i.d. or t.i.d.

E.R. TABLETS

Adults and children age 12 and over. *Initial:* 900 to 1,800 mg daily in divided doses b.i.d. or t.i.d. *Maintenance:* 450 mg b.i.d. or 300 mg t.i.d. *Maximum:* 2,400 g daily.

SLOW-RELEASE CAPSULES

Adults and children age 12 and over. 600 to 900 mg on day 1, increased to 1,200 to 1,800 mg daily in divided doses t.i.d. *Maintenance:* 900 to 1,200 mg daily in divided doses t.i.d. *Maximum:* 2,400 g daily.

SYRUP (LITHIUM CITRATE)

Adults and children age 12 and over. 8 to 16 mEq (equivalent of 300 to 600 mg of lithium carbonate) t.i.d. *Maintenance:* Equivalent of 300 mg of lithium carbonate t.i.d. or q.i.d. *Maximum:* Equivalent of 2,400 g daily of lithium carbonate.
Children up to age 12. 0.4 to 0.5 mEq (equivalent of 15 to 20 mg of lithium carbonate)/kg daily in divided doses b.i.d. or t.i.d.

Route	Onset	Peak	Duration
P.O.	1 to 3 wk	Unknown	Unknown

Mechanism of Action

May increase presynaptic degradation of the catecholamine neurotransmitters serotonin, dopamine, and norepinephrine; inhibit their release at neuronal synapses; and decrease postsynaptic receptor sensitivity. These actions may correct overactive catecholamine systems in patients with mania.

Antidepressant action may result from enhanced serotonergic activity.

Contraindications

Blood dyscrasias, bone marrow depression, brain damage, cerebrovascular disease, coma, coronary artery disease, excessive intake of other CNS depressants, hypersensitivity to lithium or its components, impaired hepatic function, myeloproliferative disorders, severe depression, severe hypertension or hypotension

Interactions

DRUGS

ACE inhibitors, NSAIDs, piroxicam: Possibly increased blood lithium level and increased risk of toxicity
acetazolamide, sodium bicarbonate, urea, xanthines: Decreased blood lithium level
calcium channel blockers, molindone: Increased risk of neurotoxicity from lithium
calcium iodide, iodinated glycerol, potassium

iodide: Possibly increased hypothyroid effects of both drugs

carbamazepine: Possibly increased therapeutic effects of carbamazepine and neurotoxic effect of lithium

chlorpromazine, other phenothiazines: Possibly impaired GI absorption and decreased blood levels of these drugs; possibly masking of early signs of lithium toxicity

desmopressin, lypressin, vasopressin: Possibly impaired antidiuretic effects of these drugs

diuretics (loop and osmotic): Increased lithium reabsorption by kidneys, possibly leading to lithium toxicity

fluoxetine, methyldopa, metronidazole: Increased risk of lithium toxicity from reduced renal clearance of lithiun

haloperidol and other antipyschotics: Increased risk of irreversible neurotoxicity and brain damage

neuromuscular blockers: Risk of prolonged paralysis or weakness

norepinephrine: Possibly decreased therapeutic effects of norepinephrine and severe respiratory depression

selective serotonin reuptake inhibitors: Increased risk of adverse effects, such as diarrhea, confusion, dizziness, agitation, and tremor

thyroid hormones: Possibly hypothyroidism

tricyclic antidepressants: Possibly severe mood swings from mania to depression

FOODS

high-sodium foods: Increased excretion and possibly decreased therapeutic effects of lithium

Adverse Reactions

CNS: Ataxia, coma, confusion, depression, dizziness, drowsiness, headache, lethargy, seizures, syncope, tremor (in hands), vertigo

CV: Arrhythmias (including bradycardia and tachycardia), ECG changes, edema

EENT: Dental caries, dry mouth, exophthalmos

ENDO: Diabetes insipidus, euthyroid goiter, hypothyroidism, myxedema

GI: Abdominal distention and pain, anorexia, diarrhea, nausea, thirst

GU: Stress incontinence, urinary frequency

HEME: Leukocytosis

MS: Muscle twitching and weakness

RESP: Dyspnea

SKIN: Acne; alopecia; dry, thin hair; pruritus; rash

Other: Cold sensitivity, weight gain or loss

Nursing Considerations

• Administer lithium after meals to slow absorption from GI tract and reduce adverse reactions. Dilute syrup with juice or other flavored drink before giving.

• Note that 5 ml of lithium citrate equals 8 mEq of lithium ion or 300 mg of lithium carbonate.

• Expect to monitor blood lithium level two or three times weekly during first month, and then weekly to monthly during maintenance therapy and when initiating or discontinuing NSAID therapy. In uncomplicated cases, plan to monitor lithium level every 2 to 3 months.

• Be aware that lithium has a narrow therapeutic range. Even a slightly high blood level is dangerous, and some patients exhibit signs of toxicity at normal levels.

• Expect prescriber to decrease dosage after acute manic episode is controlled.

• **WARNING** Be aware that lithium affects intracellular and extracellular potassium ion shift, which can cause ECG changes, such as flattened or inverted T waves; lithium also can increase the risk of cardiac arrest.

• Monitor ECGs, renal and thyroid function test results, and serum electrolyte levels, as appropriate, during lithium treatment.

• **WARNING** Be aware that lithium can cause reversible leukocytosis, which usually peaks within 7 to 10 days of initiating therapy; WBC count typically returns to baseline within 10 days after lithium is discontinued.

• Weigh patient daily to detect sudden weight changes.

• Monitor blood glucose level often in diabetic patient because lithium alters glucose tolerance.

• Palpate thyroid gland to detect enlargement because drug may cause goiter.

• Ensure that patient's fluid and sodium intake is adequate during treatment.

PATIENT TEACHING

• Advise patient to take lithium with or after meals to minimize adverse reactions.

• Instruct patient to swallow E.R. or slow-release form whole.

• Direct patient to mix syrup form with juice or other flavored drink before taking.

J
K
L

•Inform patient that frequent urination, nausea, and thirst may occur during the first few days of treatment.
•Caution patient not to stop taking lithium or adjust dosage without first consulting prescriber.
•Instruct patient to report signs of toxicity, such as diarrhea, drowsiness, muscle weakness, tremor, uncoordinated body movements, and vomiting.
•Urge patient to avoid potentially hazardous activities until drug's CNS effects are known.
•Advise patient to maintain normal fluid and sodium intake.
•Emphasize the importance of complying with scheduled checkups and laboratory tests.

lomefloxacin hydrochloride

Maxaquin

Class and Category

Chemical class: Fluoroquinolone
Therapeutic class: Antibiotic
Pregnancy category: C

Indications and Dosage

➤ *To treat mild to moderate lower respiratory tract infections caused by susceptible organisms, including* Haemophilus influenzae *and* Moraxella catarrhalis

TABLETS

Adults. 400 mg daily for 10 days.

➤ *To treat uncomplicated cystitis caused by* Escherichia coli; *to treat uncomplicated cystitis caused by* Klebsiella pneumoniae, Proteus mirabilis, *or* Staphylococcus saprophyticus

TABLETS

Adults. 400 mg daily for 3 days.

➤ *To treat complicated UTI caused by* Citrobacter diversus, *Enterobacteriaceae,* E. coli, K. pneumoniae, P. mirabilis, *or* Pseudomonas aeruginosa

TABLETS

Adults. 400 mg daily for 14 days.

➤ *To provide prophylaxis for transurethral surgery*

TABLETS

Adults. 400 mg as a single dose 2 to 6 hr before surgery.

➤ *To provide prophylaxis for transrectal biopsy*

TABLETS

Adults. 400 mg as a single dose 1 to 6 hr before surgery.

➤ *To treat gonorrhea (as alternative to ciprofloxacin or ofloxacin)*

TABLETS

Adults. 400 mg as a single dose.

DOSAGE ADJUSTMENT For patients with creatinine clearance between 11 and 39 ml/min/ 1.73 m^2, loading dose of 400 mg given on day 1 and followed by 200 mg daily.

Mechanism of Action

Inhibits the bacterial enzyme DNA gyrase, which normally is responsible for the unwinding and supercoiling of bacterial DNA before it replicates. By inhibiting this enzyme, lomefloxacin interferes with bacterial cell replication and causes cell death.

Contraindications

History of tendinitis or tendon rupture, hypersensitivity to lomefloxacin or any quinolone derivative

Interactions

DRUGS

aluminum-, calcium-, or magnesium-containing antacids; iron salts; sucralfate; zinc: Decreased absorption and blood level of lomefloxacin
cyclosporine: Possibly increased blood cyclosporine level, increased nephrotoxicity
probenecid: Decreased lomefloxacin excretion, increased risk of toxicity
warfarin: Possibly increased anticoagulant effect and risk of bleeding

Adverse Reactions

CNS: Ataxia, cerebral thrombosis, dizziness, drowsiness, hallucinations, headache, insomnia, nervousness, peripheral neuropathy, phobia, vertigo
CV: Prolonged QT interval, torsades de pointes, vasculitis
EENT: Diplopia, laryngeal edema, oral candidiasis, painful oral mucosa, taste perversion

GI: Abdominal pain, diarrhea, hepatitis, indigestion, nausea, pseudomembranous colitis, vomiting
GU: Interstitial nephritis, polyuria, renal failure, urine retention, vaginal candidiasis
HEME: Hemolytic anemia
MS: Tendinitis, tendon rupture
RESP: Pulmonary edema
SKIN: Exfolitaive dermatitis, hyperpigmentation, photosensitivity, Stevens-Johnson syndrome, toxic epidermal necrolysis
Other: Anaphylaxis

Nursing Considerations
• Know that lomefloxacin shouldn't be given to patients with QT-interval prolongation or hypokalemia or to patients taking class IA antiarrhythmic drugs (such as quinidine or procainamide) or class III antiarrhythmic drugs (such as amiodarone or sotalol) because of the increased risk of torsades de pointes.
• Expect to obtain body fluid or tissue sample for culture and sensitivity testing and to review results, if possible, before lomefloxacin therapy begins.
• If patient's culture test results are positive for gonorrhea, expect to obtain serologic test for syphilis at diagnosis and to repeat test 3 months after lomefloxacin therapy.
• Give drug with meals and a full glass of water.
• Ensure that patient maintains adequate fluid intake during therapy.
• Observe for signs of secondary infections, such as sore mouth or vaginal discharge.
• Notify prescriber if patient experiences severe or prolonged diarrhea, which may indicate pseudomembranous colitis.
• Be aware that prolonged use may lead to growth of drug-resistant organisms.
• Notify prescriber and expect to stop lomefloxacin if patient develops symptoms of peripheral neuropathy (pain, burning, tingling, numbness, weakness, or changes in sensations of light touch, pain, temperature, position, or vibration) to prevent an irreversible condition or tendon rupture that requires immediate rest and avoidance of exercise involving the affected area.
PATIENT TEACHING
• Advise patient to take lomefloxacin at the same time each day with meals and with a full glass of water.

• Caution patient not to take antacids, iron, sucralfate, or zinc 1 hour before or 2 hours after taking lomefloxacin because these preparations impair drug absorption.
• Urge patient to drink plenty of fluids during treatment.
• Instruct patient to complete the full course of therapy, even if symptoms subside.
• Advise patient to notify prescriber if symptoms don't improve within a few days after starting lomefloxacin or if severe GI distress or diarrhea develops.
• Instruct patient to notify prescriber and stop taking drug if she has tendon inflammation or pain; advise her to rest until tendinitis and tendon rupture have been ruled out.
• Urge patient to avoid direct sunlight, to wear protective clothing, and to use sunscreen because photosensitivity reactions can occur during therapy and for several days afterward.
• Explain that risk of photosensitivity can be decreased by taking lomefloxacin at least 12 hours before sun exposure. Urge patient to stop drug and notify prescriber at first sign of photosensitivity, such as skin burning, redness, swelling, blisters, rash, itching, or dermatitis.
• Inform patient that an allergic reaction may occur after a single dose. Tell patient to stop lomefloxacin and notify prescriber if rash or other allergic reaction develops.
• Caution patient to avoid hazardous activities until drug's CNS effects are known.

loracarbef

Lorabid

Class and Category
Chemical class: Carbacephem
Therapeutic class: Antibiotic
Pregnancy category: B

Indications and Dosages
➤ *To treat acute bronchitis caused by* Haemophilus influenzae, Moraxella catarrhalis, *or* Streptococcus pneumoniae
CAPSULES, ORAL SUSPENSION
Adults and adolescents. 200 to 400 mg every 12 hr for 7 days.

➤ *To treat chronic bronchitis exacerbations caused by* H. influenzae, M. catarrhalis, *or* S. pneumoniae

CAPSULES, ORAL SUSPENSION

Adults and adolescents. 400 mg every 12 hr for 7 days.

➤ *To treat pneumonia caused by* H. influenzae *or* S. pneumoniae

CAPSULES, ORAL SUSPENSION

Adults and adolescents. 400 mg every 12 hr for 14 days.

➤ *To treat pharyngitis, sinusitis, or tonsillitis caused by* Streptococcus pyogenes

CAPSULES, ORAL SUSPENSION

Adults and adolescents. 200 to 400 mg every 12 hr for 10 days.

Children. 7.5 mg/kg every 12 hr for 10 days.

➤ *To treat acute otitis media caused by* H. influenzae, M. catarrhalis, S. pneumoniae, *or* S. pyogenes

ORAL SUSPENSION

Children. 15 mg/kg every 12 hr for 10 days.

➤ *To treat uncomplicated skin and soft-tissue infections caused by* Staphylococcus aureus *or* S. pyogenes

CAPSULES, ORAL SUSPENSION

Adults and adolescents. 200 mg every 12 hr for 7 days.

ORAL SUSPENSION

Children. 7.5 mg/kg every 12 hr for 7 days.

➤ *To treat uncomplicated cystitis caused by* Escherichia coli *or* Staphylococcus saprophyticus

CAPSULES, ORAL SUSPENSION

Adults and adolescents. 200 mg daily for 7 days.

➤ *To treat uncomplicated pyelonephritis caused by* E. coli

CAPSULES, ORAL SUSPENSION

Adults and adolescents. 400 mg every 12 hr for 14 days.

DOSAGE ADJUSTMENT If creatinine clearance is 10 to 49 ml/min/1.73 m², 50% of usual dose given at normal interval or usual dose given at twice the normal interval; if clearance is less than 10 ml/min/1.73 m², usual adult dosage given every 3 to 5 days.

Contraindications

Hypersensitivity to loracarbef, other cephalosporins, or their components

Interactions

DRUGS

probenecid: Inhibited renal excretion of lo-racarbef, resulting in increased blood level

FOODS

all foods: Inhibited drug absorption

> **Mechanism of Action**
> Interferes with bacterial cell wall synthesis by inhibiting the final step in the cross-linking of peptidoglycan strands. Peptidoglycan makes the bacterial cell membrane rigid and protective. Without it, bacterial cells rupture and die.

Adverse Reactions

CNS: Dizziness, drowsiness, headache, insomnia, nervousness, seizures

EENT: Oral candidiasis

GI: Abdominal pain, anorexia, diarrhea, nausea, pseudomembranous colitis, vomiting

GU: Vaginal candidiasis

SKIN: Pruritus, rash, urticaria

Nursing Considerations

•Expect to obtain body fluid or tissue sample for culture and sensitivity testing and to review results, if possible, before giving first dose of loracarbef.

•Be aware that oral suspension is absorbed more rapidly and produces a higher peak plasma level than capsules.

•Monitor patient for signs of secondary infections, such as sore mouth and vaginal discharge.

•Watch for seizures, especially if patient has impaired renal function.

PATIENT TEACHING

•Advise patient to take loracarbef at least 1 hour before or 2 hours after meals.

•Instruct patient to complete the full course of therapy as prescribed, even if symptoms decrease.

•Instruct patient to discard unused oral solution after 14 days.

•Advise patient to report diarrhea, hives, or severe rash to prescriber.

lorazepam

Apo-Lorazepam (CAN), Ativan, Lorazepam Intensol, Novo-Lorazem (CAN), Nu-Loraz (CAN)

Class, Category, and Schedule

Chemical class: Benzodiazepine

Therapeutic class: Amnestic, antianxiety, anticonvulsant, sedative
Pregnancy category: D (parenteral), Not rated (oral)
Controlled substance schedule: IV

Indications and Dosages

➤ *To treat anxiety*
ORAL CONCENTRATE, TABLETS
Adults and adolescents. 1 to 3 mg b.i.d. or t.i.d. *Maximum:* 10 mg daily.
DOSAGE ADJUSTMENT For elderly or debilitated patients, initial dosage possibly reduced to 0.5 to 2 mg daily in divided doses.

➤ *To treat insomnia caused by anxiety*
ORAL CONCENTRATE, TABLETS
Adults and adolescents. 2 to 4 mg at bedtime.
DOSAGE ADJUSTMENT Dosage possibly reduced for elderly or debilitated patients.

➤ *To provide preoperative sedation*
I.V. INJECTION
Adults and adolescents. 0.044 mg/kg or 2 mg, whichever is less, given 2 hr before procedure. *Maximum:* 0.05 mg/kg or total of 4 mg.
I.M. INJECTION
Adults and adolescents. 0.05 mg/kg 2 hr before procedure. *Maximum:* 4 mg.

➤ *To treat status epilepticus*
I.V. INJECTION
Adults and adolescents. *Initial:* 4 mg at a rate of 2 mg/min. Repeated in 10 to 15 min if seizures don't subside. *Maximum:* 8 mg/24 hr.

Route	Onset	Peak	Duration
I.V.	5 min	Unknown	12 to 24 hr
I.M.	15 to 30 min	Unknown	12 to 24 hr

Incompatibilities
Don't mix I.V. lorazepam in same syringe as buprenorphine.

Contraindications
Acute angle-closure glaucoma, hypersensitivity to lorazepam, its components, or benzodiazepines; intra-arterial delivery; psychosis

Interactions
DRUGS
aminophylline, theophylline: Possibly reduced sedative effects of lorazepam
clozapine: Increased risk of marked sedation, excessive salivation, hypotension, ataxia, delirium, and respiratory arrest
CNS depressants: Additive CNS depression, including potentially fatal respiratory depression
digoxin: Possibly increased blood digoxin level and risk of digitalis toxicity
fentanyl: Possibly decreased therapeutic effects of fentanyl
probenecid: Possibly increased therapeutic and adverse effects of lorazepam
ACTIVITIES
alcohol use: Increased CNS depression

Mechanism of Action
May potentiate the effects of gamma-aminobutyric acid (GABA) and other inhibitory neurotransmitters by binding to specific benzodiazepine receptors in the limbic and cortical areas of the CNS. GABA inhibits excitatory stimulation, which helps control emotional behavior. The limbic system contains a highly dense area of benzodiazepine receptors, which may explain the drug's antianxiety effects. Also, lorazepam hyperpolarizes neuronal cells, thereby interfering with their ability to generate seizures.

Adverse Reactions
CNS: Amnesia, anxiety, ataxia, coma, confusion, delusions, depression, dizziness, drowsiness, euphoria, extrapyramidal symptoms, fatigue, headache, hypokinesia, irritability, malaise, nervousness, seizures, slurred speech, suicidal ideation, tremor, unsteadiness, vertigo
CV: Chest pain, palpitations, tachycardia
EENT: Blurred vision, diplopia, dry mouth, increased salivation, photophobia
ENDO: Syndrome of inappropriate ADH
GI: Abdominal pain, constipation, diarrhea, increased liver enzyme levels, jaundice, nausea, thirst, vomiting
GU: Libido changes
HEME: Agranulocytosis, pancytopenia, thrombocytopenia
RESP: Apnea, respiratory depression, worsening of sleep apnea or obstructve pulmonary disease

SKIN: Diaphoresis
Other: Anaphylaxis, injection site pain (I.M.) or phlebitis (I.V.), physical and psychological dependence, withdrawal symptoms

Nursing Considerations
•Before starting lorazepam therapy in a patient with depression, make sure he already takes an antidepressant because of the increased risk of suicide in patients with untreated depression.
•Use extreme caution when giving lorazepam to elderly patients, especially those with compromised respiratory function, because lorazepam can cause hypoventilation, sedation, unsteadiness, and respiratory depression.
•Use drug cautiously in patients with a history of alcohol or drug abuse or a personality disorder because of an increased risk of physical and psychological dependence. Also use cautiously in patients with severe hepatic insufficiency or encephalopathy because drug may worsen hepatic encephalopathy.
•For I.M. use, inject lorazepam deep into a large muscle mass, such as the gluteus maximus.
•For I.V. use, dilute lorazepam with an equal amount of sterile water for injection, sodium chloride for injection, or D₅W. Give diluted lorazepam slowly, at a rate not to exceed 2 mg/min.
•During I.V. use, monitor patient's respirations every 5 to 15 minutes and keep emergency resuscitation equipment readily available.
•**WARNING** Monitor patient's respiratory status closely because drug may cause life-threatening respiratory depression.
•Because abrupt drug discontinuation increases the risk of withdrawal symptoms, expect to taper dosage gradually, especially in epileptic patients.
PATIENT TEACHING
•Instruct patient to take lorazepam exactly as prescribed and not to stop drug without consulting prescriber because of the risk of withdrawal symptoms.
•Advise patient to avoid potentially hazardous activities until drug's CNS effects are known.
•Urge patient to avoid alcohol while taking lorazepam because it increases drug's CNS depressant effects.
•Instruct patient to report excessive drowsiness and nausea.
•Inform pregnant patient that lorazepam therapy will need to be discontinued early in the third trimester to avoid possible withdrawal symptoms in the newborn.

losartan potassium

Cozaar

Class and Category
Chemical class: Angiotensin II receptor antagonist
Therapeutic class: Antihypertensive
Pregnancy category: C (first trimester), D (later trimesters)

Indications and Dosages
➤ *To manage hypertension*
TABLETS
Adults. *Initial:* 50 mg daily. *Maintenance:* 25 to 100 mg as a single dose or in divided doses b.i.d.
➤ *To treat nephropathy in patients with type 2 diabetes and hypertension*
TABLETS
Adults. *Initial:* 50 mg daily, increased to 100 mg daily, as needed.
➤ *To reduce stroke risk in patients with hypertension and left ventricular hypertrophy*
TABLETS
Adults. *Initial:* 50 mg daily, followed by 12.5 mg hydrochlorothiazide daily. Dosage increased to 100 mg daily, as needed, followed by 25 mg hydrochlorothiazide daily, as needed.
Children age 6 and over. *Initial:* 0.7 mg/kg to a maximum of 50 mg daily. *Maximum:* 1.4 mg/kg or 100 mg daily.
DOSAGE ADJUSTMENT Initial dosage reduced to 25 mg daily for patients with impaired hepatic function or volume depletion.

Route	Onset	Peak	Duration
P.O.	Unknown	6 hr	Over 24 hr

Contraindications
Hypersensitivity to losartan or its components

Mechanism of Action

Blocks binding of angiotensin II to receptor sites in many tissues, including vascular smooth muscle and adrenal glands. Angiotensin II is a potent vasoconstrictor that also stimulates the adrenal cortex to secrete aldosterone. The inhibiting effects of angiotensin II reduce blood pressure.

Interactions

DRUGS

antihypertensives, diuretics: Possibly hypotension

cyclosporine, potassium-sparing diuretics, potassium supplements: Increased risk of hyperkalemia

indomethacin, sympathomimetics: Possibly decreased antihypertensive effect of losartan

NSAIDs: Possibly decreased renal function in patients already compromised; possibly decreased effectiveness of losartan

FOODS

high-potassium diet, potassium-containing salt substitutes: Increased risk of hyperkalemia

Adverse Reactions

CNS: Dizziness, fatigue, headache, insomnia
CV: Hypotension
EENT: Nasal congestion
GI: Diarrhea, indigestion, nausea, vomiting
HEME: Thrombocytopenia
MS: Back pain, leg pain, muscle spasms
RESP: Cough, upper respiratory tract infection
SKIN: Erythroderma
Other: Angioedema, hyperkalemia, hyponatremia

Nursing Considerations

• Be aware that losartan is more effective in some patients when given in two divided doses daily; it may be used with other antihypertensives.

• Know that patients of African descent with hypertension and left ventricular hypertrophy may not benefit from losartan to reduce stroke risk.

• **WARNING** Be aware that patients who have severe heart failure or renal artery stenosis may experience acute renal failure from losartan therapy because losartan inhibits the angiotensin-aldosterone system, on which renal function depends.

• Monitor patient's blood pressure and renal function studies to evaluate drug effectiveness.

• Periodically monitor patient's serum potassium level, as appropriate, to detect hyperkalemia.

• Monitor patient for muscle pain; rarely, rhabdomyolysis develops in patients taking other angiotensin II receptor blockers.

PATIENT TEACHING

• Instruct patient taking losartan to avoid potassium-containing salt substitutes because thay may increase the risk of hyperkalemia.

• Advise patient to avoid exercising in hot weather and drinking excessive amounts of alcohol; instruct her to notify prescriber if she experiences prolonged diarrhea, nausea, or vomiting.

lovastatin
(mevinolin)

Altoprev, Mevacor

Class and Category

Chemical class: Mevinic acid derivative
Therapeutic class: Antihyperlipidemic
Pregnancy category: X

Indications and Dosages

➤ *To reduce LDL and total cholesterol levels in patients with primary hypercholesterolemia*

TABLETS

Adults. *Initial:* 20 mg as a single dose with evening meal. *Maintenance:* 20 to 80 mg daily as a single dose or in divided doses with meals. *Maximum:* 80 mg daily.

DOSAGE ADJUSTMENT For patients who also take immunosuppressants, initial dosage decreased to 10 mg daily and maximum dosage limited to 20 mg daily.

E.R. TABLETS

Adults. *Initial:* 10 mg, 20 mg, 40 mg, or 60 mg as single dose at bedtime, increased, as needed, every 4 wk, up to maximum dose. *Maintenance:* 10 to 60 mg daily as single dose. *Maximum:* 60 mg daily.

➤ *To reduce LDL, total cholesterol, and apolipoprotein B levels in adolescents*

J
K
L

with heterozygous familial hypercholesterolemia

TABLETS

Adolescents 1 yr postmenarche (ages 10 to 17). *Initial:* 20 mg daily for LDL reduction of 20% or more, 10 mg daily for LDL reduction of less than 20%; dosage adjusted after at least 4 wk. *Maintenance:* 10 to 40 mg daily. *Maximum:* 40 mg daily.

DOSAGE ADJUSTMENT For patients who also take amiodarone or verapamil, maximum dosage limited to 40 mg daily. For patients who also take cyclosporine, gemfibrozil or other fibrates, or lipid-lowering drugs such as niacin (1 g or more daily), maximum dosage of lovastatin limited to 20 mg daily. For patients with creatinine clearance less than 30 ml/min/1.73 m^2, maximum dosage limited to 20 mg daily.

Route	Onset	Peak	Duration
P.O.	In 2 wk	Unknown	4 to 6 wk

Mechanism of Action

Interferes with the hepatic enzyme hydroxymethylglutaryl-coenzyme A reductase. By doing so, lovastatin reduces the formation of mevalonic acid (a cholesterol precursor), thus interrupting the pathway by which cholesterol is synthesized. When the cholesterol level declines in hepatic cells, LDLs are consumed, which also reduces the amount of circulating total cholesterol and serum triglycerides. The decrease in LDLs may result in a decreased level of apolipoprotein B, which is found within each LDL particle.

Contraindications

Acute hepatic disease, breastfeeding, hypersensitivity to lovastatin or its components, pregnancy, unexplained elevated liver function test results

Interactions

DRUGS

amiodarone, clarithromycin, cyclosporine, danazol, erythromycin, fibric acid derivatives, gemfibrozil and other fibrates, HIV protease inhibitors, immunosuppressants, itraconazole, ketoconazole, nefazodone, *niacin (1 g daily or more), telithromycin, verapamil:* Increased risk of severe myopathy or rhabdomyolysis

bile acid sequestrants, cholestyramine, colestipol: Decreased bioavailability of lovastatin

isradipine: Increased hepatic clearance of lovastatin

itraconazole, ketoconazole: Increased lovastatin blood level

oral anticoagulants: Increased anticoagulant effect and risk of bleeding

FOODS

all foods: Increased lovastatin absorption

grapefruit juice (more than 1 qt daily): Increased risk of myopathy or rhabdomyolysis

ACTIVITIES

alcohol use: Increased lovastatin blood level

Adverse Reactions

CNS: Dizziness, fatigue, headache, insomnia

EENT: Blurred vision, cataracts, pharyngitis, rhinitis, sinusitis

GI: Abdominal cramps and pain, constipation, diarrhea, elevated liver function test results, flatulence, indigestion, nausea, vomiting

MS: Arthritis, back pain, myalgia, myopathy, myositis, rhabdomyolysis

RESP: Cough, upper respiratory tract infection

SKIN: Dermatomyositis, erythema multiforme, pruritus, rash, Stevens-Johnson syndrome, toxic epidermal necrolysis

Other: Anaphylaxis, angioedema

Nursing Considerations

•Administer lovastatin cautiously in patients who have a history of liver disease and patients who consume large amounts of alcohol.

•Monitor patient's liver function test results before and during lovastatin therapy. If patient's serum transaminase levels rise, expect to measure them more often, as ordered. If patient's AST or ALT level reaches or exceeds three times the upper limit of normal and persists at that level, expect to discontinue drug.

•Administer lovastatin 1 hour before or 4 hours after giving bile acid sequestrant, cholestyramine, or colestipol.

•Expect patient to be prescribed a standard

low-cholesterol diet during lovastatin therapy.
•Be aware that drug exerts effects mainly on total cholesterol and LDL levels and has only slight effects on HDL and triglyceride levels.
PATIENT TEACHING
•Instruct patient who takes drug once daily to do so with evening meal to enhance absorption.
•Advise patient to report muscle aches, pains, tenderness, or weakness; severe GI distress; and vision changes.
•Urge patient to avoid consuming alcohol or more than 1 quart of grapefruit juice daily while taking drug.
•Direct patient to follow a low-cholesterol diet along with lovastatin therapy. Recommend weight loss and exercise programs as appropriate.
•Stress the importance of periodic eye examinations during therapy.
•Teach female patients appropriate contraceptive methods and the need to report suspected pregnancy immediately.

loxapine hydrochloride

Loxapac (CAN), Loxitane, Loxitane C, Loxitane IM

loxapine succinate

Loxapac (CAN), Loxitane

Class and Category
Chemical class: Dibenzoxazepine derivative
Therapeutic class: Antipsychotic
Pregnancy category: C

Indications and Dosages
➤ *To treat psychotic disorders and schizophrenia*
CAPSULES, ORAL SOLUTION
Adults. *Initial:* 10 mg b.i.d., increased over 7 days. *Maintenance:* 15 to 25 mg b.i.d. to q.i.d. *Maximum:* 250 mg daily.
DOSAGE ADJUSTMENT For elderly patients, dosage reduced to 3 to 5 mg b.i.d.
➤ *To treat acute exacerbations of psychotic disorders*
I.M. INJECTION
Adults. 12.5 to 50 mg every 4 to 6 hr or longer. *Maximum:* 250 mg daily.

Route	Onset	Peak	Duration
P.O.	20 to 30 min	1.5 to 3 hr	12 hr

Mechanism of Action
May treat psychotic disorders by blocking dopamine at postsynaptic receptors in the brain. With prolonged use, loxapine enhances antipsychotic effects by causing depolarization blockade of dopamine tracts, resulting in decreased dopamine neurotransmission.

Contraindications
Blood dyscrasias, bone marrow depression, cerebrovascular disease, coma, coronary artery disease, hypersensitivity to loxapine or its components, impaired hepatic function, myeloproliferative disorders, severe drug-induced CNS depression, severe hypertension or hypotension

Interactions
DRUGS
amphetamines, ephedrine: Decreased effects of these drugs
antacids, antidiarrheals (adsorbent): Possibly decreased absorption of oral loxapine
anticholinergics: Possibly increased anticholinergic effects
anticonvulsants: Lowered seizure threshold, increased risk of seizures
antidyskinetics: Possibly antagonized therapeutic effects of these drugs
bromocriptine: Possibly decreased therapeutic effects of bromocriptine
CNS depressants: Increased effects of CNS depression
dopamine: Possibly decreased alpha-adrenergic effects of dopamine
epinephrine: Possibly severe hypotension or tachycardia, and decreased effects of epinephrine
guanadrel, guanethidine, levodopa: Possibly decreased therapeutic effects of these drugs
MAO inhibitors, tricyclic antidepressants: Possibly increased blood levels of these drugs and increased CNS depressant and anticholinergic effects of these drugs and loxapine
metaraminol: Possibly decreased vasopressor effect of metaraminol

methoxamine: Possibly decreased vasopressor effect and duration of action of methoxamine

ACTIVITIES

alcohol use: Increased CNS depression

Adverse Reactions

CNS: Confusion, drowsiness, dystonia, involuntary motor activity, neuroleptic malignant syndrome, pseudoparkinsonism, sleep disturbance, tardive dyskinesia

CV: Orthostatic hypotension

EENT: Blurred vision, dry mouth

ENDO: Galactorrhea, gynecomastia

GI: Constipation, ileus, nausea, vomiting

GU: Menstrual irregularities, sexual dysfunction, urine retention

SKIN: Photosensitivity (mild), rash

Other: Weight gain

Nursing Considerations

• Be aware that loxapine's full antipsychotic effect may require weeks.

• Loxapine shouldn't be given to treat dementia-related psychosis in the elderly because of an increased mortality risk.

• Assess for signs of tardive dyskinesia, including involuntary protrusion of tongue and chewing movements. These signs may appear months or years after loxapine therapy begins and may not disappear with dosage reduction.

• Observe for extrapyramidal reactions or parkinsonian symptoms, such as excessive salivation, masklike facies, rigidity, and tremor, especially in first few days of treatment. Prescriber may reduce dosage to control these symptoms.

• **WARNING** Monitor patient for neuroleptic malignant syndrome, a rare but possibly fatal adverse reaction. Early evidence includes altered mental status, arrhythmias, fever, and muscle rigidity.

PATIENT TEACHING

• Instruct patient to dilute loxapine oral solution with orange or grapefruit juice just before taking. Advise her to use the calibrated dropper that accompanies the solution to ensure correct dosage.

• Direct patient to avoid taking antacids and antidiarrheals 2 hours before or after taking loxapine.

• Caution patient to avoid alcohol while taking loxapine.

• Advise patient to change position slowly to minimize the effects of orthostatic hypotension.

• Urge patient to avoid potentially hazardous activities until CNS effects of loxapine are known.

• Advise patient to avoid prolonged exposure to sun and to use sunscreen to minimize the risk of photosensitivity.

• Encourage patient to have periodic eye examinations during therapy.

lubiprostone

Amitiza

Class and Category

Chemical class: Chloride channel activator

Therapeutic class: Intestinal motility enhancer

Pregnancy category: C

Indications and Dosages

➤ *To treat chronic idiopathic constipation*

CAPSULES

Adults. 24 mcg b.i.d. with food and water.

➤ *To treat irritable bowel syndrome with constipation*

CAPSULES

Adults. 8 mcg b.i.d. with food and water.

Mechanism of Action

Enhances chloride-rich intestinal fluid secretion by locally activating chloride channels. By increasing intestinal fluid secretion, lubiprostone increases motility in the intestine, which aids the passage of stool, alleviating constipation.

Contraindications

Diarrhea, hypersensitivity to lubiprostone or its components, mechanical GI obstruction

Interactions

DRUGS

antidiarrheals: Decreased GI motility

Adverse Reactions

CNS: Asthenia, dizziness, fatigue, headache, malaise

CV: Chest discomfort or pain, edema, increased heart rate
EENT: Dry mouth, throat tightness
GI: Abdominal distention or pain, diarrhea, dyspepsia, flatulence, nausea, vomiting
MS: Muscle cramps or spasms
RESP: Dyspnea
SKIN: Rash
Other: Angioedema

Nursing Considerations
•Be aware that lubiprostone shouldn't be used in patients with severe diarrhea.
•Make sure female patients have a negative pregnancy test before starting lubiprostone therapy because safety of drug during pregnancy is unknown.
•Monitor patient closely for adverse reactions, particularly dyspnea and especially after giving first dose.
PATIENT TEACHING
•Advise patient to take drug with food to minimize risk of nausea.
•Tell women to use effective contraception while taking lubiprostone and to notify prescriber if pregnancy is suspected. Drug may need to be discontinued.
•Instruct patient to notify prescriber if severe diarrhea occurs.

lypressin

Diapid

Class and Category
Chemical class: Synthetic vasopressin analogue
Therapeutic class: Antidiuretic
Pregnancy category: C

Indications and Dosages
➤ *To control and prevent dehydration, polydipsia, and polyuria in patients with neurogenic diabetes insipidus that is unresponsive to other therapy*
NASAL SOLUTION
Adults and adolescents. 1 or 2 sprays q.i.d. If more drug is needed, interval between doses is decreased rather than increasing number of sprays/dose.

Route	Onset	Peak	Duration
Intranasal	In 1 hr	0.5 to 2 hr	3 to 4 hr

Mechanism of Action
Increases cellular permeability of collecting ducts in kidneys, leading to increased urine osmolality and decreased urine output.

Contraindications
Hypersensitivity to lypressin or its components

Interactions
DRUGS
carbamazepine, chlorpropamide, clofibrate: Possibly increased antidiuretic effect
demeclocycline, lithium, norepinephrine: Decreased antidiuretic effect of lypressin

Adverse Reactions
CNS: Headache
EENT: Conjunctivitis; nasal congestion, irritation, and itching; periorbital edema and itching; rhinorrhea
GI: Abdominal cramps, diarrhea, heartburn (if excessive intranasal use causes dripping into pharynx)
RESP: Cough, transient dyspnea (if drug is accidentally inhaled)
Other: Water intoxication

Nursing Considerations
•Assess patient for nasal congestion or upper respiratory tract infection, which can reduce lypressin absorption and require larger doses or adjunct therapy.
•Administer final spray of drug at bedtime to help control nocturia.
•WARNING Be aware that inadvertent inhalation, although rare, may cause chest tightness, continuous cough, and dyspnea.
•Observe for nasal irritation during long-term therapy.
•Monitor patient for signs and symptoms of water intoxication, including coma, confusion, drowsiness, persistent headache, seizures, urine retention, and weight gain.
PATIENT TEACHING
•Teach patient how to administer lypressin correctly by holding head upright and bottle in a vertical position and spraying 1 or 2 sprays in each nostril with each dose.
•Instruct patient to take last dose of day at bedtime to control nocturia.

J
K
L

•Instruct patient to use drug exactly as prescribed. Explain that using extra sprays
wastes drug.
•Advise patient to report abdominal cramps,
heartburn, persistent headache, severe nasal
irritation, and shortness of breath.

M

magnesium chloride

(contains 64 mg of elemental magnesium per tablet, 100 mg of elemental magnesium per enteric-coated tablet, 64 mg of elemental magnesium per E.R. tablet, and 200 mg of elemental magnesium per 1 ml of injection)

Chloromag, Mag-L-100, Slow-Mag

magnesium citrate
(citrate of magnesia)

(contains 40.5 to 47 mg elemental magnesium per 5 ml oral solution)

Citroma, Citro-Mag (CAN)

magnesium gluconate

(contains 54 mg elemental magnesium per 5 ml oral solution and 27 to 29.3 mg elemental magnesium per tablet)

Almora, Maglucate (CAN), Magonate, Magtrate

magnesium hydroxide
(milk of magnesia)

(contains 135 mg elemental magnesium per tablet, 129 to 130 mg elemental magnesium per chewable tablet, and 164 to 328 mg elemental magnesium per 5 ml liquid, liquid concentrate, or oral solution)

Phillips' Chewable Tablets, Phillips' Magnesia Tablets (CAN), Phillips' Milk of Magnesia, Phillips' Milk of Magnesia Concentrate

magnesium lactate

(contains 84 mg elemental magnesium per E.R. tablet)

Mag-Tab SR Caplets

magnesium oxide

(contains 84.5 mg elemental magnesium per capsule and 50 to 302 mg elemental magnesium per tablet)

Mag-200, Mag-Ox 400, Maox, Uro-Mag

magnesium sulfate

(contains 100 to 500 mg elemental magnesium per 1 ml of injection, 1 to 5 g elemental magnesium per 10 ml of injection, and 40 mEq per 5 mg of crystals)

Class and Category

Chemical class: Cation, electrolyte
Therapeutic class: Antacid, antiarrhythmic, anticonvulsant, electrolyte replacement, laxative
Pregnancy category: A (parenteral magnesium sulfate), Not rated (others)

Indications and Dosages

➤ *To correct magnesium deficiency caused by alcoholism, magnesium-depleting drugs, malnutrition, or restricted diet; to prevent magnesium deficiency based on U.S. and Canadian recommended daily allowances*

CAPSULES, CHEWABLE TABLETS, CRYSTALS, ENTERIC-COATED TABLETS, E.R. TABLETS, LIQUID, LIQUID CONCENTRATE, ORAL SOLUTION, TABLETS (MAGNESIUM CHLORIDE, CITRATE, GLUCONATE, HYDROXIDE, LACTATE [EXCEPT IN CHILDREN], OXIDE, SULFATE)

Dosage individualized based on severity of deficiency and normal recommended daily allowances listed below.

Adult men and children over age 10. 270 to 400 mg daily (*Canada:* 130 to 250 mg daily).
Adult women and children over age 10. 280 to 300 mg daily (*Canada:* 135 to 210 mg daily).
Pregnant women. 320 mg daily (*Canada:* 195 to 245 mg daily).
Breast-feeding women. 340 to 355 mg daily (*Canada:* 245 to 265 mg daily).
Children ages 7 to 10. 170 mg daily (*Canada:* 100 to 135 mg daily).
Children ages 4 to 6. 120 mg daily (*Canada:* 65 mg daily).
Children from birth to age 3. 40 to 80 mg/day (*Canada:* 20 to 50 mg daily).

➤ *To treat mild magnesium deficiency*

I.M. INJECTION (MAGNESIUM SULFATE)

Adults and adolescents. 1 g every 6 hr for 4 doses.

➤ *To treat severe hypomagnesemia*

I.V. INFUSION (MAGNESIUM CHLORIDE)

Adults. 4 g diluted in 250 ml of D_5W and infused at no more than 3 ml/min. *Maximum:* 40 g daily.

I.V. INFUSION (MAGNESIUM SULFATE)

Adults and adolescents. 5 g diluted in 1 L of I.V. solution and infused over 3 hr.

➤ *To provide supplemental magnesium in total parenteral nutrition*

I.V. INFUSION (MAGNESIUM SULFATE)

Adults. 1 to 3 g daily.

M

Children. 0.25 mg to 1.25 g daily.

DOSAGE ADJUSTMENT Adult dosage may be increased to 6 g daily for certain conditions, such as short-bowel syndrome.

I.M. INJECTION (MAGNESIUM SULFATE)

Adults and adolescents. Up to 250 mg/kg every 4 hr, p.r.n.

➤ *To prevent and control seizures in preeclampsia or eclampsia as well as seizures caused by epilepsy, glomerulonephritis, or hypothyroidism*

I.V. INFUSION OR INJECTION (MAGNESIUM SULFATE)

Adults. *Loading:* 4 g diluted in 250 ml of compatible solution and infused over 30 min. *Maintenance:* 1 to 2 g/hr by continuous infusion.

I.M. INJECTION (MAGNESIUM SULFATE)

Adults. 4 to 5 g every 4 hr, p.r.n.
Children. 20 to 40 mg/kg, repeated p.r.n.

➤ *To relieve indigestion with hyperacidity*

CHEWABLE TABLETS, LIQUID, LIQUID CONCENTRATE, ORAL SOLUTION TABLETS (MAGNESIUM HYDROXIDE)

Adults and adolescents. 400 to 1,200 mg (5 to 15 ml liquid or 2.5 to 7.5 ml liquid concentrate) up to 4 times daily with water, or 622 to 1,244 mg (tablets or chewable tablets) up to 4 times daily.

CAPSULES, TABLETS (MAGNESIUM OXIDE)

Adults and adolescents. 140 mg (capsules) t.i.d. or q.i.d. with water or milk, or 400 to 800 mg daily (tablets).

➤ *To relieve constipation, to evacuate colon for rectal or bowel examination*

LIQUID, LIQUID CONCENTRATE (MAGNESIUM HYDROXIDE)

Adults and children age 12 and over. 2.4 to 4.8 g (30 to 60 ml) daily as single dose or divided doses.
Children ages 6 to 11. 1.2 to 2.4 g (15 to 30 ml)/day as a single dose or in divided doses.
Children ages 2 to 5. 0.4 to 1.2 g (5 to 15 ml) daily as single dose or divided doses.

ORAL SOLUTION (MAGNESIUM CITRATE)

Adults and children age 12 and over. 11 to 25 g daily as single dose or divided doses.
Children ages 6 to 11. 5.5 to 12.5 g daily as single dose or divided doses.
Children ages 2 to 5. 2.7 to 6.25 g daily as single dose or divided doses.

CRYSTALS (MAGNESIUM SULFATE)

Adults and children age 12 and over. 10 to 30 g daily as single dose or divided doses.

DOSAGE ADJUSTMENT Dosage limited to 20 g

of magnesium sulfate every 48 hr for patients with severe renal impairment.

Children ages 6 to 11. 5 to 10 g daily as a single dose or in divided doses.
Children ages 2 to 5. 2.5 to 5 g daily as a single dose or in divided doses.

CAPSULES, TABLETS (MAGNESIUM OXIDE)

Adults. 2 to 4 g with a full glass of water or milk, usually at bedtime.

Route	Onset	Peak	Duration
P.O.*	0.5 to 3 hr	Unknown	Unknown
P.O.†	20 min	Unknown	20 to 180 min
I.M.‡	1 hr	Unknown	3 to 4 hr
I.V.‡	Immediate	Unknown	About 30 min

Mechanism of Action

Assists all enzymes involved in phosphate transfer reactions that use adenosine triphosphate (ATP). Magnesium is required for normal function of the ATP-dependent sodium-potassium pump in muscle membranes. It may effectively treat digitalis glycoside–induced arrhythmias because correction of hypomagnesemia improves the sodium-potassium pump's ability to distribute potassium into intracellular spaces and because magnesium decreases calcium uptake and potassium outflow through myocardial cell membranes.

As a laxative, magnesium exerts a hyperosmotic effect in the small intestine. It causes water retention that distends the bowel and causes the duodenum to secrete cholecystokinin. This substance stimulates fluid secretion and intestinal motility.

As an antacid, magnesium reacts with water, converting magnesium oxide to magnesium hydroxide. Magnesium hydroxide rapidly reacts with gastric acid to form water and magnesium chloride, which increases gastric pH.

As an anticonvulsant, magnesium depresses the CNS and blocks peripheral neuromuscular impulse transmission by decreasing available acetylcholine.

* For laxative effect.
† For antacid effect.
‡ For anticonvulsant effect.

Incompatibilities

Don't combine magnesium sulfate with alkali carbonates and bicarbonates, alkali hydroxides, arsenates, calcium, clindamycin phosphate, dobutamine, fat emulsions, heavy metals, hydrocortisone sodium succinate, phosphates, polymyxin B, procaine hydrochloride, salicylates, sodium bicarbonate, strontium, and tartrates.

Contraindications

Hypersensitivity to magnesium salts or any component of magnesium-containing preparations
For magnesium chloride: Coma, heart disease, renal impairment
For magnesium sulfate: Heart block, MI, preeclampsia 2 hours or less before delivery (I.V. form)
For magnesium used as laxative: Acute abdominal problem (as indicated by abdominal pain, nausea, or vomiting), diverticulitis, fecal impaction, intestinal obstruction or perforation, colostomy or ileostomy, severe renal impairment, ulcerative colitis

Interactions

DRUGS

amphotericin B, cisplatin, cyclosporine, gentamicin: Possibly magnesium wasting and need for magnesium dosage adjustment
anticholinergics: Possibly decreased absorption and therapeutic effects of these drugs
calcium salts (I.V.): Possibly neutralization of magnesium sulfate's effects
cellulose sodium phosphate: Possibly binding with magnesium, possibly decreased therapeutic effectiveness of cellulose
CNS depressants: Increased CNS depression
digoxin (I.V.): Possibly heart block and conduction changes, especially when calcium salts are also administered
digoxin, fluoroquinolones, folic acid, H$_2$-receptor blockers, iron preparations, isoniazid, ketoconazole, penicillamine, phenothiazines, phenytoin, phosphates (oral), tetracyclines: Possibly decreased absorption and blood levels of these drugs
diuretics (loop or thiazide): Possibly hypomagnesemia
edetate sodium, sodium polystyrene sulfonate: Possibly binding with magnesium
enteric-coated drugs: Possibly quicker dissolution of these drugs and increased risk of adverse GI reactions

etidronate (oral): Decreased etidronate absorption
mecamylamine: Possibly prolonged effects of mecamylamine
methenamine, streptomycin, sucralfate, tetracyclines, tobramycin (oral), urinary acidifiers: Possibly decreased therapeutic effects of these drugs
misoprostol: Increased misoprostol-induced diarrhea
neuromuscular blockers: Possibly increased neuromuscular blockade
nifedipine: Possibly increased hypotensive effects when taken with magnesium sulfate
potassium-sparing diuretics: Increased risk of hypermagnesemia
salicylates: Possibly increased excretion and lower blood levels of salicylates
sodium polystyrene sulfonate resin: Possibly metabolic alkalosis

FOODS

high-glucose intake: Increased urinary excretion of magnesium

ACTIVITIES

alcohol use: Increased urinary excretion of magnesium

Adverse Reactions

CNS: Confusion, decreased reflexes, dizziness, syncope
CV: Arrhythmias, hypotension
GI: Flatulence, vomiting
MS: Muscle cramps
RESP: Dyspnea, respiratory depression or paralysis
SKIN: Diaphoresis
Other: Allergic reaction, hypermagnesemia, injection site pain or irritation (I.M. form), laxative dependence, magnesium toxicity

Nursing Considerations

• Be aware that magnesium sulfate is the elemental form of magnesium. Oral preparations aren't all equivalent.
• Be aware that drug isn't metabolized. Drug remaining in the GI tract produces watery stool within 30 minutes to 3 hours.
• Make sure patient chews magnesium chewable tablets thoroughly before swallowing.
• Avoid giving other oral drugs within 2 hours of a magnesium-containing antacid.
• Before administering drug as a laxative, shake oral solution, liquid, or liquid concentrate well and give with a large amount of water.

M

•**WARNING** Observe for and report to prescriber early signs of hypermagnesemia: bradycardia, depressed deep tendon reflexes, diplopia, dyspnea, flushing, hypotension, nausea, slurred speech, vomiting, and weakness.

•**WARNING** Be aware that magnesium may precipitate myasthenic crisis by decreasing patient's sensitivity to acetylcholine.

•Frequently assess cardiac status of patient taking drugs that lower heart rate, such as beta blockers, because magnesium may aggravate symptoms of heart block.

•**WARNING** Be aware that magnesium chloride for injection contains the preservative benzyl alcohol, which may cause fatal toxic syndrome in neonates and premature infants.

•Provide adequate diet, exercise, and fluids for patient being treated for constipation.

•Monitor serum electrolyte levels in patients with renal insufficiency because they're at risk for magnesium toxicity.

•Be aware that magnesium salts aren't intended for long-term use.

PATIENT TEACHING

•Advise patient to chew magnesium chewable tablets thoroughly before swallowing then drink a full glass of water. Mention that these tablets have a chalky taste.

•Instruct patient to take magnesium-containing antacid between meals and at bedtime. Urge him not to take other drugs within 2 hours of the antacid.

•Tell patient to notify prescriber and avoid using a magnesium-containing laxative if he has abdominal pain, nausea, or vomiting.

•Instruct patient to refrigerate magnesium citrate solution.

•Caution patient about the risk of dependence with long-term laxative use.

•Teach patient to prevent constipation by increasing dietary fiber and fluid intake and exercising regularly.

• Inform patient that magnesium supplements used to replace electrolytes can cause diarrhea.

mannitol

Osmitrol, Resectisol

Class and Category

Chemical class: Hexahydroxy alcohol
Therapeutic class: Antiglaucoma, diagnostic agent, osmotic diuretic, urinary irrigant
Pregnancy category: B

Indications and Dosages

➤ *To reduce intracranial or intraocular pressure*

I.V. INFUSION

Adults and adolescents. 0.25 to 2 g/kg as 15% to 25% solution given over 30 to 60 min. If used before eye surgery, 1.5 to 2 g/kg 60 to 90 min before procedure. *Maximum:* 6 g/kg daily.

DOSAGE ADJUSTMENT For small or debilitated patients, dosage reduced to 0.5 g/kg.

➤ *To diagnose oliguria or inadequate renal function*

I.V. INFUSION

Adults and adolescents. 200 mg/kg or 12.5 g as 15% to 20% solution given over 3 to 5 min. Second dose given only if patient fails to excrete 30 to 50 ml of urine in 2 to 3 hr. Drug discontinued if no response after second dose. Alternatively, 100 ml of 20% solution diluted in 180 ml normal saline solution (forming 280 ml of 7.2% solution) and infused at 20 ml/min; followed by measurement of urine output. *Maximum:* 6 g/kg daily.

➤ *To prevent oliguria or acute renal failure*

I.V. INFUSION

Adults and adolescents. 50 to 100 g as 5% to 25% solution. *Maximum:* 6 g/kg daily.

➤ *To treat oliguria*

I.V. INFUSION

Adults and adolescents. 50 to 100 g as 15% to 25% solution given over 90 min to several hr. *Maximum:* 6 g/kg daily.

➤ *To promote diuresis in drug toxicity*

I.V. INFUSION

Adults and adolescents. *Loading:* 25 g. *Maintenance:* Up to 200 g as 5% to 25% solution given continuously to maintain urine output of 100 to 500 ml/hr with positive fluid balance of 1 to 2 L. *Maximum:* 6 g/kg daily.

➤ *To promote diuresis in hemolytic transfusion reaction*

I.V. INFUSION

Adults. 20 g given over 5 min and repeated if needed. *Maximum:* 6 g/kg daily.

➤ *To provide irrigation during transurethral resection of prostate gland*

IRRIGATION SOLUTION
Adults. 2.5% or 5% solution, as needed.

Route	Onset	Peak	Duration
I.V.*	1 to 3 hr	Unknown	Up to 8 hr
I.V.†	30 to 60 min	Unknown	4 to 8 hr
I.V.‡	In 15 min	Unknown	3 to 8 hr

Mechanism of Action

Elevates plasma osmolality, causing water to flow from tissues, such as the brain and eyes, and from CSF, into extracellular fluid, thereby decreasing intracranial and intraocular pressure.

As an osmotic diuretic, mannitol increases the osmolarity of glomerular filtrate, which decreases water reabsorption. This leads to increased excretion of water, sodium, chloride, and toxic substances.

As an irrigant, mannitol minimizes the hemolytic effects of water used as an irrigant and reduces the movement of hemolyzed blood from the urethra to the systemic circulation, which prevents hemoglobinemia and serious renal complications.

Incompatibilities

Don't administer mannitol through same I.V. line as blood or blood products.

Contraindications

Active intracranial bleeding (except during craniotomy), anuria, hepatic failure, hypersensitivity to mannitol or its components, pulmonary edema, severe dehydration, severe heart failure, severe pulmonary congestion, severe renal insufficiency

Interactions
DRUGS
digoxin: Increased risk of digitalis toxicity from hypokalemia
diuretics: Possibly increased therapeutic effects of mannitol

Adverse Reactions

CNS: Chills, dizziness, fever, headache, seizures
CV: Chest pain, heart failure, hypertension, tachycardia, thrombophlebitis

---

* To produce diuresis.
† To decrease intraocular pressure.
‡ To decrease intracranial pressure.

EENT: Blurred vision, dry mouth, rhinitis
GI: Diarrhea, nausea, thirst, vomiting
GU: Polyuria, urine retention
RESP: Pulmonary edema
SKIN: Extravasation with edema and tissue necrosis, rash, urticaria
Other: Dehydration, hyperkalemia, hypernatremia, hypervolemia, hypokalemia, hyponatremia (dilutional), metabolic acidosis, water intoxication

Nursing Considerations

• If crystals form in mannitol solution exposed to low temperature, place solution in hot-water bath to redissolve crystals.
• Use a 5-micron in-line filter when administering drug solution of 15% or greater.
• During I.V. infusion of mannitol, monitor vital signs, central venous pressure, and fluid intake and output every hour. Measure urine output with indwelling urinary catheter, as appropriate.
• Check weight and monitor BUN and serum creatinine electrolyte levels daily.
• Provide frequent mouth care to relieve thirst and dry mouth.

PATIENT TEACHING
• Inform patient that he may experience dry mouth and thirst during mannitol therapy.
• Instruct patient to report chest pain, difficulty breathing, or pain at I.V. site.

maprotiline hydrochloride

Ludiomil

Class and Category

Chemical class: Dibenzobicyclooctadiene derivative
Therapeutic class: Antidepressant, tricyclic antidepressant
Pregnancy category: B

Indications and Dosages

➤ *To treat mild to moderate depression*
TABLETS
Adults and adolescents. *Initial:* 75 mg daily in divided doses for 2 wk. Increased in 25-mg increments as needed and tolerated. *Maintenance:* 150 to 225 mg daily in divided doses; for prolonged therapy, possibly 75 to 150 mg daily in divided doses.

➤ *To treat hospitalized patients with*

M

severe depression

TABLETS

Adults and adolescents. *Initial:* 100 to 150 mg daily in divided doses, increased as needed and tolerated. *Maintenance:* 150 to 225 mg daily in divided doses; for prolonged therapy, possibly 75 to 150 mg daily in divided doses.

DOSAGE ADJUSTMENT For patients over age 60, initial dosage reduced to 25 mg daily and then increased by 25 mg/wk up to maintenance dosage of 50 to 75 mg daily in divided doses.

Route	Onset	Peak	Duration
P.O.	1 to 3 wk	3 to 6 wk	Unknown

Mechanism of Action

Blocks norepinephrine's reuptake at adrenergic nerve fibers. Normally, when a nerve impulse reaches an adrenergic nerve fiber, norepinephrine is released from its storage sites and metabolized in the nerve or at the synapse. Some norepinephrine reaches receptor sites on target organs and tissues, but most is taken back into the nerve and stored by way of the reuptake mechanism. By blocking norepinephrine reuptake, maprotiline increases its level at nerve synapses. An elevated norepinephrine level may improve mood and, consequently, decrease depression.

Contraindications

Hypersensitivity to maprotiline, mirtazapine, or their components; use within 14 days of MAO inhibitor therapy

Interactions

DRUGS

anticholinergics, antihistamines: Increased atropine-like adverse effects, such as blurred vision, constipation, dizziness, and dry mouth

anticonvulsants: Increased risk of CNS depression, possibly lower seizure threshhold and increased risk of seizures

bupropion, clozapine, haloperidol, loxapine, molindone, other tricyclic antidepressants, phenothiazines, pimozide, thioxanthenes, trazodone: Possibly increased anticholinergic effects, possibly lowered seizure threshhold and increased risk of seizures

cimetidine: Possibly increased blood maprotiline level

clonidine, guanadrel, guanethidine: Possibly decreased antihypertensive effects of these drugs, possibly increased CNS depression (with clonidine)

CNS depressants: Increased risk of CNS depression

estrogens, oral contraceptives containing estrogen: Possibly decreased therapeutic effects and increased adverse effects of maprotiline

MAO inhibitors: Increased risk of hyperpyrexia, hypertensive crisis, severe seizures, or death

sympathomimetics: Increased risk of arrhythmias, hyperpyrexia, hypertension, or tachycardia

thyroid hormones: Increased risk of arrhythmias

ACTIVITIES

alcohol use: Increased risk of CNS depression

Adverse Reactions

CNS: Agitation, dizziness, drowsiness, fatigue, headache, insomnia, seizures, suicidal ideation, tremor, weakness

EENT: Blurred vision, dry mouth, increased intraocular pressure

ENDO: Gynecomastia

GI: Constipation, diarrhea, epigastric distress, increased appetite, nausea, vomiting

GU: Impotence, libido changes, testicular swelling, urinary hesitancy, urine retention

HEME: Agranulocytosis

SKIN: Diaphoresis, photosensitivity, pruritus, rash

Other: Weight loss

Nursing Considerations

• Give largest dose of maprotiline at bedtime if daytime drowsiness occurs.

• Check CBC as ordered, if fever, sore throat, or other signs of agranulocytosis develop.

• Take seizure precautions according to facility policy.

• Watch patient closely (especially children, adolescents, and young adults), for suicidal tendencies, particularly when therapy starts and dosage changes, because depression may worsen temporarily during these times, possibly leading to suicidal ideation.

• Expect to taper drug dosage gradually because abrupt drug discontinuation may produce withdrawal symptoms.

PATIENT TEACHING

• Advise patient to take maprotiline exactly as prescribed. Caution him not to stop taking drug abruptly because of the risk of withdrawal symptoms, including headache, nausea, nightmares, and vertigo.

• Inform patient that he may not feel drug's effects for several weeks.

• Suggest that patient take drug with food if adverse GI reactions develop.

• Urge patient to report difficulty urinating, excessive drowsiness, fever, or sore throat.

• Advise patient to avoid potentially hazardous activities until drug's CNS effects are known.

• Caution patient to avoid alcohol and other CNS depressants while taking drug.

• Urge family or caregiver to watch patient closely for suicidal tendencies, especially when therapy starts or dosage changes and particularly if patient is a child, teenager, or young adult.

mecamylamine hydrochloride

Inversine

Class and Category

Chemical class: Ganglionic blocker, secondary amine
Therapeutic class: Antihypertensive
Pregnancy category: C

Indications and Dosages

➤ *To manage moderately severe to severe hypertension, to treat uncomplicated malignant hypertension*

TABLETS

Adults. *Initial:* 2.5 mg b.i.d. Total dosage increased by 2.5 mg every 2 days until desired response occurs. *Maintenance:* 25 mg daily in divided doses t.i.d.

Route	Onset	Peak	Duration
P.O.	0.5 to 2 hr	3 to 5 hr	6 to 12 hr

Mechanism of Action

Reduces blood pressure by blocking acetylcholine's effects at autonomic ganglia. This action decreases the effects of the sympathetic and parasympathetic nervous systems, reduces sympathetic tone in blood vessels, and causes vasodilation.

Contraindications

Chronic pyelonephritis; concurrent use of antibiotics or sulfonamides; coronary insufficiency; glaucoma; hypersensitivity to mecamylamine; mild, moderate, or labile hypertension; organic pyloric stenosis; recent MI; uncooperative behavior; uremia

Interactions

DRUGS

diuretics, other antihypertensives: Increased antihypertensive effects
urinary alkalinizers: Increased risk of mecamylamine toxicity

ACTIVITIES

alcohol use: Possibly increased effects of mecamylamine
vigorous exercise: Increased effects of mecamylamine

Adverse Reactions

CNS: Choreiform movements, confusion, dizziness, fatigue, headache, nervousness, paresthesia, seizures, syncope, tremor, weakness

CV: Hypotension, orthostatic hypotension

EENT: Blurred vision, dry mouth, mydriasis

GI: Anorexia, constipation, diarrhea, ileus, nausea, vomiting

GU: Decreased libido, impotence, urine retention

RESP: Interstitial pulmonary edema and fibrosis

Nursing Considerations

• Use mecamylamine cautiously in patients with coronary artery disease and those who have had a stroke because drug may reduce blood flow to heart and brain.

• Also use drug cautiously in patients with renal insufficiency because drug may further impair renal function and may accumulate in blood.

• Give drug after meals for more gradual absorption and more constant blood pressure control.

• Give largest doses of drug at noon and in the evening.

• Monitor blood pressure with patient standing at start of treatment to determine drug's effectiveness and need for increased dosage. Check blood pressure 3 to 5 hours after dose, during drug's peak effect.

• Expect to reduce dosage for patients with conditions that may decrease drug require-

ments, such as fever, infection, and sodium depletion.
•Monitor for orthostatic hypotension, especially in the morning, during hot weather, and after exercise.
•Assess bowel function and be alert for signs of ileus (abdominal cramps and distention, constipation, and diarrhea).
•Expect to discontinue drug gradually to prevent rebound hypertension.

PATIENT TEACHING
•Instruct patient to take mecamylamine after meals and at the same time every day.
•Urge patient not to use alcohol while taking drug.
•Instruct patient to change position slowly to minimize orthostatic hypotension.
•Inform patient that excessive sweating, vigorous exercise, hot weather, and salt depletion can cause dizziness and hypotension.
•Caution patient to avoid potentially hazardous activities until drug's CNS effects are known.
•Instruct patient to report abdominal cramps or distention, blurred vision, persistent constipation or liquid stools, severe dizziness, shortness of breath, or tremor.
•Inform male patient that drug may cause decreased libido and impotence.
•If possible, teach patient how to monitor his blood pressure daily at home and provide guidelines for calling prescriber.

meclizine hydrochloride
(meclozine hydrochloride)

Antivert, Bonamine (CAN), Bonine, Dizmiss, Dramamine II, Meclicot, Medivert, Meni-D

Class and Category
Chemical class: Piperazine derivative
Therapeutic class: Antiemetic, antivertigo
Pregnancy category: B

Indications and Dosages
➤ *To prevent and treat vertigo*
CAPSULES, CHEWABLE TABLETS, TABLETS
Adults and adolescents. 25 to 100 mg daily, p.r.n., in divided doses.

➤ *To treat motion sickness*
CAPSULES, TABLETS
Adults. 25 to 50 mg 1 hr before travel and then every 24 hr, p.r.n., for duration of trip.

Route	Onset	Peak	Duration
P.O.	1 hr	Unknown	8 to 24 hr

Mechanism of Action
May inhibit nausea and vomiting by reducing the sensitivity of the labyrinthine apparatus and blocking cholinergic synapses in the brain's vomiting center.

Contraindications
Hypersensitivity to meclizine or its components

Interactions
DRUGS
anticholinergics: Possibly potentiated anticholinergic effects
apomorphine: Possibly decreased emetic response to apomorphine
CNS depressants: Possibly potentiated CNS depression
ACTIVITIES
alcohol use: Possibly potentiated CNS depression

Adverse Reactions
CNS: Dizziness, drowsiness, euphoria, excitement, fatigue, hallucinations, headache, insomnia, nervousness, restlessness, vertigo
CV: Hypotension, palpitations, tachycardia
EENT: Blurred vision; diplopia; dry mouth, nose, and throat; tinnitus
GI: Abdominal pain, anorexia, constipation, diarrhea, nausea, vomiting
GU: Urinary frequency and hesitancy, urine retention
RESP: Bronchospasm, thickening of respiratory secretions
SKIN: Jaundice, rash, urticaria

Nursing Considerations
•Use meclizine cautiously in patients with asthma, glaucoma, or prostate gland enlargement.
•Be aware that drug may mask signs of brain tumor, intestinal obstruction, or ototoxicity.

PATIENT TEACHING
•Inform patient that meclizine works best for motion sickness when taken before travel.
•Instruct patient to chew meclizine chew-

able tablets thoroughly before swallowing them.
•Instruct patient to report blurred vision or drowsiness.
•Urge patient to avoid alcohol while taking drug.
•Caution patient to avoid potentially hazardous activities until drug's CNS effects are known.
•Advise patient to have regular eye examinations during long-term therapy.

meclofenamate sodium

Meclomen

Class and Category

Chemical class: Fenamate (anthranilic acid) derivative
Therapeutic class: Analgesic, antidysmenorrheal, anti-inflammatory, antirheumatic
Pregnancy category: Not rated

Indications and Dosages

➤ *To relieve pain and inflammation in rheumatoid arthritis and osteoarthritis*
CAPSULES
Adults and adolescents over age 14. 50 to 100 mg every 6 to 8 hr, p.r.n. *Maximum:* 400 mg/day.

➤ *To relieve mild to moderate pain*
CAPSULES
Adults and adolescents over age 14. 50 mg every 4 to 6 hr, p.r.n. Increased to 100 mg every 4 to 6 hr, if needed. *Maximum:* 400 mg daily.

➤ *To treat hypermenorrhea and primary dysmenorrhea*
CAPSULES
Adults and adolescents over age 14. 100 mg t.i.d. for up to 6 days.

Route	Onset	Peak	Duration
P.O.*	1 hr	0.5 to 2 hr	4 to 6 hr
P.O.†	Few days	2 to 3 wk	Unknown

Contraindications

Hypersensitivity to aspirin, iodides, meclofenamate, other NSAIDs, or their components

---

* For analgesic effect.
† For antirheumatic effect.

Mechanism of Action

Blocks cyclooxygenase, the enzyme needed to synthesize prostaglandins, which mediate the inflammatory response and cause local vasodilation, swelling, and pain. By inhibiting prostaglandins, this NSAID reduces inflammatory symptoms. It also relieves pain because prostaglandins promote pain transmission from the periphery to the spinal cord.

Interactions

DRUGS
acetaminophen: Increased risk of adverse renal effects with long-term use of both drugs
anticoagulants, thrombolytics: Prolonged PT and increased risk of bleeding
antihypertensives: Decreased effectiveness of antihypertensives
beta blockers: Impaired antihypertensive effect of beta blockers
cefamandole, cefoperazone, cefotetan, plicamycin, valproic acid: Hypoprothrombinemia and increased risk of bleeding
cimetidine: Altered blood meclofenamate level
colchicine, glucocorticoids, potassium supplements: Increased GI irritability and bleeding
cyclosporine, gold compounds, nephrotoxic drugs: Increased risk of nephrotoxicity
digoxin: Increased blood digoxin level
insulin, oral antidiabetic drugs: Decreased effectiveness of these drugs
lithium: Increased risk of lithium toxicity
loop diuretics: Decreased effects of these drugs
methotrexate: Increased risk of methotrexate toxicity
NSAIDs, salicylates: Increased GI irritability and risk of bleeding, decreased meclofenamate effectiveness
phenytoin: Increased blood phenytoin level
probenecid: Increased risk of meclofenamate toxicity
ACTIVITIES
alcohol use: Increased GI irritability and bleeding

Adverse Reactions

CNS: Dizziness, drowsiness, fatigue, headache, insomnia, seizures, stroke

M

CV: Hypertension, MI, peripheral edema, tachycardia
EENT: Stomatitis, tinnitus
GI: Abdominal pain; anorexia; constipation; diarrhea; diverticulitis; dyspepsia; dysphagia; elevated liver function test results; esophagitis; flatulence; gastritis; gastroenteritis; gastroesophageal reflux disease; GI bleeding, perforation, and ulceration; hepatic failure; indigestion; jaundice; melena; nausea; perforation of stomach or intestines; stomatitis; vomiting
GU: Acute renal failure, dysuria, elevated BUN and serum creatinine levels
HEME: Agranulocytosis, anemia, easy bruising, hemolytic anemia, leukopenia, neutropenia, pancytopenia, thrombocytopenia
RESP: Asthma, respiratory depression
SKIN: Erythema multiforme, pruritus, rash, Stevens-Johnson syndrome, toxic epidermal necrolysis, urticaria
Other: Anaphylaxis, angioedema

Nursing Considerations

• Use meclofenamate with extreme caution in patients with a history of ulcer disease or GI bleeding because NSAIDs such as meclofenamate increase the risk of GI bleeding and ulceration. Expect to use meclofenamate for the shortest time possible in these patients.
• Be aware that serious GI tract ulceration, bleeding, and perforation may occur without warning symptoms. Elderly patients are at greater risk. To minimize risk, give drug with food and a full glass of water. If GI distress occurs, withhold drug and notify prescriber immediately.
• Use meclofenamate cautiously in patients with hypertension, and monitor blood pressure closely throughout therapy. Drug may cause hypertension or worsen it.
• **WARNING** Monitor patient closely for thrombotic events, including MI and stroke, because NSAIDs increase the risk.
• Monitor patient—especially if he's elderly or receiving long-term meclofenamate therapy—for less common but serious adverse GI reactions, including anorexia, constipation, diverticulitis, dysphagia, esophagitis, gastritis, gastroenteritis, gastroesophageal reflux disease, hemorrhoids, hiatal hernia, melena, stomatitis, and vomiting.
• Monitor liver function test results because, in rare cases, elevations may progress to severe hepatic reactions, including fatal hepatitis, liver necrosis, and hepatic failure.
• Monitor BUN and serum creatinine levels in elderly patients, patients taking diuretics or ACE inhibitors, and patients with heart failure, impaired renal function, or hepatic dysfunction; drug may cause renal failure.
• Monitor CBC for decreased hemoglobin and hematocrit because drug may worsen anemia.
• **WARNING** If patient has bone marrow suppression or is receiving an antineoplastic drug, monitor laboratory results (including WBC count), and watch for evidence of infection because anti-inflammatory and antipyretic actions of meclofenamate may mask signs and symptoms, such as fever and pain.
• Assess patient's skin regularly for signs of rash or other hypersensitivity reaction because meclofenamate is an NSAID and may cause serious skin reactions without warning, even in patients with no history of NSAID sensitivity. At first sign of reaction, stop drug and notify prescriber.
• Expect lower doses of meclofenamate to be used for long-term therapy.

PATIENT TEACHING
• Tell patient to take drug with a full glass of water to keep it from lodging in esophagus and causing irritation. Also suggest taking drug with food or milk to avoid GI distress.
• Instruct patient to report itching, rash, severe diarrhea, and swelling in ankles or fingers.
• Caution patient to avoid potentially hazardous activities until drug's CNS effects are known.
• Caution pregnant patient not to take NSAIDs such as meclofenamate during the last trimester because NSAIDs may cause premature closure of the fetal ductus arteriosus.
• Explain that meclofenamate may increase the risk of serious adverse cardiovascular reactions; urge patient to seek immediate medical attention if signs or symptoms arise, such as chest pain, shortness of breath, weakness, and slurring of speech.
• Explain that meclofenamate may increase the risk of serious adverse GI reactions; stress the importance of seeking immediate

medical attention for such signs and symptoms as epigastric or abdominal pain, indigestion, black or tarry stools, or vomiting blood or material that looks like coffee grounds.

•Alert patient to rare but serious skin reactions to meclofenamate. Urge him to seek immediate medical attention for rash, blisters, itching, fever, or other indications of hypersensitivity.

meloxicam

Mobic

Class and Category

Chemical class: Oxicam derivative
Therapeutic class: Anti-inflammatory
Pregnancy category: C

Indications and Dosages

➤ *To relieve signs and symptoms of osteoarthritis and rheumatoid arthritis*

ORAL SUSPENSION, TABLETS

Adults. 7.5 mg daily. *Maximum:* 15 mg daily.

➤ *To relieve pauciarticular or polyarticular signs and symptoms of juvenile rheumatoid arthritis*

ORAL SUSPENSION, TABLETS

Children age 2 and over. 0.125 mg/kg daily. *Maximum:* 7.5 mg daily.

Mechanism of Action

Blocks cyclooxygenase, the enzyme needed to synthesize prostaglandins, which mediate the inflammatory response and cause local vasodilation, swelling, and pain. By inhibiting prostaglandins, the NSAID meloxicam reduces inflammatory symptoms. It also relieves pain because prostaglandins promote pain transmission from the periphery to the spinal cord.

Contraindications

Angioedema, asthma, bronchospasm, nasal polyps, rhinitis, or urticaria induced by hypersensitivity to aspirin, meloxicam, other NSAIDs, or their components

Interactions

DRUGS

ACE inhibitors: Decreased antihypertensive effect, increased risk of renal failure

aspirin: Increased risk of GI ulceration
furosemide: Decreased diuretic effect of furosemide, possibly renal impairment
lithium: Elevated blood lithium level, possibly lithium toxicity
oral anticoagulants, warfarin: Increased risk of bleeding

ACTIVITIES

alcohol use, smoking: Increased risk of GI bleeding

Adverse Reactions

CNS: Confusion, dizziness, fever, headache, insomnia, mood alteration, seizures, stroke
CV: Chest pain, edema, heart failure, hypertension, MI, tachycardia, vasculitis
EENT: Laryngitis, pharyngitis, sinusitis
GI: Abdominal pain, anorexia, colitis, constipation, diarrhea, diverticulitis, dyspepsia, dysphagia, elevated liver function test results, esophagitis, flatulence, gastritis, gastroenteritis, gastroesophageal reflux disease, GI bleeding and ulceration, hepatic failure, hepatitis, indigestion, melena, nausea, pancreatitis, perforation of stomach or intestines, stomatitis, vomiting
GU: Acute renal failure, acute urine retention (children), urinary frequency, UTI
HEME: Agranulocytosis, anemia, easy bruising, hemolytic anemia, leukopenia, neutropenia, pancytopenia, thrombocytopenia
MS: Arthralgia; back pain; joint crepitation, effusion, or swelling; muscle spasms; myalgia
RESP: Asthma, bronchospasm, cough, dyspnea, respiratory depression, upper respiratory tract infection
SKIN: Erythema multiforme, exfoliative dermatitis, photosensitivity, pruritus, rash, Stevens-Johnson syndrome, toxic epidermal necrolysis
Other: Anaphylaxis, angioedema, flulike symptoms

Nursing Considerations

•Use meloxicam with extreme caution in patients with a history of ulcer disease or GI bleeding because NSAIDs such as meloxicam increase the risk of GI bleeding and ulceration. Expect to use meloxicam for the shortest time possible in these patients.

•Be aware that serious GI tract ulceration, bleeding, and perforation may occur without warning symptoms. Elderly patients are at greater risk. To minimize risk, give drug with food and a full glass of water. If GI dis-

tress occurs, withhold drug and notify prescriber immediately.
•Use meloxicam cautiously in patients with hypertension, and monitor blood pressure closely throughout therapy. Drug may cause hypertension or worsen it.
•WARNING Monitor patient closely for thrombotic events, including MI and stroke, because NSAIDs increase the risk.
•Monitor patient—especially if he's elderly or receiving long-term meloxicam therapy—for less common but serious adverse GI reactions, including anorexia, constipation, diverticulitis, dysphagia, esophagitis, gastritis, gastroenteritis, gastroesophageal reflux disease, hemorrhoids, hiatal hernia, melena, stomatitis, and vomiting.
•Monitor liver function test results because, in rare cases, elevations may progress to severe hepatic reactions, including fatal hepatitis, liver necrosis, and hepatic failure.
•Monitor BUN and serum creatinine levels in elderly patients; patients taking diuretics, angiotensin II receptor antagonists, or ACE inhibitors; and patients with heart failure, impaired renal function, or hepatic dysfunction; drug may cause renal failure.
•Monitor CBC for decreased hemoglobin and hematocrit because drug may worsen anemia.
•WARNING If patient has bone marrow suppression or is receiving an antineoplastic drug, monitor laboratory results (including WBC count), and watch for evidence of infection because anti-inflammatory and antipyretic actions of meloxicam may mask signs and symptoms, such as fever and pain.
•Assess patient's skin regularly for signs of rash or other hypersensitivity reaction because meloxicam is an NSAID and may cause serious skin reactions without warning, even in patients with no history of NSAID sensitivity. At first sign of reaction, stop drug and notify prescriber.
•Monitor patient for adequate hydration before beginning meloxicam therapy to decrease risk of renal dysfunction.
PATIENT TEACHING
•Instruct patient to take meloxicam with food or after meals if stomach upset occurs.
•If oral suspension is prescribed, tell patient to shake container gently before use.
•Caution patient to avoid using other NSAIDs, aspirin, or products containing as-

pirin while taking meloxicam.
•Advise patient to refrain from smoking and alcohol use because these activities may increase the risk of adverse GI reactions.
•Instruct patient to notify prescriber if he develops signs or symptoms of hepatic dysfunction, such as dark yellow or brown urine, fatigue, fever, itching, lethargy, nausea, or yellowing of eyes or skin.
•Advise patient, especially if he's taking an oral anticoagulant such as warfarin, to report immediately signs of bleeding, such as easy bruising, stomach pain, blood in urine, or black tarry stools.
•Caution pregnant patient not to take NSAIDs such as meloxicam during the last trimester because they may cause premature closure of the ductus arteriosus.
•Explain that meloxicam may increase the risk of serious adverse cardiovascular reactions; urge patient to seek immediate medical attention if signs or symptoms arise, such as chest pain, shortness of breath, weakness, and slurring of speech.
•Explain that meloxicam may increase the risk of serious adverse GI reactions; stress the importance of seeking immediate medical attention for such signs and symptoms as epigastric or abdominal pain, indigestion, black or tarry stools, or vomiting blood or material that looks like coffee grounds.
•Alert patient to rare but serious skin reactions. Urge him to seek immediate medical attention for rash, blisters, itching, fever, or other indications of hypersensitivity.

memantine hydrochloride

Namenda

Class and Category
Chemical class: N-methyl-D-aspartate (NMDA) receptor antagonist
Therapeutic class: Antidementia agent
Pregnancy category: B

Indications and Dosages
➤ *To treat moderate-to-severe dementia of the Alzheimer's type*
TABLETS
Adults. *Initial:* 5 mg daily P.O., increased by 5 mg/wk, as needed, to 10 mg daily in two divided doses; then 15 mg daily with one

5-mg and one 10-mg dose daily; then 20 mg daily in two divided doses. *Maintenance:* 20 mg daily.

DOSAGE ADJUSTMENT Dosage reduction probable for patients with renal impairment.

Contraindications
Hypersensitivity to memantine, amantadine, or their components

Interactions
DRUGS
amantadine, dextromethorphan, ketamine: Possibly additive effects
carbonic anhydrase inhibitors, sodium bicarbonate: Decreased memantine clearance, leading to increased blood drug levels and risk of adverse effects
cimetidine, hydrochlorothiazide, metformin, nicotinic acid, quinidine, ranitidine, triamterene: Possibly increased blood levels of both agents

Adverse Reactions
CNS: Abnormal gait, agitation, akathisia, anxiety, confusion, delirium, delusions, depression, dizziness, drowsiness, dyskinesia, fatigue, hallucinations, headache, hyperexcitability, insomnia, neuroleptic malignant syndrome, psychosis, restlessness, seizures, somnolence, stroke, tardive dyskinesia

Mechanism of Action

Memantine blocks the action of the excitatory amino acid glutamate on N-methyl-D-aspartate (NMDA) receptor cells in the central nervous system. In Alzheimer's disease, glutamate levels are abnormally high when brain cells are both at rest and active. Normally, when certain brain cells are resting, magnesium ions block NMDA receptors and prevent the influx of sodium and calcium ions and the outflow of potassium ions. When learning and memory cells in the brain are active, glutamate engages with NMDA receptors, magnesium ions are removed from NMDA receptors, and the cells are depolarized. During depolarization, sodium and calcium ions enter brain cells and potassium ions leave. In Alzheimer's disease, excessive circulating glutamate permanently removes magnesium ions and opens ion channels. The excessive influx of calcium may damage brain cells and play a major role in Alzheimer's disease. What's more, dying brain cells release additional glutamate, worsening the cycle of brain cell destruction.

Memantine replaces magnesium on the NMDA receptors of brain cells, closing ion channels and preventing calcium influx and the resulting damage to brain cells. By preventing excessive brain cell death, memantine slows the progression of Alzheimer's disease.

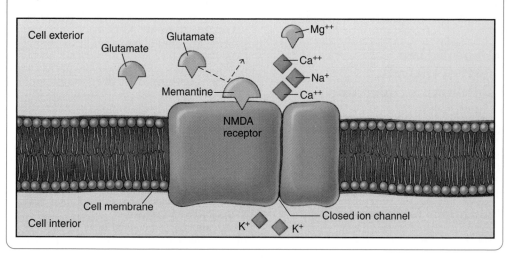

CV: AV block, chest pain, hypertension, peripheral edema, prolonged QT interval, supraventricular tachycardia, tachycardia
ENDO: Hypoglycemia
GI: Acute pancreatitis, anorexia, colitis, constipation, diarrhea, hepatic failure, ileus, nausea, vomiting
GU: Acute renal failure, impotence, urinary incontinence, UTI
HEME: Thrombocytopenia
MS: Arthralgia, back pain
RESP: Bronchitis, cough, dyspnea, upper respiratory tract infection
SKIN: Stevens-Johnson syndrome
Other: Generalized pain, flulike symptoms

Nursing Considerations
•Use memantine cautiously in patients with renal tubular acidosis or severe UTI because these conditions cause urine to become alkaline, thereby reducing memantine excretion and increasing the risk of adverse reactions.
•Use cautiously in patients with severe hepatic impairment because drug undergoes partial hepatic metabolism which may increase risk of adverse reactions.
•Monitor patient's response to memantine, and notify prescriber if serious or bothersome adverse reactions occur.

PATIENT TEACHING
•Advise patient to avoid a diet excessively high in fruits and vegetables because these foods contribute to alkaline urine, which can alter memantine clearance and increase adverse reactions.
•Caution patient to avoid hazardous activities until drug's CNS effects are known.

meperidine hydrochloride
(pethidine hydrochloride)
Demerol

Class, Category, and Schedule
Chemical class: Phenylpiperidine derivative opioid
Therapeutic class: Analgesic
Pregnancy category: C
Controlled substance schedule: II

Indications and Dosages
➤ *To relieve moderate to severe pain*
SYRUP, TABLETS, I.M. OR SUBCUTANEOUS INJECTION

Adults. 50 to 150 mg every 3 to 4 hr, p.r.n.
Children. 1.1 to 1.8 mg/kg every 3 to 4 hr, p.r.n.

➤ *To provide preoperative sedation*
I.V. INJECTION
Adults. 15 to 35 mg/hr, p.r.n.
I.M. OR SUBCUTANEOUS INJECTION
Adults. 50 to 100 mg 30 to 90 min before surgery.
Children. 1 to 2 mg/kg 30 to 90 min before surgery. *Maximum:* 100 mg every 3 to 4 hr.

➤ *As adjunct to anesthesia*
I.V. INFUSION OR INJECTION
Adults. Individualized. Repeated slow injections of 10 mg/ml solution or continuous infusion of dilute solution (1 mg/ml) titrated as needed.

➤ *To provide obstetric analgesia*
I.M. OR SUBCUTANEOUS INJECTION
Adults. 50 to 100 mg given with regular, painful contractions; repeated every 1 to 3 hr.

DOSAGE ADJUSTMENT For patients with creatinine clearance of 10 to 50 ml/min/1.73 m^2, 75% of usual dose is used; with creatinine clearance of less than 10 ml/min/1.73 m^2, 50% of usual dose is used.

Route	Onset	Peak	Duration
P.O.	15 min	1 to 1.5 hr	2 to 4 hr
I.V.	1 min	5 to 7 min	2 to 4 hr
I.M., SubQ	10 to 15 min	30 to 50 min	2 to 4 hr

Mechanism of Action
Binds with opiate receptors in the spinal cord and higher levels of the CNS. In this way, meperidine stimulates mu and kappa receptors, which alters the perception of and emotional response to pain.

Incompatibilities
Don't mix meperidine in same syringe with aminophylline, barbiturates, heparin, iodides, methicillin, morphine sulfate, phenytoin, sodium bicarbonate, sulfadiazine, or sulfisoxazole.

Contraindications
Acute asthma; hypersensitivity to meperidine, opioids, or their components; increased

intracranial pressure; severe respiratory depression; upper respiratory tract obstruction; use within 14 days of MAO inhibitor therapy

Interactions

DRUGS

acyclovir, ritonavir: Possibly increased blood meperidine level

alfentanil, CNS depressants, fentanyl, sufentanil: Increased risk of CNS and respiratory depression and hypotension

amphetamines, MAO inhibitors: Risk of increased CNS excitation or depression with possibly fatal reactions

anticholinergics: Increased risk of severe constipation

antidiarrheals (such as loperamide and difenoxin and atropine): Increased risk of severe constipation and increased CNS depression

antihypertensives: Increased risk of hypotension

buprenorphine: Possibly decreased therapeutic effects of meperidine and increased risk of respiratory depression

cimetidine: Reduced clearance and volume of distribution of meperidine

hydroxyzine: Increased risk of CNS depression and hypotension

metoclopramide: Possibly decreased effects of metoclopramide

naloxone, naltrexone: Decreased pharmacologic effects of meperidine

neuromuscular blockers: Increased risk of prolonged respiratory and CNS depression

oral anticoagulants: Possibly increased anticoagulant effect and risk of bleeding

phenytoin: Possibly enhanced hepatic metabolism of meperidine

ACTIVITIES

alcohol use: Possibly increased CNS and respiratory depression and hypotension

Adverse Reactions

CNS: Confusion, depression, dizziness, drowsiness, euphoria, headache, increased intracranial pressure, lack of coordination, malaise, nervousness, nightmares, restlessness, seizures, syncope, tremor

CV: Hypotension, orthostatic hypotension, tachycardia

EENT: Blurred vision, diplopia, dry mouth

GI: Abdominal cramps or pain, anorexia, constipation, ileus, nausea, vomiting

GU: Dysuria, urinary frequency, urine retention

RESP: Dyspnea, respiratory arrest or depression, wheezing

SKIN: Diaphoresis, flushing, pruritus, rash, urticaria

Other: Injection site pain, redness, and swelling; physical and psychological dependence

Nursing Considerations

• Use meperidine with extreme caution in patients with acute abdominal conditions, hepatic or renal disorders, hypothyroidism, prostatic hyperplasia, seizures, or supraventricular tachycardia.

• To minimize local anesthetic effect, dilute meperidine syrup with water before administration.

• Give I.V. dose slowly by direct injection or as a slow continuous infusion. Mix with D_5W, normal saline solution, or Ringer's or lactated Ringer's solution.

• Keep naloxone available when giving I.V. meperidine.

• Be aware that subcutaneous injection is painful and isn't recommended.

• Be aware that oral form of meperidine is less than half as effective as parenteral meperidine. Give I.M. form when possible, and expect to increase dosage when switching patient to oral form.

• Monitor patient's respiratory and cardiovascular status during treatment. Notify prescriber immediately and expect to discontinue drug if respiratory rate falls to less than 12 breaths/minute or if respiratory depth decreases.

• Monitor patient's bowel function to detect constipation, and assess the need for stool softeners.

• Assess for signs of physical dependence and abuse.

• Expect withdrawal symptoms to occur if drug is abruptly withdrawn after long-term use.

PATIENT TEACHING

• Inform patient that meperidine is a controlled substance and that he'll need identification to purchase it.

• Advise patient to take drug exactly as prescribed.

• Instruct patient to report constipation, severe nausea, and shortness or breath.

• Advise patient to avoid potentially hazardous activities until drug's CNS effects are known.

M

•Instruct patient to prevent postoperative atelectasis by turning, coughing, and deep-breathing.
•Urge patient to avoid alcohol, sedatives, and tranquilizers during therapy with meperidine.

mephentermine sulfate

Wyamine

Class and Category

Chemical class: Sympathomimetic amine
Therapeutic class: Vasopressor
Pregnancy category: C

Indications and Dosages

➤ *To treat hypotension secondary to spinal anesthesia*

I.V. INJECTION

Adults. 30 to 45 mg (15 mg for obstetric patients); may be repeated, as needed, to maintain blood pressure.

I.V. INFUSION

Adults. Dosage individualized based on patient response to therapy. Average dose is 1 to 5 mg/min.

Route	Onset	Peak	Duration
I.V.	Almost immediate	Unknown	15 to 30 min

Mechanism of Action

Stimulates alpha-adrenergic receptors directly and indirectly, resulting in positive inotropic and chronotropic effects. Indirect stimulation occurs by the release of norepinephrine from its storage sites in the heart and other tissues. By enhancing cardiac contraction, mephentermine improves cardiac output, thereby increasing blood pressure. Increased peripheral resistance from peripheral vasoconstriction may also contribute to increased blood pressure. Mephentermine can affect the heart rate but the change is variable, based on vagal tone. It may also stimulate beta-adrenergic receptors.

Contraindications

Hypersensitivity to mephentermine, phenothiazine-induced hypotension, use within 14 days of MAO inhibitor therapy

Interactions

DRUGS

alpha blockers and other drugs with alpha-blocking effects: Possibly decreased peripheral vasoconstrictive and hypertensive effects of mephentermine
beta blockers (ophthalmic): Decreased effects of mephentermine; increased risk of bronchospasm, wheezing, decreased pulmonary function, and respiratory failure
beta blockers (systemic): Increased risk of bronchospasm and decreased effects of both drugs
diuretics and other antihypertensives: Possibly reduced effectiveness of these drugs
doxapram: Possibly increased vasopressor effects of either drug
ergot alkaloids: Increased vasopressor effects
guanadrel, guanethidine, mecamylamine, methyldopa, reserpine: Possibly decreased effects of these drugs and increased risk of adverse effects
hydrocarbon inhalation anesthetics: Increased risk of atrial and ventricular arrhythmias
MAO inhibitors: Increased, lengthened cardiac stimulation and vasopressor effects, and possibly severe headache and hypertensive crisis
maprotiline, tricyclic antidepressants: Increased vasopressor response; increased risk of prolonged QTc interval, arrhythmias, hypertension, and hyperpyrexia
methylphenidate: Possibly increased vasopressor effect of mephentermine
nitrates: Possibly reduced antianginal effects of nitrates and decreased vasopressor effect
other sympathomimetics (such as dopamine): Possibly increased cardiac effects and adverse reactions
oxytocin: Possibly severe hypertension
thyroid hormones: Increased effects of both drugs, increased risk of coronary insufficiency in patients with coronary artery disease

Adverse Reactions

CNS: Anxiety, dizziness, drowsiness, euphoria, headache, incoherence, nervousness, psychosis, restlessness, seizures, weakness
CV: Angina, arrhythmias (including bradycardia, tachycardia, and ventricular arrhythmias), hypertension, hypotension, palpita-

tions, peripheral vasoconstriction
GI: Nausea, vomiting
RESP: Dyspnea
SKIN: Peripheral necrosis

Nursing Considerations
•Before administering mephentermine, expect to intervene, as ordered, to correct hemorrhage, hypovolemia, metabolic acidosis, or hypoxia.
•Discard vial if you observe discoloration or precipitate.
•Using D_5W or normal saline solution, prepare a 1-mg/ml solution for infusion.
•Administer drug using an infusion pump to provide a controlled rate.
•Monitor blood pressure, cardiac rate and rhythm, central venous pressure (if appropriate), and urine output during administration. Adjust infusion rate according to patient response, as ordered. Be aware that patients with a history of cardiovascular disease (including hypertension) or hyperthyroidism and chronically ill patients are at increased risk for mephentermine's adverse cardiovascular effects.
•Assess patients with angle-closure glaucoma for signs of an exacerbation, such as eye pain or blurred vision.
•Assess circulation in patients with a history of occlusive vascular disease, such as atherosclerosis and Raynaud's disease, because mephentermine may cause decreased circulation and increase the risk of necrosis or gangrene. Inspect I.V. site periodically for signs of extravasation.
•WARNING Be aware that weeping, excitability, seizures, and hallucinations are some of the symptoms of mephentermine overdose. Contact prescriber immediately if patient experiences such symptoms, and expect to provide supportive treatment.
•Be aware that mephentermine can increase contractions in pregnant women, especially during the third trimester. Expect drug to be prescribed only when benefits outweigh potential adverse effects.
•Store drug at 15° to 30° C (59° to 86° F); don't freeze.

PATIENT TEACHING
•Instruct patient receiving mephentermine to report adverse reactions, including chest pain, difficulty breathing, dizziness, irregular heartbeat, headache, and weakness.

mephenytoin
Mesantoin

Class and Category
Chemical class: Hydantoin derivative
Therapeutic class: Anticonvulsant
Pregnancy category: Not rated

Indications and Dosages
➤ *To control generalized tonic-clonic, focal, and jacksonian seizures when other drugs are ineffective*
TABLETS
Adults. *Initial:* 50 to 100 mg daily during first wk. Increased by 50 to 100 mg at 1-wk intervals until desired response is reached. *Maintenance:* 200 to 600 mg daily in equally divided doses. *Maximum:* 1.2 g daily.
Children. *Initial:* 20 to 50 mg daily. Increased by 25 to 50 mg at 1-wk intervals until desired response occurs. *Maintenance:* 100 to 400 mg daily in equally divided doses. *Maximum:* 400 mg daily.
➤ *To replace other anticonvulsants*
TABLETS
Adults. 50 to 100 mg daily during first wk. Dosage gradually increased while decreasing dosage of other drug over 3 to 6 wk.

Route	Onset	Peak	Duration
P.O.	30 min	Unknown	24 to 48 hr

M

Mechanism of Action
Limits the spread of seizure activity and the start of new seizures by:
• regulating voltage-dependent sodium and calcium channels in neurons
• inhibiting calcium movement across neuronal membranes
• enhancing sodium-potassium adenosine triphosphatase activity in neurons and glial cells.
   These actions may reflect a slowed recovery rate of inactivated sodium channels.

Contraindications
Hypersensitivity to mephenytoin, phenytoin, other hydantoins, or their components

Interactions
DRUGS
acetaminophen: Increased risk of hepatotox-

icity with long-term acetaminophen use

amiodarone: Possibly increased blood mephenytoin level and risk of toxicity

antacids: Possibly decreased mephenytoin effectiveness

antineoplastics: Increased mephenytoin metabolism

bupropion, clozapine, loxapine, MAO inhibitors, maprotiline, phenothiazines, pimozide, thioxanthenes: Possibly lowered seizure threshold and decreased therapeutic effects of mephenytoin, possibly intensified CNS depressant effects of these drugs

calcium channel blockers, fluconazole, itraconazole, ketoconazole, miconazole, omeprazole: Possibly increased blood phenytoin level

carbamazepine: Decreased blood carbamazepine level, possibly increased blood phenytoin level and risk of toxicity

chloramphenicol, cimetidine, disulfiram, isoniazid, methylphenidate, metronidazole, phenylbutazone, ranitidine, salicylates, sulfonamides, trimethoprim: Possibly impaired metabolism of these drugs and increased risk of mephenytoin toxicity

corticosteroids, cyclosporine, digoxin, disopyramide, doxycycline, furosemide, levodopa, mexiletine, quinidine: Decreased therapeutic effects of these drugs

diazoxide: Possibly decreased therapeutic effects of both drugs

estrogens, progestins: Decreased therapeutic effects of these drugs, increased blood phenytoin level

felbamate: Possibly impaired metabolism and increased blood level of phenytoin

fluoxetine: Possibly increased blood phenytoin level and risk of toxicity

folic acid: Increased mephenytoin metabolism, decreased seizure control

haloperidol: Possibly lowered seizure threshold and decreased therapeutic effects of mephenytoin; possibly decreased blood haloperidol level

insulin, oral antidiabetic drugs: Possibly increased blood glucose level and decreased therapeutic effects of these drugs

lamotrigine: Possibly decreased therapeutic effects of lamotrigine

lithium: Increased risk of lithium toxicity

methadone: Possibly increased methadone metabolism, leading to withdrawal symptoms

molindone: Possibly lowered seizure thresh-

old, impaired absorption, and decreased therapeutic effects of mephenytoin

oral anticoagulants: Possibly impaired metabolism of these drugs and increased risk of mephenytoin toxicity; possibly increased anticoagulant effect initially, but decreased effect with prolonged therapy

oral contraceptives containing estrogen and progestin: Possibly breakthrough bleeding and decreased contraceptive effectiveness

rifampin: Possibly decreased therapeutic effects of mephenytoin

streptozocin: Possibly decreased therapeutic effects of streptozocin

sucralfate: Possibly decreased mephenytoin absorption

tricyclic antidepressants: Possibly lowered seizure threshold and decreased therapeutic effects of mephenytoin; possibly decreased blood level of tricyclic antidepressants

valproic acid: Decreased blood phenytoin level, increased blood valproic acid level

vitamin D analogues: Decreased vitamin D analogue activity, risk of anticonvulsant-induced rickets and osteomalacia

xanthines: Possibly inhibited mephenytoin absorption and increased clearance of xanthines

zaleplon: Increased clearance and decreased effectiveness of zaleplon

ACTIVITIES

alcohol use: Possibly decreased mephenytoin effectiveness

Adverse Reactions

CNS: Ataxia, choreoathetoid movements, confusion, dizziness, drowsiness, excitement, fatigue, fever, headache, peripheral neuropathy, sedation, slurred speech, stuttering, tremor

EENT: Gingival hyperplasia, nystagmus

GI: Constipation, diarrhea, nausea, vomiting

HEME: Agranulocytosis, leukopenia, thrombocytopenia

MS: Muscle twitching

SKIN: Rash, Stevens-Johnson syndrome, toxic epidermal necrolysis

Other: Lymphadenopathy, systemic lupus erythematosus

Nursing Considerations

•Because of mephenytoin's potentially dangerous adverse effects, expect to use it only when other drugs are ineffective.

•Keep in mind that mephenytoin doesn't control absence seizures.

•**WARNING** Be aware that drug shouldn't be abruptly discontinued because doing so may cause status epilepticus. Plan to reduce dosage gradually or substitute another drug, as prescribed, when discontinuing mephenytoin.
•Obtain CBC and differential before treatment, after 2 weeks of treatment, and then monthly during first year of treatment, as ordered.
•Notify prescriber immediately and expect to discontinue mephenytoin and substitute another drug if depressed blood counts, enlarged lymph nodes, or rash develops.

PATIENT TEACHING
•Urge patient to take mephenytoin exactly as prescribed and not to stop it abruptly.
•Advise patient to take drug with food to enhance absorption and reduce adverse GI reactions.
•Caution patient on once-a-day therapy to be especially careful not to miss a dose.
•Advise patient to report impaired coordination, persistent headache, rash, severe GI distress, swollen gums or lymph nodes, or unusual bleeding or bruising.
•Encourage patient to maintain good oral hygiene and to have regular dental checkups to reduce the risk of gum disease.
•Instruct patient to keep medical appointments to monitor drug effectiveness and check for adverse reactions. Explain the need for periodic laboratory tests.
•Advise patient to wear medical identification stating that he has epilepsy and takes mephenytoin to prevent seizures.

mephobarbital

Mebaral

Class, Category, and Schedule
Chemical class: Barbiturate derivative
Therapeutic class: Anticonvulsant, sedative
Pregnancy category: D
Controlled substance schedule: IV

Indications and Dosages
➤ *To treat seizures*
TABLETS
Adults. 400 to 600 mg daily as a single dose or in divided doses, usually beginning with low dose and increasing over 4 to 5 days until optimum dosage is determined.
Children over age 5. 32 to 64 mg t.i.d. or q.i.d.

Children under age 5. 16 to 32 mg t.i.d. or q.i.d.
➤ *To provide sedation*
TABLETS
Adults. 32 to 100 mg t.i.d. or q.i.d.
Children. 16 to 32 mg t.i.d. or q.i.d.

Route	Onset	Peak	Duration
P.O.	30 to 60 min	Unknown	10 to 16 hr

Mechanism of Action
May reduce seizure activity by reducing transmission of monosynaptic and polysynaptic nerve impulses, which causes decreased excitability in nerve cells. As a sedative, mephobarbital inhibits upward conduction of nerve impulses to the reticular formation of the brain, which disrupts impulse transmission to the cortex. As a result, mephobarbital depresses the CNS and produces drowsiness, hypnosis, and sedation.

Contraindications
Hepatic disease or failure; history of addiction to sedatives or hypnotics; hypersensitivity to mephobarbital, other barbiturates, or their components; nephritis; porphyria; severe respiratory disease with obstruction or dyspnea

Interactions
DRUGS
acetaminophen: Possibly decreased effects of acetaminophen (with long-term mephobarbital use)
anesthetics (halogenated hydrocarbon): Increased risk of hepatotoxicity (with long-term mephobarbital use)
carbamazepine, chloramphenicol, corticosteroids, cyclosporine, dacarbazine, digoxin, disopyramide, doxycycline, griseofulvin, metronidazole, oral contraceptives, phenylbutazone, quinidine, theophyllines, vitamin D: Decreased effectiveness of these drugs
CNS depressants: Increased CNS depression
divalproex sodium, valproic acid: Increased risk of CNS depression and neurotoxicity
guanadrel, guanethidine: Increased risk of orthostatic hypotension
haloperidol: Possibly decreased blood haloperidol level and change in seizure pattern

M

hydantoins: Possibly interference with hydantoin metabolism
leucovorin: Possibly decreased anticonvulsant effect of mephobarbital
maprotiline: Possibly increased CNS depression and decreased therapeutic effects of mephobarbital
mexiletine: Possibly decreased blood mexiletine level
oral anticoagulants: Possibly decreased therapeutic effects of anticoagulants, possibly increased risk of bleeding when mephobarbital is discontinued
tricyclic antidepressants: Possibly decreased therapeutic effects of tricyclic antidepressants

ACTIVITIES
alcohol use: Increased CNS depression

Adverse Reactions

CNS: Agitation, anxiety, ataxia, confusion, delusions, depression, dizziness, drowsiness, fever, hallucinations, headache, insomnia, irritability, nervousness, nightmares, paradoxical stimulation, seizures, syncope, tremor
CV: Orthostatic hypotension
EENT: Vision changes
GI: Anorexia, constipation, hepatic dysfunction, nausea, vomiting
HEME: Agranulocytosis
MS: Arthralgia, bone pain, muscle twitching or weakness
RESP: Respiratory depression
SKIN: Exfoliative dermatitis, rash, Stevens-Johnson syndrome
Other: Physical and psychological dependence, weight loss

Nursing Considerations

• Observe patient for signs of physical and psychological dependence, especially with prolonged use of mephobarbital at high doses.
• Observe for signs of chronic barbiturate intoxication, including confusion, insomnia, poor judgment, slurred speech, and unsteady gait.
• Assess for paradoxical stimulation in patient who receives drug for acute or chronic pain.
• **WARNING** Expect to taper dosage gradually when discontinuing drug. Be aware that withdrawal symptoms can be severe and may cause death. Mild signs and symptoms, including anxiety, muscle twitching, nausea, orthostatic hypotension, and progressive weakness, may appear 8 to 12 hours after last drug dose. More severe signs include delirium and seizures.

PATIENT TEACHING
• Advise patient to take mephobarbital exactly as prescribed. Caution him not to stop taking drug abruptly because of the risk of withdrawal symptoms and, for epileptic patients, seizures.
• Instruct patient to avoid alcohol, sleeping pills, and other sedatives while taking mephobarbital because of the risk of increased CNS depression.
• Advise patient to avoid potentially hazardous activities until CNS effects of mephobarbital are known.
• Advise patient to change position slowly to minimize the effects of orthostatic hypotension.
• Urge patient to report confusion, fever, rash, or severe dizziness.

meprobamate

Apo-Meprobamate (CAN), Equanil, MB-Tab, Meprospan, Miltown, Neuramate

Class, Category, and Schedule

Chemical class: Carbamate derivative
Therapeutic class: Antianxiety
Pregnancy category: Not rated
Controlled substance schedule: IV

Indications and Dosages

➤ *To treat anxiety*
S.R. CAPSULES
Adults and adolescents. 400 to 800 mg every morning and bedtime. *Maximum:* 2,400 mg daily.
Children ages 6 to 12. 200 mg every morning and at bedtime.
TABLETS
Adults and adolescents. 1,200 to 1,600 mg/ day in divided doses t.i.d. or q.i.d. *Maximum:* 2,400 mg daily.
DOSAGE ADJUSTMENT For patients with creatinine clearance of 10 to 50 ml/min/1.73 m^2, drug administered every 12 hr; with creatinine clearance of less than 10 ml/min/ 1.73 m^2, drug administered every 18 hr.
Children ages 6 to 12. 200 to 600 mg daily in divided doses b.i.d. or t.i.d.

Route	Onset	Peak	Duration
P.O.	1 hr	Unknown	Unknown

Mechanism of Action

May act at multiple sites in the CNS, including the thalamus and limbic system. Meprobamate inhibits spinal reflexes, causing CNS relaxation; its sedative effects may account for its anticonvulsant action. It also has muscle relaxant properties.

Contraindications

Hypersensitivity to meprobromate or related drugs, such as carisoprodol; porphyria

Interactions

DRUGS
CNS depressants: Increased CNS depression
ACTIVITIES
alcohol use: Increased CNS depression

Adverse Reactions

CNS: Ataxia, dizziness, drowsiness, euphoria, headache, paradoxical stimulation, paresthesia, slurred speech, syncope, vertigo, weakness
CV: Arrhythmias, including tachycardia; hypotension; palpitations
EENT: Impaired visual accommodation
GI: Diarrhea, nausea, vomiting
SKIN: Erythematous maculopapular rash, pruritus, urticaria
Other: Physical dependence

Nursing Considerations

• Use meprobamate cautiously in patients with impaired hepatic or renal function, seizure disorders, or suicidal tendencies.
• Also use drug cautiously in patients with a history of drug dependence or abuse because meprobamate use can lead to physical dependence and abuse.
• Observe for signs of chronic drug intoxication, such as ataxia, slurred speech, and vertigo.
• **WARNING** When discontinuing drug, expect to taper dosage over 2 weeks because stopping abruptly can worsen previous symptoms, such as anxiety, or cause withdrawal symptoms, such as confusion, hallucinations, muscle twitching, tremor, and vomiting.
PATIENT TEACHING
• Instruct patient to take meprobamate ex-

actly as directed and not to stop taking it abruptly.
• Advise patient not to crush or chew S.R. capsules.
• Instruct patient to avoid hazardous activities until drug's CNS effects are known.
• Direct patient to avoid alcohol, sedatives, and other CNS depressants while taking meprobamate.
• Inform patient that meprobamate may become less effective after several months of treatment.
• Instruct patient to report development of a rash.

meropenem

Merrem I.V.

Class and Category

Chemical class: Carbapenem
Therapeutic class: Antibiotic
Pregnancy category: B

Indications and Dosages

➤ *To treat complicated appendicitis and peritonitis caused by susceptible strains of alpha-hemolytic streptococci,* Bacteroides fragilis, Bacteroides thetaiotaomicron, Escherichia coli, Klebsiella pneumoniae, Peptostreptococcus *species, or* Pseudomonas aeruginosa

I.V. INFUSION OR INJECTION
Adults and children weighing more than 50 kg (110 lb). 1 g every 8 hr infused over 15 to 30 min or given as a bolus over 3 to 5 min.
Children over age 3 months weighing less than 50 kg. 20 mg/kg every 8 hr infused over 15 to 30 min or given as a bolus over 3 to 5 min. *Maximum:* 1 g every 8 hr.
DOSAGE ADJUSTMENT For patients with creatinine clearance of 26 to 50 ml/min/1.73 m^2, dosage reduced to 1 g every 12 hr. For those with creatinine clearance of 10 to 25 ml/min/1.73 m^2, dosage reduced to 500 mg every 12 hr. For those with creatinine clearance of less than 10 ml/min/1.73 m^2, dosage reduced to 500 mg every 24 hr.

➤ *To treat complicated skin and skin structure infections caused by* Staphylococcus aureus, Streptococcus agalactiae, Streptococcus pyogenes, *viridans group* streptococci, Enterococcus faecalis *(excluding vancomycin-resistant isolates)*, Pseudomonas aeruginosa, Escherichia coli, Proteus mirabilis, Bacteroides fragilis, *and* Peptostreptococcus species

I.V. INFUSION

Adults and children weighing more than 50 kg (110 lb). 500 mg every 8 hr infused over 15 to 30 min.

Children over age 3 months weighing less than 50 kg. 10 mg/kg every 8 hr infused over 15 to 30 min. *Maximum:* 500 mg every 8 hr.

DOSAGE ADJUSTMENT For patients with creatinine clearance of 26 to 50 ml/min/1.73 m^2, dosage reduced to 500 mg every 12 hr. For those with creatinine clearance of 10 to 25 ml/min/1.73 m^2, dosage reduced to 250 mg every 12 hr. For those with creatinine clearance of less than 10 ml/min/1.73 m^2, dosage reduced to 250 mg every 24 hr.

➤ *To treat bacterial meningitis caused by* Haemophilus influenzae, Neisseria meningitidis, *or* Streptococcus pneumoniae *in children*

I.V. INFUSION OR INJECTION

Children weighing more than 50 kg. 2 g every 8 hr infused over 15 to 30 min or given as a bolus over 3 to 5 min.

Children over age 3 months weighing less than 50 kg. 40 mg/kg every 8 hr infused over 15 to 30 min or given as a bolus over 3 to 5 min. *Maximum:* 2 g every 8 hr.

Mechanism of Action

Penetrates cell walls of most gram-negative and gram-positive bacteria, inactivating penicillin-binding proteins. This action inhibits bacterial cell wall synthesis and causes cell death.

Incompatibilities

Don't mix meropenem in same solution with other drugs.

Contraindications

Hypersensitivity to meropenem, other carbapenem drugs, beta lactams, or their components

Interactions

DRUGS

probenecid: Inhibited renal excretion of meropenem

valproic acid: Possibly reduced blood level of valproic acid to subtherapeutic level

Adverse Reactions

CNS: Headache, seizures

CV: Shock

EENT: Epistaxis, glossitis, oral candidiasis

GI: Anorexia, constipation, diarrhea, elevated liver function test results, nausea, pseudomembranous colitis, vomiting

GU: Elevated BUN and serum creatinine levels, hematuria, renal failure

HEME: Agranulocytosis, hemolytic anemia, leukopenia, neutropenia, positive Coombs' test

RESP: Apnea, dyspnea

SKIN: Diaper rash from candidiasis (children), erythema multiforme, pruritus, rash, Stevens-Johnson syndrome, toxic epidermal necrolysis

Other: Anaphylaxis; angioedema; injection site inflammation, pain, phlebitis, or thrombophlebitis; sepsis

Nursing Considerations

•Obtain body fluid and tissue samples, as ordered, for culture and sensitivity testing. Expect to review test results, if possible, before giving first dose of meropenem.

•For I.V. bolus, add 10 ml of sterile water for injection to 500 mg/20-ml vial, or 20 ml of diluent to 1 g/30-ml vial of drug. Shake to dissolve.

•WARNING Be aware that fatal hypersensitivity reactions have occurred with meropenem use. Determine whether patient has had previous reactions to antibiotics or other allergens. Monitor patient closely and stop drug immediately if signs and symptoms of anaphylaxis occur. Notify prescriber, and expect to provide supportive emergency care that may include epinephrine and I.V. steroid administration, oxygen, and airway management.

•Monitor patient closely for diarrhea, which may indicate pseudomembranous colitis caused by *Clostridium difficile.* If diarrhea occurs, notify prescriber and expect to withhold meropenem and treat with fluids, electrolytes, protein, and an antibiotic effective against *C. difficile.*

•Take seizure precautions according to facility policy, especially for patients with bacterial meningitis or CNS or renal disorders because of an increased risk of seizures with meropenem.

•Monitor patient with creatinine clearance of 10 to 26 ml/min/1.73 m² for signs and symptoms of seizures, heart failure, renal failure, or shock.

PATIENT TEACHING

•Tell patient to report trouble breathing, injection site pain, and sore mouth.

•Urge patient to tell prescriber about diarrhea that's severe or lasts longer than 3 days. Remind patient that watery or bloody stools can occur 2 or more months after antibiotic therapy and can be serious, requiring prompt treatment.

mesalamine

Asacol, Canasa, Lialda, Mesasal (CAN), Pentasa, Rowasa, Salofalk (CAN)

Class and Category

Chemical class: 5-Aminosalicylic acid derivative
Therapeutic class: Anti-inflammatory
Pregnancy category: B

Indications and Dosages

➤ *To treat and maintain remission of ulcerative colitis*

DELAYED-RELEASE TABLETS (ASACOL)

Adults. *Initial:* 0.8 g t.i.d. for 6 wk. *Maintenance:* 1.6 g daily in divided doses.

DELAYED-RELEASE TABLETS (MESASAL)

Adults. 1.5 to 3 g daily in divided doses for 6 wk.

DELAYED-RELEASE TABLETS (SALOFALK)

Adults. 1 g t.i.d. or q.i.d. for 6 wk.

E.R. CAPSULES

Adults. 1 g q.i.d. for up to 8 wk.

➤ *To treat mild to moderate distal ulcerative colitis, proctitis, and proctosigmoiditis*

RECTAL SUSPENSION

Adults. 4 g (60 ml) daily at bedtime for 3 to 6 wk.

➤ *To treat active ulcerative proctitis*

SUPPOSITORIES (CANASA)

Adults. 0.5 g b.i.d. or t.i.d. for 3 to 6 wk. Or 1 g at bedtime for 3 to 6 wk.

➤ *To induce remission in patients with active mild to moderate ulcerative colitis.*

TABLETS

Adults. 2.4 or 4.8 g once daily with a meal for up to 8 wk.

Mechanism of Action

May reduce inflammation by inhibiting the enzyme cyclooxygenase and decreasing production of arachidonic acid metabolites, which may be increased in patients with inflammatory bowel disease. Cyclooxygenase is needed to form prostaglandins from arachidonic acid. Prostaglandins mediate inflammatory activity and produce signs and symptoms of inflammation. Mesalamine also may reduce inflammation by interfering with leukotriene synthesis and by inhibiting the enzyme lipoxygenase, both of which take part in inflammatory response.

Contraindications

Hypersensitivity to mesalamine, salicylates, or their components

Interactions

DRUGS

digoxin: Possibly decreased absorption and bioavailability of digoxin
lactulose: Possibly interference with delayed-release tablets or E.R. capsules
omeprazole: Increased mesalamine absorption

Adverse Reactions

CNS: Chills, dizziness, fatigue, fever, headache (severe), weakness
EENT: Rhinitis
GI: Abdominal cramps or pain (severe), anorexia, bloody diarrhea, colitis, diarrhea, elevated liver function test results, flatulence, indigestion, nausea, pancreatitis, rectal pain, vomiting
GU: Acute or chronic renal failure, nephrotoxicity
HEME: Agranulocytosis, granulocytopenia
MS: Back pain, dysarthria
RESP: Fibrosing alveolitis, pneumonitis
SKIN: Acne, alopecia, pruritus, rash
Other: Angioedema, drug fever, systemic lupus erythematosus

Nursing Considerations

•Use mesalamine cautiously in patients with sulfite sensitivity. Some drug formulations contain sulfites, which may cause hypersensitivity reactions in these patients.

•Ensure that suppository is firm before in-

M

serting it. If it's too soft, chill in refrigerator for 30 minutes or run under cold water before removing wrapper. Moisten it with water-soluble lubricant or tap water before insertion. Have patient retain suppository for 1 to 3 hours, as directed.
•Administer rectal suspension at bedtime, and have patient retain it for the prescribed time—about 8 hours, if possible. Retention time ranges from 3.5 to 12 hours.
•Be aware that rectal suspension may darken slightly over time but that this change doesn't affect potency. Discard rectal suspension that turns dark brown.
•Assess patient for evidence of acute intolerance similar to flare-up of inflammatory bowel disease: acute abdominal cramps and pain, bloody diarrhea, and, possibly, fever, headache, and rash.
•For patients with impaired renal function, expect to monitor renal function test results periodically during long-term therapy because drug may cause nephrotoxicity.
•Monitor patient's CBC with differential for eosinophilia, which may indicate an allergic reaction.

PATIENT TEACHING
•Instruct patient taking oral drug to swallow tablets or capsules whole and not to break outer coating.
•Teach patient how to administer rectal suspension or suppositories correctly. Emphasize shaking suspension bottle well before using.
•Advise patient to notify prescriber immediately about abdominal cramps or pain, bloody diarrhea, fever, headache, or rash.

mesoridazine besylate

Serentil

Class and Category

Chemical class: Alkylpiperidine phenothiazine derivative
Therapeutic class: Antipsychotic
Pregnancy category: Not rated

Indications and Dosages

➤ *To treat schizophrenia in patients who failed to respond to other antipsychotic drugs, either because those drugs were ineffective or because intolerable adverse effects prevented attainment of an effective dose*

ORAL SOLUTION, TABLETS
Adults and adolescents. 50 mg t.i.d., increased as needed and tolerated. *Maximum:* 400 mg daily.
I.M. INJECTION
Adults and adolescents. 25 mg, repeated in 30 to 60 min, as needed. *Maximum:* 200 mg/day.

Route	Onset	Peak	Duration
P.O., I.M.	Up to several wk	6 wk to 6 mo	4 to 8 hr

Mechanism of Action

Depresses brain areas that control activity and aggression—including the cerebral cortex, hypothalamus, and limbic system—by an unknown mechanism.

Contraindications

Blood dyscrasias; bone marrow depression; cerebral arteriosclerosis; coma; concurrent use of high doses of CNS depressants; concurrent use of other drugs that prolong the QTc interval, such as disopyramide, procainamide, and quinidine; congenital long-QT syndrome; coronary artery disease; hepatic dysfunction; history of arrhythmias; hypersensitivity to mesoridazine, other phenothiazines, or their components; myeloproliferative disorders; severe CNS depression; severe hypertension or hypotension; subcortical brain damage

Interactions
DRUGS

aluminum- or magnesium-containing antacids, antidiarrheals (adsorbent): Decreased mesoridazine absorption
amantadine, anticholinergics: Increased anticholinergic effects, and possibly decreased therapeutic effects of mesoridazine
aminoglycosides, ototoxic drugs: Masked symptoms of ototoxicity, such as dizziness, tinnitus, and vertigo
anticonvulsants: Possibly lowered seizure threshold
antithyroid drugs: Increased risk of agranulocytosis
appetite suppressants: Possibly antagonized anorectic effect
astemizole, cisapride, disopyramide, erythro-

mycin, pimozide, probucol, procainamide, quinidine: Increased risk of prolonged QT interval and life-threatening arrhythmias
beta blockers: Increased blood levels of both drugs, possibly resulting in additive hypotension, retinopathy, arrhythmias, and tardive dyskinesia
CNS depressants, general anesthetics: Increased CNS depression
dextroamphetamine: Possibly interference with action of either drug
levodopa: Possibly inhibited effects of levodopa
lithium: Possibly decreased absorption of mesoridazine
opioid analgesics: Possibly decreased mesoridazine effects; increased CNS and respiratory depression and orthostatic hypotension; increased risk of severe constipation
oral anticoagulants: Possibly decreased therapeutic effects of anticoagulants
sympathomimetics: Possibly decreased therapeutic effects of these drugs and increased risk of hypotension
thiazide diuretics: Possibly orthostatic hypotension, hyponatremia, and water intoxication
tricyclic antidepressants: Increased tricyclic antidepressant levels, inhibited mesoridazine metabolism, increased risk of neuroleptic malignant syndrome
ACTIVITIES
alcohol use: Increased CNS depression

Adverse Reactions
CNS: Ataxia, dizziness, drowsiness, extrapyramidal reactions (tardive dyskinesia, pseudoparkinsonism), fever, neuroleptic malignant syndrome, restlessness, seizures, slurred speech, syncope, tremor, weakness
CV: Hypotension, orthostatic hypotension, prolonged QTc interval, torsades de pointes
EENT: Blurred vision, dry mouth, hypertrophic papillae of tongue, increased salivation, photophobia
ENDO: Galactorrhea, gynecomastia
GI: Constipation, hepatotoxicity, nausea, vomiting
GU: Dysuria, ejaculation disorders, impotence, menstrual irregularities, priapism
HEME: Agranulocytosis, leukopenia, thrombocytopenia
SKIN: Contact dermatitis, decreased sweating, jaundice, photosensitivity, rash

Other: Injection site pain, weight gain

Nursing Considerations
• Before beginning mesoridazine therapy, expect to perform a 12-lead ECG to detect prolonged QTc interval. If patient's QTc interval is greater than 450 milliseconds (msec), expect to withhold drug because of the risk of life-threatening torsades de pointes.
• Wear gloves when working with liquid and parenteral forms of mesoridazine, and avoid contact with clothing or skin; drug may cause contact dermatitis.
• Discard injection solution if it's frankly discolored or contains precipitate; slightly yellow color is acceptable.
• Inject I.M. drug deep into upper outer quadrant of buttocks; massage area afterward to prevent sterile abscess.
• Implement continuous ECG monitoring, as ordered, to detect arrhythmias. Expect to discontinue mesoridazine if the QTc interval exceeds 500 msec.
• Monitor serum potassium level before and during therapy, and administer potassium supplements as prescribed.
• Assess patient for hypotension and orthostatic hypotension, especially during I.M. therapy. Notify prescriber if either develops.
• **WARNING** Monitor patient for evidence of neuroleptic malignant syndrome, a potentially fatal reaction to antipsychotic drugs, and notify prescriber if they develop. Early signs include altered mental status, fever, hypertension or hypotension, muscle rigidity, and tachycardia.
• Assess patient for signs of blood dyscrasias, including cellulitis, fever, and pharyngitis. If they develop, discontinue drug, as directed.
• Monitor patient for signs of tardive dyskinesia, even after treatment stops. Notify prescriber if they develop.
• Expect to taper drug dosage before discontinuation to avoid adverse reactions, such as dizziness, nausea, tremor, and vomiting.
PATIENT TEACHING
• Instruct patient to take mesoridazine exactly as prescribed and not to stop it abruptly.
• Inform patient that I.M. injection may be painful.
• Caution patient to avoid hazardous activities until drug's CNS effects are known.
• Advise patient to change position slowly to

M

minimize effects of orthostatic hypotension.
•Instruct patient to report fever, involuntary facial movements, sore throat, unusual bleeding or bruising, and yellowing of eyes or skin.
•Urge patient to avoid alcohol and prolonged sun exposure during therapy.
•If patient requires long-term therapy, explain the risk of tardive dyskinesia. Also advise him to have regular eye examinations.

metaproterenol sulfate

Alupent, Arm-a-Med Metaproterenol, Dey-Lute Metaproterenol

Class and Category

Chemical class: Sympathomimetic amine
Therapeutic class: Antiasthmatic, bronchodilator
Pregnancy category: C

Indications and Dosages

➤ *To treat bronchospasm*

SYRUP, TABLETS

Adults and children age 9 or over weighing more than 27 kg (59 lb). 20 mg every 6 to 8 hr.
Children ages 6 to 9 weighing 27 kg or less. 10 mg every 6 to 8 hr.

INHALATION AEROSOL

Adults and adolescents. 2 to 3 inhalations (1.3 to 1.95 mg) every 3 to 4 hr. *Maximum:* 12 inhalations daily.
Children ages 6 to 12. 1 to 3 inhalations (0.65 to 1.95 mg) every 3 to 4 hr. *Maximum:* 12 inhalations daily.

INHALATION NEBULIZER

Adults and adolescents. 0.2 to 0.3 ml of 5% solution diluted in 2.5 ml normal saline solution t.i.d. or q.i.d., p.r.n., but no more than every 4 hr.
Children ages 6 to 12. 0.1 to 0.2 ml of 5% solution diluted in normal saline solution to a total volume of 3 ml t.i.d. or q.i.d., p.r.n., but no more than every 4 hr.

Route	Onset	Peak	Duration
P.O.	15 min	1 hr	4 hr or longer
Inhalation (aerosol)	1 min	1 hr	4 hr or longer
Inhalation (nebulizer)	5 to 30 min	Unknown	4 hr or longer

Mechanism of Action

Attaches to beta$_2$ receptors on bronchial cell membranes. This stimulates the intracellular enzyme adenyl cyclase to convert adenosine triphosphate to cyclic adenosine monophosphate (cAMP). An increased intracellular level of cAMP relaxes bronchial smooth-muscle cells and inhibits histamine release.

Contraindications

Angina, cerebral arteriosclerosis, dilated heart failure, heart block from digitalis toxicity, hypersensitivity to metaproterenol or its components, labor, local anesthesia, organic brain damage, tachyarrhythmias

Interactions

DRUGS

beta blockers: Increased risk of bronchospasm
MAO inhibitors, tricyclic antidepressants: Possibly potentiated cardiovascular effects of metaproterenol
other sympathomimetics: Possibly additive effects of both drugs and risk of toxicity
theophylline: Increased risk of arrhythmias

Adverse Reactions

CNS: Dizziness, fatigue, headache, insomnia, malaise, nervousness, tremor
CV: ECG changes, hypertension, palpitations, tachycardia
EENT: Dry mouth, pharyngitis, taste perversion
GI: Diarrhea, nausea, vomiting
RESP: Asthma exacerbation, cough

Nursing Considerations

•Anticipate that a single dose of nebulized metaproterenol may not completely stop an acute asthma attack.
•Monitor for adverse reactions and signs of toxicity, especially if patient uses tablets and aerosol. Notify prescriber if they develop.
•Be aware that tolerance may occur with continued use.

PATIENT TEACHING

•Caution patient not to use metaproterenol inhaler or nebulizer more often than prescribed.
•Teach patient to use metaproterenol inhaler correctly, to hold breath during second half

of inhalation, and to wait 2 minutes between inhalations.

•Instruct parents to use spacer with their child's metered-dose inhaler.

•Advise patient to use metaproterenol 5 minutes before using corticosteroid inhaler, if prescribed, to maximize airway opening and drug effects.

•Instruct patient to notify prescriber immediately if diarrhea, increased shortness of breath, insomnia, or irregular heartbeat occurs.

•Instruct patient to notify prescriber if drug becomes less effective.

metaxalone

Skelaxin

Class and Category

Chemical class: Oxazolidinone derivative
Therapeutic class: Skeletal muscle relaxant
Pregnancy category: Not rated

Indications and Dosages

➤ *To relieve discomfort caused by acute, painful musculoskeletal conditions*

TABLETS

Adults and children over age 12. 800 mg t.i.d. or q.i.d.

Route	Onset	Peak	Duration
P.O.	Usually in 1 hr	Unknown	4 to 6 hr

Mechanism of Action

May depress the CNS, resulting in sedation, which in turn may reduce skeletal muscle spasms to provide pain relief. Metaxalone does not directly relax tense skeletal muscles.

Contraindications

Hypersensitivity to metaxalone or its components, significant renal or hepatic disease, tendency to develop drug-induced, hemolytic, or other anemias

Interactions

DRUGS

CNS depressants: Increased CNS depression

ACTIVITIES

alcohol use: Increased CNS depression

Adverse Reactions

CNS: Dizziness, drowsiness, excitement, general CNS depression, headache, insomnia, irritability, nervousness, restlessness
GI: Abdominal cramps or pain, GI upset, jaundice, hepatotoxicity, nausea, vomiting
HEME: Hemolytic anemia, leukopenia
SKIN: Pruritus, rash

Nursing Considerations

•Be aware that metaxalone may not be prescribed for women who are or may become pregnant unless the potential benefits outweigh the risks because drug's effect on fetus is unknown.

•Expect to avoid giving metaxalone with food because food may increase CNS depression, especially in elderly patients.

•Monitor patient for excessive drowsiness, which may lead to respiratory depression.

•Caution patient to consult prescriber before taking other drugs, such as sleeping pills, cold or allergy preparations, opioid analgesics, and antidepressants.

•Monitor liver function test results for elevations, especially in patients with preexisting hepatic disease.

•Monitor renal function test results, as prescribed, for signs of impaired renal function because drug is excreted by the kidneys.

•Provide rest and other pain-relief measures.

•Store drug at 15° to 30° C (59° to 86° F).

PATIENT TEACHING

•Advise patient to take metaxalone tablets exactly as prescribed and not to increase dosage or frequency.

•Instruct patient to take metaxalone tablets on an empty stomach.

•Caution patient to avoid hazardous activities, such as driving or operating machinery, until drug's CNS effects are known.

•Instruct patient to avoid alcohol and other CNS depressants during metaxalone therapy.

•Urge patient to notify prescriber if he notices a rash or itching, which may signify a hypersensitivity reaction, or if he develops signs of hepatotoxicity, such as tiredness, nausea, yellow skin, or flulike symptoms.

metformin hydrochloride

Fortamet, Gen-Metformin (CAN), Glucophage, Glucophage XR, Glumetza, Glycon (CAN), Novo-Metformin (CAN), Riomet

M

Class and Category
Chemical class: Dimethylbiguanide
Therapeutic class: Antidiabetic
Pregnancy category: B

Indications and Dosages
➤ *To reduce blood glucose level in type 2 diabetes mellitus*

ORAL SOLUTION, TABLETS

Adults and children age 10 and over. *Initial:* 500 mg b.i.d. or 850 mg daily. Dosage increased as prescribed by 500 mg/wk or by 850 mg every 2 wk until desired response occurs. Usual: 500 to 850 mg b.i.d. or t.i.d. *Maximum:* 2,550 mg daily (adults and adolescents age 17 and over); 2,000 mg daily (children ages 10 to 16).

DOSAGE ADJUSTMENT If patient takes insulin, initial dosage reduced to 500 mg daily and then increased as prescribed by 500 mg every wk until blood glucose level is controlled.

E.R. TABLETS (GLUCOPHAGE XR, GLUMETZA)

Adults and adolescents age 18 and over. *Initial:* 500 mg daily (Glucophage XR) or 1,000 mg daily (Glumetza) with evening meal. Increased as prescribed by 500 mg/wk. *Maximum:* 2,000 mg daily.

DOSAGE ADJUSTMENT If control isn't achieved with maximum once-daily E.R. dosage, regimen may be changed to 1,000 mg b.i.d. If control is not achieved after 4 wk of maximum dosage, an oral sulfonylurea may be prescribed.

E.R. TABLETS (FORTAMET)

Adults and adolescents age 17 and over. *Initial:* 500 to 1,000 mg once daily in evening. Increased in increments of 500 mg weekly, as needed. *Maximum:* 2,500 mg daily. If control isn't achieved after 4 wk at maximum dosage, an oral sulfonylurea may be prescribed.

➤ *As adjunct to insulin therapy in type 2 diabetes mellitus*

ORAL SOLUTION, TABLETS, E.R. TABLETS

Adults. *Initial:* 500 mg (Glucophage, Glucophage XR, Fortamet) or 1,000 mg (Glumetza) daily in addition to current dose of insulin. Increased by 500 mg/wk, as needed. *Maximum:* 2,000 mg for Glucophage XR and Glumetza; 2,500 mg for Glucophage and Fortamet.

DOSAGE ADJUSTMENT If patient's fasting blood glucose level drops below 120 mg/dl, insulin dosage decreased by 10% to 25%.

Subsequent insulin dosage decrease may be needed based upon patient's continued response.

Contraindications
Hypersensitivity to metformin or its components, impaired renal function, metabolic acidosis, use of iodinated contrast media within preceding 48 hours

Route	Onset	Peak	Duration
P.O. (tablets)	Unknown	Up to 2 wk	2 wk after drug discontinued

Mechanism of Action
May promote storage of excess glucose as glycogen in the liver, which reduces glucose production. Metformin also may improve glucose use by skeletal muscle and adipose tissue by increasing glucose transport across cell membranes. This drug also may increase the number of insulin receptors on cell membranes and make them more sensitive to insulin. In addition, metformin modestly decreases blood triglyceride and total cholesterol levels.

Interactions
DRUGS
calcium channel blockers, corticosteroids, estrogens, isoniazid, nicotinic acid, oral contraceptives, phenothiazines, phenytoin, sympathomimetics, thiazide and other diuretics, thyroid drugs: Possibly hyperglycemia
cationic drugs (such as amiloride, cimetidine, digoxin, morphine, procainamide, quinidine, quinine, ranitidine, triamterene, trimethoprim, vancomycin), nifedipine: Increased blood metformin level
clofibrate, MAO inhibitors, probenecid, propranolol, rifabutin, rifampin, salicylates, sulfonamides, sulfonylureas: Increased risk of hypoglycemia

FOODS
all foods: Possibly delayed metformin absorption

ACTIVITIES
alcohol use: Increased risk of hypoglycemia and lactate formation

Adverse Reactions

CNS: Headache
EENT: Metallic taste
ENDO: Hypoglycemia
GI: Abdominal distention, anorexia, constipation, diarrhea, flatulence, indigestion, nausea, vomiting
HEME: Aplastic anemia, megaloblastic anemia, thrombocytopenia
SKIN: Photosensitivity, rash
Other: Lactic acidosis, weight loss

Nursing Considerations

• Administer metformin tablets with food, which decreases and slightly delays absorption, thus reducing the risk of adverse GI reactions. Administer E.R. tablets with evening meal; don't break or crush them.
• Expect prescriber to alter dosage if patient has a condition that decreases or delays gastric emptying, such as diarrhea, gastroparesis, GI obstruction, ileus, or vomiting.
• Assess BUN and serum creatinine level, as appropriate, before and during long-term therapy in those at increased risk for lactic acidosis.
• Monitor patient's hepatic function, as ordered, because impaired hepatic function may significantly reduce the liver's ability to clear lactate, predisposing the patient to lactic acidosis.
• Monitor patient's blood glucose level to evaluate drug effectiveness. Assess for hyperglycemia and the need for insulin during times of increased stress, such as infection and surgery.
• Withhold drug, as ordered, if patient becomes dehydrated or develops hypoxemia or sepsis because these conditions increase the risk of lactic acidosis.
• Be aware that iodinated contrast media used in radiographic studies increase the risk of renal failure and lactic acidosis during metformin therapy. Expect to withhold metformin for 48 hours before and after testing.

PATIENT TEACHING
• Instruct patient to take metformin tablets with meals: at breakfast if taking drug once a day, or at breakfast and dinner if taking drug twice a day. Instruct him to take E.R. tablets once daily with evening meal and to swallow them whole without crushing or chewing them.
• Direct patient to take drug exactly as pre-

scribed and not to change the dosage or frequency unless instructed.
• Stress the importance of following prescribed diet, exercising regularly, controlling weight, and checking blood glucose level.
• Teach patient how to measure blood glucose level and recognize hyperglycemia and hypoglycemia. Urge him to notify prescriber of abnormal blood glucose level.
• Caution patient to avoid alcohol, which can increase the risk of hypoglycemia.
• Instruct patient to watch for early signs of lactic acidosis, including drowsiness, hyperventilation, malaise, and muscle pain, and notify prescriber if such signs develop.
• Advise patient to expect laboratory monitoring of glycosylated hemoglobin level every 3 months until blood glucose is controlled.

methadone hydrochloride

Dolophine, Methadose

Class, Category, and Schedule

Chemical class: Phenylheptylamine
Therapeutic class: Synthetic opiate agonist
Pregnancy category: C
Controlled substance schedule: II

Indications and Dosages

➤ *To manage opioid detoxification*

DISPERSIBLE TABLETS, ORAL CONCENTRATE, I.M. OR SUBCUTANEOUS INJECTION
Adults. *Initial:* 15 to 40 mg daily or as needed. *Usual:* Dosage individualized based on clinical response. *Maximum:* 120 mg daily.
Children. Dosage individualized based on age and size. *Maximum:* 120 mg daily.

➤ *To maintain opioid abstinence*

DISPERSIBLE TABLETS, ORAL CONCENTRATE
Adults. Dosage individualized based on clinical response. *Maximum:* 120 mg daily.
Children. Dosage individualized based on age and size. *Maximum:* 120 mg daily.

➤ *To treat severe or chronic pain*
ORAL CONCENTRATE, ORAL SOLUTION
Adults. 5 to 20 mg every 4 to 8 hr. Dosage increased or dosing interval decreased, as prescribed and as needed. *Maximum:* 120 mg/day.
Children. Dosage individualized based on age and size.

M

TABLETS, I.M. OR SUBCUTANEOUS INJECTION

Adults. 2.5 to 10 mg every 3 to 4 hr as needed. For chronic pain, dosage and dosing interval may be adjusted, as prescribed and as needed.

Children. Dosage individualized based on age and size.

DOSAGE ADJUSTMENT Elderly patients, debilitated patients, and patients with severe hepatic or renal dysfunction, hypothyroidism, Addison's disease, prostatic hyperplasia, or urethral stricture need individualized reduced dosages.

Route	Onset	Peak	Duration
P.O.	30 to 60 min	1.5 to 2 hr	4 to 6 hr
I.M.	10 to 20 min	1 to 2 hr	4 to 5 hr

Mechanism of Action

Binds with and activates opioid receptors (primarily mu receptors) in the spinal cord and in higher levels of the CNS to produce analgesia and euphoric effects.

Contraindications

Acute or postoperative pain, acute or severe asthma, chronic respiratory disease, diarrhea associated with pseudomembranous colitis or poisoning, hypersensitivity to methadone or its components, respiratory depression, severe inflammatory bowel disease

Interactions

DRUGS

ammonium chloride, ascorbic acid, potassium, sodium phosphate: May precipitate methadone withdrawal symptoms

amitriptyline, chloripramine, nortriptyline: Increased CNS and respiratory depression

anticholinergics: Possibly severe constipation leading to ileus; urine retention

antiemetics, general anesthetics, hypnotics, phenothiazines, sedatives, tranquilizers: Possibly coma, hypotension, respiratory depression, and severe sedation

antihistamines, choral hydrate, glutethimide, MAO inhibitors, methocarbamol: Increased CNS and respiratory depressant effects of methadone

antihypertensives, hypotension-producing drugs: Increased hypotension, risk of orthostatic hypotension

azole antifungals, macrolide antibiotics: Increased or prolonged opioid effect

buprenorphine: Decreased therapeutic effect of methadone, increased respiratory depression, possibly withdrawal symptoms

calcium channel blockers, class Ia and class III antiarrhythmics, diuretics, laxatives, mineralocorticoid hormones, neuroleptics, tricyclic antidepressants: Increased risk of electrolyte disturbances and prolonged QT interval

carbamazepine, phenobarbital, St. John's wort: Possibly precipitation of withdrawal symptoms

cimetidine: Increased analgesic and CNS and respiratory depressant effects of methadone

desipramine: Increased plasma desipramine level

didanosine, stavudine: Decreased plasma levels of these drugs

diuretics: Decreased diuresis

efavirenz, nevirapine, ritonavir, ritonavir and lopinavir: Decreased blood methadone level

hydroxyzine: Increased analgesic, CNS depressant, and hypotensive effects of methadone

loperamide, paregoric: Increased CNS depression, possibly severe constipation

MAO inhibitors: Possibly increased risk of severe adverse reactions

metoclopramide: Possibly antagonized metoclopramide effects on GI motility

mixed agonist-antagonist analgesics: Possibly withdrawal symptoms

naloxone: Antagonized analgesic and CNS and respiratory depressant effects of methadone, and possibly withdrawal symptoms

naltrexone: Possibly induction or worsening of withdrawal symptoms if methadone given within 7 days before naltrexone

neuromuscular blockers: Increased or prolonged respiratory depression

opioid analgesics (such as alfentanil and sufentanil): Increased CNS and respiratory depression, increased hypotension

phenytoin, rifampin: May precipitate withdrawal symptoms

selective serotonin reuptake inhibitors: Possibly increased blood methadone levels and increased risk of methadone toxicity

zidovudine: Increased blood zidovudine level and risk of toxicity

ACTIVITIES

alcohol use: Increased CNS and respiratory depression, possibly hypotension

Adverse Reactions

CNS: Agitation, amnesia, anxiety, asthenia, coma, confusion, decreased concentration, delirium, delusions, depression, dizziness, drowsiness, euphoria, fever, hallucinations, headache, insomnia, lethargy, light-headedness, malaise, psychosis, restlessness, sedation, seizures, syncope, tremor

CV: Bradycardia, cardiac arrest, cardiomyopathy, edema, heart failure, hypotension, orthostatic hypotension, palpitations, phlebitis, prolonged QT interval, shock, tachycardia, torsades de pointes, T-wave inversion on ECG, ventricular fibrillation or tachycardia

EENT: Blurred vision, diplopia, dry mouth, glossitis, laryngeal edema or laryngospasm (allergic), miosis, nystagmus, rhinitis

GI: Abdominal cramps or pain, anorexia, biliary tract spasm, constipation, diarrhea, dysphagia, elevated liver function test results, gastroesophageal reflux, hiccups, ileus and toxic megacolon (in patients with inflammatory bowel disease), indigestion, nausea, vomiting

GU: Amenorrhea, decreased ejaculate potency, decreased libido, difficult ejaculation, impotence, prolonged labor, urinary hesitancy, urine retention

HEME: Anemia, leukopenia, thrombocytopenia

MS: Arthralgia

RESP: Apnea, asthma exacerbation, atelectasis, bronchospasm, depressed cough reflex, hypoventilation, pulmonary edema, respiratory arrest and depression, wheezing

SKIN: Diaphoresis, flushing

Other: Allergic reaction; facial edema; hypokalemia; hypomagnesemia; injection site edema, pain, rash, or redness; physical and psychological dependence; weight gain; withdrawal symptoms

Nursing Considerations

•Before giving methadone, make sure opioid antagonist and equipment for administering oxygen and controlling respiration are nearby.

•Before therapy begins, assess patient's current drug use, including all prescription and OTC drugs.

•**WARNING** Give drug cautiously to patients at risk for a prolonged QT interval, such as those with cardiac hypertrophy, hypokalemia, or hypomagnesemia; those with a history of cardiac conduction abnormalities; and those taking diuretics or medications that affect cardiac conduction.

•Dilute oral concentrate with water or another liquid to a volume of at least 30 ml, but preferably to 90 ml or more, before administration. Dissolve dispersible tablets in water or another liquid before administration.

•Monitor patient for expected excessive drowsiness, unsteadiness, or confusion during first 3 to 5 days of therapy, and notify prescriber if effects continue to worsen or persist beyond this time.

•**WARNING** Monitor respiratory and circulatory status carefully and at frequent intervals during methadone therapy because respiratory depression, circulatory depression, respiratory arrest, shock, hypotension, and cardiac arrest are potential hazards of therapy. Monitor children frequently for respiratory depression and paradoxical CNS excitation because of their increased sensitivity to drug. Assess patient for excessive or persistent sedation; dosage may need to be adjusted.

•Monitor for drug tolerance, especially in patients with a history of chronic drug abuse, because methadone can cause physical and psychological dependence.

•Monitor patient for pain because maintenance dosage doesn't provide pain relief; patients who have developed a tolerance to opiate agonists, including those with chronic cancer pain, may require a higher dosage.

•Monitor patients who are pregnant or who have liver or renal impairment for increased adverse effects from methadone because drug may have a prolonged duration and cumulative effect in these patients. Methadone may prolong labor by reducing strength, duration, and frequency of uterine contractions, so expect dosage to be tapered before third trimester of pregnancy. Breast-feeding mothers on maintenance therapy put their infants at risk of withdrawal symptoms if they abruptly stop breast-feeding or discontinue methadone therapy. Methadone also accumulates in CNS tissue, increasing the risk of seizures in infants.

M

•Check plasma amylase and lipase levels in patients who develop biliary tract spasms because levels may increase up to 15 times normal. Notify prescriber immediately of any significant or sustained increase.

•Monitor patients who have head injuries or other conditions that may increase intracranial pressure (ICP) because methadone may further increase ICP.

•Assess patient for withdrawal symptoms and tolerance to therapy because physiologic dependence can occur with long-term methadone use. Avoid abrupt discontinuation because withdrawal symptoms will occur within 3 to 4 days after last dose.

•Monitor patients, especially the elderly, for cardiac arrhythmias, hypotension, hypovolemia, orthostatic hypotension, and vasovagal syncope because methadone may produce cholinergic effects in patients with cardiac disease, resulting in bradycardia and peripheral vasodilation; dosage decrease may be indicated.

•Monitor patients with prostatic hypertrophy, urethral stricture, or renal disease for urine retention and oliguria because methadone can increase tension of detrusor muscle.

•Be prepared to treat patient's symptoms of anxiety, and be aware that anxiety may be confused with symptoms of opioid abstinence and that methadone doesn't have antianxiety effects.

PATIENT TEACHING

•Instruct patient taking oral concentrate form of methadone to dilute it with water or another liquid to a volume of at least 30 ml and preferably to 90 ml or more before administration.

•Instruct patient to dissolve dispersible tablets in water or other liquid before administration.

•Advise patient to notify prescriber of all other drugs he's currently taking and to avoid alcohol and other depressants, such as sleeping pills and tranquilizers, because they may increase drug's CNS depressant effects.

•Instruct patient to take drug only as prescribed and not to change dosage without prescriber approval. Inform patient that abrupt cessation of methadone therapy can precipitate withdrawal symptoms. Urge him to notify prescriber if he develops any concerns over therapy.

•Urge patient to notify prescriber if he experiences palpitations, dizziness, light-headedness, or syncope, which may be caused by methadone-induced arrhythmias.

•Instruct patient to avoid potentially hazardous activities or those that require mental alertness because methadone therapy may cause drowsiness or sleepiness.

•Teach patient to change positions slowly to minimize the effects of orthostatic hypotension.

•Instruct patient to notify prescriber of worsening or breakthrough pain because dosage may need to be adjusted.

•Inform parents that a child on methadone maintenance therapy may become unusually excited or restless; advise them to notify prescriber of changes in child's behavior.

•Instruct female patient to notify prescriber immediately if she becomes pregnant during methadone therapy because drug may cause physical dependence in fetus and withdrawal symptoms in neonate.

•Caution patient who is breast-feeding not to stop doing so abruptly and not to stop taking methadone without prescriber's approval because infant may experience withdrawal symptoms.

methamphetamine hydrochloride

Desoxyn, Desoxyn Gradumet

Class, Category, and Schedule

Chemical class: Amphetamine
Therapeutic class: CNS stimulant
Pregnancy category: C
Controlled substance schedule: II

Indications and Dosages

➤ *To treat attention-deficit hyperactivity disorder (ADHD)*

E.R. TABLETS

Children age 6 and over. 20 to 25 mg daily.

TABLETS

Children age 6 and over. *Initial:* 5 mg once or twice daily. Increased by 5 mg every wk. *Maintenance:* 20 to 25 mg daily in divided doses b.i.d.

Route	Onset	Peak	Duration
P.O.	Unknown	Unknown	6 to 24 hr

Mechanism of Action

May produce CNS stimulation by facilitating norepinephrine's release and blocking its reuptake at adrenergic nerve terminals and by directly stimulating alpha and beta receptors in the peripheral nervous system. Methamphetamine also promotes dopamine release and blocks its reuptake in the brain's limbic regions. The drug appears to act mainly in the cerebral cortex and, possibly, the reticular activating system. These actions decrease motor restlessness, increase alertness, and diminish drowsiness and fatigue. The drug's peripheral actions include increased blood pressure and mild bronchodilation and respiratory stimulation.

Contraindications

Advanced arteriosclerosis; glaucoma; hypersensitivity to methamphetamine, sympathomimetic amines, or their components; hyperthyroidism; history of drug abuse; moderate to severe hypertension; severe agitation; symptomatic cardiovascular disease; use within 14 days of MAO inhibitor therapy

Interactions
DRUGS

ascorbic acid: Decreased methamphetamine absorption and therapeutic effect
beta blockers: Increased risk of heart block, hypotension, and severe bradycardia
CNS stimulants: Increased CNS stimulation and risk of adverse reactions
digoxin, levodopa: Increased risk of arrhythmias
diuretics, other antihypertensives: Possibly decreased antihypertensive effect
ethosuximide, phenobarbital, phenytoin: Possibly delayed absorption of these drugs
haloperidol, phenothiazines: Possibly interference with the effects of these drugs and with methamphetamine's CNS stimulant effects
inhalation anesthetics: Increased risk of ventricular arrhythmias
insulin: Altered insulin requirements
lithium: Possibly antagonized CNS stimulant effects of methamphetamine
MAO inhibitors: Possibly severe hypertension, risk of hypertensive crisis, increased vasopressor effect of methamphetamine

meperidine: Increased risk of hypotension and life-threatening interactions, such as severe respiratory depression and coma
metrizamide (intrathecal): Increased risk of seizures
thyroid hormones: Enhanced effects of both drugs
tricyclic antidepressants: Increased risk of arrhythmias and severe hypertension
urinary acidifiers: Increased metabolism and shortened pharmacologic effects of methamphetamine
urinary alkalinizers: Decreased metabolism and prolonged pharmacologic effects of methamphetamine

FOODS

caffeine: Increased methamphetamine effects

Adverse Reactions

CNS: Dizziness, euphoria, headache, hyperactivity, insomnia, irritability, mania, nervousness, psychotic episodes, restlessness, stroke, talkativeness, tremor
CV: Arrhythmias, chest pain, hypertension, hypotension, MI, palpitations, tachycardia
EENT: Accommodation abnormality, blurred vision, dry mouth, taste perversion
ENDO: Stunted growth
GI: Abdominal cramps, anorexia, constipation, diarrhea, nausea, vomiting
GU: Impotence, libido changes
SKIN: Diaphoresis, urticaria
Other: Physical and psychological dependence

Nursing Considerations

•Methamphetamine shouldn't be used in a patient (especially a child or an adolesccent) with a serious heart condition, such as a structural heart defect, cardiomyopathy, or a serious heart rhythm abnormality.
•Use methamphetamine cautiously in patients with a history of psychiatric problems or suicidal or homicidal tendencies.
•Assess for seizures in patients with a history of seizure disorders because drug may lower seizure threshold.
•Observe patient for evidence of drug tolerance and, possibly, extreme dependence, which may develop after a few weeks. Be aware that methamphetamine abuse may occur.
•Expect treatment for ADHD to include psychological, educational, and social measures in addition to drug therapy.

M

•Monitor child's growth pattern. If growth appears to be delayed, notify prescriber because methamphetamine therapy may need to be interrupted temporarily.

•Watch for signs of chronic methamphetamine intoxication, including hyperactivity, insomnia, irritability, and personality changes. Notify prescriber if such signs occur.

•Monitor patient for exertional chest pain, unexplained syncope, and other evidence that could suggest heart disease. If present, notify prescriber. A cardiac evaluation will be needed, and methamphetamine therapy may need to be stopped.

PATIENT TEACHING

•Instruct parent of patient to give methamphetamine at least 6 hours before bedtime to prevent insomnia.

•Explain the high risk of abuse with this drug. Instruct parent of patient not to increase dosage unless advised by prescriber and not to give drug to prevent fatigue.

•WARNING Advise patient to take methamphetamine exactly as prescribed because misuse may cause serious heart effects or even death.

•Caution parent that patient should not crush or chew E.R. tablets.

•Advise parent that patient should avoid caffeine, which increases drug's effects.

•Instruct parent of patient to report signs of overstimulation, such as diarrhea, hyperactivity, insomnia, and irritability.

methazolamide

MZM, Neptazane

Class and Category

Chemical class: Sulfonamide derivative
Therapeutic class: Antiglaucoma
Pregnancy category: C

Indications and Dosages

➤ *To treat open-angle glaucoma*

TABLETS

Adults. 50 to 100 mg b.i.d. or t.i.d.

Route	Onset	Peak	Duration
P.O.	2 to 4 hr	6 to 8 hr	10 to 18 hr

Contraindications

Cirrhosis; hyperchloremic acidosis; hypersensitivity to methazolamide, other carbonic anhydrase inhibitors, or their components; hypokalemia; hyponatremia; severe adrenocortical, hepatic, or renal impairment

Mechanism of Action

Inhibits the enzyme carbonic anhydrase, which normally appears in renal proximal tubule cells, choroid plexus of the brain, and ciliary processes of the eye. By inhibiting this enzyme in the eyes, methazolamide decreases aqueous humor secretion, which reduces intraocular pressure.

Interactions

DRUGS

amphetamines, anticholinergics, mecamylamine, procainamide, quinidine: Decreased renal clearance of these drugs, increased risk of toxicity

amphotericin B, corticosteroids: Increased risk of severe hypokalemia

barbiturates, carbamazepine, phenytoin, primidone: Increased risk of osteopenia

digoxin: Increased risk of hypokalemia and digitalis toxicity

ephedrine: Possibly prolonged duration of action of ephedrine

insulin, oral antidiabetic drugs: Increased risk of glycosuria and hyperglycemia

lithium: Increased lithium excretion

mannitol: Increased diuresis and further reduction of intraocular pressure

methenamine compounds: Decreased methenamine effectiveness

mexiletine: Possibly impaired renal excretion of mexiletine

neuromuscular blockers: Possibly prolonged duration of action of blockers from methazolamide-induced hypokalemia, increased risk of prolonged respiratory paralysis and depression

salicylates: Possibly CNS depression and metabolic acidosis, increased risk of methazolamide toxicity

Adverse Reactions

CNS: Confusion, depression, drowsiness, fatigue, fever, malaise, paresthesia, seizures, weakness

EENT: Hearing loss, myopia (transient), taste perversion, tinnitus

GI: Anorexia, diarrhea, nausea, vomiting
GU: Crystalluria, nephrotoxicity, renal calculi
SKIN: Photosensitivity, pruritus, rash, Stevens-Johnson syndrome, urticaria
Other: Metabolic acidosis

Nursing Considerations
•Use methazolamide cautiously in patients with obstructive pulmonary disease.
•Monitor fluid intake and output, weight, and serum electrolyte levels during methazolamide therapy.
PATIENT TEACHING
•Direct patient to take methazolamide exactly as prescribed because increasing dosage may lead to metabolic acidosis.
•Advise patient to take drug with food if GI distress occurs.
•Instruct patient to notify prescriber if rash develops.
•Caution patient to avoid hazardous activities until drug's CNS effects are known.
•Emphasize the importance of having regular eye examinations during methazolamide therapy.

methenamine hippurate
Hiprex, Urex

methenamine mandelate
Mandelamine

Class and Category
Chemical class: Formaldehyde precursor, hexamethylenetetramine
Therapeutic class: Antibiotic
Pregnancy category: C

Indications and Dosages
➤ *To prevent or suppress frequently recurring UTI caused by a wide variety of gram-negative and gram-positive bacteria (including enterococci,* Escherichia coli, Micrococcus pyogenes, *and staphylococci) in intermittently catheterized patients with neurogenic bladder*
ENTERIC-COATED TABLETS, ORAL SUSPENSION (METHENAMINE MANDELATE)
Adults and adolescents. 1 g q.i.d. before meals and at bedtime.
Children ages 6 to 12. 500 mg q.i.d., or 50 mg/kg daily in divided doses.
Children under age 6. 18.4 mg/kg q.i.d.

TABLETS (METHENAMINE HIPPURATE)
Adults and adolescents. 1 g b.i.d.
Children ages 6 to 12. 0.5 to 1 g every 12 hr.

Mechanism of Action
Hydrolyzes to formaldehyde and ammonia in an acidic environment, such as urine, producing greater amounts of formaldehyde as pH decreases. Formaldehyde has bactericidal action, possibly by denaturing proteins. To facilitate hydrolysis, methenamine is formulated with a weak organic acid, such as hippuric acid or mandelic acid.

Contraindications
Concurrent therapy with sulfonamides, hypersensitivity to methenamine, renal insufficiency, severe dehydration, severe hepatic disease

Interactions
DRUGS
bicarbonate-containing antacids, urinary alkalizers: Decreased methenamine effect
sulfonamides, such as sulfamethizole: Possibly formation of insoluble precipitate in urine
FOODS
milk, milk products, most fruits: Possibly decreased effectiveness of methenamine

Adverse Reactions
CNS: Headache
CV: Edema
EENT: Stomatitis
GI: Abdominal cramps, anorexia, diarrhea, nausea, vomiting
GU: Bladder irritation, crystalluria, dysuria, hematuria, proteinuria, urinary frequency
RESP: Pulmonary hypersensitivity (dyspnea, pneumonitis)
SKIN: Pruritus, rash, urticaria

Nursing Considerations
•Be aware that methenamine is used for prophylaxis; it isn't recommended as primary treatment for UTI.
•Be aware that drug shouldn't be given to patients whose creatinine clearance is less than 50 ml/min/1.73 m^2.
•Before giving first dose, obtain urine specimen for culture and sensitivity tests, as ordered, and to review test results if available.

M

•Plan to give methenamine mandelate around the clock to maintain a therapeutic blood level.

•Make sure patient receives adequate fluids.

•Expect to repeat culture and sensitivity tests if patient fails to improve.

PATIENT TEACHING

•Instruct patient to take methenamine with food to avoid GI distress.

•Direct patient to drink extra fluids; avoid alkaline foods, such as milk, milk products, and most fruits; and avoid antacids that contain sodium bicarbonate or carbonate during methenamine therapy.

•Instruct patient to report painful urination, rash, or severe GI distress.

•Urge patient to comply with order for urine testing before and during long-term therapy.

methicillin sodium

Staphcillin

Class and Category

Chemical: Penicillinase-resistant penicillin
Therapeutic: Antibiotic
Pregnancy category: B

Indications and Dosages

➤ *To treat general infections, such as sepsis, sinusitis, and skin and soft-tissue infections, caused by susceptible organisms (including penicillinase-producing and non–penicillinase-producing strains of* Staphylococcus epidermidis, Staphylococcus saprophyticus, *and* Streptococcus pneumoniae*)*

I.V. INFUSION, I.M. INJECTION

Adults and children weighing 40 kg (88 lb) or more. 1 g every 4 to 6 hr (I.M.) or 1 g every 6 hr (I.V.). *Maximum:* 24 g daily.

Children weighing less than 40 kg. 25 mg/kg every 6 hr.

DOSAGE ADJUSTMENT For adults and children with cystic fibrosis, dosage adjusted to 50 mg/kg every 6 hr.

➤ *To treat bacterial meningitis*

I.V. INFUSION, I.M. INJECTION

Neonates weighing 2 kg (4.4 lb) or more. 50 mg/kg every 8 hr for first wk after birth and then 50 mg/kg every 6 hr.

Neonates weighing less than 2 kg. 25 to 50 mg/kg every 12 hr for first wk after birth and then 50 mg/kg every 8 hr.

Mechanism of Action

Kills bacterial cells by inhibiting bacterial cell wall synthesis. In susceptible bacteria, the rigid, cross-linked cell wall is assembled in several steps. In the final stage of cross-linking, methicillin binds with and inactivates penicillin-binding proteins (enzymes responsible for linking cell wall strands), resulting in bacterial cell lysis and death. *Staphylococcus aureus* has developed resistance to methicillin by altering its penicillin-binding proteins.

Incompatibilities

Don't mix methicillin in same syringe or I.V. solution with other drugs. Don't mix methicillin with dextrose solutions because their low acidity may damage drug. Administer methicillin at least 1 hour before or after aminoglycosides and at different sites; otherwise, mutual inactivation can occur.

Contraindications

Hypersensitivity to methicillin sodium, other penicillins, or their components

Interactions

DRUGS

aminoglycosides: Substantial aminoglycoside inactivation

chloramphenicol, erythromycins, sulfonamides, tetracyclines: Possibly decreased therapeutic effects of methicillin

methotrexate: Increased risk of methotrexate toxicity

probenecid: Possibly decreased renal clearance, increased blood level, and increased risk of toxicity of methicillin

Adverse Reactions

CNS: Aggressiveness, agitation, anxiety, confusion, depression, headache, seizures

EENT: Oral candidiasis

GI: Abdominal pain, diarrhea, hepatotoxicity, nausea, pseudomembranous colitis, vomiting

GU: Interstitial nephritis, vaginitis

HEME: Leukopenia, neutropenia, thrombocytopenia

SKIN: Exfoliative dermatitis, pruritus, rash, urticaria

Other: Anaphylaxis; infusion site redness, swelling, and tenderness; injection site pain, redness, and swelling; serum sicknesslike reaction

Nursing Considerations
•**WARNING** Be aware that methicillin is not a first-line treatment for the indications above because of the prevalence of methicillin-resistant *Staphylococcus aureus.*
•Before giving first dose, obtain appropriate body fluid or tissue specimens for culture and sensitivity tests, as ordered, and review test results if available.
•Inject I.M. form deep into gluteal muscle.
•During I.V. use, observe infusion site closely for redness, swelling, and tenderness.
•Monitor fluid intake and output and renal function test results during therapy.
•Observe for signs of superinfection, such as diarrhea, vaginal itching, and white patches or sores in mouth or on tongue. Notify prescriber if they occur.
•Closely monitor renal function test results, including serum creatinine level; about one-third of patients experience interstitial nephritis after 10 days of methicillin therapy.
•Monitor patient's liver function test results, and watch for signs of hepatotoxicity, such as fever and nausea. Notify prescriber if they develop.

PATIENT TEACHING
•Explain that I.M. injection may be painful.
•Unless contraindicated, instruct patient to drink extra fluids during methicillin therapy.
•Advise patient to report diarrhea, injection site pain, mouth sores, or rash.

methimazole

Tapazole

Class and Category
Chemical class: Thioimidazole derivative
Therapeutic class: Antithyroid
Pregnancy category: D

Indications and Dosages
➤ *To treat mild hyperthyroidism*
TABLETS
Adults and adolescents. *Initial:* 15 mg daily as a single dose or in divided doses b.i.d. for 6 to 8 wk or until euthyroid level is reached. *Maintenance:* 5 to 30 mg daily as a single dose or in divided doses b.i.d.
Children. *Initial:* 0.4 mg/kg daily as a single dose or in divided doses b.i.d. *Maintenance:* 0.2 mg/kg daily as a single dose or in divided doses b.i.d.

➤ *To treat moderate hyperthyroidism*
TABLETS
Adults and adolescents. *Initial:* 30 to 40 mg/day as a single dose or in divided doses b.i.d. for 6 to 8 wk or until euthyroid level is reached. *Maintenance:* 5 to 30 mg daily as a single dose or in divided doses b.i.d.
Children. *Initial:* 0.4 mg/kg daily as a single dose or in divided doses b.i.d. *Maintenance:* 0.2 mg/kg daily as a single dose or in divided doses b.i.d.

➤ *To treat severe hyperthyroidism*
TABLETS
Adults and adolescents. *Initial:* 60 mg daily as a single dose or in divided doses b.i.d. for 6 to 8 wk or until euthyroid level is reached. *Maintenance:* 5 to 30 mg daily as a single dose or in divided doses b.i.d.
Children. *Initial:* 0.4 mg/kg daily as a single dose or in divided doses b.i.d. *Maintenance:* 0.2 mg/kg daily as a single dose or in divided doses b.i.d.

➤ *As adjunct to treat thyrotoxicosis*
SUPPOSITORIES
Adults and adolescents. 15 to 20 mg every 4 hr on first day and then adjusted based on patient response.
Children. 0.4 mg/kg daily as a single dose or in divided doses b.i.d.

Route	Onset	Peak	Duration
P.O.	5 days	7 wk	Unknown

Mechanism of Action
Directly interferes with thyroid hormone synthesis in the thyroid gland by inhibiting iodide incorporation into thyroglobulin. Iodination of thyroglobulin is an important step in synthesizing the thyroid hormones thyroxine and triiodothyronine. Eventually, thyroglobulin is depleted and the circulating thyroid hormone level drops.

Contraindications
Breast-feeding; hypersensitivity to methimazole, other antithyroid drugs, or their components

Interactions
DRUGS
amiodarone, iodine, potassium iodide: De-

creased response to methimazole
digoxin: Possibly increased blood digoxin
level
oral anticoagulants: Possibly a need for altered anticoagulant dosage

Adverse Reactions

CNS: Drowsiness, headache, paresthesia,
vertigo
CV: Edema
EENT: Loss of taste
ENDO: Hypothyroidism
GI: Diarrhea, indigestion, nausea, vomiting
HEME: Agranulocytosis, aplastic anemia,
leukopenia, thrombocytopenia
MS: Arthralgia, myalgia
SKIN: Alopecia, jaundice, pruritus, rash,
skin discoloration, urticaria
Other: Lupus-like symptoms, lymphadenopa-
thy

Nursing Considerations

•Closely monitor thyroid function test results during methimazole therapy.
•Check CBC results to detect abnormalities
caused by inhibition of myelopoiesis.
•Watch for signs of hypothyroidism, such as
cold intolerance, depression, and edema.
•Be aware that hyperthyroidism may increase metabolic clearance of beta blockers
and theophylline and that dosages of these
drugs may need to be reduced as the patient's thyroid condition becomes corrected.
PATIENT TEACHING
•Instruct patient to take drug with meals to
avoid adverse GI reactions.
•Explain about possible hair loss or thinning
during and for months after therapy.
•Instruct patient to notify prescriber immediately about cold intolerance, fever, sore
throat, tiredness, and unusual bleeding or
bruising.

methocarbamol

Carbacot, Robaxin, Robaxin 750, Skelex

Class and Category

Chemical class: Carbamate derivative of
guaifenesin
Therapeutic class: Skeletal muscle relaxant
Pregnancy category: C

Indications and Dosages

➤ *To relieve discomfort caused by acute,*
painful musculoskeletal conditions
TABLETS
Adults and adolescents. *Initial:* 1,500 mg
q.i.d. for 2 to 3 days; for severe discomfort,
8,000 mg daily. *Maintenance:* 750 mg every
4 hr, 1,000 mg q.i.d., or 1,500 mg t.i.d.
I.V. INJECTION (100 MG/ML)
Adults and adolescents. Up to 3,000 mg daily
administered at 8-hr intervals for 3 consecutive days. Regimen repeated as prescribed
after patient is drug-free for 48 hr.
I.M. INJECTION (100 MG/ML)
Adults and adolescents. 1,000 to 3,000 mg/
day administered at 8-hr intervals for 3 consecutive days. Regimen repeated as prescribed after patient is drug-free for 48 hr.
➤ *To provide supportive therapy for teta-*
nus
TABLETS
Adults and adolescents. 24,000 mg daily
given by NG tube.
I.V. INFUSION OR INJECTION (100 MG/ML)
Adults and adolescents. 1,000 to 3,000 mg by
infusion or 1,000 to 2,000 mg by direct injec-
tion every 6 hr. *Maximum:* 300 mg (3 ml)/min.
Children. 15 mg/kg every 6 hr.

Route	Onset	Peak	Duration
P.O.	30 min	Unknown	Unknown
I.V.	Immediate	Unknown	Unknown

Mechanism of Action

May depress the CNS, which leads to sedation and reduced skeletal muscle
spasms. Methocarbamol also alters the
perception of pain.

Contraindications

Hypersensitivity to methocarbamol or its
components, renal disease (injectable form)

Interactions

DRUGS
CNS depressants: Increased CNS depression
ACTIVITIES
alcohol use: Increased CNS depression

Adverse Reactions

CNS: Dizziness, drowsiness, fever, headache,
light-headedness, seizures (I.V.), syncope,
vertigo, weakness

CV: Bradycardia, hypotension, and thrombophlebitis (parenteral)
EENT: Blurred vision, conjunctivitis, diplopia, metallic taste, nasal congestion, nystagmus
GI: Nausea
GU: Black, brown, or green urine
SKIN: Flushing, pruritus, rash, urticaria
Other: Anaphylaxis (parenteral), angioedema, injection site irritation or pain (I.M.), injection site sloughing (I.V.)

Nursing Considerations
•If needed, crush methocarbamol tablets and mix with water for administration by NG tube.
•Administer I.V. form directly through infusion line at 3 ml/min. To prepare solution, add 10 ml to no more than 250 ml of D_5W or normal saline solution. Infuse at no more than 300 mg (3 ml)/ min to avoid hypotension and seizures.
•Keep patient recumbent during I.V. methocarbamol administration and for at least 15 minutes afterward. Then have him rise slowly.
•Monitor I.V. site regularly for signs of phlebitis.
•Inject I.M. form deep into large muscle, such as the gluteus. Give no more than 5 ml/dose every 8 hours. One dose is usually adequate.
•Don't give methocarbamol by subcutaneous route.
•Keep epinephrine, antihistamines, and corticosteroids available in case patient experiences anaphylactic reaction.
•Be aware that the parenteral dosage form shouldn't be used in patients with renal dysfunction because the polyethylene glycol 300 vehicle is nephrotoxic.

PATIENT TEACHING
•Tell patient to take drug exactly as prescribed.
•Advise patient to take drug with food or milk to avoid nausea.
•Inform patient that urine may turn green, black, or brown until mehtocarbamol is discontinued.
•Advise patient to avoid potentially hazardous activities until drug's CNS effects are known.
•Instruct patient to avoid alcohol and other CNS depressants during therapy.

methotrexate
(amethopterin)
Rheumatrex

methotrexate sodium
Folex, Folex PFS, Mexate, Mexate-AQ

Class and Category
Chemical class: Folic acid analogue
Therapeutic class: Antipsoriatic, antirheumatic
Pregnancy category: X

Indications and Dosages
➤ *To treat severe psoriasis unresponsive to other therapy*
TABLETS (METHOTREXATE)
Adults. 2.5 to 5 mg every 12 hr for 3 doses/ wk, increased as ordered by 2.5 mg/wk. *Maximum:* 20 mg/wk.
I.V. OR I.M. INJECTION (METHOTREXATE SODIUM)
Adults. 10 mg/wk. *Maximum:* 25 mg/wk.
➤ *To treat severe rheumatoid arthritis unresponsive to other therapy*
TABLETS (METHOTREXATE)
Adults. 2.5 to 5 mg every 12 hr for 3 doses/ wk, increased as ordered by 2.5 mg/wk. *Maximum:* 20 mg/wk.

Route	Onset	Peak	Duration
P.O., I.V., I.M.	3 to 6 wk	Unknown	Unknown

M

Mechanism of Action
May exert immunosuppressive effects by inhibiting replication and function of T and possibly B lymphocytes. Methotrexate also slows rapidly growing cells, such as epithelial skin cells in psoriasis. This action may result from the drug's inhibition of dihydrofolate reductase, the enzyme that reduces folic acid to tetrahydrofolic acid. Inhibition of tetrahydrofolic acid interferes with DNA synthesis and cell reproduction in rapidly proliferating cells.

Contraindications
Breast-feeding, hypersensitivity to methotrexate or its components, pregnancy

Interactions
DRUGS
bone marrow depressants: Possibly increased bone marrow depression
co-trimoxazole: Possibly increased bone marrow suppression
folic acid: Possibly decreased effectiveness of methotrexate
hepatotoxic drugs: Increased risk of hepatotoxicity
chloramphenicol, neomycin, tetracycline: Possibly decreased absorption of methotrexate
NSAIDs, penicillins, phenylbutazone, phenytoin, probenecid, salicylates, sulfonamides: Increased risk of methotrexate toxicity
oral anticoagulants: Increased risk of bleeding
sulfonamides: Increased risk of hepatotoxicity
theophylline: Possibly increased risk of theophylline toxicity
vaccines: Risk of disseminated infection with live-virus vaccines, risk of suppressed response to killed-virus vaccines
ACTIVITIES
alcohol use: Increased risk of hepatotoxicity

Adverse Reactions
CNS: Aphasia, cerebral thrombosis, chills, dizziness, drowsiness, fatigue, fever, headache, hemiparesis, leukoencephalopathy, malaise, paresis, seizures
CV: Chest pain, deep vein thrombosis, hypotension, pericardial effusion, pericarditis, thromboembolism
ENDO: Gynecomastia
EENT: Blurred vision, conjunctivitis, gingivitis, glossitis, pharyngitis, stomatitis, transient blindness, tinnitus
GI: Abdominal pain, anorexia, cirrhosis, diarrhea, elevated liver function test results, enteritis, GI bleeding and ulceration, hepatitis, hepatotoxicity, nausea, pancreatitis, vomiting
GU: Cystitis, hematuria, infertility, menstrual dysfunction, nephropathy, renal failure, tubular necrosis, vaginal discharge
HEME: Anemia, aplastic anemia, leukopenia, neutropenia, pancytopenia, thrombocytopenia
MS: Arthralgia, dysarthia, myalgia, stress fracture
RESP: Dry nonproductive cough, dyspnea, interstitial pneumonitis, pneumonia, pulmonary fibrosis or failure, pulmonary infiltrates

SKIN: Acne, alopecia, altered skin pigmentation, ecchymosis, erythema multiforme, exfoliative dermatitis, furunculosis, necrosis, photosensitivity, pruritus, psoriatic lesions, rash, Stevens-Johnson syndrome, telangiectasia, toxic epidermal necrolysis, ulceration, urticaria
Other: Anaphylaxis, increased risk of infection, lymphadenopathy, lymphoproliferative disease

Nursing Considerations
•Follow facility policy for preparing and handling drug; parenteral form poses a risk of carcinogenicity, mutagenicity, and teratogenicity. Avoid skin contact.
•Monitor results of CBC, chest X-ray, liver and renal function tests, and urinalysis before and during treatment.
•Unless contraindicated, increase patient's fluid intake to 2 to 3 L daily to reduce the risk of adverse GU reactions.
•Assess patient for signs of bleeding and infection.
•**WARNING** Expect renal impairment to severely alter drug elimination.
•Be aware that high doses of methotrexate can impair renal elimination by forming crystals that obstruct the flow of urine. To prevent drug precipitation, alkalinize patient's urine with sodium bicarbonate tablets, as ordered.
•Follow standard precautions because drug can cause immunosuppression.
•If patient becomes dehydrated from vomiting, notify prescriber and expect to withhold drug until patient recovers.
•If patient receives high doses of drug, keep leucovorin readily available to use as antidote.
•Be aware that methotrexate resistance may develop with prolonged use.
PATIENT TEACHING
•Prepare a calendar of treatment days for patient, and stress the importance of following instructions exactly.
•Instruct patient to avoid alcohol during methotrexate therapy.
•Encourage frequent mouth care to reduce the risk of mouth sores.
•Instruct patient to use sunblock when exposed to sunlight.
•Advise patient to notify prescriber about bruising, chills, cough, fever, dark or bloody

urine, mouth sores, shortness of breath, sore throat, and yellow skin or eyes.
•Urge women of childbearing age to use reliable contraception during methotrexate therapy.

methoxypolyethylene glycol-epoetin beta

Mircera

Class and Category
Chemical class: Continuous erythropoietin receptor activator
Therapeutic class: Antianemic
Pregnancy category: C

Indications and Dosages
➤ *To treat anemia associated with chronic renal failure in dialysis-dependent and dialysis-independent patients*

I.V. INJECTION, SUBCUTANEOUS INJECTION
Adults not currently being treated with an erythropoiesis-stimulating agent. *Initial:* 0.6 mcg/kg every 2 wk with dosage increased or decreased by 25% monthly as needed. *Maintenance:* 1.2 mcg/kg every 4 wk.
Adults stabilized on less than 8,000 units/wk of epoetin alfa or 40 mcg/wk of darbepoetin alfa. 60 mcg every 2 wk or 120 mcg every 4 wk.
Adults stabilized on 8,000 to 16,000 units/wk of epoetin alfa or 40 to 80 mcg/wk of darbepoetin alfa. 100 mcg every 2 wk or 200 mcg every 4 wk.
Adults stabilized on more than 16,000 units/wk of epoetin alfa or more than 80 mcg/wk of darbepoetin alfa. 180 mcg every 2 wk or 360 mcg every 4 wk.
DOSAGE ADJUSTMENT If hemoglobin increase is greater than 1 g/dl during any 2-wk period or hemoglobin is increasing and approaching 12 g/dl, dosage reduced by 25%. If hemoglobin continues to increase despite this reduction, drug discontinued until hemoglobin begins to decrease; then drug restarted at a dose 25% less than previously given. If hemoglobin doesn't increase by 1 g/dl after 4 wk of therapy, dosage increased by 25%.

Route	Onset	Peak	Duration
I.V., SubQ	7 to 15 days	72 hr	4 wk

Mechanism of Action
Stimulates release of reticulocytes from bone marrow into the bloodstream, where they develop into mature RBCs.

Incompatiblities
Don't mix methoxypolyethylene glycol-epoetin beta with any other drug.

Contraindications
Hemoglobin greater than 12 g/dl, hypersensitivity to methoxypolyethylene glycol-epoetin beta or its components, red cell aplasia, uncontrolled hypertension

Adverse Reactions
CNS: Headache, seizures, stroke
CV: Chest pain, congestive heart failure, deep vein thrombosis, hypertension, hypotension, MI, tachycardia, vascular access thrombosis
EENT: Nasopharyngitis
GI: Constipation, diarrhea, GI bleeding, vomiting
GU: UTI
HEME: Pure red cell aplasia, severe anemia
MS: Back or limb pain, muscle spasms
RESP: Cough, upper respiratory tract infection
SKIN: Erythema, pruritus, rash
Other: Anaphylaxis, antibody formation to drug

Nursing Considerations
•Use drug cautiously in patients who have conditions that could decrease or delay response to drug, such as aluminum intoxication, folic acid deficiency, hemolysis, infection, inflammation, iron deficiency, malignant neoplasm, osteitis (birrosa cystica), or vitamin B_{12} deficiency.
•Also use drug cautiously in patients with a cardiovascular disorder caused by hypertension, a history of seizures, vascular disease, or a hematologic disorder, such as hypercoagulation, myelodysplastic syndrome or sickle cell disease.
•Be aware that if the patient's blood pressure is difficult to control even with drug therapy or dietary measures, dose of methoxypolyethylene glycol-epoetin beta should be reduced or the drug withheld until blood pressure is controlled.

M

•Don't shake vial during preparation to avoid denaturing glycoprotein, inactivating drug. Protect vials and prefilled syringes from light by storing in the original cartons.
•Discard unused portion of single-dose vial because it contains no preservatives.
•**WARNING** Target hemoglobin shouldn't exceed 12 g/dl because it increases risk of life-threatening adverse cardiovascular effects.
•Monitor drug effectiveness by checking hemoglobin every 2 weeks until it has stabilized between 10 and 12 g/dl and maintenance dose has been established. Then expect hemoglobin to be monitored at least monthly unless dosage adjustment is needed.
•Expect to give an iron supplement because iron requirements rise when erythropoiesis consumes existing iron stores.
•Notify prescriber if patient has sudden loss of response to drug, evidenced by severe anemia and a low reticulocyte count. Anti-erythropoietin antibody-related anemia may be present, which requires that drug and any other erythropoietic proteins be stopped.
•Take seizure precautions, especially during the first couple months of therapy.
•Risk of hypertensive or thrombotic complications increases if hemoglobin rises more than 1 g/dl over 2 weeks.
PATIENT TEACHING
•Teach patient how to administer drug and how to dispose of needles properly. Caution against reusing needles.
•Stress importance of complying with dosage regimen and keeping follow-up medical and laboratory appointments.
•Review possible adverse reactions, and urge patient to notify prescriber about chest pain, headache, hives, rapid heartbeat, rash, seizures, shortness of breath, or swelling.
•Advise patient that the risk of seizures is highest during the first couple of months of methoxypolyethylene glycol-epoetin beta therapy. Urge him to avoid hazardous activities during this time.
•Encourage patient to eat iron-rich foods.

methscopolamine bromide

Pamine, Pamine Forte

Class and Category
Chemical class: Quaternary ammonium de-

rivative of scopolamine
Therapeutic class: Anticholingeric
Pregnancy category: C

Indications and Dosages
➤ *As adjunct to treat peptic ulcer*
TABLETS
Adults. For mild to moderate symptoms, 2.5 mg 30 min before meals and 2.5 to 5 mg at bedtime; for severe symptoms, 5 mg 30 min. before meals and at bedtime.

Route	Onset	Peak	Duration
P.O.	1 hr	Unknown	4 to 6 hr

Mechanism of Action
Reduces volume and total acid content of gastric secretions, which may have a beneficial effect in treating peptic ulcer. Drug also reduces GI motility and inhibits salivation, which may produce additional beneficial effects.

Contraindications
Glaucoma, hypersensitivity to methscopolamine bromide or its components, intestinal atony (elderly or debilitated patients), myasthenia gravis, obstructive disease of GI or GU tract, paralytic ileus, severe ulcerative colitis, toxic megacolon complicating ulcerative colitis, unstable cardiovascular status in acute hemorrhage

Interactions
DRUGS
antacids: Possibly decreased methscopolamine absorption
anticholinergics, antipsychotics, tricyclic antidepressants: Possibly increased anticholinergic effects

Adverse Reactions
CNS: Confusion, dizziness, drowsiness, headache, insomnia, nervousness, weakness
CV: Palpitations, tachycardia
EENT: Blurred vision, cycloplegia, dry mouth, increased intraocular pressure, loss of taste, pupil dilation
ENDO: Suppression of lactation
GI: Bloating, constipation, nausea, vomiting
GU: Impotence, urinary hesitancy, urine retention
SKIN: Decreased sweating, urticaria
Other: Anaphylaxis

Nursing Considerations
•Use with caution in elderly patients and in patients with autonomic neuropathy, congestive heart failure, coronary artery disease, hepatic or renal disease, hypertension, hyperthyroidism, prostatic hypertrophy, tachycardia, or ulcerative colitis.
•Notify prescriber if diarrhea occurs because it may be an early sign of incomplete intestinal obstruction.

PATIENT TEACHING
•Advise patient to avoid excessive exposure to heat to reduce the risk of heat prostration and heatstroke because methscopolamine decreases sweating.
•Caution patient to avoid antacids because they may interfere with drug's absorption.
•Advise patient to avoid hazardous activities until drug's CNS effects are known.

methsuximide

Celontin

Class and Category
Chemical class: Succinimide derivative
Therapeutic class: Anticonvulsant
Pregnancy category: Not rated

Indications and Dosages
➤ *To treat absence seizures unresponsive to other drugs*

CAPSULES
Adults and children. *Initial:* 300 mg daily. Increased by 150 to 300 mg daily every 1 to 2 wk until control is achieved with minimal adverse reactions. *Maximum:* 1.2 g daily in divided doses.

Mechanism of Action
Elevates seizure threshold and reduces frequency of seizures by depressing the motor cortex and elevating the threshold of CNS response to convulsive stimuli. Methsuximide is metabolized to the active metabolite *N*-demethylmethsuximide, which may add to the anticonvulsant effects of the drug.

Contraindications
Hypersensitivity to methsuximide, succinimides, or their components

Interactions
DRUGS
carbamazepine, phenobarbital, phenytoin, primidone: Possibly decreased blood methsuximide level
CNS depressants: Possibly increased CNS depression
haloperidol: Altered seizure pattern; possibly decreased blood haloperidol level
loxapine, MAO inhibitors, maprotiline, molindone, phenothiazines, pimozide, thioxanthenes, tricyclic antidepressants: Possibly lowered seizure threshold and reduced therapeutic effect of methsuximide

ACTIVITIES
alcohol use: Possibly increased CNS depression

Adverse Reactions
CNS: Aggressiveness, ataxia, decreased concentration, dizziness, drowsiness, fatigue, fever, headache, insomnia, irritability, mental depression, nightmares, seizures
EENT: Periorbital edema, pharyngitis
GI: Abdominal and epigastric pain, abdominal cramps, abnormal liver function test results, anorexia, diarrhea, hiccups, nausea, vomiting
GU: Microscopic hematuria, proteinuria
HEME: Agranulocytosis, aplastic anemia, eosinophilia, leukopenia, pancytopenia
MS: Muscle pain
SKIN: Erythematous and pruritic rash, Stevens-Johnson syndrome, systemic lupus erythematosus, urticaria
Other: Lymphadenopathy

Nursing Considerations
•Monitor CBC and platelet count and assess patient for signs of infection, such as cough, fever, and pharyngitis, because methsuximide may cause blood dyscrasias.
•Monitor liver function test results and urinalysis results in patients with a history of hepatic or renal disease; methsuximide may cause functional changes in the liver and kidneys.
•When giving drug to patient with a history of mixed-type epilepsy, institute seizure precautions because drug may increase risk of generalized tonic-clonic seizures.
•Expect the dosage to be carefully and slowly adjusted according to patient's response and needs and withdrawn slowly to avoid precipitating seizures.

• Plan to use the 150-mg capsule when making dosage adjustments for small children.
• Notify prescriber if patient develops depression or aggressiveness.

PATIENT TEACHING

• Advise patient to take a missed dose as soon as he remembers unless it's nearly time for the next dose. Warn him not to double the dose.
• Instruct patient to take the drug with milk or food to reduce gastric irritation.
• Advise patient to notify prescriber if he develops cough, fever, or pharyngitis.
• Urge patient to avoid alcohol because of the increased risk of CNS depression.
• Instruct patient to avoid hazardous activities until drug's adverse effects are known.
• Caution patient not to stop taking drug abruptly to avoid the risk of absence seizures.

methyldopa

Aldomet, Apo-Methyldopa (CAN), Dopamet (CAN), Nu-Medopa (CAN)

methyldopate hydrochloride

Aldomet

Class and Category

Chemical class: 3,4-dihydroxyphenylalanine (DOPA) analogue
Therapeutic class: Antihypertensive
Pregnancy category: B (oral form), C (parenteral form)

Indications and Dosages

➤ *To manage hypertension, to treat hypertensive crisis*

ORAL SUSPENSION, TABLETS (METHYLDOPA)

Adults. *Initial:* 250 mg b.i.d. or t.i.d. for first 48 hr, increased as ordered after 2 days. *Maintenance:* 500 to 2,000 mg daily in divided doses b.i.d. to q.i.d. *Maximum:* 3,000 mg daily.
Children. *Initial:* 10 mg/kg daily in divided doses b.i.d. to q.i.d. for first 48 hr, increased as ordered after 2 days. *Maximum:* 65 mg/kg or 3,000 mg daily.

I.V. INFUSION (METHYLDOPATE HYDROCHLORIDE)

Adults. 250 to 500 mg diluted in D₅W and infused over 30 to 60 min every 6 hr. *Maximum:* 1,000 mg every 6 hr.

Children. 20 to 40 mg/kg infused over 30 to 60 min every 6 hr. *Maximum:* 65 mg/kg or 3,000 mg daily.

Route	Onset	Peak	Duration
P.O.	Unknown	4 to 6 hr*	12 to 24 hr†
I.V.	Unknown	4 to 6 hr	10 to 16 hr

Mechanism of Action

Is decarboxylated in the body to produce alpha-methylnorepinephrine, a metabolite that stimulates central inhibitory alpha-adrenergic receptors. This action may reduce blood pressure by decreasing sympathetic stimulation of the heart and peripheral vascular system.

Incompatibilities

Don't administer methyldopa through same I.V. line as barbiturates or sulfonamides.

Contraindications

Active hepatic disease, hypersensitivity to methyldopa or its components, impaired hepatic function from previous methyldopa therapy, use within 14 days of MAO inhibitor therapy

Interactions

DRUGS

antihypertensives: Increased hypotension
appetite suppressants, NSAIDs, tricyclic antidepressants: Possibly decreased therapeutic effects of methyldopa
central anesthetics: Possibly need for reduced anesthetic dosage
CNS depressants: Possibly increased CNS depression
haloperidol: Increased risk of adverse CNS effects
levodopa: Possibly decreased therapeutic effects of levodopa and increased risk of adverse CNS effects
lithium: Increased risk of lithium toxicity
MAO inhibitors: Possibly hallucinations, headaches, hyperexcitability, and severe hypertension
oral anticoagulants: Possibly increased therapeutic effects of anticoagulants
sympathomimetics: Possibly decreased thera-

---

* For single dose; 2 to 3 days for multiple doses.
† For single dose; 24 to 48 hr for multiple doses.

peutic effects of methyldopa and increased vasopressor effects of sympathomimetics
ACTIVITIES
alcohol use: Possibly increased CNS depression

Adverse Reactions
CNS: Decreased concentration, depression, dizziness, drowsiness, fever, headache, involuntary motor activity, memory loss (transient), nightmares, paresthesia, parkinsonism, sedation, vertigo, weakness
CV: Angina, bradycardia, edema, heart failure, myocarditis, orthostatic hypotension
EENT: Black or sore tongue, dry mouth, nasal congestion
ENDO: Gynecomastia
GI: Constipation, diarrhea, flatulence, hepatic necrosis, hepatitis, nausea, pancreatitis, vomiting
GU: Decreased libido, impotence
HEME: Agranulocytosis, hemolytic anemia, leukopenia, positive Coombs' test, positive tests for ANA and rheumatoid factor, thrombocytopenia
SKIN: Eczema, rash, urticaria
Other: Weight gain

Nursing Considerations
• For I.V. infusion, add methyldopate to 100 ml of D$_5$W and administer over 30 to 60 minutes.
• Expect to monitor CBC and differential results before and periodically during methyldopa therapy.
• Monitor blood pressure regularly during therapy.
• Monitor results of Coombs' test; a positive result after several months of treatment indicates that patient has hemolytic anemia. Expect prescriber to discontinue drug.
• Assess for weight gain and edema. If they develop, administer a diuretic, as prescribed.
• Notify prescriber if patient experiences signs of heart failure (dyspnea, edema, hypertension) or involuntary, rapid, jerky movements.
• Be aware that hypertension may return within 48 hours after stopping drug.
PATIENT TEACHING
• Instruct patient to take methyldopa exactly as prescribed and not to skip a dose. Explain that hypertension can return within 48 hours after stopping drug.

• Suggest that patient take drug at bedtime to minimize daytime drowsiness.
• Instruct patient to weigh himself daily and to report a gain of more than 5 lb (2.3 kg) in 2 days.
• Advise patient to change position slowly to minimize effects of orthostatic hypotension.
• Direct patient to notify prescriber about bruising, chest pain, fever, involuntary jerky movements, prolonged dizziness, rash, and yellow eyes or skin.
• Caution patient not to discontinue drug abruptly; doing so may precipitate withdrawal symptoms, such as headache, hypertension, increased sweating, nausea, and tremor.

methylnaltrexone bromide

Relistor

Class and Category
Chemical class: Noroxymorphone methobromide
Therapeutic class: Peripheral mu-opioid receptor antagonist
Pregnancy category: B

Indications and Dosages
➤ *To treat opioid-induced constipation in patients receiving palliative care and not responsive to laxative therapy.*
SUBCUTANEOUS INJECTION
Adults weighing more than 114 kg (251 lb): 0.15 mg/kg every other day as needed. *Maximum:* 0.15 mg/kg daily.
Adults weighing 62 to 114 kg (136 to 251 lb): 12 mg every other day as needed. *Maximum:* 12 mg daily.
Adults weighing 38 to less than 62 kg (84 to less than 136 lb): 8 mg every other day as needed. *Maximum:* 8 mg daily.
Adults weighing less than 38 kg: 0.15 mg/kg every other day as needed. *Maximum:* 0.15 mg/kg daily.
DOSAGE ADJUSTMENT For patients with severe renal failure (creatinine clearance less than 30 ml/min/1.73 m^2), dosage reduced by half.

Route	Onset	Peak	Duration
SubQ	Unknown	0.5 hr	Unknown

Mechanism of Action

Binds to peripherally acting mu-opioid receptors in the GI tract, preventing opioid- induced slowing of GI transit time and motility. When transit time and motility is restored to normal, constipation is relieved.

Contraindications

Hypersensitivity to methylnaltrexone bromide or its components, I.V. administration, mechanical GI obstruction

Adverse Reactions

CNS: Dizziness
GI: Abdominal pain, diarrhea, flatulence, nausea

Nursing Considerations

•To determine volume of drug to give patients who weigh more than 114 kg (251 lb) or less than 38 kg (84 lb), multiply patient's weight in pounds by 0.0034 and round up the volume to the nearest 0.1 ml. Or. multiply patient's weight in kilograms by 0.0075 and round up the volume to the nearest 0.1 ml. For patients who weigh 62 to 114 kg (136 to 251 lb), injection volume administered should be 0.6 ml. For patients who weigh 38 to less than 62 kg (84 to less than 136 lb), injection volume administered should be 0.4 ml.
•Inspect vial before giving drug to make sure solution is clear and colorless to pale yellow.
•Give drug only as subcutaneous injection into patient's upper arm, abdomen, or thigh and no more than once in 24 hours. Make sure to rotate injection sites.
•Once drug is drawn into syringe, it should be given immediately. However, if needed, it may be stored at room temperature for up to 24 hours.
•Notify prescriber about severe or persistent diarrhea, and expect drug to be discontinued.

PATIENT TEACHING
•Teach patient or caregiver how to prepare and administer methylnaltrexone subcutaneously. Stress importance of rotating injection sites.
•Inform patient that a bowel movement may occur within 30 minutes after drug has been administered.

•Advise patient that if severe or persistent diarrhea occurs, prescriber should be notified and drug discontinued.
•Reassure patient that drug is not a controlled substance.
•Tell patient to stop taking methylnaltrexone if she stops taking opioid pain medication.

methylphenidate hydrochloride

Concerta, Daytrana Ritalin LA, Metadate, Metadate CD, Metadate ER, Methylin, Methylin ER, PMS-Methylphenidate (CAN), Riphenidate (CAN), Ritalin, Ritalin-LA, Ritalin SR (CAN), Ritalin-SR

Class, Category, and Schedule

Chemical class: Piperidine derivative
Therapeutic class: CNS stimulant
Pregnancy category: C
Controlled substance schedule: II

Indications and Dosages

➤ *To treat attention-deficit hyperactivity disorder (ADHD)*
CAPSULES, E.R. TABLETS, ORAL SOLUTION, S.R. TABLETS, TABLETS
Adults and adolescents. 5 to 20 mg b.i.d. or t.i.d. *Maximum:* 90 mg daily.
Children ages 6 to 12. 5 mg b.i.d. before breakfast and lunch; increased by 5 to 10 mg daily at 1-wk intervals. *Maximum:* 60 mg daily.
E.R. ONCE-DAILY TABLETS (CONCERTA)
Adults and adolescents. 18 mg daily; increased in 18-mg increments at 1-wk intervals. *Maximum:* 72 mg daily, not to exceed 2 mg/kg daily.
Children ages 6 to 12. 18 mg daily. *Maximum:* 54 mg daily.
E.R. ONCE-DAILY CAPSULES (METADATE CD)
Children age 6 and over. 20 mg daily. Dosage titrated to 40 or 60 mg daily based on individual response. *Maximum:* 60 mg daily.
DOSAGE ADJUSTMENT Dosage reduced or drug stopped if no improvement in 1 mo. When maintenance dosage is achieved with tablets, may be switched to E.R. or S.R. tablets.
TRANSDERMAL PATCH
Children ages 6 to 12. *Initial:* 10-mg (12.5-cm^2) patch worn 9 hr daily; after 1 wk, increased to 15-mg (18.75-cm^2) patch worn 9 hr daily; after 1 more wk, increased to

20-mg (25-cm^2) patch worn 9 hr daily; after 1 more wk, increased to 30-mg (37.5-cm^2) patch worn 9 hr daily. *Maximum:* 30-mg (37.5-cm^2) patch worn 9 hr daily.

➤ *To treat narcolepsy*
ORAL SOLUTION, TABLETS
Adults and adolescents. 5 to 20 mg b.i.d. or t.i.d. *Maximum:* 90 mg daily.

Route	Onset	Peak	Duration
P.O. (tablets)	Unknown	Unknown	3 to 6 hr
P.O. (E.R., S.R.)	Unknown	Unknown	About 8 hr
P.O. (E.R. once-daily)	Unknown	Unknown	About 12 hr

Mechanism of Action

Blocks the reuptake mechanism of dopaminergic neurons in the cerebral cortex and subcortical structures of the brain, including the thalamus, decreasing motor restlessness and improving concentration.

Methylphenidate also may trigger sympathomimetic activity. This action produces increased motor activity, alertness, mild euphoria, and decreased fatigue in patients with narcolepsy.

Contraindications

Angina pectoris, anxiety, cardiac arrhythmias, depression, fructose intolerance, glaucoma, glucose-galactose malabsorption, heart failure, hypersensitivity to methylphenidate or its components, hyperthyroidism, motor tics, recent MI, severe agitation, severe hypertension, sucrase-isomaltase insufficiency, tension, thyrotoxicosis, Tourette's syndrome or family history of it, use of halogenated anethestics, use within 14 days of an MAO inhibitor

Interactions
DRUGS
anticholinergics: Possibly increased anticholinergic effects of both drugs
anticonvulsants, oral anticoagulants, phenylbutazone, tricyclic antidepressants: Inhibited metabolism and increased blood levels of these drugs
diuretics, antihypertensives: Decreased therapeutic effects of these drugs
halogenated anesthetics: Possibly sudden decrease in blood pressure during surgery
MAO inhibitors: Possibly increased adverse effects of methylphenidate, possibly severe hypertension
FOODS
caffeine: Increased methylphenidate effects

Adverse Reactions

CNS: Agitation, aggressiveness, anxiety, confusion, depression, dizziness, dyskinesia, emotional lability, fever, hallucinations, headache, hyperactivity, insomnia, irritability, ischemic neurologic defects (reversible), mania, motor tics, nervousness, paresthesia, psychosis, sedation, seizures, stroke, suicidal ideation, transient mood depression, tension, tremor, Tourette's syndrome, vertigo
CV: Angina, arrhythmias, bradycardia, chest pain, extrasystoles, hypertension, hypotension, MI, palpitations, Raynaud's phenomenon, sudden death, tachycardia
EENT: Accommodation abnormality, blurred vision, diplopia, dry mouth or throat, mydriasis, pharyngitis, rhinitis, sinusitis, vision changes
ENDO: Dysmenorrhea, growth suppression in children with long-term use
GI: Abdominal pain, anorexia, constipation, diarrhea, dyspepsia, hepatotoxicity, nausea, vomiting
GU: Decreased libido
HEME: Anemia, decreased platelet count, leukopenia, pancytopenia, thrombocytopenia, thrombocytopenic purpura
MS: Arthralgia, myalgia, muscle tightness or twitching
RESP: Increased cough, upper respiratory tract infection
SKIN: Allergic contact dermatitis, alopecia, application site reactions (transdermal patch), diaphoresis, erythema multiforme, exfoliative dermatitis, pruritus, rash, urticaria
Other: Anaphylaxis, angioedema, physical and psychological dependence, weight loss

Nursing Considerations

•WARNING Be aware that methylphenidate may induce CNS stimulation and psychosis and may worsen behavior disturbances and thought disorders in patients who already have psychosis. Use drug cautiously in patients with psychosis.

•Keep in mind that, when signs and symptoms of ADHD occur with acute stress reactions or with pre-existing structural cardiac abnormalities or other serious heart problems, treatment with methylphenidate usually isn't indicated because of possible worsened reaction or sudden death.

•Monitor children and adolescents for first-time psychotic or manic symptoms. If present, notify prescriber and expect drug to be discontinued.

•**WARNING** Know that the E.R. tablet form (Concerta) shouldn't be administered to patients with esophageal motility disorders; drug may cause GI obstruction because the tablet doesn't change shape in GI tract.

•Monitor blood pressure and pulse rate to detect hypertension and excessive stimulation. Notify prescriber if you detect such signs. For patient with hypertension, expect to increase antihypertensive dosage or add another antihypertensive to existing regimen.

•**WARNING** Watch for signs of physical or psychological dependence. Methylphenidate's abuse potential is similar to that of amphetamines; use cautiously in patients with a history of drug abuse.

•Stopping drug abruptly after long-term use may unmask dysphoria, paranoia, severe depression, or suicidal thoughts.

•Monitor growth in children. Report failure to grow or gain weight, and expect to stop drug.

•Watch patient closely (especially children, adolescents, and young adults), for suicidal tendencies, particularly when therapy starts and dosage changes, because depression may worsen temporarily during these times possibly leading to suicidal ideation.

PATIENT TEACHING

•Stress need to take drug exactly as prescribed because misuse may cause serious adverse cardiovascular reactions, including sudden death.

•If patient uses transdermal form, teach him to apply patch to a clean, dry location in his hip area 2 hours before an effect is needed and to remove it 9 hours after application.

•Caution patient to avoid applying patch to skin that is oily, damaged, or irritated and to avoid the waistline, where clothing may dislodge patch. Tell patient to rotate application sites between hips.

•Instruct patient to apply patch immediately after opening the pouch and removing the protective liner. Tell him to press patch firmly in place with the palm of his hand for about 30 seconds. Reassure patient that exposing site to water shouldn't cause patch to fall off. If a patch does fall off, explain that a new patch may be applied but that the total exposure time for the day shouldn't exceed 9 hours.

•Tell patient not to chew or crush E.R. tablets.

•Advise patient to take tablets at least 6 hours before bedtime to avoid insomnia and to take E.R. once-daily tablets in the morning.

•Advise patient taking E.R. once-daily tablets (Concerta) that he may notice intact tablet in stool. Explain that drug is slowly released from nonabsorbable tablet shell.

•Tell patient taking capsule form to swallow it whole or sprinkle contents onto a tablespoon of applesauce and take immediately, followed by a liquid such as water.

•Direct patient to notify prescriber about excessive nervousness, fever, insomnia, palpitations, rash, or vomiting.

•Warn patient with seizure disorder that drug may cause seizures.

•Inform parents of children on long-term therapy that drug may delay growth.

•Urge family or caregiver to watch patient closely for suicidal tendencies, especially when therapy starts or dosage changes and particularly if patient is a child, teenager, or young adult.

methylprednisolone

Medrol, Meprolone

methylprednisolone acetate

depMedalone, Depoject, Depo-Medrol, Depopred, Depo-Predate, Methylcotolone

methylprednisolone sodium succinate

A-methaPred, Solu-Medrol

Class and Category

Chemical class: Synthetic glucocorticoid
Therapeutic class: Anti-inflammatory, im-

munosuppressant
Pregnancy category: Not rated

Indications and Dosages

➤ *To treat ulcerative colitis*

I.V. INFUSION (METHYLPREDNISOLONE SODIUM SUCCINATE)

Adults. 40 to 120 mg 3 to 7 times/wk for 2 or more wk. Later doses given I.V. or I.M., based on patient's condition and response.
Children. 0.14 to 0.84 mg/kg daily in divided doses every 12 to 24 hr.

➤ *To treat a wide range of immune and inflammatory disorders, including allergic rhinitis, asthma, Crohn's disease, and systemic lupus erythematosus*

TABLETS (METHYLPREDNISOLONE)

Adults. 4 to 48 mg daily as a single dose or in divided doses.
Children. 0.42 to 1.67 mg/kg daily in divided doses t.i.d. or q.i.d.

I.V. INFUSION, I.M. INJECTION (METHYLPREDNISOLONE SODIUM SUCCINATE)

Adults. *Initial:* 10 to 40 mg infused over several min. Later doses given I.V. or I.M., based on patient's condition and response.
Children. 0.14 to 0.84 mg/kg every 12 to 24 hr.

I.M. INJECTION (METHYLPREDNISOLONE ACETATE)

Adults. 40 to 120 mg daily to every 2 wk, according to clinical response.
Children. 0.14 to 0.84 mg/kg every 12 to 24 hr.

INTRA-ARTICULAR, INTRALESIONAL, OR SOFT-TISSUE INJECTION (METHYLPREDNISOLONE ACETATE)

Adults. 4 to 80 mg every 1 to 5 wk, according to clinical response.

➤ *To treat adrenal hyperplasia*

I.M. INJECTION (METHYLPREDNISOLONE ACETATE)

Adults. 40 mg every 2 wk.
Children. 0.14 to 0.84 mg/kg every 12 to 24 hr.

➤ *To treat acute exacerbations of multiple sclerosis*

TABLETS (METHYLPREDNISOLONE)

Adults. 160 mg daily for 7 days followed by 64 mg every other day for 1 mo.

I.V. OR I.M. INJECTION (METHYLPREDNISOLONE ACETATE, METHYLPREDNISOLONE SODIUM SUCCINATE)

Adults. 160 mg daily for 1 wk followed by 64 mg every other day for 1 mo.

➤ *To treat adrenocortical insufficiency*

TABLETS (METHYLPREDNISOLONE), I.M. INJECTION (METHYLPREDNISOLONE SODIUM SUCCINATE)

Children. 0.18 mg/kg daily in divided doses t.i.d.

I.M. INJECTION (METHYLPREDNISOLONE ACETATE)

Children. 0.12 mg/kg every 3 days or 0.039 to 0.059 mg/kg daily.

Route	Onset	Peak	Duration
P.O.	In 60 min	1 to 2 hr	1.25 to 1.5 days
I.V.	Rapid	30 min	Unknown
I.M.	6 to 48 hr	4 to 8 days	1 to 4 wk

Mechanism of Action

Binds to intracellular glucocorticoid receptors and suppresses inflammatory and immune responses by inhibiting accumulation of neutrophils and monocytes at inflammation sites, stabilizing lysosomal membranes, suppressing the antigen response of macrophages and helper T cells, and inhibiting the synthesis of inflammatory response mediators, such as cytokines, interleukins, and prostaglandins.

Incompatibilities

Don't mix methylprednisolone with any drug without first consulting pharmacist. Don't dilute methylprednisolone acetate with any other drug.

Contraindications

Fungal infection, hypersensitivity to methylprednisolone or its components, idiopathic thrombocytopenic purpura (I.M.)

Interactions

DRUGS

acetaminophen: Increased risk of hepatotoxicity
amphotericin B, carbonic anhydrase inhibitors: Possibly severe hypokalemia
anabolic steroids, androgens: Increased risk of edema and worsening of acne
anticholinergics: Possibly increased intraocular pressure
asparaginase: Increased risk of hyperglycemia and toxicity
aspirin, NSAIDs: Increased risk of adverse GI effects and bleeding
cyclosporine: Increased risk of seizures
digoxin: Possibly hypokalemia-induced arrhythmias and digitalis toxicity
ephedrine, phenobarbital, phenytoin, ri-

M

fampin: Decreased blood methylprednisolone level

estrogens, oral contraceptives: Possibly increased therapeutic and toxic effects of methylprednisolone

insulin, oral antidiabetic drugs: Possibly increased blood glucose level

isoniazid: Possibly decreased therapeutic effects of isoniazid

mexiletine: Possibly decreased blood mexiletine level

neuromuscular blockers: Possibly increased neuromuscular blockade, causing respiratory depression or apnea

oral anticoagulants, thrombolytics: Increased risk of GI ulceration and hemorrhage, possibly decreased therapeutic effects of these drugs

potassium-depleting drugs, such as thiazide diuretics: Possibly severe hypokalemia

potassium supplements: Possibly decreased effects of these supplements

somatrem, somatropin: Possibly decreased therapeutic effects of these drugs

streptozocin: Increased risk of hyperglycemia

troleandomycin: Increased blood methylprednisolone level

vaccines: Decreased antibody response and increased risk of neurologic complications

ACTIVITIES

alcohol use: Increased risk of adverse GI effects and bleeding

Adverse Reactions

CNS: Ataxia, behavioral changes, depression, dizziness, euphoria, fatigue, headache, increased intracranial pressure with papilledema, insomnia, malaise, mood changes, paresthesia, restlessness, seizures, steroid psychosis, syncope, vertigo

CV: Arrhythmias (from hypokalemia), edema, fat embolism, heart failure, hypertension, hypotension, thromboembolism, thrombophlebitis

EENT: Exophthalmos, glaucoma, increased intraocular pressure, nystagmus, posterior subcapsular cataracts

ENDO: Adrenal insufficiency, cushingoid symptoms (moon face, buffalo hump, central obesity, supraclavicular fat pad enlargement), diabetes mellitus, growth suppression in children, hyperglycemia, negative nitrogen balance from protein catabolism

GI: Abdominal distention, hiccups, increased appetite, melena, nausea, pancreatitis, peptic ulcer, ulcerative esophagitis, vomiting

GU: Amenorrhea, glycosuria, menstrual irregularities, perineal burning or tingling

HEME: Easy bruising, leukocytosis

MS: Arthralgia; aseptic necrosis of femoral and humeral heads; compression fractures; muscle atrophy, twitching, or weakness; myalgia; osteoporosis; spontaneous fractures; steroid myopathy; tendon rupture

SKIN: Acne; altered skin pigmentation; diaphoresis; erythema; hirsutism; necrotizing vasculitis; petechiae; purpura; rash; scarring; sterile abscess; striae; subcutaneous fat atrophy; thin, fragile skin; urticaria

Other: Anaphylaxis, hypocalcemia, hypokalemia, hypokalemic alkalosis, impaired wound healing, masking of signs of infection, metabolic alkalosis, suppressed skin test reaction, weight gain

Nursing Considerations

• Give methylprednisolone tablets with food to minimize indigestion and GI irritation. For once-daily dosing, administer in the morning to coincide with normal cortisol secretion. Expect prescriber to add an antacid or H$_2$-receptor antagonist to regimen.

• Discard parenteral products that are discolored or contain particles.

• Inject I.M. form deep into gluteal muscle.

• Arrange for low-sodium diet with added potassium, as prescribed.

• Protect patient from falling, especially elderly patient at risk for fractures from osteoporosis.

• Closely monitor for signs of infection because drug may mask them.

• Assess for possible depression or psychotic episodes during therapy.

• Monitor blood glucose level; dosage of insulin or oral antidiabetic drug may need to be adjusted in diabetic patient.

•**WARNING** To avoid possibly fatal acute adrenocortical insufficiency, expect to taper long-term therapy when discontinuing it.

PATIENT TEACHING

• Caution patient not to stop taking methylprednisolone abruptly or to change dosage without consulting prescriber.

• Tell patient to take a missed dose as soon as he remembers unless it's nearly time for the next dose. Caution against double-dosing.

• Urge patient to notify prescriber immedi-

ately about dark or tarry stools; signs of impending adrenocortical insufficiency, such as anorexia, dizziness, fainting, fatigue, fever, joint pain, muscle weakness, or nausea; and sudden weight gain or swelling.
•Instruct patient not to obtain vaccinations unless approved by prescriber.
•Urge patient to take vitamin D, calcium supplements, or both if recommended by prescriber.
•Inform patient that insomnia and restlessness usually resolve after 1 to 3 weeks.
•Caution patient to avoid people with contagious diseases.
•Explain the need for regular exercise or physical therapy to maintain muscle mass.
•Advise patient to carry medical identification that documents his need for long-term corticosteroid therapy.

metoclopramide hydrochloride

Apo-Metoclop (CAN), Maxeran (CAN), Metoclopramide Intensol, Octamide, PMS-Metoclopramide (CAN), Reglan

Class and Category

Chemical class: Benzamide
Therapeutic class: Antiemetic, upper GI stimulant
Pregnancy category: B

Indications and Dosages

➤ *To treat diabetic gastroparesis*
ORAL SOLUTION, ORAL SOLUTION CONCENTRATE, TABLETS
Adults and adolescents. 10 mg 30 min before meals and at bedtime up to q.i.d.
I.V. OR I.M. INJECTION
Adults and adolescents. 10 mg t.i.d. or q.i.d. for severe symptoms; dosage adjusted as needed.

➤ *To treat gastroesophageal reflux disease*
ORAL SOLUTION, ORAL SOLUTION CONCENTRATE, TABLETS
Adults and adolescents. 10 to 15 mg 30 min before meals and at bedtime.

➤ *To prevent chemotherapy-induced vomiting*
I.V. INFUSION
Adults and adolescents. 3 mg/kg before chemotherapy and then 0.5 mg/kg/hr for 8 hr.

I.V. INJECTION
Adults and adolescents. 1 to 2 mg/kg 30 min before chemotherapy and then repeated every 2 to 3 hr, as needed.
Children. 1 mg/kg as a single dose, repeated in 1 hr. *Maximum:* 2 mg/kg.

➤ *To prevent postoperative nausea and vomiting*
I.M. INJECTION
Adults and adolescents. 10 to 20 mg near end of procedure.
DOSAGE ADJUSTMENT Reduced by half if creatinine clearance is less than 40 ml/min/ 1.73 m^2.

Route	Onset	Peak	Duration
P.O.	30 to 60 min	Unknown	1 to 2 hr
I.V.	1 to 3 min	Unknown	1 to 2 hr
I.M.	10 to 15 min	Unknown	1 to 2 hr

Mechanism of Action
Antagonizes the inhibitory effect of dopamine on GI smooth muscle. This causes gastric contraction, which promotes gastric emptying and peristalsis, thus reducing gastroesophageal reflux. Metoclopramide also blocks dopaminergic receptors in the chemoreceptor trigger zone, preventing nausea and vomiting.

Incompatibilities
Don't administer metoclopramide through same I.V. line as calcium gluconate, cephalothin sodium, chloramphenicol sodium, cisplatin, erythromycin lactobionate, furosemide, methotrexate, penicillin G potassium, or sodium bicarbonate.

Contraindications
Concurrent use of butyrophenones, phenothiazines, or other drugs that may cause extrapyramidal reactions; GI hemorrhage, mechanical obstruction, or perforation; hypersensitivity to metoclopramide or its components; pheochromocytoma; seizure disorders

Interactions
DRUGS
anticholinergics, opioid analgesics: Possibly decreased therapeutic effects of metoclopramide

M

apomorphine: Possibly decreased antiemetic effect of apomorphine, possibly increased CNS depression
bromocriptine, pergolide: Possibly decreased therapeutic effects of these drugs
cimetidine: Possibly decreased absorption and therapeutic effects of cimetidine
CNS depressants: Possibly increased CNS depression
cyclosporine: Increased blood cyclosporine level
digoxin: Decreased gastric digoxin absorption
levodopa: Possibly decreased levodopa effects
MAO inhibitors: Increased risk of severe hypertension if patient has essential hypertension
mexiletine: Possibly faster mexiletene absorption
succinylcholine: Possibly prolonged therapeutic action of succinylcholine
ACTIVITIES
alcohol use: Increased risk of excessive sedation

Adverse Reactions

CNS: Agitation, anxiety, depression, dizziness, drowsiness, extrapyramidal reactions (motor restlessness, parkinsonism, tardive dyskinesia), fatigue, headache, insomnia, irritability, lassitude, neuroleptic malignant syndrome, panic reaction, restlessness
CV: AV block, fluid retention, heart failure, hypertension, hypotension, supraventricular tachycardia
EENT: Dry mouth
ENDO: Galactorrhea, gynecomastia
GI: Constipation, diarrhea, nausea
GU: Menstrual irregularities
HEME: Agranulocytosis
SKIN: Rash
Other: Restless leg syndrome

Nursing Considerations

•Use metoclopramide cautiously in patients with hypertension because it may increase catecholamine levels.
•Use drug cautiously in elderly patients because they have an increased risk of tardive dyskinesia and parkinsonian effects. Expect to stop drug if these symptoms develop.
•Monitor patient with NADH-cytochrome b5 reductase deficiency because metoclopramide increases the risk of methemoglobinemia and sulfhemoglobinemia and patient can't receive methylene blue.

•Assess patient for signs of intestinal obstruction, such as abnormal bowel sounds, diarrhea, nausea, and vomiting, before administering metoclopramide. Notify prescriber if you detect them.
•For I.V. use, you need not dilute doses of 10 mg or less. Give drug over 1 to 2 minutes. For doses larger than 10 mg, dilute in 50 ml of normal saline solution, half-normal (0.45) saline solution, D_5W, or lactated Ringer's solution and infuse over at least 15 minutes.
•Avoid rapid I.V. delivery because it may cause anxiety, restlessness, and drowsiness.
•**WARNING** Notify prescriber if patient displays signs of toxicity, such as disorientation, drowsiness, and extrapyramidal reactions.
•Monitor patient, especially one with heart failure or cirrhosis, for possible signs of fluid retention or volume overload due to transient increase in plasma aldosterone level.
•Monitor patient closely for neuroleptic malignant syndrome, a rare but potentially fatal disorder characterized by hyperthermia, muscle rigidity, altered level of consciousness, irregular pulse or blood pressure, tachycardia, diaphoresis, and arrhythmias.
•Store drug in a light-resistant container; discard if discolored or contains particulate.
PATIENT TEACHING
•Advise against activities that require alertness for about 2 hours after each dose.
•Urge patient to avoid alcohol and CNS depressants while taking metoclopramide because they may increase CNS depression.
•Tell patient to immediately report involuntary movements of face, eyes, tongue, or hands.
•Explain that stopping metoclopramide may cause withdrawal symptoms that include dizziness, nervousness, and headache.

metolazone

Diulo, Mykrox, Zaroxolyn

Class and Category

Chemical class: Quinazoline derivative
Therapeutic class: Antihypertensive, diuretic
Pregnancy category: B

Indications and Dosages

➤ *To manage mild to moderate hypertension*
EXTENDED TABLETS
Adults. 2.5 to 5 mg daily.

PROMPT TABLETS (MYKROX)
Adults. 0.5 mg daily. *Maintenance:* 0.5 to
1 mg daily. *Maximum:* 1 mg daily.

➤ *To manage edema from heart failure or
renal disease*

EXTENDED TABLETS
Adults. 5 to 20 mg daily.

Route	Onset	Peak	Duration
P.O.	1 hr	2 hr	12 to 24 hr

Mechanism of Action

Promotes renal excretion of water and sodium by inhibiting their reabsorption in
distal convoluted tubules. The resulting reduction in plasma and extracellular fluid
volume reduces blood pressure. Metolazone
also helps reduce blood pressure by decreasing peripheral vascular resistance.

Contraindications

Anuria; hepatic coma; hypersensitivity to
metolazone, other sulfonamide derivatives,
quinethazones, thiazides, or their components; renal failure

Interactions
DRUGS

allopurinol: Increased risk of hypersensitivity
to allopurinol
amiodarone: Increased risk of arrhythmias
from hypokalemia
amphotericin B: Increased risk of electrolyte
imbalances
anesthetics: Increased effects of anesthetics
antigout drugs: Increased blood uric acid
level and risk of gout attack
antihypertensives: Increased hypotension
antineoplastics: Prolonged antineoplastic-
induced leukopenia
calcium salts: Increased risk of hypercalcemia
cholestyramine, colestipol: Decreased metolazone absorption
diazoxide: Increased risk of hyperglycemia
digoxin: Increased risk of electrolyte imbalances and digoxin-induced arrhythmias
diuretics: Additive effects of both drugs, possibly leading to severe hypovolemia and electrolyte imbalances
dopamine: Increased diuretic effect
insulin, oral antidiabetic drugs: Decreased
effectiveness of these drugs, increased risk of

hyperglycemia
lithium: Increased risk of lithium toxicity
methenamine: Decreased metolazone effectiveness from urinary alkalinization
methyldopa: Possibly hemolytic anemia
neuromuscular blockers: Increased risk of
hypokalemia and neuromuscular blockade,
increased risk of respiratory depression
NSAIDs, sympathomimetics: Possibly decreased metolazone effectiveness
oral anticoagulants: Decreased anticoagulation
vitamin D: Increased vitamin D action, increased risk of hypercalcemia

Adverse Reactions

CNS: Anxiety, chills, depression, dizziness,
drowsiness, headache, insomnia, neuropathy, paresthesia, restlessness, syncope,
weakness
CV: Chest pain, cold extremities, orthostatic
hypotension, palpitations, peripheral edema,
vasculitis, venous thrombosis
EENT: Bitter taste, blurred vision, dry
mouth, epistaxis, pharyngitis, sinus congestion, tinnitus
ENDO: Hyperglycemia
GI: Abdominal pain, anorexia, cholecystitis,
constipation, diarrhea, hepatic dysfunction,
hepatitis, indigestion, nausea, pancreatitis,
vomiting
GU: Decreased libido, glycosuria, impotence
HEME: Agranulocytosis, aplastic anemia,
leukopenia, thrombocytopenia
MS: Arthralgia, gout, myalgia
RESP: Cough
SKIN: Dry skin, necrosis, petechiae, photo-
sensitivity, pruritus, rash, urticaria
Other: Hypochloremia, hypokalemia, hypo-
natremia, hypovolemia, metabolic alkalosis

Nursing Considerations

•WARNING Be aware that Mykrox prompt
tablets shouldn't be substituted for Diulo or
Zaroxolyn extended tablets because they
aren't equivalent.
•Anticipate giving metolazone with a loop
diuretic if patient responds poorly to loop
diuretic alone.
•To monitor drug's diuretic effect, measure
fluid intake and output and daily weight.
•If response to 1 mg of Mykrox is inadequate, expect to add another drug rather
than increase dosage.
•Monitor blood chemistry test results and

M

assess for signs and symptoms of hypochloremia, hypokalemia, and, possibly, mild metabolic alkalosis.
•Monitor serum calcium and uric acid levels, especially if patient has a history of gout or renal calculi. Metolazone may slightly increase calcium reabsorption and decrease uric acid excretion.

PATIENT TEACHING
•Inform patient that metolazone controls but doesn't cure hypertension. Discuss possible need for lifelong therapy and consequences of uncontrolled hypertension.
•Instruct patient to take drug at the same time each day.
•Direct patient to take drug with food or milk to minimize adverse GI reactions.
•Advise patient to change position slowly to minimize effects of orthostatic hypotension.
•Urge patient to notify prescriber about persistent, severe diarrhea, nausea, or vomiting, which can cause dehydration and increase the risk of orthostatic hypotension.
•Stress the importance of weight and diet control, especially limiting sodium intake.
•Inform diabetic patient that metolazone may increase blood glucose level and that he should check his blood glucose level often.

metoprolol succinate

Toprol-XL

metoprolol tartrate

Apo-Metoprolol (CAN), Betaloc (CAN), Betaloc Durules (CAN), Lopresor (CAN), Lopresor SR (CAN), Lopressor, Novometoprol (CAN)

Class and Category
Chemical class: Beta$_1$-adrenergic antagonist
Therapeutic class: Antianginal, antihypertensive, MI prophylaxis and treatment
Pregnancy category: C

Indications and Dosages
➤ *To manage hypertension, alone or with other antihypertensives*
E.R. TABLETS (METOPROLOL SUCCINATE)
Adults. *Initial:* 25 to 100 mg daily, adjusted weekly as prescribed. *Maximum:* 400 mg daily.
E.R. TABLETS (METOPROLOL TARTRATE)
Adults. *Maintenance:* 100 to 400 mg daily to maintain blood pressure control after therapeutic level has been achieved with immediate-release tablets.
TABLETS (METOPROLOL TARTRATE)
Adults. *Initial:* 100 mg daily, adjusted weekly as prescribed. *Maximum:* 450 mg daily as a single dose or in divided doses.

➤ *To treat acute MI or evolving acute MI*
TABLETS (METOPROLOL TARTRATE), I.V. INJECTION (METOPROLOL TARTRATE)
Adults. *Initial:* 5 mg by I.V. bolus every 2 min for 3 doses followed by 50 mg P.O. for patients who tolerate total I.V. dose (or 25 to 50 mg P.O. for patients who can't tolerate total I.V. dose) every 6 hr for 48 hr, starting 15 min after final I.V. dose; after 48 hr, 100 mg b.i.d. followed by maintenance dosage. *Maintenance:* 100 mg P.O. b.i.d. for at least 3 mo.

➤ *To treat angina pectoris and chronic stable angina*
E.R. TABLETS (METOPROLOL SUCCINATE)
Adults. 100 mg daily, increased weekly as prescribed. *Maximum:* 400 mg daily as a single dose or in divided doses.
E.R. TABLETS (METOPROLOL TARTRATE)
Adults. *Initial:* 100 mg daily, adjusted weekly as prescribed. *Maximum:* 450 mg daily.
TABLETS (METOPROLOL TARTRATE)
Adults. *Initial:* 50 mg b.i.d., adjusted weekly as prescribed. *Maximum:* 450 mg daily.

➤ *To treat stable, symptomatic (New York Heart Association [NYHA] Class II or III), ischemic, hypertensive, or cardiomyopathic heart failure*
E.R. TABLETS (METOPROLOL SUCCINATE)
Adults. *Initial:* 25 mg daily (NYHA Class II) or 12.5 mg daily (NYHA Class III or more severe heart failure) for 2 wk. Then dosage doubled every 2 wk as tolerated. *Maximum:* 200 mg daily.

Route	Onset	Peak	Duration
P.O.	60 min	1 to 2 hr	Unknown
P.O. (E.R.)	Unknown	6 to 12 hr	Unknown
I.V.	Unknown	20 min	Unknown

Contraindications
Acute heart failure; pulse less than 45 beats/minute; cardiogenic shock; hypersensitivity to metoprolol, its components, or other beta blockers; pheochromocytoma; second- or

third-degree AV block; severe peripheral arterial disorders; sick sinus syndrome

Mechanism of Action

Inhibits stimulation of beta$_1$-receptor sites, located mainly in the heart, resulting in decreased cardiac excitability, cardiac output, and myocardial oxygen demand. These effects help relieve angina. Metoprolol also helps reduce blood pressure by decreasing renal release of renin.

Interactions

DRUGS

aluminum salts, barbiturates, calcium salts, cholestyramine, colestipol, NSAIDs, rifampin, salicylates, sulfinpyrazone: Decreased therapeutic effects of metoprolol
amiodarone, digoxin, diltiazem, verapamil: Increased risk of complete AV block
calcium channel blockers: Increased risk of heart failure and increased effects of both drugs
cimetidine: Increased blood metoprolol level
clonidine: Increased risk of hypotension; increased risk of rebound hypertension when clonidine is discontinued
digoxin: Decreased heart rate and slowed atrioventricular conduction
estrogens: Possibly decreased antihypertensive effect of metoprolol
general anesthetics: Increased risk of hypotension and heart failure
insulin, oral antidiabetic drugs: Decreased blood glucose control, possibly masking of signs and symptoms of hypoglycemia (by metoprolol)
lidocaine: Increased risk of lidocaine toxicity
MAO inhibitors: Risk of hypertension
neuromuscular blockers: Possibly enhanced and prolonged neuromuscular blockade
other antihypertensives: Additive hypotensive effect
phenothiazines: Possibly increased blood levels of both drugs
propafenone: Increased blood level and half-life of metoprolol
sympathomimetics, xanthines: Possibly decreased therapeutic effects of both drugs

FOODS

all foods: Increased bioavailability of metoprolol

Adverse Reactions

CNS: Anxiety, confusion, depression, dizziness, drowsiness, fatigue, hallucinations, headache, insomnia, weakness
CV: Angina, arrhythmias (including AV block and bradycardia), chest pain, decreased HDL level, increased triglyceride levels, gangrene of extremity, heart failure, hypertension, orthostatic hypotension
EENT: Nasal congestion, rhinitis, taste disturbance
GI: Constipation, diarrhea, hepatitis, nausea, vomiting
GU: Impotence
HEME: Leukopenia, thrombocytopenia
MS: Arthralgia, back pain, myalgia
RESP: Bronchospasm, dyspnea
SKIN: Diaphoresis, photosensitivity, rash, urticaria, worsening of psoriasis

Nursing Considerations

• Use metoprolol with extreme caution in patients with bronchospastic disease who don't respond to or can't tolerate other antihypertensive therapy. Expect to give smaller doses more often to avoid higher plasma levels that occur with longer dosage intervals.
• Use cautiously in patients with hypertension or angina who have congestive heart failure because beta blockers such as metoprolol can further depress myocardial contractility, causing heart failure to worsen.
• For patient with acute MI who can't tolerate initial dosage or who delays treatment, start with maintenance dosage, as prescribed and tolerated.
• Before starting therapy for heart failure, expect to give a diuretic, an ACE inhibitor, and digoxin to stabilize patient.
• Be aware that the metoprolol dosage for heart failure is highly individualized. Monitor patient for signs and symptoms of worsening heart failure during dosage increases. If heart failure worsens, expect to increase the diuretic dosage and possibly decrease the metoprolol dosage or temporarily discontinue drug, as prescribed. Be aware that the metoprolol dosage shouldn't be increased until signs and symptoms of worsening heart failure have been stabilized.
• If patient with heart failure develops symptomatic bradycardia, expect to decrease the metoprolol dosage.
• **WARNING** If dosage exceeds 400 mg daily,

monitor patient for bronchospasm and dyspnea because metoprolol competitively blocks beta$_2$-adrenergic receptors in bronchial and vascular smooth muscles.

•**WARNING** When substituting metoprolol for clonidine, expect to gradually reduce clonidine dosage and increase metoprolol dosage over several days. Giving these drugs together causes additive hypotensive effects.

•Patients who take metoprolol may be at risk for AV block. If AV block results from depressed AV node conduction, prepare to administer appropriate drug, as prescribed, or assist with insertion of temporary pacemaker.

•Check for signs of poor glucose control in patient with diabetes mellitus. Metoprolol may interfere with therapeutic effects of insulin and oral antidiabetic drugs. It also may mask evidence of hypoglycemia, such as palpitations, tachycardia, and tremor.

•Monitor patient with peripheral vascular disease for evidence of arterial insufficiency (pain, pallor, and coldness in affected extremity) because metoprolol can precipitate or aggravate peripheral vascular disease.

•Be aware that abrupt withdrawal of drug can precipitate thyroid storm in patient with hyperthyroidism or thyrotoxicosis.

•**WARNING** Expect to taper dosage when drug is discontinued; stopping abruptly can cause myocardial ischemia, MI, ventricular arrhythmias, or severe hypertension, especially in patients with cardiac disease.

PATIENT TEACHING

•Instruct patient to take metoprolol with food at the same time each day—once daily for E.R. tablets. Inform him that he may halve tablets but not chew or crush them.

•Advise patient to notify prescriber if pulse rate falls below 60 beats/minute or is significantly lower than usual.

•Urge diabetic patient to check his blood glucose level often during metoprolol therapy.

•Caution patient not to stop metoprolol abruptly.

metronidazole

Apo-Metronidazole (CAN), Flagyl, Flagyl I.V. RTU, Metric 21, MetroGel, MetroGel-Vaginal, Nidagel (CAN), Novonidazol (CAN), Protostat, Trikacide (CAN)

metronidazole hydrochloride

Flagyl I.V.

Class and Category

Chemical class: Nitroimidazole derivative
Therapeutic class: Antibiotic, antiprotozoal
Pregnancy category: B

Indications and Dosages

➤ *To treat systemic anaerobic infections caused by* Bacteroides fragilis, Clostridium difficile, Clostridium perfringens, Eubacterium, Fusobacterium, Peptococcus, Peptostreptococcus, *and* Veillonella *species*

CAPSULES, TABLETS

Adults and adolescents. 7.5 mg/kg up to 1,000 mg every 6 hr for 7 days or longer. *Maximum:* 4,000 mg daily.

Children. 7.5 mg/kg every 6 hr or 10 mg/kg every 8 hr.

I.V. INFUSION

Adults and adolescents. *Initial:* 15 mg/kg and then 7.5 mg/kg up to 1,000 mg every 6 hr for 7 days or longer. *Maximum:* 4,000 mg daily.

Children. 7.5 mg/kg every 6 hr or 10 mg/kg every 8 hr.

➤ *To treat amebiasis (*Entamoeba histolytica*)*

CAPSULES, TABLETS

Adults. 500 to 750 mg t.i.d. for 5 to 10 days.

Children. 11.6 to 16.7 mg/kg t.i.d. for 10 days.

➤ *To treat trichomoniasis (*Trichomonas vaginalis*)*

CAPSULES, TABLETS

Adults. 2,000 mg as a single dose, 1,000 mg b.i.d. for 24 hr, or 250 mg t.i.d. for 7 days.

Children. 5 mg/kg t.i.d. for 7 days.

➤ *To prevent perioperative bowel infection*

I.V. INFUSION

Adults and adolescents. 15 mg/kg 1 hr before surgery and then 7.5 mg/kg 6 and 12 hr after initial dose.

➤ *To treat acne in patients with rosacea*

TOPICAL GEL

Adults. Thin film applied to affected area b.i.d. for 9 wk.

➤ *To treat bacterial vaginosis*

VAGINAL CREAM

Adults. 500 mg (1 applicatorful) once or twice daily for 10 to 20 days.

VAGINAL GEL
Adults. 37.5 mg (1 applicatorful) once or twice daily for 5 days.
VAGINAL TABLETS
Adults. 500 mg at bedtime for 10 to 20 days.

Mechanism of Action
Undergoes intracellular chemical reduction during anaerobic metabolism. After metronidazole is reduced, it damages DNA's helical structure and breaks its strands, which inhibits bacterial nucleic acid synthesis and causes cell death.

Incompatibilities
Don't administer I.V. metronidazole with aluminum needles or hubs or through same I.V. line as other drugs.

Contraindications
Breast-feeding, hypersensitivity to metronidazole or its components, trichomoniasis during first trimester of pregnancy

Interactions
DRUGS
cimetidine: Possibly delayed elimination and increased blood level of metronidazole
disulfiram: Possibly combined toxicity, resulting in confusion and psychotic reactions
neurotoxic drugs: Increased risk of neurotoxicity
oral anticoagulants: Possibly increased anticoagulant effect
phenobarbital: Increased metabolism and decreased blood level and half-life of metronidazole
phenytoin: Decreased phenytoin clearance
ACTIVITIES
alcohol use: Possibly disulfiram-like effects

Adverse Reactions
CNS: Ataxia, dizziness, encephalopathy, fever, headache, light-headedness, peripheral neuropathy, seizures (high doses)
EENT: Dry mouth, lacrimation (topical form), metallic taste, pharyngitis
GI: Abdominal cramps or pain, anorexia, diarrhea, nausea, pancreatitis, vomiting
GU: Darkened urine, vaginal candidiasis (oral, parenteral, and topical forms); burning or irritation of sexual partner's penis, candidal cervicitis or vaginitis, dysuria, urinary

frequency, vulvitis (vaginal form)
HEME: Leukopenia
MS: Back pain
SKIN: Burning sensation, stinging sensation, dry skin (topical form); erythema, pruritus, rash, urticaria (oral and parenteral forms)
Other: Injection site edema, pain, or tenderness

Nursing Considerations
• Give I.V. drug by slow infusion over 1 hour; don't give by direct I.V. injection.
• Discontinue primary I.V. infusion during metronidazole infusion.
• **WARNING** If patient has adverse CNS reactions, such as seizures or peripheral neuropathy, tell prescriber and stop drug immediately.
• Monitor patient with severe liver disease because slowed metronidazole metabolism may cause drug to accumulate in body and increase the risk of adverse effects.
• If skin irritation occurs, apply topical metronidazole gel less frequently or discontinue it, as ordered.
• Monitor CBC and culture and sensitivity tests if therapy lasts longer than 10 days or if second course of treatment is needed.
PATIENT TEACHING
• Instruct female patient to notify prescriber if she is pregnant, intends to get pregnant, or is breast-feeding.
• Direct patient to take metronidazole at evenly spaced intervals throughout the day and with food to minimize adverse GI reactions.
• Urge patient to complete the entire course of therapy.
• Caution patient to avoid alcohol during therapy and for at least 3 days afterward.
• Advise patient to avoid hazardous activities until drug's CNS effects are known.
• If patient reports dry mouth, suggest ice chips or sugarless hard candy or gum; suggest a dental visit if dryness lasts longer than 2 weeks.
• Instruct patient to notify prescriber if no improvement occurs within a few days of taking tablets or capsules.
• Direct patient using topical gel to wash hands and affected area with a mild, nonirritating cleaner; to rinse well and pat dry; and then to apply a thin film of drug and wash hands again.

• Advise patient with rosacea to keep topical gel away from his eyes. If drug gets into his eyes, urge him to wash them immediately with large amounts of cool tap water and to call prescriber if eyes continue to hurt or burn.

• Instruct patient with rosacea to notify prescriber if no improvement occurs after 3 weeks of topical use; full therapeutic effect may take 9 weeks.

• Teach patient how to fill, insert, and clean vaginal cream or gel applicator after use. Instruct her to wash her hands before and after administration.

• To help vaginal tablets dissolve, instruct patient to run tap water over unwrapped tablet for a few seconds before insertion.

• Inform patient with trichomoniasis that her male sexual partners should wear condoms during her treatment and that they may need treatment themselves to prevent reinfection.

• Caution patient that vaginal cream and tablets (not gel) may contain oils that damage latex condoms.

• Urge patient to follow up with prescriber to make sure infection is gone.

metyrosine

Demser

Class and Category

Chemical class: Alpha-methyl tyrosine
Therapeutic class: Antipheochromocytoma agent
Pregnancy category: C

Indications and Dosages

➤ *To control hypertension and related symptoms until pheochromocytomectomy is performed, to treat chronic malignant pheochromocytoma*

CAPSULES

Adults and adolescents. *Initial:* 250 mg q.i.d., increased as ordered by 250 to 500 mg daily. *Maintenance:* 2,000 to 3,000 mg daily in divided doses q.i.d. Preoperative dosage given for at least 7 days. *Maximum:* 4,000 mg daily in divided doses.

Contraindications

Hypersensitivity to metyrosine or its components

Mechanism of Action

Blocks the activity of tyrosine hydroxylase, the enzyme that controls the rate of catecholamine synthesis. This action decreases production of the catecholamines epinephrine and norepinephrine, which, in patients with pheochromocytoma, are produced in excessive amounts.

Interactions

DRUGS

CNS depressants: Increased sedation
haloperidol, phenothiazines: Increased extrapyramidal effects

ACTIVITIES

alcohol use: Increased sedation

Adverse Reactions

CNS: Anxiety, confusion, depression, disorientation, extrapyramidal reactions (difficulty speaking, drooling, parkinsonism, tremor, trismus), hallucinations, headache, sedation
CV: Peripheral edema
EENT: Dry mouth, nasal congestion, pharyngeal edema
ENDO: Galactorrhea, gynecomastia
GI: Abdominal pain, diarrhea, elevated serum AST level, nausea, vomiting
GU: Crystalluria, dysuria (transient), ejaculation failure, hematuria, impotence, urolithiasis
HEME: Anemia, eosinophilia, thrombocytopenia, thrombocytosis
SKIN: Urticaria

Nursing Considerations

• Expect patient taking metyrosine to experience moderate to severe sedation at low and high dosages. Sedation begins during first 24 hours, peaks after 2 to 3 days, and tends to wane during next few days. It usually subsides after 1 week unless dosage is increased or exceeds 2 g daily.

• Obtain urine specimens as ordered to check for crystalluria and urolithiasis. If crystalluria develops, increase fluid intake to achieve daily urine output of 2,000 ml or more with doses above 2 g daily. If crystalluria persists, reduce dosage or stop drug, as ordered.

• Expect to adjust dosage, as prescribed, based on clinical response and urine catecholamine level.

•If signs and symptoms aren't adequately controlled by metyrosine, expect to add an alpha-adrenergic blocker, such as phenoxybenzamine, as prescribed.

PATIENT TEACHING
•Inform patient about metyrosine's sedative effects. Advise him to avoid alcohol and CNS depressants, which may increase sedation.
•Instruct patient to increase fluid intake, as appropriate.
•Urge patient to report drooling, severe diarrhea, trembling and shaking of hands and fingers, or trouble speaking.
•Inform patient that he may experience changes in sleep pattern for 2 to 3 days after stopping drug.
•Advise patient to keep regular visits with prescriber to monitor progress.

mexiletine hydrochloride

Mexitil

Class and Category

Chemical class: Lidocaine analogue
Therapeutic class: Class IB antiarrhythmic
Pregnancy category: C

Indications and Dosages

➤ *To treat life-threatening ventricular arrhythmias*

CAPSULES

Adults. *Initial:* 200 mg every 8 hr, adjusted, as ordered, by 50 to 100 mg/dose every 2 to 3 days, as tolerated. If patient tolerates 300 mg or less every 8 hr, total dosage may be divided and given every 12 hr. If patient continues to experience arrhythmias, dosage frequency may be changed to q.i.d. *Maximum:* 1,200 mg daily when given every 8 hr (400 mg/dose); 900 mg daily when given every 12 hr (450 mg/dose).

➤ *To rapidly control life-threatening ventricular arrhythmias*

CAPSULES

Adults. *Initial:* 400 mg followed by 200 mg after 8 hr. *Maintenance:* 200 mg every 8 hr, adjusted, as ordered, by 50 to 100 mg/dose every 2 to 3 days, as tolerated. If patient tolerates 300 mg or less every 8 hr, total dosage may be divided and given every 12 hr. If patient continues to experience arrhythmias, dosage frequency may be changed to q.i.d.

DOSAGE ADJUSTMENT For patients with severe hepatic disease or heart failure, dosage reduced and adjusted every 2 or 3 days.

Route	Onset	Peak	Duration
P.O.	0.5 to 2 hr	2 to 3 hr	8 to 12 hr

Mechanism of Action

Produces antiarrhythmic effect by inhibiting fast sodium channels in myocardial cell membranes, especially in the His-Purkinje system. This action decreases the duration of the action potential and effective refractory period of the His-Purkinje system. The myocardium, which becomes refractory again after the resting membrane potential is restored, is less likely to generate and respond to ectopic ventricular impulses.

Contraindications

Cardiogenic shock, second- or third-degree AV block without a pacemaker

Interactions

DRUGS

aluminum- or magnesium-containing antacids: Delayed mexiletine absorption
antiarrhythmics: Increased cardiac effects
cimetidine: Possibly increased or decreased blood mexiletine level
hepatic enzyme inducers: Accelerated metabolism and decreased blood level of mexiletine
metoclopramide: Accelerated mexiletine absorption
rifampin: Decreased blood mexiletine level
theophylline: Increased blood theophylline level
urine acidifiers: Accelerated renal excretion of mexiletine
urine alkalinizers: Delayed mexiletine excretion

FOODS

caffeine: Possibly decreased clearance and increased effects of caffeine
foods that may acidify urine (such as cheese, cranberries, eggs, fish, grains, meats, plums, poultry, and prunes): Accelerated renal excretion of mexiletine
foods that may alkalinize urine (such as milk and all vegetables and fruits except cranberries, plums, and prunes): Delayed renal excretion of mexiletine

M

ACTIVITIES
smoking: Reduced mexiletine half-life

Adverse Reactions
CNS: Confusion, dizziness, fatigue, headache, lack of coordination, light-headedness, nervousness, paresthesia, seizures, sleep disturbance, syncope, tremor, weakness
CV: Atrial arrhythmias, atrioventricular conduction disorders, bradycardia, cardiogenic shock, chest pain, heart failure, hypotension, palpitations, PVCs, ventricular arrhythmias (increased)
EENT: Blurred vision, dry mouth, tinnitus
GI: Constipation, diarrhea, heartburn, nausea, vomiting
HEME: Agranulocytosis, leukopenia, thrombocytopenia
RESP: Dyspnea
SKIN: Rash

Nursing Considerations
•If mexiletine is replacing another antiarrhythmic, expect to give the first dose 6 to 12 hours after last dose of quinidine sulfate or disopyramide, 3 to 6 hours after last dose of procainamide, or 8 to 12 hours after last dose of tocainide, as prescribed.
•If mexiletine is replacing parenteral lidocaine, expect to reduce or withdraw lidocaine 1 to 2 hours after starting mexiletine, as prescribed.
•Monitor continuous ECG and serum mexiletine level.
•Assess patient for thrombocytopenia, which may occur within a few days after mexiletine therapy starts. Expect platelet count to return to normal within 1 month after mexiletine therapy stops.
PATIENT TEACHING
•Instruct patient to take mexiletine at evenly spaced intervals, to avoid missing doses, and to take drug as prescribed, even if he's feeling well.
•Advise patient to take drug with food to reduce adverse GI reactions.
•Inform patient that nausea and vomiting may occur within 2 hours after dose but tend to lessen as treatment continues.
•Advise patient to avoid hazardous activities until drug's CNS effects are known.
•Teach patient how to take his pulse, and advise him to contact prescriber if rate falls below 50 beats/minute or if rhythm is irregular.

•Urge patient to notify prescriber immediately about chest pain, chills, fast or irregular heartbeat, fever, shortness of breath, and unusual bleeding or bruising.
•Advise patient to avoid dramatically increasing intake of foods that may acidify urine (cheese, cranberries, eggs, fish, grains, meats, plums, poultry, prunes) or alkalinize urine (milk, all vegetables, all fruits except cranberries, plums, and prunes).
•Encourage patient to keep regular visits with prescriber to monitor progress.

mezlocillin sodium

Mezlin

Class and Category
Chemical class: Acyclaminopenicillin
Therapeutic class: Antibiotic
Pregnancy category: B

Indications and Dosages
➤ *To treat moderate to severe infections, including bacteremia, bone and joint infections, gynecologic infections (such as endometritis, pelvic cellulitis, and pelvic inflammatory disease), intra-abdominal infections (such as cholangitis, cholecystitis, hepatic abscess, intra-abdominal abscess, and peritonitis), lower respiratory tract infections (such as pneumonia and lung abscess), meningitis, septicemia caused by susceptible bacteria, or skin and soft-tissue infections (such as cellulitis and diabetic foot ulcer); to manage febrile neutropenia*

I.V. INFUSION, I.M. INJECTION
Adults and adolescents. 3 g every 4 hr or 4 g every 6 hr.

➤ *To treat life-threatening infections of the types listed above*
I.V. INFUSION, I.M. INJECTION
Adults and adolescents. Up to 350 mg/kg daily. *Maximum:* 24,000 mg daily.
Children and infants. 50 mg/kg every 4 hr (or infused over 30 min every 4 hr).
Neonates over age 7 days weighing 2,000 g (4.4 lb) or less. 75 mg/kg I.V. every 8 hr.
Neonates age 7 days or less weighing 2,000 g or less. 75 mg/kg I.V. every 12 hr.
Neonates age 7 days or less weighing more than 2,000 g. 75 mg/kg I.V. every 6 hr.

➤ *To treat uncomplicated UTI*

I.V. INFUSION, I.M. INJECTION

Adults. 1.5 to 2 g every 6 hr.

➤ *To treat complicated UTI*

I.V. INFUSION

Adults. 3 g every 6 hr.

DOSAGE ADJUSTMENT Dosing interval extended to 6 to 8 hr if needed for patients with creatinine clearance of 10 to 30 ml/min/1.73 m^2. Dosing interval extended and dosage reduced to 1.5 to 2 g for patients with creatinine clearance below 10 ml/min/1.73 m^2.

➤ *To treat uncomplicated gonorrhea caused by susceptible strains of* Neisseria gonorrhoeae

I.V. INFUSION, I.M. INJECTION

Adults. 1 to 2 g as a single dose given with 1 g of probenecid P.O. (or probenecid given up to 30 min before mezlocillin).

➤ *To prevent infection from potentially contaminated surgical procedures*

I.V. INFUSION

Adults. 4 g 30 min before surgery and then 4 g every 6 hr for 2 more doses.

➤ *To prevent infection in cesarean section*

I.V. INFUSION

Adults. 4 g as soon as umbilical cord is clamped; then 4 g every 4 hr for 2 more doses, starting 4 hr after initial dose.

Mechanism of Action

Inhibits bacterial cell wall synthesis. In susceptible bacteria, the rigid, cross-linked cell wall is assembled in several stages. Mezlocillin exerts its effects in the final stage of the cross-linking process by binding with and inactivating penicillin-binding proteins (enzymes responsible for linking cell wall strands). This action causes bacterial cell lysis and death.

Incompatibilities

Administer mezlocillin at separate sites and at least 1 hour before or after administering aminoglycosides. Don't mix mezlocillin in the same I.V. bag, bottle, or tubing with other drugs.

Contraindications

Hypersensitivity to mezlocillin, other penicillins, or their components

Interactions

DRUGS

aminoglycosides: Substantial aminoglycoside inactivation

chloramphenicol, erythromycins, sulfonamides, tetracyclines: Possibly decreased therapeutic effects of mezlocillin

methotrexate: Increased risk of methotrexate toxicity

probenecid: Increased blood level and prolonged half-life of mezlocillin

Adverse Reactions

CNS: Depression, headache, seizures

EENT: Oral candidiasis

GI: Abdominal pain, diarrhea, pseudomembranous colitis, nausea, vomiting

GU: Vaginitis

HEME: Leukopenia, neutropenia

SKIN: Exfoliative dermatitis, pruritus, rash, urticaria

Other: Anaphylaxis; hypokalemia; injection site pain, redness, and swelling; serum sicknesslike reaction

Nursing Considerations

•**WARNING** Before starting mezlocillin, make sure that patient has had no previous hypersensitivity reactions to penicillins.

•Anticipate that mezlocillin therapy will last for at least 2 days after signs and symptoms have resolved—typically 7 to 10 days, depending on severity of infection. Complicated infections may need longer treatment. Group A beta-hemolytic streptococcal infections usually are treated for at least 10 days to reduce the risk of rheumatic fever or glomerulonephritis.

•For I.M. injection, reconstitute each gram of mezlocillin with 3 to 4 ml of sterile water for injection and shake vigorously. Inject no more than 2 g into a large muscle, such as the gluteus maximus, over 12 to 15 seconds to minimize discomfort.

•Although drug may be given I.M., expect to use intermittent I.V. infusion, as directed, for serious infections.

•For I.V. use, reconstitute each gram of mezlocillin with 9 to 10 ml of sterile water for injection, D$_5$W, or sodium chloride for injection and shake vigorously. Inject directly into I.V. tubing over 3 to 5 minutes.

•For intermittent infusion, further dilute to desired volume (50 to 100 ml) with an appropriate I.V. solution and administer over

M

30 minutes. Discontinue other infusions during mezlocillin administration.
•Be aware that mezlocillin powder and reconstituted solution may darken slightly but that potency isn't affected.
•Periodically monitor serum potassium level in patient on long-term therapy, as ordered.
•During long-term therapy, monitor for signs and symptoms of superinfection, such as oral candidiasis and vaginitis.

PATIENT TEACHING
•Instruct patient taking mezlocillin to notify prescriber immediately about increased bruising or other bleeding tendencies.
•Advise patient to report diarrhea and to check with prescriber before taking an antidiarrheal medicine because of the risk of masking pseudomembranous colitis.

micafungin sodium

Mycamine

Class and Category

Chemical class: Semisynthetic lipopeptide echinocandin
Therapeutic class: Antifungal
Pregnancy category: C

Indications and Dosages

➤ *To treat esophageal candidiasis*
I.V. INFUSION
Adults. 150 mg infused over 1 hr daily.

➤ *To prevent* Candida *infection in patients undergoing hematopoietic stem cell transplantation*
I.V. INFUSION
Adults. 50 mg infused over 1 hr daily.

➤ *To treat candidemia, acute disseminated candidiasis, and* Candida *peritonitis and abscesses*
I.V. INFUSION
Adults. 100 mg infused over 1 hr daily.

Contraindications

Hypersensitivity to micafungin, its components, or other echinocandins

Incompatibilities

Mixing or infusing with other drugs may cause micafungin to precipitate.

Interactions

DRUGS
immunosuppressants: Possibly additive adverse hematologic effects
itraconazole, nifedipine, sirolimus: Increased plasma levels of these drugs

Mechanism of Action

Inhibits synthesis of 1,3-beta-D-glucan, which is an essential component of the *Candida* fungal cell wall. Without 1,3-beta-D-glucan, the fungal cell dies.

Adverse Reactions

CNS: Anxiety, delirium, dizziness, dysgeusia, fatigue, fever, headache, insomnia, intracranial hemorrhage, rigors, seizures, somnolence
CV: Arrhythmia, atrial fibrillation, bradycardia, cardiac arrest, deep venous thrombosis, hypertension, hypotension, MI, peripheral edema, phlebitis, tachycardia, shock, vasodilation
EENT: Epistaxis, mucosal inflammation
ENDO: Hypoglycemia, hyperglycemia
GI: Abdominal pain, anorexia, constipation, diarrhea, dyspepsia, elevated liver enzyme levels, hepatic dysfunction, hiccups, hyperbilirubinemia, jaundice, nausea, vomiting
GU: Acute renal failure, anuria, elevated serum creatinine and blood urea levels, oliguria, renal tubular necrosis
HEME: Anemia, coagulopathy, eosinophilia, hemolytic anemia, leukopenia, lymphopenia, neutropenia, pancytopenia, thrombocytopenia
MS: Arthralgia, back pain
RESP: Apnea, cough, cyanosis, dyspnea, hypoxia, pneumonia, pulmonary embolism
SKIN: Erythema, erythema multiforme, flushing, necrosis, pruritus, rash, urticaria
Other: Acidosis, anaphylaxis, angioedema, bacteremia, hyperkalemia, hypernatremia, hypocalcemia, hypokalemia, hypomagnesemia, hyponatremia, hypophosphatemia, injection site reactions including phlebitis and thrombophlebitis, sepsis

Nursing Considerations

•Use cautiously in patients with hepatic or renal insufficiency.
•Reconstitute micafungin by adding 5 ml normal saline solution to each 50-mg vial being used (to yield 10 mg micafungin/ml) or 5 ml normal saline solution to each 100-mg vial (to yield 20 mg micafungin/ml). Swirl vial gently to minimize excessive foaming. Add reconstituted solution to 100 ml normal

saline solution, and administer solution over 1 hour. Protect diluted solution from light, although you need not cover the infusion drip chamber or tubing.

•Always flush an existing intravenous line with normal saline solution before administering micafungin through that line.

•Monitor infusion rate carefully because infusions that took less than 1 hour to infuse have been associated with more frequent hypersensitivity reactions.

•**WARNING** Monitor patient closely for hypersensitivity reactions including anaphylaxis and angioedema. Discontinue infusion immediately if present, notify prescriber, and provide supportive care, as prescribed.

•Monitor patient's liver and renal function closely throughout therapy because liver and renal abnormalities may occur in patients receiving micafungin.

•Monitor hematologic status closely because a variety of hematologic abnormalities may occur. If abnormalities are detected, monitor patient closely. If patient's condition worsens, expect micafungin to be discontinued.

PATIENT TEACHING

•Instruct patient to report any infusion site discomfort immediately.

•Tell patient to report any unusual or persistent signs and symptoms to prescriber.

midazolam hydrochloride

Versed

Class, Category, and Schedule

Chemical class: Benzodiazepine
Therapeutic class: Sedative-hypnotic
Pregnancy category: D
Controlled substance schedule: IV

Indications and Dosages

➤ *To induce preoperative sedation or amnesia, to control preoperative anxiety*

ORAL SOLUTION

Children ages 6 months to 16 years. 0.25 to 0.5 mg/kg as a single dose 30 to 45 min before surgery. *Usual:* 0.5 mg/kg. *Maximum:* 20 mg.

I.V. INJECTION

Adults age 60 and over. 1.5 mg over 2 min immediately before procedure. After 2-min waiting period, dosage adjusted to desired

level in 25% increments, as ordered. *Maximum:* 1 mg in 2 min.

Adults under age 60 and adolescents. Up to 2.5 mg over 2 min immediately before procedure. After 2-min waiting period, dosage adjusted to desired level in 25% increments, as ordered. *Maximum:* 5 mg.

Children ages 6 to 12. *Initial:* 0.025 to 0.05 mg/kg, up to 0.4 mg/kg, if needed. *Maximum:* 10 mg.

Children ages 6 months to 5 years. *Initial:* 0.05 to 0.1 mg/kg, up to 0.6 mg/kg, if needed. *Maximum:* 6 mg.

I.M. INJECTION

Adults age 60 and over. 0.02 to 0.05 mg/kg as a single dose 30 to 60 min before surgery.

Adults under age 60 and adolescents. 0.07 to 0.08 mg/kg as a single dose 30 to 60 min before surgery.

Children ages 6 months to 12 years. 0.1 to 0.15 mg/kg, up to 0.5 mg/kg for more anxious patients. *Maximum:* 10 mg.

➤ *To relieve agitation and anxiety in mechanically ventilated patients*

I.V. INFUSION

Adults. *Initial:* 0.01 to 0.05 mg/kg infused over several min, repeated at 10- to 15-min intervals until adequate sedation occurs. *Maintenance:* 0.02 to 0.1 mg/kg/hr initially, adjusted to desired level in 25% to 50% increments, as ordered. After achieving desired level of sedation, infusion rate decreased by 10% to 25% every few hr, as ordered, until minimum effective infusion rate is determined.

Children. *Initial:* 50 to 200 mcg/kg over 2 to 3 min followed by 1 to 2 mcg/kg/min by continuous infusion. *Maintenance:* 0.4 to 6 mcg/kg/min.

Infants over age 32 weeks. 1 mcg/kg/min by continuous infusion.

Infants under age 32 weeks. 0.5 mcg/kg/min by continuous infusion.

Route	Onset	Peak	Duration
I.V.*	1.5 to 5 min	Rapid	2 to 6 hr
I.M.*	5 to 15 min	15 to 60 min	2 to 6 hr
I.M.†	30 to 60 min	Unknown	Unknown

* For sedation.
† For amnesia.

Mechanism of Action

May exert its sedating effect by increasing the activity of gamma-aminobutyric acid, a major inhibitory neurotransmitter in the brain. As a result, midazolam produces a calming effect, relaxes skeletal muscles, and—at high doses—induces sleep.

Contraindications

Acute angle-closure glaucoma; alcohol intoxication; coma; hypersensitivity to midazolam, other benzodiazepines, or their components; shock

Interactions

DRUGS

antihypertensives: Increased risk of hypotension

cimetidine, diltiazem, erythromycin, fluconazole, indinavir, itraconazole, ketoconazole, ranitidine, ritonavir, saquinavir, verapamil: Intense and prolonged sedation caused by reduced midazolam metabolism

CNS depressants: Possibly increased CNS and respiratory depression and hypotension

rifampin: Decreased blood midazolam level

FOODS

grapefruit, grapefruit juice: Possibly increased blood midazolam level and risk of toxicity

ACTIVITIES

alcohol use: Possibly intense, prolonged sedative effect and increased respiratory depression and hypotension

Adverse Reactions

CNS: Agitation, delirium, or dreaming during emergence from anesthesia; anxiety; ataxia; chills; combativeness; confusion; dizziness; drowsiness; euphoria; excessive sedation; headache; insomnia; lethargy; nervousness; nightmares; paresthesia; prolonged emergence from anesthesia; restlessness; retrograde amnesia; sleep disturbance; slurred speech; weakness; yawning

CV: Cardiac arrest, hypotension, nodal rhythm, PVCs, tachycardia, vasovagal episodes

EENT: Blurred vision, diplopia, or other vision changes; increased salivation; laryngospasm; miosis; nystagmus; toothache

GI: Hiccups, nausea, retching, vomiting

RESP: Airway obstruction, bradypnea, bronchospasm, coughing, decreased tidal volume, dyspnea, hyperventilation, respiratory arrest, shallow breathing, tachypnea, wheezing

SKIN: Pruritus, rash, urticaria

Other: Injection site burning, edema, induration, pain, redness, and tenderness

Nursing Considerations

• Before administering midazolam, determine whether patient consumes alcohol or takes antihypertensives, antibiotics, or protease inhibitors because these substances can produce an intense and prolonged sedative effect when taken during midazolam therapy.

• **WARNING** Be aware that I.V. midazolam is given only in hospital or ambulatory care settings that allow continuous monitoring of respiratory and cardiac function. Keep resuscitative drugs and equipment at hand.

• As needed, combine midazolam injection with D₅W, normal saline solution, or lactated Ringer's solution. With D₅W and normal saline, solution is stable 24 hours. With lactated Ringer's, solution is stable 4 hours.

• As needed, mix injection in same syringe with atropine sulfate, meperidine hydrochloride, morphine sulfate, or scopolamine hydrobromide. The resulting solution is stable for 30 minutes.

• Assess level of consciousness frequently because the range between sedation and unconsciousness or disorientation is narrow with midazolam.

• Be aware that recovery time is usually 2 hours but may be up to 6 hours.

PATIENT TEACHING

• Inform patient that he may not remember procedure because midazolam produces amnesia.

• Advise patient to avoid hazardous activities until drug's adverse CNS effects, such as dizziness and drowsiness, have worn off.

• Instruct patient to avoid alcohol and other CNS depressants for 24 hours after receiving drug, unless directed otherwise by prescriber.

midodrine hydrochloride

ProAmatine

Class and Category

Chemical class: Desglymidodrine prodrug
Therapeutic class: Antihypotensive, vasopressor
Pregnancy category: C

Indications and Dosages
➤ *To treat symptomatic orthostatic hypotension*
TABLETS
Adults. 10 mg t.i.d. in 3- to 4-hr intervals.
DOSAGE ADJUSTMENT Initial dose possibly reduced to 2.5 mg for patients with renal impairment.

Route	Onset	Peak	Duration
P.O.	Unknown	30 min	2 to 3 hr

Mechanism of Action
Is broken down into the active metabolite desglymidodrine. Desglymidodrine directly stimulates alpha-adrenergic receptors in arteries and veins. This action increases total peripheral vascular resistance, which in turn increases systolic and diastolic blood pressure.

Contraindications
Acute renal disease, hypersensitivity to midodrine or its components, initial supine systolic pressure above 180 mm Hg, persistent and excessive supine hypertension, pheochromocytoma, severe heart disease, thyrotoxicosis, urine retention

Interactions
DRUGS
beta blockers, digoxin: Enhanced or precipitated bradycardia, AV block, arrhythmias
cimetidine, flecainide, metformin, procainamide, quinidine, ranitidine, triamterene: Possibly decreased renal clearance of these drugs
dihydroergotamine, ephedrine, phenylephrine, phenylpropanolamine, pseudoephedrine: Increased vasopressor effects
doxazosin, prazosin, terazosin: Antagonized midodrine effects
fludrocortisone acetate: Increased risk of supine hypertension

Adverse Reactions
CNS: Anxiety, asthenia, chills, confusion, delusions, dizziness, feeling of pressure or fullness in head, headache, hyperesthesia, insomnia, nervousness, paresthesia, somnolence
CV: Hypertension (sitting and supine), vasodilation
EENT: Canker sore, dry mouth, vision changes
GI: Flatulence, indigestion, nausea
GU: Dysuria, urinary frequency and urgency, urine retention
MS: Back pain, leg cramps
SKIN: Dry skin, erythema multiforme, facial flushing, piloerection, rash, scalp pruritus

Nursing Considerations
• Monitor hepatic and renal function, as ordered, before and during midodrine therapy.
• Give drug at 3- to 4-hour intervals, if ordered and needed to control symptoms. Don't give after evening meal, less than 4 hours before bed, or more often than every 3 hours.
• **WARNING** Monitor for severe, persistent systolic supine hypertension, which may develop with single doses up to 20 mg.
• Avoid placing patient flat in bed for any length of time. Elevate head of bed when he's supine.
• Monitor supine and sitting blood pressure frequently during midodrine therapy.
PATIENT TEACHING
• Instruct patient to take midodrine every 3 to 4 hours during daytime but not to take final dose after evening meal or within 4 hours of going to bed.
• Advise patient to elevate head of bed when he lies supine. Caution him not to remain flat for any length of time.
• Direct patient to notify prescriber immediately about headache, increased dizziness, urine retention, or vision changes.
• Encourage patient to keep follow-up appointments to monitor blood pressure and hepatic and renal function.

miglitol
Glyset

Class and Category
Chemical class: Desoxynojirimycin derivative
Therapeutic class: Alpha-glucosidase inhibitor, antidiabetic drug
Pregnancy category: B

Indications and Dosages
➤ *To manage type 2 diabetes mellitus*
TABLETS
Adults. *Initial:* 25 mg t.i.d. with first bite of each meal. Alternatively, 25 mg daily, gradually increased to 25 mg t.i.d. *Maximum:* 100 mg t.i.d.

DOSAGE ADJUSTMENT After 4 to 8 wk, dosage increased, if ordered, to 50 mg t.i.d. for about 3 mo; then dosage adjusted based on glycosylated hemoglobin (HbA$_{1C}$) level.

Route	Onset	Peak	Duration
P.O.	Rapid	2 to 3 hr	Unknown

Mechanism of Action
Inhibits intestinal glucoside hydrolase enzymes, which normally hydrolyze oligosaccharides and disaccharides to glucose and other monosaccharides. This action delays carbohydrate digestion and absorption and reduces the postprandial blood glucose level.

Contraindications
Acute or chronic bowel disorder, diabetic ketoacidosis, hypersensitivity to miglitol or its components

Interactions
DRUGS
digestive enzyme preparations, intestinal adsorbents (activated charcoal): Decreased miglitol effects
digoxin: Decreased blood digoxin level
propranolol, ranitidine: Decreased bioavailability of these drugs

Adverse Reactions
GI: Abdominal pain, diarrhea, flatulence, hepatotoxicity
HEME: Low serum iron level
SKIN: Rash (transient)

Nursing Considerations
• Use miglitol cautiously in patient with serum creatinine level above 2 mg/dl.
• Be aware that some patients with type 2 diabetes also may receive a sulfonylurea as an adjunct to miglitol therapy.
• Give miglitol with first bite of each meal. Drug must have arrived at site of enzymatic action when carbohydrates reach small intestine.
• Review patient's HbA$_{1C}$ level, as appropriate, to monitor long-term glucose control.
• Monitor patient for evidence of overdose, such as transient increases in abdominal discomfort, diarrhea, and flatulence (but not hypoglycemia).

PATIENT TEACHING
• Explain that miglitol is an adjunct to diet, which is the primary treatment for type 2 diabetes mellitus.
• Instruct patient to take drug with first bite of each meal.
• Describe signs and symptoms of hypoglycemia and pathophysiology of diabetes to patient and family members.
• If miglitol is the only drug patient takes to control blood glucose level, explain that it won't cause hypoglycemia.
• If patient takes a sulfonylurea or insulin with miglitol, recommend that he keep a source of glucose readily available to reverse hypoglycemia.
• Explain the importance of monitoring blood and urine glucose levels.
• Explain that adverse GI reactions usually decrease in frequency and intensity over time.
• Teach obese patient about weight loss, calorie restriction, diet, and regular exercise, as indicated.

milnacipran hydrochloride

Savella

Class and Category
Chemical class: Selective norepinephrine and serotonin reuptake inhibitor
Therapeutic class: Anti-fibromyalgia
Pregnancy category: C

Indications and Dosages
➤ *To manage fibromyalgia*
TABLETS
Adults and adolescents age 17 and over. *Initial:* 12.5 mg on day one; 12.5 mg b.i.d. on days 2 and 3; 25 mg b.i.d. on days 4 through 7; and then 50 mg b.i.d., increased, if needed to 100 mg b.i.d. *Maximum:* 100 mg b.i.d.
DOSAGE ADJUSTMENT For patients with severe renal impairment (creatinine clearance of 5 to 29 ml/min/1.73 m^2), maintenance dosage reduced by half.

Route	Onset	Peak	Duration
P.O.	Unknown	2 to 4 hr	Unknown

Contraindications
Hypersensitivity to milnacipran or its com-

ponents, uncontrolled narrow-angle glaucoma, use within 14 days of an MAO inhibitor

Mechanism of Action

Inhibits reuptake of norepinephrine and serotonin by CNS neurons without affecting uptake of dopamine or other neurotransmitters, thereby increasing the amount of norepinephrine and serotonin available in nerve synapses. Elevated norepinephrine and serotonin levels may improve symptoms of fibromyalgia, including by central analgesic effect.

Interactions

DRUGS

aspirin, NSAIDs, warfarin: Increased risk of bleeding
clomipramine: Increased risk of euphoria and postural hypotension
clonidine: Possibly inhibited antihypertensive effect
CNS-active drugs: Possibly increased CNS effects
digoxin (I.V.): Possibly increased risk of postural hypotension and tachycardia
epinephrine, norepinephrine: Increased risk of arrhythmias and paroxysmal hypertension
lithium: Increased risk of serotonin syndrome
MAO inhibitors: Possibly hyperpyretic episodes, hypertensive crisis, serotonin syndrome, and severe seizures
serotonergic drugs such as SSRIs, triptans, and tramadol: Incrased risk of hypertension and coronary artery vasoconstriction

ACTIVITIES

alcohol use: Increased risk of liver impairment

Adverse Reactions

CNS: Anxiety, chills, delirium, depression, dizziness, fatigue, fever, hallucinations, headache, hypoesthesia, insomnia, irritability, loss of consciousness, migraine, neuroleptic malignant sydrome, parkinsonism, paresthesia, seizures, serotonin syndrome, suicidal ideation, tremor
CV: Chest pain, hypercholesterolemia, hypertension, hypertensive crisis, increased heart rate, palpitations, peripheral edema, somnolence, supraventricular tachycardia, tachycardia

EENT: Accommodation abnormality, blurred vision, dry mouth, mydriasis
ENDO: Hot flashes, hyperprolactinemia
GI: Abdominal distention or pain, anorexia, constipation, diarrhea, dyspepsia, elevated liver enzymes, gastroesophageal reflux, flatulence, hepatitis, jaundice, liver dysfunction, nausea, vomiting
GU: Acute renal failure, cystitis, decreased libido, dysuria, ejaculation disorder, erectile dysfunction, prostatitis, scrotal or testicular pain, testicular swelling, urinary hesitation, urine retention, urethral pain, UTI
HEME: Leukeopenia, neutropenia, thrombocytopenia
MS: Rhabdomyolysis
RESP: Dyspnea, upper respiratory infection
SKIN: Erythema multiforme, flushing, hyperhidrosis, night sweats, pruritus, rash, Stevens-Johnson syndrome
Other: Hyponatremia, weight gain or loss

Nursing Considerations

•Because milnacipran may aggravate liver disease, drug should not be given to patients with alcohol addiction or chronic liver disease.
•Use cautiously in patients with mild to moderate renal impairment and patients with significant hypertension or cardiac disease. Also use cautiously in patients with a history of dysuria, especially men with prostatic hypertrophy, prostatitis, and other lower urinary tract obstructive disorders.
•At least 14 days should elapse between stopping an MAO inhibitor and starting milnacipran therapy. At least 5 days should elapse between stopping milnacipran and starting an MAO inhibitor.
•Measure patient's blood pressure and heart rate before starting and periodically throughout milnacipran therapy because drug can raise blood pressure and heart rate. If hypertension or tachycardia occurs and persists, notify prescriber and expect dosage to be reduced or drug discontinued.
•Watch closely for suicidal tendencies, especially when therapy starts and dosage changes.
•**WARNING** Monitor patient closely for serotonin syndrome, a rare but serious adverse effect of selective serotonin reuptake inhibitors such as milnacipran. Signs and symptoms include agitation, confusion, diaphoresis, diarrhea, fever, hyperactive reflexes, poor

coordination, restlessness, shaking, talking or acting with uncontrolled excitement, tremor, and twitching. If symptoms occur, notify prescriber immediately, expect to discontinue drug, and provide supportive care.

•Monitor patient's liver function. If jaundice or signs and symptoms of liver dysfunction occur, notify prescriber and expect drug to be discontinued.

•Watch for hypersensitivity reactions, especially in patients who have an aspirin sensitivity, because drug contains the yellow dye tartrazine.

•Check patient's serum sodium level, as ordered, because drug may cause hyponatremia, especially in elderly patients, patients taking diuretics, and patients who are volume depleted.

•Expect to taper drug when no longer needed, as ordered, to minimize adverse reactions.

PATIENT TEACHING
•Urge family or caregiver to watch patient closely for suicidal tendencies, especially when therapy starts or dosage changes.

•Caution patient against stopping drug abruptly because serious adverse effects may result.

•Instruct patient to alert all prescribers that he takes milnacipran.

•Tell patient to have his blood pressure monitored regularly throughout milnacipran therapy.

•Advise patient to avoid activities, such as driving, that require alertness until the CNS effects of milnacipran are known.

•Caution patient to avoid aspirin and NSAIDs, if possible, while taking milnacipran.

milrinone lactate

Primacor

Class and Category
Chemical class: Bipyridine derivative
Therapeutic class: Inotropic, vasodilator
Pregnancy category: C

Indications and Dosages
➤ *To provide short-term treatment of acute heart failure*
I.V. INFUSION
Adults. *Loading:* 50 mcg/kg over 10 min (at

least 0.375 mcg/kg/min). *Usual:* 0.375 to 0.75 mcg/kg/min. *Maximum:* 1.13 mg/kg daily.

DOSAGE ADJUSTMENT Dosage adjusted according to cardiac output, pulmonary artery wedge pressure (PAWP), and clinical response. If creatinine clearance is 30 to 39 ml/min/1.73 m², infusion rate reduced to 0.33 mcg/kg/min; if 20 to 29 ml/min/1.73 m², to 0.28 mcg/kg/min; if 10 to 19 ml/min/1.73 m², to 0.23 mcg/kg/min; and if less than 9 ml/min/1.73 m², to 0.2 mcg/kg/min.

Route	Onset	Peak	Duration
I.V.	5 to 15 min	Unknown	3 to 6 hr

Incompatibilities
Don't administer milrinone through same I.V. line as furosemide because precipitate will form. Don't add other drugs to premixed milrinone flexible containers.

Contraindications
Hypersensitivity to milrinone or its components

Interactions
DRUGS
antihypertensives: Possibly hypotension

Adverse Reactions
CNS: Headache, tremor
CV: Angina, hypotension, supraventricular arrhythmias, ventricular ectopic activity, ventricular fibrillation, ventricular tachycardia, torsades de pointes
GI: Liver function test abnormalities
HEME: Thrombocytopenia
RESP: Bronchospasm
SKIN: Rash
Other: Anaphylactic shock, hypokalemia, infusion site reactions (pain, swelling, redness)

Nursing Considerations
•Make sure ECG equipment is available for continuous monitoring during milrinone therapy.

•Discard drug if it's discolored or contains particles.

•For loading dose, directly infuse undiluted drug into I.V. line with a compatible infusing solution. For continuous infusion, dilute drug with half-normal (0.45) saline solution, normal saline solution, or D₅W. Dilution isn't needed when using premixed milrinone flexi-

Mechanism of Action

An inotropic drug, milrinone increases the force of myocardial contraction—and cardiac output—by blocking the enzyme phosphodiesterase. Normally, this enzyme is activated by hormones binding to cell membrane receptors. As shown below left, phosphodiesterase normally degrades intracellular cAMP, which restricts calcium movement into myocardial cells. By inhibiting phosphodiesterase, as shown below right, milrinone slows the rate of cAMP degradation, increasing the intracellular cAMP level and the amount of calcium that enters myocardial cells. In blood vessels, increased cAMP causes smooth-muscle relaxation, which improves cardiac output by reducing preload and afterload.

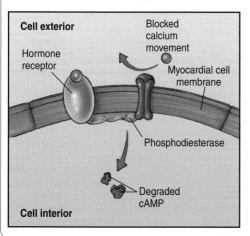

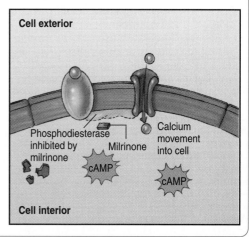

ble containers.
• Check platelet count before and periodically during infusion, as ordered. Expect to discontinue drug if platelet count falls below 150,000/mm^3.
• Administer loading dose using a controlled-rate infusion device. For continuous infusion, use a calibrated electronic infusion device.
• Monitor cardiac output, pulmonary artery wedge pressure, blood pressure, heart rate, weight, and fluid status during therapy to determine drug effectiveness.
• Monitor renal and liver function test results and serum electrolyte levels. Notify prescriber of abnormalities.
• If severe hypotension develops, notify prescriber immediately and expect to stop drug.
• Expect patient to receive digoxin before starting milrinone, which can increase ventricular response rate.

PATIENT TEACHING
• Reassure patient that you will be present and that he will be monitored constantly during therapy.

minocycline

Minocin

minocycline hydrochloride

Alti-Minocycline (CAN), Apo-Minocycline (CAN), Dynacin, Gen-Minocycline (CAN), Minocin, Novo-Minocycline (CAN), Vectrin

Class and Category

Chemical class: Tetracycline
Therapeutic class: Antibiotic, antiprotozoal
Pregnancy category: D

Indications and Dosages

➤ *To treat bartonellosis, brucellosis, chancroid, granuloma inguinale, inclusion conjunctivitis, lymphogranuloma venereum, nongonococcal urethritis, plague, psittacosis, Q fever, relapsing fever, respiratory tract infections (including pneumonia), rickettsial pox, Rocky Mountain spotted fever, tulare-*

M

mia, typhus, and UTI caused by gram-negative organisms (including Bartonella bacilliformis, Brucella *species,* Haemophilus ducreyi, Haemophilus influenzae, Vibrio cholerae, *and* Yersinia pestis*), susceptible gram-positive organisms (including certain strains of* Streptococcus pneumoniae)*, and other organisms (including* Actinomyces *species,* Bacillus anthracis, Borrelia recurrentis, Chlamydia *species,* Mycoplasma pneumoniae, *and* Rickettsiae)*; as adjunct to treat intestinal amebiasis and as alternative to treat listeriosis caused by* Listeria monocytogenes, *syphilis caused by* Treponema pallidum, *and yaws caused by* Treponema pertenue *for nonpregnant patients allergic to penicillin*

CAPSULES, ORAL SUSPENSION
Adults and adolescents. *Initial:* 200 mg. *Maintenance:* 100 mg every 12 hr. Or 100 to 200 mg initially followed by 50 mg every 6 hr.
Children over age 8. *Initial:* 4 mg/kg. *Maintenance:* 2 mg/kg every 12 hr.

I.V. INJECTION
Adults and adolescents. *Initial:* 200 mg. *Maintenance:* 100 mg every 12 hr. *Maximum:* 400 mg daily.
Children over age 8. *Initial:* 4 mg/kg. *Maintenance:* 2 mg/kg every 12 hr.
DOSAGE ADJUSTMENT If patient has renal impairment, don't exceed 200 mg daily.

➤ *As adjunct to treat inflammatory acne vulgaris that's unresponsive to oral tetracycline or erythromycin*
CAPSULES, ORAL SUSPENSION
Adults and adolescents. 50 mg once daily to t.i.d.

➤ *To treat uncomplicated gonorrhea caused by* Neisseria gonorrhoeae *in nonpregnant patients allergic to penicillin*
CAPSULES, ORAL SUSPENSION
Adults and adolescents. *Initial:* 200 mg. *Maintenance:* 100 mg every 12 hr for at least 4 days.

➤ *To treat uncomplicated gonococcal urethritis in men*
CAPSULES, ORAL SUSPENSION
Adults and adolescents. 100 mg b.i.d. for 5 days.

➤ *To treat asymptomatic meningococcal*

carriers with Neisseria meningitidis *in nasopharynx*
CAPSULES, ORAL SUSPENSION
Adults and adolescents. 100 mg every 12 hr for 5 days.
Children over age 8. *Initial:* 4 mg/kg. *Maintenance:* 2 mg/kg every 12 hr for 5 days.

➤ *To treat infections caused by* Mycobacterium marinum
CAPSULES, ORAL SUSPENSION
Adults. 100 mg every 12 hr for 6 to 8 wk.

Route	Onset	Peak	Duration
P.O.	Unknown	2 to 4 hr	6 to 12 hr
I.V.	Unknown	Unknown	6 to 12 hr

Mechanism of Action
Inhibits bacterial protein synthesis by competitively binding to the 30S ribosomal subunit of the mRNA-ribosome complex of certain organisms.

Incompatibilities
Don't mix minocycline in same syringe with solution that contains calcium because precipitate will form.

Contraindications
Hypersensitivity to minocycline, other tetracyclines, or their components

Interactions
DRUGS
aluminum-, calcium-, or magnesium-containing antacids; calcium supplements; choline and magnesium salicylates; iron-containing preparations; magnesium-containing laxatives; sodium bicarbonate: Possibly formation of nonabsorbable complex, impaired minocycline absorption
cholestyramine, colestipol: Possibly impaired cholestyramine or colestipol absorption
cimetidine: Possibly decreased GI absorption and effectiveness of minocycline
digoxin: Possibly increased blood digoxin level and risk of digitalis toxicity
insulin: Possibly decreased need for insulin
iron salts: Possibly decreased GI absorption and antimicrobial effect of minocycline
lithium: Possibly increased or decreased blood lithium level
methoxyflurane: Increased risk of nephrotox-

icity

oral anticoagulants: Possibly potentiated anticoagulant effects

oral contraceptives containing estrogen: Decreased contraceptive effectiveness, increased risk of breakthrough bleeding

penicillin: Interference with bactericidal action of penicillin

vitamin A: Possibly benign intracranial hypertension

Adverse Reactions

CNS: Dizziness, fever, headache, light-headedness, unsteadiness, vertigo

CV: Pericarditis

EENT: Blurred vision, darkened or discolored tongue, glossitis, papilledema, tooth discoloration, vision changes

GI: Abdominal cramps or pain, anorexia, diarrhea, dysphagia, enterocolitis, esophageal irritation and ulceration, hepatitis, hepatotoxicity, indigestion, nausea, pancreatitis, pseudomembranous colitis, vomiting

GU: Genital candidiasis, nephrotoxicity

HEME: Eosinophilia, hemolytic anemia, neutropenia, thrombocytopenia, thrombocytopenic purpura

MS: Arthralgia, myopathy (transient)

RESP: Pulmonary infiltrates (with eosinophilia)

SKIN: Erythema multiforme, exfoliative dermatitis, brown pigmentation of skin and mucous membranes, erythematous and maculopapular rash, jaundice, onycholysis, photosensitivity, pruritus, purpura (anaphylactoid), Stevens-Johnson syndrome, urticaria

Other: Anaphylaxis, angioedema, serum sicknesslike reaction, systemic lupus erythematosus exacerbation

Nursing Considerations

•Use minocycline cautiously in patients with renal or hepatic dysfunction and in those taking other hepatotoxic drugs because drug may cause nephrotoxicity or hepatotoxicity.

•**WARNING** Notify prescriber if patient is breast-feeding because minocycline appears in breast milk and may have toxic effects.

•Monitor blood, renal, and hepatic tests before and during long-term therapy.

•Shake oral suspension well before use.

•To prepare drug for I.V. use, reconstitute each 100-mg vial with 5 to 10 ml of sterile water for injection. Further dilute in 500 to 1,000 ml of normal saline solution, D_5W,

dextrose 5% in normal saline solution, or Ringer's or lactated Ringer's solution. Administer final dilution immediately, but avoid rapid administration.

•Store reconstituted drug at room temperature and use within 24 hours.

•Assess patient for signs of superinfection; if they appear, notify prescriber, discontinue minocycline, and start appropriate therapy, as ordered.

•Monitor patient for development of foul smelling diarrhea, which suggests *Clostridium difficile*. If present, notify prescriber, obtain stool culture, and expect to withhold minocycline and provide supportive care, as indicated and ordered.

•Monitor PT in patient who also takes an anticoagulant during minocycline therapy.

PATIENT TEACHING

•Instruct patient to shake oral suspension well and to use calibrated measuring device.

•Advise patient to take minocycline with a full glass of water, with food or milk, and in an upright position to minimize esophageal and GI irritation.

•Direct patient to take a missed dose as soon as he remembers unless it's nearly time for the next dose. Caution against double-dosing.

•Instruct patient not to take minocycline within 2 hours of an antacid or 3 hours of an iron preparation.

•Urge patient to complete full course of treatment even if he feels better beforehand.

•Instruct patient to notify prescriber if no improvement occurs in a few days.

•Advise patient to avoid prolonged exposure to sun or sunlamps during therapy.

•Counsel female patient to avoid becoming pregnant because minocycline should be avoided, if possible, during tooth development (last half of gestation up to age 8). Drug may permanently turn teeth yellow, gray, or brown and cause enamel hypoplasia. It also may slow skeletal growth and cause congenital anomalies, including limb reduction.

•Encourage patient who uses an oral contraceptive to use additional contraceptive method during minocycline therapy.

•Instruct patient to notify prescriber immediately about blurred vision, dizziness, headache, known or suspected pregnancy, and unsteadiness.

M

• Explain that diarrhea may occur up to 2 months after completing therapy; urge patient to notify prescriber if it occurs.

minoxidil (oral)

Loniten

minoxidil (topical)

Apo-Gain (CAN), Gen-Minoxidil (CAN), Minox (CAN), Minoxigaine (CAN), Rogaine (CAN), Rogaine ES for Men, Rogaine for Men, Rogaine for Women

Class and Category

Chemical class: Piperidinopyrimidine derivative
Therapeutic class: Antihypertensive (oral), hair-growth stimulant (topical)
Pregnancy category: C

Indications and Dosages

➤ *To manage severe symptomatic hypertension or hypertension with target organ damage that's unresponsive to other treatment*

TABLETS
Adults and adolescents. *Initial:* 5 mg as a single dose or divided doses b.i.d. Increased, as directed, after at least 3 days. *Maintenance:* 10 to 40 mg daily. *Maximum:* 100 mg daily.
Children. *Initial:* 0.2 mg/kg daily. Increased, as directed, after at least 3 days. *Maintenance:* 0.25 to 1 mg/kg daily as a single dose or in divided doses b.i.d. *Maximum:* 50-mg starting dose, 50 mg daily.
DOSAGE ADJUSTMENT Dosage possibly reduced for elderly patients and for patients who have renal failure or are undergoing dialysis.

➤ *To treat alopecia*
TOPICAL 2%
Adults up to age 65. 1 ml applied b.i.d. to area of desired hair growth.
TOPICAL 5%
Adult men up to age 65. 1 ml applied b.i.d. to area of desired hair growth.

Route	Onset	Peak	Duration
P.O.	30 min	2 to 3 hr	24 to 48 hr
Topical 2%	4 mo	1 yr	Unknown
Topical 5%	2 mo	1 yr	Unknown

Mechanism of Action

Reduces blood pressure by inhibiting intracellular phosphodiesterase, an enzyme that facilitates hydrolysis of cAMP and cGMP. This action decreases the intracellular cAMP level, relaxes arterial smooth muscles, and lowers blood pressure. Oral minoxidil produces greater dilation in arteries than in veins. It also reduces peripheral resistance and increases heart rate, cardiac output, and stroke volume.

Topical minoxidil may cause hair regrowth by increasing cutaneous blood flow and stimulating resting hair follicles.

Contraindications

Acute MI; dissecting aortic aneurysm; hypersensitivity to minoxidil or its components, including propylene glycol; pheochromocytoma; skin irritation or abrasions (topical)

Interactions

DRUGS
guanethidine: Possibly severe hypotension, increased risk of orthostatic hypotension (oral)
nitrates, other hypotension-producing drugs, potent parenteral antihypertensives: Possibly severe hypotension
NSAIDs, sympathomimetics: Decreased antihypertensive effects
topical petrolatum, topical steroids: Increased absorption of topical minoxidil if used on same area
topical retinoids: Increased absorption of topical minoxidil and, possibly, formation of granulation tissue

Adverse Reactions

CNS: Fatigue, paresthesia (oral); light-headedness, neuritis (topical); headache (both)
CV: ECG changes, heart failure, pericardial tamponade, pericarditis, rebound hypertension (oral); cardiac tamponade, hypotension, palpitations, reflex hypertension (topical); angina, edema, fast or irregular heartbeat, pericardial effusion (both)
EENT: Vision changes (topical)
ENDO: Breast tenderness (oral)
GI: Abdominal distention, ascites, nausea, vomiting (oral)
GU: Elevated BUN and serum creatinine levels (oral); sexual dysfunction (topical)

HEME: Leukopenia; thrombocytopenia; transient decrease in hematocrit, hemoglobin, and erythrocyte counts (oral)
RESP: Dyspnea, pulmonary hypertension (oral)
SKIN: Flushing, hyperpigmentation, Stevens-Johnson syndrome (oral); allergic contact dermatitis, alopecia, dry or flaky skin, eczema, erythema, folliculitis, scalp burning (topical); hypertrichosis, rash (both)
Other: Facial edema (topical); sodium and water retention, weight gain (both)

Nursing Considerations

•**WARNING** Be aware that patient who receives guanethidine should be hospitalized before starting oral minoxidil therapy so that his blood pressure can be monitored.
•Be aware that drug isn't usually prescribed for mild hypertension.
•For rapid management of hypertension, expect to adjust dosage up to every 6 hours and to monitor patient as prescribed. Also expect to give a beta blocker and diuretic.
•Monitor progress by measuring blood pressure frequently and weight daily. Evaluate for signs of fluid and sodium retention and for other systemic adverse reactions.
•Watch for signs of pericardial effusion. Be prepared to stop oral minoxidil, if ordered.
•Expect to discontinue oral minoxidil gradually because abrupt discontinuation may lead to rebound hypertension.
•Apply topical drug only on healthy scalp. Avoid using on sunburned or abraded scalp.
•Use gloves when applying solution.
•Avoid inhaling mist from spray applicator.
•Expect minoxidil to be least effective in men with mainly frontal hair loss.
•Expect topical form to have little effect on blood pressure in patients who don't have hypertension.

PATIENT TEACHING
•Inform patient that oral minoxidil controls but doesn't cure hypertension.
•Advise him to take tablets at the same time every day.
•Teach patient how to take his radial pulse, and advise him to measure it daily. Instruct him to notify prescriber if it exceeds normal rate by 20 beats/minute or more.
•Stress the importance of daily blood pressure and weight measurements.
•Instruct patient to notify prescriber immediately about bloating, breathing problems, a fast or irregular heartbeat, flushed or red skin, swelling of feet or lower legs, or weight gain of more than 5 lb (2.3 kg) in 1 day.
•Advise patient to have regular checkups with prescriber to monitor progress.
•Urge patient to consult prescriber before taking other prescription or OTC drugs.
•Reassure patient that body hair thickening and darkening reverses after oral minoxidil is discontinued.
•For patient using topical minoxidil, teach proper application technique and provide manufacturer's written instructions. Advise him to wear gloves when applying drug and to make sure hair and scalp are dry first.
•Instruct patient to start applying drug at center of balding area, to let dry for 2 to 4 hours, and not to use hairdryer to help it dry faster.
•Warn patient to avoid applying drug to abraded, irritated, or sunburned areas of scalp; to avoid inhaling mist when using a spray applicator; and to avoid getting drug in his eyes, nose, or mouth. If accidental contact does occur, advise him to flush the area with large amounts of cool tap water.
•Instruct patient not to shampoo his hair for at least 4 hours after application and to avoid using other skin products on treated skin. Direct him to avoid using minoxidil 24 hours before and after applying chemical hair products, such as dyes and relaxers.
•Caution patient not to use more drug or apply it more often than prescribed and not to apply it to other body areas. Explain the risk of adverse systemic reactions with excessive topical use.
•Tell patient to keep topical minoxidil away from heat or flame because it's flammable.
•Inform patient that minoxidil may stain clothing, hats, or bed linens before it's dry.
•Instruct patient to notify prescriber if burning, itching, or redness develops after application. For severe reactions, advise patient to wash drug off and consult prescriber before applying it again.
•Urge patient to consult prescriber if hair loss continues after 2 weeks or if growth fails to increase in 4 months.
•Inform patient that new hair growth may be lost 3 to 4 months after stopping topical minoxidil and that progressive hair loss will resume.

M

mirtazapine

Remeron, Remeron SolTab

Class and Category

Chemical class: Piperazinoazepine
Therapeutic class: Antidepressant
Pregnancy category: C

Indications and Dosages

➤ *To treat major depression*

DISINTEGRATING TABLETS, TABLETS

Adults. *Initial:* 15 mg daily, preferably at bedtime. Increased as needed and tolerated at 1- to 2-wk intervals. *Maximum:* 45 mg daily.

Route	Onset	Peak	Duration
P.O.	1 to 2 wk	6 wk or longer	Unknown

Mechanism of Action

May inhibit neuronal reuptake of norepinephrine and serotonin. By doing so, this tetracyclic antidepressant increases the action of these neurotransmitters in nerve cells. Increased neuronal serotonin and norepinephrine levels may elevate mood.

Contraindications

Hypersensitivity to mirtazapine or its components, use within 14 days of an MAO inhibitor

Interactions

DRUGS

antihypertensives: Increased hypotensive effects of these drugs or enhanced mirtazapine effects
anxiolytics, hypnotics, other CNS depressants (including sedatives): Increased CNS depression
MAO inhibitors: Possibly hyperpyrexia, hypertension, seizures

ACTIVITIES

alcohol use: Increased CNS depression

Adverse Reactions

CNS: Agitation, amnesia, anxiety, apathy, asthenia, ataxia, cerebral ischemia, chills, confusion, delirium, delusions, depersonalization, depression, dizziness, dream disturbances, drowsiness, dyskinesia, dystonia, emotional lability, euphoria, extrapyramidal reactions, fever, hallucinations, hostility, hyperkinesia, hyperreflexia, hypoesthesia, hypokinesia, lack of coordination, malaise, mania, migraine headache, neurosis, paranoia, paresthesia, seizures, somnolence, syncope, tremor, vertigo
CV: Angina, bradycardia, edema, hypercholesterolemia, hypertension, hypertriglyceridemia, hypotension, MI, orthostatic hypotension, peripheral edema, PVCs, vasodilation
EENT: Accommodation disturbances, conjunctivitis, dry mouth, earache, epistaxis, eye pain, glaucoma, gingival bleeding, glossitis, hearing loss, hyperacusis, keratoconjunctivitis, lacrimation, pharyngitis, sinusitis, stomatitis
ENDO: Breast pain
GI: Abdominal distention and pain, anorexia, cholecystitis, colitis, constipation, elevated ALT level, eructation, increased appetite, nausea, thirst, vomiting
GU: Amenorrhea, cystitis, dysmenorrhea, dysuria, hematuria, impotence, increased libido, leukorrhea, renal calculi, urinary frequency and incontinence, urine retention, UTI, vaginitis
HEME: Agranulocytosis, neutropenia
MS: Arthralgia, back pain, dysarthria, muscle twitching, myalgia, myasthenia, neck pain and rigidity
RESP: Asthma, bronchitis, cough, dyspnea, pneumonia
SKIN: Acne, alopecia, dry skin, exfoliative dermatitis, photosensitivity, pruritus, rash
Other: Dehydration, facial edema, flulike symptoms, herpes simplex, weight change

Nursing Considerations

• Administer mirtazapine before bedtime.
• Expect disintegrating tablet to dissolve on patient's tongue within 30 seconds.
• **WARNING** Don't give drug within 14 days of an MAO inhibitor to avoid serious, possibly fatal, reaction.
• If patient takes drug for depression, watch closely for suicidal tendencies, especially when therapy starts or dosage changes, because depression may temporarily worsen.
• Monitor patient closely for infection (fever, pharyngitis, stomatitis), which may be linked to a low WBC count. If these signs occur, notify prescriber and expect to stop drug.
• Expect mirtazapine therapy to last 6 months or longer for acute depression.

PATIENT TEACHING

• Instruct patient not to swallow disintegrat-

ing tablet. Tell him to hold tablet on tongue and allow it to dissolve. Inform him that tablet will dissolve within 30 seconds.
•Inform phenylketonuric patient that mirtazapine disintegrating tablets contain phenlyalanine 2.6 mg per 15-mg tablet, 5.2 mg per 30-mg tablet, and 7.8 mg per 45-mg tablet.
•Instruct patient to avoid alcohol and other CNS depressants during mirtazapine therapy and for up to 7 days after drug is discontinued.
•Advise patient to avoid potentially hazardous activities until drug's CNS effects are known.
•Direct patient to change position slowly to minimize the effects of orthostatic hypotension.
•Instruct patient to notify prescriber immediately about chills, fever, mouth irritation, sore throat, and other signs of infection.
•Encourage patient to visit prescriber regularly during therapy to monitor progress.

misoprostol

Cytotec

Class and Category

Chemical class: Prostaglandin E_1 analogue
Therapeutic class: Antiulcer, gastric antisecretory
Pregnancy category: X

Indications and Dosages

➤ *To prevent NSAID-induced gastric ulcers*
TABLETS
Adults. 200 mcg q.i.d. or 400 mcg b.i.d. with food, with last dose at bedtime every day.
DOSAGE ADJUSTMENT Dosage reduced to 100 mcg q.i.d. if patient can't tolerate 200-mcg dose.

Route	Onset	Peak	Duration
P.O.	30 min	60 to 90 min	3 to 6 hr

Mechanism of Action

May protect the stomach from NSAID-induced mucosal damage by increasing gastric mucus production and mucosal bicarbonate secretion. Misoprostol also inhibits gastric acid secretion caused by such stimuli as food, coffee, and histamine.

Contraindications

Breast-feeding, hypersensitivity to prostaglandins or their analogues, in pregnant women (to prevent NSAID-induced gastric ulcers)

Interactions
DRUGS
magnesium-containing antacids: Increased misoprostol-induced diarrhea

Adverse Reactions
CNS: Headache, syncope
CV: Arrhythmias, chest pain, edema, hypertension, hypotension, increased cardiac enzyme levels, MI, phlebitis, thromboembolism
GI: Abdominal pain, constipation, diarrhea, flatulence, indigestion, nausea, vomiting
GU: Dysmenorrhea, hypermenorrhea, menstrual irregularities, vaginal bleeding
SKIN: Diaphoresis

Nursing Considerations
•**WARNING** Ask female patient if she is or may be pregnant. If so, notify prescriber because misoprostol may cause uterine bleeding, contractions, and spontaneous abortion as well as teratogenic effects in the fetus.
•Use drug cautiously in patients with cerebrovascular disease, coronary artery disease, or uncontrolled epilepsy because of the risk of severe complications.
•Also use misoprostol cautiously in patients with inflammatory bowel disease because drug may worsen intestinal inflammation and cause diarrhea. If diarrhea causes severe dehydration, misoprostol may be discontinued.

PATIENT TEACHING
•Caution female patient about the risk of taking misoprostol during pregnancy, and urge her to use reliable contraception during therapy. Urge her to notify prescriber immediately if she is or might be pregnant.
•Instruct patient to take misoprostol with meals and at bedtime.
•Advise patient that he may take NSAIDs, if prescribed, during misoprostol therapy.
•Explain that diarrhea is dose related and usually resolves after 8 days. Tell patient to avoid magnesium-containing antacids because they may worsen diarrhea and to call prescriber if diarrhea lasts more than 8 days.
•Urge female patient to notify prescriber immediately about postmenopausal bleeding; she may need diagnostic tests.

M

mitoxantrone hydrochloride

Novantrone

Class and Category

Chemical class: Anthracenedione
Therapeutic class: Antineoplastic
Pregnancy category: D

Indications and Dosages

➤ *To reduce neurologic disability and frequency of relapses in patients with secondary (chronic) progressive, progressive relapsing, or worsening relapsing-remitting multiple sclerosis (patients whose neurologic status is significantly abnormal between relapses)*

I.V. INFUSION
Adults. 12 mg/m^2 over 5 to 15 min every 3 mo.
Maximum: Cumulative dose of 140 mg/m^2.

➤ *As adjunct to treat pain related to advanced hormone-refractory prostate cancer*

I.V. INFUSION
Adults. 12 to 14 mg/m^2 over 5 to 15 min every 21 days.

➤ *As adjunct to treat acute nonlymphocytic leukemia (ANLL)*

I.V. INFUSION
Adults. *Initial:* 12 mg/m^2 over at least 3 min on days 1 to 3 with 100 mg/m^2 of cytarabine as a continuous 24-hr infusion on days 1 to 7. If patient's antileukemic response is inadequate or incomplete, a second induction course is given at the same dosage. *Maintenance:* 6 wk after induction, 12 mg/m^2 over at least 3 min on days 1 and 2 with 100 mg/m^2 of cytarabine as a continuous 24-hr infusion on days 1 to 5. A second maintenance course is given 4 wk after the first if needed and tolerated.

Incompatibilities

Don't mix mitoxantrone in the same infusion as heparin (because a precipitate may form); don't mix with any other drugs.

Contraindications

Hypersensitivity to mitoxantrone or its components

Interactions

DRUGS
allopurinol, colchicine, probenecid, sulfin-pyrazone: Possibly interference with antihyperuricemic action of these drugs
blood-dyscrasia–causing drugs (such as cephalosporins and sulfasalazine): Increased risk of leukopenia and thrombocytopenia
bone marrow depressants, such as carboplatin and lomustine: Possibly additive bone marrow depression
daunorubicin, doxorubicin: Increased risk of cardiotoxicity
methotrexate and other antineoplastics: Risk of developing leukemia
vaccines, killed virus: Decreased antibody response to vaccine
vaccines, live virus: Increased risk of replication of and adverse effects of vaccine virus, decreased antibody response to vaccine

Mechanism of Action

Binds to DNA, causing cross-linkage and strand breakage, interfering with RNA synthesis, and inhibiting topoisomerase II, an enzyme that uncoils and repairs damaged DNA. Mitoxantrone produces a cytocidal effect on proliferating and nonproliferating cells and doesn't appear to be cell-cycle specific. It's known to inhibit B-cell, T-cell, and macrophage proliferation and impair antigen function.

Adverse Reactions

CNS: Headache, seizures
CV: Arrhythmias, chest pain, congestive heart failure, decreased left ventricular ejection fraction, ECG changes
EENT: Blue-colored cornea, conjunctivitis, mucositis, stomatitis
GI: Abdominal pain, diarrhea, GI bleeding, nausea, vomiting
GU: Blue-green urine, renal failure
HEME: Acute myelogenous leukemia, leukopenia, other leukemias, thrombocytopenia
MS: Myelodysplasia
RESP: Cough, dyspnea
SKIN: Alopecia, extravasation, jaundice
Other: Allergic reaction, anaphylaxis, hyperuricemia, infection, infusion site pain or redness

Nursing Considerations

•Before mitoxantrone therapy and before each dose, expect patient to have an ECG and evaluation of his left ventricular ejection fraction. Expect to obtain hematocrit, hemoglobin level, and CBC with platelet count. If patient's left ventricular ejection fraction drops below normal, expect drug to be discontinued.

•Be aware that drug shouldn't be given to patient with multiple sclerosis whose neutrophil count is less than 1,500/mm^3.

•Obtain liver function test results, as ordered, before each course of therapy. Expect that drug won't be given to patient with multiple sclerosis and abnormal liver function.

•Assess patient for cardiac dysfunction throughout therapy. Notify prescriber of any significant changes, and expect drug to be discontinued.

•Anticipate obtaining pregnancy test before each course of therapy for women of childbearing age who have multiple sclerosis.

•Follow facility policy for handling antineoplastics. Be aware that manufacturer recommends goggles, gloves, and a gown during drug preparation and administration.

•Before infusing drug, dilute it in at least 50 ml of normal saline solution or D$_5$W.

•**WARNING** Be aware that drug shouldn't be given intrathecally because paralysis may occur.

•If mitoxantrone solution contacts your skin or mucosa, wash thoroughly with warm water. If it contacts your eyes, irrigate them thoroughly with water or normal saline solution.

•Discard unused diluted solution because it contains no preservatives. After penetration of the stopper, store undiluted drug for up to 7 days at room temperature or 14 days under refrigeration. Avoid freezing drug.

•If extravasation occurs, stop the infusion immediately and notify prescriber. Reinsert the I.V. line in another vein and resume the infusion. Although mitoxantrone is a nonvesicant, observe the extravasation site for signs of necrosis or phlebitis.

•Monitor patients with chickenpox or recent exposure to it and patients with herpes zoster for severe, generalized disease.

•Watch for evidence of cardiotoxicity, such as arrhythmias and chest pain, in patient with heart disease. Risk increases when cumulative dose reaches 140 mg/m^2 in cancer patient, 100 mg/m^2 in multiple sclerosis patient.

•Monitor blood uric acid level for hyperuricemia in patients with a history of gout or renal calculi. Expect to administer allopurinol, as prescribed, to patients with leukemia or lymphoma who have elevated blood uric acid level to prevent uric acid nephropathy.

•**WARNING** If severe or life-threatening nonhematologic or hematologic toxicity occurs during the first induction course, expect to withhold the second course until it resolves.

•If patient develops thrombocytopenia, take precautions according to facility policy.

•Assess patient for evidence of infection, such as fever, if leukopenia occurs. Expect to obtain appropriate specimens for culture and sensitivity testing.

•Be aware that patients receiving mitoxantrone in combination with other antineoplastics or radiation therapy are at risk for developing secondary leukemia, including acute myelogenous leukemia.

PATIENT TEACHING

•Advise patient to complete dental work, if possible, before treatment begins or defer it until blood counts return to normal; drug may delay healing and cause gingival bleeding. Teach patient proper oral hygiene, and advise use of a toothbrush with soft bristles.

•Urge patient to drink plenty of fluid to increase urine output and uric acid excretion.

•Advise patient to contact prescriber immediately if GI upset occurs, but to continue taking drug unless otherwise directed.

•Stress the importance of complying with the dosage regimen and keeping follow-up medical and laboratory appointments.

•Explain that urine may appear blue-green for 24 hours after treatment and that the whites of the eyes may appear blue. Stress that these effects are temporary and harmless. Explain that hair loss is possible, but that hair should return after therapy ends.

•Caution patient not to receive immunizations unless approved by prescriber. Also, advise persons who live in same household as patient to avoid receiving immunization with oral polio vaccine. Tell patient to avoid persons who recently received the oral polio vaccine or to wear a mask over his nose and mouth.

•Instruct patient to avoid persons with infections if bone marrow depression occurs. Advise patient to contact prescriber if fever,

chills, cough, hoarseness, lower back or side pain, or painful or difficult urination occurs; these changes may signal an infection.
•Tell patient to contact prescriber immediately if he notices unusual bleeding or bruising, black or tarry stools, blood in urine or stool, or pinpoint red spots on his skin.
•Urge patient not to touch his eyes or the inside of his nose unless he has just washed his hands.
•Stress the need to avoid accidental cuts, as from a razor or fingernail clippers, because they may cause excessive bleeding or infection.
•Caution patient to avoid contact sports or activities that may cause bruising or injury.
•Urge patient to comply with yearly examinations after therapy ends to check for late-occurring drug-induced heart problems.

modafinil

Provigil

Class, Category, and Schedule
Chemical class: Benzhydryl sulfinylacetamide derivative
Therapeutic class: CNS stimulant
Pregnancy category: C
Controlled substance schedule: IV

Indications and Dosages
➤ *To improve daytime wakefulness in patients with narcolepsy, obstructive sleep apnea hypopnea syndrome, and shift work sleep disorder*
TABLETS
Adults and adolescents age 16 and over. 200 mg daily in the morning or 1 hr before starting work shift *Maximum:* 400 mg daily.
DOSAGE ADJUSTMENT For patients with severe hepatic impairment, dosage should be reduced by 50%.

Mechanism of Action
May inhibit the release of gamma-aminobutyric acid (GABA), the most common inhibitory neurotransmitter, or CNS depressant, in the brain. Modafinil also increases the release of glutamate, an excitatory neurotransmitter, or CNS stimulant, in the thalamus and hippocampus. These two actions may improve wakefulness.

Contraindications
Hypersensitivity to modafinil or its components

Interactions
DRUGS
amitriptyline, citalopram, clomipramine, diazepam, imipramine, propranolol, tolbutamide, topiramate: Possibly prolonged elimination time and increased blood levels of these drugs
carbamazepine: Possibly decreased modafinil effectiveness and decreased blood carbamazepine level
cimetidine, clarithromycin, erythromycin, fluconazole, fluoxetine, fluvoxamine, itraconazole, ketoconazole, nefazodone, sertraline: Possibly inhibited metabolism, decreased clearance, and increased blood level of modafinil
contraceptive-containing implants or devices, oral contraceptives: Possibly contraceptive failure
cyclosporine: Possibly decreased blood cyclosporine level and increased risk of organ transplant rejection
dexamethasone, phenobarbital and other barbiturates, primidone, rifabutin, rifampin: Possibly decreased blood level and effectiveness of modafinil
dextroamphetamine, methylphenidate: Possibly 1-hour delay in modafinil absorption when these drugs are administered together
fosphenytoin, mephenytoin, phenytoin: Possibly decreased effectiveness of modafinil, increased blood phenytoin level, and increased risk of phenytoin toxicity
theophylline: Possibly decreased blood level and effectiveness of theophylline
triazolam: Possibly decreased effectiveness of triazolam
warfarin: Possibly decreased warfarin metabolism and increased risk of bleeding
FOODS
all foods: 1-hour delay in modafinil absorption and possibly delayed onset of action
caffeine: Increased CNS stimulation
grapefruit juice: Possibly decreased modafinil metabolism

Adverse Reactions
CNS: Aggressiveness, agitation, anxiety, confusion, delusions, depression, hallucinations, headache, insomnia, mania, nervousness, psychosis, suicidal ideation
GI: Nausea

HEME: Agranulocytosis
SKIN: Drug rash with eosinophilia and systemic symptoms (DRESS), rash, Stevens-Johnson syndrome, toxic epidermal necrolysis
Other: Anaphylaxis, angioedema, infection, multi-organ hypersensitivity

Nursing Considerations
•Modafinil shouldn't be given to patients with mitral valve prolapse syndrome or a history of left ventricular hypertrophy because drug may cause ischemic changes.
•Use cautiously in patients with recent MI or unstable angina because effect of drug is unknown in these disorders.
•Use cautiously in patients with a history of psychosis, depression, or mania because these conditions may worsen during therapy and may require modafinil to be stopped.
•WARNING Monitor patient with a history of alcoholism, stimulant abuse, or other substance abuse for compliance with modafinil therapy. Observe for signs of misuse or abuse, including frequent prescription refill requests, increased frequency of dosing, or drug-seeking behavior. Also watch for evidence of excessive modafinil dosage, including aggressiveness, anxiety, confusion, decreased prothrombin time, diarrhea, irritability, nausea, nervousness, palpitations, sleep disturbances, and tremor.
•Be aware that modafinil, like other CNS stimulants, may alter mood, perception, thinking, judgment, feelings, motor skills, and signs that patient needs sleep.
•If giving drug to patient with a history of psychosis, emotional instability, or psychological illness with psychotic features, be prepared to perform baseline behavioral assessments or frequent clinical observation.
•Stop modafinil at first sign of rash, and notify prescriber. Although rare, rash may indicate a potentially life-threatening event.
•Monitor patient for signs and symptoms of multisystem organ hypersensitivity, such as fever, rash, myocarditis, hepatitis, hematologic abnormalities, pruritus, asthenia, or any other serious abnormality because multiorgan hypersensitivity may vary in its presentation. Notify prescriber if suspected, and expect to discontinue drug and provide supportive care, as ordered.
•Watch closely for suicidal tendencies, especially in patients with a psychiatric history.

PATIENT TEACHING
•Inform patient that modafinil can help, but not cure, narcolepsy and that drug's full effects may not be seen right away.
•Advise patient to avoid taking modafinil within 1 hour of eating because food may delay drug's absorption and onset of action. If he drinks grapefruit juice, encourage him to drink a consistent amount daily.
•Instruct patient to stop taking modafinil and to notify prescriber if he develops a rash, fever, or other serious effect.
•Urge patient to report chest pain, depression, anxiety, or evidence of psychosis or mania to prescriber.
•Inform patient that drug can affect his concentration and function and can hide signs of fatigue. Urge him not to drive or perform activities that require mental alertness until drug's full CNS effects are known.
•Because alcohol may decrease alertness, advise patient to avoid it while taking modafinil.
•Encourage a regular sleeping pattern.
•Caution patient to avoid excessive intake of foods, beverages, and over-the-counter drugs that contain caffeine because caffeine may lead to increased CNS stimulation.
•Inform female patient that modafinil can decrease the effectiveness of certain contraceptives, including birth control pills and implantable hormonal contraceptives. If she uses such contraceptives, urge her to use an alternate birth control method during modafinil therapy and for up to 1 month after she stops taking the drug.
•Advise patient to keep follow-up appointments with prescriber so that her progress can be monitored.
•Urge family or caregiver to watch patient closely for abnormal behaviors, including suicidal tendencies, especially if patient has a psychiatric history.

moexipril hydrochloride

Univasc

Class and Category
Chemical class: Prodrug of moexiprilat
Therapeutic class: Antihypertensive
Pregnancy category: C (first trimester), D (later trimesters)

Indications and Dosages

➤ *To manage hypertension without diuretic therapy*

TABLETS

Adults. *Initial:* 7.5 mg daily 1 hr before a meal. *Maintenance:* 7.5 to 30 mg as a single dose or in divided doses b.i.d. 1 hr before meals. *Maximum:* 30 mg/day.

DOSAGE ADJUSTMENT For patients with creatinine clearance of less than 40 ml/min/ 1.73 m^2, initial dosage reduced to 3.75 mg daily and increased, as ordered, to maximum of 15 mg daily.

➤ *To manage hypertension with diuretic therapy*

TABLETS

Adults. *Initial:* 3.75 mg daily 1 hr before a meal. Increased gradually, as ordered, until blood pressure is controlled.

Route	Onset	Peak	Duration
P.O.	1 hr	3 to 6 hr	24 hr

Mechanism of Action

Is converted to the active metabolite moexiprilat, which reduces blood pressure by inhibiting ACE activity. ACE normally catalyzes the conversion of angiotensin I to angiotensin II—a vasoconstrictor that stimulates aldosterone secretion by the adrenal cortex and directly suppresses renin release. Inhibited ACE activity results in decreased peripheral arterial resistance, increased plasma renin activity, and decreased aldosterone secretion. Decreased aldosterone secretion causes water and sodium excretion.

Contraindications

History of angioedema with previous ACE inhibitor use, hypersensitivity to moexipril or its components

Interactions

DRUGS

allopurinol, bone marrow depressants, corticosteroids (systemic), cytostatic drugs, procainamide: Increased risk of possibly fatal neutropenia or agranulocytosis

antacids: Possibly decreased moexipril bioavailability

cyclosporine, heparin, potassium-containing drugs, potassium-sparing diuretics, potassium supplements: Increased risk of hyperkalemia

digoxin: Possibly increased blood digoxin level

diuretics, other hypotension-producing drugs: Hypotension, risk of renal failure (from sodium or volume depletion caused by diuretics), possibly decreased secondary aldosteronism and hypokalemia caused by diuretics

lithium: Increased blood lithium level and risk of lithium toxicity

NSAIDs (especially indomethacin), sympathomimetics: Decreased antihypertensive effect of moexipril

phenothiazines: Increased pharmacologic effects of moexipril

FOODS

all foods: Decreased moexipril absorption

low-salt milk, salt substitutes: Possibly hyperkalemia

ACTIVITIES

alcohol use: Possibly hypotension

Adverse Reactions

CNS: Anxiety, chills, confusion, dizziness, drowsiness, fatigue, fever, headache, malaise, mood changes, nervousness, sleep disturbance, stroke, syncope

CV: Angina, arrhythmias, chest pain, hypotension, MI, orthostatic hypotension, palpitations, peripheral edema

EENT: Dry mouth, hoarseness, laryngeal edema, mouth or tongue swelling, pharyngitis, rhinitis, sinusitis, taste perversion, tinnitus

GI: Abdominal distention or pain, anorexia, constipation, diarrhea, dysphagia, elevated liver function test results, hepatitis, increased appetite, nausea, pancreatitis, vomiting

GU: Azotemia, elevated BUN and serum creatinine and uric acid levels, interstitial nephritis, oliguria, proteinuria, renal insufficiency, urinary frequency

HEME: Agranulocytosis, bone marrow depression, elevated erythrocyte sedimentation rate, hemolytic anemia, leukocytosis, leukopenia, neutropenia, thrombocytopenia

MS: Arthralgia, leg heaviness or weakness, myalgia, myositis

RESP: Bronchospasm, cough, dyspnea, upper respiratory tract infection

SKIN: Alopecia, diaphoresis, flushing, onycholysis, pallor, pemphigus, photosensitivity, pruritus, rash, Stevens-Johnson syndrome, urticaria
Other: Anaphylaxis, angioedema (of arms, face, larynx, legs, lips, mucous membranes, tongue), flulike symptoms, hyperkalemia, hyponatremia, positive ANA titer

Nursing Considerations
•**WARNING** Contact prescriber if patient is or may be pregnant. Moexipril may cause fetal or neonatal harm or death if used during second or third trimester.
•Be aware that patient who already takes a diuretic should be medically supervised for several hours after first dose of moexipril.
•Administer drug 1 hour before meals.
•Monitor blood pressure, leukocyte count, and liver and renal function test results during moexipril therapy.
•Be aware that black patients may be less responsive to drug's antihypertensive effect if moexipril is used alone to control blood pressure.

PATIENT TEACHING
•Urge female patient to notify prescriber immediately if she is or may be pregnant.
•Instruct patient to take moexipril at the same time each day, 1 hour before meals.
•Direct patient to take a missed dose as soon as he remembers unless it's nearly time for the next dose. Caution against doubling the dose.
•**WARNING** Instruct patient to stop drug and seek immediate medical attention for hoarseness; swelling of tongue, glottis, larynx, face, hands, or feet; or sudden difficulty swallowing or breathing.
•Caution patient not to stop drug without consulting prescriber even if he feels better.
•Inform patient about possible dizziness, especially after first dose and if he takes a diuretic.
•Advise patient to change position slowly to minimize effects of orthostatic hypotension.
•Caution patient to avoid potentially hazardous activities until drug's CNS effects are known.
•Instruct patient to notify prescriber if he faints or experiences persistent dizziness.
•Instruct patient to report evidence of infection (such as chills, fever, and sore throat), diarrhea, nausea, or vomiting, which may lead to dehydration-induced hypotension.
•Advise patient to avoid alcohol during moexipril therapy because it may cause hypotension.
•Instruct patient to check with prescriber before taking OTC drugs.
•Urge patient to avoid potassium supplements and potassium-containing salt substitutes unless prescriber allows them.
•Advise patient to visit prescriber regularly to monitor progress.
•Discuss the importance of weight control and low-salt diet in managing hypertension.

molindone hydrochloride
Moban, Moban Concentrate

Class and Category
Chemical class: Dihydroindolone derivative
Therapeutic class: Antipsychotic drug
Pregnancy category: Not rated

Indications and Dosages
➤ *To manage symptoms of psychotic disorders*
ORAL SOLUTION, TABLETS
Adults and children age 12 and over. *Initial:* 50 to 75 mg daily in divided doses t.i.d. or q.i.d. Dosage increased to 100 mg daily in 3 to 4 days as needed. *Maintenance:* For mild psychosis, 5 to 15 mg t.i.d. or q.i.d.; for moderate psychosis, 10 to 25 mg t.i.d. or q.i.d.; for severe psychosis, 225 mg daily in divided doses. *Maximum:* 225 mg daily.
DOSAGE ADJUSTMENT Initial dosage reduced for elderly or debilitated patients.

Route	Onset	Peak	Duration
P.O.	Unknown	Unknown	24 to 36 hr

Mechanism of Action
Occupies dopamine receptor sites in the reticular activating and limbic systems in the CNS. By blocking dopamine activity in these areas, molindone reduces the symptoms of psychosis, helping the patient to think and behave more coherently.

Contraindications
Hypersensitivity to molindone, its components, or other antipsychotic drugs, includ-

ing haloperidol, loxapine, phenothiazines, and thioxanthenes

Interactions

DRUGS

amphetamines: Decreased amphetamine effectiveness, decreased antipsychotic effectiveness of molindone

anesthetics, barbiturates, benzodiazepines, CNS depressants, opioid analgesics: Possibly prolonged and intensified CNS depressant effects

antacids, antidiarrheals: Decreased molindone absorption

anticholinergics, antidyskinetics, antihistamines: Possibly increased anticholinergic effects

beta blockers: Possibly increased effect of beta blocker

bromocriptine: Possibly decreased therapeutic effects of bromocriptine and increased serum prolactin level

extrapyramidal reaction–causing drugs, such as amoxapine, haloperidol, loxapine, metoclopramide, olanzapine, phenothiazines, pimozide, rauwolfia alkaloids, risperidone, tacrine, and thioxanthenes: Increased severity of extrapyramidal effects

insulin, oral antidiabetic drugs: Possibly increased serum glucose level

levodopa: Inhibited antidyskinetic effects of levodopa, possibly decreased antipsychotic effects of molindone

lithium: Increased risk of neurotoxicity, increased extrapyramidal effects

MAO inhibitors, maprotiline, trazodone, tricyclic antidepressants: Possibly prolonged and intensified sedative or anticholinergic effects of all drugs

phenytoin, tetracycline: Interference with absorption of phenytoin and tetracycline

ACTIVITIES

alcohol use: Prolonged and intensified CNS depression

Adverse Reactions

CNS: Depression, drowsiness, euphoria, extrapyramidal reactions (such as akathisia, dystonia, motor restlessness, pseudoparkinsonism, and tardive dyskinesia), headache, hyperactivity, lack of coordination, neuroleptic malignant syndrome, tiredness

CV: Orthostatic hypotension, tachycardia, unstable blood pressure

EENT: Blinking or eyelid spasm, blurred vision, dry mouth, inability to move eyes, nasal congestion

ENDO: Breast engorgement, lactation

GI: Constipation, nausea

GU: Decreased libido, menstrual irregularities, urine retention

MS: Muscle spasms of back, face, and neck; muscle twitching; twisting movements of the body; weakness or stiffness of limbs

RESP: Dyspnea

SKIN: Diaphoresis, pallor, rash

Other: Heatstroke

Nursing Considerations

• Molindone shouldn't be used to treat dementia-related psychosis in the elderly because of an increased mortality risk.

• **WARNING** Assess patient for signs and symptoms of neuroleptic malignant syndrome, such as diaphoresis, dyspnea, fatigue, fever, incontinence, pallor, severe muscle stiffness, tachycardia, and unstable blood pressure; notify prescriber immediately if they occur. Expect to discontinue drug and begin intensive medical treatment. Monitor patient carefully for recurrence if antipsychotic therapy resumes.

• Molindone shouldn't be given to patients who have severe CNS depression or who are comatose because of drug's CNS depressant effects.

• Monitor elderly patients for orthostatic hypotension and symptoms of tardive dyskinesia, including blinking or eyelid spasms, involuntary movements of the limbs, and unusual facial expressions, because these patients may be sensitive to drug's anticholinergic and extrapyramidal effects. Expect to reduce dosage or discontinue drug.

• Give oral solution undiluted or mixed with water, carbonated beverage, fruit juice, or milk.

PATIENT TEACHING

• Instruct patient to follow treatment regimen and to notify prescriber before discontinuing drug because gradual dosage reduction may be needed.

• Instruct patient not to take drug within 2 hours of taking an antacid. Advise him to take drug with food or a full glass of milk or water to reduce gastric irritation.

• Instruct patient to take oral solution undiluted or mixed with water, carbonated beverage, fruit juice, or milk.

•Urge patient to avoid alcohol consumption because of possible additive effects and hypotension.

•Advise patient, especially an elderly patient, to rise slowly from a supine or seated position to avoid feeling dizzy, light-headed, or faint.

•Explain that drug may reduce the body's response to heat. Tell patient to avoid temperature extremes, such as hot showers, tubs, or saunas. Urge caution during exercise.

•Caution patient not to take OTC drugs for colds or allergies during therapy because they can increase the risk of heatstroke and increase anticholinergic effects, such as blurred vision, constipation, dry mouth, and urine retention.

•Inform patient and family members that maximum clinical improvement in symptoms may take several weeks or months.

mometasone furoate monohydrate

Nasonex

Class and Category

Chemical class: Glucocorticoid
Therapeutic class: Antiasthmatic, anti-inflammatory
Pregnancy category: C

Indications and Dosages

➤ *To manage symptoms of seasonal or perennial allergic rhinitis*

NASAL SPRAY

Adults and children 12 years and over. 100 mcg (2 sprays) in each nostril daily. **Children ages 2 to 12.** 50 mcg (1 spray) in each nostril daily.

➤ *To maintain asthma control*

ORAL INHALATION

Adults and children age 12 and over who have been taking bronchodilators alone or inhaled corticosteroids. *Initial:* 220 mcg (1 inhalation) once daily in evening. *Maximum:* 440 mcg (2 inhalations) daily given as 220 mcg (1 inhalation) b.i.d. or 440 mcg (1 inhalation) once daily.

Adults and children age 12 and over who have taken oral corticosteroids. 440 mcg (2 inhalations) b.i.d.

Children ages 4 to 11. 110 mcg (1 inhalation) once daily in evening.

Mechanism of Action

Inhibits the activity of cells and mediators active in the inflammatory response, possibly by decreasing influx of inflammatory cells into nasal passages and thereby decreasing nasal inflammation.

Contraindications

Hypersensitivity to mometasone or its components; recent septal ulcers, nasal surgery, or nasal trauma; status asthmaticus or other asthma episodes that require emergency care

Adverse Reactions

CNS: Headache
CV: Chest pain
EENT: Cataracts, conjunctivitis, dry mouth, earache, epistaxis, glaucoma, nasal irritation, oral and pharyngeal candidiasis, otitis media, pharyngitis, rhinitis, sinusitis, throat tightness, unpleasant taste
ENDO: Adrenal insufficiency, growth suppression
GI: Diarrhea, dyspepsia, nausea, vomiting
GU: Dysmenorrhea
MS: Arthralgia, decreased bone mineral density, myalgia, pain
RESP: Asthma, bronchitis, bronchospasm, increased cough, upper respiratory tract infection, wheezing
SKIN: Urticaria
Other: Angioedema, flulike symptoms, viral infection

Nursing Considerations

•Use mometasone cautiously if patient has tubercular infection; untreated fungal, bacterial, or systemic viral infection; or ocular herpes simplex.

•If patient takes an oral corticosteroid, expect to taper it slowly 1 week after changing to mometasone. If patient takes prednisone, expect to reduce it by no more than 2.5 mg daily at weekly intervals, beginning at least 1 week after mometasone therapy starts. Monitor patient for symptoms of systemically active corticosteroid withdrawal such as joint and muscle pain, lassitude, and depression despite maintenance or even improvement of respiratory symptoms.

•WARNING Assess patient switched from systemic corticosteroid to mometasone for adrenal insufficiency (fatigue, hypotension,

M

lassitude, nausea, vomiting, weakness) during initial treatment and during stress, trauma, surgery, infection or an electrolyte-depleting condition. Notify prescriber immediately if signs or symptoms arise because adrenal insufficiency may be life-threatening. Hypothalamic-pituitary-adrenal axis function may take several months to recover after systemic corticosteroids are discontinued. Abrupt withdrawal of mometasone also may precipitate adrenal insufficiency.

•Notify prescriber immediately if patient has bronchospasm after mometasone oral inhalation, and expect to administer a fast-acting inhaled bronchodilator, discontinue mometasone, and use an alternate drug.

•Closely monitor a child's growth pattern; drug may stunt growth.

•Report oropharyngeal candidiasis, and expect patient to receive appropriate antifungal therapy while remaining on mometasone therapy. If candidiasis is severe, however, mometasone therapy may need to be temporarily halted.

PATIENT TEACHING

•For nasal spray, instruct patient to shake container before each use. Instruct her to blow her nose, tilt her head slightly forward, and insert tube into a nostril, pointing toward inner corner of eye, away from nasal septum. Tell her to hold the other nostril closed and spray while inhaling gently. Then have her repeat the procedure in the other nostril.

•For oral inhalation, give patient these instructions for using the inhaler: Remove cap only after placing inhaler in an upright position. Twist cap in a counterclockwise direction while holding the colored base, making sure the indented arrow (found on the white portion of the inhaler directly above the colored base) is pointing to the dose counter. Removing the cap loads the inhaler with the drug, and the dose counter on the base will count down by one. Take a full breath in and out, and then place the mouthpiece in your mouth. Firmly close your lips around the mouthpiece, taking care not to cover the ventilation holes on the inhaler. Then take a fast, deep breath. You may not taste, smell, or feel anything with the inhalation. After taking the breath, remove the inhaler from your mouth and hold your breath for about 10 seconds. Don't exhale into the inhaler.

Wipe the mouthpiece dry, if needed, and replace the cap right away, turning it clockwise as you press down. You should hear a click when the cap is fully closed. Write down the date inhaler is opened, and discard it 45 days from that date or when dose counter reads 00, whichever comes first.

•Instruct patient to gargle or rinse after each use of oral inhaler to help prevent mouth and throat dryness, relieve throat irritation, and prevent oropharyngeal infection.

•**WARNING** Caution patient not to use mometasone oral inhalation to relieve acute bronchospasm and to notify prescriber if rescue inhaler is required more often or doesn't seem to be as effective.

•If patient switches from an oral corticosteroid to mometasone, advise her to carry or wear medical identification indicating the need for supplemental systemic corticosteroids during stress or severe asthma attack and to seek emergency care if either occurs.

•Instruct patient to contact prescriber if symptoms persist or worsen after 3 weeks.

•Caution patient to avoid exposure to chickenpox and measles and, if exposed, to contact prescriber immediately.

montelukast sodium

Singulair

Class and Category

Chemical class: Leukotriene receptor antagonist
Therapeutic class: Antiasthmatic
Pregnancy category: B

Indications and Dosages

➤ *To prevent or treat asthma*

ORAL GRANULES

Children ages 12 to 23 mo. 4 mg daily in the evening. *Maximum:* 4 mg daily.

CHEWABLE TABLETS

Children ages 6 to 14. 5 mg daily in the evening. *Maximum:* 5 mg daily.

Children ages 2 to 5. 4 mg daily in the evening. *Maximum:* 4 mg daily.

TABLETS

Adults and adolescents age 15 and over. 10 mg daily in the evening. *Maximum:* 10 mg daily.

➤ *To treat seasonal allergic rhinitis*

ORAL GRANULES

Children ages 2 to 5. 4 mg daily.
CHEWABLE TABLETS
Children ages 6 to 14. 5 mg daily.
Children ages 2 to 5. 4 mg daily.
TABLETS
Adults and adolescents age 15 and over.
10 mg daily.

➤ *To treat perennial allergic rhinitis*
ORAL GRANULES
Children ages 6 months to 5 years. 4 mg
daily.
CHEWABLE TABLETS
Children ages 6 to 14. 5 mg daily.
Children ages 2 to 5. 4 mg daily.
TABLETS
Adults and adolescents age 15 and over.
10 mg daily.

➤ *To prevent exercise-induced broncho-*
constriction
TABLETS
Adults and adolescents age 15 and over.
10 mg at least 2 hr before exercise. *Maximum:* 10 mg in 24 hr.

Route	Onset	Peak	Duration
P.O.	Unknown	Unknown	24 hr

Mechanism of Action

Antagonizes receptors for cysteinyl leukotrienes, which are produced by arachidonic
acid metabolism and released from mast
cells, eosinophils, and other cells. When
cysteinyl leukotrienes bind to their receptor
sites in bronchial airways, they increase endothelial membrane permeability, which
leads to airway edema, smooth-muscle contraction, and altered activity of the cells involved in asthma's inflammatory process.
Montelukast blocks these effects.

Interactions
DRUGS
phenobarbital: Decreased amount of circulating montelukast

Adverse Reactions
CNS: Anxiousness, asthenia, dizziness, fatigue, fever, headache, hypoesthesia, paresthesia, suicidal ideation
EENT: Dental pain, epistaxis, nasal congestion (in all patients); laryngitis, otitis media,
pharyngitis, sinusitis

GI: Abdominal pain, cholestatic hepatitis,
dyspepsia, elevated liver function test results, hepatotoxicity, indigestion, infectious
gastroenteritis (in all patients); diarrhea,
nausea (in children)
GU: Pyuria
RESP: Cough, upper respiratory tract infection
SKIN: Erythema nodosum, pruritus, rash,
urticaria
Other: Anaphylaxis, angioedema (in all patients); flulike syndrome, viral infection (in
children)

Nursing Considerations
•WARNING Be aware that drug shouldn't be
given for acute asthma attack or status asthmaticus.
•Be aware that montelukast shouldn't be
abruptly substituted for inhaled or oral corticosteroids; expect to taper corticosteroid
dosage gradually, as directed.
•Monitor patient for adverse reactions, such
as cardiac and pulmonary symptoms, eosinophilia, and vasculitis, in patient undergoing
corticosteroid withdrawal. Notify prescriber
if such reactions occur.
•Watch patient closely for suicidal tendencies throughtout montelukast therapy.

PATIENT TEACHING
•Advise patient to take montelukast daily as
prescribed, even when he feels well. Urge
him not to decrease dosage or stop taking
other prescribed asthma drugs unless instructed by prescriber.
•Caution patient not to use drug for acute
asthma attack or status asthmaticus; make
sure he has appropriate short-acting rescue
drug available.
•Tell parents administering oral granules to
pour contents directly into the child's mouth
or mix with ice cream or cold or room temperature applesauce, carrots, or rice—but not
liquids or other foods—just before administration. Liquids may be given after drug has
been administered. Once packet is opened,
the full dose must be administered within
15 minutes. Drug must not be stored for future use if mixed with food.
•Instruct patient to notify prescriber if he
needs to use a short-acting inhaled bronchodilator more often than usual, or more
often than prescribed, to control symptoms.
•Teach patient to use a peak flowmeter to

M

determine his personal best expiratory volume.

• Caution patient with aspirin sensitivity to avoid aspirin and NSAIDs during montelukast therapy. Montelukast may not effectively reduce bronchospasm in such a patient.

• Inform patient (or parents of child) with phenylketonuria that chewable tablet contains phenylalanine.

• Instruct patient to notify prescriber if she is or could be pregnant.

• Urge family or caregiver to watch patient closely for abnormal behaviors, including suicidal tendencies, while patient is taking montelukast.

morphine sulfate

Astramorph PF, Avinza, DepoDur, Duramorph, Epimorph (CAN), Kadian, M-Eslon (CAN), Morphine Extra-Forte (CAN), Morphine Forte (CAN), Morphine H.P. (CAN), Morphitec (CAN), MS Contin, MSIR, MS/L, MS/L Concentrate, MS/S, OMS Concentrate, Oramorph SR, Rescudose, RMS Uniserts, Roxanol, Roxanol 100, Roxanol UD, Statex (CAN)

Class, Category, and Schedule
Chemical class: Phenanthrene derivative
Therapeutic class: Analgesic
Pregnancy category: C
Controlled substance schedule: II

Indications and Dosages
➤ *To relieve acute or chronic moderate to severe pain; as adjunct to treat pulmonary edema caused by left-sided heart failure; to supplement general, local, or regional anesthesia*

CAPSULES, ORAL SOLUTION, SYRUP, TABLETS
Adults. *Initial:* 10 to 30 mg every 4 hr, p.r.n.
Children. Individualized dosage based on patient's age, size, and need.

I.V. INFUSION
Adults. *Initial:* 15 mg (or more) followed by 0.8 to 10 mg/hr, increased as needed for effectiveness. *Maintenance:* 0.8 to 80 mg/hr.
Children. 0.01 to 0.04 mg/kg/hr postoperatively, 0.025 to 2.6 mg/kg/hr for severe chronic cancer pain, or 0.03 to 0.15 mg/kg/hr for sickle cell crisis.
Neonates. *Initial:* 0.010 mg/kg/hr (10 mcg/kg/hr) postoperatively. *Maintenance:* 0.015 to

0.02 mg/kg/hr (15 to 20 mcg/kg/hr).

I.V. INJECTION
Adults. 2.5 to 15 mg injected slowly.
Children. 0.5 to 0.1 mg/kg given slowly.

I.M. OR SUBCUTANEOUS INJECTION
Adults. *Initial:* 10 mg (based on 70-kg [154-lb] adult) every 4 hr. *Maintenance:* 5 to 20 mg.
Children. *Initial:* 0.1 to 0.2 mg/kg every 4 hr. *Maximum:* 15 mg/dose.

EPIDURAL INFUSION (PRESERVATIVE-FREE)
Adults. *Initial:* 2 to 4 mg/24 hr, increased by 1 to 2 mg/24 hr, as directed.

EPIDURAL INJECTION (PRESERVATIVE-FREE)
Adults. *Initial:* 5 mg into lumbar region. If pain isn't relieved after 1 hr, 1- to 2-mg doses given at appropriate intervals to relieve pain. *Maximum:* 10 mg/24 hr.

INTRATHECAL INJECTION (PRESERVATIVE-FREE)
Adults. 0.2 to 1 mg as a single dose.

SUPPOSITORIES
Adults. 10 to 30 mg every 4 hr, p.r.n.
Children. Individualized dosage based on patient's age, size, and need.

➤ *To relieve chronic moderate to severe pain that requires opioids for more than a few days*

E.R. CAPSULES
Adults. Individualized dosage given every 12 to 24 hr.

E.R. TABLETS
Adults. 30 mg every 12 hr. Dosage increased based on patient's response.

➤ *To relieve MI pain*

I.V. INJECTION
Adults. 1 to 4 mg by slow I.V. injection. Repeated up to every 5 min, if needed. *Maximum:* 2 to 15 mg.

➤ *To provide preoperative analgesia*

I.M. OR SUBCUTANEOUS INJECTION
Adults. 5 to 20 mg given 45 to 60 min before surgery.
Children. 0.05 to 0.1 mg/kg given 45 to 60 min before surgery. *Maximum:* 10 mg.

➤ *To provide analgesia during labor*

I.M. OR SUBCUTANEOUS INJECTION
Adults. 10 mg, with subsequent doses based on patient's response.

Mechanism of Action
Binds with and activates opioid receptors (mainly mu receptors) in brain and spinal cord to produce analgesia and euphoria.

Route	Onset	Peak	Duration
P.O.	Unknown	1 to 2 hr	4 to 5 hr
P.O. (E.R.)	Unknown	Unknown	8 to 12 hr
I.V.	Unknown	20 min	4 to 5 hr
I.M.	10 to 30 min	30 to 60 min	4 to 5 hr
SubQ	10 to 30 min	50 to 90 min	4 to 5 hr
Epidural	15 to 60 min	Unknown	Up to 24 hr
Intrathecal	15 to 60 min	Unknown	Up to 24 hr
P.R.	20 to 60 min	Unknown	Unknown

Contraindications

For all drug forms: Asthma, hypersensitivity to morphine or its components, labor (premature delivery), prematurity (in infants), respiratory depression, upper airway obstruction

For oral solution: Acute abdominal disorders, acute alcoholism, alcohol withdrawal syndrome, arrhythmias, brain tumor, head injuries, heart failure caused by chronic lung disease, increased intracranial or cerebrospinal pressure, recent biliary tract surgery, respiratory insufficiency, seizure disorders, severe CNS depression, surgical anastomosis, use within 14 days of an MAO inhibitor

For I.V., I.M., or subcutaneous injection: Acute alcoholism, alcohol withdrawal syndrome, arrhythmias, brain tumor, heart failure caused by chronic lung disease, seizure disorders

For epidural or intrathecal injection: Anticoagulant therapy, bleeding tendency, injection site infection, parenteral corticosteroid treatment (or other treatment or condition that prohibits drug administration by intrathecal or epidural route) within 2 weeks

Interactions

DRUGS

amitriptyline, clomipramine, nortriptyline: Increased CNS and respiratory depression
anticholinergics: Possibly severe constipation leading to ileus, urine retention
antidiarrheals (such as loperamide and paregoric): CNS depression, possibly severe constipation

antihistamines, chloral hydrate, glutethimide, MAO inhibitors, methocarbamol: Increased CNS and respiratory depressant effects of morphine
antihypertensives, hypotension-producing drugs: Increased hypotension, risk of orthostatic hypotension
buprenorphine: Decreased therapeutic effects of morphine, increased respiratory depression, possibly withdrawal symptoms
cimetidine: Increased analgesic and CNS and respiratory depressant effects of morphine
CNS depressants (antiemetics, general anesthetics, hypnotics, phenothiazines, sedatives, tranquilizers): Possibly coma, hypotension, respiratory depression, severe sedation
diuretics: Decreased diuretic efficacy
hydroxyzine: Increased analgesic, CNS depressant, and hypotensive effects of morphine
metoclopramide: Possibly antagonized metoclopramide effect on GI motility
mixed agonist-antagonist analgesics: Possibly withdrawal symptoms
naloxone: Antagonized analgesic and CNS and respiratory depressant effects of morphine, possibly withdrawal symptoms
naltrexone: Possibly induction or worsening of withdrawal symptoms if morphine given within 7 to 10 days before naltrexone
neuromuscular blockers: Increased or prolonged respiratory depression
opioid analgesics (such as alfentanil and sufentanil): Increased CNS and respiratory depression, increased hypotension
zidovudine: Decreased zidovudine clearance

ACTIVITIES

alcohol use: Increased CNS and respiratory depression, increased hypotension

Adverse Reactions

CNS: Amnesia, anxiety, coma, confusion, decreased concentration, delirium, delusions, depression, dizziness, drowsiness, euphoria, fever, hallucinations, headache, insomnia, lethargy, light-headedness, malaise, psychosis, restlessness, sedation, seizures, syncope, tremor, unarousable, unresponsiveness
CV: Bradycardia, cardiac arrest, hypotension, orthostatic hypotension, palpitations, shock, tachycardia
EENT: Blurred vision, diplopia, dry mouth, laryngeal edema or laryngospasm (allergic), miosis, nystagmus, rhinitis

M

GI: Abdominal cramps or pain, anorexia, biliary tract spasm, constipation, diarrhea, dysphagia, elevated liver function test results, gastroesophageal reflux, hiccups, ileus and toxic megacolon (in patients with inflammatory bowel disease), intestinal obstruction, indigestion, nausea, vomiting

GU: Decreased ejaculate potency, decreased libido, difficult ejaculation, impotence, menstrual irregularities, oliguria, prolonged labor, urinary hesitancy, urine retention

HEME: Anemia, leukopenia, thrombocytopenia

MS: Arthralgia

RESP: Apnea, asthma exacerbation, atelectasis, bronchospasm, depressed cough reflex, hypoventilation, pulmonary edema, respiratory arrest and depression, wheezing

SKIN: Diaphoresis, flushing, pallor, pruritus, urticaria

Other: Allergic reaction; anaphylaxis; facial edema; injection site edema, pain, rash, or redness; physical and psychological dependence; withdrawal symptoms

Nursing Considerations

• Use cautiously in patients about to undergo surgery of the biliary tract and patients with acute pancreatitis secondary to biliary tract disease because morphine may cause spasm of the sphincter of Oddi.

• Store morphine sulfate at room temperature.

• Before giving morphine, make sure opioid antagonist and equipment for giving oxygen and controlling respiration are available.

• Before therapy, assess patient's drug use, including all prescription and OTC drugs.

• Expect prescriber to start patient who has never received opioids on immediate-release form and then switch to E.R. form if therapy must last longer than a few days.

• Give oral form with food or milk to minimize adverse GI reactions, if needed. Solution can be mixed with fruit juice to improve taste.

• If needed, open E.R. capsules and sprinkle contents on applesauce (at room temperature or cooler) just before giving to patient. Make sure patient doesn't chew or crush capsules or dissolve capsule's pellets in his mouth.

• Be aware that E.R. forms of morphine aren't interchangeable.

• Discard injection solution that is discolored or darker than pale yellow or that contains precipitates that don't dissolve with shaking.

•**WARNING** Don't use highly concentrated solutions (such as 10 to 25 mg/ml) for single-dose I.V., I.M., or subcutaneous administration. These solutions are intended for use in continuous, controlled microinfusion devices.

• For direct I.V. injection, dilute appropriate dose with 4 to 5 ml of sterile water for injection. Inject 2.5 to 15 mg directly into tubing of free-flowing I.V. solution over 4 to 5 minutes. Rapid I.V. injection may increase adverse reactions.

• For continuous I.V. infusion, dilute drug in D_5W and administer with infusion-control device. Adjust dose and rate based on patient response, as prescribed.

• Avoid I.M. route for long-term therapy because of injection site irritation.

• During subcutaneous injection, take care to avoid injecting drug intradermally.

• For intrathecal injection, expect prescriber to give no more than 2 ml of 0.5-mg/ml solution or 1 ml of 1-mg/ml solution. Expect intrathecal dosage to be about one-tenth of epidural dosage.

• If rectal suppository is too soft to insert, chill it in refrigerator for 30 minutes or run wrapped suppository under cold tap water.

•**WARNING** Monitor respiratory and cardiovascular status carefully and frequently during morphine therapy. Be alert for respiratory depression and hypotension.

• Monitor patient with seizure disorder for increased seizure activity because morphine may worsen the disorder.

• Monitor patient for excessive or persistent sedation; dosage may need to be adjusted.

• If patient is receiving a continuous morphine infusion, watch for and notify prescriber about new neurologic signs or symptoms. Inflammatory masses (such as granulomas) have caused serious neurologic reactions, including paralysis.

• Expect morphine to cause physical and psychological dependence; watch for drug tolerance and withdrawal symptoms, such as body aches, diaphoresis, diarrhea, fever, piloerection, rhinorrhea, sneezing, and yawning.

• If tolerance to morphine develops, expect prescriber to increase dosage.

• Morphine may have a prolonged duration and cumulative effect in patients with impaired hepatic or renal function. It also may prolong labor by reducing strength, duration, and frequency of uterine contractions.

•When discontinuing morphine in patients receiving more than 30 mg daily, expect prescriber to reduce daily dose by about one-half for 2 days and then by 25% every 2 days thereafter until total dose reaches initial amount recommended for patients who haven't received opioids (15 to 30 mg daily). This regimen minimizes the risk of withdrawal symptoms.

PATIENT TEACHING
•Instruct patient to take morphine exactly as prescribed and not to change dosage without consulting prescriber.
•Explain that patient may take tablets or capsules with food or milk to relieve GI distress and may mix oral solution with juice to improve taste.
•Urge patient not to break, chew, or crush E.R. capsules and tablets to avoid rapid release and, possibly, toxicity.
•For patient who has difficulty swallowing, suggest that he open E.R. capsules and sprinkle contents on food or liquids. Urge him to take drug immediately and not let capsule contents dissolve in his mouth.
•Instruct patient to moisten rectal suppository before inserting it.
•Urge patient to avoid alcohol and other CNS depressants during morphine therapy.
•Advise patient to avoid potentially hazardous activities during morphine therapy.
•Tell patient to change positions slowly to minimize the orthostatic hypotension.
•Instruct patient to notify prescriber about worsening or breakthrough pain.
•Inform patient that morphine may be habit-forming. Urge him to notify prescriber if he experiences anxiety, decreased appetite, excessive tearing, irritability, muscle aches or twitching, rapid heart rate, or yawning.
•Advise female patient to notify prescriber if she becomes pregnant. Regular morphine use during pregnancy may cause physical dependence in fetus and withdrawal in neonate.

moxifloxacin hydrochloride

Avelox, Avelox IV

Class and Category
Chemical class: Fluoroquinolone
Therapeutic class: Antibiotic

Pregnancy category: C

Indications and Dosages
➤ *To treat acute sinusitis caused by* Haemophilus influenzae, Moraxella catarrhalis, *or* Streptococcus pneumoniae; *to treat mild to moderate community-acquired pneumonia caused by* Chlamydia pneumoniae, H. influenzae, M. catarrhalis, Mycoplasma pneumoniae, *or* S. pneumoniae *(including penicillin- or multi-drug-resistant strains)*

TABLETS, I.V. INFUSION
Adults. 400 mg every 24 hr for 10 days.

➤ *To treat acute exacerbation of chronic bronchitis caused by* H. influenzae, H. parainfluenzae, Klebsiella pneumoniae, M. catarrhalis, S. pneumoniae, *or* Staphylococcus aureus

TABLETS, I.V. INFUSION
Adults. 400 mg every 24 hr for 5 days.

➤ *To treat uncomplicated skin and soft-tissue infections caused by* S. aureus *or* Streptococcus pyogenes

TABLETS, I.V. INFUSION
Adults. 400 mg every 24 hr for 7 days.

➤ *To treat complicated skin and skin structure infections caused by* S. aureus, E. coli, K. pneumoniae, *or* Enterobacter cloacae

TABLETS, I.V. INFUSION
Adults. 400 mg every 24 hr for 7 to 21 days.

➤ *To treat complicated intra-abdominal infections, including polymicrobial infections such as abscesses caused by* E.coli, Bacteroides fragilis, Streptococcus anginosus, Streptococcus constellatus, Enterococcus faecalis, Proteus mirabilis, Clostridium perfringens, Bacteroides thetaiotaomicron, *or* Peptostreptococcus *species*

TABLETS, I.V. INFUSION
Adults. 400 mg every 24 hr for 5 to 14 days with initial dosage given as I.V. infusion.

Incompatibilities
Do not infuse I.V. form of moxifloxacin simultaneously through the same I.V. line with other I.V. substances, additives, or drugs.

Contraindications
Hypersensitivity to moxifloxacin, other fluoroquinolones, or their components

M

Mechanism of Action

Inhibits synthesis of the bacterial enzyme DNA gyrase by counteracting the excessive supercoiling of DNA during replication or transcription. Inhibition of DNA gyrase causes rapid- and slow-growing bacterial cells to die.

Interactions

DRUGS

aluminum- or magnesium-containing antacids; drug formulations with divalent or trivalent cations, such as didanosine chewable buffered tablets or powder for oral solution; metal cations, such as iron; multivitamins containing iron or zinc; sucralfate: Possibly substantial interference with moxifloxacin absorption, causing low blood moxifloxacin level

class Ia antiarrhythmics, such as quinidine; class III antiarrhythmics, such as sotalol; other drugs known to prolong QTc interval, such as disopyramide and pentamidine: Possibly prolonged QTc interval

corticosteroids: Increased risk of Achilles and other tendon ruptures

NSAIDs: Increased risk of CNS stimulation and seizures

warfarin: Possibly increased anticoagulation

Adverse Reactions

CNS: Dizziness, fever, headache, psychosis, psychotic reaction, seizures, syncope

CV: Hypertension, hypotension, palpitations, peripheral edema, tachycardia, vasculitis, vasodilation, ventricular tachyarrhythmias

EENT: Altered taste

GI: Abdominal pain, abnormal liver function test results, acute hepatic necrosis or failure, cholestatic hepatitis, diarrhea, dyspepsia, hepatitis, jaundice, nausea, pseudomembranous colitis, vomiting

GU: Acute renal insufficiency or failure, interstitial nephritis

HEME: Agranulocytosis, aplastic anemia, eosinophilia, hemolytic anemia, leukopenia, pancytopenia, prolonged PT, thrombocytopenia

MS: Arthralgia, myalgia, tendon inflammation, pain, or rupture

RESP: Allergic pneumonitis

SKIN: Photosensitivity, rash, Stevens-Johnson syndrome, toxic epidermal necrolysis

Other: Anaphylaxis, anaphylactic shock, angioedema, serum sickness

Nursing Considerations

•Obtain a fluid or tissue specimen for culture and sensitivity, as ordered. Expect to begin therapy before results are available.

•**WARNING** Before starting moxifloxacin therapy, determine if patient receives a class Ia antiarrhythmic, such as quinidine; a class III antiarrhythmic, such as sotalol; or other drugs that prolong the QTc interval. Be aware that these drugs should be avoided in patients taking moxifloxacin because they may prolong the QTc interval and lead to life-threatening ventricular tachycardia or torsades de pointes.

•Infuse drug over 60 minutes with ready-to-use flexible bags with 400 mg of moxifloxacin in 250 ml of 0.8% saline. Don't dilute further.

•If giving through Y-type tubing or piggyback method, stop other solutions during moxifloxacin infusion, and flush the line before and after infusion with a compatible solution, such as normal; saline solution, 1M sodium chloride, 5% dextrose, sterile water for injection, 10% dextrose, or lactated Ringer's. Also flush line before and after giving other drugs in the same I.V. line.

•Don't refrigerate I.V. moxifloxacin ready-to-use bags because precipitation will occur. Discard any unused portion; premixed bags are for single-use only.

•Expect to obtain a 12-lead ECG to assess patient for a prolonged QTc interval. Ask patient if he or a blood relative has a history of prolonged QTc interval. Monitor elderly patients closely because they may have increased risk of prolonged QT interval.

•If patient has hypokalemia, expect to correct it before beginning moxifloxacin therapy to prevent arrhythmias.

•Determine if patient has a history of a CNS disorder, such as cerebral arteriosclerosis or epilepsy, because drug may lower the seizure threshold. Notify prescriber before therapy starts, and take seizure precautions.

•If profuse, watery diarrhea develops, contact prescriber and expect to obtain a stool specimen to rule out pseudomembranous colitis caused by *Clostridium difficile.* If diarrhea occurs, notify prescriber and expect to withhold moxifloxacin and treat with fluids, electrolytes, protein, and an antibiotic effective against *C. difficile.*

•Monitor patient's serum potassium level, as ordered, during therapy to assess for hypokalemia.

•Keep emergency resuscitation equipment readily available, and observe for evidence of hypersensitivity, such as angioedema, dyspnea, and urticaria. If you suspect anaphylaxis, prepare to give epinephrine, corticosteroids, and diphenhydramine, as prescribed.

PATIENT TEACHING

•Urge patient to notify prescriber immediately about palpitations or fainting because they may indicate a serious arrhythmia.

•Teach patient to take drug at least 4 hours before and 8 hours after aluminum- or magnesium-containing antacids, didanosine chewable buffered tablets or oral solution prepared from powder, multivitamins containing iron or zinc, or sucralfate.

•Urge patient to drink plenty of fluids while taking moxifloxacin.

•Caution patient to stop taking moxifloxacin and notify prescriber if he has trouble breathing, a rash, or other signs of an allergic reaction.

•Urge patient to stop any exercise and contact prescriber immediately if he develops tendon inflammation, pain, or rupture.

•Caution patient to avoid activities of mental alertness until adverse CNS effects are known.

•Urge patient to tell prescriber if diarrhea develops, even more than 2 months after moxifloxacin therapy ends.

•Caution patient to complete the prescribed course of therapy even if he feels better before it's completed.

•Tell patient to avoid excessive exposure to sunlight or artificial ultraviolet light because severe sunburn may result. Instruct patient to notify prescriber if sunburn develops because moxifloxacin may need to be discontinued.

mycophenolate mofetil
CellCept, CellCept Oral Suspension

mycophenolate mofetil hydrochloride
CellCept Intravenous

mycophenolic acid
Myfortic

Class and Category
Chemical class: 2-morpholinoethyl ester of mycophenolic acid
Therapeutic class: Immunosuppressant
Pregnancy category: D

Indications and Dosages

➤ *To prevent organ rejection in patients receiving allogenic kidney transplants*

CAPSULES, ORAL SUSPENSION, TABLETS, I.V. INFUSION

Adults. 1 g (over 2 hr for I.V. infusion) b.i.d.

E.R. TABLETS

Adults. 720 mg b.i.d.

SUSPENSION

**Children with body surface area less than 1.25 m². ** 600 mg/m² b.i.d. *Maximum:* 2 g (10 ml) daily.

CAPSULES

Children with body surface area of 1.25 m² to 1.5 m². 750 mg b.i.d.

CAPSULES, TABLETS

Children with body surface area greater than 1.5 m². 1 g b.i.d.

➤ *To prevent organ rejection in patients receiving allogenic heart transplants*

CAPSULES, ORAL SUSPENSION, TABLETS, I.V. INFUSION

Adults. 1.5 g (over 2 hr for I.V. infusion) b.i.d.

➤ *To prevent organ rejection in patients receiving allogenic liver transplants*

I.V. INFUSION

Adults. 1 g infused over 2 hr b.i.d.

CAPSULES, ORAL SUSPENSION, TABLETS

Adults. 1.5 g b.i.d.

Incompatibilities
Don't mix or administer mycophenolate mofetil hydrochloride in the same infusion catheter with other I.V. drugs or admixtures.

Contraindications
Hypersensitivity to mycophenolate mofetil, mycophenolic acid, or any of its components; hypersensitivity to polysorbate 80 (I.V. form)

M

Mechanism of Action

Hydrolyzes to form mycophenolic acid (MPA), which inhibits guanosine nucleotide synthesis and proliferation of T and B lymphocytes. MPA also suppresses antibody formation by B lymphocytes and prevents glycosylation of lymphocyte and monocyte glycoproteins involved in adhesion to endothelial cells. MPA also may inhibit leukocytes from sites of inflammation and graft rejection, which may explain how mycophenolate mofetil prolongs allogeneic transplant survival.

Interactions

DRUGS

acyclovir, ganciclovir, probenecid: Increased plasma levels of both drugs
antacids with magnesium and aluminum hydroxides, sevelamer: Decreased absorption of oral mycophenolate mofetil
azathioprine: Increased bone marrow suppression
cholestyramine, cyclosporine, norfloxacin, metronidazole, rifampin: Decreased plasma level of mycophenolate mofetil
live vaccines: Decreased effectiveness of live vaccines
oral contraceptives: Possibly decreased effectiveness of oral contraceptives

Adverse Reactions

CNS: Agitation, anxiety, chills, confusion, delirium, depression, dizziness, emotional lability, fever, hallucinations, headache, hypertonia, hypesthesia, insomnia, malaise, meningitis, nervousness, neuropathy, paresthesia, progressive multifocal leukoencephalopathy, psychosis, seizure, somnolence, syncope, thinking abnormality, tremor, vertigo
CV: Angina pectoris, arrhythmias, arterial thrombosis, atrial fibrillation or flutter, bradycardia, cardiac arrest, CV disorder, congestive heart failure, extrasystole, generalized edema, hemorrhage, hypercholesterolemia, hyperlipemia, hypertension, hypotension, increased lactic dehydrogenase, increased SGOT and SGPT, increased venous pressure, infectious endocarditis, orthostatic hypotension, palpitations, pericardial effusion, peripheral edema, peripheral vascular disorder, pulmonary edema or hypertension, supraventricular tachycardia, thrombosis, vasodilation, vasospasm, ventricular extrasystole, ventricular tachycardia
EENT: Amblyopia, cataract, conjunctivitis, deafness, dry mouth, ear disorder or pain, epistaxis, eye hemorrhage, gingivitis, gum hyperplasia, lacrimation disorder, mouth ulceration, oral moniliasis, pharyngitis, rhinitis, sinusitis, stomatitis, tinnitus, vision abnormality, voice alteration
ENDO: Cushing's syndrome, diabetes mellitus, hypercalcemia, hypocalcemia, hypoglycemia, hypothyroidism, parathyroid disorder
GI: Abdomen enlargement or pain, anorexia, ascites, cholangitis, cholestatic jaundice, colitis, constipation, diarrhea, dyspepsia, dysphagia, esophagitis, flatulence, gastritis, gastroenteritis, gastrointestinal hemorrhage, gastrointestinal infection, gastrointestinal moniliasis, hepatitis, hernia, ileus, jaundice, liver damage, liver function test abnormalities, melena, nausea, pancreatitis, peritonitis, rectal disorder, stomach ulcer, vomiting
GU: Albuminuria; bilirubinemia; dysuria; hematuria; hydronephrosis; impotence; increased BUN or creatinine levels; kidney tubular necrosis; nocturia; oliguria; pain; prostatic disorder; pyelonephritis; renal failure; scrotal edema, urinary tract disorder or infection; urine abnormality, frequency, incontinence, or retention
HEME: anemia, coagulation disorder, hypochromic anemia, increased prothrombin time or thromboplastin time, leukocytosis, leukopenia, polyhemia, thrombocytopenia
MS: Arthralgia; back, neck or pelvic pain; joint disorder; leg cramps; myalgia; myasthenia; osteoporosis
RESP: Apnea; asthma; atelectasis; bronchitis; cough; dyspnea; hemoptysis; hyperventilation; hypoxia; lung edema; pleural effusion; pneumonia; pneumothorax; pulmonary fibrosis; respiratory acidosis, moniliasis, neoplasm, or pain; sputum increase
SKIN: Abscess; acne; cellulite; ecchymosis; fungal dermatitis; pallor; petechia; pruritus; rash; benign neoplasm, carcinoma, hypertrophy, or ulcer; sweating; vesiculobullous rash
Other: Abnormal healing, accidental injury, acidosis, alkalosis, alopecia, cyst, dehydration, facial edema, flulike syndrome, gout, hiccup, hirsutism, hyperkalemia, hyperuricemia, hypervolemia, hypochloremia, hypokalemia, hypomagnesemia, hypona-

tremia, hypoproteinemia, hypophosphatemia, increased alkaline phosphatase, increased gamma glutamyl transpeptidase, infection, lymphoma, malignancies, sepsis, thirst, weight gain or loss

Nursing Considerations

• Before starting mycophentolate therapy in a woman of childbearing potential, make sure she has a negative pregnancy test within 1 week of starting therapy, using a test with a sensitivity of at least 25 mIU/ml. Therapy shouldn't start until results are confirmed.
• Expect to give I.V. form within 24 hours of transplantation and for no longer than 14 days. Expect to switch patient to oral form as soon as possible, as ordered.
• Expect to administer oral form of drug as soon as possible following transplantation.
• When preparing oral suspension or I.V. form, avoid inhalation or direct contact with skin or mucous membranes. If contact occurs, wash area thoroughly with soap and water and rinse eyes with water.
• To prepare oral suspension, tap closed bottle several times to loosen powder and then measure 94 ml of water in a graduated cylinder. Add half of the water to the bottle and shake for about 1 minute. Then add reminder of water and shake again for 1 minute. Remove child-resistant cap and push bottle adapter into neck of bottle. Close bottle tightly with child-resistant cap. Be aware that the suspension bottle may become cold immediately after reconstitution.
• Know that oral suspension can be administered by 8F or larger nasogastric tube.
• When giving oral suspension, don't mix with any other drugs. Ask patient about history of phenylketonuria before initial administration because oral suspension contains aspartame.
• Don't open or crush capsules. If necessary, use the oral suspension.
• Handle I.V. form similarly to a chemotherapeutic drug because mycophenolate mofetil is genotoxic and embryotoxic and may have mutagenic properties.
• Know that I.V. form must be reconstituted and diluted to 6 mg/ml using 5% dextrose injection USP. Inject 14 ml of 5% dextrose injection USP into each vial (2 vials will be needed for each 1-g dose; 3 vials for each 1.5-g dose), then shake gently. Further dilute

a 1-g dose by adding 2 reconstituted vials to 140 ml of 5% dextrose injection USP; dilute a 1.5-g dose by adding 3 reconstituted vials to 210 ml of 5% dextrose injection USP.
• Be aware that I.V. should be administered within 4 hours of constitution as an infusion over no less than 2 hours. Never administer by rapid or bolus I.V. injection.
• Know that cyclosporine and corticosteroids should be used with mycophenolate mofetil therapy.
• Obtain CBC weekly during first month of therapy, twice monthly for the second and third months of therapy, and then monthly through the first year, as ordered.
• Monitor patient closely for adverse reactions because drug has many adverse effects, some of which can be serious or severe.
• Expect to stop drug or reduce the dose and provide supportive care, as ordered, if neutropenia develops.
• **WARNING** Mycophenolate mofetil therapy has been associated with progressive multifocal leukoencephalopathy that can be life-threatening. Monitor patient for hemiparesis, apathy, confusion, cognitive deficiencies, and ataxia. Report suspicions of disorder immediately to prescriber.

PATIENT TEACHING

• Advise women of childbearing age that two forms of contraceptives should be used simultaneously before beginning mycophenolate mofetil therapy and for 6 weeks following discontinuation of therapy because of potential for fetal harm. Inform women who use oral contraceptives that drug may decrease effectiveness of oral contraceptives. Urge patient to notify prescriber immediately if pregnancy occurs.
• Before therapy starts, tell patient about increased risk of lymphomas or other malignancies. Tell patient to report any unusual signs or symptoms to prescriber.
• Tell patient to take oral form of drug on an empty stomach.
• Instruct patient not to crush tablets or capsules or open capsules.
• Inform patient not to receive live vaccines during therapy. Urge him to avoid people who have received such vaccines or to wear a protective mask when he's around them.
• Tell patient to report any serious or ongoing adverse reactions, especially neurologic abnormalities, to prescriber immediately.

M

• Caution patient to avoid contact with people who have infections because drug causes immunosuppression.

• Urge patient to report any signs of infection, unexpected bruising or bleeding, or any other sign of bone marrow depression immediately.

• Tell patient that frequent laboratory tests may be needed during therapy. Stress that having these tests done is essential to continuing therapy.

• Advise patient to avoid exposure to direct sunlight and UV light and to wear sunscreen when outdoors because of increased risk for skin cancer.

• Advise patient not to take antacids at the same time as oral mycophenolate mofetil because some antacids can decrease drug's absorption.

• Stress importance of follow-up care to monitor the drug's effectiveness and possible adverse effects because of the increased risk for cancer and infections as a result of immunosuppression. Inform patient of the need for periodic laboratory tests.

N·O

nabumetone

Relafen

Class and Category

Chemical class: Naphthylalkanone derivative
Therapeutic class: Anti-inflammatory, antirheumatic
Pregnancy category: C (first trimester), Not rated (later trimesters)

Indications and Dosages

➤ *To relieve symptoms of acute and chronic osteoarthritis and rheumatoid arthritis*

TABLETS

Adults. *Initial:* 1 g daily as a single dose or in divided doses b.i.d., increased to 1.5 to 2 g daily in divided doses b.i.d. *Maintenance:* Adjusted according to clinical response. *Maximum:* 2 g daily.

Mechanism of Action

Blocks activity of cyclooxygenase, the enzyme needed to synthesize prostaglandins, which mediate the inflammatory response and cause local vasodilation, swelling, and pain. Prostaglandins also promote pain transmission from the periphery to the spinal cord. By blocking cyclooxygenase and inhibiting prostaglandins, the NSAID nabumetone reduces inflammatory symptoms and relieves pain.

Contraindications

Angioedema, asthma, bronchospasm, nasal polyps, rhinitis, or urticaria induced by aspirin, iodides, or other NSAIDs

Interactions

DRUGS

acetaminophen (long-term use): Increased risk of adverse renal effects
anticoagulants, thrombolytics: Increased risk of GI bleeding
antihypertensives: Decreased antihypertensive effectiveness
beta blockers: Decreased antihypertensive effects of beta blockers
bone marrow depressants, such as aldesleukin and cisplatin: Increased risk of leukopenia and thrombocytopenia
cefamandole, cefoperazone, cefotetan, plicamycin, valproic acid: Increased risk of hypoprothrombinemia and bleeding
colchicine, other NSAIDs, salicylates: Increased GI irritability and bleeding
cyclosporine, gold compounds, nephrotoxic drugs: Increased risk of nephrotoxicity
digoxin: Increased blood digoxin level and risk of digitalis toxicity
diuretics: Decreased diuretic effectiveness
glucocorticoids, potassium supplements: Increased GI irritability and bleeding
insulin, oral antidiabetic drugs: Increased effectiveness of these drugs; risk of hypoglycemia
lithium: Increased risk of lithium toxicity
methotrexate: Increased risk of methotrexate toxicity
probenecid: Increased risk of nabumetone toxicity

ACTIVITIES

alcohol use: Increased GI irritability and bleeding

Adverse Reactions

CNS: Drowsiness, fatigue, fever, headache, nervousness, seizures, stroke, vertigo
CV: Edema, hypertension, MI, tachycardia
EENT: Dry mouth, pharyngitis, stomatitis, tinnitus
GI: Abdominal pain, anorexia, constipation, diarrhea, diverticulitis, dyspepsia, dysphagia, esophagitis, flatulence, gastritis, gastroenteritis, gastroesophageal reflux disease, GI bleeding and ulceration, hepatic dysfunction, indigestion, jaundice, melena, nausea, perforation of stomach or intestines, stomatitis, vomiting
GU: Albuminuria, azotemia, interstitial nephritis, nephrotic syndrome
HEME: Agranulocytosis, anemia, eosinophilia, granulocytopenia, hemolytic anemia, leukopenia, neutropenia, pancytopenia, thrombocytopenia
MS: Muscle spasms, myalgia
RESP: Asthma, pneumonitis, respiratory depression
SKIN: Alopecia, erythema multiforme, photosensitivity, pruritus, rash, Stevens-Johnson syndrome, toxic epidermal necrolysis
Other: Anaphylaxis, angioedema

N
O

Nursing Considerations

•Use nabumetone with extreme caution in patients with a history of ulcer disease or GI bleeding because NSAIDs such as nabumetone increase the risk of GI bleeding and ulceration. Expect to use nabumetone for the shortest time possible in these patients.

•Be aware that serious GI tract ulceration, bleeding, and perforation may occur without warning symptoms. Elderly patients are at greater risk. To minimize risk, give drug with food. If GI distress occurs, withhold drug and notify prescriber immediately.

•Use nabumetone cautiously in patients with hypertension, and monitor blood pressure closely throughout therapy. Drug may cause hypertension or worsen it.

•WARNING Monitor patient closely for thrombotic events, including MI and stroke, because NSAIDs increase the risk.

•Monitor patient—especially if he's elderly or receiving long-term nabumetone therapy—for less common but serious adverse GI reactions, including anorexia, constipation, diverticulitis, dysphagia, esophagitis, gastritis, gastroenteritis, gastroesophageal reflux disease, hemorrhoids, hiatal hernia, melena, stomatitis, and vomiting.

•Monitor liver function test results because, in rare cases, elevations may progress to severe hepatic reactions, including fatal hepatitis, liver necrosis, and hepatic failure.

•Monitor BUN and serum creatinine levels in elderly patients, patients taking diuretics or ACE inhibitors, and patients with heart failure, impaired renal function, or hepatic dysfunction; nabumetone may cause renal failure.

•Monitor CBC for decreased hemoglobin and hematocrit; drug may worsen anemia.

•WARNING If patient has bone marrow suppression or is receiving treatment with an antineoplastic, monitor laboratory results (including WBC count), and watch for evidence of infection because anti-inflammatory and antipyretic actions of nabumetone may mask signs and symptoms, such as fever and pain.

•Assess patient's skin regularly for signs of rash or other hypersensitivity reaction because nabumetone is an NSAID and may cause serious skin reactions without warning, even in patients with no history of NSAID sensivitity. At first sign of reaction, stop drug and notify prescriber.

•Assess patient for severe hepatic reactions, including jaundice. Stop drug, as prescribed, if symptoms persist.

PATIENT TEACHING

•Instruct patient to take nabumetone with food to reduce GI distress.

•Advise patient to take drug with a full glass of water and to remain upright for 15 to 30 minutes afterward to prevent drug from lodging in the esophagus and causing irritation.

•Tell patient not to increase dosage or frequency of use without consulting prescriber.

•Urge patient to avoid alcohol to reduce risk of GI bleeding.

•Inform patient that regular laboratory tests are needed to check for drug toxicity during long-term therapy.

•Caution pregnant patient not to take NSAIDs such as nabumetone during the last trimester because they may cause premature closure of the ductus arteriosus.

•Explain that nabumetone may increase the risk of serious adverse cardiovascular reactions; urge patient to seek immediate medical attention if signs or symptoms arise, such as chest pain, shortness of breath, weakness, and slurring of speech.

•Explain that nabumetone may increase the risk of serious adverse GI reactions; stress the importance of seeking immediate medical attention for such signs and symptoms as epigastric or abdominal pain, indigestion, black or tarry stools, or vomiting blood or material that looks like coffee grounds.

•Alert patient to rare but serious skin reactions. Urge her to seek immediate medical attention for rash, blisters, itching, fever, or other indications of hypersensitivity.

nadolol

Corgard, Syn-Nadolol (CAN)

Class and Category

Chemical class: Nonselective beta blocker
Therapeutic class: Antianginal, antihypertensive
Pregnancy category: C

Indications and Dosages

➤ *To manage hypertension, alone or with other antihypertensives*

TABLETS

Adults. *Initial:* 40 mg daily, increased by

40 to 80 mg daily every 7 days, as prescribed. *Maintenance:* 40 to 80 mg daily. *Maximum:* 320 mg daily.

➤ *To manage angina pectoris as long-term therapy*

TABLETS

Adults. *Initial:* 40 mg daily, increased by 40 to 80 mg daily every 3 to 7 days, as prescribed. *Maintenance:* 40 to 80 mg daily. *Maximum:* 240 mg daily.

DOSAGE ADJUSTMENT Interval possibly increased to every 24 to 36 hr if creatinine clearance is 31 to 50 ml/min/1.73 m^2; to every 24 to 48 hr if it's 10 to 30 ml/min/1.73 m^2; or to every 40 to 60 hr if it's less than 10 ml/min/1.73 m^2.

Route	Onset	Peak	Duration
P.O.	Up to 5 days	4 hr	24 hr

Mechanism of Action

Selectively blocks alpha$_1$ and beta$_2$ receptors in vascular smooth muscle and beta$_1$ receptors in the heart, thereby reducing peripheral vascular resistance and blood pressure. Potent beta blockade decreases cardiac excitability, cardiac output, and myocardial oxygen demand, thus reducing angina. It also prevents reflex tachycardia, which typically occurs with most alpha blockers.

Contraindications

Asthma; bronchospasm; cardiogenic shock; heart failure; hypersensitivity to nadolol, other beta blockers, or their components; second- or third-degree AV block; severe COPD; sinus bradycardia

Interactions

DRUGS

allergen immunotherapy, allergenic extracts for skin testing: Increased risk of serious systemic reactions or anaphylaxis
amiodarone: Increased risk of conduction abnormalities and negative inotropic effects
beta blockers, digoxin: Increased risk of bradycardia
calcium channel blockers: Increased risk of bradycardia
cimetidine: Possibly increased effects of nadolol

clonidine, guanabenz: Impaired blood pressure control
diazoxide, nitroglycerin: Increased risk of hypotension
estrogens, NSAIDs: Possibly reduced antihypertensive effect of nadolol
general anesthetics: Increased risk of hypotension and myocardial depression
insulin, oral antidiabetic drugs: Possibly increased risk of hyperglycemia and impaired recovery from hypoglycemia, masking of signs of hypoglycemia
lidocaine: Increased risk of lidocaine toxicity
neuromuscular blockers: Possibly prolonged action of these drugs
phenothiazines: Possibly increased blood levels of both drugs
reserpine: Increased risk of bradycardia and hypotension
sympathomimetics with alpha- and beta-adrenergic effects, such as pseudoephedrine: Possibly hypertension, excessive bradycardia, and heart block
xanthines, such as theophyllines: Possibly decreased therapeutic effects of both drugs

Adverse Reactions

CNS: Anxiety, depression, dizziness, drowsiness, fatigue, headache, paresthesia, syncope, vertigo, weakness, yawning
CV: Bradycardia, chest pain, edema, heart block, heart failure, hypotension, orthostatic hypotension, ventricular arrhythmias
EENT: Nasal congestion, taste perversion
GI: Dyspepsia, elevated liver function test results, hepatic necrosis, hepatitis, nausea, vomiting
GU: Ejaculation failure, impotence
RESP: Cough, dyspnea, wheezing
SKIN: Jaundice, pruritus, scalp tingling

Nursing Complications

• Use nadolol cautiously in patients with diabetes mellitus because it may prolong or worsen hypoglycemia by interfering with glycogenolysis.
• Anticipate that drug may worsen psoriasis and, in patients with myasthenia gravis, muscle weakness and diplopia.
• **WARNING** Withdraw drug gradually over 2 weeks, or as ordered, to avoid MI caused by unopposed beta stimulation or thyroid storm caused by underlying hyperthyroidism. Expect drug to mask tachycardia caused by hyperthyroidism.

N
O

PATIENT TEACHING
•Teach patient how to take her radial pulse, and direct her to do so before each dose of nadolol.
•Instruct patient to notify prescriber if pulse rate falls below 60 beats/minute.
•Caution patient not to stop taking nadolol abruptly or change dosage. Tell her to take a missed dose as soon as possible unless it's within 8 hours of the next scheduled dose.
•Advise patient with diabetes to check blood glucose level often because nadolol may mask signs of hypoglycemia, such as tachycardia.
•Review signs of impending heart failure, and urge patient to notify prescriber immediately if they occur.

nafarelin acetate

Synarel

Class and Category

Chemical class: Decapeptide, gonadotropin-releasing hormone analogue
Therapeutic class: Antiendometriotic, gonadal hormone inhibitor
Pregnancy category: X

Indications and Dosages

➤ *To treat endometriosis*
NASAL INHALATION
Adults. 1 spray (200 mcg) into a nostril every morning and 1 spray into other nostril every evening for up to 6 mo. If amenorrhea doesn't occur in 2 mo, dosage increased, as prescribed, to 800 mcg daily in divided doses.

➤ *To treat gonadotropin-dependent precocious puberty*
NASAL INHALATION
Children at puberty. 2 sprays (400 mcg) into each nostril every morning and evening.
Maximum: 1,800 mcg daily in divided doses t.i.d.

Route	Onset	Peak	Duration
Nasal	60 to 120 days*	20 days†	3 to 6 mo†

* For gonadal hormone inhibitor effects, 4 wk.
† For antiendometriotic effects.

Mechanism of Action

Stimulates the release of the gonadotropins luteinizing hormone (LH) and follicle-stimulating hormone (FSH), which temporarily increase ovarian steroidogenesis. Within 1 month, however, repeated administration of nafarelin halts pituitary gland stimulation and decreases LH and FSH secretion. This action decreases the estrogen level, which improves symptoms of endometriosis. In children, repeated nafarelin administration returns LH and FSH to prepubescent levels, stopping development of secondary sex characteristics and slowing bone growth.

Contraindications

Breastfeeding; hypersensitivity to gonadotropin-releasing hormones, gonadotropin-releasing hormone analogues, nafarelin, or their components; pregnancy; undiagnosed vaginal bleeding

Interactions

DRUGS
nasal decongestants: Possibly impaired nafarelin absorption

Adverse Reactions

CNS: Asthenia, depression, fever, headache, mood changes, paresthesia
CV: Chest pain, edema, hot flashes, palpitations
EENT: Eye pain, rhinitis
ENDO: Galactorrhea, gynecomastia, transient increase in pubic hair growth
GU: Hypermenorrhea, hypertrophy of female genitalia, impotence, libido changes, menstrual irregularities, ovarian cysts, uterine bleeding, vaginal dryness, vaginal spotting between menses
MS: Arthralgia, decreased bone density, myalgia
RESP: Dyspnea
SKIN: Acne, hirsutism, rash, seborrhea, skin discoloration (brown)
Other: Body odor

Nursing Considerations

•Be aware that pregnancy must be ruled out before nafarelin therapy starts and that drug isn't recommended for use by breastfeeding women.

•Expect to start treatment for endometriosis between days 2 and 4 of menstrual cycle. Menses should cease after 6 weeks of treatment. Continued menses may indicate lack of compliance.

•Be aware that bone loss may increase if endometriosis treatment lasts longer than 6 months. Safety of retreatment after 6 months is unknown.

•Avoid giving nasal decongestant within 2 hours after nafarelin administration because it may impair nafarelin absorption.

•Be aware that prescriber will regularly monitor serum hormone levels in patient with gonadotropin-dependent precocious puberty, especially during first 6 to 8 weeks of therapy, to ensure rapid suppression of pituitary function.

PATIENT TEACHING
•Instruct patient to comply with prescriber's instructions for administering nafarelin to obtain desired drug effects.

•Instruct patient to tilt her head back while administering nafarelin to enhance absorption; urge her to try not to sneeze afterward.

•Caution patient not to change dosage without consulting prescriber.

•Counsel patient to use nonhormonal contraception and to notify prescriber if she is or could be pregnant.

•Direct patient not to use nasal decongestant within 2 hours after using nafarelin. If rhinitis occurs, urge her to contact prescriber for instructions.

•Teach patient how to cope with adverse reactions to help maximize compliance.

•Inform patient with endometriosis that drug should cause menses to stop. Urge her to notify prescriber if periods fail to stop even though she's taking drug exactly as prescribed.

•Advise patient with endometriosis to avoid alcohol and tobacco during therapy because they increase bone loss.

•Inform patient with gonadotropin-dependent precocious puberty that signs of puberty will persist during first month of treatment. If they don't resolve within 2 months, advise patient or parents to notify prescriber.

•Tell patient with gonadotropin-dependent precocious puberty that prescriber will as-sess bone growth velocity and bone age during first 3 to 6 months of therapy.

•Reassure parents of child with precocious puberty that child will resume growing when treatment stops.

nafcillin sodium

Nafcil, Nallpen, Unipen

Class and Category
Chemical class: Penicillin
Therapeutic class: Antibiotic
Pregnancy category: B

Indications and Dosages
➤ *To treat infections caused by penicillinase-producing* Staphylococcus aureus

CAPSULES, TABLETS
Adults and adolescents. 250 to 1,000 mg every 4 to 6 hr. *Maximum:* 6,000 mg daily.
Children over age 1 month. 6.25 to 12.5 mg/ kg every 6 hr.
Neonates. 10 mg/kg every 6 to 8 hr.

I.V. INFUSION
Adults and adolescents. 500 to 1,500 mg every 4 hr. *Maximum:* 20,000 mg daily.
Children from birth to age 12. 10 to 20 mg/ kg every 4 hr, or 20 to 40 mg/kg every 8 hr.

I.M. INJECTION
Adults and adolescents. 500 mg every 4 to 6 hr. *Maximum:* 12,000 mg daily.
Children over age 1 month. 25 mg/kg every 12 hr.
Neonates. 10 mg/kg every 12 hr.

➤ *To treat streptococcal pharyngitis*
CAPSULES, TABLETS
Children. 250 mg every 8 hr.

➤ *To treat bone and joint infections, endocarditis, meningitis, and pericarditis caused by susceptible organisms*

I.V. INFUSION
Adults and adolescents. 1,500 to 2,000 mg every 4 to 6 hr. *Maximum:* 20,000 mg daily.

I.V. INFUSION, I.M. INJECTION
Children from birth to age 12. 10 to 20 mg/ kg every 4 hr or 20 to 40 mg/kg every 8 hr. For meningitis in neonates weighing up to 2 kg (4.4 lb), 25 to 50 mg/kg every 12 hr for first week after birth and then 50 mg/kg every 8 hr. For neonates weighing 2 kg or more, 50 mg/kg every 8 hr during first week after birth and then 50 mg/kg every 6 hr.

N O

Mechanism of Action

Binds to certain penicillin-binding proteins in bacterial cell walls, thereby inhibiting the final stage of bacterial cell wall synthesis. The result is cell lysis. Nafcillin's action is bolstered by its chemical composition; its unique side chain resists destruction by beta-lactamases.

Incompatibilities

Don't mix nafcillin in same I.V. bag as aminoglycosides; they're chemically incompatible.

Contraindications

Hypersensitivity to nafcillin, other penicillins, or their components

Interactions

DRUGS

aminoglycosides: Substantial mutual inactivation

chloramphenicol, erythromycins, sulfonamides, tetracyclines: Possibly decreased therapeutic effects of nafcillin

hepatotoxic drugs: Increased risk of hepatotoxicity

methotrexate: Increased risk of methotrexate toxicity

probenecid: Increased blood nafcillin level

FOODS

all foods: Decreased nafcillin absorption

Adverse Reactions

CNS: Depression, headache, seizures

EENT: Oral candidiasis

GI: Abdominal pain, diarrhea, nausea, pseudomembranous colitis, vomiting

GU: Vaginitis

HEME: Leukopenia, neutropenia

SKIN: Exfoliative dermatitis, pruritus, rash, urticaria

Other: Anaphylaxis; hypokalemia; injection site pain, redness, and swelling; serum sicknesslike reaction

Nursing Considerations

• Obtain body fluid or tissue samples for culture and sensitivity testing, as prescribed, and obtain test results, if possible, before giving nafcillin, as ordered.

• Give capsules or tablets at least 1 hour before meals or 2 hours afterward.

• For I.M. injection, use only reconstituted solutions from vials. Inject deep into large muscle, preferably upper outer quadrant of gluteus maximus or lateral part of thigh.

• For intermittent I.V. infusion, infuse over 30 to 60 minutes.

• Give nafcillin at least 1 hour before or after aminoglycosides, especially if patient has renal disease.

• When giving nafcillin to patient at risk for hypertension or fluid overload, be aware that each gram contains 2.5 mEq of sodium.

• **WARNING** Avoid giving nafcillin to premature neonate if drug was reconstituted with bacteriostatic water that contains benzyl alcohol. Doing so can cause potentially fatal metabolic acidosis and circulatory, CNS, renal, and respiratory dysfunction.

• Monitor serum nafcillin levels closely in children, as ordered, because the liver and biliary tract, principal routes of nafcillin elimination, function immaturely in children.

• Watch for evidence of superinfection, such as oral candidiasis and pseudomembranous colitis, especially in elderly, immunocompromised, or debilitated patients who receive large doses of nafcillin. If profuse, watery diarrhea develops, contact prescriber and expect to obtain a stool specimen to rule out pseudomembranous colitis caused by *Clostridium difficile.* If diarrhea occurs, notify prescriber and expect to withhold nafcillin and treat with fluids, electrolytes, protein, and an antibiotic effective against *C. difficile.*

PATIENT TEACHING

• Instruct patient to take nafcillin capsules or tablets on an empty stomach.

• Urge patient to complete entire prescription, even if she feels better.

• Advise patient to notify prescriber if she experiences chills, fever, GI distress, or rash.

• Urge patient to tell prescriber if diarrhea develops, even 2 or ore months after nafcillin therapy ends.

nalbuphine hydrochloride

Nubain

Class and Category

Chemical class: Phenanthrene derivative

Therapeutic class: Analgesic, anesthesia adjunct
Pregnancy category: B

Indications and Dosages

➤ *To relieve moderate to severe pain*

I.V., I.M., OR SUBCUTANEOUS INJECTION
Adults weighing 70 kg (154 lb). 10 mg every 3 to 6 hr, p.r.n. Dosage adjusted for patients weighing more or less.

➤ *As adjunct to anesthesia*

I.V. INJECTION
Adults. 0.3 to 3 mg/kg over 10 to 15 min followed by 0.25 to 0.5 mg/kg, as needed.
DOSAGE ADJUSTMENT For patients who have repeatedly received an opioid agonist, initial dose possibly reduced to 25% of usual dosage. For patients in whom tolerance to drug's effects hasn't developed, maximum usually is 20 mg/dose or 160 mg daily.

Route	Onset	Peak	Duration
I.V.	2 to 3 min	30 min	3 to 4 hr
I.M.	In 15 min	1 hr	3 to 6 hr
SubQ	In 15 min	Unknown	3 to 6 hr

Mechanism of Action

Binds with and stimulates mu and kappa opiate receptors in the spinal cord and higher levels in the CNS. In this way, nalbuphine alters the perception of and emotional response to pain.

Incompatibilities

Don't administer nalbuphine with diazepam or pentobarbital. Use separate I.V. line or flush line well before and after administration.

Contraindications

Hypersensitivity to nalbuphine or its components

Interactions

DRUGS
alfentanil, CNS depressants, fentanyl, sufentanil: Increased risk of hypotension and CNS and respiratory depression
anticholinergics: Increased risk of severe constipation and urine retention
antidiarrheals, such as difenoxin and atropine, loperamide, and paregoric: Increased

risk of severe constipation and increased CNS depression
antihypertensives: Increased risk of hypotension
buprenorphine: Possibly decreased therapeutic effects of nalbuphine and increased risk of respiratory depression
hydroxyzine: Increased risk of CNS depression and hypotension
MAO inhibitors: Risk of possibly fatal increased CNS excitation or depression
metoclopramide: Possibly antagonized effects of metoclopramide
naloxone, naltrexone: Decreased pharmacologic effects of nalbuphine
neuromuscular blockers: Increased risk of prolonged CNS and respiratory depression

ACTIVITIES
alcohol use: Increased risk of coma, hypotension, profound sedation, and respiratory depression

Adverse Reactions

CNS: Confusion, depression, dizziness, euphoria, fatigue, hallucinations, headache, nervousness, restlessness, seizures, syncope, tiredness, weakness
CV: Hypertension, hypotension, tachycardia
EENT: Blurred vision, diplopia, dry mouth
GI: Abdominal cramps, anorexia, constipation, nausea, vomiting
GU: Decreased urine output, ureteral spasm
RESP: Dyspnea, pulmonary edema, respiratory depression, wheezing
SKIN: Diaphoresis, flushing, pruritus, rash, sensation of warmth, urticaria
Other: Injection site burning, pain, redness, swelling, and warmth

Nursing Considerations

• Use nalbuphine cautiously in patients taking other drugs that can cause respiratory depression.
• Keep resuscitation equipment and naloxone readily available to reverse nalbuphine's effects, if needed.
• For direct I.V. injection through an I.V. line with a compatible infusing solution, give drug slowly—no more than 10 mg over 3 to 5 minutes. Inject into free-flowing normal saline solution, D₅W, or lactated Ringer's solution.
• During prolonged use, expect to give a stool

softener to minimize constipation.

•If patient is opioid-dependent, expect drug to cause withdrawal symptoms, such as abdominal cramps, anorexia, anxiety, backache, bone or joint pain, confusion, depression, diaphoresis, dysphoria, erythema, fear, fever, irritability, labile blood pressure and pulse, lacrimation, muscle spasms, myalgia, mydriasis, nasal congestion, nausea, opioid craving, piloerection, restlessness, rhinorrhea, sensation of crawling skin, sleep disturbances, tremor, uneasiness, vomiting, and yawning.

•**WARNING** Be aware that drug may obscure neurologic assessment findings if patient has a cerebral aneurysm, head injury, or increased intracranial pressure.

PATIENT TEACHING

•Advise patient to avoid hazardous activities until nalbuphine's CNS effects are known.

•Counsel patient against making important decisions while receiving drug because it may cloud her judgment.

nalidixic acid

NegGram

Class and Category

Chemical class: Naphthyridine derivative quinolone

Therapeutic class: Antibiotic

Pregnancy category: Not rated (first trimester), B (later trimesters)

Indications and Dosages

➤ *To treat UTI caused by gram-negative bacteria, such as most* Enterobacter *species,* Escherichia coli, Klebsiella *species,* Morganella morganii, Proteus mirabilis, Proteus vulgaris, *and* Providencia rettgeri

ORAL SUSPENSION, TABLETS

Adults and children age 12 and over. *Initial:* 1,000 mg every 6 hr for 1 to 2 wk. *Maintenance:* 500 mg every 6 hr. *Maximum:* 4,000 mg daily.

Children ages 3 months to 12 years. *Initial:* 55 mg/kg daily in divided doses q.i.d. for 1 to 2 wk. *Maintenance:* 33 mg/kg daily in divided doses q.i.d.

Contraindications

Hypersensitivity to nalidixic acid or its com-

ponents, porphyria, seizure disorder, use with melphalan or other related chemotherapeutic alkylating drugs

Mechanism of Action

Inhibits the enzyme DNA gyrase, which is responsible for the unwinding and supercoiling of bacterial DNA before it replicates. By inhibiting this enzyme, nalidixic acid causes bacterial cells to die.

Interactions

DRUGS

aluminum-, calcium-, and magnesium-containing antacids; didanosine; multivitamins containing iron or zinc; sucralfate: Possibly interference with nalidixic acid absorption

chloramphenicol, nitrofurantoin, tetracycline: Decreased effects of nalidixic acid

cyclosporine: Possibly increased blood cyclosporine level

melphalan: Possibly increased risk of serious GI toxicity

oral anticoagulants: Increased anticoagulant effects

probenecid: Decreased effects of nalidixic acid and increased risk of adverse reactions

theophylline: Possibly increased blood theophylline level

FOODS

caffeine: Decreased clearance and prolonged half-life of caffeine

Adverse Reactions

CNS: Confusion, drowsiness, hallucinations, headache, increased intracranial pressure with bulging fontanels (in infants and children), light-headedness, malaise, paresthesia, peripheral neuropathy, psychosis, restlessness, seizures, tremor, weakness

EENT: Altered color perception, blurred vision, diplopia, halo vision, photophobia

GI: Abdominal pain, diarrhea, nausea, pseudomembranous colitis, vomiting

HEME: Eosinophilia, hemolytic anemia, leukopenia, thrombocytopenia

MS: Tendon rupture

SKIN: Jaundice, photosensitivity, pruritus, rash, Stevens-Johnson syndrome, urticaria

Other: Anaphylaxis, metabolic acidosis

Nursing Considerations

•Be aware that nalidixic acid shouldn't be

given to patient with creatinine clearance below 10 ml/min/1.73 m² because of the increased risk of drug toxicity and should be used cautiously in patients with liver disease, epilepsy, glucose-6-phosphate dehydrogenase deficiency, or severe cerebral arteriosclerosis or renal failure.

•Avoid giving drug within 2 hours of giving didanosine; multivitamin that contains iron or zinc; sucralfate; or antacid that contains aluminum, calcium, or magnesium.

•If nalidixic acid therapy exceeds 2 weeks, monitor patient's blood counts and renal and liver function test results periodically, as ordered.

•**WARNING** Stop nalidixic acid at first sign of hypersensitivity, including rash, because it may indicate anaphylaxis. Reaction may occur with first dose. Expect to give epinephrine and supportive care.

•If patient also takes cyclosporine or theophylline, monitor blood level of these drugs and adjust dosage, as prescribed.

•If patient has a history of seizures or cerebral arteriosclerosis, monitor for seizures during nalidixic acid therapy.

•Notify prescriber if patient has symptoms of peripheral neuropathy (pain, burning, tingling, numbness, weakness, or altered sensations of light touch, pain, temperature, position sense, or vibration sense), which could be permanent; or tendon rupture, which requires immediate rest. In each case, expect to stop nalidixic acid.

PATIENT TEACHING

•Encourage patient to drink plenty of fluids during therapy unless directed otherwise by prescriber.

•Urge patient to complete entire course of therapy, even if she feels better before it's finished.

•Advise patient to protect skin from sunlight.

•Urge patient to notify prescriber immediately about vision changes or such adverse CNS reactions as confusion, drowsiness, hallucinations, psychosis, and seizures.

•Urge patient to stop drug and notify prescriber if rash or other evidence of hypersensitivity develops.

•Tell patient to take drug at least 2 hours before or after aluminum-, calcium-, or magnesium-containing antacids; didanosine chewable buffered tablets or oral solution prepared from powder; multivitamins that contain iron or zinc; or sucralfate.

•Caution patient to avoid hazardous tasks until CNS effects of drug are known.

•Instruct patient to limit caffeine intake while taking nalidixic acid.

•Tell patient to stop drug and notify prescriber if she develops tendon pain or inflammation or abnormal changes in motor or sensory function.

•Urge patient to notify prescriber if diarrhea develops, even up to 2 months after nalidixic acid therapy stops.

naloxone hydrochloride

Narcan

Class and Category

Chemical class: Thebaine derivative
Therapeutic class: Opioid antagonist
Pregnancy category: B

Indications and Dosages

➤ *To treat known or suspected opioid overdose*

I.V. INJECTION

Adults and children age 5 and over weighing more than 20 kg (44 lb). 0.4 to 2 mg repeated every 2 to 3 min, p.r.n. If no response after 10 mg, patient may not have opioid-induced respiratory depression.

Infants and children under age 5. 0.01 mg/kg as a single dose; if no improvement, another 0.1 mg/kg, as prescribed. Or, 0.1 mg/kg repeated every 2 to 3 min, as needed

I.V., I.M., OR SUBCUTANEOUS INJECTION

Neonates. 0.01 mg/kg repeated I.V. every 2 to 3 min, as prescribed, until desired response occurs. Or, initial I.V. dose of 0.1 mg/kg.

➤ *To treat postoperative opioid-induced respiratory depression*

I.V. INJECTION

Adults and adolescents. *Initial:* 0.1 to 0.2 mg every 2 to 3 min until desired response occurs. Additional doses given every 1 to 2 hr, if needed, based on patient response.

Children. *Initial:* 0.005 to 0.01 mg every 2 to 3 min until desired response occurs. Additional doses given every 1 to 2 hr, if needed, based on patient response.

➤ *To reverse opioid-induced asphyxia*

I.V. , I.M., OR SUBCUTANEOUS INJECTION

Neonates. *Initial:* 0.01 mg/kg every 2 to

N O

3 min until desired response occurs. Additional doses given every 1 to 2 hr, if needed, based on patient response.

➤ *As adjunct to treat hypotension caused by septic shock*

I.V. INFUSION OR INJECTION

Adults. 0.03 to 0.2 mg/kg over 5 min followed by continuous infusion of 0.03 to 0.3 mg/kg/hr for 1 to 24 hr, as needed, based on patient response.

Route	Onset	Peak	Duration
I.V.	1 to 2 min	5 to 15 min	45 min or longer
I.M., SubQ	2 to 5 min	5 to 15 min	45 min or longer

Mechanism of Action

Briefly and competitively antagonizes mu, kappa, and sigma receptors in the CNS, thus reversing the analgesia, hypotension, respiratory depression, and sedation caused by most opioids. Mu receptors are responsible for analgesia, euphoria, miosis, and respiratory depression. Kappa receptors are responsible for analgesia and sedation. Sigma receptors control dysphoria and other delusional states.

Incompatibilities

Don't mix naloxone with any other solution unless you verify that drugs are compatible; drug is incompatible with alkaline, bisulfite, and metabisulfite solutions.

Contraindications

Hypersensitivity to naloxone or its components

Interactions

DRUGS

butorphanol, nalbuphine, pentazocine: Reversal of these drugs' analgesic and adverse effects

opioid analgesics: Reversal of these drugs' analgesic and adverse effects, possibly withdrawal symptoms in opioid-dependent patients

Adverse Reactions

CNS: Excitement, irritability, nervousness, restlessness, seizures, tremor, violent behavior

CV: Hypertension (severe), hypotension, ventricular fibrillation, ventricular tachycardia
GI: Nausea, vomiting
RESP: Pulmonary edema
SKIN: Diaphoresis
Other: Withdrawal symptoms

Nursing Considerations

• Keep resuscitation equipment readily available during naloxone administration.
• Administer drug by I.V. route whenever possible.
• Give repeat doses as prescribed, depending on patient's response.
• Anticipate that rapid reversal of opioid effects can cause diaphoresis, nausea, and vomiting.
• **WARNING** Monitor for withdrawal symptoms, especially when giving naloxone to opioid-dependent patient. Symptoms may include abdominal cramps, anorexia, anxiety, backache, bone or joint pain, confusion, depression, diaphoresis, dysphoria, erythema, fear, fever, irritability, labile blood pressure and pulse, lacrimation, muscle spasms, myalgia, mydriasis, nasal congestion, nausea, opioid craving, piloerection, restlessness, rhinorrhea, sensation of crawling skin, sleep disturbances, tremor, uneasiness, vomiting, and yawning.
• Expect patient with hepatic or renal dysfunction to have increased circulating blood naloxone level.

PATIENT TEACHING

• Inform patient or family that naloxone will reverse opioid-induced adverse reactions.
• Urge opioid-dependent patient to seek drug rehabilitation.

naltrexone hydrochloride

ReVia, Vivitrol

Class and Category

Chemical class: Thebaine derivative
Therapeutic class: Opioid antagonist
Pregnancy category: C

Indications and Dosages

➤ *To treat opioid dependence*

TABLETS

Adults. *Initial:* 25 mg, repeated within 1 hr, if needed and if no withdrawal symptoms occur. *Maintenance:* 50 to 150 mg daily or 350 mg/wk by intermittent dosing regimen.

➤ *As adjunct to treat alcoholism*
TABLETS
Adults. 50 mg daily (up to 100 mg daily for some patients) for 12 wk.
I.M. INJECTION
Adults. 380 mg every 4 wk or once monthly.

Route	Onset	Peak	Duration
P.O.	15 to 30 min	In 12 hr	24 hr*
I.M.	Unknown	2 hr	Unknown

Mechanism of Action

Displaces opioid agonists from—or blocks them from binding with—mu, kappa, and delta receptors. Opioid receptor blockade reverses the euphoric effect of opioids. Naltrexone also inhibits the effects of endogenous opioids, thus reducing alcohol craving.

Contraindications

Acute hepatitis, acute opioid withdrawal, concurrent use of opioid analgesics (including opioid agonists, such as methadone or levo-alpha-acetyl-methadol [LAAM]), failure of naloxone challenge test, hepatic failure, hypersensitivity to naltrexone or its components, opioid dependence, positive urine screen for opioids

Interactions

DRUGS
opioid analgesics: Reversal of the analgesic and adverse effects of these drugs, possibly withdrawal symptoms in opioid-dependent patients
thioridazine: Increased somnolence and lethargy

Adverse Reactions

CNS: Anxiety, chills, confusion, depression, dizziness, fatigue, fever, hallucinations, headache, insomnia, irritability, nervousness, restlessness, somnolence, suicidal ideation, syncope
CV: Chest pain, edema, hypertension, tachycardia
EENT: Blurred vision, burning eyes, conjunctivitis, dry mouth, eyelid swelling,

---

* For 50 mg; 48 hr for 100 mg; 72 hr for 150 mg.

hoarseness, pharyngitis, rhinitis, sneezing, tinnitus
GI: Abdominal cramps, anorexia, constipation, diarrhea, GI ulceration, hepatotoxicity with excessive doses, nausea, thirst, vomiting
GU: Difficult ejaculation, urinary frequency
MS: Arthralgia, back pain or stiffness, joint sitffness, muscle cramps, myalgia
RESP: Cough, dyspnea, eosinophilic pneumonia, upper respiratory tract infection
SKIN: Pruritus, rash
Other: Injection site reactions, such as pain, tenderness, induration, swelling, erythema, pruritus

Nursing Considerations

• Use naltrexone cautiously in patients with severe renal impairment, thrombocytopenia, hemophilia, or severe hepatic failure.
• To avoid withdrawal symptoms, wait 7 to 10 days after last opioid dose, as prescribed, before starting naltrexone. Because urine testing isn't always conclusive, prepare patient for naloxone challenge test if there are any doubts about patient's abstinence.
• Give oral drug with food or antacids to decrease adverse GI reactions.
• Dilute parenteral form using only diluent supplied in carton. Inject in gluteal muscle using only needle supplied in carton. Don't substitute any components for components in carton. Store entire dose pack in refrigerator; unrefrigerated drug can be stored at room temperature for no more than 7 days.
• Inspect injection site for reactions, such as tenderness, induration, swelling, or redness. Ask if patient feels pain or itching at the site. Report any such findings to prescriber because abscesses and site necrosis may occur and require surgical intervention.
• **WARNING** Never give parenteral form intravenously.
• Patients who receive naltrexone and need pain management are more likely to have longer, deeper respiratory depression and histamine-release reactions (such as facial swelling, itching, generalized erythema, and bronchoconstriction) if given an opioid analgesic. Expect alternative analgesics to be used, such as regional analgesia, conscious sedation with a benzodiazepine, nonopioid analgesics, or general anesthesia. If an opioid analgesic must be used, monitor patient closely.
• Watch patient closely for suicidal tenden-

cies throughout naltrexone therapy.
•Anticipate that some patients may need treatment for up to 1 year.

PATIENT TEACHING

•**WARNING** Caution patient against taking opioids during naltrexone therapy or in the future because she'll be more sensitive to them. In fact, strongly warn patient that taking large doses of heroin or any other opioid (including methadone or LAAM) while taking naltrexone could lead to coma, serious injury, or death.

•Explain that patient may have nausea after first injection but that it is usually mild and subsides within a few days. Most patients don't have nausea with repeat doses.

•Tell patient to report adverse reactions promptly, especially dyspnea, coughing, wheezing, abdominal pain, and jaundice.

•Urge family or caregiver to watch patient closely for abnormal behaviors, including suicidal tendencies, even after patient stops taking naltrexone.

•Inform patient that naltrexone doesn't eliminate or diminish alcohol withdrawal symptoms.

•Urge patient to have comprehensive rehabilitation in addition to receiving naltrexone.

•Inform patient about nonopioid treatments for cough, diarrhea, and pain.

•Instruct patient to carry medical identification that lists naltrexone therapy.

•Instruct women of childbearing age to notify prescriber if pregnancy is suspected.

nandrolone decanoate

Deca-Durabolin, Hybolin Decanoate, Kabolin

Class, Category, and Schedule

Chemical class: Testosterone derivative
Therapeutic class: Antianemic
Pregnancy category: X
Controlled substance schedule: III

Indications and Dosages

➤ *To manage anemia caused by chronic renal failure*

I.M. INJECTION

Adults and adolescents age 14 and over.
50 to 100 mg every 1 to 4 wk for females; 50 to 200 mg every 1 to 4 wk for males.
Children ages 2 to 13. 25 to 50 mg every 3 to 4 wk.

Mechanism of Action

Increases production of erythropoietin, a precursor of RBCs. Nandrolone also increases hemoglobin level and RBC volume.

Contraindications

Breast cancer in females with hypercalcemia; breast or prostate cancer in males; hypersensitivity to nandrolone, anabolic steroids, or their components; known or suspected pregnancy; nephrosis; nephrotic phase of nephritis; severe hepatic dysfunction

Interactions

DRUGS

corticosteroids: Increased risk of edema and severe acne
drugs with sodium: Increased risk of edema
hepatotoxic drugs: Increased risk of hepatotoxicity
insulin, oral antidiabetic drugs: Possibly hypoglycemia
NSAIDs, oral anticoagulants, salicylates: Increased anticoagulant effects
somatrem, somatropin: Possibly accelerated epiphyseal maturation

FOODS

food with sodium: Increased risk of edema

Adverse Reactions

CNS: Excitement, depression, insomnia
CV: Edema, hyperlipidemia
ENDO: Feminization in postpubertal males (epididymitis, gynecomastia, impotence, oligospermia, priapism, testicular atrophy); glucose intolerance; virilism in females (acne, clitoral enlargement, decreased breast size, deepened voice, diaphoresis, emotional lability, flushing, hirsutism, hoarseness, libido changes, male-pattern baldness, menstrual irregularities, nervousness, oily hair or skin, vaginitis, weight gain); virilism in prepubertal males (acne, decreased ejaculatory volume, epididymitis, penis enlargement, prepubertal closure of epiphyseal plates, priapism, unnatural growth of body and facial hair)
GI: Diarrhea, elevated liver function test results, hepatocellular carcinoma, nausea, vomiting
GU: Urinary frequency
HEME: Unusual bleeding
SKIN: Jaundice

Other: Injection site induration and pain, physical and psychological dependence

Nursing Considerations

•Provide adequate calories and protein, as ordered, to maintain a positive nitrogen balance. Also provide adequate iron intake to ensure optimal response to nandrolone.
•Weigh patient daily to detect fluid retention, which can lead to edema. If patient retains fluid, expect to place her on sodium-restricted diet or diuretic therapy, as ordered.
•Assess boys under age 7 for secondary sexual characteristics, and notify prescriber.
•Assess patient for signs of virilism, and notify prescriber if they develop.
•Monitor diabetic patient for decreased glucose control; notify prescriber of hyperglycemia.
•Be aware that some people use nandrolone as a sports aid; long-term use may lead to abuse, addiction, and such adverse reactions as antisocial behavior, cardiovascular complications, hepatotoxicity, and libido changes.
•If no improvement occurs after 6 months, expect prescriber to discontinue nandrolone.

PATIENT TEACHING
•Review signs of virilism, and urge patient to notify prescriber if they develop. Explain that some changes may be permanent.
•To prevent vaginitis, advise women to wash after intercourse and to wear cotton underwear.
•Instruct patient to notify prescriber immediately about menstrual changes.
•Advise patient to notify prescriber about sudden weight gain—a sign of edema, which may cause significant problems in patients with cardiac or renal disorders.
•Inform adolescent males that they may need a semen evaluation every 3 to 4 months.
•Instruct diabetic patient to monitor blood glucose level often, to watch for signs of hyperglycemia, and to report significant changes.

naproxen

Apo-Naproxen (CAN), EC-Naprosyn, Naprosyn, Naprosyn-E (CAN), Naxen (CAN), Novo-Naprox (CAN), Nu-Naprox (CAN)

naproxen sodium

Aleve, Anaprox, Anaprox DS, Apo-Napro-Na (CAN), Naprelan, Naprosyn-SR (CAN), Novo-Naprox Sodium (CAN)

Class and Category

Chemical class: Propionic acid derivative
Therapeutic class: Analgesic, anti-inflammatory, antipyretic
Pregnancy category: C

Indications and Dosages

➤ *To relieve mild to moderate musculoskeletal inflammation, including ankylosing spondylitis, osteoarthritis, and rheumatoid arthritis*

DELAYED-RELEASE TABLETS, ORAL SUSPENSION, TABLETS (NAPROXEN)

Adults. 250 to 500 mg b.i.d. *Maximum:* 1,500 mg daily for limited periods, as prescribed.

E.R. TABLETS (NAPROXEN SODIUM)

Adults. 750 to 1,000 mg daily. *Maximum:* 1,500 mg daily.

TABLETS (NAPROXEN SODIUM)

Adults. 275 to 550 mg b.i.d. *Maximum:* 1,650 mg daily for limited periods, as prescribed.

SUPPOSITORIES (NAPROXEN SODIUM)

Adults. 500 mg at bedtime in addition to daytime P.O. administration. *Maximum:* 1,500 mg daily (P.O. and suppository combined).

➤ *To relieve symptoms of juvenile rheumatoid arthritis and other inflammatory conditions in children*

ORAL SUSPENSION, TABLETS (NAPROXEN)

Children. 10 mg/kg daily in divided doses b.i.d.

➤ *To relieve symptoms of acute gouty arthritis*

DELAYED-RELEASE TABLETS, ORAL SUSPENSION, TABLETS (NAPROXEN)

Adults. *Initial:* 750 mg, then 250 mg every 8 hr until symptoms subside.

E.R. TABLETS (NAPROXEN SODIUM)

Adults. *Initial:* 1,000 to 1,500 mg on day 1; then 1,000 mg daily until symptoms subside. *Maximum:* 1,500 mg daily.

TABLETS (NAPROXEN SODIUM)

Adults. *Initial:* 825 mg, then 275 mg every 8 hr until symptoms subside.

➤ *To relieve mild to moderate pain, including acute tendinitis and bursitis, arthralgia, dysmenorrhea, and myalgia*

N
O

DELAYED-RELEASE TABLETS (NAPROXEN)
Adults. *Initial:* 1,000 mg daily. *Maximum:* 1,500 mg daily.
E.R. TABLETS (NAPROXEN SODIUM)
Adults. *Initial:* 1,100 mg daily, increased as prescribed. *Maximum:* 1,500 mg daily.
ORAL SUSPENSION, TABLETS (NAPROXEN)
Adults. *Initial:* 500 mg, then 250 mg every 6 to 8 hr, p.r.n. *Maximum:* 1,250 mg daily.
TABLETS (NAPROXEN SODIUM)
Adults. *Initial:* 550 mg, then 275 mg every 6 to 8 hr, p.r.n. *Maximum:* 1,375 mg daily.
➤ *To relieve fever and mild to moderate musculoskeletal inflammation or pain*
TABLETS (OTC NAPROXEN SODIUM)
Adults. 220 mg every 8 to 12 hr; or 440 mg and 220 mg 12 hr later. *Maximum:* 660 mg daily for 10 days unless directed otherwise.
DOSAGE ADJUSTMENT For patients over age 65, 220 mg every 12 hr. *Maximum:* 440 mg for 10 days unless directed otherwise.

Route	Onset	Peak	Duration
P.O. (naproxen)*	1 hr[†]	2 to 4 hr[†‡]	7 to 12 hr[†]
P.O. (naproxen sodium)*	30 min[†]	1 hr[†‡]	7 to 12 hr[†]

Mechanism of Action

Blocks cyclooxygenase, the enzyme needed to synthesize prostaglandins, which mediate the inflammatory response and cause local vasodilation, swelling, and pain. Thus, naproxen, an NSAID, reduces symptoms of inflammation and relieves pain. Antipyretic action probably stems from its effect on the hypothalamus, which increases peripheral blood flow, causing vasodilation and heat dissipation.

Contraindications

Angioedema, asthma, bronchospasm, nasal polyps, rhinitis, or urticaria induced by aspirin, iodides, or other NSAIDs; hypersensitivity to naproxen or its components

---

* For antirheumatism, onset is in 14 days, peak is unknown, and duration is 2 to 4 wk.
[†] For analgesia.
[‡] For gout, 1 to 2 days.

Interactions
DRUGS
ACE inhibitors: Decreased antihypertensive effects; increased risk of renal dysfunction
acetaminophen: Increased risk of adverse renal effects with combined long-term use
aluminum hydroxide or magnesium oxide antacids, cholestyramine, sucralfate: Possibly delayed absorption of naproxen
anticoagulants, thrombolytics: Prolonged PT, increased risk of bleeding
antihypertensives: Decreased effectiveness of antihypertensive
aspirin: Decreased aspirin effectiveness from lowered plasma and peak aspirin levels
beta blockers: Decreased antihypertensive effects of these drugs
bone marrow depressants, such as aldesleukin and cisplatin: Increased risk of leukopenia and thrombocytopenia
cefamandole, cefoperazone, cefotetan, plicamycin, valproic acid: Increased risk of hypoprothrombinemia and bleeding
cimetidine: Altered blood naproxen level
colchicine, glucocorticoids, other NSAIDs, potassium supplements, salicylates: Increased GI irritability and bleeding
cyclosporine, gold compounds, nephrotoxic drugs: Increased risk of nephrotoxicity
digoxin: Increased blood digoxin level and risk of digitalis toxicity
diuretics: Decreased diuretic effectiveness
furosemide: Decreased natriuretic effect
insulin, oral antidiabetic drugs: Increased effectiveness of these drugs; risk of hypoglycemia
lithium: Increased risk of lithium toxicity
methotrexate: Increased risk of methotrexate toxicity
naproxen-containing products: Increased risk of toxicity
phenytoin: Increased blood phenytoin level
probenecid: Increased risk of naproxen toxicity
ACTIVITIES
alcohol use, smoking: Increased risk of naproxen-induced GI ulceration

Adverse Reactions
CNS: Aseptic meningitis, chills, cognitive impairment, decreased concentration, depression, dizziness, dream disturbances, drowsiness, fever, headache, insomnia, lightheadedness, malaise, seizures, stroke, vertigo
CV: Edema, heart failure, hypertension, MI, palpitations, tachycardia, vasculitis

EENT: Papilledema, papillitis, retrobulbar optic neuritis, stomatitis, tinnitus, vision or hearing changes
ENDO: Hyperglycemia, hypoglycemia
GI: Abdominal pain, anorexia, colitis, constipation, diarrhea, diverticulitis, dyspepsia, dysphagia, elevated liver function test results, esophagitis, flatulence, gastritis, gastroenteritis, gastroesophageal reflux disease, GI bleeding and ulceration, heartburn, hematemesis, hepatitis, indigestion, melena, nausea, pancreatitis, peptic ulceration, perforation of stomach or intestines, stomatitis, vomiting
GU: Elevated serum creatinine level, glomerulonephritis, hematuria, infertility (in women), interstitial nephritis, menstrual irregularities, nephrotic syndrome, renal failure, renal papillary necrosis
HEME: Agranulocytosis, anemia, aplastic anemia, eosinophilia, granulocytopenia, hemolytic anemia, leukopenia, neutropenia, pancytopenia, thrombocytopenia
MS: Muscle weakness, myalgia
RESP: Asthma, dyspnea, eosinophilic pneumonitis, respiratory depression
SKIN: Alopecia, diaphoresis, ecchymosis, erythema multiforme, photosensitivity, pruritus, pseudoporphyria, purpura, rash, Stevens-Johnson syndrome, systemic lupus erythematosus, toxic epidermal necrolysis, urticaria
Other: Anaphylaxis, angioedema, hyperkalemia

Nursing Considerations
• Use naproxen with extreme caution in patients with a history of ulcer disease or GI bleeding because NSAIDs such as naproxen increase the risk of GI bleeding and ulceration. Expect to use naproxen for the shortest time possible in these patients.
• Be aware that serious GI tract ulceration, bleeding, and perforation may occur without warning symptoms. Elderly patients are at greater risk. To minimize risk, give drug with food. If GI distress occurs, withhold drug and notify prescriber immediately.
• Use naproxen cautiously in patients with hypertension, and monitor blood pressure closely. Drug may cause hypertension or worsen it. Because of naproxen's sodium content, watch for fluid retention.
• Rehydrate a dehydrated patient before giving drug. If patient has renal disease, monitor

renal function closely during therapy.
• Naproxen isn't recommended for patients with advanced renal disease.
• **WARNING** Monitor patient closely for thrombotic events, including MI and stroke, because NSAIDs increase the risk.
• Monitor patient—especially if she's elderly or receiving long-term naproxen therapy—for less common but serious adverse GI reactions, including anorexia, constipation, diverticulitis, dysphagia, esophagitis, gastritis, gastroenteritis, gastroesophageal reflux disease, hemorrhoids, hiatal hernia, melena, stomatitis, and vomiting.
• Monitor liver function test results because, in rare cases, elevations may progress to severe hepatic reactions, including fatal hepatitis, liver necrosis, and hepatic failure.
• Monitor BUN and serum creatinine levels in elderly patients, patients taking diuretics or ACE inhibitors, and patients with heart failure, impaired renal function, or hepatic dysfunction; naproxen may cause renal failure.
• Monitor CBC for decreased hemoglobin and hematocrit because drug may worsen anemia.
• **WARNING** If patient has bone marrow suppression or is receiving treatment with an antineoplastic drug, monitor laboratory results (including WBC count), and watch for evidence of infection because anti-inflammatory and antipyretic actions of naproxen may mask signs and symptoms, such as fever and pain.
• Assess patient's skin regularly for signs of rash or other hypersensitivity reaction because naproxen is an NSAID and may cause serious skin reactions without warning, even in patients with no history of NSAID sensivitity. At first sign of reaction, stop drug and notify prescriber.
• Assess drug effectiveness in ankylosing spondylitis, as evidenced by decreased night pain, morning stiffness, and pain at rest; in osteoarthritis: decreased joint pain or tenderness and increased mobility, range of motion, and ability to perform daily activities; in rheumatoid arthritis: increased mobility and decreased joint swelling and morning stiffness; in acute gouty arthritis: decreased heat, pain, swelling, and tenderness in affected joints.
• Tell prescriber if patient complains of vi-

N
O

sion changes; patient may need ophthalmic exam.

PATIENT TEACHING
• Caution patient not to exceed recommended dosage because serious adverse reactions may occur.
• Tell patient to swallow delayed-release tablets whole and not to break, crush, or chew them.
• Advise patient to take drug with food to reduce GI distress.
• Tell patient to take drug with a full glass of water and to remain upright for 15 to 30 minutes after taking it to prevent drug from lodging in esophagus and causing irritation.
• Caution patient to avoid hazardous activities until drug's CNS effects are known.
• Urge patient to keep scheduled appointments with prescriber to monitor progress.
• Tell pregnant patient to avoid taking naproxen-containing products late in pregnancy.
• Advise against taking naproxen for more than 10 days without consulting prescriber.
• Explain that naproxen may increase the risk of serious adverse cardiovascular reactions; urge patient to seek immediate medical attention if signs or symptoms arise, such as chest pain, shortness of breath, weakness, and slurring of speech.
• Inform patient that naproxen may increase the risk of serious adverse GI reactions; stress the importance of seeking immediate medical attention for such signs and symptoms as epigastric or abdominal pain, indigestion, black or tarry stools, or vomiting blood or material that looks like coffee grounds.
• Alert patient to rare but serious skin reactions. Urge her to seek immediate medical attention for rash, blisters, itching, fever, or other indications of hypersensitivity.

naratriptan hydrochloride

Amerge

Class and Category
Chemical class: Selective serotonin 5-HT receptor agonist
Therapeutic class: Antimigraine
Pregnancy category: C

Indications and Dosages
➤ *To relieve acute migraine with or without aura*

TABLETS
Adults. 1 to 2.5 mg as a single dose, repeated in 4 hr p.r.n. if only partial relief obtained. *Maximum:* 5 mg daily.
DOSAGE ADJUSTMENT For patients with mild to moderate renal or hepatic impairment, maximum dosage reduced to 2.5 mg daily.

Mechanism of Action
Binds to receptors on intracranial blood vessels and sensory nerves in the trigeminal-vascular system to stimulate negative feedback, which halts serotonin release. Thus, naratriptan selectively constricts inflamed and dilated cranial vessels in the carotid circulation and inhibits production of proinflammatory neuropeptides.

Contraindications
Basilar or hemiplegic migraine; cerebrovascular, peripheral vascular, or coronary artery disease (ischemic or vasospastic); hypersensitivity to naratriptan or its components; hypertension (uncontrolled); severe hepatic or renal dysfunction; use within 24 hours of another 5-HT agonist or an ergotamine-containing or ergot-type drug, such as dihydroergotamine or methysergide

Interactions
DRUGS
ergot-containing drugs: Possibly prolonged or additive vasospastic reactions
fluoxetine, fluvoxamine, paroxetine, sertraline: Possibly weakness, hyperreflexia, and incoordination
oral contraceptives: Possibly reduced clearance and increased blood level of naratriptan
other selective serotonin 5-HT receptor agonists (including rizatriptan, sumatriptan, and zolmitriptan): Possibly additive effects

Adverse Reactions
CNS: Dizziness, drowsiness, fatigue, malaise, paresthesia
CV: Chest pain, pressure, or heaviness
EENT: Decreased salivation, otitis media, pharyngitis, photophobia, rhinitis, throat tightness
GI: Nausea, vomiting

Nursing Considerations
• **WARNING** Because naratriptan therapy can cause coronary artery vasospasm, monitor patient with coronary artery disease for signs or symptoms of angina while taking drug. Because naratriptan may also cause peripheral vasospastic reactions, such as ischemic bowel disease, monitor patient for abdominal pain and bloody diarrhea.
• Monitor patient for hypertension during naratriptan therapy. Naratriptan may increase systolic blood pressure by as much as 32 mm Hg.
• Be prepared to perform a complete neurovascular assessment in any patient who reports an unusual headache or who fails to respond to first dose of naratriptan.

PATIENT TEACHING
• Inform patient that naratriptan is used to treat acute migraine attacks and that it won't prevent or reduce the number of migraines.
• Advise patient not to take more than maximum prescribed during any 24-hour period.
• If patient has no relief from initial dose of naratriptan, instruct her to notify prescriber rather than taking another dose in 4 hours because she may need a different drug.
• Advise patient to seek reevaluation by prescriber if she experiences more than four headaches during any 30-day period while taking naratriptan.

natalizumab

Tysabri

Class and Category
Chemical class: Recombinant humanized IgG4K monoclonal antibody
Therapeutic class: Anti-multiple sclerotic
Pregnancy category: C

Indications and Dosages
➤ *To delay physical disability and reduce frequency of clinical exacerbations in relapsing forms of multiple sclerosis; to induce and maintain remission in moderately to severely active Crohn's disease with evidence of inflammation in patients who had inadequate response to or are unable to tolerate conventional therapy and inhibitors of tumor necrosis factor alpha*

I.V. INFUSION
Adults. 300 mg infused over 1 hr every 4 wk.

Route	Onset	Peak	Duration
I.V.	Unknown	24 wk	Unknown

Mechanism of Action
Inhibits migration of leukocytes out of the vascular space, increasing the number of circulating leukocytes. It does this by binding to integrins on the surface of leukocytes (except neutrophils) and inhibiting adhesion of leukocytes to their counter receptors. In multiple sclerosis, lesions probably occur when activated inflammatory cells, including T-lymphocytes cross the blood-brain barrier.

Contraindications
History of or presence of progressive multifocal leukoencephalopathy, hypersensitivity to natalizumab or its components

Interactions
DRUGS
antineoplastics, immunosuppresants, immunomodulating agents: Increased risk of life-threatening infection

Adverse Reactions
CNS: Depression, dizziness, fatigue, headache, progressive multifocal leukoencephalopathy (PML), rigors, somnolence, suicidal ideation, vertigo
CV: Chest discomfort, peripheral edema
EENT: Sinusutis, tonsillitis, tooth infection
GI: Abdominal discomfort, abnormal liver function test results, cholelithiasis, diarrhea, gastroenteritis, hepatotoxicity, jaindice, nausea
GU: Amenorrhea; dysmenorrhea; irregular menstruation; ovarian cysts; UTI; urinary incontinence, frequency, or urgency; vaginitis
MS: Arthralgia, back or limb pain, joint swelling, muscle cramp
RESP: Cough, pneumonia or other respiratory tract infection
SKIN: Dermatitis, night sweats, pruritus, rash, urticaria
Other: Acute hypersensitivity reaction, anaphylaxis, antibody formation, flulike illness, herpes, serious infection, weight gain or loss

N
O

Nursing Considerations
•Make sure patient has enrolled in the TOUCH Prescribing Program before giving natalizumab. Once patient has signed and initialed the TOUCH program enrollment form, place the original signed form in the patient's medical record, send a copy to Biogen Idec, and give a copy to the patient.
•Be aware that all serious opportunistic and atypical infections must be reported to Biogen Idec at 1-800-456-2255 and the FDA's MedWatch Program at 1-800-FDA-1088.
•Make sure patient with multiple sclerosis has had an MRI of the brain before starting natalizumab therapy. It will help distinguish evidence of multiple sclerosis from PML symptoms if they occur after therapy starts.
•Dilute natalizumab concentrate 300 mg/ 15 ml in 100 ml of normal saline injection. Gently invert solution to mix completely. Do not shake.
•Following dilution, infuse drug immediately over 1 hour. After infusion, flush line with normal saline injection.
•Do not give natalizumab by I.V. push or bolus injection.
•If not infused right away, refrigerate drug and use within 8 hours.
•Observe patient during and for 1 hour after infusion for hypersensitivity reaction, evidenced by urticaria, dizziness, fever, rash, rigors, pruritus, nausea, flushing, hypotension, dyspnea, and chest pain. Reaction is more likely to occur if natalizumab therapy was interrupted. If hypersensitivity reaction occurs, notify prescriber; expect to withhold drug and provide supportive care.
•**WARNING** Monitor patient closely for evidence of PML, a viral brain infection that may be disabling or fatal, because natalizumab increases the risk. If patient has unexplained neurologic changes, notify prescriber, withhold natalizumab, and prepare patient for a gadolinium-enhanced brain MRI and possible cerebrospinal fluid analysis, as ordered.
•Expect that patient will be reevaluated 3 months after first infusion, 6 months after first infusion, and every 6 months thereafter.
•Assess patient for evidence of infection because natalizumab may adversely affect immune system, increasing risk of infection. If infection occurs, expect to obtain appropriate specimens for culture and sensitivity and to treat accordingly.
•Be aware that if patient with Crohn's disease has no therapeutic response after 12 weeks, natalizumab should be discontinued. If patient is on chronic oral corticosteroid therapy, expect tapering of oral corticosteroid dose to begin. If patient can't be tapered off oral corticosteroids within 6 months of starting natalizumab therapy, expect natalizumab to be discontinued. Likewise, if patient needs additional steroid use that extends beyond 3 months in a calendar year to control the signs and symptoms of Crohn's disease, expect natalizumab to be discontinued.
•Assess patient's liver function regularly, as ordered, because natalizumab may cause significant liver damage. Expect drug to be discontinued if patient becomes jaundiced or liver enzymes become elevated.

PATIENT TEACHING
•Instruct patient on benefits and risks of natalizumab therapy, and provide medication guide for patient to read.
•Encourage patient to ask questions before signing the enrollment form.
•Emphasize need to report any worsening symptoms that persist over several days.
•Tell patient to inform all health care providers that he is receiving natalizumab therapy.
•Stress the need to have follow-up visits 3 months after first infusion, 6 months after first infusion, and at least every 6 months thereafter.
•Instruct patient to report signs and symptoms of an allergic reaction such as urticaria, dizziness, fever, rash, rigors, pruritus, nausea, flushing, hypotension, dyspnea, and chest pain.
•Instruct patient to avoid people who have infections. Advise him to report fever, cough, lower-back or side pain, or other unexplained signs and symptoms because they may indicate infection.

nateglinide

Starlix

Class and Category
Chemical class: Amino acid derivative
Therapeutic class: Antidiabetic
Pregnancy category: C

Indications and Dosages

➤ *To control blood glucose level in type 2 diabetes mellitus as monotherapy or with metformin or a thiazolidinedione*

TABLETS

Adults. 120 mg t.i.d. 1 to 30 min before meals.

DOSAGE ADJUSTMENT Dosage reduced to 60 mg t.i.d. in patients with near-goal glycosylated hemoglobin (HbA_{1c}) level.

Route	Onset	Peak	Duration
P.O.	20 min	1 hr	4 hr

Contraindications

Diabetic ketoacidosis, hypersensitivity to nateglinide or its components, type 1 diabetes mellitus

Interactions

DRUGS

corticosteroids, sympathomimetics, thiazide diuretics, thyroid products: Possibly reduced hypoglycemic effects of nateglinide

MAO inhibitors, nonselective beta-adrenergic blockers, NSAIDs, salicylates: Possibly additive hypoglycemic effects of nateglinide

Adverse Reactions

CNS: Dizziness

ENDO: Hypoglycemia

GI: Cholestatic hepatitis, diarrhea, elevated liver enzyme levels, jaundice

MS: Accidental trauma, arthropathy, back pain

RESP: Bronchitis, cough, upper respiratory tract infection

SKIN: Pruritus, rash, urticaria

Other: Flulike symptoms

Nursing Considerations

• Administer nateglinide 1 to 30 minutes before meals to reduce the risk of hypoglycemia.

• Monitor fasting glucose and HbA_{1c} levels

Mechanism of Action

Nateglinide stimulates the release of insulin from functioning beta cells of the pancreas. In patients with type 2 diabetes mellitus, a lack of functioning beta cells diminishes blood levels of insulin and causes glucose intolerance. By interacting with the adenosine triphosphatase (ATP)–potassium channel on the beta cell membrane, nateglinide prevents potassium (K^+) from leaving the cell. This causes the beta cell to depolarize and the cell membrane's calcium channel to open. Consequently, calcium (Ca^{++}) moves into the cell and insulin moves out of it. The extent of insulin release is glucose dependent; the lower the glucose level, the less insulin is secreted from the cell.

By promoting insulin secretion in patients with type 2 diabetes mellitus, nateglinide improves glucose tolerance.

N
O

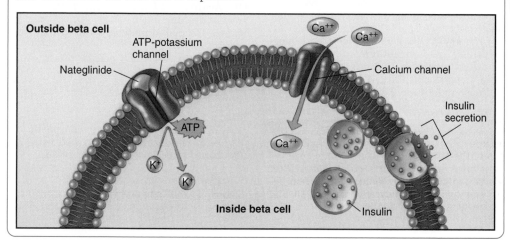

Outside beta cell — ATP-potassium channel — Nateglinide — Ca^{++} — Ca^{++} — Calcium channel — ATP — K^+ — K^+ — Ca^{++} — Ca^{++} — Insulin secretion — Inside beta cell — Insulin

periodically, as ordered, to evaluate treatment effectiveness.
•Monitor patient frequently in event of fever, infection, trauma, or surgery because transient loss of glucose control may occur, requiring an alteration in therapy.

PATIENT TEACHING
•Instruct patient to take nateglinide 1 to 30 minutes before meals. Advise her to skip scheduled dose if she skips a meal to reduce the risk of hypoglycemia.
•Teach patient how to measure blood glucose level and recognize hyperglycemia and hypoglycemia. Advise her to notify prescriber if blood glucose level is abnormal.
•Inform patient that strenuous exercise,insufficient caloric intake, and consumption of alcohol increase the risk of hypoglycemia.
•Advise patient to monitor blood glucose level as prescribed and to keep follow-up appointments to monitor HbA$_{1c}$ level because drug may become less effective over time.

nebivolol hydrochloride

Bystolic

Class and Category
Chemical class: Beta-adrenergic blocker
Therapeutic class: Antihypertensive
Pregnancy category: C

Indications and Dosages
➤ *To treat hypertension*
TABLETS
Adults. *Initial:* 5 mg once daily, increased at 2-wk intervals, as needed. *Maximum:* 40 mg once daily.
DOSAGE ADJUSTMENT For patients with moderate renal impairment (creatinine clearance less than 30 ml/min/1.73 m^2) or moderate hepatic impairment (Child-Pugh Class B), initial dose reduced to 2.5 mg.

Route	Onset	Peak	Duration
P.O.	Unknown	1.5 to 4 hr	Unknown

Contraindications
Advanced AV block, cardiogenic shock, decompensated cardiac failure, hypersensitivity to nebivolol or its components, sick sinus syndrome (unless permanent pacemaker is in place), severe bradycardia, severe hepatic impairment

Mechanism of Action
May prevent arterial dilation and inhibit renin secretion, although precise mechanism of action isn't known. Negative chronotropic effects may slow resting heart rate, and negative inotropic effects may reduce cardiac output, myocardial contractility, and myocardial oxygen consumption during stress or exercise. All of these actions may work together to lower systolic and diastolic blood pressure.

Interactions
DRUGS
antiarrhythmias such as disopyramide, beta blockers, digoxin, diltiazem: Increased effect on AV conduction and myocardial depression; increased risk of bradycardia
fluoxetine, paroxetine, propafenone, quinidine: Increased hypertensive effect of nebivolol
guanethidine, reserpine: Possibly excessive reduction of sympathetic activity

Adverse Reactions
CNS: Asthenia, dizziness, fatigue, headache, insomnia, paresthesia, somnolence, syncope, vertigo
CV: Allergic vasculitis, AV block, bradycardia, chest pain, hypercholesterolemia, hyperuricemia, MI, peripheral edema, peripheral ischemia, Raynaud's phenomenon
GI: Abdominal pain, diarrhea, elevated liver enzymes, nausea, vomiting
GU: Acute renal failure, elevated BUN level, erectile dysfunction
HEME: Decreased platelet count, thrombocytopenia
RESP: Acute pulmonary edema, bronchospasm, dyspnea
SKIN: Pruritus, psoriasis, rash, urticaria
Other: Angioedema

Nursing Considerations
•Know that patients with bronchospastic disease usually shouldn't be treated with beta blocker therapy such as nebivolol.
•Use nebivolol cautiously in patients with impaired hepatic or renal function.
•Expect to administer an alpha blocker, as ordered, before starting nebivolol therapy in patients with pheochromocytoma.
•Monitor blood pressure and pulse rate

often, especially at start of nebivolol therapy and during dosage adjustments. Also monitor fluid intake and output and daily weight, and watch for evidence of heart failure, such as dyspnea, edema, fatigue, and jugular vein distention. If heart failure occurs or worsens, expect drug to be discontinued.

•Be aware that drug shouldn't be stopped abruptly because MI, myocardial ischemia, severe hypertension, or ventricular arrhythmias may result.

•Expect to temporarily withhold nebivolol before surgery. If drug will be continued during perioperative period, monitor patient closely for protracted severe hypotension and difficulty restarting and keeping a heartbeat.

•Assess distal circulation and peripheral pulses in a patient with peripheral vascular disease because drug can worsen it.

•Be aware that nebivolol may mask tachycardia from hyperthyroidism and that abrupt withdrawal can cause thyroid storm. Drug also can decrease blood glucose level, prolong or mask symptoms of hypoglycemia, and promote hyperglycemia in patient with diabetes mellitus; or worsen psoriasis.

•Monitor patient closely for hypersensitivity reactions that may occur with beta blockers, especially patients with a history of severe anaphylactic reactions who may not be responsive to the usual doses of epinephrine used to treat allergic reactions.

PATIENT TEACHING

•Instruct patient to take nebivolol exactly as prescribed and not to stop taking it abruptly.

•Tell patient to weigh herself daily during nebivolol therapy and to notify prescriber if she gains more than 2 lb (0.9 kg) in 1 day or 5 lb. (2.3 kg) in 1 week.

•Advise patient to rise slowly from a seated or lying position to minimize effects of orthostatic hypotension.

•Advise patient to avoid hazardous activities until drug's CNS effects are known.

•Instruct patient to contact prescriber about bleeding or bruising, cough at night, dizziness, edema, rash, shortness of breath, or slow pulse rate.

•Advise diabetic patient to monitor her blood glucose level more often during nebivolol therapy because drug may mask symptoms of hypoglycemia.

•Inform patient with psoriasis that drug may aggravate this condition.

nefazodone hydrochloride

Serzone

Class and Category

Chemical class: Phenylpiperazine derivative
Therapeutic class: Antidepressant
Pregnancy category: C

Indications and Dosages

➤ *To treat major depression*

TABLETS

Adults. *Initial:* 100 mg b.i.d., increased by 100 to 200 mg daily every wk, as prescribed. *Maintenance:* 150 to 300 mg b.i.d. *Maximum:* 600 mg daily.

DOSAGE ADJUSTMENT Initial dosage possibly reduced to 50 mg b.i.d. for elderly or debilitated patients; then dosage adjusted as ordered, based on patient response.

Route	Onset	Peak	Duration
P.O.	Several wk	Unknown	Unknown

Mechanism of Action

May inhibit serotonin reuptake at presynaptic neurons, which may increase the neuronal level of serotonin, an inhibitory neurotransmitter thought to regulate mood. Nefazodone also may act as a postsynaptic serotonin receptor antagonist, further increasing the amount of synaptic serotonin that's available.

Contraindications

Concurrent use of astemizole, cisapride, or terfenadine; hypersensitivity to nefazodone, other phenylpiperazine antidepressants, or their components; restarting nefazodone therapy that was discontinued because of liver injury; use within 14 days of MAO inhibitor therapy

Interactions

DRUGS

alprazolam, buspirone, carbamazepine, cyclosporine, modafinil, triazolam: Increased blood levels of these drugs
antihypertensives: Increased risk of hypotension
astemizole, cisapride, terfenadine: Increased blood levels of these drugs, prolonged QT in-

terval, and, possibly, serious cardiovascular effects, including death from ventricular tachycardia

cilostazol: Decreased cilostazol clearance, increased adverse effects of cilostazol, such as headache

dextromethorphan, sibutramine, tramadol, trazodone: Increased risk of serotonin syndrome

digoxin: Increased blood digoxin level, increased risk of digitalis toxicity

haloperidol: Decreased haloperidol clearance

indinavir: Inhibited indinavir metabolism

levobupivacaine: Increased blood levobupivacaine level, possibly toxicity

lovastatin, simvastatin: Increased risk of rhabdomyolysis and myositis

MAO inhibitors: Possibly fatal reactions, including autonomic instability (with rapidly fluctuating vital signs), hyperthermia, mental status changes (such as severe agitation progressing to delirium and coma), muscle rigidity, and myoclonus

methadone: Increased blood level and adverse effects of methadone, additive CNS effects

nevirapine: Increased nefazodone metabolism, inhibited nevirapine metabolism

ritonavir: Inhibited nefazodone and ritonavir metabolism

sildenafil: Decreased sildenafil clearance

tacrolimus: Decreased tacrolimus clearance and increased adverse effects, including delirium and renal failure

ACTIVITIES

alcohol use: Increased risk of CNS depression

Adverse Reactions

CNS: Abnormal gait, apathy, asthenia, ataxia, chills, confusion, decreased concentration, delusions, depersonalization, dizziness, dream disturbances, euphoria, fever, hallucinations, headache, hostility, hypotonia, insomnia, light-headedness, malaise, memory loss, myoclonic jerks, neuralgia, paranoia, paresthesia, somnolence, suicidal ideation, syncope, tremor, vertigo

CV: Angina, hypertension, hypotension, peripheral edema, orthostatic hypotension, tachycardia, vasodilation, ventricular arrhythmias

EENT: Abnormal vision, blurred vision, conjunctivitis, diplopia, dry eyes and mouth, earache, epistaxis, eye pain, gingivitis, hali-

tosis, hyperacusis, laryngitis, mydriasis, neck rigidity, periodontal abscess, pharyngitis, photophobia, stomatitis, taste perversion, tinnitus, visual field defects

ENDO: Breast pain, gynecomastia, lymphadenopathy

GI: Abdominal distention, colitis, constipation, diarrhea, elevated liver function test results, eructation, esophagitis, gastritis, gastroenteritis, hernia, hepatotoxicity, hiccups, increased appetite, indigestion, life-threatening hepatic failure, nausea, peptic ulcer, rectal bleeding, thirst, vomiting

GU: Abnormal ejaculation; amenorrhea; cystitis; hematuria; hypermenorrhea; impotence; libido changes; nocturia; pelvic pain; polyuria; renal calculi; urinary frequency, incontinence, or urgency; urine retention; UTI; vaginal bleeding; vaginitis

HEME: Anemia, leukopenia

MS: Arthralgia, arthritis, bursitis, dysarthria, gout, muscle stiffness, tenosynovitis

RESP: Asthma, bronchitis, cough, dyspnea, pneumonia

SKIN: Acne, alopecia, dry skin, ecchymosis, eczema, maculopapular rash, photosensitivity, pruritus, rash, urticaria

Other: Allergic reaction, dehydration, infection, serotonin syndrome, weight loss

Nursing Considerations

•**WARNING** Be aware that nefazodone should not be given with astemizole, cisapride, MAO inhibitors, or terfenadine; serious, even fatal, reactions may occur.

•**WARNING** Be aware that life-threatening hepatic failure has occurred during nefazodone therapy, resulting in need for transplant or even death. Monitor patient for signs of hepatic failure, such as jaundice, malaise, and elevated liver function test results.

•Assess for signs of serotonin syndrome, such as abdominal cramps, aggressive behavior, agitation, chills, diarrhea, headache, insomnia, lack of coordination, nausea, palpitations, paresthesia, poor concentration, and worsening of obsessive thoughts.

•Monitor patient closely for suicidal tendencies, especially when therapy starts or dosage changes, because depression may worsen temporarily. Follow facility policy.

PATIENT TEACHING

•Instruct patient to take nefazodone exactly as prescribed and not to alter dosage.

•Urge patient to immediately report evidence of hepatic failure, such as jaundice, dark urine, lack of appetite, nausea, or abdominal pain.
•Inform patient that antidepressant effects may not occur for several weeks and that treatment may last 6 months or longer.
•Caution patient to avoid alcohol during nefazodone therapy.
•Advise patient to avoid hazardous activities until drug's CNS effects are known.
•Suggest that patient try sugarless gum or hard candy for dry mouth. Urge her to notify prescriber if dry mouth persists.
•Urge family or caregiver to watch patient closely for suicidal tendencies, especially when therapy starts or dosage changes.

neomycin sulfate

Mycifradin, Neo-Fradin

Class and Category

Chemical class: Aminoglycoside
Therapeutic class: Antibiotic
Pregnancy category: D

Indications and Dosages

➤ *To suppress intestinal bacterial growth in preoperative bowel preparation*

TABLETS (24-HR REGIMEN)

Adults. 1 g every hr for 4 doses and then 1 g every 4 hr for remainder of 24 hr before surgery. Or, for 8 a.m. surgery, 1 g of neomycin with erythromycin at 1 p.m., 2 p.m., and 11 p.m. the day before surgery.
Children. 25 mg/kg at 1 p.m., 2 p.m., and 11 p.m. the day before surgery.

TABLETS (2- TO 3-DAY REGIMEN)

Adults and children. 88 mg/kg every 4 hr in 6 equally divided doses for 2 to 3 days before surgery.

➤ *As adjunct in hepatic encephalopathy*

TABLETS

Adults. 4 to 12 g daily in divided doses every 6 hr for 5 to 6 days.
Children. 50 to 100 mg/kg daily in divided doses every 6 hr for 5 to 6 days.

➤ *To treat infectious diarrhea caused by enteropathic* Escherichia coli

TABLETS

Adults and children. 50 mg/kg daily in divided doses q.i.d. for 2 to 3 days.

Mechanism of Action

Is transported into bacterial cells, where it competes with messenger RNA to bind with a specific receptor protein on the 30S ribosomal subunit of DNA. This action causes abnormal, nonfunctioning proteins to form. A lack of functional proteins causes bacterial cell death.

Contraindications

Hypersensitivity or serious reaction to neomycin, other aminoglycosides, or their components; inflammatory or ulcerative GI disease; intestinal obstruction

Interactions

DRUGS

digoxin, spironolactone: Possibly reduced absorption rate of these drugs
dimenhydrinate: Possibly masked symptoms of neomycin-induced ototoxicity
methotrexate: Possibly decreased absorption and bioavailability of methotrexate
neuromuscular blockers: Potentiated neuromuscular blockade, increased risk of prolonged respiratory depression
oral anticoagulants: Possibly potentiated anticoagulant effects

Adverse Reactions

EENT: Ototoxicity
GI: Diarrhea, malabsorption syndrome (decreased serum carotene level and xylose absorption, increased fecal fat and flatulence), nausea, pseudomembranous colitis, vomiting
GU: Nephrotoxicity

Nursing Considerations

•Monitor patient's BUN and serum creatinine levels to assess renal function before and during neomycin therapy. Expect to decrease dosage or stop drug if nephrotoxicity develops.
•Monitor blood neomycin level, as directed, to assess for therapeutic range of 5 to 10 mcg/ml.
•**WARNING** Neomycin is highly ototoxic and may cause hearing loss and tinnitus.
•Watch for evidence of pseudomembranous colitis, such as severe abdominal cramps and severe, watery diarrhea.
•Anticipate that neomycin's curare-like effect may worsen muscle weakness in patients

N
O

with neuromuscular disorders, such as myasthenia gravis and parkinsonism.

PATIENT TEACHING
• Urge patient to complete the full course of neomycin therapy.
• Unless contraindicated, urge patient to drink plenty of fluids to prevent nephrotoxicity.
• Urge patient undergoing bowel preparation to comply with recommended regimen, including low-residue diet, bisacodyl enema administration, and neomycin use.
• Advise patient to notify prescriber about hearing loss or ringing in ears.

neostigmine bromide

Prostigmin

neostigmine methylsulfate

Prostigmin

Class and Category

Chemical class: Quaternary ammonium compound
Therapeutic class: Anticholinesterase, curare antidote
Pregnancy category: C

Indications and Dosages

➤ *To treat symptoms of myasthenia gravis*
TABLETS (NEOSTIGMINE BROMIDE)
Adults. *Initial:* 15 mg every 3 to 4 hr. Dosage adjusted based on clinical response. *Maintenance:* 150 mg daily in divided doses based on clinical response.
Children. 2 mg/kg daily in 6 to 8 divided doses.

I.M. OR SUBCUTANEOUS INJECTION (NEOSTIGMINE METHYLSULFATE)
Adults. *Initial:* 0.5 mg. Dosage adjusted based on clinical response.
Children. 0.01 to 0.04 mg/kg every 2 to 3 hr.

➤ *To reverse nondepolarizing neuromuscular blockade*
I.V. INJECTION (NEOSTIGMINE METHYLSULFATE)
Adults. 0.5 to 2 mg by slow push, repeated as needed up to 5 mg; 0.6 to 1.2 mg of atropine or 0.2 to 0.6 mg of glycopyrrolate is given with or a few minutes before neostigmine, as ordered.
Children. 0.04 mg/kg by slow push; 0.02 mg of atropine/kg is given I.M. or subcuta-

neously with each dose or alternate doses.

➤ *To prevent postoperative, nonobstructive urine retention and abdominal distention (adynamic ileus)*
I.M. OR SUBCUTANEOUS INJECTION (NEOSTIGMINE METHYLSULFATE)
Adults. 0.25 mg immediately after surgery and repeated every 4 to 6 hr for 2 to 3 days.

➤ *To treat postoperative, nonobstructive urine retention and abdominal distention (adynamic ileus)*
I.M. OR SUBCUTANEOUS INJECTION (NEOSTIGMINE METHYLSULFATE)
Adults. 0.5 mg; injections repeated every 3 hr for at least 5 doses if patient has voided or bladder has emptied within 1 hr.

Route	Onset	Peak	Duration
P.O.	45 to 75 min*	Unknown	3 to 6 hr
I.V.	4 to 8 min†	30 min	2 to 4 hr
I.M.	20 to 30 min†	30 min	2 to 4 hr

Mechanism of Action

Inhibits the action of cholinesterase, an enzyme that destroys acetylcholine at myoneuronal junctions, thereby increasing acetylcholine accumulation at myoneuronal junctions and facilitating nerve impulse transmission across the junctions. This action:
• helps prevent or relieve urine retention by increasing detrusor muscle tone in the bladder and causing bladder contractions strong enough to induce urination
• prevents or treats postoperative abdominal distention by increasing gastric motility and tone
• improves muscle strength and increases muscle response to repetitive nerve stimulation in myasthenia gravis.

Contraindications

Hypersensitivity to neostigmine, other anticholinesterases, bromides, or their components; mechanical obstruction of intestinal or urinary tract; peritonitis

---

* For adynamic ileus, 2 to 4 hr.
† For adynamic ileus, 10 to 30 min.

Interactions
DRUGS

aminoglycosides, anesthetics, capreomycin, colistimethate, colistin, lidocaine, lincomycins, polymyxin B, quinine: Increased risk of neuromuscular blockade
anticholinergics: Possibly masked signs of cholinergic crisis
guanadrel, guanethidine, mecamylamine, trimethaphan: Possibly antagonized effects of neostigmine, possibly decreased antihypertensive effects
neuromuscular blockers: Possibly prolonged action of depolarizing—and antagonized action of nondepolarizing—neuromuscular blockers
procainamide, quinidine: Possibly antagonized effects of neostigmine
quinine: Decreased neostigmine effectiveness

Adverse Reactions
CNS: Dizziness, drowsiness, headache, seizures, syncope, weakness
CV: Arrhythmias (AV block, bradycardia, nodal rhythm, tachycardia), cardiac arrest, ECG changes, hypotension
EENT: Increased salivation, lacrimation, miosis, vision changes
GI: Abdominal cramps, diarrhea, flatulence, increased peristalsis, nausea, vomiting
GU: Urinary frequency
MS: Arthralgia, dysarthria, muscle spasms
RESP: Bronchospasm, dyspnea, increased bronchial secretions, respiratory arrest or depression
SKIN: Flushing, diaphoresis, rash, urticaria

Nursing Considerations
•Be aware that 15 mg of oral neostigmine bromide is equivalent to 0.5 mg of parenteral neostigmine methylsulfate.
•If also giving atropine, be sure to administer it before neostigmine, as prescribed.
•When giving neostigmine I.V., make sure patient is well ventilated and airway remains patent until normal respiration is assured.
•If patient has myasthenia gravis, give drug night and day, as ordered, with larger portions of daily dose during periods of increased fatigue. If patient's condition becomes refractory to neostigmine, expect to reduce dosage or discontinue drug, as prescribed, for a few days.
•WARNING Monitor patient for evidence of neostigmine overdose, which can cause possibly fatal cholinergic crisis (increased muscle weakness, including respiratory muscles). Expect to stop neostigmine and atropine, as ordered.

PATIENT TEACHING
•Instruct patient to take neostigmine exactly as prescribed.
•Advise patient to take drug with food or milk to reduce adverse GI reactions.
•Suggest that patient with myasthenia gravis keep a daily record of doses and adverse reactions during therapy.
•Instruct patient to schedule activities to minimize fatigue.

nesiritide

Natrecor

Class and Category
Chemical class: Human B-type natriuretic peptide
Therapeutic class: Arterial and venous smooth muscle cell relaxant
Pregnancy category: C

Indications and Dosages
➤ *To reduce dyspnea at rest or with minimal activity in patients with acute decompensated congestive heart failure*
I.V. INFUSION, I.V. INJECTION
Adults. 2-mcg/kg bolus and then continuous infusion of 0.01 mcg/kg/min for up to 48 hr.

Route	Onset	Peak	Duration
I.V.	In 15 min	1 hr	3 hr

Mechanism of Action
Binds to the guanylate cyclase receptor of vascular smooth muscle and endothelial cells. This action increases intracellular levels of cyclic guanosine monophosphate, which leads to arterial and venous smooth muscle cell relaxation. Ultimately, nesiritide reduces pulmonary capillary wedge pressure and systemic arterial pressure in patients with congestive heart failure, which decreases the heart's workload and subsequently relieves dyspnea.

Incompatibilities
Don't infuse nesiritide through same I.V. line as bumetanide, enalaprilat, ethacrynate so-

dium, furosemide, heparin, hydralazine, or insulin because these drugs are chemically and physically incompatible with nesiritide. Don't infuse drugs that contain the preservative sodium metabisulfite through same I.V. line as nesiritide.

Contraindications

Hypersensitivity to nesiritide or its components; primary therapy for cardiogenic shock; systolic blood pressure less of than 90 mm Hg

Interactions
DRUGS

ACE inhibitors: Increased risk of symptomatic hypotension

Adverse Reactions

CNS: Anxiety, dizziness, headache, insomnia
CV: Angina, bradycardia, hypotension, PVCs, ventricular tachycardia
GI: Abdominal pain, nausea, vomiting
GU: Elevated serum creatinine level
MS: Back pain

Nursing Considerations

•**WARNING** Be aware that nesiritide isn't recommended for patients suspected to have low cardiac filling pressures or patients for whom vasodilating drugs aren't appropriate, such as those with constrictive pericarditis, pericardial tamponade, restrictive or obstructive cardiomyopathy, significant valvular stenosis, or other conditions in which cardiac output depends on venous return.
•Reconstitute 1.5-mg vial by adding 5 ml of diluent removed from a 250-ml plastic I.V. bag containing preservative-free D_5W, normal saline solution, dextrose 5% in half-normal (0.45) saline solution, or dextrose 5% in quarter-normal (0.2) saline solution.
•Don't shake vial. Rock it gently so that all surfaces, including the stopper, are in contact with the diluent to ensure complete reconstitution. Inspect drug for particulate matter and discoloration; if present, discard drug.
•Withdraw entire contents of reconstituted solution and add it to the same 250-ml plastic I.V. bag used to withdraw diluent to yield a solution of about 6 mcg/ml. Invert the I.V. bag several times to ensure complete mixing.
•After preparing the infusion bag, withdraw

the bolus volume from the infusion bag and administer it over about 60 seconds. Immediately after the bolus, infuse drug at 0.1 ml/kg/hr, which will deliver 0.01 mcg/kg/min.
•Prime I.V. tubing with 25 ml of solution before connecting to the I.V. line and before administering the bolus dose or starting the infusion.
•Flush the I.V. line between doses of nesiritide and incompatible drugs.
•Because nesiritide binds to heparin and therefore could bind to the heparin lining of a heparin-coated catheter, don't give it through a central heparin-coated catheter.
•Store reconstituted vials at room temperature (20° to 25° C [68° to 77° F]) or refrigerate (2° to 8° C [36° to 46° F]) for up to 24 hours.
•Because nesiritide contains no antimicrobial preservatives, discard the reconstituted solution after 24 hours.
•Monitor blood pressure and heart rate and rhythm frequently during therapy.
•If hypotension occurs, notify prescriber and expect to reduce dosage or discontinued the drug. Implement measures to support blood pressure as prescribed.
•Assess patient's breath sounds and respiratory rate, rhythm, depth, and quality frequently during drug therapy.
•Monitor serum creatinine level during drug therapy and notify prescriber of abnormal results.
•Store unopened drug at controlled room temperature or refrigerate. Keep in carton until time of use.
PATIENT TEACHING
•Instruct patient to notify you or another nurse if she becomes dizzy because this may indicate hypotension.
•Reassure patient that her blood pressure, heart rate, and breathing will be monitored frequently.

netilmicin sulfate

Netromycin

Class and Category

Chemical class: Aminoglycoside
Therapeutic class: Antibiotic
Pregnancy category: D

Indications and Dosages

➤ *To treat serious systemic infections, such as intra-abdominal infections, lower respiratory tract infections, septicemia, and skin and soft-tissue infections, caused by* Enterobacter aerogenes, Escherichia coli, Klebsiella pneumoniae, Proteus mirabilis, Pseudomonas aeruginosa, Serratia *species, and* Staphylococcus aureus

I.V. INFUSION, I.M. INJECTION

Adults and children age 12 and over. 1.3 to 2.2 mg/kg every 8 hr or 2 to 3.25 mg/kg every 12 hr for 7 to 14 days. *Maximum:* 7.5 mg/kg daily.

Children ages 6 weeks to 12 years. 1.8 to 2.7 mg/kg every 8 hr or 2.7 to 4 mg/kg every 12 hr for 7 to 14 days.

Infants up to age 6 weeks. 2 to 3.25 mg/kg every 12 hr for 7 to 14 days.

➤ *To treat complicated UTI caused by* Citrobacter *species,* Enterobacter *species,* E. coli, K. pneumoniae, P. mirabilis, P. aeruginosa, Serratia *species, and* Staphylococcus *species*

I.V. INFUSION, I.M. INJECTION

Adults and adolescents. 1.5 to 2 mg/kg every 12 hr for 7 to 14 days. *Maximum:* 7.5 mg/kg daily.

Mechanism of Action

Is transported into bacterial cells, where it competes with messenger RNA to bind with a specific receptor protein on the 30S ribosomal subunit of DNA. This action causes abnormal, nonfunctioning proteins to form. A lack of functional proteins causes bacterial cell death.

Incompatibilities

Don't mix netilmicin with beta-lactam antibiotics (penicillins and cephalosporins) because substantial mutual inactivation may result. If prescribed concurrently, administer these drugs at separate sites.

Contraindications

Hypersensitivity to netilmicin, other aminoglycosides, or their components

Interactions

DRUGS

capreomycin, other aminoglycosides: Increased risk of nephrotoxicity, neuromuscular blockade, and ototoxicity

cephalosporins, nephrotoxic drugs: Increased risk of nephrotoxicity

loop diuretics, ototoxic drugs: Increased risk of ototoxicity

methoxyflurane, polymyxins (parenteral): Increased risk of nephrotoxicity and neuromuscular blockade

neuromuscular blockers: Increased neuromuscular blockade

Adverse Reactions

CNS: Disorientation, dizziness, encephalopathy, headache, myasthenia gravis–like syndrome, neuromuscular blockade (acute muscle paralysis and apnea), paresthesia, peripheral neuropathy, seizures, vertigo, weakness

CV: Hypotension, palpitations

EENT: Blurred vision, hearing loss, nystagmus, tinnitus

GI: Diarrhea, elevated liver function tests results, nausea, vomiting

GU: Elevated BUN and serum creatinine levels, nephrotoxicity, oliguria, proteinuria

HEME: Anemia, eosinophilia, leukopenia, prolonged PT, thrombocytopenia, thrombocytosis

MS: Muscle twitching

RESP: Apnea

SKIN: Allergic dermatitis, erythema, pruritus, rash

Other: Angioedema; hyperkalemia; injection site hematoma, induration, and pain

Nursing Considerations

• To prepare netilmicin for I.V. use, dilute each dose in 50 to 200 ml of suitable diluent, such as normal saline solution, D_5W, or lactated Ringer's solution, and give slowly over 30 to 60 minutes.

• Ensure adequate hydration during therapy to maintain adequate renal function.

• Monitor blood netilmicin level; optimum peak level is 6 to 10 mcg/ml and trough level is 0.5 to 2 mcg/ml.

• Check patient's BUN and serum creatinine levels, urine specific gravity, and creatinine clearance during netilmicin therapy, as ordered.

• Anticipate higher risk of nephrotoxicity in elderly patients, those with impaired renal function, and those who receive high doses or prolonged netilmicin therapy.

• Reduce dosage or discontinue drug, as ordered, if signs of drug-induced auditory or vestibular toxicity develop; the damage may be permanent.

PATIENT TEACHING
• Encourage patient to drink plenty of fluids during netilmicin therapy.
• Instruct patient to notify prescriber immediately about dizziness, hearing loss, muscle twitching, nausea, numbness and tingling, ringing or buzzing in ears, seizures, significant changes in amount of urine or frequency of urination, and vomiting.
• Urge patient to keep follow-up appointments to monitor progress.

nicardipine hydrochloride

Cardene, Cardene IV, Cardene SR

Class and Category

Chemical class: Dihydropyridine derivative
Therapeutic class: Antianginal, antihypertensive
Pregnancy category: C

Indications and Dosages

➤ *To manage angina pectoris and Prinzmetal's angina, to manage hypertension*

CAPSULES
Adults and adolescents. 20 to 40 mg t.i.d., increased every 3 days, as prescribed.

E.R. CAPSULES
Adults. 30 mg b.i.d.

I.V. INFUSION
Adults. 0.5 to 2.2 mg/hr by continuous infusion.

➤ *To control acute hypertension*

I.V. INFUSION
Adults. *Initial:* 5 mg/hr by continuous infusion; increased by 2.5 mg/hr every 5 to 15 min, as prescribed. *Maximum:* 15 mg/hr.

Route	Onset	Peak	Duration
P.O.	20 min	1 to 2 hr	Unknown
P.O. (E.R.)	20 min	1 to 2 hr	12 hr
I.V.	Immediate	Unknown	Unknown

Incompatibilities

Don't mix nicardipine with sodium bicarbonate or LR solution, and don't administer through same I.V. line.

Mechanism of Action

May slow extracellular calcium movement into myocardial and vascular smooth-muscle cells by deforming calcium channels in cell membranes, inhibiting ion-controlled gating mechanisms, and interfering with calcium release from the sarcoplasmic reticulum. By decreasing the intracellular calcium level, nicardipine inhibits smooth-muscle cell contraction and dilates coronary and systemic arteries. As with other calcium channel blockers, these actions lead to decreased myocardial oxygen requirements and reduced peripheral resistance, blood pressure, and afterload.

Contraindications

Advanced aortic stenosis, hypersensitivity to any calcium channel blocker, second- or third-degree AV block in patient without artificial pacemaker

Interactions

DRUGS
anesthetics (hydrocarbon inhalation): Possibly hypotension
beta blockers, other antihypertensives, prazocin: Increased risk of hypotension
calcium supplements: Possibly impaired action of nicardipine
cimetidine: Increased nicardipine bioavailability
digoxin: Transiently increased blood digoxin level, increased risk of digitalis toxicity
disopyramide, flecainide: Increased risk of bradycardia, conduction defects, and heart failure
estrogens: Possibly increased fluid retention and decreased therapeutic effects of nicardipine
lithium: Increased risk of neurotoxicity
NSAIDs, sympathomimetics: Possibly decreased therapeutic effects of nicardipine
procainamide, quinidine: Possibly prolonged QT interval

FOODS
grapefruit, grapefruit juice: Possibly increased bioavailability of nicardipine
high-fat meals: Decreased blood nicardipine level

ACTIVITIES
alcohol use: Increased hypotensive effect

Adverse Reactions

CNS: Anxiety, asthenia, ataxia, confusion, dizziness, drowsiness, headache, nervousness, paresthesia, psychiatric disturbance, syncope, tremor, weakness
CV: Arrhythmias (bradycardia, tachycardia), chest pain, heart failure, hypotension, orthostatic hypotension, palpitations, peripheral edema
EENT: Altered taste, blurred vision, dry mouth, epistaxis, gingival hyperplasia, pharyngitis, rhinitis, tinnitus
ENDO: Gynecomastia, hyperglycemia
GI: Anorexia, constipation, diarrhea, elevated liver function test results, indigestion, nausea, thirst, vomiting
GU: Dysuria, nocturia, polyuria, sexual dysfunction, urinary frequency
HEME: Anemia, leukopenia, thrombocytopenia
MS: Joint stiffness, muscle spasms
RESP: Bronchitis, cough, upper respiratory tract infection
SKIN: Dermatitis, diaphoresis, erythema multiforme, flushing, photosensitivity, pruritus, rash, Stevens-Johnson syndrome, urticaria
Other: Hypokalemia, weight gain

Nursing Considerations

•Check blood pressure and pulse rate before nicardipine therapy begins, during dosage changes, and periodically throughout therapy. During prolonged therapy, periodically assess ECG tracings for arrhythmias and other changes.
•Dilute each 25-mg ampule of nicardipine with 240 ml of solution to yield 0.1 mg/ml. Mixture is stable at room temperature for 24 hours.
•If using premixed nicardipine for intravenous infusion, check strength carefully because drug comes as single strength (20 mg nicardipine in 200 ml of solution, providing 0.1 mg/ml) or double strength (40 mg nicardipine in 200 ml of solution, providing 0.2 mg/ml).
•Administer continuous infusion by I.V. pump or controller, and adjust according to patient's blood pressure, as prescribed.
•Change peripheral I.V. site every 12 hours, if feasible.
•Give first dose of oral nicardipine 1 hour before stopping I.V. infusion, as prescribed.

•Monitor fluid intake and output and daily weight for signs of fluid retention, which may precipitate heart failure. Also assess for signs of heart failure, such as crackles, dyspnea, jugular vein distention, peripheral edema, and weight gain.
•During prolonged therapy, periodically monitor liver and renal function test results. Expect elevated liver function test results to return to normal after drug is discontinued.
•Monitor serum potassium level during prolonged therapy. Hypokalemia increases the risk of arrhythmias.
•Because of drug's negative inotropic effect on some patients, closely monitor patients who take a beta blocker or have heart failure or significant left ventricular dysfunction.
•**WARNING** Expect to taper dosage gradually before discontinuing drug. Otherwise, angina or dangerously high blood pressure could result.

PATIENT TEACHING

•Urge patient to take nicardipine as prescribed, even if she feels well.
•Instruct patient to swallow E.R. capsules whole, not to chew, crush, cut, or open them.
•Advise patient not to take drug within 1 hour of eating a high-fat meal or grapefruit product. Urge her not to alter the amount of grapefruit products in her diet without consulting prescriber.
•**WARNING** Caution patient against stopping nicardipine abruptly because angina or dangerously high blood pressure could result.
•Teach patient how to take her pulse, and urge her to notify prescriber immediately if it falls below 50 beats/minute.
•Teach patient how to measure her blood pressure, and advise her to do so weekly if nicardipine was prescribed for hypertension. Suggest that she keep a log of blood pressure readings to take to follow-up visits.
•Advise patient to change position slowly to minimize effects of orthostatic hypotension.
•Urge patient to avoid potentially hazardous activities until drug's CNS effects are known.
•Advise patient to notify prescriber immediately about chest pain that's not relieved by rest or nitroglycerin, constipation, irregular heartbeats, nausea, pronounced dizziness, severe or persistent headache, and swelling of hands or feet.
•Encourage patient to comply with suggested lifestyle changes, such as alcohol modera-

N
O

tion, low-sodium or low-fat diet, regular exercise, smoking cessation, stress management, and weight reduction.

•Inform patient that saunas, hot tubs, and prolonged hot showers may cause dizziness or fainting.

•Instruct patient to avoid prolonged sun exposure and to use sunscreen when going outdoors.

niclosamide

Niclocide

Class and Category

Chemical class: Salicylanilide derivative
Therapeutic class: Anthelmintic
Pregnancy category: B

Indications and Dosages

➤ *To treat beef* (Taenia saginata), *fish* (Diphyllobothrium latum), *or pork* (Taenia solium) *tapeworm infestations*

CHEWABLE TABLETS
Adults. 2 g as a single dose; repeated in 7 days, if needed. *Maximum:* 2 g daily.
Children weighing more than 34 kg (75 lb). 1.5 g as a single dose; repeated in 7 days, if needed. *Maximum:* 2 g daily.
Children weighing 11 (24 lb) to 34 kg. 1 g as a single dose; repeated in 7 days, if needed. *Maximum:* 2 g daily.

➤ *To treat dwarf tapeworm* (Hymenolepsis nana) *infestations*

CHEWABLE TABLETS
Adults. 2 g daily for 7 days; repeated in 7 to 14 days, if needed.
Children weighing more than 34 kg. 1.5 g on day 1 and then 1 g daily for the next 6 days; repeated in 7 to 14 days, if needed. *Maximum:* 2 g daily.
Children weighing 11 to 34 kg. 1 g on day 1 and then 500 mg daily for the next 6 days; repeated in 7 to 14 days, if needed. *Maximum:* 2 g daily.

Contraindications

Age under 2 years; hypersensitivity to niclosamide, other anthelmintics, or their components

Interactions

ACTIVITIES
alcohol use: Decreased niclosamide effects

Mechanism of Action

May alter anaerobic energy production in tapeworms by inhibiting oxidative phosphorylation in their mitochondria, which decreases the synthesis of ATP. Niclosamide causes the scolex (headlike segment) and proximal segment of the tapeworm to detach from the intestinal wall, which leads to parasite evacuation from the intestines through normal peristalsis.

Adverse Reactions

CNS: Dizziness, drowsiness, headache, lightheadedness
EENT: Taste perversion
GI: Abdominal distress, anorexia, constipation, diarrhea, nausea, vomiting
SKIN: Anal pruritus, rash

Nursing Considerations

•To identify infestation, collect several stool specimens before starting niclosamide therapy, as ordered, because eggs and parasite segments are released irregularly.

•If patient can't chew tablets thoroughly, crush them and give with small amount of water.

•For young child, crush tablets to fine powder and mix with small amount of water to make paste.

•Be aware that treatment isn't considered successful until stools have shown no eggs or parasites for at least 3 months.

PATIENT TEACHING
•Instruct patient to take niclosamide after a light meal.

•For young child, instruct parent to crush tablets to fine powder and mix with small amount of water to make paste.

•Urge patient to complete entire course of niclosamide therapy.

•Advise patient to avoid hazardous activities until drug's CNS effects are known.

•Advise patient to store niclosamide in a cool, dry, dark place. Caution against storing in bathroom, near kitchen sink, or in other damp places because heat and moisture break down drug.

•Inform patient that stool may need to be examined on day 7 of treatment and again 1 and 3 months after treatment.

•Instruct patient to wash her hands thoroughly, to wash all bedding, and to use

meticulous personal and environmental hygiene to decrease the risk of autoinfection.
• Caution patient against eating undercooked fish, pork, or beef.

nicotine for inhalation

Nicotrol Inhaler

nicotine nasal solution

Nicotrol NS

nicotine polacrilex

Nicorette, Nicorette Plus (CAN), Thrive

nicotine transdermal system

Habitrol, Nicoderm, NicoDerm CQ, Nicotrol, ProStep

Class and Category

Chemical class: Pyridine alkaloid
Therapeutic class: Smoking cessation adjunct
Pregnancy category: C (nicotine polacrilex), D (other forms of nicotine)

Indications and Dosages

➤ *To relieve nicotine withdrawal symptoms, including craving*

CHEWING GUM

Adults. *Initial:* 2 or 4 mg p.r.n. or every 1 to 2 hr, adjusted to complete withdrawal by 4 to 6 mo. *Maximum:* 30 pieces of 2-mg gum daily or 20 pieces of 4-mg gum daily.

NASAL SOLUTION

Adults. 1 to 2 sprays (1 to 2 mg) in each nostril/hr. *Maximum:* 5 mg/hr or 40 mg daily for up to 3 mo.

ORAL INHALATION

Adults and adolescents. 6 to 16 cartridges (24 to 64 mg) daily for up to 12 wk; then dosage gradually reduced over 12 wk or less. *Maximum:* 16 cartridges (64 mg) daily for 6 mo.

TRANSDERMAL SYSTEM

Adults. *Initial:* 14 to 22 mg daily, adjusted to lower-dose systems over 2 to 5 mo.

DOSAGE ADJUSTMENT For adolescents and for adults weighing less than 45 kg (100 lb) and who smoke less than 10 cigarettes daily or have heart disease, initial dosage reduced to 11 to 14 mg daily and adjusted to lower-dose systems over 2 to 5 mo.

Mechanism of Action

Binds selectively to nicotinic-cholinergic receptors at autonomic ganglia, in the adrenal medulla, at neuromuscular junctions, and in the brain. By providing a lower dose of nicotine than cigarettes, this drug reduces nicotine craving and withdrawal symptoms.

Contraindications

Hypersensitivity to nicotine, its components, or components of transdermal system; life-threatening arrhythmias; nonsmokers; recovery from acute MI; severe angina pectoris; skin disorders (transdermal); temporomandibular joint disease (chewing gum)

Interactions

DRUGS

acetaminophen, beta blockers, imipramine, insulin, oxazepam, pentazocine, theophylline: Possibly increased therapeutic effects of these drugs (chewing gum, nasal spray, transdermal system)
alpha blockers, bronchodilators: Possibly increased therapeutic effects of these drugs (chewing gum, transdermal system)
bupropion: Potentiated therapeutic effects of nicotine, possibly increased risk of hypertension
sympathomimetics: Possibly decreased therapeutic effects of these drugs (chewing gum, transdermal system)
theophylline, tricyclic antidepressants: Possibly altered pharmacologic actions of these drugs (oral inhalation)

FOODS

acidic beverages (citrus juices, coffee, soft drinks, tea, wine): Decreased nicotine absorption from gum if beverages consumed within 15 minutes before or while chewing gum
caffeine: Increased effects of caffeine (chewing gum, nasal spray, transdermal system)

Adverse Reactions

CNS: Dizziness, dream disturbances, drowsiness, headache, irritability, light-headedness, nervousness (chewing gum, transdermal system); amnesia, confusion, difficulty speaking, headache, migraine headache, paresthesia (nasal spray); chills, fever, headache, paresthesia (oral inhalation)

CV: Arrhythmias (all forms); hypertension (chewing gum, transdermal system); peripheral edema (nasal spray)

EENT: Increased salivation, injury to teeth or dental work, mouth injury, pharyngitis, stomatitis (chewing gum); altered taste, dry mouth (chewing gum, transdermal system); altered smell and taste, burning eyes, dry mouth, earache, epistaxis, gum disorders, hoarseness, lacrimation, mouth and tongue swelling, nasal blisters, nasal irritation or ulceration, pharyngitis, rhinitis, sinus problems, sneezing, vision changes (nasal spray); altered taste, lacrimation, pharyngitis, rhinitis, sinusitis, stomatitis (oral inhalation)

GI: Eructation (chewing gum); abdominal pain, constipation, diarrhea, flatulence, increased appetite, indigestion, nausea, vomiting (chewing gum, transdermal system); abdominal pain, constipation, diarrhea, flatulence, hiccups, indigestion, nausea (nasal spray); diarrhea, flatulence, hiccups, indigestion, nausea, vomiting (oral inhalation)

GU: Dysmenorrhea (chewing gum, transdermal system); menstrual irregularities (nasal spray)

MS: Jaw and neck pain (chewing gum); arthralgia, myalgia (chewing gum, transdermal system); arthralgia, back pain, myalgia (nasal spray); back pain (oral inhalation)

RESP: Cough (chewing gum, transdermal system); bronchitis, bronchospasm, chest tightness, cough, dyspnea, increased sputum production (nasal spray); chest tightness, cough, dyspnea, wheezing (oral inhalation)

SKIN: Diaphoresis, erythema, pruritus, rash, urticaria (chewing gum, transdermal system); acne, flushing of face, pruritus, purpura, rash (nasal spray); pruritus, rash, urticaria (oral inhalation)

Other: Allergic reaction (chewing gum, transdermal system); physical dependence (nasal spray); flulike symptoms, generalized pain, withdrawal symptoms (oral inhalation)

Nursing Considerations
•When administering nicotine by oral inhalation, expect optimal effect to result from continuous puffing for 20 minutes.
•To avoid possible burns, remove patch before patient has an MRI.

PATIENT TEACHING
•Instruct patient to read and follow package instructions to obtain best results with nicotine product.
•Advise patient to notify prescriber about other drugs she takes.
•Stress that patient must stop smoking as soon as nicotine treatment starts to avoid toxicity.
•For chewing gum therapy, instruct patient to wait at least 15 minutes after drinking coffee, juice, soft drink, tea, or wine. Advise her to chew gum until she detects a tingling sensation or peppery taste and then to place the gum between her cheek and gum until tingling or peppery taste subsides. Then direct her to move the gum to a different site until tingling or taste subsides, repeating until she no longer feels the sensation—usually about 30 minutes. Caution against swallowing the gum.
•For nasal spray, tell patient to tilt her head back and spray into a nostril. Caution against sniffing, swallowing, or inhaling spray because nicotine is absorbed through nasal mucosa.
•Warn patient that prolonged use of nasal form may cause dependence.
•For oral inhalation, tell patient to use 6 to 16 cartridges daily to prevent or relieve withdrawal symptoms and craving. Starting with 1 or 2 cartridges daily yields poor success. Direct patient to inhale through device like a cigarette, puffing often for 20 minutes.
•For transdermal system, tell patient not to open package until just before use because nicotine is lost in the air. Advise her to apply system to clean, hairless, dry site on upper outer arm or upper body. Instruct her to change systems and rotate sites every 24 hours and not to use the same site for 7 days. To avoid possible burns, advise patient to remove patch before undergoing any MRI procedure.
•**WARNING** Urge patient to keep all unused nicotine forms safely away from children and pets and to discard used forms carefully. (Enough nicotine may remain in used systems to poison children and pets.) Instruct her to contact a poison control center immediately if she suspects that a child has ingested nicotine.
•Explain to patient with asthma or COPD that nicotine may cause bronchospasm.
•Inform patient that it may take several attempts to successfully stop smoking. Urge her to join a smoking cessation program.

nifedipine

Adalat, Adalat CC, Adalat PA (CAN), Adalat XL (CAN), Apo-Nifed (CAN), Novo-Nifedin (CAN), Nu-Nifed (CAN), Procardia, Procardia XL

Class and Category

Chemical class: Dihydropyridine derivative
Therapeutic class: Antianginal, antihypertensive
Pregnancy category: C

Indications and Dosages

➤ *To manage angina*
CAPSULES (ADALAT, APO-NIFED, NOVO-NIFEDIN, NU-NIFED, PROCARDIA)

Adults. *Initial:* 10 mg t.i.d., increased over 1 to 2 wk as needed. *Maintenance:* 10 to 20 mg t.i.d. *Maximum:* 180 mg daily, 30 mg/dose.

E.R. TABLETS (ADALAT XL, PROCARDIA XL)

Adults. *Initial:* 30 to 60 mg daily, increased or decreased over 7 to 14 days based on patient response. *Maximum:* 90 mg daily.

➤ *To manage hypertension*
E.R. TABLETS (ADALAT CC)

Adults. *Initial:* 30 mg daily. *Maintenance:* 30 to 60 mg daily, increased or decreased over 7 to 14 days based on patient response. *Maximum:* 90 mg daily.

E.R. TABLETS (ADALAT PA)

Adults. *Initial:* 10 to 20 mg b.i.d., increased every 3 wk based on patient response. *Maintenance:* 20 mg b.i.d. *Maximum:* 80 mg daily.

E.R. TABLETS (ADALAT XL)

Adults. *Initial:* 30 to 60 mg daily, increased or decreased over 7 to 14 days based on patient response. *Maintenance:* 60 to 90 mg daily. *Maximum:* 120 mg daily.

E.R. TABLETS (PROCARDIA XL)

Adults. 30 to 60 mg daily, increased or decreased over 7 to 14 days based on patient response. *Maximum:* 120 mg daily.

DOSAGE ADJUSTMENT Dosage may be reduced for elderly patients and those with heart failure or impaired hepatic or renal function.

Route	Onset	Peak	Duration
P.O. (cap)	20 min	Unknown	Unknown

Contraindications

Hypersensitivity to a calcium channel blocker, second- or third-degree AV block without artificial pacemaker, sick sinus syndrome

Mechanism of Action

May slow movement of calcium into myocardial and vascular smooth-muscle cells by deforming calcium channels in cell membranes, inhibiting ion-controlled gating mechanisms, and disrupting calcium release from sarcoplasmic reticulum. Decreasing intracellular calcium level inhibits smooth-muscle cell contraction and dilates arteries, which decreases myocardial oxygen demand, peripheral resistance, blood pressure, and afterload.

Interactions

DRUGS

anesthetics (hydrocarbon inhalation): Possibly hypotension
antiviral drugs, cimetidine, dalfopristin, diltiazem, erythromycin, fluconazole, itraconazole, ketoconazole, nefazodone, other antihypertensives, prazocin, quinupristin, timolol, valproic acid, verapamil: Increased risk of hypotension
benazepril: Possibly increased heart rate and hypotensive effect
beta blockers: Increased risk of profound hypotension, heart failure, and worsening of angina
calcium supplements: Possibly interference with action of nifedipine
carbamazepine, NSAIDs, phenobarbitone, phenytoin, rifampin, rifapentine, St. John's wort, sympathomimetics: Possibly decreased therapeutic effects of nifedipine
digoxin: Transiently increased blood digoxin level, increased risk of digitalis toxicity
disopyramide, flecainide: Increased risk of bradycardia, conduction defects, and heart failure
doxazocin: Decreased doxazocin effectiveness; increased nifedipine effectiveness
estrogens: Possibly increased fluid retention and decreased therapeutic effects of nifedipine
lithium: Increased risk of neurotoxicity
metformin: Increased metformin absorption and plasma level
tacrolimus: Decreased tacrolimus metabolism

FOODS

grapefruit, grapefruit juice: Possibly increased bioavailability of nifedipine
high-fat meals: Possibly delayed nifedipine absorption

N
O

ACTIVITIES

alcohol use: Additive hypotensive effect

Adverse Reactions

CNS: Anxiety, ataxia, confusion, dizziness, drowsiness, headache, nervousness (possibly extreme), nightmares, paresthesia, psychiatric disturbance, syncope, tremor, weakness

CV: Arrhythmias (bradycardia, tachycardia), chest pain, heart failure, hypotension, palpitations, peripheral edema

EENT: Altered taste, blurred vision, dry mouth, epistaxis, gingival hyperplasia, nasal congestion, pharyngitis, sinusitis, tinnitus

ENDO: Gynecomastia, hyperglycemia

GI: Anorexia, constipation, diarrhea, dyspepsia, elevated liver function test results, hepatitis, nausea, vomiting

GU: Dysuria, nocturia, polyuria, sexual dysfunction, urinary frequency

HEME: Anemia, leukopenia, positive Coombs' test, thrombocytopenia

MS: Joint stiffness, muscle cramps

RESP: Chest congestion, cough, dyspnea, respiratory tract infection, wheezing

SKIN: Dermatitis, diaphoresis, erythema multiforme, flushing, photosensitivity, pruritus, rash, urticaria

Nursing Considerations

• When starting and stopping nifedipine therapy, taper it, as prescribed, over 7 to 14 days.
• For closely monitored hospitalized patient with angina, dosage may be increased 10 mg every 4 to 6 hours to control chest pain.
• Because of drug's negative inotropic effect on some patients, frequently monitor heart rate and rhythm and blood pressure in patients who take a beta blocker or have heart failure or significant left ventricular dysfunction.
• Monitor fluid intake and output and daily weight; fluid retention may lead to heart failure. Also assess for signs of heart failure, such as crackles, dyspnea, jugular vein distention, peripheral edema, and weight gain.

PATIENT TEACHING

• Instruct patient to swallow E.R. tablets whole, not to crush, chew, or break them. Inform her that their empty shells may appear in stool.
• Urge patient to take nifedipine exactly as prescribed, even when she's feeling well. Advise her to notify prescriber if she misses two or more doses.

• Urge patient not to take drug within 1 hour of a high-fat meal or grapefruit. Urge her not to alter the amount of grapefruit in her diet without consulting prescriber.
• **WARNING** Caution patient against stopping nifedipine abruptly because angina or dangerously high blood pressure could result.
• Teach patient how to measure her pulse rate and blood pressure, and advise her to call prescriber if they drop below accepted levels. Suggest that she keep a log of weekly measurements and take it to follow-up visits.
• Instruct patient to notify prescriber immediately about chest pain, difficulty breathing, ringing in ears, and swollen gums.
• Advise patient to avoid hazardous activities until drug's CNS effects are known.
• Urge patient to avoid alcoholic beverages because they may worsen dizziness, drowsiness, and hypotension.
• Teach patient to minimize constipation by increasing her intake of fluids, if allowed, and dietary fiber.
• Emphasize the need to comply with prescribed lifestyle changes, such as alcohol moderation, low-fat or low-sodium diet, regular exercise, smoking cessation, stress reduction, and weight reduction.
• Stress the need for good oral hygiene and regular dental visits.
• Caution patient that hot tubs, saunas, and prolonged hot showers may cause dizziness and fainting.
• Advise patient to avoid prolonged sun exposure and to wear sunscreen outdoors.

nisoldipine

Sular

Class and Category

Chemical class: Dihydropyridine derivative
Therapeutic class: Antihypertensive
Pregnancy category: C

Indications and Dosages

➤ *To manage hypertension*

E.R. TABLETS

Adults. 20 mg daily, increased by 10 mg every 7 days, as prescribed. *Maintenance:* 20 to 40 mg daily. *Maximum:* 60 mg daily.

DOSAGE ADJUSTMENT For patients over age 65 and patients with hepatic impairment, initial dosage reduced to 10 mg daily.

Mechanism of Action

May slow extracellular calcium movement into myocardial and vascular smooth-muscle cells by deforming calcium channels in cell membranes, inhibiting ion-controlled gating mechanisms, and interfering with calcium release from the sarcoplasmic reticulum. By decreasing the intracellular calcium level, nisoldipine inhibits smooth-muscle cell contraction and dilates coronary and systemic arteries. As with other calcium channel blockers, these actions lead to decreased myocardial oxygen requirements and reduced peripheral resistance, blood pressure, and afterload.

Contraindications

Hypersensitivity to any calcium channel blocker, second- or third-degree AV block without artificial pacemaker, sick sinus syndrome

Interactions

DRUGS

beta blockers: Possibly increased risk of hypotension
CYP3A4 inducers such as carbamazepine, phenytoin: Decreased nisoldipine levels and effectiveness
CYP3A4 inhibitors such as azole antifungals, cimetidine, quinidine: Increased blood nisoldipine level; increased risk of adverse reactions
NSAIDs: Decreased antihypertensive effect of nisoldipine

FOODS

grapefruit, grapefruit juice: Possibly increased bioavailability of nisoldipine
high-fat meals: Possibly delayed nisoldipine absorption

ACTIVITIES

alcohol use: Additive hypotensive effect

Adverse Reactions

CNS: Dizziness, headache
CV: Angina, hypotension, palpitations, peripheral edema, vasodilation
EENT: Pharyngitis, sinusitis
GI: Constipation, nausea
RESP: Bronchospasm, dyspnea
SKIN: Ras
Other: Allergic-type reaction

Nursing Considerations

• Monitor pulse rate and rhythm and blood pressure before starting nisoldipine therapy, during dosage adjustments, and periodically throughout therapy.
• Don't break or crush E.R. tablets.
• For optimal absorption, give drug 1 hour before or 2 hours after meals.
• Monitor fluid intake and output and daily weight to assess for signs of fluid retention, which may lead to heart failure. Also assess for signs of heart failure, such as crackles, dyspnea, jugular vein distention, peripheral edema, and weight gain.
• Monitor patient for an allergic-type reaction that may include bronchospasm, especially if patient has aspirin sensitivity, because drug contains FD&C yellow no. 5 dye.

PATIENT TEACHING

• Instruct patient to swallow E.R. nisoldipine tablets whole, not to break, crush, or chew them.
• Advise patient to take drug 1 hour before or 2 hours after meals. Urge her not to alter the amount of grapefruit products in her diet without consulting prescriber.
• Urge patient to continue taking drug as prescribed, even if she feels well.
• **WARNING** Caution patient against stopping drug abruptly because blood pressure could rise dangerously high.
• Instruct patient to notify prescriber about constipation, difficulty breathing, dizziness, irregular heartbeat, nausea, severe headache, and swelling of hands or feet.
• Teach patient and family how to measure blood pressure, and instruct them to notify prescriber if systolic blood pressure falls below 90 mm Hg. Suggest that patient keep a log of weekly measurements and take it to follow-up visits.
• Advise patient to change positions slowly to minimize the effects of orthostatic hypotension. Inform her that hot tubs, saunas, and prolonged hot showers may worsen this adverse reaction.
• Caution patient to avoid hazardous activities until drug's CNS effects are known.
• Urge patient to avoid alcohol and OTC alcohol-containing drugs without consulting prescriber. Many OTC preparations can raise blood pressure.
• Emphasize the need to adhere to prescribed lifestyle changes, such as alcohol modera-

N
O

tion, low-fat and low-sodium diet, regular exercise, smoking cessation, stress reduction, and weight reduction.

nitazoxanide

Alinia

Class and Category
Chemical class: Benzamide
Therapeutic class: Antiprotozoal
Pregnancy category: B

Indications and Dosages
➤ *To treat diarrhea caused by* Cryptosporidium parvum
ORAL SUSPENSION, TABLETS
Adults and children age 12 and over. 500 mg every 12 hr with meals for 3 days.
ORAL SUSPENSION
Children ages 4 to 11. 200 mg (10 ml) every 12 hr with meals for 3 days.
Children ages 12 months to 47 months. 100 mg (5 ml) every 12 hr with meals for 3 days.
➤ *To treat diarrhea caused by* Giardia lamblia
ORAL SUSPENSION, TABLETS
Children age 12 and over. 500 mg every 12 hr with meals for 3 days
ORAL SUSPENSION
Children ages 4 to 11. 200 mg (10 ml) every 12 hr with meals for 3 days.
Children ages 12 months to 47 months. 100 mg (5 ml) every 12 hr with meals for 3 days.

Route	Onset	Peak	Duration
P.O.	1 to 4 hr	Unknown	Unknown

Mechanism of Action
May destroy *Cryptosporidium parvum* and *Giardia lamblia* by interfering with enzyme-dependent electron transfer required for their anaerobic energy metabolism. Other unidentified mechanisms may also be involved. With loss of protozoal activity in the intestines, diarrhea ceases.

Contraindications
Hypersensitivity to nitazoxanide or its components

Interactions
DRUGS
other highly plasma protein–bound drugs with narrow therapeutic indices (such as warfarin and phenytoins): Possibly increased risk of toxicity of these drugs

Adverse Reactions
CNS: Headache
GI: Abdominal pain, anorexia, diarrhea, nausea, vomiting

Nursing Considerations
• Use nitazoxanide cautiously in children with impaired hepatic function, biliary disease, or renal insufficiency.
• Prepare suspension by first tapping bottle until powder flows freely. Add 24 ml of tap water to the powder and shake vigorously to suspend powder. Add another 24 ml of water and shake vigorously again. Keep bottle of reconstituted suspension tightly capped.
• Use oral suspension for children age 11 and under because tablets contain more nitazoxanide than is recommended for children under age 12.
PATIENT TEACHING
• Tell parents of patient to give nitazoxanide with meals.
• Advise parents to keep reconstituted nitazoxanide bottle tightly closed and to shake the bottle well before each use.
• Instruct parents to discard any unused drug after 7 days from first opening bottle.
• Inform parents of diabetic patient that oral nitazoxanide suspension contains 1.48 grams of sucrose/5 ml. Tell them that they should make sure to monitor the patient's blood glucose level closely.
• Tell parents that discoloration of eye or urine, although uncommon, may occur and is harmless.

nitrofurantoin

Apo-Nitrofurantoin (CAN), Furadantin, Macrobid, Macrodantin, Novo-Furantoin (CAN)

Class and Category
Chemical class: Nitrofuran derivative
Therapeutic class: Antibiotic
Pregnancy category: B (except near term)

Indications and Dosages
➤ *To treat acute cystitis*

CAPSULES, ORAL SUSPENSION, TABLETS

Adults. 50 to 100 mg every 6 hr. *Maximum:* 600 mg daily or 10 mg/kg daily.
Children over age 1 month. 0.75 to 1.75 mg/ kg every 6 hr.

E.R. CAPSULES

Adults and children age 12 and over. 100 mg every 12 hr for 7 days.

➤ *To suppress chronic cystitis*

CAPSULES, ORAL SUSPENSION, TABLETS

Adults. 50 to 100 mg at bedtime. *Maximum:* 600 mg daily or 10 mg/kg daily.
Children over age 1 month. 1 mg/kg daily at bedtime.

Mechanism of Action

Inactivates or alters bacterial ribosomal proteins and other macromolecules. This action of nitrofurantoin inhibits bacterial protein synthesis, aerobic energy metabolism, DNA synthesis, RNA synthesis, and cell wall synthesis. Nitrofurantoin is bacteriostatic at low doses and bactericidal at higher doses.

Contraindications

Age under 1 month, anuria, creatinine clearance of less than 60 ml/min/1.73 m^2, hypersensitivity to nitrofurantoin or parabens, oliguria, pregnancy near term

Interactions

DRUGS

hepatotoxic drugs: Increased risk of hepatotoxicity
magnesium trisilicate: Decreased nitrofurantoin absorption
methyldopa, procainamide, hemolytics: Increased risk of toxic effects from nitrofurantoin
nalidixic acid: Possibly impaired therapeutic effects of this drug
neurotoxic drugs: Increased risk of neurotoxicity
probenecid, sulfinpyrazone: Increased blood nitrofurantoin level and increased risk of toxicity

Adverse Reactions

CNS: Chills, confusion, depression, headache, neurotoxicity, peripheral neuropathy
EENT: Optic neuritis, parotitis, tooth discoloration

GI: Abdominal pain, anorexia, diarrhea, hepatitis, nausea, pancreatitis, pseudomembranous colitis, vomiting
GU: Rust-colored to brown urine
HEME: Aplastic anemia, granulocytopenia, hemolytic anemia, leukopenia, megaloblastic anemia, methemoglobinemia, thrombocytopenia
MS: Arthralgia, myalgia
RESP: Asthma (in asthmatic patients), cyanosis, pneumonitis (acute)
SKIN: Alopecia, erythema multiforme, exfoliative dermatitis, jaundice, pruritus, rash, urticaria
Other: Anaphylaxis, angioedema, drug-induced fever

Nursing Considerations

•Obtain a specimen of the patient's urine for culture and sensitivity tests, as ordered; review test results if possible before giving nitrofurantoin.
•Give drug with food or milk to avoid staining teeth.
•Don't crush or break capsules.
•Shake oral nitrofurantoin suspension before pouring dose, and mix with food or milk, as needed.
•Monitor patient for evidence of superinfection, such as abdominal pain, diarrhea, and fever. If patient develops diarrhea, it may indicate pseudomembranous colitis caused by *Clostridium difficile*. Notify prescriber and expect to withhold nitrofurantoin and treat with fluids, electrolytes, protein, and an antibiotic effective against *C. difficile*.
•Monitor elderly patients for pulmonary and hepatic abnormalities because rare but severe reactions have occurred with nitrofurantoin use in the elderly.

PATIENT TEACHING

•Instruct patient to shake nitrofurantoin oral suspension before measuring dose and to take drug with food or milk.
•Caution patient against taking any preparations that contain magnesium trisilicate during therapy.
•Inform patient that urine may turn brown, orange, or rust-colored during therapy.
•Instruct patient to complete the prescribed course of therapy even if symptoms subside before course is completed.
•Urge patient to tell prescriber about diarrhea that's severe or lasts longer than 3 days.

N
O

Explain that watery or bloody stools can occur 2 or more months after nitrofurantoin therapy and can be serious, requiring prompt treatment.

nitroglycerin
(glyceryl trinitrate)

Deponit, Minitran, Nitro-Bid, Nitrocot, Nitro-Dur, Nitrogard, Nitroglyn E-R, Nitroject, Nitrol, Nitrolingual, NitroMist, Nitrong SR, Nitro-par, Nitrostat, Nitro-time, Transderm-Nitro, Tridil

Class and Category
Chemical class: Nitrate
Therapeutic class: Antianginal, antihypertensive, vasodilator
Pregnancy category: C

Indications and Dosages
➤ *To prevent or treat angina*

E.R. BUCCAL TABLETS
Adults. 1 mg every 5 hr while awake.

E.R. CAPSULES
Adults. 2.5, 6.5, or 9 mg every 12 hr. Frequency of doses increased to every 8 hr based on patient's response.

E.R. TABLETS
Adults. 2.6 or 6.5 mg every 12 hr. Frequency of doses increased to every 8 hr based on patient's response.

S.L. TABLETS
Adults. 0.3 to 0.6 mg, repeated every 5 min. *Maximum:* 3 tabs in 15 min or 10 mg daily.

TRANSDERMAL OINTMENT
Adults. 1" to 2" (15 to 30 mg) every 8 hr. Frequency of doses increased to every 6 hr if angina occurs between doses. *Maximum:* 5" (75 mg)/application.

TRANSDERMAL PATCH
Adults. 0.1 to 0.8 mg/hr, worn 12 to 14 hr.

TRANSLINGUAL SPRAY
Adults. For treatment, 1 or 2 metered doses (0.4 or 0.8 mg) onto or under tongue, repeated every 5 min as needed. For prevention, 1 or 2 metered doses (0.4 or 0.8 mg) onto or under tongue 5 to 10 minutes before activities that could lead to acute attack.

➤ *To prevent or treat angina, to manage hypertension or heart failure*

I.V. INFUSION
Adults. 5 mcg/min, increased by 5 mcg/min every 3 to 5 min to 20 mcg/min, as prescribed, and then by 10 to 20 mcg/min every 3 to 5 min until desired effect occurs.

Route	Onset	Peak	Duration
P.O. (buccal)	3 min	Unknown	5 hr
P.O. (E.R.)	20 to 45 min	Unknown	8 to 12 hr
I.V.	1 to 2 min	Unknown	3 to 5 min
S.L.	1 to 3 min	Unknown	30 to 60 min
Trans-dermal (ointment)	In 30 min	Unknown	4 to 8 hr
Trans-dermal (patch)	In 30 min	Unknown	8 to 24 hr
Trans-lingual	2 to 4 min	Unknown	30 to 60 min

Mechanism of Action
May interact with nitrate receptors in vascular smooth-muscle cell membranes. This interaction reduces nitroglycerin to nitric oxide, which activates the enzyme guanylate cyclase, increasing intracellular formation of cGMP. The increased cGMP level may relax vascular smooth muscle by forcing calcium out of muscle cells, causing vasodilation. Venous dilation decreases venous return to the heart, reducing left ventricular end-diastolic pressure and pulmonary artery wedge pressure. Arterial dilation decreases systemic vascular resistance, systolic arterial pressure, and mean arterial pressure. Thus, nitroglycerin reduces preload and afterload, decreasing myocardial workload and oxygen demand. It also dilates coronary arteries, increasing blood flow to ischemic myocardial tissue.

Incompatibilities
Don't administer I.V. nitroglycerin through I.V. bags or tubing made of polyvinyl chloride. Don't mix drug with other solutions.

Contraindications
Acute MI (S.L.), angle-closure glaucoma, cerebral hemorrhage, concurrent use of phos-

phodiesterase inhibitors, constrictive pericarditis (I.V.), head trauma, hypersensitivity to adhesive in transdermal form, hypersensitivity to nitrates, hypotension (I.V.), hypovolemia (I.V.), inadequate cerebral circulation (I.V.), increased intracranial pressure, orthostatic hypotension, pericardial tamponade, severe anemia

Interactions
DRUGS
acetylcholine, norepinephrine: Possibly decreased therapeutic effects of these drugs
heparin: Possibly decreased anticoagulant effect of heparin (I.V. nitroglycerin)
opioid analgesics, other antihypertensives, vasodilators: Possibly increased orthostatic hypotension
phosphodiesterase inhibitors, such as sildenafil: Possibly severe hypotensive effect of nitroglycerin
sympathomimetics: Possibly decreased antianginal effect of nitroglycerin and increased risk of hypotension
ACTIVITIES
alcohol use: Possibly increased orthostatic hypotension

Adverse Reactions
CNS: Agitation, anxiety, dizziness, headache, insomnia, restlessness, syncope, weakness
CV: Arrhythmias (including tachycardia), edema, hypotension, orthostatic hypotension, palpitations
EENT: Blurred vision, burning or tingling in mouth (buccal, S.L. forms), dry mouth
GI: Abdominal pain, diarrhea, indigestion, nausea, vomiting
GU: Dysuria, impotence, urinary frequency
HEME: Methemoglobinemia
MS: Arthralgia
RESP: Bronchitis, pneumonia
SKIN: Contact dermatitis (transdermal forms), flushing of face and neck, rash

Nursing Considerations
• Use nitroglycerin cautiously in elderly patients, especially those who are volume depleted or taking several medications, because of the increased risk of hypotension and falls. Hypotension may be accompanied by angina and paradoxical slowing of the heart rate. Notify prescriber if these occur, and provide appropriate treatment, as ordered.

• Plan a nitroglycerin-free period of about 10 hours each day, as prescribed, to maintain therapeutic effects and avoid tolerance.
• Place E.R. buccal tablets in buccal pouch with patient in sitting or lying position.
• Don't break or crush E.R. tablets or capsules. Have patient swallow them whole with a full glass of water.
• Place S.L. tablet under patient's tongue and make sure it dissolves completely.
• Be sure to remove cotton from S.L. tablet container to allow quick access to the drug.
• When applying transdermal ointment, apply correct amount on dose-measuring paper. Then place paper on hairless area of body and spread in a thin even layer over an area at least 2 inches by 3 inches. Don't place on cuts or irritated areas. Wash your hands after application. Rotate sites. Store at room temperature.
• Open transdermal patch package immediately before use. Apply patch to hairless area, and press edges to seal. Rotate sites. Store at room temperature. If patient needs cardioversion or defibrillation, remove transdermal patch.
• Don't shake translingual spray container before administering. Have patient inhale and hold her breath, and then spray drug under or on her tongue.
• Be aware that I.V. nitroglycerin should be diluted only in D_5W or normal saline solution and shouldn't be mixed with other infusions. The pharmacist should add drug to a glass bottle, not a container made of polyvinyl chloride. Don't use a filter because plastic absorbs drug. Administer with infusion pump.
• Check vital signs before every dosage adjustment and frequently during therapy.
• Frequently monitor heart and breath sounds, level of consciousness, fluid intake and output, and pulmonary artery wedge pressure, if possible.
• Store premixed containers in the dark; don't freeze them.
• **WARNING** Assess patient for signs and symptoms of overdose, such as confusion, diaphoresis, dyspnea, flushing, headache, hypotension, nausea, palpitations, tachycardia, vertigo, vision changes, and vomiting. Treat as prescribed by removing nitroglycerin source, if possible; elevating the legs above heart

level; and administering an alpha-adrenergic agonist, such as phenylephrine, as prescribed, to treat severe hypotension.

PATIENT TEACHING

•Teach patient to recognize signs and symptoms of angina pectoris, including chest fullness, pain, and pressure, possibly with sweating and nausea. Pain may radiate down left arm or into neck or jaw. Inform female patients and those with diabetes mellitus or hypertension that they may experience only fatigue and shortness of breath.

•Instruct patient to read and follow package instructions to obtain full benefits of drug.

•To prevent drug tolerance, inform patient that prescriber may order a 10- to 12-hour drug-free period at night (or at another time if she has chest pain at night or in the morning).

•Instruct patient to swallow E.R. tablets or capsules whole—not to break, crush, or chew them—with a full glass of water.

•For sublingual or buccal use, advise patient to place a tablet under her tongue or in her buccal pouch when angina starts and then to sit or lie down. Instruct her not to swallow drug, but to let it dissolve. Explain that moisture in her mouth helps drug absorption. If angina doesn't subside, instruct patient to place another tablet under her tongue or in her buccal pouch after 5 minutes and to repeat, if needed, for three doses total. If pain doesn't subside after 20 minutes, urge patient to call 911 or another emergency service.

•Advise patient to carry S.L. tablets in their original brown bottle in a purse or jacket pocket, but not one that will be affected by body heat. Instruct her to store drug in a dry place at room temperature and to discard cotton from container. Advise her to discard and replace S.L. tablets after 6 months.

•Advise patient using transdermal ointment or patch to rotate sites to avoid skin sensitization.

•Inform patient that swimming or bathing doesn't affect transdermal forms but that hot tubs, saunas, prolonged hot showers, electric blankets, and magnetic therapy over site may increase drug absorption and cause dizziness and hypotension.

•Caution against inhaling translingual spray. Before first use, tell patient to press actuator button 10 times to prime container and then hold container upright with forefinger on top of actuator button. Tell her to open her mouth, bring container as close as possible, press actuator button firmly to release spray onto or under her tongue, and release button and immediately close her mouth. Remind her to replace plastic cover on container and to not spit out the drug or rinse her mouth for 5 to 10 minutes. Tell her to reprime container by pressing actuator button twice if container hasn't been used for more than 6 weeks. Remind patient to periodically check level of fluid in container. If it reaches the top or middle hole on side of container, more should be obtained. Caution patient not to let level of liquid get to bottom of hole.

•Inform patient that nitroglycerin commonly causes headache, which typically resolves after a few days of continuous therapy. Suggest taking acetaminophen, as needed.

•Advise patient to notify prescriber immediately about blurred vision, dizziness, and severe headache.

•Suggest that patient change positions slowly to minimize orthostatic hypotension.

•Advise patient to avoid hazardous activities until drug's CNS effects are known.

•Urge patient to avoid alcohol and erectile dysfunction drugs during therapy.

nitroprusside sodium

Nipride, Nitropress

Class and Category

Chemical class: Cyanonitrosylferrate
Therapeutic class: Antihypertensive, vasodilator
Pregnancy category: C

Indications and Dosages

➤ *To treat hypertensive crisis and manage severe heart failure*

I.V. INFUSION

Adults and children. *Initial:* 0.25 to 0.3 mcg/kg/min, increased gradually every few minutes until blood pressure reaches desired level. *Maintenance:* 3 mcg/kg/min (range, 0.25 to 10 mcg/kg/min). *Maximum:* 10 mcg/kg/min for 10 min.

Route	Onset	Peak	Duration
I.V.	1 to 2 min	Immediate	1 to 10 min

Mechanism of Action

May interact with nitrate receptors in vascular smooth-muscle cell membranes. This action reduces nitroprusside to nitric oxide and then activates intracellular guanylate cyclase, which increases the cGMP level. The increased cGMP level may relax vascular smooth muscle by forcing calcium out of muscle cells. Smooth-muscle relaxation causes arteries and veins to dilate, which reduces peripheral vascular resistance and blood pressure.

Incompatibilities

Don't mix nitroprusside with any other drug.

Contraindications

Acute heart failure with decreased peripheral vascular resistance, congenital optic atrophy, decreased cerebral perfusion, hypersensitivity to nitroprusside or its components, hypertension from aortic coarctation or AV shunting, tobacco-induced amblyopia

Interactions

DRUGS

dobutamine: Increased cardiac output, decreased pulmonary artery wedge pressure
ganglionic blockers, general anesthetics, hypotension-producing drugs: Increased hypotensive effect
sympathomimetics: Decreased antihypertensive effect of nitroprusside

Adverse Reactions

CNS: Anxiety, dizziness, headache, increased intracranial pressure, nervousness, restlessness
CV: Hypotension, tachycardia
ENDO: Hypothyroidism
GI: Abdominal pain, ileus, nausea, vomiting
HEME: Methemoglobinemia
MS: Muscle twitching
SKIN: Diaphoresis, flushing, rash
Other: Infusion site phlebitis

Nursing Considerations

• Obtain baseline vital signs before administering nitroprusside.
• WARNING Don't give drug undiluted. Reconstitute with 2 ml of D_5W, and add solution to 250 to 500 ml of D_5W to produce 200 mcg/ml or 100 mcg/ml, respectively.
• Be aware that solution is stable at room temperature for 24 hours when protected from light. Don't use reconstituted solution if it contains particles or is blue, green, red, or darker than faint brown.
• Use an infusion pump. Place opaque covering over infusion container because drug is metabolized by light. I.V. tubing doesn't need to be covered.
• Keep patient supine when starting drug or titrating dose up or down.
• Monitor blood pressure continuously with intra-arterial pressure monitor. Record blood pressure every 5 minutes at start of infusion and every 15 minutes thereafter.
• If patient has severe heart failure, expect to administer an inotropic drug, such as dopamine or dobutamine, as prescribed.
• WARNING For patient who receives prolonged nitroprusside therapy or short-term high-dose therapy, monitor for signs of thiocyanate toxicity (ataxia, blurred vision, delirium, dizziness, dyspnea, headache, hyperreflexia, loss of consciousness, nausea, tinnitus, vomiting). Toxicity can cause arrhythmias, metabolic acidosis, severe hypotension, and death.
• Monitor serum thiocyanate level at least every 72 hours; levels above 100 mcg/ml are associated with toxicity.
• WARNING Assess patient for evidence of cyanide toxicity (absence of reflexes, coma, distant heart sounds, hypotension, metabolic acidosis, mydriasis, pink skin, shallow respirations, and weak pulse). If you detect such evidence, discontinue nitroprusside, as ordered, and give 4 to 6 mg/kg of sodium nitrite over 2 to 4 minutes to convert hemoglobin to methemoglobin. Follow with 150 to 200 mg/kg of sodium thiosulfate. Repeat this regimen at one-half the original doses after 2 hours, as ordered.

PATIENT TEACHING

• Advise patient to change position slowly to minimize dizziness from sudden, severe hypotension.

nizatidine

Apo-Nizatidine (CAN), Axid, Axid AR

Class and Category

Chemical class: Ethenediamine derivative
Therapeutic class: Antiulcer
Pregnancy category: B

Indications and Dosages

➤ *To manage active duodenal ulcer*

CAPSULES

Adults and adolescents. 300 mg at bedtime or 150 mg b.i.d. for 8 wk.

DOSAGE ADJUSTMENT Dosage reduced to 150 mg daily for patients with creatinine clearance of 20 to 50 ml/min/1.73 m^2; to 150 mg every other day for those with creatinine clearance less than 20 ml/min/1.73 m^2.

➤ *To prevent recurrence of duodenal ulcer*

CAPSULES

Adults and adolescents. 150 mg at bedtime.

DOSAGE ADJUSTMENT Dosage reduced to 150 mg every other day for patients with creatinine clearance of 20 to 50 ml/min/1.73 m^2; to 150 mg every 3 days for those with creatinine clearance less than 20 ml/min/1.73 m^2.

➤ *To manage acute benign gastric ulcer*

CAPSULES

Adults and adolescents. 300 mg at bedtime or 150 mg b.i.d.

➤ *To manage gastroesophageal reflux disease*

CAPSULES

Adults and adolescents. 150 mg b.i.d.

➤ *To prevent or relieve acid indigestion or heartburn*

TABLETS

Adults and adolescents. 75 mg 30 min to 1 hr before meals.

Route	Onset	Peak	Duration
P.O.	Unknown	Unknown	10 to 12 hr*

Mechanism of Action

Inhibits basal and nocturnal secretion of gastric acid by reversibly and competitively blocking H$_2$ receptors, especially those in gastric parietal cells. Nizatidine also inhibits gastric acid secretion in response to stimuli, including food and caffeine.

Contraindications

Hypersensitivity to nizatidine or other H$_2$-receptor antagonists

---

* For nocturnal acid secretion; up to 4 hr for food-stimulated acid secretion.

Interactions

DRUGS

antacids: Decreased nizatidine bioavailability
itraconazole, ketoconazole: Decreased absorption of these drugs
salicylates: Increased blood level of these drugs
sucralfate: Possibly decreased nizatidine absorption

Adverse Reactions

CNS: Agitation, anxiety, confusion, depression, dizziness, fatigue, fever, hallucinations, headache, insomnia, somnolence
CV: Arrhythmias, chest pain, vasculitis
EENT: Amblyopia, dry mouth, laryngeal edema, pharyngitis, rhinitis, sinusitis
ENDO: Gynecomastia
GI: Abdominal pain, constipation, diarrhea, hepatitis, nausea, vomiting
GU: Decreased libido, hyperuricemia not associated with gout or nephrolithiasis, impotence
HEME: Anemia, aplastic anemia, eosinophilia, hemolytic anemia, leukopenia, neutropenia, pancytopenia, thrombocytopenia
MS: Back pain, myalgia
RESP: Bronchospasm, cough
SKIN: Alopecia, diaphoresis, erythema multiforme, exfoliative dermatitis, jaundice, pruritus, rash, Stevens-Johnson syndrome, toxic epidermal necrolysis, urticaria
Other: Anaphylaxis, angioedema, serum sicknesslike reaction

Nursing Considerations

• Monitor CBC, BUN and serum creatinine levels, and liver function test results before and periodically during nizatidine therapy.
• Don't give within 1 hour of an antacid.

PATIENT TEACHING

• Instruct patient not to take nizatidine within 1 hour of an antacid.
• Urge patient to take drug exactly as prescribed, even if she feels better. Inform her that ulcer may take up to 8 weeks to heal.
• If patient smokes, urge her to stop because smoking increases gastric acid production.
• Teach patient to minimize constipation by drinking plenty of fluids (if allowed), eating high-fiber foods, and exercising regularly.
• Instruct patient to notify prescriber immediately about abdominal pain, easy bruising, extreme fatigue, yellow skin or sclera, trouble swallowing food, bloody vomitus, or bloody or tarry stools.

•Urge patient not to take nizatidine with other acid reducers.

norepinephrine bitartrate
(levarterenol bitartrate)

Levophed

Class and Category
Chemical class: Catecholamine
Therapeutic class: Cardiac stimulant, vasopressor
Pregnancy category: C

Indications and Dosages
➤ *To treat acute hypotension, cardiogenic shock, and septic shock*

I.V. INFUSION
Adults. *Initial:* 0.5 to 1 mcg/min. Increased, as ordered, until systolic blood pressure reaches desired level. *Maintenance:* 2 to 12 mcg/min.
Children. 0.1 mcg/kg/min. *Maximum:* 1 mcg/kg/min.

➤ *To treat refractory shock*

I.V. INFUSION
Adults. Up to 30 mcg/min.

Route	Onset	Peak	Duration
I.V.	Rapid	Unknown	1 to 2 min

Mechanism of Action
At more than 4 mcg/min, directly stimulates alpha-adrenergic receptors and inhibits adenyl cyclase, which inhibits cAMP production. Inhibition of cAMP contricts arteries and veins and increases peripheral vascular resistance and systolic blood pressure. At less than 2 mcg/min, norepinephrine directly stimulates beta-adrenergic receptors in the myocardium and increases adenyl cyclase activity, producing positive inotropic and chronotropic effects.

Contraindications
Concurrent use of hydrocarbon inhalation anesthetics, hypersensitivity to norepinephrine or its components, hypovolemia, mesenteric or peripheral vascular thrombosis

Interactions
DRUGS
alpha blockers: Decreased vasopressor effects of norepinephrine
beta blockers: Decreased cardiac-stimulating effect of norepinephrine, possibly decreased therapeutic effects of both drugs
digoxin: Increased risk of arrhythmias, possibly potentiated inotropic effect
doxapram: Possibly increased vasopressor effects of both drugs
ergonovine, ergotamine, methylergonovine, methysergide, oxytocin: Possibly increased vasoconstriction
general anesthetics: Risk of arrhythmias
guanadrel, guanethidine: Increased vasopressor response to norepinephrine, possibly severe hypertension
MAO inhibitors: Possibly life-threatening arrhythmias, hyperpyrexia, severe headache, severe hypertension, and vomiting
maprotiline, tricyclic antidepressants: Possibly potentiated cardiovascular and pressor effects of norepinephrine, including arrhythmias, severe hypertension, and hyperpyrexia
methylphenidate: Possibly potentiated vasopressor effect of norepinephrine
nitrates: Possibly decreased therapeutic effects of both drugs
phenoxybenzamine: Possibly arrhythmias or hypotension
sympathomimetics: Increased risk of adverse cardiovascular effects
thyroid hormones: Increased risk of coronary insufficiency

Adverse Reactions
CNS: Anxiety, dizziness, headache, insomnia, nervousness, tremor, weakness
CV: Angina, bradycardia, ECG changes, edema, hypertension, hypotension, palpitations, peripheral vascular insufficiency (including gangrene), PVCs, sinus tachycardia
GI: Nausea, vomiting
GU: Decreased renal perfusion
RESP: Apnea, dyspnea
SKIN: Pallor
Other: Infusion site sloughing and tissue necrosis, metabolic acidosis

Nursing Considerations
•Dilute norepinephrine concentrate for infusion in D_5W, dextrose 5% in normal saline solution, or normal saline solution. Dilutions typically range from 16 to 32 mcg/ml.
•Make sure solution contains no particles and isn't discolored before administering.
•Give drug with a flow-control device.

N
O

•Check blood pressure every 2 to 3 minutes, preferably by direct intra-arterial monitoring, until stabilized and then every 5 minutes.
•**WARNING** Because extravasation can cause severe tissue damage and necrosis, expect prescriber to give multiple subcutaneous injections of phentolamine (5 to 10 mg diluted in 10 to 15 ml of normal saline solution) around extravasated infusion site.
•If blanching occurs along vein, change infusion site and notify prescriber at once.
•Monitor continuous ECG during therapy.

PATIENT TEACHING
•Urge patient to immediately report burning, leaking, or tingling around the I.V. site.

norfloxacin

Noroxin

Class and Category

Chemical class: Fluoroquinolone
Therapeutic class: Antibiotic
Pregnancy category: C

Indications and Dosages

➤ *To treat uncomplicated UTI caused by* Escherichia coli, Klebsiella pneumoniae, *or* Proteus mirabilis

TABLETS
Adults. 400 mg every 12 hr for 3 days.

➤ *To treat uncomplicated UTI caused by* Citrobacter freundii, Enterobacter aerogenes, Enterobacter cloacae, Enterococcus faecalis, Proteus *species,* Pseudomonas aeruginosa, Staphylococcus aureus, Staphylococcus epidermidis, Staphylococcus saprophyticus, *or* Streptococcus agalactiae

TABLETS
Adults. 400 mg every 12 hr for 7 to 10 days.

➤ *To treat complicated UTI caused by* E. coli, E. faecalis, K. pneumoniae, P. aeruginosa, P. mirabilis, *or* Serratia marcescens

TABLETS
Adults. 400 mg every 12 hr for 10 to 21 days. *Maximum:* 800 mg daily.

➤ *To treat uncomplicated gonorrhea*

TABLETS
Adults. 800 mg as a single dose.

➤ *To treat prostatitis caused by* E. coli

TABLETS
Adults. 400 mg every 12 hr for 28 days.
DOSAGE ADJUSTMENT Dosage reduced to 400 mg daily for patients with creatinine clearance of 30 ml/min/1.73 m^2 or less.

> ### Mechanism of Action
> Inhibits the enzyme DNA gyrase, which unwinds and supercoils bacterial DNA before it replicates. By inhibiting this enzyme, norfloxacin interferes with bacterial cell replication and causes cell death.

Contraindications

Hypersensitivity to norfloxacin, other fluoroquinolones, or their components

Interactions

DRUGS
aluminum-, calcium-, or magnesium-containing antacids; ferrous sulfate; magnesium-containing laxatives; sucralfate; zinc: Possibly decreased absorption and blood level of norfloxacin
caffeine, clozapine, ropinirole, tacrine, theophylline, tizanidine: Possibly increased blood level of these drugs
class Ia antiarrhythmics, such as quinidine; class III antiarrhythmics, such as sotalol; other drugs known to prolong QTc interval, such as disopyramide and pentamidine: Possibly prolonged QTc interval
cyclosporine: Possibly increased serum creatinine and blood cyclosporine levels
didanosine: Possibly decreased norfloxacin absorption
glyburide: Risk of severe hypoglycemia
nitrofurantoin: Possibly decreased norfloxacin effectiveness
NSAIDs: Possibly increased risk of CNS stimulation and seizures
probenecid: Decreased norfloxacin excretion and risk of toxicity
warfarin: Possibly increased anticoagulant effect and risk of bleeding

FOODS
caffeine: Reduced clearance of caffeine leading to accumulation of caffeine in blood

Adverse Reactions

CNS: Ataxia, confusion, dizziness, drowsiness, fever, Guillian-Barré syndrome, headache, hypoesthesia, insomnia, paresthesia, peripheral neuropathy, psychosis, seizures, tremors

CV: Prolonged QT interval, torsades de pointes, vasculitis

EENT: Decreased taste sensation. diplopia, hearing loss, stomatitis, taste perversion, tinnitus, visual changes

GI: Abdominal cramps or pain, acute hepatic necrosis or failure, diarrhea, elevated liver function test results, hepatitis, jaundice, nausea, pancreatitis, pseudomembranous colitis, vomiting

GU: Interstitial nephritis, renal failure, vaginal candidiasis

HEME: Agranulocytosis, aplastic anemia, hemolytic anemia, leukopenia, neutropenia, pancytopenia, thrombocytopenia

MS: Arthralgia; myasthenia gravis exacerbation; myalgia; tendinitis; tendon inflammation, pain, or rupture

RESP: Allergic pneumonitis, dyspnea

SKIN: Blisters, diaphoresis, erythema, erythema multiforme, exfoliative dermatitis, photosensitivity, pruritus, rash, Stevens-Johnson syndrome, toxic epidermal necrolysis, urticaria

Other: Anaphylaxis, angioedema, serum sickness

Nursing Considerations

•Obtain urine specimen for culture and sensitivity tests before starting drug, if possible.

•Determine if patient has a history of a CNS disorder because drug may lower the seizure threshold. Notify prescriber before starting drug, and institute seizure precautions.

•**WARNING** Before starting therapy, determine if patient takes a class Ia antiarrhythmic, such as quinidine; a class III antiarrhythmic, such as sotalol; or other drugs that prolong the QTc interval. Also find out if patient has hypokalemia or an underlying QT-interval prolonging condition. These drugs and conditions, especially in the elderly, may prolong the QTc interval and lead to life-threatening ventricular tachycardia or torsades de pointes in a patient taking norfloxacin.

•Give drug on an empty stomach 2 hours before or after antacids, didanosine, sucralfate, or vitamins that contain iron or zinc.

•Keep emergency resuscitation equipment readily available, and watch for signs of hypersensitivity, such as angioedema, dyspnea, jaundice, rash, and urticaria. If you suspect anaphylaxis, prepare to give epinephrine, corticosteroids, and diphenhydramine, as prescribed.

•If patient has myasthenia gravis, assess her frequently for a change in respiratory status because norfloxacin may lead to life-threatening weakness of respiratory muscles.

•Notify prescriber if patient has symptoms of peripheral neuropathy (pain, burning, tingling, numbness, weakness, or altered sensations of light touch, pain, temperature, position sense, or vibration sense), which could be permanent. Expect to stop nofloxacin.

•Monitor patients prone to tendinitis, such as the elderly, athletes, and those taking corticosteroids, for complaints of tendon pain, inflammation, or rupture. If present, notify prescriber and expect to discontinue norfloxacin, place patient on bedrest with no exercise of affected limb, and obtain diagnostic tests to confirm rupture.

•Monitor patient for diarrhea, which may indicate pseudomembranous colitis caused by *Clostridium difficile*. If diarrhea occurs, notify prescriber and expect to withhold norfloxacin and treat with fluids, electrolytes, protein, and an antibiotic effective against *C. difficile*.

PATIENT TEACHING

•Instruct patient to take norfloxacin on an empty stomach with a large glass of water to prevent crystalluria. Urge her to drink several glasses of water daily during therapy.

•Instruct patient to take drug at least 2 hours before or after eating, drinking milk, or taking antacids, didanosine, sucralfate, or vitamins that contain iron or zinc.

•Advise patient to avoid hazardous activities until drug's CNS effects are known.

•Tell patient to stop drug and report tendon pain or inflammation or abnormal changes in motor or sensory function.

•Advise patient to protect skin from sunlight and to report first sign of photosensitivity.

•Tell patient to take drug exactly as prescribed, even if symptoms subside.

•Urge patient to tell prescriber about diarrhea that's severe or lasts longer than 3 days. Remind patient that watery or bloody stools can occur 2 or more months after antibiotic therapy and can be serious, requiring prompt treatment.

N
O

nortriptyline hydrochloride

Aventyl, Pamelor

Class and Category

Chemical class: Dibenzocycloheptene derivative
Therapeutic class: Antidepressant
Pregnancy category: D

Indications and Dosages

➤ *To treat depression*

CAPSULES, ORAL SOLUTION

Adults. *Initial:* 25 mg t.i.d. or q.i.d. *Maximum:* 150 mg daily.
Adolescents. 25 to 50 mg daily or 1 to 3 mg/kg daily in divided doses.
Children ages 6 to 12. 10 to 20 mg daily or 1 to 3 mg/kg daily in divided doses.
DOSAGE ADJUSTMENT Dosage possibly reduced to 30 to 50 mg daily (in divided doses or at bedtime) for elderly patients.

Route	Onset	Peak	Duration
P.O.	2 to 3 wk	Unknown	Unknown

Mechanism of Action

May interfere with reuptake of serotonin (and possibly other neurotransmitters) at presynaptic neurons, thus enhancing serotonin's effects at postsynaptic receptors. By restoring normal neurotransmitter levels at nerve synapses, this tricyclic antidepressant may elevate mood.

Contraindications

Acute recovery phase of stroke or MI; hypersensitivity to nortriptyline, other tricyclic antidepressants, or their components; use within 14 days of MAO inhibitor therapy

Interactions

DRUGS

amantadine, anticholinergics, antidyskinetics, antihistamines: Possibly increased anticholinergic effects, confusion, hallucinations, nightmares; increased CNS depression
anticonvulsants: Possibly increased CNS depression and risk of seizures, possibly decreased anticonvulsant effectiveness
antithyroid drugs: Possibly agranulocytosis
barbiturates, carbamazepine: Possibly decreased level and effects of nortriptyline
bupropion, clozapine, cyclobenzaprine, haloperidol, loxapine, maprotiline, molindone, phenothiazines, thioxanthenes: Possibly increased sedative and anticholinergic effects and possibly increased risk of seizures
cimetidine, fluoxetine: Possibly increased blood nortriptyline level and risk of toxicity
clonidine: Possibly decreased antihypertensive effect and increased CNS depression
disulfiram: Possibly delirium
ethchlorvynol: Possibly delirium, increased CNS depression
guanadrel, guanethidine: Possibly decreased antihypertensive effect of these drugs
MAO inhibitors: Increased risk of hypertensive crisis, severe seizures, and death
oral anticoagulants: Possibly increased anticoagulant activity
pimozide, probucol: Possibly arrhythmias
sympathomimetics, including ophthalmic epinephrine and vasoconstrictive local anesthetics: Increased risk of arrhythmias, hyperpyrexia, hypertension, and tachycardia
thyroid hormones: Possibly increased therapeutic and toxic effects of both drugs

ACTIVITIES

alcohol use: Increased CNS and respiratory depression, hypertension, alcohol effects

Adverse Reactions

CNS: Ataxia, confusion, delirium, dizziness, drowsiness, excitation, hallucinations, headache, insomnia, nervousness, nightmares, parkinsonism, stroke, suicidal ideation, tremor
CV: Arrhythmias, orthostatic hypotension
EENT: Blurred vision, dry mouth, increased intraocular pressure, taste perversion
GI: Constipation, diarrhea, heartburn, ileus, increased appetite, nausea, vomiting
GU: Sexual dysfunction, urine retention
HEME: Bone marrow depression
RESP: Wheezing
SKIN: Diaphoresis, urticaria
Other: Weight gain

Nursing Considerations

• Expect to stop MAO inhibitor therapy 10 to 14 days before starting nortriptyline therapy.
• Watch patient closely (especially children, adolescents, and young adults), for suicidal tendencies, particularly when therapy starts and dosage changes because depression may

worsen temporarily during these times, possibly leading to suicidal ideation.
•Oral solution (10 mg/5 ml) is 4% alcohol.
•Give nortriptyline with food to reduce GI reactions.
•Monitor blood nortriptyline level; therapeutic range is 50 to 150 ng/ml.
•Monitor ECG tracing to detect arrhythmias.

PATIENT TEACHING
•Explain that oral solution contains alcohol.
•Discourage alcohol use during therapy.
•Explain that improvement may take weeks.
•Advise patient to avoid potentially hazardous activities until drug's CNS effects are known.
•Urge family or caregiver to watch patient closely for suicidal tendencies, especially when therapy starts or dosage changes and particularly if patient is a child, teenager, or young adult.
•Instruct patient to change position slowly to minimize orthostatic hypotension.
•Suggest that patient minimize constipation by drinking plenty of fluids (if allowed), eating high-fiber foods, and exercising regularly.

nystatin

Mycostatin, Nadostine (CAN), Nilstat, Nystex, Nystop, Pedi-Dri

Class and Category
Chemical class: Amphoteric polyene macrolide
Therapeutic class: Antifungal
Pregnancy category: Not rated (lozenges, oral suspension, tablets, topical), A (vaginal)

Indications and Dosages
➤ *To treat oropharyngeal candidiasis (thrush)*

LOZENGES (PASTILLES)
Adults and children over age 5. 200,000 to 400,000 units dissolved in mouth 4 or 5 times daily for up to 14 days.

ORAL SUSPENSION
Adults and children. 400,000 to 600,000 units swished and swallowed q.i.d. until at least 48 hr after symptoms subside.
Infants. 200,000 units to each side of mouth q.i.d. until at least 48 hr after symptoms subside.
Neonates. 100,000 units applied to each side

of mouth q.i.d. until at least 48 hr after symptoms subside.

TABLETS
Adults and adolescents. 500,000 to 1,000,000 units t.i.d. until at least 48 hr after symptoms subside.
Children age 5 and over. 500,000 units q.i.d. until at least 48 hr after symptoms subside.
➤ *To treat cutaneous and mucocutaneous candidiasis*

CREAM, OINTMENT, POWDER
Adults and children. 100,000 units (1 g) on affected area b.i.d. or t.i.d. for at least 2 wk.
➤ *To treat vulvovaginal candidiasis*

VAGINAL TABLETS
Adults and adolescents. 100,000 units (1 tab) once or twice daily for 14 days.

Mechanism of Action
Binds to sterols in fungal cell membranes, impairing membrane integrity. Cells lose intracellular potassium and other cellular contents and, eventually, die.

Contraindications
Hypersensitivity to nystatin or its components

Adverse Reactions
ENDO: Hyperglycemia (lozenge, oral suspension)
GI: Abdominal pain, diarrhea, nausea, vomiting (oral forms)
GU: Vaginal burning or itching (vaginal form)
SKIN: Irritation (topical forms)

Nursing Considerations
•Prepare nystatin powder for oral suspension for each dose; it has no preservatives.
•Gently rub nystatin cream or ointment into skin at affected area. Keep area dry and avoid occlusive dressings.
•Don't get topical form in patient's eyes.
•When treating candidal infection of feet, dust patient's shoes, socks, and feet.
•For vaginal form, use applicator supplied by manufacturer.

PATIENT TEACHING
•Instruct patient to let nystatin lozenges dissolve slowly in her mouth, not to chew or swallow them.
•Tell patient to swish oral suspension in her mouth as long as possible before swallowing.

N
O

•Advise patient to gently rub ointment or cream into skin at affected area, to keep area dry, and to avoid occlusive dressings.
•Caution patient to keep topical form away from her eyes.
•Advise patient with candidal infection of feet to dust her shoes, socks, and feet with nystatin.
•For vaginal form, tell patient to insert it with applicator supplied by manufacturer.

octreotide acetate

Sandostatin, Sandostatin LAR Depot

Class and Category

Chemical class: Cyclic octapeptide, somatostatin analogue
Therapeutic class: Antidiarrheal, hormone suppressant
Pregnancy category: B

Indications and Dosages

➤ *To control symptoms associated with vasoactive intestinal peptide tumors (watery diarrhea) and metastatic carcinoid tumors (diarrhea and flushing)*

I.M. INJECTION

Adults currently receiving subcutaneous injections. 20 mg every 4 wk for 2 mo, with subcutaneous doses continued for 2 to 4 wk after I.M. injections start. If patient has positive response to initial 2-mo regimen, dosage reduced to 10 mg every 4 wk. If symptoms persist or increase after initial 2-mo regimen, dosage increased to 30 mg every 4 wk, as prescribed.

SUBCUTANEOUS INJECTION

Adults. *Initial:* 200 to 300 mcg daily in divided doses b.i.d. to q.i.d. for first 2 wk. *Maintenance:* Individualized. *Maximum:* 450 mcg daily.

➤ *To treat symptoms of acromegaly, to suppress the release of growth hormone from pituitary tumors*

I.V. OR SUBCUTANEOUS INJECTION

Adults. *Initial:* 50 mcg t.i.d. *Usual:* 100 mcg t.i.d. *Maximum:* 1,500 mcg daily.

I.M. INJECTION

Adults currently receiving subcutaneous injections. 20 mg every 4 wk for 3 mo, then adjusted as prescribed in response to serum growth hormone level. *Maximum:* 40 mg every 4 wk.

Route	Onset	Peak	Duration
SubQ	Unknown	Unknown	Up to 12 hr

Mechanism of Action

Controls many types of secretory diarrhea by inhibiting secretion of serotonin and pituitary and GI hormones (including insulin, glucagon, growth hormone, thyrotropin, and, possibly, thyroid-stimulating hormone) as well as vasoactive intestinal peptides and pancreatic polypeptides (including gastrin, secretin, and motilin). Inhibiting serotonin and peptides increases intestinal absorption of water and electrolytes, decreases pancreatic and gastric acid secretions, and increases intestinal transit time by slowing gastric motility.

By inhibiting hormones involved in vasodilation, octreotide increases splanchnic arterial resistance and decreases GI blood flow, hepatic vein wedge pressure, hepatic blood flow, portal vein pressure, and intravariceal pressure, thus raising seated and standing blood pressures. By inhibiting serotonin secretion, octreotide eases symptoms of acromegaly, including diarrhea, flushing, wheezing, and urinary excretion of 5-hydroxyindoleacetic acid.

Incompatibilities

Don't mix octreotide in same syringe with fat emulsions or total parenteral nutrition solutions.

Contraindications

Hypersensitivity to octreotide or its components

Interactions

DRUGS

beta blockers, calcium channel blockers: Additive cardiovascular effects of these drugs
bromocriptine: Increased blood bromocriptine level
cisapride: Decreased effectiveness of both drugs
cyclosporine: Decreased blood cyclosporine level
diuretics: Increased risk of fluid and electrolyte imbalances
insulin, oral antidiabetic drugs: Increased risk of hypoglycemia

quinidine, terfenadine: Decreased metabolic clearance and increased blood levels of these drugs

vitamin B₁₂: Decreased blood levels of vitamin B_{12}

Adverse Reactions

CNS: Dizziness, drowsiness, fatigue, headache, intracranial hemorrhage, migraine, paranoia, seizures, suicidal ideation
CV: Arrhythmias (including conduction abnormalities), edema, hypertension, hypotension, MI, orthostatic hypotension, Raynaud's syndrome
EENT: Deafness, epistaxis, glaucoma, retinal vein thrombosis, sinusitis, vision changes
ENDO: Hyperglycemia, hypoglycemia, hypothyroidism, pituitary apoplexy
GI: Abdominal pain, acute cholecystitis, ascending cholangitis, biliary obstruction, cholelithiasis, cholestatic hepatitis, constipation, diarrhea, elevated liver enzymes, flatulence, gastric or peptic ulcer, GI hemorrhage, intestinal obstruction, nausea, pancreatitis, vomiting
GU: Decreased libido, hematuria, increased urine output, renal failure
HEME: Anemia, pancytopenia, thrombocytopenia
MS: Arthropathy, back pain, myalgia
RESP: Status asthmaticus, pulmonary hypertension, upper respiratory tract infection
SKIN: Alopecia, petechiae, pruritus, rash, urticaria
Other: Anaphylaxis, angioedema, dehydration, electrolyte imbalances, flulike symptoms, injection site irritation or pain

Nursing Considerations

•Give octreotide by I.V. injection only in an emergency, as prescribed.
•To prepare depot injection (long-acting suspension form), let powder and diluent warm to room temperature and then reconstitute according to manufacturer's instructions. Gently inject 2 ml of supplied diluent down side of vial without disturbing depot powder. Let diluent saturate powder. After 2 to 5 minutes, check sides and bottom of vial without inverting it. Once powder is completely saturated, swirl—don't shake—vial for 30 to 60 seconds to form suspension. Use immediately after reconstituting.
•Don't give depot injection by subcutaneous route; give only by I.M. route and only to patients who respond to and tolerate subcutaneous drug, as prescribed.
•To minimize pain, use smallest injection volume to deliver desired dose and rotate injection sites.
•Avoid using deltoid site for I.M. injection because injection site reactions and pain may result. Intragluteal injection is recommended.
•**WARNING** To avoid worsening of symptoms, expect to continue subcutaneous injections when switching to I.M. injections, as prescribed.
•Be aware that octreotide increases risk of acute cholecystitis, ascending cholangitis, biliary obstruction, cholestatic hepatitis, and pancreatitis.
•Monitor vital signs, bowels sounds, and stool consistency. Assess for abdominal pain and signs of gallbladder disease.
•Monitor serum liver enzyme levels, as appropriate.
•Monitor patient for signs of electrolyte imbalances and dehydration.
•Carefully monitor diabetic patient for altered glucose control.
•Monitor patient's thyroid function, as ordered, because octreotide suppresses secretion of thyroid-stimulating hormone, which may cause hypothyroidism.
•If patient has periodic flare-ups of symptoms, expect to give additional subcutaneous octreotide temporarily, as prescribed.
PATIENT TEACHING
•Advise patient to change position slowly to minimize effects of orthostatic hypotension.
•Instruct patient to notify prescriber about adverse reactions, especially abdominal pain, which may indicate pancreatitis.
•Urge diabetic patient to check blood glucose level often.
•Caution female patient of childbearing age that drug may restore fertility and, if pregnancy isn't desired, that contraception should be used during octreotide therapy.

ofloxacin

Floxin

Class and Category

Chemical class: Fluoroquinolone
Therapeutic class: Antibiotic
Pregnancy category: C

Indications and Dosages

➤ *To treat acute, uncomplicated cystitis caused by* Escherichia coli *or* Klebsiella pneumoniae

TABLETS, I.V. INFUSION

Adults. 200 mg every 12 hr for 3 days.

➤ *To treat uncomplicated cystitis caused by* Citrobacter diversus, Enterobacter aerogenes, Proteus mirabilis, *or* Pseudomonas aeruginosa

TABLETS, I.V. INFUSION

Adults. 200 mg every 12 hr for 7 days.

➤ *To treat complicated UTI caused by* C. diversus, E. coli, K. pneumoniae, P. mirabilis, *or* P. aeruginosa

Adults. 200 mg every 12 hr for 10 days.

➤ *To treat uncomplicated gonorrhea*

TABLETS, I.V. INFUSION

Adults and adolescents. 400 mg as single dose.

➤ *To treat urethritis or cervicitis caused by* Chlamydia trachomatis *or* Neisseria gonorrhoeae

TABLETS, I.V. INFUSION

Adults and adolescents. 300 mg b.i.d. for 7 days as an alternative to doxycycline or azithromycin.

➤ *To treat pelvic inflammatory disease caused by susceptible organisms*

TABLETS

Adults and adolescents. 400 mg b.i.d. with metronidazole P.O. for 10 to 14 days.

I.V. INFUSION

Adults and adolescents. 400 mg every 12 hr with metronidazole I.V. and then switched to oral therapy, as prescribed, after 24 hr. Complete course of therapy lasts 14 days.

➤ *To treat prostatitis caused by* E. coli

TABLETS, I.V. INFUSION

Adults. 300 mg every 12 hr for 6 wk.

➤ *To treat lower respiratory tract infections caused by* Haemophilus influenzae *or* Streptococcus pneumoniae *and skin and soft-tissue infections caused by* Staphylococcus aureus *or* Streptococcus pyogenes

TABLETS, I.V. INFUSION

Adults. 400 mg every 12 hr for 10 days.

DOSAGE ADJUSTMENT If creatinine clearance is 20 to 50 ml/min/1.73 m^2, dosing interval possibly reduced to every 24 hr; if clearance is less than 10 ml/min/1.73 m^2, dosage possibly reduced by 50% and given every 24 hr.

Mechanism of Action

Inhibits synthesis of the bacterial enzyme DNA gyrase by counteracting the excessive supercoiling of DNA during replication or transcription. Inhibition of DNA gyrase causes rapid- and slow-growing bacterial cells to die.

Incompatibilities

Don't mix ofloxacin with other I.V. drugs or additives.

Contraindications

Hypersensitivity to ofloxacin, other fluoroquinolones, or their components

Interactions

DRUGS

aluminum-, calcium-, or magnesium-containing antacids; didanosine; ferrous sulfate; magnesium-containing laxatives; multivitamins; sevelamer; sucralfate; zinc: Decreased absorption of oral ofloxacin

probenecid: Decreased ofloxacin excretion, increased risk of toxicity

procainamide: Decreased renal clearance of procainamide

warfarin: Possibly increased anticoagulant activity and risk of bleeding

Adverse Reactions

CNS: Aggressiveness, agitation, ataxia, dizziness, drowsiness, emotional lability, exacerbation of extrapyramidal disorders and myasthenia gravis, fever, headache, incoordination, insomnia, light-headedness, mania, peripheral neuropathy, psychotic reactions, restlessness, stroke, suicidal ideation, syncope

CV: Arrhythmias, prolonged QT interval, severe hypotension, torsades de pointes, vasculitis

EENT: Blurred vision; diplopia; disturbances in taste, smell, hearing, and equilibrium

ENDO: Hyperglycemia, hypoglycemia

GI: Abdominal cramps or pain, acute hepatic necrosis or failure, diarrhea, hepatitis, jaundice, nausea, pseudomembranous colitis, vomiting

GU: Acute renal insufficiency or failure, interstitial nephritis, renal calculi, vaginal candidiasis

HEME: Agranulocytosis, aplastic or he-

molytic anemia, leukopenia, pancytopenia, thrombocytopenia
MS: Arthralgia; myalgia; rhabdomyolysis; tendinitis; tendon inflammation, pain, or rupture
RESP: Allergic pneumonitis, pulmonary edema
SKIN: Blisters, diaphoresis, erythema, erythema multiforme, exfoliative dermatitis, photosensitivity, pruritus, rash, Stevens-Johnson syndrome, toxic epidermal necrolysis, urticaria
Other: Acidosis, anaphylaxis, infusion site phlebitis, serum sickness

Nursing Considerations
•Because of increased risk of prolonged QT interval, ofloxacin shouldn't be used if patient has had a prolonged QT interval, has an uncorrected electrolyte disorder, or takes a Class IA or III antiarrhythmic. Monitor elderly patients closely because risk of prolonged QT interval may be increased in this group.
•For I.V. infusion, dilute drug in normal saline solution or D_5W to at least 4 mg/ml, and infuse over 60 minutes to minimize the risk of hypotension. Discard unused portion.
•Monitor patient closely for hypersensitivity, which may occur as early as first dose. Reaction may include angioedema, bronchospasm, dyspnea, itching, rash, jaundice, shortness of breath, and urticaria. If these signs or symptoms appear, notify prescriber immediately and expect to discontinue drug.
•Notify prescriber if patient has symptoms of peripheral neuropathy (pain, burning, tingling, numbness, weakness, or altered sensations of light touch, pain, temperature, position sense, or vibration sense), which could be permanent; tendon rupture (pain and inflammation), which may occur more often in patients (especially elderly ones) taking corticosteroids and requires immediate rest; or a severe photosensitivity reaction. In each case, expect to stop ofloxacin.
•Maintain adequate hydration to prevent development of highly concentrated urine and crystalluria.
•Expect an increased risk of toxicity in severe hepatic disease, including cirrhosis.
•Be aware that ofloxacin may stimulate the CNS and aggravate seizure disorders.
•If diarrhea develops, notify prescriber because it may indicate pseudomembranous colitis. Ofloxacin may need to be discontinued and additional therapy started.
•Be alert for secondary fungal infection.
PATIENT TEACHING
•Encourage patient to take each oral dose with a full glass of water.
•Tell patient to complete full course of ofloxacin therapy exactly as prescribed, even if he feels better before it's complete.
•Urge patient not to take antacids, iron or zinc preparations, or other drugs (such as sucralfate and didanosine), within 2 hours of ofloxacin to prevent decreased or delayed drug absorption.
•Advise patient to avoid hazardous activities until CNS effects of drug are known.
•Tell patient to limit exposure to sun and ultraviolet light to prevent phototoxicity.
•Advise patient to notify prescriber immediately about burning skin, hives, itching, rash, rapid heart rate, abnormal motor or sensory function, and tendon pain.
•Urge patient to seek medical attention immediately for trouble breathing or swallowing, which may signal an allergic reaction.
•Instruct a diabetic patient who takes insulin or an antidiabetic to notify prescriber immediately if he develops a hypoglycemic reaction; ofloxacin will have to be stopped.
•Advise patient to notify prescriber if diarrhea develops, even up to 2 months after ofloxacin therapy ends. Additional therapy may be needed.

olanzapine
Zydis, Zyprexa

Class and Category
Chemical class: Thienobenzodiazepine derivative
Therapeutic class: Antipsychotic
Pregnancy category: C

Indications and Dosages
➤ *To treat psychosis*
ORALLY DISINTEGRATING TABLETS, TABLETS
Adults. *Initial:* 5 to 10 mg daily. *Usual:* 10 mg daily. *Maximum:* 20 mg daily.
➤ *To treat manic phase of acute bipolar disorder*
ORALLY DISINTEGRATING TABLETS, TABLETS
Adults. *Initial:* 10 to 15 mg daily; may be in-

creased or decreased by 5 mg every 24 hr as needed and prescribed. *Usual:* 5 to 20 mg daily for 3 to 4 wk. *Maximum:* 20 mg daily.

➤ *As adjunct to treat acute bipolar disorder*

ORALLY DISINTEGRATING TABLETS, TABLETS

Adults. *Initial:* 10 mg daily with lithium or valproate sodium; may be increased or decreased by 5 mg every 24 hr, as needed and prescribed. *Usual:* 5 to 20 mg/day for 6 wk. *Maximum:* 20 mg daily.

DOSAGE ADJUSTMENT Initial dosage possibly reduced to 5 mg for debilitated patients, those prone to hypotension, and female nonsmokers over age 65.

➤ *To treat agitation associated with schizophrenia and bipolar I mania*

I.M. INJECTION

Adults. 5 to10 mg p.r.n. Repeat as needed every 2 to 4 hr.

DOSAGE ADJUSTMENT Dosage decreased to 5 mg for elderly patients and 2.5 mg for debilitated patients, those prone to hypotension, and female nonsmokers over age 65.

Route	Onset	Peak	Duration
P.O.	1 wk	Unknown	Unknown
I.M.	Unknown	Unknown	Unknown

Mechanism of Action

May achieve its antipsychotic effects by antagonizing dopamine and serotonin receptors. Anticholinergic effects may result from competitive binding to and antagonism of the muscarinic receptors M_1 through M_5.

Contraindications

Blood dyscrasias, bone marrow depression, cerebral arteriosclerosis, coma, coronary artery disease, hepatic dysfunction, high-dose CNS depressants, hypersensitivity to olanzapine or its components, hypertension, hypotension, myeloproliferative disorders, severe CNS depression, subcortical brain damage

Interactions

DRUGS

anticholinergics: Increased anticholinergic effects, altered thermoregulation

antihypertensives: Increased effects of both drugs, increased risk of hypotension

benzodiazepines (parenteral): Increased risk of excessive sedation and cardiorespiratory depression

carbamazepine, omeprazole, rifampin: Increased olanzapine clearance

CNS depressants: Additive CNS depression, potentiated orthostatic hypotension

diazepam: Increased CNS depressant effects

fluvoxamine: Decreased olanzapine clearance

levodopa: Decreased levodopa efficacy

lorazepam (parenteral): Possibly increased somnolence with I.M. injection of olanzapine

ACTIVITIES

alcohol use: Additive CNS depression, potentiated orthostatic hypotension

smoking: Decreased blood olanzapine level

Adverse Reactions

CNS: Abnormal gait, agitation, akathisia, altered thermoregulation, amnesia, anxiety, asthenia, dizziness, euphoria, fatigue, fever, headache, hypertonia, insomnia, nervousness, neuroleptic malignant syndrome, restlessness, somnolence, stuttering, suicidal ideation, tardive dyskinesia, tremor

CV: Chest pain, hyperlipidemia, hypertension, hypotension, orthostatic hypotension, peripheral edema, tachycardia

EENT: Amblyopia, dry mouth, increased salivation, pharyngitis, rhinitis

ENDO: Hyperglycemia, prolactin elevation

GI: Abdominal pain, constipation, dysphagia, hepatitis, increased appetite, nausea, thirst, vomiting

GU: Urinary incontinence, UTI

HEME: Neutropenia

MS: Arthralgia; back, joint, or limb pain; muscle spasms and twitching

RESP: Cough

SKIN: Ecchymosis, photosensitivity, pruritus, urticaria

Other: Anaphylaxis, angioedema, flulike symptoms, weight gain

Nursing Considerations

•WARNING Be aware that olanzapine shouldn't be used for elderly patients with dementia-related psychosis because drug increases risk of death in these patients.

•Reconstitute parenteral olanzapine by dissolving contents of vial in 2.1 ml of sterile water to yield 5 mg/ml. Solution should be

clear yellow. Use within 1 hour.
•Inject I.M. olanzapine slowly and deep into muscle mass.
•Keep patient recumbent after I.M. injection of olanzapine if drowsiness, dizziness, bradycardia, or hypoventialtion occurs. Don't let patient sit or stand up until blood pressure and heart rate have returned to baseline.
•Monitor patient's blood pressure routinely during therapy because olanzapine may cause orthostatic hypotension.
•Be aware that olanzapine may worsen such conditions as angle-closure glaucoma, benign prostatic hyperplasia, and seizures.
•Assess daily weight to detect fluid retention.
•Notify prescriber if patient develops tardive dyskinesia or urinary incontinence.
•Be alert for and immediately report to prescriber signs of neuroleptic malignant syndrome.
•Watch patient closely (especially children, adolescents, and young adults), for suicidal tendencies, particularly when therapy starts and dosage changes, because depression may worsen temporarily during these times, possibly leading to suicidal ideation.
•Monitor patient's lipid levels throughout therapy, as ordered, because olanzapine may cause significant elevations.
•Monitor patient's blood glucose level routinely because olanzapine use may increase risk of hyperglycemia.

PATIENT TEACHING
•Advise patient to avoid alcohol and smoking during olanzapine therapy.
•Teach patient to open the orally disintegrating tablet sachet by peeling back the foil on the blister and not to push tablet through the foil. Immediately after opening the blister, tell him to use dry hands to remove tablet and place it in his mouth. Explain that tablet will disintegrate rapidly in his saliva so that he can easily swallow it without liquid.
•Caution patient with phenylketonuria that disintegrating olanzapine tablets contain phenylalanine.
•Urge patient to avoid potentially hazardous activities until drug's CNS effects are known.
•Instruct patient to change position slowly to minimize effects of orthostatic hypotension.
•Urge family or caregiver to watch patient closely for suicidal tendencies, especially

when therapy starts or dosage changes and particularly if patient is a child, teenager, or young adult.

olmesartan medoxomil

Benicar

Class and Category
Chemical class: Angiotensin II receptor antagonist
Therapeutic class: Antihypertensive
Pregnancy category: C (first trimester), D (later trimesters)

Indications and Dosages
➤ *To manage or as adjunct to manage hypertension*
TABLETS
Adults. *Initial:* 20 mg daily, increased in 2 wk to 40 mg daily, if needed.
DOSAGE ADJUSTMENT Lower starting dosage is recommended for patients with possible depletion of intravascular volume, such as those treated with diuretics, especially if impaired renal function is present.

Contraindications
Hypersensitivity to olmesartan medoxomil or its components

Adverse Reactions
CNS: Ashenia, dizziness, fatigue, headache, insomnia, vertigo
CV: Chest pain, hypercholesterolemia, hyperlipidemia, hypertriglyceridemia, peripheral edema, tachycardia
EENT: Pharyngitis, rhinitis, sinusitis
ENDO: Hyperglycemia, hyperuricemia
GI: Abdominal pain, diarrhea, gastroenteritis, indigestion, nausea, vomiting
GU: Acute renal failure, elevated BUN and serum creatinine levels, hematuria, UTI
MS: Arthralgia, arthritis, back pain, myalgia, rhabdomyolysis, skeletal pain
RESP: Bronchitis, cough, upper respiratory tract infection
SKIN: Alopecia, pruritus, rash, urticaria
Other: Angioedema, hyperkalemia, increased CK level, flulike symptoms, pain

Nursing Considerations
•Expect to provide treatment such as normal saline solution I.V., as prescribed, to correct known or suspected hypovolemia before be-

Mechanism of Action

Olmesartan medoxomil blocks angiotensin II from binding to receptor sites in many tissues, including vascular smooth muscle and adrenal glands. Angiotensin II, a potent vasoconstrictor, is then free to stimulate the adrenal cortex to secrete aldosterone, and the inhibiting effects of angiotensin II reduce blood pressure.

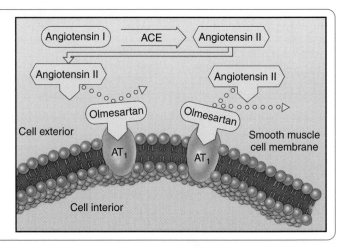

ginning olmesartan therapy.
•Monitor patient for increased BUN and serum creatinine levels, especially in a patient with impaired renal function, because drug may cause acute renal failure. If increased levels are significant or persist, notify prescriber immediately.
•Monitor blood pressure frequently to assess effectiveness of therapy. If blood pressure isn't controlled with olmesartan alone, expect to administer a diuretic, such as hydrochlorothiazide, as prescribed.
•WARNING Monitor patient's blood pressure frequently if he receives a diuretic or other antihypertensive during olmesartan therapy because of an increased risk of hypotension.
•Expect to discontinue drug temporarily if patient experiences hypotension. Place patient in supine position immediately and prepare to administer normal saline solution I.V., as prescribed. Expect to resume drug therapy after blood pressure stabilizes.
•If patient also receives a diuretic, provide adequate hydration, as appropriate, to help prevent hypovolemia. Monitor him for signs and symptoms of hypovolemia, such as hypotension with dizziness and fainting.

PATIENT TEACHING
•Advise patient to avoid exercise in hot weather and excessive alcohol use to reduce the risk of dehydration and hypotension. Also instruct him to notify prescriber if he has prolonged diarrhea, nausea, or vomiting.
•Caution patient to avoid hazardous activi-

ties until drug's CNS effects are known.
•Explain the importance of regular exercise, proper diet, and other lifestyle changes in controlling hypertension.
•Advise female patient to notify prescriber immediately about known or suspected pregnancy. Explain that if she becomes pregnant, prescriber may replace olmesartan with another antihypertensive that is safe to use during pregnancy.

olsalazine sodium

Dipentum

Class and Category
Chemical class: Salicylate derivative
Therapeutic class: Bowel disease suppressant
Pregnancy category: C

Indications and Dosages
➤ *To maintain remission of ulcerative colitis*
CAPSULES, TABLETS
Adults and adolescents. 500 mg b.i.d.

Contraindications
Hypersensitivity to olsalazine, salicylates, or their components

Interactions
DRUGS
6-mercaptopurine, thioguanine: Increased risk of myelosuppression
low-molecular-weight heparins or hepari-

noids: Increased risk of bleeding after neuraxial anesthesia
oral anticoagulants: Possibly prolonged PT
varicella vaccine: Increased risk of Reye's syndrome

Mechanism of Action
Exerts an anti-inflammatory action in the GI tract after being converted by colonic bacteria to mesalamine (5-aminosalicylic acid), which inhibits cyclooxygenase. Inhibition of cyclooxygenase reduces prostaglandin production in the intestinal mucosa. This in turn reduces production of arachidonic acid metabolites, which may be increased in patients with inflammatory bowel disease. Olsalazine also exerts an anti-inflammatory effect by indirectly inhibiting leukotriene synthesis, which normally catalyzes the production of arachidonic acid.

Adverse Reactions
CNS: Anxiety, depression, dizziness, drowsiness, fatigue, headache, insomnia, lethargy, paresthesia, vertigo
CV: Myocarditis, pericarditis, second-degree AV block
ENDO: Hot flashes
EENT: Dry eyes and mouth, lacrimation, stomatitis, tinnitus
GI: Abdominal pain, anorexia, diarrhea, dyspepsia, elevated liver enzymes, hepatitis, hepatotoxicity, nausea, vomiting
GU: Dysuria, hematuria, interstitial nephritis, nephrotic syndrome, urinary frequency
HEME: Aplastic or hemolytic anemia, lymphopenia, neutropenia, pancytopenia
MS: Arthralgia, joint pain, muscle spasms, myalgia
RESP: Dyspnea, interstitial lung disease
SKIN: Acne, alopecia, erythema nodosum, photosensitivity, pruritus, rash
Other: Dehydration

Nursing Considerations
• Assess patient for aspirin allergy before giving olsalazine.
• If patient has severe allergies or asthma, watch closely for worsening symptoms during olsalazine therapy, and notify prescriber immediately if they occur.
• Assess quantity and consistency of stools and frequency of bowel movements before, during, and after therapy.
• Give drug with food to decrease adverse GI reactions.
• Monitor skin for adequate hydration.
• Assess patient for abdominal pain and hyperactive bowel sounds.
• Monitor renal and hepatic status in patient with underlying renal or hepatic dysfunction because drug may further impair these functions.

PATIENT TEACHING
• Instruct patient to take olsalazine with food.
• Urge patient to continue taking drug as prescribed, even if symptoms improve.
• Advise patient to watch for signs of dehydration.

omalizumab
Xolair

Class and Category
Chemical class: Recombinant IgG1K anti-IgE monoclonal antibody
Therapeutic class: Antiallergenic
Pregnancy category: B

Indications and Dosages
➤ *To treat moderate to severe persistent asthma in patients with positive skin test or in vitro reactivity to a perennial aeroallergen whose symptoms have been inadequately controlled with inhaled corticosteroids*

SUBCUTANEOUS INJECTION
Adults and adolescents age 12 and over.
150 to 375 mg every 2 or 4 wk. Dose and frequency determined by body weight and blood IgE levels.

DOSAGE ADJUSTMENT Dosage adjusted for significant changes in body weight.

Mechanism of Action
Helps reduce inflammation by binding to circulating IgE and preventing it from binding to mast cells. This action inhibits degranulation and blocks release of histamine and other chemical mediators. In asthma, inflammation results when antigen reexposure causes mast cells to degranulate and release histamine and other chemical mediators.

N
O

Contraindications

Hypersensitivity to omalizumab or its components

Adverse Reactions

CNS: Dizziness, fatigue, headache, vertigo
EENT: Earache, pharyngitis, sinusitis
MS: Arm or leg pain, arthralgia, fractures
RESP: Upper respiratory tract infection
SKIN: Dermatitis, pruritus, urticaria
Other: Anaphylaxis; generalized pain; injection site bruising, burning, hive or mass formation, induration, inflammation, itching, pain, redness, stinging, and warmth; malignancies; viral infection

Nursing Considerations

•Record patient's weight and obtain blood IgE levels, as ordered, before starting omalizumab therapy; dosage and dosing frequency are based on these factors.
•Reconstitute using sterile water for injection, and allow 15 to 20 minutes on average for lyophilized product to dissolve. Draw 1.4 ml sterile water for injection into a 3-ml syringe with a 1" 18G needle. Place omalizumab vial upright and inject sterile water into vial using aseptic technique. Gently swirl the upright vial for about 1 minute to evenly wet the powder. Do not shake. Every 5 minutes, gently swirl for 5 to 10 seconds until solution contains no gel-like particles. Discard if powder takes longer than 40 minutes to dissolve, and start with a new vial. Once reconstituted, solution should be clear or slightly opalescent and may have a few small bubbles or foam around the edge of the vial. Use omalizumab within 8 hours if refrigerated or 4 hours if stored at room temperature.
•To remove reconstituted omalizumab from vial, invert vial for 15 seconds to let solution drain toward stopper. Using a new 3-ml syringe with a 1" 18-gauge needle, insert needle into inverted vial and position needle tip at the very bottom of the solution in the vial stopper. Then pull plunger all the way back to end of syringe barrel in order to remove all the solution from the inverted vial. To obtain a full 150-mg dose (1 vial containing 1.2 ml of reconstituted omalizumab), you must withdraw all product from the vial before expelling any air or excess solution from the syringe.
•Do not administer more than 150 mg of omalizumab per injection site.
•Be prepared to inject omalizumab over 5 to 10 seconds because solution is slightly viscous.
•**WARNING** Monitor patient closely for hypersensitivity reactions, particularly for first 2 hours after administration. Although rare, anaphylaxis has occurred as early as first dose and more than 1 year after starting regular treatment. Keep emergency medication and equipment readily available.
•**WARNING** Monitor patient closely for signs of cancer. Report any abnormal findings to prescriber.

PATIENT TEACHING

•Instruct patient to notify prescriber immediately about possible hypersensitivity, such as rash, hives, or difficulty breathing.
•Caution patient that any improvement in his asthma may take time.
•Encourage patient to comply with regularly scheduled prescriber visits.
•Inform patient of risk of malignancy and suggest routine cancer screening.
•Instruct patient that omalizumab is not used to treat acute bronchospasm or status asthmaticus.
•Tell patient not to abruptly discontinue any prescribed systemic or inhaled corticosteroid when starting omalizumab therapy because steroid dosage must be tapered gradually under prescriber's supervision.
•If female patient becomes pregnant within 8 weeks before or during omalizumab therapy, urge her to enroll in the Xolair Pregnancy Exposure Registry at 1-866-496-5247. Also, tell her to notify prescriber because drug may need to be changed.

omega-3-acid ethyl esters

Lovaza

Class and Category

Chemical class: Ethyl esters of omega-3 fatty acids
Therapeutic class: Lipid regulator
Pregnancy category: C

Indications and Dosages

➤ *As adjunct to diet to reduce triglyceride level that exceeds 500 mg/dl*

CAPSULES

Adults. 4 g once daily or 2 g b.i.d.

Mechanism of Action

Omega-3-acid ethyl esters are essential fatty acids that may inhibit very-low-density lipoprotein and triglyceride synthesis in the liver. With less triglyceride synthesis, plasma triglyceride levels decrease.

Contraindications

Hypersensitivity to omega-3-acid ethyl esters or their components

Interactions

DRUGS

anticogulants: Possibly increased bleeding time

Adverse Reactions

CV: Angina pectoris
EENT: Halitosis, nosebleeds, taste perversion
GI: Diarrhea, dyspepsia, eructation, nausea, vomiting
HEME: Prolonged bleeding time
MS: Back pain
SKIN: Bruising, rash
Other: Flulike symptoms

Nursing Considerations

•Be aware that drugs known to increase triglyceride levels—such as beta blockers, thiazide diuretics and estrogens—should be discontinued or changed, if possible, before omega-3 ethyl ester therapy starts.
•Expect to check patient's triglyceride level before starting and periodically throughout omega-3-acid ethyl ester therapy to determine effectiveness.
•Administer drug with meals.
•Expect to stop omega-3-acid ethyl ester therapy after 2 months if patient's trigylceride level doesn't decrease as expected.

PATIENT TEACHING

•Explain to patient the importance of dietary measures, an exercise program, and controlling other factors—such as blood glucose level—that may contribute to elevated triclyceride levels.
•Advise patient to take drug with meals.
•Explain that patient will need periodic laboratory tests to evaluate therapy.
•Instruct patient to seek immediate medical attention if chest pain occurs.

omeprazole

Losec (CAN), Prilosec, Zegerid

Class and Category

Chemical class: Substituted benzimidazole
Therapeutic class: Antiulcer
Pregnancy category: C

Indications and Dosages

➤ *To treat gastroesophageal reflux disease (GERD) without esophageal lesions, to prevent erosive esophagitis*

DELAYED-RELEASE CAPSULES, DELAYED-RELEASE TABLETS, ORAL SUSPENSION

Adults. 20 mg daily for 4 wk.

➤ *To treat GERD with erosive esophagitis*

DELAYED-RELEASE CAPSULES, DELAYED-RELEASE TABLETS, ORAL SUSPENSION

Adults. 20 mg daily for 4 to 8 wk.

➤ *To treat pediatric GERD and other acid-related disorders*

DELAYED-RELEASE CAPSULES

Children age 2 and over weighing 20 kg (44 lb) or less. 10 mg daily.
Children age 2 and over weighing more than 20 kg. 20 mg daily.

➤ *To provide short-term treatment of active benign gastric ulcer*

DELAYED-RELEASE CAPSULES

Adults. 40 mg daily for 4 to 8 wk.

DELAYED-RELEASE TABLETS

Adults. 20 mg daily for 4 to 8 wk, increased to 40 mg daily, p.r.n.

➤ *To treat duodenal or gastric ulcer associated with* Helicobacter pylori

DELAYED-RELEASE CAPSULES, ORAL SUSPENSION

Adults. 40 mg daily with clarithromycin for 14 days, followed by 20 mg daily alone for another 14 days. Or, 20 mg b.i.d. with amoxicillin for 14 days. Or, 20 mg b.i.d. with amoxicillin and clarithromycin for 10 days.

DELAYED-RELEASE TABLETS

Adults. 20 mg b.i.d. with clarithromycin and amoxicillin or metronidazole for 7 days, followed by 20 mg daily for up to 3 wk (for duodenal ulcer) or 20 to 40 mg daily for up to 12 wk (for gastric ulcer).

➤ *To provide long-term treatment of gastric hypersecretory conditions, such as multiple endocrine adenoma syndrome, systemic mastocytosis, and Zollinger-Ellison syndrome*

N
O

DELAYED-RELEASE CAPSULES, DELAYED-RELEASE TABLETS
Adults. 60 mg daily or in divided doses, as prescribed. *Maximum:* 120 mg t.i.d.

Route	Onset	Peak	Duration
P.O.	1 hr	In 2 hr	72 to 96 hr

Contraindications
Hypersensitivity to omeprazole, other proton pump inhibitors, or their components

Interactions
DRUGS
alprazolam, astemizole, carbamazepine, cisapride, cyclosporine, diazepam, diltiazem, erythromycin, felodipine, lidocaine, lovastatin, midazolam, quinidine, simvastatin, terfenadine, triazolam, verapamil, voriconazole: Decreased clearance and increased blood levels of these drugs
ampicillin, iron salts, itraconazole, ketoconazole, vitamin B_{12}: Impaired absorption of these drugs
atazanavir: Decreased plasma atazanavir level
cilostazol: Increased blood cilostazol level
clarithromycin: Increased blood levels of omeprazole and clarithromycinl
digoxin: Increased digoxin bioavailability, possibly digitalis toxicity
levobupivacaine: Increased risk of levobupivacaine toxicity
methotrexate: Possibly delayed methotrexate elimination
nifedipine: Decreased nifedipine clearance, increased risk of hypotension
phenytoin: Decreased phenytoin clearance, increased risk of phenytoin toxicity
sucralfate: Decreased omeprazole absorption
tacrolimus: Possibly increased tacrolimus level
warfarin: Possibly increased risk of abnormal bleeding

Mechanism of Action
Omeprazole interferes with gastric acid secretion by inhibiting the hydrogen-potassium-adenosine triphosphatase (H^+K^+-ATPase) enzyme system, or proton pump, in gastric parietal cells. Normally, the proton pump uses energy from the hydrolysis of adenosine triphosphate to drive hydrogen (H^+) and chloride (Cl^-) out of parietal cells and into the stomach lumen in exchange for potassium (K^+), which leaves the stomach lumen and enters the parietal cells. After this exchange, H^+ and Cl^- combine in the stomach to form hydrochloric acid (HCl), as shown below left. Omeprazole irreversibly blocks the exchange of intracellular H^+ and extracellular K^+, as shown below right. By preventing H^+ from entering the stomach lumen, omeprazole prevents additional HCl from forming.

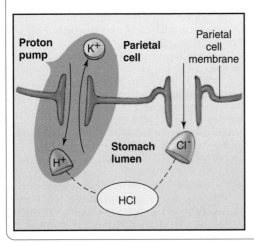

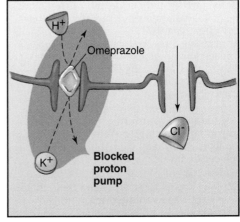

Adverse Reactions

CNS: Agitation, asthenia, dizziness, drowsiness, fatigue, headache, psychic disturbances, somnolence

CV: Chest pain, hypertension, peripheral edema

EENT: Anterior ischemic optic neuropathy, optic atrophy or neuritis, stomatitis

ENDO: Hypoglycemia

GI: Abdominal pain, constipation, diarrhea, dyspepsia, elevated liver function test results, flatulence, hepatic dysfunction or failure, indigestion, nausea, pancreatitis, vomiting

GU: Interstitial nephritis

HEME: Agranulocytosis, anemia, hemolytic anemia, leukopenia, leukocytosis, neutropenia, pancytopenia, thrombocytopenia

MS: Back pain

RESP: Cough

SKIN: Erythema multiforme, photosensitivity, pruritus, rash, Stevens-Johnson syndrome, toxic epidermal necrolysis, urticaria

Other: Anaphylaxis, angioedema, hyponatremia

Nursing Considerations

•Give omeprazole before meals, preferably in the morning for once-daily dosing. If necessary, also give an antacid, as prescribed.

•If needed, open capsule and sprinkle enteric-coated granules on applesauce or yogurt or mix with water or acidic fruit juice, such as apple or cranberry juice. Give immediately.

•To give drug via NG tube, mix granules in acidic juice because enteric coating dissolves in alkaline pH.

•Because drug can interfere with absorption of vitamin B_{12}, monitor for macrocytic anemia.

•Be aware that long-term use of omeprazole may increase the risk of gastric carcinoma.

PATIENT TEACHING

•Tell patient to take drug before eating—usually before breakfast—and to swallow delayed-release capsules or tablets whole. If needed, patient may sprinkle contents of capsule onto 1 tablespoon of applesauce and swallow immediately without chewing pellets. Tell him to follow with a glass of cool water and not to keep any leftover mixture.

•If patient takes the oral suspension, tell him to empty the package into a small cup containing 2 tablespoons of water (no other beverage should be used), stir the mixture well, drink it immediately, refill the cup with water, and drink again.

•Encourage patient to avoid alcohol, aspirin products, ibuprofen, and foods that may increase gastric secretions during therapy. Tell him to notify all prescribers about prescription drug use.

•Advise patient to notify prescriber immediately about abdominal pain or diarrhea.

•Urge female patient of childbearing age to use effective contraception during therapy and to inform prescriber immediately if she becomes or suspects she may be pregnant.

ondansetron hydrochloride

Zofran, Zofran ODT

Class and Category

Chemical class: Carbazole
Therapeutic class: Antiemetic
Pregnancy category: B

Indications and Dosages

➤ *To prevent chemotherapy-induced nausea and vomiting*

DISINTEGRATING TABLETS, ORAL SOLUTION, TABLETS

Adults and children age 12 and over. *Initial:* 8 mg given 30 min before chemotherapy. *Postchemotherapy:* 8 mg given 8 hr after initial dose, then 8 mg every 12 hr for 1 to 2 days.

Children ages 4 to 12. *Initial:* 4 mg given 30 min before chemotherapy. *Postchemotherapy:* 4 mg given 4 and 8 hr after initial dose, then 4 mg every 8 hr for 1 to 2 days.

I.V. INFUSION

Adults. 32 mg infused over 15 min starting 30 min before chemotherapy; or three 0.15-mg/kg doses, each infused over 15 min, starting with the first dose given 30 min before chemotherapy and second and third doses given 4 and 8 hours after first dose.

Children ages 6 months to 18 years. Three 0.15-mg/kg doses, each infused over 15 min, starting with first dose given 30 min before chemotherapy and second and third doses given 4 and 8 hours after first dose.

N
O

➤ *To prevent postoperative nausea and*
  vomiting

DISINTEGRATING TABLETS, ORAL SOLUTION, TABLETS

Adults. 16 mg as a single dose 1 hr before
anesthesia induction.

I.V. INJECTION

Adults and children age 12 and over. 4 mg as
a single dose over 2 to 5 min just before
anesthesia induction or if nausea or vomiting
develops shortly after surgery.

**Children ages 2 to 12 weighing more than
40 kg (88 lb).** 4 mg as a single dose over 2 to
5 min just before anesthesia induction or if
nausea or vomiting develops shortly after
surgery.

**Children ages 1 month to 12 years weighing
less than 40 kg.** 0.1 mg/kg as a single dose
over 2 to 5 min just before or immediately
after anesthesia induction or if nausea or
vomiting develops shortly after surgery.

I.M. INJECTION

Adults and children age 12 and over. 4 mg as
a single dose just before anesthesia induction
or if nausea or vomiting develops shortly
after surgery.

➤ *To prevent nausea and vomiting after*
  radiation therapy

DISINTEGRATING TABLETS, ORAL SOLUTION, TABLETS

Adults and children age 12 and over. *Initial:*
8 mg as a single dose given 1 to 2 hr before
radiation therapy. *Posttherapy:* 8 mg every
8 hr, as needed and tolerated.

DOSAGE ADJUSTMENT For patients with hepatic impairment, maximum dosage limited
to 8 mg daily I.V. or P.O.

Mechanism of Action

Blocks serotonin receptors centrally in the
chemoreceptor trigger zone and peripherally at vagal nerve terminals in the intestine. This action reduces nausea and vomiting by preventing serotonin release in
the small intestine (the probable cause of
chemotherapy- and radiation-induced
nausea and vomiting) and by blocking
signals to the CNS. Ondansetron may also
bind to other serotonin receptors and to
mu-opioid receptors.

Incompatibilities

Don't give ondansetron in same I.V. line as
acyclovir, allopurinol, aminophylline, ampho-

tericin B, ampicillin, ampicillin and sulbac-
tam, amsacrine, cefepime, cefoperazone,
furosemide, ganciclovir, lorazepam, methylprednisolone, mezlocillin, piperacillin, or
sargramostim. Alkaline solutions and highly
concentrated fluorouracil solutions are physically incompatible.

Contraindications

Hypersensitivity to ondansetron or its components

Interactions

DRUGS

cisplatin, cyclophosphamide: Possibly altered
blood levels of these drugs

ACTIVITIES

alcohol use: Increased stimulant and sedative
effects, including mood and physical sensations

Adverse Reactions

CNS: Agitation, akathisia, anxiety, ataxia,
dizziness, drowsiness, fever, headache, hypotension, restlessness, seizures, syncope,
somnolence, weakness

CV: Arrythmias, chest pain, hypotension,
pulmonary embolism, shock, tachycardia,
transient prolonged QT interval

EENT: Accommodation disturbances, altered
taste, blurred vision, dry mouth, laryngeal
edema, laryngospasm, transient blindness

GI: Abdominal pain, anorexia, constipation,
diarrhea, elevated liver function test results,
flatulence, indigestion, intestinal obstruction,
thirst

RESP: Bronchospasm, shortness of breath

SKIN: Flushing, hyperpigmentation, maculopapular rash, pruritus

Other: Anaphylaxis, angioedema, injection
site burning, pain, and redness

Nursing Considerations

•**WARNING** Be aware that oral disintegrating
tablets may contain aspartame, which is metabolized to phenylalanine and must be used
cautiously in patients with phenylketonuria.

•Place disintegrating tablet on patient's
tongue immediately after opening package. It
dissolves in seconds.

•Use calibrated container or oral syringe to
measure dose of oral solution.

•Give up to 4 mg I.V. diluted in 50 ml of
D$_5$W or normal saline solution.

•**WARNING** Be aware that ondansetron may

mask symptoms of adynamic ileus or gastric distention after abdominal surgery.

PATIENT TEACHING
• Advise patient to use calibrated container or oral syringe to measure oral solution.
• Instruct patient to place ondansetron disintegrating tablet on his tongue immediately after opening package and to let it dissolve on his tongue before swallowing.
• Advise patient to immediately report signs of hypersensitivity, such as rash.
• Reassure patient with transient blindness that it will resolve within a few minutes to 48 hours.

orlistat

Xenical

Class and Category
Chemical class: Lipase inhibitor
Therapeutic class: Antiobesity
Pregnancy category: B

Indications and Dosages
➤ *To promote weight loss in patients with a body mass index above 30 kg (66 lb)/m² —27 kg (59.4 lb)/m² in patients with diabetes mellitus, hyperlipidemia, or hypertension—and to reduce the risk of weight regain*

GELCAPS
Adults. 120 mg t.i.d. with fat-containing meals.

Contraindications
Cholestasis, chronic malabsorption syndrome, hypersensitivity to orlistat or its components

Interactions
DRUGS
cyclosporine: Altered cyclosporine absorption
fat-soluble vitamins: Decreased vitamin absorption, especially vitamin E and beta-carotene
pravastatin: Potentiated lipid-lowering effect

Adverse Reactions
CNS: Anxiety, depression, dizziness, fatigue, headache, sleep disturbance
CV: Pedal edema
EENT: Gingival or tooth disorder, otitis
GI: Abdominal discomfort or pain, cholelithiasis, diarrhea (infectious), fatty or

Mechanism of Action
In the GI tract, orlistat binds with and inactivates gastric and pancreatic enzymes known as lipases, as shown. Normally, lipase enzymes convert ingested triglycerides into absorbable free fatty acids and monoglycerides. By inactivating lipase, orlistat allows undigested triglycerides to pass through the GI tract and exit the body in feces. Blocking the absorption of some of these fats lowers the number of calories the person receives from food, which promotes weight loss.

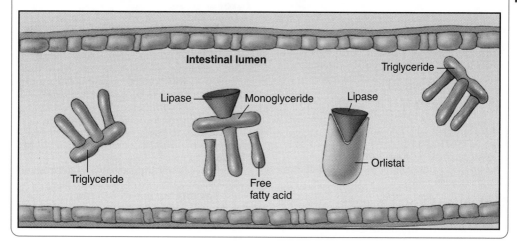

oily stool, fecal incontinence or urgency, flatulence with discharge, increased frequency of bowel movements, nausea, pancreatitis, rectal pain, vomiting
GU: Menstrual irregularities, UTI, vaginitis
MS: Arthralgia, arthritis, back pain, leg pain, myalgia, tendinitis
RESP: Respiratory tract infection
SKIN: Dry skin, pruritus, rash, urticaria
Other: Anaphylaxis, angioedema, flulike symptoms

Nursing Considerations
• Give orlistat with or up to 1 hour after meals that contain fat.
• Consult prescriber if you think that patient has an eating disorder, such as anorexia nervosa or bulimia.

PATIENT TEACHING
• Instruct patient to take orlistat with or shortly after meals that contain fat.
• Advise patient to take a multivitamin that contains fat-soluble vitamins and beta-carotene at least 2 hours before or after taking drug, if indicated.
• Inform patient about orlistat's adverse GI effects, but explain that reducing dietary fat may decrease them. Instruct him to notify prescriber if they become too unpleasant.
• Help patient plan a reduced-fat diet (less than 30% of daily calories) and an exercise program to promote weight loss.
• Advise patient to weigh himself daily, at the same time each day and wearing similar clothes, to check his progress in losing weight.

orphenadrine citrate
Aniflex, Banflex, Flexoject, Miolin, Mio-Rel, Myotrol, Norflex, Orfro, Orphenate

orphenadrine hydrochloride
Disipal (CAN)

Class and Category
Chemical class: Tertiary amine
Therapeutic class: Skeletal muscle relaxant
Pregnancy category: C

Indications and Dosages
➤ *To relieve muscle spasms in painful musculoskeletal conditions*

E.R. TABLETS (ORPHENADRINE CITRATE)
Adults and adolescents. 100 mg b.i.d. in the morning and evening.
TABLETS (ORPHENADRINE HYDROCHLORIDE)
Adults and adolescents. 50 mg t.i.d. *Maximum:* 250 mg daily.
I.V. OR I.M. INJECTION (ORPHENADRINE CITRATE)
Adults and adolescents. 60 mg every 12 hr, p.r.n.
DOSAGE ADJUSTMENT Dosage reduced to 25 to 50 mg t.i.d. or q.i.d. if patient also receives aspirin and caffeine.

Route	Onset	Peak	Duration
P.O.	In 1 hr	Unknown	4 to 6 hr*
I.V.	Immediate	Unknown	4 to 6 hr
I.M.	30 min	Unknown	4 to 6 hr

Mechanism of Action
May reduce muscle spasms by acting on the cerebral motor centers or the medulla. Postganglionic anticholinergic effects and some antihistaminic and local anesthetic action contribute to skeletal muscle relaxation.

Contraindications
Angle-closure glaucoma; hypersensitivity to orphenadrine or its components; myasthenia gravis; obstruction of bladder neck, duodenum, or pylorus; prostatic hypertrophy; stenosing peptic ulcers

Interactions
DRUGS
amantadine, amitriptyline, amoxapine, antimuscarinics, atropine, bupropion, carbinoxamine, chlorpromazine, clemastine, clomipramine, clozapine, cyclobenzaprine, diphenhydramine, disopyramide, doxepin, imipramine, maprotiline, mesoridazine, methdilazine, nortriptyline, phenothiazines, procainamide, promazine, promethazine, protriptyline, thioridazine, triflupromazine, trimeprazine, trimipramine: Possibly additive anticholinergic effects
CNS depressants: Increased CNS depression
haloperidol: Increased schizophrenic symptoms, possibly tardive dyskinesia

---

* 12 hr for extended-release.

propoxyphene: Increased risk of anxiety, confusion, and tremor

ACTIVITIES

alcohol use: Increased CNS depression

Adverse Reactions

CNS: Agitation, confusion, dizziness, drowsiness, light-headedness, syncope, tremor

CV: Palpitations, tachycardia

EENT: Blurred vision, dry eyes and mouth, increased contact lens awareness

GI: Abdominal distention, constipation, nausea, vomiting

GU: Urine retention

Nursing Considerations

•Be aware that orphenadrine shouldn't be given to patients with tachycardia or cardiac insufficiency.

•Administer I.V. form over 5 minutes with patient in supine position. Have patient remain in this position for 5 to 10 minutes to minimize adverse reactions. Then assist him to sitting position.

•Be aware that drug can aggravate myasthenia gravis and cause tachycardia.

•Anticipate that drug's anticholinergic effects may cause blurred vision, dry eyes, and increased contact lens awareness.

PATIENT TEACHING

•Advise patient to avoid hazardous activities until orphenadrine's CNS effects are known.

•Inform patient that dry mouth may occur but can be relieved with such measures as increased intake of fluid, ice chips, and sugarless candy or gum.

•Suggest that patient (especially one who wears contact lenses) use artificial tears to avoid discomfort from dry eyes.

oxacillin sodium

Bactocill, Prostaphlin

Class and Category

Chemical class: Penicillin
Therapeutic class: Antibiotic
Pregnancy category: B

Indications and Dosages

➤ *To treat bacteremia, bone and joint infections (such as osteomyelitis and infectious arthritis), CNS infections (such as ventriculitis and meningitis), endocarditis, septicemia, skin and soft-tissue infections, upper and lower respiratory tract infections, and UTI caused by penicillinase-producing strains of staphylococcus or other susceptible organisms*

CAPSULES, ORAL SOLUTION

Adults and children weighing 40 kg (88 lb) or more. 500 to 1,000 mg every 4 to 6 hr. *Maximum:* 6 g daily.

Children weighing less than 40 kg. 50 to 100 mg/kg daily in divided doses every 4 to 6 hr.

➤ *To treat mild to moderate infections caused by penicillinase-producing strains of staphylococcus or other susceptible organisms*

I.V. INFUSION, I.M. INJECTION

Adults and children weighing 40 kg or more. 250 to 500 mg every 4 to 6 hr.

Infants and children weighing less than 40 kg. 50 mg/kg daily in divided doses every 4 to 6 hr.

Neonates over age 7 days weighing more than 2,000 g. 25 to 50 mg/kg every 6 hr.

Neonates over age 7 days weighing less than 2,000 g. 25 to 50 mg/kg every 8 hr.

Neonates age 7 days and under weighing more than 2,000 g. 25 to 50 mg/kg every 8 hr.

Neonates age 7 days and under weighing 2,000 g or less. 25 to 50 mg/kg every 12 hr.

➤ *To treat severe infections caused by penicillinase-producing strains of staphylococcus or other susceptible organisms*

I.V. INFUSION, I.M. INJECTION

Adults and children weighing 40 kg or more. 1,000 mg every 4 to 6 hr.

Infants and children weighing less than 40 kg. 100 to 200 mg/kg daily in divided doses every 4 to 6 hr.

Neonates over age 7 days weighing more than 2,000 g. 25 to 50 mg/kg every 6 hr.

Neonates over age 7 days weighing less than 2,000 g. 25 to 50 mg/kg every 8 hr.

Neonates age 7 days and under weighing more than 2,000 g. 25 to 50 mg/kg every 8 hr.

Neonates age 7 days and under weighing 2,000 g or less. 25 to 50 mg/kg every 12 hr.

➤ *To treat endocarditis caused by methicillin-susceptible* Staphylococcus aureus *in patients without a prosthetic valve*

I.V. INFUSION

Adults. 2 g every 4 hr for 4 to 6 wk.

➤ *To treat endocarditis caused by methi-cillin-susceptible* S. aureus *in patients with a prosthetic valve*

I.V. INFUSION

Adults. 2 g every 4 hr for at least 6 wk.

Mechanism of Action

Inhibits bacterial cell wall synthesis. In susceptible bacteria, the rigid, cross-linked cell wall is assembled in several steps. Oxacillin exerts its effects in the final stage of the cross-linking process by binding with and inactivating penicillin-binding proteins (enzymes responsible for linking the cell wall strands). This action causes bacterial cell lysis and death.

Incompatibilities

Don't give oxacillin at same time or in same admixture as aminoglycosides because they are chemically and physically incompatible and will inactivate each other.

Contraindications

Hypersensitivity to oxacillin, penicillins, or their components

Interactions

DRUGS

aminoglycosides: Inactivation of both drugs
chloramphenicol, erythromycins, sulfon-amides, tetracyclines: Decreased therapeutic effects of oxacillin
oral contraceptives: Decreased contraceptive efficacy
probenecid: Increased blood oxacillin level

FOODS

all foods: Altered absorption of oxacillin

Adverse Reactions

CNS: Anxiety, depression, fatigue, hallucina-tions, headache, seizures
EENT: Oral candidiasis
GI: Diarrhea, nausea, pseudomembranous colitis, vomiting
GU: Interstitial nephritis, vaginal candidiasis
HEME: Agranulocytosis, anemia, granulocy-topenia, neutropenia
SKIN: Exfoliative dermatitis, pruritus, rash, urticaria
Other: Anaphylaxis

Nursing Considerations

•Administer oxacillin at least 1 hour before

other antibiotics.
•Give oral forms on an empty stomach, preferably 1 hour before or 2 hours after a meal, to prevent impaired absorption.
•Before reconstitution, tap bottle several times to loosen powder. For I.M. injection, reconstitute with sterile water for injection, half-normal (0.45) saline solution, or normal saline solution. Shake until solution is clear.
•For I.V. infusion, reconstitute only with normal saline solution or D₅W.
•When giving drug to patient at risk for hy-pertension or fluid overload, be aware that each gram of oxacillin contains 4.02 mEq of sodium.
•Monitor patient closely for diarrhea, which may indicate pseudomembranous colitis caused by *Clostridium difficile.* If diarrhea occurs, notify prescriber and expect to with-hold oxacillin and treat with fluids, electro-lytes, protein, and an antibiotic effective against *C. difficile.*

PATIENT TEACHING

•Advise patient to take oxacillin on an empty stomach.
•Instruct patient to notify prescriber imme-diately should a rash develop.
•Advise female patient who uses an oral contraceptive to use an additional contracep-tive method during oxacillin therapy.
•Urge patient to tell prescriber about diar-rhea that's severe or lasts longer than 3 days. Remind patient that watery or bloody stools can occur 2 or more months after antibiotic therapy and can be serious, requiring prompt treatment.

---

oxandrolone

Oxandrin

Class, Category, and Schedule

Chemical class: Testosterone derivative
Therapeutic class: Appetite stimulant
Pregnancy category: X
Controlled susbstance schedule: III

Indications and Dosages

➤ *To promote weight gain after chronic in-fection, extensive surgery, failure to maintain weight despite no evidence of pathology, or severe trauma; to offset protein catabolism from prolonged use of corticosteroids*

TABLETS

Adults. 2.5 to 20 mg in divided doses given b.i.d. to q.i.d. for 2 to 4 wk; intermittent therapy repeated as prescribed. *Maximum:* 20 mg daily.

Children. 0.1 mg/kg daily; intermittent therapy repeated as prescribed.

DOSAGE ADJUSTMENT Dosage shouldn't exceed 5 mg b.i.d. for elderly patients.

Mechanism of Action

Promotes tissue-building processes and reverses catabolic or tissue-depleting processes by promoting protein anabolism.

Contraindications

Breast cancer (males); breast cancer with hypercalcemia (females); hypersensitivity to oxandrolone, anabolic steroids, or their components; nephrosis; pregnancy; prostate cancer

Interactions
DRUGS

corticosteroids: Increased risk of edema and severe acne
hepatotoxic drugs: Increased risk of hepatotoxicity
insulin, oral antidiabetic drugs: Possibly hypoglycemia
NSAIDs, oral anticoagulants, salicylates: Increased anticoagulant effects
sodium-containing drugs: Increased risk of edema
somatrem, somatropin: Possibly accelerated epiphyseal closure
warfarin: Increased warfarin half-life and risk of bleeding

FOODS

high-sodium foods: Increased risk of edema

Adverse Reactions

CNS: Depression, excitement, insomnia
CV: Decreased serum HDL level, edema, hyperlipidemia, hypertension
ENDO: Feminization in postpubertal males (epididymitis, gynecomastia, impotence, oligospermia, priapism, testicular atrophy); glucose intolerance; virilism in females (acne, clitoral enlargement, decreased breast size, deepened voice, diaphoresis, emotional lability, flushing, hirsutism, hoarseness, libido changes, male-pattern baldness, menstrual irregularities, nervousness, oily skin or hair, vaginal bleeding, vaginitis, weight gain), virilism in prepubertal males (acne, decreased ejaculatory volume, penis enlargement, prepubertal closure of epiphyseal plates, unnatural growth of body and facial hair)
GI: Diarrhea, elevated liver function test results, hepatocellular carcinoma, nausea, vomiting
GU: Benign prostatic hyperplasia, prostate cancer, urinary frequency, urine retention (elderly males)
HEME: Iron deficiency anemia, leukemia, prolonged bleeding time
SKIN: Jaundice
Other: Fluid retention, hypercalcemia (females), physical and psychological dependence, sodium retention

Nursing Considerations

• Use oxandrolone cautiously in patients with heart disease because drug has hypercholesterolemic effects.
• Provide adequate calories and protein, as ordered, to maintain a positive nitrogen balance during oxandrolone therapy.
• Anticipate an increased risk of fluid and sodium retention in patients with cardiac, hepatic, or renal dysfunction.
• Weigh patient daily to detect fluid retention. If patient has fluid retention, expect a sodium-restricted diet or diuretics.
• **WARNING** Be aware that oxandrolone may suppress spermatogenesis in males and cause permanent virilization in females.
• Monitor blood glucose level frequently in patient with diabetes mellitus.
• If patient takes an oral anticoagulant, check INR or PT as ordered.

PATIENT TEACHING

• Advise patient to consume a diet high in protein and calories to achieve maximum therapeutic effect of oxandrolone.
• Urge patient to weigh himself daily during therapy and to notify prescriber immediately about swelling or unexplained weight gain.
• Explain that drug may alter libido.
• Inform woman that drug may cause permanent physical changes, such as clitoral enlargement, deepened voice, and hair growth.
• Advise female patient of childbearing age that she must use contraception during oxandrolone therapy and should notify prescriber immediately about suspected or

known pregnancy.

•Instruct diabetic patient to monitor blood glucose level frequently.

•If patient takes warfarin, advise bleeding precautions (such as an electric shaver and soft toothbrush). Tell patient to notify prescriber immediately if bleeding occurs.

oxaprozin

Daypro

Class and Category

Chemical class: Proprionic acid derivative
Therapeutic class: Anti-inflammatory, antirheumatic
Pregnancy category: C (first trimester), Not rated (later trimesters)

Indications and Dosages

➤ *To treat rheumatoid arthritis*

TABLETS

Adults. 1,200 mg daily. Dosage adjusted based on response. *Maximum:* 1,800 mg daily or 26 mg/kg daily (whichever is less) in divided doses b.i.d. or t.i.d.

➤ *To treat osteoarthritis*

TABLETS

Adults. 600 to 1,200 mg daily. *Maximum:* 1,800 mg daily or 26 mg/kg (whichever is less) in divided doses b.i.d. or t.i.d.

DOSAGE ADJUSTMENT Initial loading dose of 1,200 to 1,800 mg possibly given to speed onset of action. Initial dose limited to 600 mg daily for patients with renal impairment.

Route	Onset	Peak	Duration
P.O.	In 7 days	Unknown	Unknown

Mechanism of Action

Blocks cyclooxygenase, the enzyme needed to synthesize prostaglandins, which mediate the inflammatory response and cause local vasodilation, swelling, and pain. By blocking cyclooxygenase and prostaglandins, the NSAID oxaprozin relieves pain.

Contraindications

Angioedema, asthma, bronchospasm, nasal polyps, rhinitis, or urticaria induced by aspirin, iodides, or other NSAIDs

Interactions

DRUGS

ACE inhibitors, antihypertensives: Decreased antihypertensive response, possibly impaired renal function

acetaminophen: Increased risk of adverse renal effects with long-term use of both drugs

anticoagulants, thrombolytics: Prolonged PT, increased risk of bleeding

beta blockers: Decreased antihypertensive effect

bone marrow depressants: Increased risk of leukopenia and thrombocytopenia

cefamandole, cefoperazone, cefotetan, plicamycin, valproic acid: Increased risk of hypoprothrombinemia and bleeding

cimetidine: Decreased oxaprozin clearance

corticosteroids, potassium supplements: Increased risk of adverse GI effects

digoxin: Increased blood digoxin level and risk of digitalis toxicity

diuretics: Possibly decreased diuretic effect

insulin, oral antidiabetic drugs: Increased effectiveness of these drugs; risk of hypoglycemia

lithium: Increased blood lithium level

methotrexate: Increased blood methotrexate level and risk of methotrexate toxicity

other NSAIDs, salicylates: Increased GI irritability and bleeding

probenecid: Increased risk of oxaprozin toxicity

ACTIVITIES

alcohol use, smoking: Increased risk of adverse GI effects

Adverse Reactions

CNS: Aseptic meningitis, cerebral hemorrhage, confusion, dizziness, drowsiness, fatigue, headache, insomnia, ischemic stroke, nervousness, sedation, transient ischemic attacks, vertigo, weakness

CV: Deep vein thrombosis, hypertension, hypotension, MI, peripheral edema

EENT: Tinnitus

ENDO: Hypoglycemia

GI: Abdominal pain, constipation, diarrhea, dyspepsia, elevated liver function test results, GI bleeding or ulceration, hepatitis, jaundice, liver failure, nausea, perforation of stomach or intestine, vomiting

GU: Acute renal failure, dysuria, interstitial nephritis, urinary frequency

HEME: Agranulocytosis, anemia, aplastic anemia, leukopenia, pancytopenia, thrombocytopenia

SKIN: Alopecia, erythema multiforme, exfo-

liative dermatitis, maculopapular rash, photosensitivity, Stevens-Johnson syndrome, toxic epidermal necrolysis
Other: Anaphylaxis, angioedema

Nursing Considerations
•Use oxaprozin with extreme caution in patients with a history of ulcer disease or GI bleeding because NSAIDs such as oxaprozin increase the risk of GI bleeding and ulceration. Expect to use oxaprozin for the shortest time possible in these patients.
•Be aware that serious GI tract ulceration, bleeding, and perforation may occur without warning symptoms. Elderly patients are at greater risk. To minimize risk, give drug with food. If GI distress occurs, withhold drug and notify prescriber immediately.
•Use oxaprozin cautiously in patients with hypertension, and monitor blood pressure closely throughout therapy. Drug may cause hypertension or worsen it.
•**WARNING** Monitor patient closely for thrombotic events, including MI and stroke, because NSAIDs increase the risk.
•**WARNING** If patient has bone marrow suppression or is receiving antineoplastic drug therapy, monitor laboratory results (including WBC count), and watch for evidence of infection because anti-inflammatory and antipyretic actions of oxaprozin may mask signs and symptoms, such as fever and pain.
•Especially if patient is elderly or taking oxaprozin long-term, watch for less common but serious adverse GI reactions, including anorexia, constipation, diverticulitis, dysphagia, esophagitis, gastritis, gastroenteritis, gastroesophageal reflux disease, hemorrhoids, hiatal hernia, melena, stomatitis, and vomiting.
•Monitor liver function test results because, in rare cases, elevated levels may progress to severe hepatic reactions, including fatal hepatitis, liver necrosis, and hepatic failure.
•Monitor BUN and serum creatinine levels in patients with heart failure, impaired renal function, or hepatic dysfunction; those taking diuretics or ACE inhibitors; and elderly patients because drug may cause renal failure.
•Monitor CBC for decreased hemoglobin level and hematocrit because drug may worsen anemia.
•Assess patient's skin routinely for rash or other signs of hypersensitivity reaction because oxaprozin and other NSAIDs may cause serious skin reactions without warning, even in patients with no history of NSAID hypersensitivity. Stop drug at first sign of reaction, and notify prescriber.

PATIENT TEACHING
•Instruct patient to take oxaprozin exactly as prescribed.
•Advise patient to take drug with a full glass of water and to stay upright for 15 to 30 minutes afterward to prevent drug from lodging in esophagus and causing irritation.
•Urge patient to avoid alcohol as well as aspirin and other NSAIDs during oxaprozin therapy to avoid bleeding complications.
•Advise patient to avoid excessive sun exposure to reduce the risk of photosensitivity.
•Caution patient to avoid hazardous activities until drug's CNS effects are known.
•Inform patient that risk of bleeding may continue up to 2 weeks after stopping drug.
•Explain that oxaprozin may increase the risk of serious adverse cardiovascular reactions; urge patient to seek immediate medical attention if signs or symptoms arise, such as chest pain, shortness of breath, weakness, and slurring of speech.
•Inform patient that oxaprozin also may increase the risk of serious adverse GI reactions; stress need to seek immediate medical attention for such signs and symptoms as epigastric or abdominal pain, indigestion, black or tarry stools, or vomiting blood or material that looks like coffee grounds.
•Alert patient to rare but serious skin reactions. Urge him to seek immediate medical attention for rash, blisters, itching, fever, or other indications of hypersensitivity.

oxazepam

Apo-Oxazepam (CAN), Novoxapam (CAN), Serax

Class, Category, and Schedule
Chemical class: Benzodiazepine
Therapeutic class: Antianxiety, sedative hypnotic
Pregnancy category: Not rated
Controlled substance schedule: IV

Indications and Dosages
➤ *To treat anxiety*
CAPSULES, TABLETS
Adults. 10 to 15 mg t.i.d. or q.i.d. for mild to

moderate anxiety; up to 30 mg t.i.d. or q.i.d. for severe anxiety.

➤ *To help manage acute alcohol with-drawal symptoms*

CAPSULES, TABLETS
Adults. 15 to 30 mg t.i.d. or q.i.d.
DOSAGE ADJUSTMENT For elderly or debilitated patients, initial dose of 10 mg t.i.d. increased cautiously to 15 mg t.i.d. or q.i.d.

Mechanism of Action
May potentiate the effects of gamma-aminobutyric acid (GABA) and other inhibitory neurotransmitters by binding to specific benzodiazepine receptors in limbic and cortical areas of the CNS. GABA inhibits excitatory stimulation, which helps control emotional behavior. The limbic system contains highly dense areas of benzodiazepine receptors, which may explain oxazepam's antianxiety effects.

Contraindications
Acute angle-closure glaucoma; concurrent use of itraconazole or ketoconazole; hypersensitivity to oxazepam, benzodiazepines, or their components; psychoses

Interactions
DRUGS
cimetidine, oral contraceptives: Impaired metabolism and elimination of oxazepam
clozapine: Increased risk of respiratory depression and arrest
CNS depressants: Increased risk of apnea and CNS depression
levodopa: Decreased therapeutic effects of levodopa
probenecid: Increased therapeutic effects of oxazepam and risk of oversedation

ACTIVITIES
alcohol use: Increased risk of apnea and CNS depression

Adverse Reactions
CNS: Anxiety (in daytime), ataxia, confusion, depression, dizziness, drowsiness, fatigue, headache, insomnia, nightmares, sleep disturbance, slurred speech, syncope, talkativeness, tremor, vertigo
GI: Nausea
Other: Drug tolerance, physical and psychological dependence, withdrawal symptoms

Nursing Considerations
•**WARNING** Be aware that oxazepam may cause physical and psychological dependence.
•Be aware that drug shouldn't be stopped abruptly after prolonged use; doing so may cause seizures or withdrawal symptoms, such as insomnia, irritability, and nervousness.
•Be aware that withdrawal symptoms can occur when therapy lasts only 1 or 2 weeks.
•**WARNING** Monitor respiratory status in patients with pulmonary disease (such as severe COPD), respiratory depression, or sleep apnea; drug may worsen ventilatory failure.
•Expect an increased risk of falls among elderly patients from impaired cognition and motor function. Take safety precautions.
•Be aware that drug may worsen acute intermittent porphyria, myasthenia gravis, and severe renal impairment.
•Expect patient with late-stage Parkinson's disease to experience decreased cognition or coordination and, possibly, increased psychosis.

PATIENT TEACHING
•Instruct patient to take oxazepam exactly as prescribed and not to stop taking it without consulting prescriber.
•Caution patient about possible drowsiness and reduced coordination.
•Urge patient to avoid alcohol, which increases oxazepam's sedative effects.

oxcarbazepine

Trileptal

Class and Category
Chemical class: Tricyclic iminostilbene derivative
Therapeutic class: Anticonvulsant
Pregnancy category: C

Indications and Dosages
➤ *As adjunct to treat partial seizures*
ORAL SUSPENSION, TABLETS
Adults and adolescents over age 16. *Initial:* 300 mg b.i.d. Dosage increased by 600 mg/day every wk. *Usual:* 1,200 mg daily. *Maximum:* 2,400 mg daily.
Children ages 4 to 16. *Initial:* 4 to 5 mg/kg b.i.d. to maximum initial dose of 600 mg daily. *Usual:* 900 mg daily for children weighing 20 to 29 kg (44 to 64 lb); 1,200 mg daily for those weighing 29.1 to 39 kg (65 to 86 lb);

1,800 mg daily for those weighing more than 39 kg. *Maximum:* 1,800 mg daily.

DOSAGE ADJUSTMENT For patients with creatinine clearance of less than 30 ml/min/1.73 m², usual initial dosage reduced by 50%.

➤ *As monotherapy to treat partial seizures*

ORAL SUSPENSION, TABLETS

Adults and adolescents over age 16. *Initial:* 300 mg b.i.d. Dosage increased by 300 mg/ day every 3 days as needed. *Usual:* 1,200 mg daily. *Maximum:* 2,400 mg daily.

Children ages 4 to 16. *Initial:* 4 to 5 mg/kg b.i.d., increased by 5 mg/kg daily every third day to maximum maintenance dosage, as needed. *Maximum:* 900 mg daily for children weighing 20 to 24.9 kg (44 to 55 lb); 1,200 mg daily for those weighing 25 to 34.9 kg (55 to 77 lb); 1,500 mg daily for those weighing 35 to 49.9 kg (77 to 110 lb); 1,800 mg daily for those weighing 50 to 59.9 kg (110 to 132 lb); 2,100 mg daily for those weighing 60 to 70 kg (132 to 154 lb).

➤ *To convert to monotherapy in treating partial seizures*

ORAL SUSPENSION, TABLETS

Adults and adolescents over age 16. *Initial:* 300 mg b.i.d. Dosage increased by 600 mg daily every wk over 2 to 4 wk, as needed, while dosage of other anticonvulsant is reduced. *Usual:* 1,200 mg daily. *Maximum:* 2,400 mg daily.

Children ages 4 to 16. *Initial:* 4 to 5 mg/kg b.i.d., increased by 10 mg/kg daily weekly as needed to maximum maintenance dosage while dosage of other anticonvulsant is reduced over 3 to 6 wk. *Maximum:* 900 mg daily for children weighing 20 to 24.9 kg (44 to 55 lb); 1,200 mg daily for those weighing 25 to 34.9 kg (55 to 77 lb); 1,500 mg daily for those weighing 35 to 49.9 kg (77 to 110 lb); 1,800 mg daily for those weighing 50 to 59.9 kg (110 to 132 lb); 2,100 mg daily for those weighing 60 to 70 kg (132 to 154 lb).

Mechanism of Action

May prevent or halt seizures by closing or blocking sodium channels in the neuronal cell membrane. By preventing sodium from entering the cell, oxcarbazepine may slow nerve impulse transmission, thus decreasing the rate at which neurons fire.

Contraindications

Hypersensitivity to carbamazepine, oxcarbazepine, or their components

Interactions

DRUGS

carbamazepine, phenobarbital, phenytoin, valproic acid: Decreased blood oxcarbazepine level, possibly increased blood levels of phenobarbital and phenytoin

felodipine, verapamil: Decreased blood levels of these drugs

oral contraceptives: Decreased effectiveness

ACTIVITIES

alcohol use: Possibly additive CNS depressant effects

Adverse Reactions

CNS: Abnormal gait, ataxia, dizziness, fatigue, fever, headache, somnolence, tremor

EENT: Abnormal vision, diplopia, nystagmus, rhinitis

GI: Abdominal pain, indigestion, nausea, vomiting

SKIN: Rash, Stevens-Johnson syndrome, toxic epidermal necrolysis

Other: Anaphylalxis, hyponatremia

Nursing Considerations

•Patient with an allergic reaction to carbamazepine may have hypersensitivity to oxcarbazepine.

•Monitor serum sodium level for signs of hyponatremia, especially during first 3 months.

•Monitor therapeutic oxcarbazepine levels during initiation and titration, and expect to adjust dosage accordingly.

•Implement seizure precautions as needed.

•Monitor patient's skin closely. If a reaction develops, notify prescriber immediately because skin reactions caused by oxcarbazepine may be serious or life-threatening.

•WARNING Monitor patient closely for evidence of multi-organ hypersensitivity, such as fever, rash, organ dysfunction, lymphadenopathy, hepatitis, liver function abnormalities, hematologic abnormalities, pruritus, nephritis, oliguria, hepato-renal syndrome, arthralgia, and asthenia. If suspected, notify prescriber and expect to stop giving drug. Provide supportive care, as prescribed.

PATIENT TEACHING

•Teach patient to shake suspension well and prepare the dose immediately afterwards. Tell him to then withdraw the prescribed

amount using the supplied oral dosing syringe. Instruct him to mix the dose in a small glass of water just before taking it, or tell him that he can swallow drug directly from the syringe. Instruct him to close the bottle and rinse the syringe with warm water and allow it to dry thoroughly.
•Inform patient that he may experience dizziness, double vision, and unsteady gait.
•Instruct patient not to drink alcohol during oxcarbazepine therapy.
•Alert patient to the possibility of hypersensitivity or serious skin reactions and the need to report them to prescriber.
•Warn patient to notify prescriber immediately if he develops a fever; rash; swelling of face, eyes, lips, tongue; difficulty swallowing or breathing; or other symptoms because drug may need to be stopped and emergency medical care given.
•Alert female patients of childbearing age that oxcarbazepine may render hormonal contraceptives ineffective. Urge patient to use an additional or a different contraceptive during oxcarbazepine therapy.

oxtriphylline

Apo-Oxtriphylline (CAN), Choledyl, Choledyl SA

Class and Category

Chemical class: Xanthine derivative
Therapeutic class: Bronchodilator
Pregnancy category: C

Indications and Dosages

➤ *To treat acute asthma, bronchospasm due to chronic bronchitis or COPD*

DELAYED-RELEASE TABLETS

Adults and children age 6 and over. 300 mg daily for 3 days; then increased to 400 mg daily for 3 days. *Maintenance:* 600 mg daily in divided doses every 6 to 8 hr.

E.R. TABLETS

Adults and children age 6 and over. 300 mg daily for 3 days; then increased to 400 mg daily for 3 days. *Maintenance:* 600 mg daily in divided doses every 12 hr.

Contraindications

Hypersensitivity to oxtriphylline, xanthines, or their components; peptic ulcer; seizure disorder unless controlled by an anticonvulsant

Mechanism of Action

Inhibits phosphodiesterase enzymes, causing bronchodilation. Normally, these enzymes inactivate cAMP and cGMP, which are responsible for bronchial smooth-muscle relaxation. Other mechanisms of action may include calcium translocation, prostaglandin antagonism, catecholamine stimulation, inhibition of cGMP metabolism, and adenosine receptor antagonism.

Interactions

DRUGS

activated charcoal, aminoglutethimide, barbiturates, ketoconazole, rifampin, sulfinpyrazone, sympathomimetics: Decreased blood theophylline level
allopurinol, beta blockers (nonselective), calcium channel blockers, cimetidine, corticosteroids, disulfiram, ephedrine, influenza virus vaccine, interferon, macrolides, mexiletine, oral contraceptives, quinolones, thiabendazole: Increased blood theophylline level
benzodiazepines, propofol: Possibly antagonized sedative effects of these drugs
carbamazepine, isoniazid, loop diuretics: Possibly altered blood theophylline level
halothane anesthetics: Increased risk of cardiotoxicity
hydantoins: Possibly decreased blood hydantoin level
ketamine: Increased risk of seizures
lithium: Decreased blood lithium level
neuromuscular blockers: Possibly reversal of neuromuscular blockade
tetracyclines: Possibly increased adverse effects of theophylline

FOODS

all foods: Altered bioavailability and absorption of E.R. oxtriphylline
charcoal broiled beef; low-carbohydrate, high-protein diet: Increased theophylline elimination
high-carbohydrate, low-protein diet: Decreased elimination and prolonged half-life of theophylline

ACTIVITIES

alcohol use: Increased CNS effects, especially with elixir
smoking (1 or more packs daily): Decreased effects of oxtriphylline

Adverse Reactions

CNS: Anxiety, dizziness, headache, insomnia, restlessness, seizures
CV: Hypotension, palpitations, sinus tachycardia
EENT: Unpleasant taste
GI: Anorexia, diarrhea, nausea, vomiting
RESP: Tachypnea
SKIN: Alopecia, flushing, rash

Nursing Considerations

•Be aware that oxtriphylline contains 64% anhydrous theophylline, so dosage is based on equivalent of 5 to 6 mg of anhydrous theophylline/kg.
•Be aware that food delays absorption of delayed-release and E.R. forms and that large volumes of fluid may increase absorption.
•Know that delayed-release and E.R. preparations vary in their absorption rate.
•Monitor blood theophylline level because toxicity may develop at a level only slightly above therapeutic.

PATIENT TEACHING
•If patient complains of GI discomfort, suggest taking drug with or just after meals.
•Urge patient to stop smoking and to notify prescriber about changes in smoking habits. Also instruct him to avoid alcohol during oxtriphylline therapy.
•Encourage patient to keep follow-up appointments for laboratory studies.

oxybutynin chloride

Ditropan, Ditropan XL, Gelnique 10%

Class and Category

Chemical class: Tertiary amine
Therapeutic class: Antispasmodic
Pregnancy category: B

Indications and Dosages

➤ *To treat overactive bladder, including neurogenic bladder, with urinary frequency, urgency, or incontinence from involuntary contraction of detrusor muscle*

E.R. TABLETS
Adults. *Initial:* 5 mg daily, adjusted by 5 mg/wk, as prescribed. *Maximum:* 30 mg daily.
SYRUP, TABLETS
Adults. 5 mg b.i.d. or t.i.d. *Maximum:* 5 mg q.i.d. or 20 mg daily.

Children age 5 and over. 5 mg b.i.d. *Maximum:* 15 mg t.i.d.
TRANSDERMAL SYSTEM
Adults. System supplying 3.9 mg daily, applied twice weekly.
TOPICAL GEL
Adults. 1 sachet (containing 100 mg/g oxybutynin chloride gel) applied once daily to dry, intact skin on the abdomen, upper arms, shoulders, or thighs.
DOSAGE ADJUSTMENT For elderly patients, possibly 2.5 mg b.i.d. initially, increased to maximum of 5 mg t.i.d., as prescribed.

Route	Onset	Peak	Duration
P.O.	30 to 60 min	3 to 6 hr	6 to 10 hr
Trans-dermal	Unknown	24 to 48 hr	96 hr

Mechanism of Action

Exerts antimuscarinic (atropine-like) and potent direct antispasmodic (papaverine-like) actions on smooth muscle in the bladder and decreases detrusor muscle contractions. The result is increased bladder capacity and a decreased urge to void.

Contraindications

Acute hemorrhage, angle-closure glaucoma, gastric retention (gel form), GI obstruction, hypersensitivity to oxybutynin or its components, ileus, intestinal atony in elderly or debilitated patients, myasthenia gravis, obstructive uropathy, toxic megacolon with ulcerative colitis, urine retention (gel form)

Interactions

DRUGS
amantadine, amitriptyline, amoxapine, antimuscarinics, brompheniramine, bupropion, carbinoxamine, chlorpheniramine, chlorpromazine, clemastine, clomipramine, clozapine, cyclobenzaprine, dimenhydrinate, diphenhydramine, disopyramide, doxepin, doxylamine, imipramine, maprotiline, mesoridazine, methdilazine, nortriptyline, procainamide, promazine, promethazine, protriptyline, thioridazine, triflupromazine, trimeprazine, trimipramine: Increased anticholinergic effects
CNS depressants: Increased sedation
ketoconazole: Possibly altered total absorption rate and blood level of ketoconazole

N
O

opioid agonists: Increased depressive effects on GI motility and bladder function
parasympathomimetics: Decreased antimuscarinic action of oxybutynin

ACTIVITIES
alcohol use: Increased sedation

Adverse Reactions

CNS: Agitation, asthenia, confusion, dizziness, drowsiness, fatigue, hallucinations, headache, insomnia, nervousness, psychosis, restlessness, seizures, somnolence
CV: Arrhythmias, hypertension, hypotension, palpitations, peripheral edema, tachycardia, vasodilation
EENT: Blurred vision; cycloplegia; dry eyes, mouth, nose, and throat; keratoconjunctivitis sicca; eye irritation; mydriasis; nasopharyngitis; rhinitis; sinusitis
ENDO: Hyperglycemia, suppression of lactation
GI: Abdominal pain, constipation, decreased GI motility, diarrhea, dysphagia, esophagitis, flatulence, gastroesophageal reflux, indigestion, nausea, vomiting
GU: Cystitis, dysuria, impotence, urinary hesitancy, urine retention, UTI
MS: Arthralgia, arthritis, back pain
RESP: Asthma, bronchitis, cough, upper respiratory tract infection
SKIN: Decreased sweating, dry skin, flushing, pruritus, rash, urticaria
Other: Application site reactions (anesthesia, dermatitis, erythema, irritation, papules, pruritus), flulike symptoms, fungal infections, heatstroke

Nursing Considerations

•Use oxybutynin cautiously in patients with diarrhea because it may signal incomplete GI obstruction, especially in patients with colostomy or ileostomy. Also use cautiously in patients with dementia because drug may aggravate symptoms.
•Use cautiously in patients with myasthenia gravis or GI disorders because drug may adversely affect these conditions.
•Assess urinary symptoms before and after treatment.
•Make sure patient swallows E.R. tablets whole and doesn't crush, chew, or divide them. Expect to see portions of drug in stool.
•Apply transdermal system to dry, intact skin of abdomen, hip, or buttock; rotate sites to avoid the same site for at least 7 days.

•Apply gel form to dry, intact skin on the patient's abdomen, upper arms, shoulders, or thighs. Rotate application sites.
•**WARNING** Watch for adverse cardiovascular reactions in patients with arrhythmias, coronary artery disease, heart failure, or hypertension because drug's antimuscarinic effects may increase their risk.
•Decreased GI motility can cause adynamic ileus; assess for abdominal pain and ileus.
•Be aware that drug may aggravate benign prostatic hyperplasia, gastroesophageal reflux disease, and hyperthyroidism.
•Monitor patient for anticholinergic CNS effects, such as hallucinations, agitation, confusion and somnolence, especially in the first few months of therapy or when dosage is increased. If such effects occur, notify prescriber and expect dosage to be reduced or drug discontinued.

PATIENT TEACHING
•Instruct patient to take oxybutynin on an empty stomach. If adverse GI reactions develop, suggest taking drug with food or milk.
•Advise patient to swallow tablets whole and not to chew, crush, or break them.
•Instruct patient how to apply transdermal system or gel. Tell her to apply to clean, dry skin, avoiding areas that have been recently shaved or have open sores or rashes. Remind patient to wash hands after handling product.
•Warn patient that gel is flammable and that she should avoid open fire or smoking until gel has dried. Also tell patient that she should avoid bathing, swimming, showering, exercising, or immersing application site in water for 1 hour after application and to cover site with clothing once gel has dried.
•Warn of possible decreased alertness, and advise patient against performing hazardous activities until drug's CNS effects are known.
•Caution patient to avoid strenuous exercise and excessive sun exposure because of increased risk of heatstroke.
•Urge patient to avoid alcohol during therapy.

oxycodone hydrochloride

OxyContin, Roxicodone, Supeudol (CAN)

Class, Category, and Schedule
Chemical class: Phenanthrene derivative

Therapeutic class: Analgesic
Pregnancy category: Not rated
Controlled substance schedule: II

Indications and Dosages

➤ *To relieve moderate to severe pain*
ORAL SOLUTION
Adults. 5 mg every 3 to 6 hr, p.r.n., and increased as needed.
TABLETS
Adults. 5 mg every 3 to 6 hr or 10 mg every 6 to 8 hr, p.r.n.

➤ *To manage pain for more than a few days*
CONTROLLED-RELEASE TABLETS, E.R. TABLETS
Adults who haven't received opioids before. *Initial:* 10 to 20 mg every 12 hr, adjusted every 1 to 2 days, as prescribed, based on total amount of oxycodone needed daily to control pain.
Adults who currently receive an opioid agonist or fixed-ratio combination drugs (opioid agonist plus acetaminophen, aspirin, or NSAID). Half the 24-hr oxycodone dose every 12 hr, as prescribed. Be prepared to manage breakthrough pain with immediate-release tablets, p.r.n., and adjust every 1 to 2 days, as prescribed.
Adults who use fentanyl transdermal patch. 10 mg oxycodone for each 25 mcg/hr of fentanyl patch dosage every 12 hr, beginning 12 to 18 hr after removing patch.
DOSAGE ADJUSTMENT To provide supplemental analgesia for adults receiving controlled-release oxycodone, one-fourth to one-third the 12-hr controlled-release dose given as tablet every 3 to 6 hr, p.r.n.

Route	Onset	Peak	Duration
P.O.	10 to 15 min	1 hr	3 to 4 hr

Mechanism of Action

Alters the perception of and emotional response to pain at the spinal cord and higher levels of the CNS by blocking the release of inhibitory neurotransmitters, such as gamma-aminobutyric acid and acetylcholine.

Contraindications

Hypercapnia, hypersensitivity to oxycodone or its components, ileus, use within 14 days of MAO inhibitor therapy

Interactions
DRUGS
anticholinergics: Possibly severe constipation and ileus
antidiarrheals: Possibly severe constipation and additive CNS depression
antihypertensives: Possibly exaggerated antihypertensive effects and risk of orthostatic hypotension
butorphanol, pentazocine: Possibly acute withdrawal symptoms in opioid-dependent patients, decreased analgesic effects
carbamazepine, phenytoin, primidone, rifampin: Possibly need for increased oxycodone dosage to achieve analgesia and prevent withdrawal symptoms in opioid-dependent patients
cimetidine: Possibly apnea, confusion, disorientation, and seizures from respiratory depression and impaired CNS function
CNS depressants: Possibly increased CNS and respiratory depression and orthostatic hypotension
MAO inhibitors: Possibly fatal reactions, including cardiac arrest, coma, respiratory depression, seizures, and severe hypertension
nalbuphine, nalmefene, naloxone, naltrexone: Blocked oxycodone effects, withdrawal symptoms in opioid-dependent patients
ACTIVITIES
alcohol use: Additive CNS effects

Adverse Reactions
CNS: Abnormal dreams, anxiety, asthenia, chills, dizziness, drowsiness, euphoria, excitation, headache, insomnia, nervousness, sedation, seizures, somnolence, syncope, twitching
CV: Bradycardia, chest pain, hypotension, orthostatic hypotension, palpitations
EENT: Blurred vision, dry eyes or mouth, lens opacities, miosis
ENDO: Syndrome of inappropriate antidiuretic hormone secretion
GI: Abdominal pain, anorexia, constipation, diarrhea, dyspepsia, elevated liver function test results, gastritis, hiccups, nausea, vomiting
GU: Amenorrhea, decreased libido, erectile dysfunction, oliguria, urinary hesitancy, urine retention
RESP: Dyspnea, respiratory depression
SKIN: Diaphoresis, pruritus, rash
Other: Anaphylaxis, drug tolerance, hypona-

N
O

tremia, physical and psychological dependence, withdrawal symptoms

Nursing Considerations
•WARNING Be aware that oxycodone has a high potential for abuse.
•WARNING Be aware that abuse of crushed controlled-release tablets poses a hazard of overdose and death. If you suspect abuse and determine that patient also is abusing alcohol or illicit substances, notify prescriber immediately because the risk of overdose and death is increased. If you suspect parenteral abuse, be aware that tablet excipients, especially talc, may result in local tissue necrosis, infection, pulmonary granulomas, endocarditis, and valvular heart injury.
•Assess baseline neurologic status before each dose in patient with head injury because oxycodone may obscure progression of his condition.
•Assess patient's pain level regularly, and give drug as prescribed before pain becomes severe.
•Be prepared to adjust dosage for patient who hasn't previously received opioids until he can tolerate drug's effects.
•Expect to give controlled-release tablets only to opioid-tolerant patients who need at least 160 mg daily.
•Assess patient for possible respiratory depression or paradoxical excitation during dosage titration.
•Assess patient for abdominal pain because oxycodone may mask underlying GI disorders.

PATIENT TEACHING
•WARNING Strongly warn patient to swallow oxycodone tablets whole and not to break, chew, or crush them because taking broken, chewed, or crushed tablets leads to rapid release and absorption of a potentially fatal dose.
•Instruct patient not to take oxycodone more often than prescribed and not to stop taking drug abruptly after long-term use.
•Instruct patient to avoid alcohol and potentially hazardous activities during oxycodone therapy.
•Tell patient to notify prescriber about signs of possible toxicity or hypersensitivity, such as excessive light-headedness, extreme dizziness, itching, swelling, and trouble breathing.

oxymetholone
Anadrol-50, Anapolon-50 (CAN)

Class, Category, and Schedule
Chemical class: Testosterone derivative
Therapeutic class: Antianemic, antiangioedema (hereditary)
Pregnancy category: X
Controlled substance schedule: III

Indications and Dosages
➤ *To treat acquired and congenital aplastic anemias, anemias caused by deficient RBC production, bone marrow failure anemias, hypoplastic anemias caused by myelotoxic drugs, and myelofibrosis; to prevent or treat hereditary angioedema*

TABLETS
Adults and children. 1 to 2 mg/kg daily for 3 to 6 mo. *Maximum:* 5 mg/kg daily.

Mechanism of Action
Combats anemia by increasing production of erythropoietin, a precursor of RBCs. Oxymetholone also increases the hemoglobin level and RBC volume.

Contraindications
Breast or prostate cancer in men, hypercalcemia in women with breast cancer, hypersensitivity to oxymetholone or anabolic steroids, nephrosis, nephrotic phase of nephritis, pregnancy, severe hepatic dysfunction

Interactions
DRUGS
corticosteroids: Increased risk of edema and severe acne
hepatotoxic drugs: Increased risk of hepatotoxicity
insulin, oral antidiabetic drugs: Possibly hypoglycemia
NSAIDs, oral anticoagulants, salicylates: Increased anticoagulant effects
sodium-containing drugs: Increased risk of edema
somatrem, somatropin: Possibly accelerated epiphyseal maturation
FOODS
high-sodium foods: Increased risk of edema

Adverse Reactions
CNS: Depression, excitement, insomnia

CV: Decreased serum HDL level, edema, hyperlipidemia, hypertension
ENDO: Feminization in postpubertal males (epididymitis, gynecomastia, impotence, oligospermia, priapism, testicular atrophy), glucose intolerance, virilism in females (acne, clitoral enlargement, decreased breast size, deepened voice, diaphoresis, emotional lability, flushing, hirsutism, hoarseness, libido changes, male-pattern baldness, menstrual irregularities, nervousness, oily hair or skin, vaginal bleeding, vaginitis, weight gain), virilism in prepubertal males (acne, decreased ejaculatory volume, penis enlargement, prepubertal closure of epiphyseal plates, unnatural growth of body and facial hair)
GI: Diarrhea, elevated liver function test results, hepatocellular carcinoma, nausea, vomiting
GU: Benign prostatic hyperplasia, prostate cancer, urinary frequency, urine retention (elderly men)
HEME: Iron deficiency anemia, leukemia, prolonged bleeding time
SKIN: Jaundice
Other: Fluid retention, hypercalcemia (females), physical and psychological dependence, sodium retention

Nursing Considerations
• Be aware that oxymetholone shouldn't be used in patients with a history of hypercalcemia because drug may exacerbate this condition or in patients with prostate problems because drug may promote benign or cancerous tumor growth.
• Anticipate increased risk of fluid and sodium retention in patients with cardiac, hepatic, or renal dysfunction. Monitor for signs and symptoms of fluid retention.
• Monitor daily weight. Expect to place patient with fluid retention on sodium-restricted diet or diuretics, as prescribed.
• **WARNING** Be aware that oxymetholone may suppress spermatogenesis in males and cause permanent virilization in females.

PATIENT TEACHING
• Advise patient to consume a diet high in protein and calories to achieve maximum therapeutic effect of oxymetholone.
• Instruct patient to check his weight daily during oxymetholone therapy and to notify prescriber immediately about swelling or unexplained weight gain.

• Inform patient that drug may cause libido changes.
• Advise diabetic patient to monitor blood glucose levels frequently because drug may increase hypoglycemic effect of antidiabetic drugs.
• Inform female patient that drug may cause permanent physical changes, such as clitoral enlargement, deepened voice, and unnatural hair growth.
• Advise female patient of childbearing age to use contraception during therapy and to notify prescriber immediately about suspected or known pregnancy.

oxymorphone hydrochloride

Numorphan, Opana, Opana ER

Class, Category, and Schedule
Chemical class: Phenanthrene derivative
Therapeutic class: Analgesic
Pregnancy category: Not rated
Controlled substance schedule: II

Indications and Dosages
➤ *To relieve moderate to severe pain*
TABLETS
Adults. *Initial:* 5 to 20 mg every 4 to 6 hr, p.r.n.

➤ *To relieve moderate to severe pain in patients requiring continuous, around-the-clock opioid treatment for an extended time*
E.R. TABLETS
Adults. *Initial:* 5 mg every 12 hr, increased as needed in 5- to 10-mg increments every 3 to 7 days.
DOSAGE ADJUSTMENT For patients with creatinine clearance less than 50 ml/min/1.73 m^2 or elderly patients, dosage started at lowest level and titrated slowly. For patients receiving other CNS depressants, dosage started at ⅓ to ½ the usual starting dose.

➤ *To relieve moderate to severe pain, to relieve anxiety in patients with dyspnea from pulmonary edema caused by acute left ventricular dysfunction*
I.V. INJECTION
Adults. *Initial:* 0.5 mg, repeated every 3 to 6 hr, p.r.n.

N
O

I.M. or subcutaneous injection
Adults. *Initial:* 1 to 1.5 mg, repeated every 3 to 6 hr, p.r.n.
Suppositories
Adults. 5 mg every 4 to 6 hr, p.r.n.

➤ *To relieve obstetric pain during labor*
I.M. injection
Adults. 0.5 to 1 mg as a single dose.

Route	Onset	Peak	Duration
I.V.	5 to 10 min	15 to 30 min	3 to 4 hr
I.M.	10 to 15 min	30 to 90 min	3 to 6 hr
SubQ	10 to 20 min	30 to 90 min	3 to 6 hr
P.R.	15 to 30 min	2 hr	3 to 6 hr

Mechanism of Action

Alters the perception of and emotional response to pain at the spinal cord and higher levels of the CNS by blocking the release of inhibitory neurotransmitters, such as gamma-aminobutyric acid and acetylcholine.

Contraindications

Acute or severe asthma; hypercarbia; hypersensitivity to oxymorphone, other morphine analogues, or their components; ileus; moderate to severe hepatic impairment; pulmonary edema from a chemical respiratory irritant; severe respiratory depression; upper airway obstruction

Interactions
Drugs
anticholingerics: Increased risk of urine retention, severe constipation
antidiarrheals, antiperistaltics: Increased risk of severe constipation, CNS depression
antihypertensives, diuretics, hypotension-producing drugs: Increased hypotensive effects
buprenorphine: Reduced oxymorphone effectiveness if buprenorphine is given first, possibly withdrawal symptoms in oxymorphone-dependent patients
CNS depressants: Additive CNS depressant effects, increased risk of habituation
hydroxyzine, other opioid analgesics: Increased analgesia, CNS depression, and hypotensive effects
MAO inhibitors: Increased risk of unpredictable, severe, sometimes fatal adverse reactions
metoclopramide: Antagonized effects of metoclopramide on GI motility
naloxone: Antagonized analgesic, CNS, and respiratory depressant effects of oxymorphone
naltrexone: Withdrawal symptoms in oxymorphone-dependent patients
neuromuscular blockers: Additive respiratory depression
Activities
alcohol use: Additive CNS depressant effects, increased risk of habituation

Adverse Reactions
CNS: Agitation, asthenia, CNS depression, confusion, delusions, depersonalization, dizziness, drowsiness, euphoria, fatigue, hallucinations, headache, insomnia, lightheadedness, nervousness, nightmares, restlessness, seizures, somnolence, tiredness, tremor, weakness
CV: Bradycardia, hypertension, hypotension, palpitations, tachycardia
EENT: Blurred vision, diplopia, dry mouth, laryngeal edema, laryngospasm, miosis, tinnitus
GI: Abdominal cramps or pain, anorexia, biliary colic, constipation, hepatotoxicity, ileus, nausea, vomiting
GU: Decreased urine output, dysuria, urinary frequency and hesitancy, urine retention
MS: Muscle rigidity (with large doses), uncontrolled muscle movements
RESP: Apnea, atelectasis, bradypnea, bronchospasm, dyspnea, irregular breathing, respiratory depression, wheezing
SKIN: Dermatitis, diaphoresis, erythema, flushing of face, pruritus, urticaria
Other: Angioedema, injection site burning, pain, redness, and swelling

Nursing Considerations
• Use with extreme caution in patients with increased intracranial pressure or head injury because oxymorphone may obscure neurologic signs of increasing severity.
• Use cautiously in patients with mild hepatic impairment because drug is metabolized in the liver; impaired renal function because drug is excreted by the kidneys; and biliary tract disease because drug may cause spasm of the sphincter of Oddi.

- •Use cautiously in patients receiving mixed agonist-antagonist opioid analgesics because these drugs may reduce analgesic effect of oxymorphone or may cause withdrawal symptoms.
- •Use cautiously in elderly patients because plasma oxymorphone levels are higher in elderly than in younger patients.
- •Be aware that oral hydromorphone shouldn't be used "as needed" or for first 24 hours after surgery in patients not already taking opioids because of the risk of oversedation and respiratory depression.
- •If patient is being converted from one form of drug to another, watch closely for analgesic effectiveness and adverse reactions. For conversion from oral immediate-release form to oral extended-release form, expect that you may give half the patient's total daily dose every 12 hours. For conversion from parenteral oxymorphone to oral form, expect hat you may give 10 times the patient's total daily parenteral dose as tablets, divided into equal doses and given over 24 hours.
- •Taper dosage, as ordered, before stopping therapy to prevent withdrawal in physically dependent patients.
- •Monitor vital signs during oxymorphone therapy to detect respiratory depression and hypotension, especially in elderly patients, debilitated patients, and those with conditions accompanied by hypoxia, when even moderate doses may severely decrease pulmonary ventilation.
- •Monitor urinary and bowel status; constipation may become so severe that it causes ileus.
- •Offer fluids to relieve dry mouth.

PATIENT TEACHING
- •Instruct patient to take oxymorphone exactly as prescribed and not to stop taking it abruptly; warn that drug can cause physical dependence.
- •Stress the importance of taking drug before pain becomes severe.
- •Instruct patient prescribed tablet form to take it on an empty stomach.
- •Tell patient prescribed extended-release tablet form not to break, chew, dissolve, or crush tablets before taking them because going so will lead to a rapid drug release and increased risk of a potentially fatal dose.
- •Instruct patient to store suppositories in refrigerator.

- •Encourage patient to increase fluid and fiber intake during therapy to prevent constipation.
- •Stress need to avoid alcohol and CNS depressants during therapy because of risk of severe life-threatening adverse reactions.
- •Caution patient to avoid potentially hazardous activities until drug's CNS effects are known.
- •Advise female patient to stop drug and notify prescriber about known or suspected pregnancy.

oxytetracycline
Terramycin I.M.

oxytetracycline hydrochloride
Terramycin

Class and Category
Chemical class: Tetracycline derived from *Streptomyces rimosus*
Therapeutic class: Antibiotic, antiprotozoal
Pregnancy category: D

Indications and Dosages
➤ *To treat systemic bacterial and protozoal infections, such as bronchitis, chlamydial infection, Lyme disease, nongonococcal urethritis, rickettsial infection, traveler's diarrhea, and UTI*
CAPSULES (OXYTETRACYCLINE HYDROCHLORIDE)
Adults and adolescents. 250 to 500 mg every 6 hr. *Maximum:* 4,000 mg daily.
Children ages 8 to 12. 6.25 to 12.5 mg/kg every 6 hr.
I.M. INJECTION (OXYTETRACYCLINE)
Adults and adolescents. 100 mg every 8 hr, 150 mg every 12 hr, or 250 mg daily. *Maximum:* 500 mg daily.
Children ages 8 to 12. 5 to 8.3 mg/kg every 8 hr or 7.5 to 12.5 mg/kg every 12 hr. *Maximum:* 250 mg daily.
DOSAGE ADJUSTMENT Dosage possibly reduced for patients with renal impairment.

➤ *To treat brucellosis*
CAPSULES (OXYTETRACYCLINE HYDROCHLORIDE)
Adults and adolescents. 500 mg every 6 hr for 3 wk with 1,000 mg of streptomycin I.M. every 12 hr in wk 1 and daily in wk 2. *Maximum:* 4,000 mg daily.

➤ *To treat uncomplicated gonorrhea*
CAPSULES (OXYTETRACYCLINE HYDROCHLORIDE)
Adults and adolescents. *Initial:* 1,500 mg, then 500 mg every 6 hr to total of 9,000 mg for full course of treatment.
➤ *To treat syphilis*
CAPSULES (OXYTETRACYCLINE HYDROCHLORIDE)
Adults and adolescents. 500 to 1,000 mg every 6 hr for 10 to 15 days to total of 30 to 40 g for full course of treatment.

Mechanism of Action
Binds with ribosomal subunits of susceptible bacteria and alters the cytoplasmic membrane, inhibiting bacterial protein synthesis and rendering the organism ineffective.

Contraindications
Hypersensitivity to tetracyclines or their components

Interactions
DRUGS
antacids, calcium supplements, cholestyramine, choline salicylates, colestipol, iron supplements, magnesium salicylates: Possibly decreased absorption of oxytetracycline
digoxin: Increased blood digoxin level
lithium: Altered blood lithium level
methoxyflurane: Increased risk of nephrotoxicity
oral anticoagulants: Increased anticoagulant effects
oral contraceptives: Decreased contraceptive effectiveness, increased risk of breakthrough bleeding and pregnancy
penicillins: Decreased bactericidal effects of penicillins
sodium bicarbonate: Possibly decreased absorption of oral oxytetracycline
vitamin A: Increased risk of benign intracranial hypertension
FOODS
all foods, especially dairy products: Possibly interference with oxytetracycline absorption

Adverse Reactions
CNS: Dizziness, light-headedness, tiredness, unsteadiness, weakness
EENT: Darkened, discolored, or sore tongue; stomatitis, tooth discoloration (in infants and children under age 8)
GI: Abdominal cramps, diarrhea, indigestion, nausea, thirst, vomiting
GU: Urinary frequency
SKIN: Photosensitivity
Other: Superinfection

Nursing Considerations
•**WARNING** Be aware that oxytetracycline shouldn't be given to premature infants because it may impair skeletal growth or to children under age 8 because it may permanently discolor teeth and cause enamel hypoplasia.
•For an adult patient, administer I.M. injection in the upper outer quadrant of the buttocks or mid-lateral thigh; the deltoid muscle may be used but only if well developed. In children, administer injection only in the mid-lateral thigh.
•Be aware that patient should be switched from parenteral to oral form as soon as possible.
PATIENT TEACHING
•Instruct patient to take oxytetracycline capsules 1 hour before meals and 3 hours before or after other drugs and dairy products.
•Advise patient to take drug with a full glass of water and in an upright position to minimize adverse GI reactions.
•Urge patient to complete entire course of oxytetracycline therapy, even if he feels better beforehand.
•Caution patient to avoid potentially hazardous activities until drug's CNS effects are known.
•Advise patient to avoid excessive sun exposure and to protect skin when outdoors.
•Urge female patient who uses oral contraceptives to use an additional form of birth control during oxytetracycline therapy.
•Advise patient to discard outdated capsules because drug may become toxic.

➤━━━━━━━━━━━━━━━◄

P

paliperidone

Invega

Class and Category

Chemical class: Benzisoxazole derivative
Therapeutic class: Antipsychotic (Atypical)
Pregnancy category: C

Indications and Dosages

➤ *To treat schizophrenia*

E.R. TABLETS

Adults. *Initial:* 6 mg once daily in the morning; then increased or decreased in increments of 3 mg daily every 6 or more days, as needed. *Maximum:* 12 mg daily.

DOSAGE ADJUSTMENT For patients with mild renal impairment (creatinine clearance 50 to 79 ml/min/1.73 m^2), maximum dosage is 6 mg daily. For patients with moderate to severe renal impairment (creatinine clearance less than 50 ml/min/1.73 m^2), maximum dosage is 3 mg daily.

Route	Onset	Peak	Duration
P.O.	Unknown	24 hr	Unknown

Mechanism of Action

The main active metabolite of risperidone, paliperidone selectively blocks serotonin and dopamine receptors in the mesocortical tract of the CNS to suppress psychotic symptoms.

Contraindications

AV block, cardiac arrhythmias, congenital heart disease, history of congenital long-QT syndrome; hypersensitivity to paliperidone, risperidone, or its components

Interactions

DRUGS

antiarrhythmics of class IA (such as quinidine, procainamide) and class III (such as amiodarone, sotalol), antibiotics (such as gatifloxacin, moxifloxacin), antipsychotics (such as chlorpromazine, thioridazine): Increased risk of QT-interval prolongation

antihypertensives: Increased antihypertensive effects
bromocriptine, levodopa, pergolide: Possibly antagonized effects of these drugs
carbamazepine: Decreased blood paliperidone level
CNS depressants: Additive CNS depression
paroxetine: Possible increased blood paliperidone level

ACTIVITIES

alcohol use: CNS depression

Adverse Reactions

CNS: Agitation, akathisia, anxiety, asthenia, dizziness, dyskinesia, dystonia, extrapyramidal disorder, fatigue, fever, headache, hyperkinesia, hypertonia, neuroleptic malignant syndrome, parkinsonism, somnolence, syncope, tardive dyskinesia, tremor
CV: Bundle branch block, first-degree heart block, hypertension, orthostatic hypotension, palpitations, prolonged QT interval, tachycardia, venous thrombosis
EENT: Blurred vision, dry mouth, salivary hypersecretion, swollen tongue
ENDO: Hyperglycemia
GI: Dyspepsia, nausea, upper abdominal pain
HEME: Thrombocytopenia
MS: Back or limb pain
RESP: Cough, dyspnea
Other: Anaphylaxis, weight gain

Nursing Considerations

• Paliperidone shouldn't be used to treat dementia-related psychosis in the elderly because of an increased mortality risk.
• Paliperidone shouldn't be given to any patient with a condition that severely narrows the GI tract because tablet doesn't change its shape as it passes and could cause a blockage.
• **WARNING** Immediately notify prescriber and expect to stop drug if patient shows signs of neuroleptic malignant syndrome (altered mental status, autonomic instability, hyperpyrexia, muscle rigidity), which can be fatal.
• Monitor patient for involuntary, dyskinetic movements. Notify prescriber if present, and expect to stop therapy. In some cases, therapy may need to continue despite tardive dyskinesia.
• Monitor blood glucose level because drug increases risk of hyperglycemia and possible ketoacidosis or hyperosmolar coma.

P

•Dosage adjustments of paliperidone may be needed when carbamazepine therapy is started or discontinued because of carbamazepine's interaction with paliperidone.

PATIENT TEACHING
•Instruct patient to take the tablet whole with liquid. Caution against chewing, splitting, or crushing tablet because it's designed to release drug at a controlled rate.
•Explain that shell of tablet will be eliminated in stool and that patient need not worry if he sees tablet in stool.
•Urge patient to rise from a sitting or lying position slowly to minimize effects of orthostatic hypotension.
•Caution patient to avoid hazardous activities until CNS effects of drug are known.
•Advise patient to avoid activities that may cause overheating, such as exercising strenuously, being exposed to extreme heat, or becoming dehydrated.

palonosetron hydrochloride

Aloxi

Class and Category
Chemical class: Selective serotonin subtype 3 (5-HT₃) receptor antagonist
Therapeutic class: Antiemetic
Pregnancy category: B

Indications and Dosages
➤ *To prevent acute and delayed nausea and vomiting from chemotherapy*
CAPSULES
Adults. 0.5 mg 1 hr before start of chemotherapy.
I.V. INJECTION
Adults. 0.25 mg over 30 sec approximately 30 min before start of chemotherapy.

➤ *To prevent postoperative nausea and vomiting for up to 24 hr after surgery*
I.V. INJECTION
Adults. 0.75 mg over 10 sec immediately before induction of anesthesia.

Incompatibilities
Palonosetron shouldn't be mixed with any other drug.

Contraindications
Hypersensitivity to palonosetron or its components

Adverse Reactions
CNS: Anxiety, dizziness, drowsiness, fatigue, headache, insomnia, weakness
CV: Bradycardia, hypotension, prolonged QT interval, tachycardia
GI: Abdominal pain, constipation, diarrhea
SKIN: Dermatitis, pruritus, rash
Other: Hyperkalemia, hypersensitivity reaction, injection site reaction (burning, induration, discomfort, pain)

Mechanism of Action
Chemotherapy-induced nausea and vomiting may occur when a chemotherapeutic drug irritates the small intestine's mucosa, causing enterochromaffin cells within the mucosa to release serotonin (5-HT₃). Then, 5-HT₃ stimulates sympathetic receptors on afferent vagal nerve endings and the vagus nerve initiates the vomiting reflex.

Palonosetron selectively blocks 5-HT₃ receptors in afferent vagal nerve endings, preventing the vagus nerve from inducing the vomiting reflex and thereby averting or reducing the nausea and vomiting associated with chemotherapy. Palonosetron may also block 5-HT₃ receptors centrally, in the chemoreceptor trigger zone of the brain's area postrema.

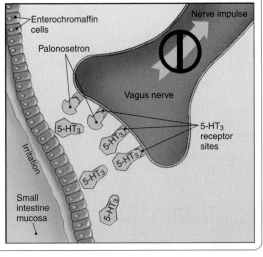

Nursing Considerations

• Use palonosetron cautiously in patients who have or may develop prolonged cardiac conduction intervals—especially QT interval—such as those with congenital QT syndrome, hypokalemia, or hypomagnesemia; those taking a diuretic known to induce electrolyte abnormalities, an antiarrhythmic, or another drug that may prolong QT interval; and those who have received cumulative high-dose anthracycline therapy. With these patients, obtain a baseline ECG before giving palonosetron; repeat the ECG 15 minutes or 24 hours after giving drug, as ordered. Notify prescriber of any delayed conduction.
• Flush I.V. line with normal saline solution before and after giving I.V. palonosetron.
• Closely monitor any patient hypersensitive to other selective serotonin receptor antagonists for a similar reaction. If a reaction occurs, notify prescriber immediately.

PATIENT TEACHING

• Advise patient to avoid hazardous activities until drug's CNS effects are known.
• Instruct patient to notify prescriber of any hypersensitivity reaction, such as rash or allergic dermatitis.

pamidronate disodium

Aredia

Class and Category

Chemical class: Bisphosphonate
Therapeutic class: Antihypercalcemic, bone resorption inhibitor
Pregnancy category: D

Indications and Dosages

➤ *To treat cancer-induced hypercalcemia that's inadequately managed by oral hydration alone*

I.V. INFUSION

Adults. 60 to 90 mg over 2 to 24 hr as a single dose when corrected serum calcium level is 12 to 13.5 mg/dl; 90 mg over 2 to 24 hr when corrected serum calcium level is greater than 13.5 mg/dl. May be repeated as prescribed after 7 days if hypercalcemia recurs.
DOSAGE ADJUSTMENT For patients with renal failure, dosage is limited to 30 mg over 4 to 24 hr, as prescribed. For patients with cardiac or renal failure, drug is given in a smaller volume of fluid or at a slower rate, as prescribed.

➤ *To treat moderate to severe Paget's disease of bone*

I.V. INFUSION

Adults. 30 mg daily over 4 hr on 3 consecutive days for a total dose of 90 mg. Repeated as needed and tolerated.

➤ *To treat osteolytic bone metastases of breast cancer*

I.V. INFUSION

Adults. 90 mg over 2 hr every 3 to 4 wk.

➤ *To treat osteolytic bone metastases of multiple myeloma*

I.V. INFUSION

Adults. 90 mg over 4 hr every mo.

Mechanism of Action

Inhibits bone resorption, possibly by impairing attachment of osteoclast precursors to mineralized bone matrix, thus reducing the rate of bone turnover in Paget's disease and osteolytic metastases. Pamidronate also reduces the flow of calcium from resorbing bone into the bloodstream.

Incompatibilities

Don't mix pamidronate with calcium-containing infusion solutions, such as Ringer's solution.

Contraindications

Hypersensitivity to pamidronate, other bisphosphonates, or their components

Interactions

DRUGS

calcium-containing preparations; vitamin D preparations, such as calcifediol and calcitriol: Antagonized pamidronate effects when used to treat hypercalcemia
thalidomide: Increased risk of renal dysfunction in patients with multiple myeloma

Adverse Reactions

CNS: Confusion, fever, psychosis, visual hallucinations
CV: Hypotension
EENT: Conjunctivitis
GI: Abdominal cramps, anorexia, GI bleeding, indigestion, nausea, vomiting
GU: Azotemia, focal segmental glomerulosclerosis, nephrotic syndrome, hematuria, renal toxicity leading to failure

P

HEME: Leukopenia, lymphopenia
MS: Bone pain, muscle spasms or stiffness, osteonecrosis (mainly of jaw)
RESP: Dyspnea
SKIN: Pruritus, rash
Other: Anaphylaxis, angioedema, flulike symptoms, hyperkalemia, hypernatremia, hypocalcemia, hypokalemia, hypomagnesemia, hypophosphatemia, injection site pain and swelling, reactivation of herpes simplex and zoster infections

Nursing Considerations
• Make sure patient has had a dental checkup before invasive dental procedures during pamidronate therapy, especially if patient has cancer; is receiving chemotherapy, head or neck radiation, or a corticosteroid; or has poor oral hygiene because the risk of osteonecrosis is increased in these patients.
• **WARNING** Do not give more than 90 mg at any one time because of increased risk of serious adverse effect on kidneys.
• Monitor patient for hypocalcemia, especially if patient has had thyroid surgery.
• Stay alert for fever during the first 3 days of pamidronate therapy, especially in patients receiving high doses. If fever develops, obtain the patient's CBC with differential, as ordered.
• Obtain serum creatinine level before each treatment. Notify prescriber of abnormal results because drug may need to be withheld or dosage adjusted until creatinine level returns to normal.
• Assess patient with anemia, leukopenia, or thrombocytopenia for worsening of the condition during first 2 weeks of therapy.
PATIENT TEACHING
• Stress the importance of complying with prescribed administration schedule for pamidronate.
• Advise patient to avoid calcium and vitamin D supplements during pamidronate therapy.
• Instruct patient on proper oral hygiene and on need to notify prescriber about invasive dental procedures.

pancreatin

Donnazyme: 500 mg pancreatin, 1,000 units lipase, 12,500 units protease, 12,500 units amylase

Hi-Vegi-Lip: 2,400 mg pancreatin, 4,800 units lipase, 60,000 units protease, 60,000 units amylase
4X Pancreatin: 2,400 mg pancreatin, 12,000 units lipase, 60,000 units protease, 60,000 units amylase
8X Pancreatin: 7,200 mg pancreatin, 22,500 units lipase, 180,000 units protease, 180,000 units amylase
Pancrezyme 4X: 2,400 mg pancreatin, 12,000 units lipase, 60,000 units protease, 60,000 units amylase

Class and Category
Chemical class: Pancreatic enzyme
Therapeutic class: Digestant, pancreatic enzyme replacement
Pregnancy category: C

Indications and Dosages
➤ *To treat pancreatic insufficiency, including steatorrhea*
CAPSULES, TABLETS
Adults. 8,000 to 24,000 units of lipase with meals or snacks, adjusted as prescribed, according to need for steatorrhea control. For severe insufficiency, up to 36,000 units of lipase with meals or snacks.

Mechanism of Action
Releases the enzymes pancreatin, lipase, amylase, and protease, mainly in the duodenum and upper jejunum. These enzymes facilitate the hydrolysis of fats into glycerol and fatty acids, starches into dextrins and sugars, and proteins into peptides. Pancreatin acts locally in the GI tract but is quickly inactivated by gastric acid.

Contraindications
Acute exacerbation of chronic pancreatic disease; acute pancreatitis; hypersensitivity to pancreatin, pancrelipase, or pork

Interactions
DRUGS
acarbose, miglitol: Decreased effectiveness of these drugs
aluminum hydroxide, H₂-receptor antagonists, omeprazole, sodium bicarbonate: Increased gastric pH, prolonged enzymatic action of pancreatin
calcium carbonate– and magnesium hydrox-

ide–containing antacids: Decreased pancreatin effectiveness
iron supplements: Decreased iron absorption

Adverse Reactions
EENT: Stomatitis
GI: Abdominal cramps or pain, diarrhea, intestinal obstruction, nausea
SKIN: Rash, urticaria
Other: Hyperuricemia

Nursing Considerations
•**WARNING** Don't administer pancreatin to patient who is allergic to pork.
•Assess patient for GI disturbances and hyperuricemia when giving high doses of pancreatin.
•If patient opens capsules and sprinkles contents on food, watch for signs or symptoms of sensitization (chest tightness, dyspnea, nasal congestion, wheezing), which may result from repeated inadvertent inhalation of powder.
•Be aware that brands of pancreatin aren't interchangeable because the same doses don't contain equivalent amounts of drug.
PATIENT TEACHING
•Instruct patient to take pancreatin before or with meals or snacks to maximize effectiveness.
•To prevent capsule or tablet from lodging in esophagus, advise patient to take drug with a beverage while sitting upright, to swallow it quickly, and to follow with 1 or 2 mouthfuls of solid food.
•Caution patient not to chew tablets; doing so may irritate mouth, lips, and tongue.
•If patient has trouble swallowing capsules, advise her to open the capsule and sprinkle its contents on food without inhaling them.
•Caution patient not to take antacids that contain calcium carbonate or magnesium hydroxide during therapy.

pancrelipase

Cotazym: 8,000 units lipase, 30,000 units protease, 30,000 units amylase
Cotazym-S: 5,000 units of lipase, 20,000 units protease, 20,000 units amylase
Ilozyme: 11,000 units lipase, 30,000 units protease, 30,000 units amylase
Ku-Zyme HP: 8,000 units lipase, 30,000 units

protease, 30,000 units amylase
Pancrease: 4,500 units lipase, 25,000 units protease, 20,000 units amylase
Pancrease MT 4: 4,000 units lipase, 12,000 units protease, 12,000 units amylase
Pancrease MT 10: 10,000 units lipase, 30,000 units protease, 30,000 units amylase
Pancrease MT 16: 16,000 units lipase, 48,000 units protease, 48,000 units amylase
Pancrease MT 20: 20,000 units lipase, 44,000 units protease, 56,000 units amylase
Protilase: 4,000 units lipase, 25,000 units protease, 20,000 units amylase)
Ultrase MT 12: 12,000 units lipase, 39,000 units protease, 39,000 units amylase
Ultrase MT 20: 20,000 units lipase, 65,000 units protease, 65,000 units amylase
Viokase Tablets: 8,000 units lipase, 30,000 units protease, 30,000 units amylase
Viokase Powder: 16,800 units lipase, 70,000 units protease, 70,000 units amylase
Zymase: 12,000 units lipase, 24,000 units protease, 24,000 units amylase

Class and Category
Chemical class: Porcine pancreatic enzyme
Therapeutic class: Pancreatic enzyme replacement
Pregnancy category: C

Indications and Dosages
➤ *To treat pancreatic insufficiency, including steatorrhea*
CAPSULES, DELAYED-RELEASE CAPSULES, POWDER, TABLETS
Adults and adolescents. 33,000 to 44,000 units of lipase before or with meals or snacks; adjusted as prescribed. For patients with severe deficiency, possibly up to 88,000 units of lipase with meals or snacks or dosing frequency increased to every hr.
Children ages 7 to 12. 4,000 to 12,000 units of lipase with meals and snacks; adjusted as needed and tolerated.
Children ages 1 to 6. 4,000 to 8,000 units of lipase with meals and 4,000 units of lipase with each snack; adjusted as needed and tolerated.
Infants ages 6 to 11 months. 2,000 units of lipase with meals; adjusted as needed and tolerated.

Contraindications
Acute exacerbation of chronic pancreatic disease; acute pancreatitis; hypersensitivity to pancreatin, pancrelipase, or pork

Mechanism of Action
Releases high levels of the enzymes lipase, amylase, and protease, mainly in the duodenum and upper jejunum. These enzymes facilitate the hydrolysis of fats into glycerol and fatty acids, starches into dextrins and sugars, and proteins into peptides.

Interactions
DRUGS
acarbose, miglitol: Decreased effectiveness of these drugs
aluminum hydroxide, H₂-receptor antagonists, omeprazole, sodium bicarbonate: Increased gastric pH, prolonged enzymatic action of pancrelipase
calcium carbonate– and magnesium hydroxide–containing antacids: Decreased pancrelipase effectiveness
iron supplements: Decreased iron absorption

Adverse Reactions
EENT: Stomatitis
GI: Abdominal cramps or pain, diarrhea, intestinal obstruction, nausea
HEME: Anemia
SKIN: Rash, urticaria
Other: Hyperuricemia

Nursing Considerations
•WARNING Don't administer pancrelipase to patient who is allergic to pork.
•Be aware that brands of pancrelipase aren't interchangeable because the same doses don't contain equivalent amounts of drug.
•Mix powder with fluid or soft, nondairy food.
•If needed, open delayed-release capsules and mix contents (enteric-coated spheres, microspheres, or microtablets) with liquid or soft food that requires no chewing. Give immediately because enteric coating will dissolve after prolonged contact with foods at a pH greater than 6.
•If patient opens capsules and sprinkles contents on food, assess for signs of sensitization (chest tightness, dyspnea, nasal congestion, wheezing), which may result from repeated inadvertent inhalation of powder.
•Give drug before or with meals and snacks, and follow with a glass of water or juice.
•Expect drug to cause stomatitis if held in mouth.

•Check stool for fecal fat content, as ordered.
•Monitor patient for iron deficiency anemia because serum iron level may decline during pancrelipase therapy.
PATIENT TEACHING
•Instruct patient to take pancrelipase before or with meals and snacks and to follow with a glass of water or juice.
•Instruct patient not to chew capsules (or capsule contents) or crush tablets and to swallow immediately because drug may cause irritation if held in mouth.
•Urge patient not to inhale powder from delayed-release capsules; doing so may cause chest tightness, shortness of breath, stuffy nose, trouble breathing, and wheezing.
•Inform patient that sneezing and tearing also may result from contact with powder.
•Caution patient not to use antacids because they may decrease drug effectiveness.
•Inform patient that her stool may smell foul.

pantoprazole sodium
Pantoloc (CAN), Protonix

Class and Category
Chemical class: Substituted benzimidazole
Therapeutic class: Antiulcer, gastric acid proton pump inhibitor
Pregnancy category: B

Indications and Dosages
➤ *To treat gastroesophageal reflux disease (GERD)*
DELAYED-RELEASE TABLETS
Adults. 40 mg daily for up to 8 wk. Repeated for another 4 to 8 wk if healing doesn't occur.
I.V. INFUSION
Adults. 40 mg daily infused over 2 min or 15 min for 7 to 10 days, followed by oral doses.

➤ *To maintain healing of erosive esophagitis and reduce relapse of daytime and nighttime symptoms in patients with GERD*
DELAYED-RELEASE TABLETS
Adults. 40 mg daily for up to 12 mo.

➤ *To treat pathological hypersecretion associated with Zollinger-Ellison syndrome or other neoplastic conditions*
I.V. INFUSION
Adults. 80 mg every 12 hr infused over 2 min

or 15 min; adjusted based on patient's acid output measurements up to 80 mg every 8 hr.

Route	Onset	Peak	Duration
P.O.	1 day	1 wk	1 wk
I.V.	1 day	Unknown	1 wk

Mechanism of Action

Interferes with gastric acid secretion by inhibiting the hydrogen-potassium-adenosine triphosphatase (H^+-K^+-ATPase) enzyme system, or proton pump, in gastric parietal cells. Normally, the proton pump uses energy from the hydrolysis of ATPase to drive H^+ and chloride (Cl^-) out of parietal cells and into the stomach lumen in exchange for potassium (K^+), which leaves the stomach lumen and enters parietal cells. After this exchange, H^+ and Cl^- combine in the stomach to form hydrochloric acid (HCl). Pantoprazole irreversibly inhibits the final step in gastric acid production by blocking the exchange of intracellular H^+ and extracellular K^+, thus preventing H^+ from entering the stomach and additional HCl from forming.

Incompatibilities

Midazolam and products containing zinc may cause precipitation or discoloration.

Contraindications

Hypersensitivity to pantoprazole, substituted benzimidazoles (omeprazole, lansoprazole, rabeprazole sodium), or their components

Interactions

DRUGS

ampicillin, cyanocobalamin, digoxin, iron salts, ketoconazole: Possibly impaired absorption of these drugs
atazanavir: Significantly decreased atazanavir level
warfarin: Increased INR, PT, and bleeding risk

Adverse Reactions

CNS: Anxiety, asthenia, confusion, dizziness, headache, hypertonia, hypokinesia, insomnia, malaise, migraine, speech disorder vertigo
CV: Chest pain, hypercholesterolemia, hyperlipidemia
EENT: Anterior ischemic optic neuropathy, blurred vision, increased salivation, pharyngitis, rhinitis, sinusitis, tinnitus
ENDO: Hyperglycemia
GI: Abdominal pain, atrophic gastritis, constipation, diarrhea, elevated liver function tests results, flatulence, gastroenteritis, hepatotoxicity, indigestion, nausea, pancreatitis, vomiting
GU: Elevated serum creatinine level, interstitial nephritis
HEME: Pancytopenia
MS: Arthralgia, back or neck pain, rhabdomyolysis
RESP: Bronchitis, dyspnea, increased cough, upper respiratory tract infection
SKIN: Erythema multiforme, rash, Stevens-Johnson syndrome, toxic epidermal necrolysis
Other: Anaphylaxis, angioedema, elevated creatine kinase and phosphokinase levels, flulike symptoms, generalized pain, hyperuricemia, infection, injection site reaction

Nursing Considerations

• Ensure the continuity of gastric acid suppression during transition from oral to I.V. pantoprazole (or vice versa) because even a brief interruption of effective suppression can lead to serious complications.
• Don't give pantoprazole within 4 weeks of testing for *Helicobacter pylori* because antibiotics, proton pump inhibitors, and bismuth preparations suppress *H. pylori* and may lead to false-negative results. Be aware that drug may cause false-positive results in urine screening tests for tetrahydrocannabinol. Obtain guidelines regarding pantoprazole use from prescriber before testing.
• Flush I.V. line with D_5W, normal saline solution, or lactated Ringer's injection before and after giving drug.
• When giving I.V. over 2 minutes, reconstitute with 10 ml of normal saline injection. Solution may be stored up to 2 hours at room temperature.
• When giving I.V. over 15 minutes, reconstitute with 10 ml normal saline injection. Then, further reconstitute with 100 ml (for GERD) or 80 ml (for pathological hypersecretion in Zollinger-Ellison syndrome) of D_5W, normal saline injection, or lactated Ringer's injection. Solution may be stored up to 2 hours before further dilution and up to 22 hours before use.
• Monitor PT or INR during therapy, as ordered, if patient takes an oral anticoagulant.

P

•Be aware that, if drug is given for more than 3 years, patient may not be able to absorb vitamin B_{12} because of hypochlorhydria or achlorhydria. Treatment for cyanocobalamin deficiency may be needed.

PATIENT TEACHING
•Instruct patient to swallow pantoprazole tablets whole and not to chew or crush them.
•Advise patient to expect relief of symptoms within 2 weeks of starting therapy.
•Advise patient who takes warfarin to follow bleeding precautions and to notify prescriber immediately if bleeding occurs.

paricalcitol

Zemplar

Class and Category

Chemical class: Sterol derivative, vitamin D analogue
Therapeutic class: Antihyperparathyroid
Pregnancy category: Not rated

Indications and Dosages

➤ *To prevent and treat secondary hyperparathyroidism in patients with chronic renal failure stage 3 or 4*

I.V. INJECTION

Adults. *Initial:* 0.04 to 0.1 mcg/kg (2.8 to 7 mcg) no more than every other day at any time during dialysis. *Maintenance:* If initial dosage doesn't produce a satisfactory response, 2 to 4 mcg given every 2 to 4 wk. *Maximum:* 0.24 mcg/kg/dose or up to 16.8 mcg/dose.

Children age 5 and over. *Initial:* 0.04 mcg/kg three times weekly if baseline intact parathyroid hormone (iPTH) level is less than 500 pg/ml, or 0.08 mcg/kg three times weekly if baseline iPTH level equals or exceeds 500 pg/ml. *Maintenance:* If initial dosage isn't adequate, adjust in 0.04-mcg/kg increments as needed.

DOSAGE ADJUSTMENT If serum PTH level remains the same or increases, dosage is increased. If serum PTH level decreases by less than 30%, dosage is increased. If serum PTH level decreases by 30% to 60%, dosage is maintained. If serum PTH level decreases by more than 60%, dosage is decreased. If serum PTH level is 1.5 to 3 times the upper limit of normal, dosage is maintained.

DOSAGE ADJUSTMENT Dosage is immediately reduced or stopped if serum calcium level is elevated or serum calcium-phosphorus product exceeds 75. Dosage restarted at a lower dose when these levels return to normal.

CAPSULES

Adults. *Initial:* If baseline iPTH level is less than 500 pg/ml, 1 mcg daily or 2 mcg three times weekly, doses separated by at least 1 day. If iPTH level exceeds 500 pg/ml, 2 mcg daily or 4 mcg three times weekly, doses separated by at least 1 day. *Maintenance:* Dosage adjusted in 1-mcg increments based on iPTH level relative to baseline.

Route	Onset	Peak	Duration
I.V.	Unknown	Unknown	15 hr

Mechanism of Action

Reduces serum PTH level by an unknown mechanism. In chronic renal failure, decreased renal synthesis of vitamin D leads to chronic hypocalcemia. In response, parathyroid glands secrete PTH to stimulate vitamin D synthesis, but serum calcium levels can't normalize because of renal failure.

Contraindications

Evidence of vitamin D toxicity, hypercalcemia, hypersensitivity to paricalcitol or components

Interactions

DRUGS
atazanavir, clarithromycin, indinavir, itraconazole, ketoconazole, nefazodone, nelfinavir, ritonavir, saquinavir, telithromycin, voriconazole: Increased effects of oral paricalcitol
drugs, such as cholestyramine, that impair absorption of fat-soluble vitamins: Possibly impaired absorption of oral paricalcitol

Adverse Reactions

CNS: Arthritis, asthenia, chills, depression, dizziness, fever, headache, insomnia, lightheadedness, malaise, neuropathy, syncope, vertigo
CV: Cardiomyopathy, chest pain, congestive heart failure, edema, hypertension, hypotension, MI, orthostatic hypotension, palpitations
EENT: Amblopia, bronchitis, dry mouth, epistaxis, pharyngitis, retinal abnormality, rhinitis, sinusitis, taste perversion

ENDO: Hypoglycemia
GI: Abdominal pain, constipation, diarrhea, dyspepsia, gastritis, gastroenteritis, GI bleeding, nausea, vomiting
GU: Abnormal kidney function, uremia, UTI
MS: Back pain, leg cramps, myalgia
RESP: Increased cough, pneumonia
SKIN: Ecchymosis, hypertrophy, pruritus, rash (including vesiculobullous), ulceration, urticaria
Other: Acidosis, allergic reaction, dehydration, generalized edema, gout, hyperkalemia, hyperphosphatemia, hypervolemia, hypokalemia, infections, influenza, sepsis

Nursing Considerations
•Before giving drug, look for particles and discoloration; if present, discard drug.
•Give as I.V. bolus; discard unused portion.
•Monitor serum calcium and phosphorus levels, as ordered, twice weekly to guide dosage adjustments and then monthly.
•**WARNING** Paricalcitol may lead to vitamin D toxicity and hypercalcemia. Look for early evidence, including arthralgia, constipation, dry mouth, headache, metallic taste, myalgia, nausea, somnolence, vomiting, and weakness. Also look for late evidence, including albuminuria, anorexia, arrhythmias, azotemia, conjunctivitis (calcific), decreased libido, elevated BUN and serum ALT and AST levels, vascular calcification, hypercholesterolemia, hypertension, hyperthermia, irritability, mild acidosis, nephrocalcinosis, nocturia, pancreatitis, photophobia, polydipsia, polyuria, pruritus, rhinorrhea, and weight loss.
•If toxicity occurs, notify prescriber immediately and expect to decrease or stop drug. Place patient on bed rest and give fluids, low-calcium diet, and a laxative, as prescribed. If patient has a hypercalcemic crisis and dehydration, expect to infuse normal saline solution and a loop diuretic to prompt renal calcium excretion.
•Expect to check patient's serum PTH level every 3 months.
•If patient also takes digoxin, monitor her for evidence of digitalis glycoside toxicity, which is potentiated by hypercalcemia.
•Store drug at 25° C (77° F).
PATIENT TEACHING
•Advise patient to follow a diet high in calcium and low in phosphorus.
•Explain that patient may need phosphate binders to control serum phosphorus level.
•Review the early evidence of hypercalcemia and vitamin D toxicity. Tell patient to contact prescriber immediately if it develops.
•Urge patient to avoid hazardous activities until drug's adverse CNS effects are known.
•If patient takes digoxin, explain evidence of toxicity and the need to contact prescriber immediately if it develops.

paroxetine hydrochloride
Paxil, Paxil CR

paroxetine mesylate
Pexeva

Class and Category
Chemical class: Phenylpiperidine derivative
Therapeutic class: Antidepressant, antiobsessional, antipanic
Pregnancy category: D

Indications and Dosages
➤ *To treat major depression*
C.R. TABLETS
Adults. *Initial:* 25 mg daily, increased as prescribed and tolerated by 12.5 mg daily every wk. *Maximum:* 62.5 mg daily.
ORAL SUSPENSION, TABLETS
Adults. *Initial:* 20 mg daily, increased as prescribed and tolerated by 10 mg daily every wk. *Maximum:* 50 mg daily.

➤ *To treat obsessive-compulsive disorder*
ORAL SUSPENSION, TABLETS
Adults. *Initial:* 20 mg daily, increased as prescribed and tolerated by 10 mg daily every wk. *Usual:* 20 to 60 mg daily. *Maximum:* 60 mg daily.

➤ *To treat panic disorder*
C.R. TABLETS
Adults. *Initial:* 12.5 mg daily, increased by 12.5 mg daily every wk as needed. *Maximum:* 75 mg daily.
ORAL SUSPENSION, TABLETS
Adults. *Initial:* 10 mg daily, increased as prescribed and tolerated by 10 mg daily every wk. *Usual:* 10 to 60 mg daily. *Maximum:* 60 mg daily.

➤ *To treat social anxiety disorder*
C.R. TABLETS
Adults. *Initial:* 12.5 mg daily, increased by 12.5 mg daily every wk as needed. *Maxi-*

P

mum: 37.5 mg daily.

ORAL SUSPENSION, TABLETS (HYDROCHLORIDE)

Adults. *Initial:* 20 mg daily, increased as prescribed and tolerated by 10 mg daily every wk. *Usual:* 20 to 60 mg daily. *Maximum:* 60 mg daily.

➤ *To treat generalized anxiety disorder*

ORAL SUSPENSION, TABLETS (HYDROCHLORIDE)

Adults. *Initial:* 20 mg daily, increased as prescribed and tolerated by 10 mg daily every wk. *Usual:* 20 to 50 mg daily. *Maximum:* 60 mg daily.

➤ *To treat posttraumatic stress disorder*

ORAL SUSPENSION, TABLETS (HYDROCHLORIDE)

Adults. *Initial:* 20 mg daily, increased as prescribed and tolerated by 10 mg daily every wk. *Usual:* 20 to 50 mg daily. *Maximum:* 50 mg daily.

➤ *To treat premenstrual dysphoric disorder*

C.R. TABLETS

Adults. *Initial:* 12.5 mg daily in the morning, increased as needed after 1 wk to 25 mg daily. Or, 12.5 mg daily in the morning only during luteal phase of menstrual cycle (2-wk period before onset of monthly cycle), increased as needed after 1 wk to 25 mg daily in the morning during luteal phase of menstrual cycle.

DOSAGE ADJUSTMENT For patients who are elderly, debilitated, or have creatinine clearance less than 30 ml/min/1.73 m^2, initially 10 mg daily; maximum, 40 mg daily. Avoid C.R. form. For patients taking C.R. tablets with creatinine clearance less than 30 ml/min/1.73 m^2, initially 12.5 mg daily; maximum, 50 mg daily.

Route	Onset	Peak	Duration
P.O.	1 to 4 wk	Unknown	Unknown

Mechanism of Action

Exerts antidepressant, antiobsessional, and antipanic effects by potentiating serotonin activity in the CNS and inhibiting serotonin reuptake at presynaptic neuronal membrane. Blocked serotonin reuptake increases levels and prolongs activity of serotonin at synaptic receptor sites.

Contraindications

Hypersensitivity to paroxetine or its components, pimozide therapy, use within 14 days of an MAO inhibitor, thioridazine therapy

Interactions

DRUGS

antacids: Hastened release of C.R. paroxetine

aspirin, NSAIDs, warfarin: Increased anticoagulant activity and risk of bleeding

astemizole: Increased risk of arrhythmias

atomoxetine; risperidone; other drugs metabolized by CYP2D6, such as amitriptyline, desipramine, fluoxetine, imipramine, phenothiazines, tamoxifen, type IC antiarrhythmics: Increased plasma levels of these drugs

barbiturates, primidone: Decreased blood paroxetine level

cimetidine: Possibly increased blood paroxetine level

cisapride, isoniazid, MAO inhibitors, procarbazine: Possibly serotonin syndrome

codeine, haloperidol, metoprolol, perphenazine, propranolol, risperidone, thioridazine: Decreased metabolism and increased effects of these drugs

cyproheptadine: Decreased paroxetine effects

dextromethorphan: Decreased dextromethorphan metabolism and increased risk of toxicity

digoxin: Possibly decreased digoxin effects

encainide, flecainide, propafenone, quinidine: Potentiated toxicity of these drugs

fosamprenavir, ritonavir: Decreased plasma paroxetine level

lithium: Possibly increased blood paroxetine level, increased risk of serotonin syndrome

methadone: Decreased methadone metabolism, increased risk of adverse effects

phenytoin: Possibly phenytoin toxicity

pimozide: Increased risk of prolonged QT interval

procyclidine: Increased blood procyclidine level and anticholinergic effects

serotonergic drugs such as linezolid, St. John's wort, tramadol, triptans, and tryptophan: Increased risk of serotonin syndrome

tamoxifen: Decreased tamoxifen effectiveness

theophylline: Possibly increased blood theophylline level and risk of toxicity

thioridazine: Increased thioridazine level, possibly leading to prolonged QT interval and life-threatening ventricular arrhythmias

tramadol: Increased risk of serotonin syndrome and seizures

tricyclic antidepressants: Increased metabolism and blood antidepressant levels; increased risk of toxicity, including seizures

Adverse Reactions

CNS: Agitation, akathisia, asthenia, confusion, decreased concentration, dizziness, drowsiness, emotional lability, hallucinations, headache, insomnia, mania, neuroleptic malignant syndrome, psychomotor agitation, restlessness, serotonin syndrome, somnolence, suicidal ideation, tremor
CV: Palpitations, tachycardia
EENT: Blurred vision, dry mouth, rhinitis, taste perversion
GI: Abdominal cramps or pain, anorexia, constipation, diarrhea, flatulence, nausea, vomiting
GU: Decreased libido, difficult ejaculation, impotence, sexual dysfunction, urine retention
MS: Back pain, myalgia, myasthenia, myopathy
SKIN: Diaphoresis, rash
Other: Weight gain or loss

Nursing Considerations

• Shake oral suspension well. Measure with an oral syringe or calibrated device.
• Don't give enteric-coated form with antacids.
• Watch for akathisia (inner sense of restlessness) and psychomotor agitation, especially during the first few weeks of therapy.
• Watch patient closely (especially children, adolescents, and young adults), for suicidal tendencies, particularly when therapy starts and dosage changes, because depression may worsen temporarily during these times, possibly leading to suicidal ideation.
• Watch for mania, which may result from any antidepressant in a susceptible patient.
• Monitor patient closely for evidence of GI bleeding, especially if patient also takes a drug known to cause GI bleeding, such as aspirin, an NSAID, or warfarin.
• **WARNING** Monitor patient closely for serotonin syndrome exhibited by agitation, hallucinations, coma, tachycardia, labile blood pressure, hyperthermia, hyperreflexia, incoordination, nausea, vomiting, or diarrhea. Notify prescriber immediately because serotonin syndrome may be life-threatening. Be prepared to provide supportive care.
• **WARNING** Be aware that serotonin syndrome in its most severe form may resemble neuroleptic malignant syndrome, which includes hyperthermia, muscle rigidity, autonomic instability with possibly rapid changes in vital signs and mental status. Stop drug immediately, and provide supportive care.
• To minimize adverse reactions, expect to taper drug rather than stopping abruptly.

PATIENT TEACHING

• Advise patient to take paroxetine in the morning to minimize insomnia and to take it with food if adverse GI reactions develop.
• Instruct patient to avoid taking C.R. paroxetine within 2 hours of an antacid.
• Tell patient to swallow C.R. tablets whole and not to cut, crush, or chew them.
• Suggest that patient avoid hazardous activities until drug's CNS effects are known.
• Tell family or caregiver to observe patient closely for suicidal tendencies, especially when therapy starts or dosage changes and especially if patient is a child, teenager, or young adult.
• Explain that full effect may take 4 weeks.
• Urge patient to avoid alcohol during paroxetine therapy; its effects on drug are unknown.
• Tell patient not to take aspirin or NSAIDs during therapy because they increase the risk of bleeding. If patient takes warfarin, tell her to adopt bleeding precautions and to notify prescriber at once if bleeding occurs.
• Inform patient that episodes of acute depression may persist for months or longer and that they require continued follow-up.
• Instruct patient not to stop drug abruptly but to taper dosage as instructed.
• Alert female patients of childbearing age that paroxetine may cause birth defects and persistent pulmonary hypertension in the newborn if taken during the first trimester of pregnancy. Stress the need for effective contraception and to notify prescriber if pregnancy occurs or is suspected.
• Caution patient to alert all prescribers about paroxetine therapy because of potentially serious drug interactions.

pegfilgrastim

Neulasta

Class and Category

Chemical class: Recombinant granulocyte colony-stimulating factor conjugate
Therapeutic class: Antineutropenic, hematopoietic stimulator
Pregnancy category: C

Indications and Dosages

➤ *To reduce the risk of infection, as manifested by febrile neutropenia, after myelosuppressive chemotherapy*

Adults. 6 mg with each chemotherapy cycle.

Contraindications
Hypersensitivity to filgrastim, pegfilgrastim, or their components or to proteins derived from *Escherichia coli*

Mechanism of Action
Induces formation of neutrophil progenitor cells by binding to receptors on granulocytes, which then divide. Pegfilgrastim also potentiates the effects of mature neutrophils, thus reducing fever and the risk of infection from severe neutropenia. It is pharmacologically identical to human granulocyte colony-stimulating factor.

Interactions
DRUGS
lithium: Increased neutrophil production

Adverse Reactions
CNS: Fever
GI: Elevated liver function test results, splenic rupture, splenomegaly
GU: Elevated uric acid level
HEME: Leukocytosis, sickle cell crisis
MS: Bone pain
RESP: Acute respiratory distress syndrome, dyspnea, hypoxia, pulmonary infiltrates
SKIN: Acute febrile neutrophilic dermatosis (Sweet's syndrome), erythema, flushing, rash, urticaria
Other: Anaphylaxis, angioedema, antibody formation to pegfilgrastim, injection site reactions (pain, induration, erythema)

Nursing Considerations
•Avoid giving pegfilgrastim for 14 days before and 24 hours after cytotoxic chemotherapy.
•Check CBC, hematocrit, and platelet count before and periodically during therapy.
•Let drug warm to room temperature before injection. Use prefilled syringe and needles.
•Don't shake the solution.
•Discard drug that contains particles, is discolored, or was stored more than 48 hours at room temperature.
•**WARNING** If signs of allergy occur, stop pegfilgrastim infusion and notify prescriber at once. If anaphylaxis occurs, give antihistamine, epinephrine, corticosteroid, and bronchodilator, as ordered.

•**WARNING** Be aware that patients receiving filgrastim (parent drug) have had splenic rupture and acute respiratory distress syndrome. Assess patient for fever, respiratory distress, and upper abdominal or shoulder tip pain.
•Assess patients with sickle cell disease for signs of sickle cell crisis; urge hydration.
•Give nonopioid and opioid analgesics, as ordered, if patient experiences bone pain.
•Store drug at 2° to 8° C (36° to 46° F), and protect from freezing and light.
•Be aware that needle cover contains dry natural rubber and should not be handled by persons with a latex allergy.

PATIENT TEACHING
•Urge patient to promptly report possibly serious reactions (trouble breathing, rash, chest tightness, left upper abdominal pain, shoulder tip pain) and evidence of infection (fever, chills).
•If patient will be giving herself the drug, teach her how to prepare, give, and store it.
•Alert her that needle cover contains dry natural rubber and should not be handled if she has a latex allergy.
•Tell patient to rotate injection sites among thigh, abdomen (except for 2″ around navel), buttocks, and outer, upper arms. Caution her to avoid tender, hard, red, or bruised areas.
•Urge patient to discard used needles and syringes in a puncture-resistant container and not to reuse them.
•Stress the importance of follow-up tests.
•Advise patient to store pegfilgrastim in refrigerator and not to freeze it. Tell her to discard drug if left unrefrigerated for more than 48 hours.

pegvisomant

Somavert

Class and Category
Chemical class: Human growth hormone (GH) receptor antagonist
Therapeutic class: Growth suppressant
Pregnancy category: B

Indications and Dosages
➤ *To treat acromegaly in patients with an inadequate response to surgery, radiation, or other medical treatment or for whom such treatment is inappropriate*

Mechanism of Action

In acromegaly, elevated blood levels of growth hormone (GH) overstimulate the liver to produce excessive amounts of insulin-like growth factors (IGFs), such as IGF-1. Excessive IGFs before puberty stimulate the linear growth of bones, causing the patient's unusual height and extremely long arms and legs. After puberty, the excessive hormone secretion causes periosteal bone proliferation, resulting in widening of the hands and feet, and coarsening of the facial features, as well as other complications.

Pegvisomant selectively blocks GH cell surface receptors. As a result, the liver delivers less IGF-1 and other proteins to the blood, preventing the overgrowth of bone and other tissues.

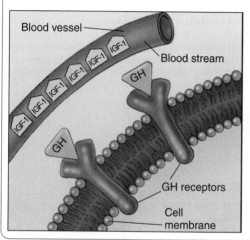

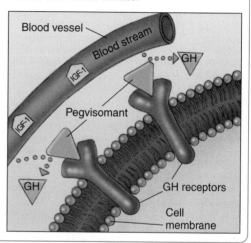

SUBCUTANEOUS INJECTION
Adults. *Initial:* 40 mg as loading dose on day 1; then 10 mg daily. *Maintenance:* Adjusted every 4 to 6 wk in 5-mg increments if insulin-like growth factor-I (IGF-I) levels are abnormal. *Maximum:* 30 mg daily.

Contraindications

Hypersensitivity to pegvisomant, its components, or latex

Interactions

DRUGS

Insulin, oral antidiabetics: Enhanced action of insulin and oral antidiabetics, possibly resulting in hypoglycemia
Opioids: Decreased serum pegvisomant levels

Adverse Reactions

CNS: Dizziness, paresthesia
CV: Chest pain, hypertension, peripheral edema
EENT: Ear infection, sinusitis
GI: Diarrhea, elevated liver function test results, nausea
MS: Back pain

RESP: Upper respiratory tract infection
SKIN: Blisters
Other: Cold, flulike symptoms, injection site lipohypertrophy and pain, weight gain

Nursing Considerations

•Obtain liver enzyme levels before starting pegvisomant, as ordered. If they're elevated but 3 times or less normal, expect to monitor them monthly for 6 months, quarterly for 6 months, and then twice yearly for the next year. If they're more than 3 times normal, expect to withhold drug until the cause of elevation has been determined.
•Reconstitute drug by injecting 1 ml of diluent provided (sterile water for injection) into vial, aiming the stream against vial wall. Hold vial between the palms of both hands and roll gently to dissolve powder. Don't shake. Give within 6 hours of reconstitution, and discard any remaining amount.
•Watch for evidence of liver dysfunction during therapy. If liver enzyme levels rise to 3 to 5 times normal but patient has no evi-

dence of liver dysfunction (jaundice, bilirubinuria, fatigue, nausea, vomiting, right-upper-quadrant pain, ascites, unexplained edema, easy bruising) or increases in serum total bilirubin level, expect therapy to continue but liver enzymes to be monitored weekly and a complete hepatic workup to be done. If enzyme levels are at least 5 times above normal or transaminase level is at least 3 times above normal with increased total bilirubin (with or without evidence of hepatic dysfunction), notify prescriber immediately and expect to stop drug. If patient develops evidence of hepatic dysfunction, regardless of liver enzyme levels, notify prescriber immediately, and expect a complete liver workup to be performed. If liver damage is confirmed, expect drug to be stopped.

•Monitor patient's IGF-1 levels every 4 to 6 weeks, as ordered, until they've normalized and then every 6 months. Notify prescriber if levels are decreased or elevated. Be aware that GH levels should not be used to make dosage adjustments because pegvisomant interferes with laboratory measurement of GH.

PATIENT TEACHING
•Teach patient how to reconstitute and administer pegvisomant.
•Tell patient about the need for frequent laboratory studies and their importance to properly adjust drug dosage and detect drug-related abnormalities.
•Advise patient to stop drug immediately and notify prescriber if her skin or whites of her eyes become yellow or she has other evidence of liver dysfunction, such as dark urine, light-colored stools, little or no appetite for several days, nausea, tiredness, or abdominal pain.
•Instruct woman of childbearing age to report known or suspected pregnancy.
•Caution patient to tell prescriber about all other drugs she's taking.

penbutolol sulfate

Levatol

Class and Category

Chemical class: Nonselective beta-adrenergic blocker
Therapeutic class: Antihypertensive
Pregnancy category: Not rated

Indications and Dosages

➤ *To manage hypertension*
TABLETS
Adults. 20 mg daily.
DOSAGE ADJUSTMENT For elderly patients, dosage individualized according to sensitivity to drug.

Route	Onset	Peak	Duration
P.O.	Unknown	1.5 to 3 hr	Unknown

Mechanism of Action

May reduce blood pressure by competing with beta-adrenergic receptor agonists, which helps reduce cardiac output, decrease sympathetic outflow to peripheral blood vessels, and inhibit renin release by the kidneys.

Contraindications

Asthma, bradycardia (fewer than 45 beats/min), cardiogenic shock, heart failure, hypersensitivity to penbutolol or its components, second- or third-degree AV block

Interactions

DRUGS
allergen immunotherapy, allergenic extracts for skin testing: Increased risk of serious systemic reaction or anaphylaxis
amiodarone: Additive depressant effect on cardiac conduction, negative inotropic effects
anesthetics (hydrocarbon inhalation): Increased risk of myocardial depression and hypotension
calcium channel blockers, clonidine, diazoxide, guanabenz, other hypotension-producing drugs, reserpine: Additive hypotension and possibly other beta blocker effects
cimetidine: Possibly increased blood penbutolol level
estrogens: Decreased antihypertensive effect of penbutolol
fentanyl and its derivatives: Possibly increased risk of initial bradycardia after induction doses of fentanyl derivative (with long-term penbutolol use)
insulin, oral antidiabetic drugs: Possibly impaired glucose control and masking of hypoglycemia symptoms such as tachycardia
lidocaine: Decreased lidocaine clearance, increased risk of lidocaine toxicity
MAO inhibitors: Increased risk of significant

hypertension

neuromuscular blockers: Possibly potentiated and prolonged action of these drugs

NSAIDs: Possibly decreased hypotensive effect of penbutolol

other beta blockers: Additive beta blocker effects

phenothiazines: Increased blood levels of both drugs

phenytoin (parenteral): Additive cardiac depressant effects

sympathomimetics, xanthines: Possibly inhibited effects of penbutolol and these drugs

Adverse Reactions

CNS: Anxiety, depression, dizziness, drowsiness, fatigue, insomnia, light-headedness, nervousness, syncope, weakness

CV: Bradycardia, chest pain, edema, peripheral vascular insufficiency

EENT: Nasal congestion

GI: Constipation, diarrhea, epigastric pain, nausea, vomiting

GU: Impotence

RESP: Bronchospasm, dyspnea

Nursing Considerations

•Expect varied drug effectiveness in elderly patients, who may be more sensitive to penbutolol's antihypertensive effects because of reduced drug clearance by kidneys.

•**WARNING** Avoid stopping therapy abruptly because doing so may precipitate myocardial infarction, myocardial ischemia, severe hypertension, or ventricular arrhythmias, particularly in patients with cardiovascular disease. Watch for tachycardia because drug may also mask certain signs of hyperthyroidism. Be aware that abrupt withdrawal of drug in patients with hyperthyroidism or thyrotoxicosis can precipitate thyroid storm.

•Monitor blood pressure and cardiac output, as appropriate, in patients who have a history of systolic heart failure or left ventricular dysfunction because drug's negative inotropic effect can depress cardiac output.

•Monitor patients with diabetes mellitus who take antidiabetic drugs because penbutolol can prolong hypoglycemia or promote hyperglycemia. Be aware that penbutolol can also mask signs of hypoglycemia, especially tachycardia, palpitations, and tremor.

•Watch for impaired circulation in elderly patients with age-related peripheral vascular disease or patients with Raynaud's phenomenon. Elderly patients are also at increased risk for beta blocker–induced hypothermia.

•Monitor drug refill frequency to help determine patient compliance.

PATIENT TEACHING

•Instruct patient to take penbutolol at the same time every day and not to change dosage without consulting prescriber.

•Advise patient not to stop taking drug abruptly, but to taper dosage gradually under prescriber's supervision.

•Instruct patient with diabetes mellitus to regularly monitor blood glucose level and test urine for ketones.

•Advise patient to consult prescriber before taking OTC drugs, especially cold remedies.

•Urge patient to avoid hazardous activities until CNS effects of drug are known.

•Instruct patient to inform prescriber of chest pain, fainting, light-headedness, or shortness of breath, any of which may indicate the need for a dosage change.

•Inform patient that penbutolol doesn't cure hypertension. Encourage her to follow recommended diet and lifestyle changes.

penicillamine

Cuprimine, Depen

Class and Category

Chemical class: Degradation product of penicillin

Therapeutic class: Antirheumatic, antiurolithic, chelating agent

Pregnancy category: D

Indications and Dosages

➤ *To treat cystinuria*

CAPSULES, TABLETS

Adults and adolescents. 500 mg q.i.d.

Children. 7.5 mg/kg q.i.d.

➤ *To treat rheumatoid arthritis*

CAPSULES, TABLETS

Adults and adolescents. *Initial:* 125 or 250 mg daily. Dosage increased by 125 or 250 mg daily every 2 to 3 mo. *Maximum:* 1,500 mg daily.

➤ *To treat Wilson's disease*

CAPSULES, TABLETS

Adults and adolescents. Dosage individualized up to 2 g daily in divided doses q.i.d. by

P

measuring urinary copper excretion.

DOSAGE ADJUSTMENT For elderly patients, 125 mg daily initially, then increased by 125 mg daily every 2 to 3 mo, up to maximum of 750 mg daily; for pregnant women, maximum dose of 1 g daily; for women undergoing planned cesarean section, dosage limited to 250 mg daily during last 6 wk of pregnancy and until wound healing completed.

Route	Onset	Peak	Duration
P.O.	2 to 3 mo*	Unknown	Unknown

Mechanism of Action

Combines with copper to form a ring-shaped complex that is excreted in urine, thereby reducing copper levels in the body. Penicillamine also lowers urine cystine levels by binding with cystine to form penicillamine-cysteine disulfide, which is more soluble than cystine and more easily excreted in urine. The decrease in urine cystine levels also helps prevent the formation of cystine calculi and may help existing cystine calculi dissolve over time. In addition, penicillamine improves lymphocyte function by reducing IgM rheumatoid factor and immune complexes in serum and synovial fluid, which may play a role in the treatment of rheumatoid arthritis.

Contraindications

Hypersensitivity to penicillin, penicillamine, or their components; penicillamine-related aplastic anemia or agranulocytosis; renal insufficiency (for patients with rheumatoid arthritis)

Interactions

DRUGS

4-aminoquinolines, bone marrow depressants, gold compounds, immunosuppressants (excluding glucocorticoids), phenylbutazone: Possibly increased risk of serious hematologic or renal adverse reactions
iron supplements: Possibly decreased effectiveness of penicillamine

---

* For rheumatoid arthritis; 1 to 3 mo for Wilson's disease.

pyridoxine: Decreased effectiveness of pyridoxine, possibly increased risk of anemia or peripheral neuritis reaction

Adverse Reactions

CNS: Agitation, anxiety, fever, mental changes, myasthenic syndrome, neuropathy
EENT: Altered or loss of taste, optic neuritis, stomatitis, tinnitus
GI: Anorexia, diarrhea, hepatic dysfunction, intrahepatic cholestasis, mild epigastric pain, pancreatitis, nausea, toxic hepatitis, vomiting
GU: Glomerulonephropathy, hematuria, proteinuria, renal failure
HEME: Agranulocytosis, aplastic anemia, hemolytic anemia, leukopenia, thrombocytopenia
MS: Arthralgia, dystonia, muscle weakness
SKIN: Pemphigus, pruritus, rash, urticaria
Other: Lupuslike symptoms, lymphadenopathy

Nursing Considerations

•Use penicillamine cautiously in elderly patients because they're at greater risk for rash, altered taste, and renal impairment.
•Administer penicillamine 1 hour before or 2 hours after meals and at least 1 hour before or after any other drug, food, or milk. Give last dose of day at least 3 hours after evening meal to ensure maximum absorption.
•For patient who has difficulty swallowing capsules or tablets, open capsule and mix contents in 15 to 30 ml of pureed fruit or fruit juice to mask drug's sulfur odor. Alternatively, request pharmacist to prepare an elixir for oral administration.
•Expect to administer 25 mg of pyridoxine, as prescribed, to patients being treated with penicillamine because penicillamine increases intake requirements for this vitamin.
•Watch for febrile reactions in patients who developed a fever during previous penicillamine therapy. Expect drug to be discontinued if patient develops drug-induced fever.
•Assess skin and mucous membranes for possible sensitivity reactions, such as skin lesions and mouth ulcers. Be prepared to discontinue drug as prescribed.
•Expect to monitor urine laboratory test results, as ordered, twice weekly during the first month of therapy, then every 2 weeks for the next 5 months, and monthly thereafter. Watch for proteinuria or hematuria,

which may precipitate nephrotic syndrome, especially in patients with renal disease or history of renal insufficiency. Also, weigh patient daily, observe for signs of edema, and monitor intake and output because penicillamine may worsen underlying renal disease.

•**WARNING** Monitor patient's WBC and differential cell count, hemoglobin, and platelet count, as ordered, and assess patient's skin, lymph nodes, and body temperature for abnormalities twice weekly during first month of therapy, then every 2 weeks for the next 5 months, and monthly thereafter because drug may cause potentially serious hematologic reactions.

•Because of the potential for cross-sensitivity between penicillamine and penicillin, monitor for symptoms of an allergic reaction in patients with a history of penicillin allergy.

•Notify prescriber if patient complains of decreased sense of taste, especially for salty and sweet foods. Expect normal taste sensation to be restored (except in patients with Wilson's disease) with administration of 5 to 10 mg of copper a day, as prescribed.

•Monitor patients with diabetes mellitus for reduced insulin requirements to prevent the risk of nighttime hypoglycemia because penicillamine may promote the formation of anti-insulin antibodies.

•Check liver function tests, as ordered, every 6 months (every 3 months for first year if patient has Wilson's disease) throughout penacillamine therapy because drug may cause serious hepatic dysfunction.

PATIENT TEACHING
•Advise patient to take penicillamine on an empty stomach.

•Instruct adult male and nonpregnant female patients with cystinuria to increase their fluid intake and follow the prescribed low-methionine diet to minimize cystine production and enhance drug's effectiveness. Encourage patient to drink about 1 pint of fluid at bedtime and again during the night because this is when urine is more concentrated.

•Tell patient to notify prescriber immediately if he develops a fever, sore throat, chills, bruising, or bleeding because drug may need to be stopped.

•Instruct patient being treated for Wilson's disease to follow a diet low in copper, avoiding such foods as broccoli, chocolate, copper-enriched cereals, liver, molasses, mushrooms,

nuts, and shellfish. Inform her that it may take 1 to 3 months of therapy for her condition to improve.

•Advise patient to consult prescriber before having dental work done during penicillamine therapy because drug can promote mouth ulcers.

•Instruct patient to avoid consuming iron during penicillamine therapy because iron can decrease drug's effectiveness.

•Explain that sense of taste may decrease during penicillamine therapy. Advise patient to notify prescriber if it becomes intolerable.

•Inform patient with rheumatoid arthritis that improvement may take 2 to 3 months of therapy.

•Caution female patient to notify prescriber immediately if she becomes or may be pregnant because dosage may need to be reduced to prevent serious birth defects.

penicillin G benzathine
Bicillin C-R, Bicillin C-R 900/300, Bicillin L-A, Megacillin (CAN), Permapen

penicillin G potassium
Megacillin (CAN), Pentids, Pfizerpen

penicillin G procaine
Ayercillin (CAN), Crysticillin 300 AS, Pfizerpen-AS, Wycillin

penicillin G sodium
penicillin V potassium
Apo-Pen-VK (CAN), Beepen-VK, Betapen-VK, Ledercillin VK, Nadopen-V 200 (CAN), Nadopen-V 400 (CAN), Novo-Pen-VK (CAN), Nu-Pen VK (CAN), Pen Vee (CAN), Pen Vee K, V-Cillin K (CAN), Veetids

Class and Category
Chemical class: Penicillin
Therapeutic class: Antibiotic
Pregnancy category: B

Indications and Dosages
➤ *To treat systemic infections caused by gram-positive organisms (including* Bacillus anthracis, Corynebacterium diphtheriae, *enterococci,* Listeria monocytogenes, Staphylococcus aureus, *and*

S. epidermidis), *gram-negative organisms (including* Neisseria gonorrhoeae, N. meningitidis, Pasteurella multocida, *and* Streptobacillus moniliformis *[rat-bite fever]), and gram-positive anaerobes (including* Actinomyces israelii *[actinomycosis],* Clostridium perfringens, C. tetani, Peptococcus *species,* Peptostreptococcus *species, and spirochetes, especially* Treponema carateum *[pinta],* T. pallidum, *and* T. pertenue *[yaws]*)

ORAL SOLUTION, TABLETS (PENICILLIN G POTASSIUM)
Adults and adolescents. 200,000 to 500,000 units (125 to 312 mg) every 4 to 6 hr. *Maximum:* 2 million units daily.
Children. 4,167 to 15,000 units/kg every 4 hr, 6,250 to 22,500 units/kg every 6 hr, or 8,333 to 30,000 units/kg every 8 hr.

TABLETS (PENICILLIN V POTASSIUM)
Adults and adolescents. 200,000 to 800,000 units (125 to 500 mg) every 6 to 8 hr. *Maximum:* 11,520,000 units (7,200 mg) daily
Children. 4,167 to 13,280 units (2.5 to 8.3 mg)/kg every 4 hr, 6,250 to 20,000 units (3.75 to 12.5 mg)/kg every 6 hr, or 8,333 to 26,720 units (5 to 16.7 mg)/kg every 8 hr.

I.V. INFUSION, I.M. INJECTION (PENICILLIN G POTASSIUM, PENICILLIN G SODIUM)
Adults and adolescents. 1 to 5 million units every 4 to 6 hr. *Maximum:* 80 million units daily.
Children. 8,333 to 16,667 units/kg every 4 hr or 12,500 to 25,000 units/kg every 6 hr.
Premature and full-term neonates. 30,000 units/kg every 12 hr.

I.M. INJECTION (PENICILLIN G PROCAINE)
Adults and adolescents. 600,000 to 1,200,000 units daily in divided doses every 12 to 24 hr.

➤ *To treat moderately severe to severe streptococcal infections*
I.M. INJECTION (PENICILLIN G BENZATHINE)
Adults and children weighing more than 45 kg (100 lb). 1.2 million units as a single injection.
Children weighing 27 to 45 kg (59 to 100 lb). 900,000 units as a single injection.
Children weighing less than 27 kg. 300,000 to 600,000 units as a single injection.

➤ *To treat congenital syphilis*
I.M. INJECTION (PENICILLIN G BENZATHINE: BICILLIN L-A ONLY)
Children under age 2. 50,000 units/kg as a single injection.

➤ *To treat syphilis of less than 1 year's duration*
I.M. INJECTION (PENICILLIN G BENZATHINE: BICILLIN L-A ONLY)
Adults and adolescents. 2.4 million units as a single injection.
Children. 50,000 units/kg up to adult dosage as a single injection. *Maximum:* 2.4 million units/dose.

➤ *To treat syphilis of more than 1 year's duration*
I.M. INJECTION (PENICILLIN G BENZATHINE: BICILLIN L-A ONLY)
Adults and adolescents. 2.4 million units every wk for 3 wk.
Children. 50,000 units/kg every wk for 3 wk.

➤ *To treat bacterial meningitis*
I.V. INFUSION, I.M. INJECTION (PENICILLIN G POTASSIUM)
Adults. 50,000 units/kg every 4 hr or 24 million units daily in divided doses every 2 to 4 hr.

Mechanism of Action
Inhibits the final stage of bacterial cell wall synthesis by competitively binding to penicillin-binding proteins inside the cell wall. Penicillin-binding proteins are responsible for various steps in bacterial cell wall synthesis. By binding to these proteins, penicillin leads to cell wall lysis.

Contraindications
Hypersensitivity to penicillin or its components

Incompatibilities
Don't mix any penicillin in the same syringe or container with aminoglycosides because aminoglycosides will be inactivated. Don't mix penicillin G with drugs that may result in a pH below 5.5 or above 8.

Interactions
DRUGS
ACE inhibitors, potassium-containing drugs, potassium-sparing diuretics: Increased risk of hyperkalemia (penicillin G potassium)
chloramphenicol, erythromycin, sulfonamides,

tetracycline, thrombolytics: Possibly interference with penicillin's bactericidal effect
cholestyramine, colestipol: Possibly impaired absorption of oral penicillin G
methotrexate: Decreased methotrexate clearance, increased risk of toxicity
oral contraceptives: Decreased contraceptive effectiveness (with penicillin V)
probenecid: Increased blood penicillin level
Foods
acidic beverages, such as fruit juices: Possibly altered effects of oral penicillin G

Adverse Reactions
CNS: Confusion, dizziness, dysphasia, hallucinations, headache, lethargy, sciatic nerve irritation, seizures
CV: Labile blood pressure, palpitations
EENT: Black "hairy" tongue, oral candidiasis, stomatitis, taste perversion
GI: Abdominal pain, diarrhea, elevated liver function test results (transient), indigestion, nausea, pseudomembranous colitis
GU: Interstitial nephritis (acute), vaginal candidiasis
MS: Muscle twitching
SKIN: Rash
Other: Electrolyte imbalances; injection site necrosis, pain, or redness

Nursing Considerations
•Obtain body tissue and fluid samples for culture and sensitivity tests as ordered before giving first dose. Expect to begin drug therapy before test results are known.
•Reconstitute vials of penicillin for injection with sterile water for injection, D_5W, or sodium chloride for injection.
•Administer penicillin at least 1 hour before other antibiotics.
•Inject I.M. form deep into large muscle mass. Apply ice to relieve pain.
•**WARNING** Give penicillin G benzathine and penicillin G procaine only by deep I.M. injection; I.V. injection may be fatal, and intra-arterial injection may cause extensive tissue and organ necrosis.
•Be aware that I.M. drug is absorbed slowly, which may make allergic reactions difficult to treat.
•Assess patient for signs of secondary infection, such as profuse, watery diarrhea. If such diarrhea develops, contact prescriber and expect to obtain a stool specimen to rule out pseudomembranous colitis caused by

Clostridium difficile. If diarrhea occurs, notify prescriber and expect to withhold penicillin and treat with fluids, electrolytes, protein, and an antibiotic effective against *C. difficile.*
•Monitor serum sodium level and assess for early signs of heart failure in patients receiving high doses of penicillin G sodium.
•When giving penicillin G potassium to patient at risk for hypertension or fluid overload, be aware that each gram of penicillin G potassium also contains 1.02 mEq of sodium.
Patient Teaching
•Instruct patient to report previous allergies to penicillins and to notify prescriber immediately about adverse reactions, including fever.
•Advise patient who uses oral contraceptives to use an additional form of contraception during penicillin V therapy.
•Urge patient to tell prescriber if diarrhea develops, even 2 months or more after penicillin therapy ends.

pentamidine isethionate

NebuPent, Pentacarinat (CAN), Pentam 300, Pneumopent (CAN)

Class and Category
Chemical class: Diamidine derivative
Therapeutic class: Antiprotozoal
Pregnancy category: C

Indications and Dosages
➤ *To prevent* Pneumocystis jiroveci (carinii) *pneumonia*
Oral inhalation (NebuPent, Pentacarinat)
Adults and adolescents. 300 mg every 4 wk or 150 mg every 2 wk, using nebulizer and continuing until chamber is empty (30 to 45 min).
Oral inhalation (Pneumopent)
Adults and adolescents. *Initial:* 60 mg every 24 to 72 hr for 5 doses over 2 wk, using ultrasonic nebulizer and continuing until nebulizer chamber is empty (about 15 min). *Maintenance:* 60 mg every 2 wk, using ultrasonic nebulizer and continuing until nebulizer chamber is empty.
➤ *To treat* P. jiroveci (carinii) *pneumonia*
I.V. infusion, I.M. injection
Adults and children. 4 mg/kg daily for 14 to 21 days, given deep I.M. or by I.V. infusion over 1 to 2 hr.

P

DOSAGE ADJUSTMENT Dosage possibly reduced or I.V. infusion time or dosing interval extended for patients with renal failure.

Mechanism of Action

May bind to DNA and inhibit DNA replication in *Pneumocystis jiroveci (carinii)*. Pentamidine also may inhibit dihydrofolate reductase, an enzyme needed to convert dihydrofolic acid to tetrahydrofolic acid in this organism. This action inhibits the formation of coenzymes that are essential to the growth and replication of *P. jiroveci*.

Incompatibilities

Don't mix pentamidine with other drugs or with saline solutions because precipitation may occur.

Contraindications

History of anaphylactic reaction to pentamidine or its components (inhalation form)

Interactions

DRUGS

bone marrow depressants, drugs that cause blood dyscrasias: Increased risk of adverse hematologic effects
didanosine: Increased risk of pancreatitis
erythromycin (I.V.): Increased risk of torsades de pointes
foscarnet: Increased risk of severe but reversible hypocalcemia, hypomagnesemia, and nephrotoxicity
nephrotoxic drugs: Increased risk of nephrotoxicity

Adverse Reactions

CNS: Chills, confusion, dizziness, fatigue, fever, hallucinations, headache (I.V., I.M. forms)
CV: Arrhythmias, edema, hypotension, prolonged QT interval, torsades de pointes, ventricular tachycardia (I.V., I.M. forms)
EENT: Bitter or metallic taste (all forms), pharyngitis (inhalation form)
ENDO: Diabetes mellitus, hyperglycemia (I.V., I.M. forms); hypoglycemia (all forms)
GI: Abdominal pain, anorexia, diarrhea, elevated liver function test results, nausea, vomiting (I.V., I.M. forms); pancreatitis (all forms)

GU: Elevated serum creatinine level (I.V., I.M. forms); renal insufficiency (inhalation form)
HEME: Anemia, leukopenia, thrombocytopenia, unusual bleeding or bruising (I.V., I.M. forms)
MS: Myalgia (I.V., I.M. forms)
RESP: Bronchospasm, chest pain or congestion, cough, dyspnea, extrapulmonary pneumocystosis, pneumothorax (inhalation form)
SKIN: Night sweats (I.V., I.M. forms); rash (all forms)
Other: Hyperchloremic acidosis; hyperkalemia; hypocalcemia; hypomagnesemia; infusion site sterile abscess (I.V. form); injection site induration, pain, and phlebitis (I.M. form)

Nursing Considerations

• Store pentamidine at room temperature, protected from light. Use within 24 hours after reconstitution.
• For I.V. use, dissolve contents of 300-mg vial with 3 to 5 ml of sterile water for injection or D₅W. Further dilute in 50 to 250 ml of D₅W and infuse over 1 to 2 hours.
• For I.M. use, dissolve contents of vial in 3 ml of sterile water for injection and inject deep into large muscle mass. Be aware that I.M. administration increases the risk of sterile abscess formation at injection site.
• When giving drug I.V. or I.M., keep patient supine and monitor blood pressure frequently during and after administration. Keep emergency resuscitation equipment readily available.
• Assess for hypoglycemia and arrhythmias in patient receiving I.V. or I.M. pentamidine. Although uncommon, these adverse reactions can be severe.
• For inhalation, reconstitute contents of vial with 6 ml sterile water for injection (NebuPent or Pentacarinat) or 3 to 5 ml sterile water for injection or inhalation (Pneumopent). Reconstitute immediately before use. Don't use normal saline solution because it causes precipitation. Place reconstituted drug in Respirgard II nebulizer, and set flow rate at 5 to 7 L/min for NebuPent or Pentacarinat. Don't mix with any other drugs. For Pneumopent, place reconstituted drug in Fisoneb ultrasonic nebulizer and set flow rate at the mid-flow mark.
• Administer aerosolized pentamidine with patient in supine or recumbent position for best distribution of drug.

•If patient who uses inhalation form has a history of asthma or smoking, notify prescriber if bronchospasm or a cough develops. She may need an aerosolized bronchodilator before each dose of pentamidine.

•Monitor CBC; platelet count; liver function test results; BUN, serum creatinine and calcium, and blood glucose levels; and ECG tracing throughout therapy, as ordered.

•Monitor blood glucose level because pentamidine use can induce insulin release from pancreas, causing severe hypoglycemia that can last from 1 day to several weeks.

•Be aware that hyperglycemia and diabetes mellitus can occur up to several months after discontinuation of parenteral therapy.

PATIENT TEACHING

•Stress importance of complying with the prescribed administration schedule when pentamidine is used to prevent *P. jiroveci (carinii)* pneumonia.

•Advise patient to avoid potentially hazardous activities until drug's CNS effects are known.

•Instruct patient to notify prescriber about unusual bleeding or bruising and to take precautions to avoid bleeding, such as using a soft-bristled toothbrush and an electric shaver.

•Caution patient about possible hypoglycemic effects of pentamidine therapy.

•Advise patient to have follow-up laboratory studies to test for diabetes mellitus, which can occur up to several months after stopping pentamidine therapy.

pentazocine lactate

Talwin

Class, Category, and Schedule
Chemical class: Synthetic opioid
Therapeutic class: Analgesic
Pregnancy category: C
Controlled substance schedule: IV

Indications and Dosages
➤ *To relieve moderate to severe pain*
I.V., I.M., OR SUBCUTANEOUS INJECTION
Adults. *Initial:* 30 mg every 3 to 4 hr, p.r.n. *Maximum:* 30 mg/single dose I.V., 60 mg/single dose I.M. or subcutaneously, or 360 mg/ 24 hr for all parenteral forms.

➤ *To relieve obstetric pain*
I.V. INJECTION
Adults. 20 mg when contractions become regular; repeated 2 or 3 times every 2 to 3 hr, as prescribed.

I.M. INJECTION
Adults. 30 mg as a single dose.

Route	Onset	Peak	Duration
I.V.	2 to 3 3 min	15 to 30 min	2 to 3 hr
I.M., SubQ	15 to 20 min	30 to 60 min	2 to 3 hr

Mechanism of Action
Binds with opioid receptors, primarily kappa and sigma receptors, at many CNS sites to alter the perception of and emotional response to pain.

Incompatibilities
Don't mix pentazocine in same syringe with a soluble barbiturate because precipitation will occur.

Contraindications
Hypersensitivity to pentazocine or its components

Interactions
DRUGS
anticholinergics: Increased risk of urine retention and severe constipation
antidiarrheals, antiperistaltics: Increased risk of severe constipation and CNS depression
antihypertensives, diuretics, other hypotension-producing drugs: Additive hypotensive effects
buprenorphine: Decreased pentazocine effectiveness, increased respiratory depression
CNS depressants: Increased CNS depression, increased risk of habituation
hydroxyzine, other opioid analgesics: Increased analgesia, CNS depression, and hypotensive effects
MAO inhibitors: Increased risk of unpredictable, severe, even fatal adverse reactions
metoclopramide: Antagonized metoclopramide effects on GI motility
naloxone: Antagonized analgesic, CNS, and respiratory depressant effects of pentazocine
naltrexone: Withdrawal symptoms in patients physically dependent on pentazocine
neuromuscular blockers: Increased respiratory depression

P

ACTIVITIES
alcohol use: Additive CNS depression and increased risk of habituation

Adverse Reactions

CNS: Chills, dizziness, drowsiness, euphoria, fatigue, headache, insomnia, light-headedness, nervousness, nightmares, paresthesia, restlessness, weakness
CV: Hypotension, tachycardia
EENT: Blurred vision, diplopia, dry mouth, laryngeal edema, laryngospasm
GI: Constipation, hepatotoxicity, nausea, vomiting
GU: Decreased urine output, dysuria, urinary frequency, urine retention
MS: Muscle rigidity (with large doses)
RESP: Atelectasis, bronchospasm, dyspnea, hypoventilation, wheezing
SKIN: Diaphoresis, erythema multiforme, facial flushing, pruritus, rash, Stevens-Johnson syndrome, toxic epidermal necrolysis, urticaria
Other: Facial edema; injection site burning, pain, redness, or swelling; physical and psychological dependence

Nursing Considerations

• Use pentazocine with extreme caution in patients who have head injury, intracranial lesion, or increased intracranial pressure because drug may mask neurologic evidence.
• Use pentazocine cautiously in patients who are physically dependent on opioid agonists because drug may prompt withdrawal symptoms; in patients with acute MI because drug's cardiovascular effects can increase cardiac workload; in patients with renal or hepatic dysfunction because drug is metabolized in the liver and excreted in urine; and in patients with respiratory conditions because drug depresses the respiratory system.
• When administering repeated parenteral doses, use I.M. or I.V. route when possible and as prescribed because subcutaneous route may cause severe tissue damage at injection site. Rotate I.M. sites to avoid tissue damage.
• After giving parenteral form, expect to taper dosage gradually, as prescribed, to reduce the risk of withdrawal symptoms.

PATIENT TEACHING
• Caution patient that prolonged use of pentazocine may result in drug dependence.
• Advise patient to avoid potentially hazardous activities until drug's CNS effects are known.
• Caution patient not to use alcohol or OTC drugs without consulting prescriber.
• Advise patient to report possible allergic reaction, such as a rash or itching.

pentobarbital sodium

Nembutal, Nova Rectal (CAN), Novopentobarb (CAN)

Class, Category, and Schedule

Chemical class: Barbiturate
Therapeutic class: Anticonvulsant, sedative-hypnotic
Pregnancy category: D
Controlled substance schedule: II (oral, parenteral), III (rectal)

Indications and Dosages

➤ *To provide daytime sedation*

ELIXIR
Adults. 20 mg t.i.d. or q.i.d.
Children. 2 to 6 mg/kg daily.
SUPPOSITORIES
Adults. 30 mg b.i.d. to q.i.d.
Children. 2 mg/kg t.i.d.

➤ *To provide short-term treatment of insomnia*

CAPSULES, ELIXIR
Adults. 100 mg at bedtime.
I.V. INJECTION
Adults. *Initial:* 100 mg, with additional small doses at 1-min intervals, as prescribed. *Maximum:* 500 mg.
I.M. INJECTION
Adults. 150 to 200 mg at bedtime.
SUPPOSITORIES
Adults and adolescents over age 14. 120 to 200 mg at bedtime.
Children ages 12 to 14. 60 to 120 mg at bedtime.
Children ages 5 to 12. 60 mg at bedtime.
Children ages 1 to 4. 30 to 60 mg at bedtime.
Infants ages 2 months to 1 year. 30 mg at bedtime.

➤ *To provide preoperative sedation*

CAPSULES, ELIXIR
Adults. 100 mg before surgery.
Children. 2 to 6 mg/kg before surgery. *Maximum:* 100 mg/dose.
I.M. INJECTION
Adults. 150 to 200 mg before surgery.
Children. 2 to 6 mg/kg before surgery. *Maximum:* 100 mg/dose.

SUPPOSITORIES

Children ages 12 to 14. 60 to 120 mg before surgery.

Children ages 5 to 12. 60 mg before surgery.

Children ages 1 to 4. 30 to 60 mg before surgery.

Infants ages 2 months to 1 year. 30 mg before surgery.

➤ *To provide emergency treatment of seizures associated with eclampsia, meningitis, status epilepticus, tetanus, or toxic reactions to local anesthetics or strychnine*

I.V. INJECTION

Adults. 100 mg, with additional small doses at 1-min intervals, as prescribed. *Maximum:* 500 mg.

Children. 50 mg, with additional small doses at 1-min intervals, as prescribed, until desired effect occurs.

I.M. INJECTION

Children. 50 mg, with additional small doses at 1-min intervals, as prescribed, until desired effect occurs.

DOSAGE ADJUSTMENT Dosage possibly reduced for elderly or debilitated patients and those with hepatic dysfunction.

Route	Onset	Peak	Duration
P.O., P.R.	15 to 60 min	1 to 4 hr	3 to 4 hr
I.V.	In 1 min	Unknown	15 min
I.M.	10 to 25 min	Unknown	3 to 4 hr

Mechanism of Action

Inhibits ascending conduction in the reticular formation, which controls CNS arousal to produce drowsiness, hypnosis, and sedation. Pentobarbital also decreases the spread of seizure activity in the cortex, thalamus, and limbic system. It promotes an increased threshold for electrical stimulation in the motor cortex, which may contribute to anticonvulsant effects.

Contraindications

Hepatic disease; history of addiction to hypnotics or sedatives; hypersensitivity to pento-

barbital, barbiturates, or their components; nephritis; porphyria; severe respiratory disease with airway obstruction or dyspnea

Interactions

DRUGS

acetaminophen: Possibly decreased effects of acetaminophen (long-term pentobarbital use)

carbamazepine, chloramphenicol, corticosteroids, cyclosporine, dacarbazine, digoxin, disopyramide, doxycycline, griseofulvin, metronidazole, oral contraceptives, phenylbutazone, quinidine, theophyllines, vitamin D: Decreased effectiveness of these drugs

CNS depressants: Increased CNS depression and risk of habituation

divalproex sodium, valproic acid: Increased risk of CNS toxicity and neurotoxicity

guanadrel, guanethidine: Possibly increased risk of orthostatic hypotension

halogenated hydrocarbon anesthetic: Increased risk of hepatotoxicity (with long-term pentobarbital use)

haloperidol: Possibly decreased blood haloperidol level, possibly altered seizure pattern or frequency

hydantoins: Possibly interference with hydantoin metabolism

leucovorin: Possibly decreased anticonvulsant effect of pentobarbital

maprotiline: Possibly enhanced CNS depression and decreased therapeutic effects of pentobarbital

mexiletine: Possibly decreased blood mexiletine level

oral anticoagulants: Possibly decreased therapeutic effects of these drugs, possibly increased risk of bleeding when pentobarbital is discontinued

tricyclic antidepressants: Possibly decreased therapeutic effects of these drugs

ACTIVITIES

alcohol use: Increased CNS depression

Adverse Reactions

CNS: Agitation, anxiety, ataxia, confusion, delusions, depression, dizziness, drowsiness, fever, hallucinations, headache, insomnia, irritability, nervousness, nightmares, paradoxical stimulation, seizures, syncope, tremor

CV: Orthostatic hypotension

EENT: Vision changes

GI: Anorexia, constipation, hepatic dysfunction, nausea, vomiting

HEME: Agranulocytosis

P

MS: Arthralgia, bone pain, muscle twitching or weakness
RESP: Respiratory depression
SKIN: Exfoliative dermatitis, rash, Stevens-Johnson syndrome
Other: Physical and psychological dependence, weight loss

Nursing Considerations

• Use pentobarbital with extreme caution in patients with depression, a history of drug abuse, or suicidal tendencies.
• Use drug cautiously in elderly or debilitated patients and those with acute or chronic pain because it may induce paradoxical stimulation.
• When using I.V. route, inject drug at 50 mg/min or less to avoid adverse respiratory and circulatory reactions.
• If patient shows premonitory signs of hepatic coma, withhold drug and notify prescriber immediately.
• Monitor I.V. site closely and avoid extravasation. Drug is highly alkaline and may cause local tissue damage and necrosis.

PATIENT TEACHING
• Inform patient that pentobarbital is habit-forming, and stress the importance of taking it exactly as prescribed.
• Instruct patient who takes elixir form to use a calibrated measuring device and to close container tightly after use.
• Instruct patient who uses suppositories to refrigerate them.
• Advise patient to avoid potentially hazardous activities until drug's CNS effects are known.
• Urge patient to avoid alcohol and other CNS depressants because they may increase drug's adverse CNS effects.

pentosan polysulfate sodium

Elmiron

Class and Category

Chemical class: Low-molecular-weight heparin-like compound
Therapeutic class: Local anti-inflammatory (bladder-specific)
Pregnancy category: B

Indications and Dosages

➤ *To relieve bladder discomfort or pain caused by interstitial cystitis*

CAPSULES
Adults. 100 mg t.i.d. for up to 3 mo, possibly followed by another 3 mo if no improvement and no adverse reactions occur.

Mechanism of Action

Adheres to the mucosal membrane of the bladder wall and may block irritating solutes from reaching the cells, thereby decreasing local pain and discomfort.

Contraindications

Hypersensitivity to pentosan, other structurally related compounds, or their components

Interactions

DRUGS
alteplase (recombinant), aspirin (high doses), heparin, oral anticoagulants, streptokinase: Increased risk of hemorrhage

Adverse Reactions

CNS: Depression, dizziness, emotional lability, headache
GI: Abdominal pain, diarrhea, hepatic dysfunction, indigestion, nausea, rectal hemorrhage
HEME: Unusual bleeding or bruising
SKIN: Alopecia, rash

Nursing Considerations

• Use pentosan with extreme caution in patients with conditions that increase bleeding risk, such as aneurysm, diverticula, GI ulceration, hemophilia, polyps, and thrombocytopenia (especially heparin-induced).
• Use drug cautiously in patients with hepatic dysfunction because drug is desulfated in the liver and spleen.
• Monitor for abnormal bleeding, such as unexplained bruises and epistaxis, because drug is a weak anticoagulant.

PATIENT TEACHING
• Instruct patient to take pentosan with a full glass of water at least 1 hour before or 2 hours after meals.
• Explain the pattern of exacerbations and remissions with interstitial cystitis. Reassure patient that symptoms should improve within 3 months after starting therapy.
• Advise patient to take bleeding precautions during therapy, such as using an electric shaver and a soft-bristled toothbrush.

•If alopecia develops, explain that it's usually confined to a single area.

pentoxifylline

Trental

Class and Category
Chemical class: Xanthine derivative
Therapeutic class: Blood viscosity reducer
Pregnancy category: C

Indications and Dosages
➤ *To treat peripheral vascular disease*
E.R. TABLETS
Adults. 400 mg t.i.d. with meals.
DOSAGE ADJUSTMENT Dosage possibly reduced to 400 mg b.i.d. for patients who experience adverse GI or CNS reactions.

Route	Onset	Peak	Duration
P.O.	2 to 4 wk	Unknown	Unknown

Mechanism of Action
Relieves symptoms of peripheral vascular disease through several actions. Pentoxifylline:
• reduces blood viscosity by decreasing the plasma fibrinogen level and inhibiting RBC and platelet aggregation
• improves erythrocyte flexibility by inhibiting phosphodiesterase and increasing the amount of cAMP in RBCs
• decreases peripheral vascular resistance and improves microcirculatory blood flow and tissue oxygenation.

Contraindications
Hypersensitivity to pentoxifylline, methylxanthines (such as caffeine, theophylline, and theobromine), or their components; recent cerebral or retinal hemorrhage

Interactions
DRUGS
antihypertensives: Potentiated antihypertensive effects
cefamandole, cefoperazone, cefotetan, heparin, oral anticoagulants, other platelet aggregation inhibitors, plicamycin, thrombolytics, valproic acid: Increased risk of bleeding
cimetidine: Increased blood pentoxifylline level, increased risk of adverse effects
sympathomimetics, xanthines: Enhanced CNS stimulation
ACTIVITIES
smoking: Possibly decreased therapeutic effects of pentoxifylline

Adverse Reactions
CNS: Asceptic meningitis, dizziness, headache
GI: Indigestion, nausea, vomiting

Nursing Considerations
•Use pentoxifylline cautiously in elderly patients and those with hepatic or renal dysfunction.
•Administer drug with meals and also with an antacid, if needed, to reduce adverse GI reactions.
PATIENT TEACHING
•Instruct patient to swallow pentoxifylline E.R. tablets whole and not to crush, break, or chew them.
•Advise patient to take drug with meals to reduce GI irritation. If adverse GI reactions occur anyway, advise her to also take an antacid with meals.
•Although symptoms may not improve for several weeks, urge patient to continue taking drug as prescribed to achieve maximum therapeutic effect.
•Instruct patient not to smoke during therapy because smoking constricts blood vessels and may reduce drug effectiveness.
•Urge patient to notify prescriber about adverse reactions; dosage may need reduction.

perindopril erbumine

Aceon

Class and Category
Chemical class: Perindoprilat prodrug
Therapeutic class: Antihypertensive
Pregnancy category: D

Indications and Dosages
➤ *To manage hypertension*
TABLETS
Adults. *Initial:* 4 mg daily as a single dose or in divided doses b.i.d., increased as prescribed until blood pressure is controlled or maximum dosage is reached. *Maintenance:* 4 to 8 mg daily. *Maximum:* 8 mg daily.
DOSAGE ADJUSTMENT If patient takes a di-

uretic, initial dosage possibly reduced to 2 to 4 mg daily; if patient has renal failure, initial dosage possibly reduced to 2 mg daily.

➤ *To reduce risk of cardiovascular death or nonfatal MI in patients with stable coronary artery disease*

TABLETS

Adults. *Initial:* 4 mg daily for 2 wk; then increased to 8 mg daily. *Maintenance:* 8 mg daily.

DOSAGE ADJUSTMENT If patient is elderly, 2 mg daily for 1 wk, increased to 4 mg daily for 1 wk and then to 8 mg daily if tolerated.

Mechanism of Action

Is converted to the active metabolite perindoprilat, which competes with angiotensin I binding sites, blocking conversion of angiotensin I to angiotensin II, a potent vasoconstrictor. As a result, this ACE inhibitor reduces vasoconstriction and blood pressure. Decreased angiotensin II also reduces aldosterone secretion, increasing renal excretion of water and sodium.

Contraindications

History of angioedema with ACE inhibitor treatment; hypersensitivity to perindopril, other ACE inhibitors, or their components

Interactions

DRUGS

diuretics: Increased risk of hypotension
lithium: Increased blood lithium level and risk of toxicity
potassium-sparing diuretics, potassium supplements: Increased risk of hyperkalemia
sodium aurothiomalate: Increased risk of nitritoid reaction with facial flushing, nausea, vomiting, and hypotension

Adverse Reactions

CNS: Amnesia, anxiety, dizziness, fatigue, fever, headache, hypertonia, migraine, syncope, vertigo
CV: Chest pain, ECG changes, heart murmur, hypotension, orthostatic hypotension, palpitations, PVCs
EENT: Conjunctivitis, earache, epistaxis, hoarseness, pharyngitis, rhinitis, sinusitis, sneezing, tinnitus
GI: Abdominal pain, diarrhea, elevated liver function test results, flatulence, increased appetite, indigestion
GU: Flank pain, renal calculi, urinary frequency and urgency, vaginitis
HEME: Hematoma, leukopenia, neutropenia
MS: Arthritis, back pain, gout, limb pain, myalgia, neck pain
RESP: Cough
SKIN: Canker sores, diaphoresis, dry skin, ecchymosis, erythema, pruritus, rash
Other: Angioedema, facial edema

Nursing Considerations

• Use cautiously with heart failure, renal artery stenosis, or renal dysfunction.
• Also use cautiously in elderly patients, and watch closely for adverse effects such as dizziness or vertigo, because these patients have an increased risk of falling.
• Monitor patients with hepatic dysfunction for enhanced therapeutic drug effects because drug's bioavailability is increased.
• Monitor serum potassium level to detect hyperkalemia, especially in patients with renal insufficiency or diabetes mellitus and those who use a potassium-containing salt substitute or take a potassium-sparing diuretic or potassium supplement.

PATIENT TEACHING

• Instruct patient to take perindopril exactly as prescribed, even if she feels well.
• **WARNING** Urge patient to stop taking drug and notify prescriber immediately if she experiences signs of angioedema.
• Advise patient to notify prescriber at once about fever, sore throat, or other signs that may indicate neutropenia.
• Urge patient to avoid taking potassium supplements and using potassium-containing salt substitutes unless prescriber approves.
• Instruct patient to avoid hazardous activities until drug's CNS effects are known.
• Advise woman to promptly report suspected, known, or intended pregnancy. Drug will need to be discontinued.

perphenazine

Apo-Perphenazine (CAN), PMS Perphenazine (CAN), Trilafon, Trilafon Concentrate

Class and Category

Chemical class: Piperazine phenothiazine
Therapeutic class: Antiemetic, antipyschotic
Pregnancy category: Not rated

Indications and Dosages

➤ *To treat psychotic disorders*

ORAL SOLUTION

Hospitalized adults and adolescents. 8 to 16 mg b.i.d. to q.i.d., adjusted as prescribed and tolerated. *Maximum:* 64 mg daily.

TABLETS

Adults and adolescents. 4 to 16 mg b.i.d. to q.i.d., adjusted as prescribed and tolerated. *Maximum:* 64 mg daily.

I.M. INJECTION

Adults and adolescents. 5 to 10 mg every 6 hr, adjusted as prescribed and tolerated. *Maximum:* 15 mg daily for outpatients, 30 mg daily for hospitalized patients.

➤ *To treat severe nausea and vomiting*

TABLETS

Adults and adolescents. 8 to 16 mg daily in divided doses, decreased as appropriate. *Maximum:* 24 mg daily.

I.V. INFUSION OR INJECTION

Adults and adolescents. 1 mg every 1 to 2 min, up to 5 mg total.

I.M. INJECTION

Adults and adolescents. 5 mg, increased to 10 mg as ordered for rapid control of severe vomiting. *Maximum:* 15 mg daily for outpatients, 30 mg daily for hospitalized patients.

DOSAGE ADJUSTMENT Initial dose possibly reduced and gradually increased for elderly, emaciated, or debilitated patients. Adolescents may need low adult dosage.

Route	Onset	Peak	Duration
P.O.	Several wk	4 to 7 days	Unknown
I.M.	Unknown	1 to 2 hr	6 hr

Mechanism of Action

Depresses areas of the brain that control activity and aggression, including the cerebral cortex, hypothalamus, and limbic system, by an unknown mechanism. Perphenazine also prevents nausea and vomiting by inhibiting or blocking dopamine receptors in the medullary chemoreceptor trigger zone and peripherally by blocking the vagus nerve in the GI tract.

Incompatibilities

Don't mix perphenazine oral solution with beverages that contain caffeine or tannins (such as coffee, colas, and teas) or pectinates (such as apple juice) because they're physically incompatible.

Contraindications

Blood dyscrasias; bone marrow depression; cerebral arteriosclerosis; coma; concurrent use of CNS depressants (large doses); coronary artery disease; hepatic impairment; hypersensitivity to perphenazine, other phenothiazines, or their components; myeloproliferative disorders; severe CNS depression; severe hypertension or hypotension; subcortical brain damage

Interactions

DRUGS

aluminum- and magnesium-containing antacids, antidiarrheals (adsorbent): Decreased absorption of oral perphenazine

amantadine, anticholinergics, antidyskinetics, antihistamines: Increased adverse anticholinergic effects

amphetamines: Decreased therapeutic effects of both drugs

anticonvulsants: Decreased seizure threshold, inhibited metabolism and toxicity of anticonvulsant

antithyroid drugs: Increased risk of agranulocytosis

apomorphine: Additive CNS depression, decreased emetic response to apomorphine if perphenazine is given first

appetite suppressants (except phenmetrazine): Antagonized anorectic effect of appetite suppressants

beta blockers: Increased blood levels of both drugs and risk of arrhythmias, hypotension, irreversible retinopathy, and tardive dyskinesia

bromocriptine: Possibly interference with bromocriptine's effects

CNS depressants: Increased CNS and respiratory depression and hypotensive effects

dopamine: Antagonized peripheral vasoconstriction with high doses of dopamine

ephedrine: Decreased vasopressor response to ephedrine

epinephrine: Blocked alpha-adrenergic effects of epinephrine, possibly causing severe hypotension and tachycardia

hepatotoxic drugs: Increased risk of hepatotoxicity

hypotension-causing drugs: Increased risk of severe orthostatic hypotension

P

levodopa: Inhibited antidyskinetic effects of levodopa
lithium: Possibly neurotoxicity (disorientation, extrapyramidal symptoms, unconsciousness)
maprotiline, selective serotonin reuptake inhibitors, tricyclic antidepressants: Prolonged and intensified sedative and anticholinergic effects of these drugs or perphenazine
metrizamide: Decreased seizure threshold
opioid analgesics: Increased CNS and respiratory depression, increased risk of orthostatic hypotension and severe constipation
ototoxic drugs, especially antibiotics: Possibly masking of some symptoms of ototoxicity, such as dizziness, tinnitus, and vertigo
probucol, other drugs that prolong QT interval: Prolonged QT interval, which may increase risk of ventricular tachycardia
thiazide diuretics: Possibly hyponatremia and water intoxication

ACTIVITIES
alcohol use: Increased CNS and respiratory depression, hypotensive effects, and risk of heatstroke

Adverse Reactions

CNS: Behavioral changes, cerebral edema, dizziness, drowsiness, extrapyramidal reactions (such as akathisia, dystonia, pseudoparkinsonism), fever, headache, neuroleptic malignant syndrome, seizures, suicidal ideation, syncope, tardive dyskinesia (persistent)
CV: Bradycardia, cardiac arrest, hypertension, hypotension, orthostatic hypotension, tachycardia
EENT: Blurred vision, dry mouth, glaucoma, laryngeal edema, miosis, mydriasis, nasal congestion, ocular changes (corneal opacification, retinopathy)
ENDO: Decreased libido, galactorrhea, gynecomastia, syndrome of inappropriate ADH secretion
GI: Anorexia, constipation, diarrhea, fecal impaction, nausea, vomiting
GU: Bladder paralysis, ejaculation failure, menstrual irregularities, polyuria, urinary frequency, urinary incontinence, urine retention
HEME: Agranulocytosis, eosinophilia, hemolytic anemia, leukopenia, pancytopenia, thrombocytopenic purpura
RESP: Asthma
SKIN: Diaphoresis, eczema, erythema, exfolia-
tive dermatitis, hyperpigmentation, jaundice, pallor, photosensitivity, pruritus, urticaria
Other: Anaphylaxis, angioedema

Nursing Considerations
•Perphenazine shouldn't be used to treat dementia-related psychosis in the elderly because of an increased mortality risk.
•Use perphenazine cautiously in patients with depression or hepatic, pulmonary, or renal dysfunction and in elderly patients, who are at increased risk for increased plasma concentrations and tardive dyskinesia.
•For I.V. use, dilute drug to 0.5 mg/ml with sodium chloride for injection. Protect solution from light. Slight yellowing is acceptable, but discard solution if it's markedly discolored or contains precipitate.
•Obtain blood samples for CBC and liver and renal function tests, as ordered, to detect adverse reactions.
•Monitor temperature frequently, and notify prescriber if it rises; a significant increase suggests drug intolerance.
•Monitor blood pressure of patient who takes large doses of perphenazine, especially if surgery is indicated, because of the increased risk of hypotension.
•Watch patient closely (especially children, adolescents, and young adults), for suicidal tendencies, particularly when perphenazine therapy starts and dosage changes, because depression may worsen temporarily during these times, possibly leading to suicidal ideation.

PATIENT TEACHING
•Instruct patient to take perphenazine exactly as prescribed to ensure optimal effectiveness and minimize adverse reactions.
•Remind patient who takes oral solution to use a calibrated measuring device.
•Instruct patient taking oral solution to dilute every 5 ml (teaspoon) of drug in 2 fluid oz of water, milk, tomato juice, fruit juice (except apple), soup, or carbonated beverage. Caution against using beverages that contain caffeine or tannins (cola, coffee, tea).
•Caution patient not to spill oral solution on skin or clothing because it can cause contact dermatitis and damage clothing.
•Urge patient to avoid alcohol and other CNS depressants during perphenazine therapy and to avoid potentially hazardous ac-

tivities until drug's CNS effects are known.
•Advise patient to avoid excessive sun exposure and to protect skin when outdoors.
•Instruct patient to notify prescriber about persistent or severe adverse reactions.
•Urge patient to comply with long-term follow-up to detect adverse reactions and determine possible need for perphenazine dosage adjustments.
•Urge family or caregiver to watch patient closely for suicidal tendencies, especially when therapy starts or dosage changes and particularly if patient is a child, teenager, or young adult.

phenazopyridine hydrochloride

Azo-Standard, Baridium, Eridium, Geridium, Phenazo (CAN), Phenazodine, Pyridiate, Pyridium, Urodine, Urogesic, Viridium

Class and Category
Chemical class: Azo dye
Therapeutic class: Urinary analgesic
Pregnancy category: B

Indications and Dosages
➤ *To relieve burning and pain on urination, and urinary frequency and urgency*
TABLETS
Adults and adolescents. 200 mg t.i.d. with or without food for no longer than 2 days.
Children. 4 mg/kg t.i.d. with food for no longer than 2 days.

Mechanism of Action
Exerts a topical or local anesthetic effect on the mucosa of the urinary tract as drug is excreted in urine. Phenazopyridine's exact mechanism is unknown.

Contraindications
Hypersensitivity to phenazopyridine or its components, renal insufficiency

Adverse Reactions
CNS: Headache
GI: Indigestion, nausea, vomiting
GU: Reddish orange urine
SKIN: Pruritus, rash
Other: Discoloration of body fluids

Nursing Considerations
•Notify prescriber if yellowish skin or sclerae develop in patient taking phenazopyridine because this may indicate drug accumulation from impaired renal excretion. Expect prescriber to discontinue drug.
•Be aware that phenazopyridine treatment should be limited to 2 days in patients with UTI.
PATIENT TEACHING
•Instruct patient not to take phenazopyridine for longer than 2 days and to notify prescriber if symptoms persist beyond that time.
•If GI distress develops, advise patient to take drug with meals.
•Inform patient that drug turns urine orange to red and may discolor other body fluids, such as tears.
•Advise patient not to wear contact lenses during therapy because they may become stained.

phenelzine sulfate

Nardil

Class and Category
Chemical class: Hydrazine derivative
Therapeutic class: Antidepressant
Pregnancy category: C

Indications and Dosages
➤ *To treat depression*
TABLETS
Adults. *Initial:* 1 mg/kg daily, increased gradually as prescribed and tolerated. *Maintenance:* 45 mg daily. *Maximum:* 90 mg daily.
DOSAGE ADJUSTMENT For elderly patients, initially may be reduced to 0.8 to 1 mg/kg daily in divided doses, increased as ordered and tolerated to maximum of 60 mg daily.

Route	Onset	Peak	Duration
P.O.	7 to 10 days	4 to 8 wk	10 days

Contraindications
Cardiovascular disease; cerebrovascular disease; heart failure; hepatic disease; history of headaches; hypersensitivity to phenelzine or its components; hypertension; pheochromocytoma; severe renal impairment; use of anesthetics, antihypertensives, bupropion, buspirone, carbamazepine, CNS depressants,

P

Mechanism of Action

Phenelzine relieves symptoms of unipolar depressive disorders by inhibiting the enzyme monoamine oxidase (MAO). Normally, MAO breaks down monoamine neurotransmitters, such as serotonin, as shown below left. By inhibiting this enzyme, phenelzine increases the concentration of serotonin in the vesicles of monoamine nerve endings, allowing more serotonin to be released and engage with receptors on postsynaptic cells, as shown below right. A serotonin deficiency may be responsible in part for endogenous depression.

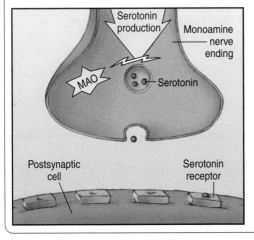

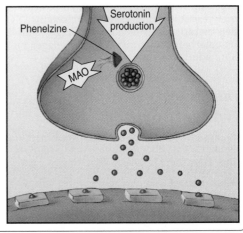

cyclobenzaprine, dextromethorphan, meperidine, selective serotonin-reuptake inhibitors, sympathomimetics, or tricyclic antidepressants; use within 14 days of other MAO inhibitor

Interactions

DRUGS

anticholinergics, antidyskinetics, antihistamines: Increased anticholinergic effect, prolonged CNS depression (antihistamines)
anticonvulsants: Increased CNS depression, possibly altered pattern of seizures
beta blockers: Increased risk of bradycardia
bromocriptine: Possibly interference with bromocriptine effects
bupropion: Increased risk of bupropion toxicity
buspirone: Increased risk of hypertension
caffeine-containing drugs: Increased risk of dangerous arrhythmias and severe hypertension
carbamazepine, cyclobenzaprine, maprotiline, other MAO inhibitors: Increased risk of hyperpyretic crisis, hypertensive crisis, severe seizures, and death; altered pattern of seizures (with carbamazepine)

CNS depressants: Increased CNS depression
dextromethorphan: Increased risk of excitation, hypertension, and hyperpyrexia
diuretics: Increased hypotensive effect
doxapram: Increased vasopressor effects of either drug
fluoxetine: Increased risk of agitation, confusion, GI symptoms, hyperpyretic episodes, hypertensive crisis, potentially fatal serotonin syndrome, restlessness, and severe seizures.
guanadrel, guanethidine: Increased risk of hypertension
haloperidol, loxapine, molindone, phenothiazines, pimozide, thioxanthenes: Prolonged and intensified anticholinergic, hypotensive, and sedative effects of these drugs or phenelzine
insulin, oral antidiabetic drugs: Increased hypoglycemic effects
levodopa: Increased risk of sudden, moderate to severe hypertension
local anesthetics (with epinephrine or levonordefrin): Possibly severe hypertension
meperidine, other opioid analgesics: In-

creased risk of coma, hyperpyrexia, hypotension, immediate excitation, rigidity, seizures, severe hypertension, severe respiratory depression, sweating, vascular collapse, and death

methyldopa: Increased risk of hallucinations, headache, hyperexcitability, and severe hypertension

methylphenidate: Increased CNS stimulant effect of methylphenidate

metrizamide: Decreased seizure threshold, increased risk of seizures

oral anticoagulants: Increased anticoagulant activity

paroxetine, sertraline, trazodone, tricyclic antidepressants: Increased risk of potentially fatal serotonin syndrome

phenylephrine (nasal or ophthalmic): Potentiated vasopressor effect of phenylephrine

rauwolfia alkaloids: Increased risk of moderate to severe hypertension, CNS depression (when phenelzine is added to rauwolfia alkaloid therapy), CNS excitation and hypertension (when rauwolfia alkaloid is added to phenelzine therapy)

spinal anesthetics: Increased risk of hypotension

succinylcholine: Possibly increased neuromuscular blockade of succinylcholine

sympathomimetics: Prolonged and intensified cardiac stimulant and vasopressor effects

tryptophan: Increased risk of confusion, disorientation, hyperreflexia, hyperthermia, hyperventilation, mania or hypomania, and shivering

FOODS

foods and beverages high in tyramine or other pressor amines, such as aged cheese; beer; fava beans or other broad beans; cured meat or sausage; liqueurs; overripe fruit; red and white wine; reduced-alcohol and alcohol-free beer and wine; sauerkraut; sherry; smoked or pickled fish, meats, and poultry; yeast or protein extracts: Increased risk of sudden, severe hypertension

ACTIVITIES

alcohol use: Increased CNS depressant effects and hypertensive crisis

Adverse Reactions

CNS: Agitation, dizziness, drowsiness, headache, overstimulation, restlessness, sedation, sleep disturbance, suicidal ideation, weakness

CV: Bradycardia, edema, hypertensive crisis, orthostatic hypotension, palpitations, tachycardia

EENT: Blurred vision, dry mouth, photophobia

ENDO: Hypoglycemia in diabetic patients

GI: Abdominal pain, constipation, diarrhea, elevated liver function test results, increased appetite, nausea

GU: Impotence, priapism, sexual dysfunction, urinary frequency, urine retention

MS: Muscle twitching

SKIN: Diaphoresis, rash

Other: Hypernatremia, weight gain

Nursing Considerations

• Use phenelzine cautiously in patients with epilepsy because drug may alter seizure threshold.

• Use phenelzine cautiously in patients with diabetes mellitus because insulin sensitivity may increase, predisposing patient to hypoglycemia.

• Expect to observe some therapeutic effect within 7 to 10 days, but keep in mind that full effect may not occur for 4 to 8 weeks.

• Monitor cardiovascular status closely for changes in heart rate (especially if patient receives more than 30 mg daily) and signs of life-threatening hypertensive crisis. Question patient frequently about headaches and palpitations. If either occurs, notify prescriber and expect to discontinue drug.

• Keep phentolamine readily available to treat hypertensive crisis. Give 5 mg by slow I.V., as prescribed, to reduce blood pressure without causing excessive hypotension. Use external cooling measures, as prescribed, to manage fever.

• To avoid hypertensive crisis, expect to wait 10 to 14 days, as prescribed, when switching patient from one MAO inhibitor to another or when switching from a dibenzazepine-related drug, such as amitriptyline or perphenazine.

• Watch closely for suicidal tendencies, especially in children, adolescents, and young adults and especially when therapy starts or dosage changes.

PATIENT TEACHING

• Inform patient and family members that therapeutic effects of phenelzine may take several weeks to appear and that she should continue taking drug as prescribed.

P

•Caution patient to rise slowly from a lying or sitting position to minimize effects of orthostatic hypotension.

• **WARNING** Instruct patient to avoid the following foods, beverages, and drugs during phenelzine therapy and for 2 weeks afterward: alcohol-free and reduced-alcohol beer and wine; appetite suppressants; beer; broad beans; cheese (except cottage and cream cheese); chocolate and caffeine in large quantities; dry sausage (including Genoa salami, hard salami, pepperoni, and Lebanon bologna); hay fever drugs; inhaled asthma drugs; liver; meat extract; OTC cold and cough preparations (including those containing dextromethorphan), nasal decongestants (tablets, drops, or spray); pickled herring; products that contain tryptophan; protein-rich foods that may have undergone protein changes by aging, pickling, fermenting, or smoking; sauerkraut; sinus drugs; weight-loss preparations; yeast extracts (including brewer's yeast in large quantities); yogurt; and wine.

•Advise patient to inform all health care providers (including dentists) that she takes an MAO inhibitor because certain drugs are contraindicated within 2 weeks of therapy.

•Urge patient to avoid potentially hazardous activities until drug's CNS effects are known.

•Stress the importance of reporting headaches and other unusual, persistent, or severe symptoms.

•Tell family or caregiver to watch closely for suicidal tendencies, especially in children, adolescents, and young adults and especially when therapy starts or dosage changes.

•Urge patient with diabetes who's taking insulin or an oral antidiabetic to check blood glucose level often during therapy because phenelzine may affect glucose control.

phenobarbital

Ancalixir (CAN), Barbita, Solfoton

phenobarbital sodium

Luminal

Class, Category, and Schedule

Chemical class: Barbiturate
Therapeutic class: Anticonvulsant, sedative-hypnotic

Pregnancy category: D
Controlled substance schedule: IV

Indications and Dosages

➤ *To treat seizures*

CAPSULES, ELIXIR, TABLETS

Adults. 60 to 250 mg daily as a single dose or in divided doses.
Children. 1 to 6 mg/kg daily as a single dose or in divided doses.

I.V. INJECTION

Adults. 100 to 320 mg, repeated as needed and as prescribed. *Maximum:* 600 mg daily.
Children. *Initial:* 10 to 20 mg/kg as a single dose. *Maintenance:* 1 to 6 mg/kg daily.

➤ *To treat status epilepticus*

I.V. INFUSION OR INJECTION

Adults. 10 to 20 mg/kg given slowly and repeated as needed and as prescribed.
Children. 15 to 20 mg/kg over 10 to 15 min.

➤ *To provide short-term treatment of insomnia*

CAPSULES, ELIXIR, TABLETS

Adults. 100 to 320 mg at bedtime.

I.V., I.M., OR SUBCUTANEOUS INJECTION

Adults. 100 to 325 mg at bedtime.

➤ *To provide daytime sedation*

CAPSULES, ELIXIR, TABLETS

Adults. 30 to 120 mg daily in divided doses b.i.d. or t.i.d.
Children. 2 mg/kg t.i.d.

I.V., I.M., OR SUBCUTANEOUS INJECTION

Adults. 30 to 120 mg daily in divided doses b.i.d. or t.i.d.

➤ *To provide preoperative sedation*

CAPSULES, ELIXIR, TABLETS

Children. 1 to 3 mg/kg before surgery.

I.M. INJECTION

Adults. 130 to 200 mg 60 to 90 min before surgery.

I.V. OR I.M. INJECTION

Children. 1 to 3 mg/kg 60 to 90 min before surgery.

DOSAGE ADJUSTMENT Dosage possibly reduced for elderly or debilitated patients to minimize confusion, depression, and excitement.

Route	Onset	Peak	Duration
P.O.	20 to 60 min	Unknown	Unknown
I.V.	5 min	30 min	4 to 6 hr
I.M., SubQ	5 to 20 min	Unknown	4 to 6 hr

Mechanism of Action

Inhibits ascending conduction of impulses in the reticular formation, which controls CNS arousal to produce drowsiness, hypnosis, and sedation. Phenobarbital also decreases the spread of seizure activity in the cortex, thalamus, and limbic system. It promotes an increased threshold for electrical stimulation in the motor cortex, which may contribute to its anticonvulsant properties.

Contraindications

Hepatic disease; history of addiction to hypnotics or sedatives; hypersensitivity to phenobarbital, other barbiturates, or their components; nephritis; porphyria; severe respiratory disease with airway obstruction or dyspnea

Interactions

DRUGS

acetaminophen: Decreased acetaminophen effectiveness with long-term phenobarbital therapy
amphetamines: Delayed intestinal absorption of phenobarbital
anesthetics (halogenated hydrocarbon): Possibly hepatotoxicity
anticonvulsants (hydantoin): Unpredictable effects on metabolism of anticonvulsant
anticonvulsants (succinimide), including carbamazepine: Decreased blood levels and elimination half-lives of these drugs
calcium channel blockers: Possibly excessive hypotension
carbonic anhydrase inhibitors: Enhanced osteopenia induced by phenobarbital
chloramphenicol, corticosteroids, cyclosporine, dacarbazine, digoxin, metronidazole, quinidine: Decreased effectiveness of these drugs from enhanced metabolism
CNS depressants: Additive CNS depression
cyclophosphamide: Possibly reduced half-life and increased leukopenic activity of cyclophosphamide
disopyramide: Possibly ineffectiveness of disopyramide
doxycycline, fenoprofen: Shortened half-life of these drugs
griseofulvin: Possibly decreased absorption and effectiveness of griseofulvin
guanadrel, guanethidine: Possibly increased orthostatic hypotension

haloperidol: Decreased seizure threshold, decreased blood haloperidol level
ketamine (high doses): Increased risk of hypotension and respiratory depression
leucovorin: Interference with phenobarbital's anticonvulsant effect
levothyroxine, oral contraceptives, phenylbutazone, tricyclic antidepressants: Decreased effectiveness of these drugs
loxapine, phenothiazines, thioxanthenes: Decreased seizure threshold
MAO inhibitors: Prolonged phenobarbital effects, possibly altered pattern of seizure activity
maprotiline: Increased CNS depression, decreased seizure threshold at high doses, decreased phenobarbital effectiveness
methoxyflurane: Possibly hepatotoxicity and nephrotoxicity
methylphenidate: Increased risk of phenobarbital toxicity
mexiletine: Decreased blood mexiletine level
oral anticoagulants: Decreased anticoagulant activity, increased risk of bleeding when phenobarbital is discontinued
pituitary hormones (posterior): Increased risk of arrhythmias and coronary insufficiency
primidone: Altered pattern of seizures, increased CNS effects of both drugs
valproate, valproic acid: Decreased phenobarbital metabolism, increased risk of barbiturate toxicity
vitamin D: Decreased phenobarbital effectiveness
xanthines: Increased xanthine metabolism, antagonized hypnotic effect of phenobarbital

ACTIVITIES

alcohol use: Additive CNS depression

Adverse Reactions

CNS: Anxiety, depression, dizziness, drowsiness, headache, irritability, lethargy, mood changes, paradoxical stimulation, sedation, vertigo
CV: Hypotension, sinus bradycardia
EENT: Miosis, ptosis
GI: Constipation, diarrhea, nausea, vomiting
GU: Decreased libido, impotence, sexual dysfunction
MS: Arthralgia, bone tenderness
RESP: Bronchospasm, respiratory depression
SKIN: Dermatitis, photosensitivity, rash, urticaria
Other: Injection site phlebitis (I.V.), physical and psychological dependence

P

Nursing Considerations
•Be aware that phenobarbital shouldn't be given during third trimester of pregnancy because repeated use can cause dependence in neonate. It also shouldn't be given to breastfeeding women because it may cause CNS depression in infants.
•Use I.V. route cautiously in patients with CV disease, hypotension, pulmonary disease, or shock because drug may cause adverse hemodynamic or respiratory effects.
•Because drug can cause respiratory depression, assess respiratory rate and depth before use, especially in patient with bronchopneumonia, pulmonary disease, respiratory tract infection, or status asthmaticus.
•Give elixir undiluted or mix with water, milk, or fruit juice. Use a calibrated device to measure doses.
•If necessary, crush tablets and mix with food or fluids.
•Reconstitute sterile powder with at least 10 ml of sterile water for injection. Don't use reconstituted solution if it fails to clear within 5 minutes. Further dilute prescribed dose with normal saline solution or D₅W and infuse over 30 to 60 minutes.
•Don't administer more rapidly than 60 mg/min by I.V. injection.
•During I.V. use, monitor blood pressure, respiratory rate, and heart rate and rhythm. Anticipate increased risk of hypotension, even at recommended rate. Keep resuscitation equipment readily available.
•During I.M. use, don't inject more than 5 ml into any one I.M. site to prevent sterile abscess formation.
•Be aware that drug may cause physical and psychological dependence.
•Anticipate that phenobarbital's CNS effects may exacerbate major depression, suicidal tendencies, or other mental disorders.
•Take safety precautions for elderly patients, as appropriate, because they're more likely to experience confusion, depression, and excitement as adverse CNS reactions.
•Anticipate that phenobarbital may cause paradoxical stimulation in children.
•Be aware that drug may trigger signs and symptoms in patients with acute intermittent porphyria.

PATIENT TEACHING
•Instruct patient to take phenobarbital elixir undiluted or to mix it with water, milk, or fruit juice. Advise her to use a calibrated device to measure doses.
•If patient has trouble swallowing tablets, suggest crushing and adding to food or fluid.
•Caution patient about possible drowsiness and reduced alertness. Advise her to avoid potentially hazardous activities until drug's CNS effects are known.
•Urge patient to avoid alcohol during therapy.
•Inform parents that a child may react with paradoxical excitement. Tell them to notify prescriber if this occurs.
•Instruct woman to report suspected, known, or intended pregnancy. Advise against breast-feeding during therapy.

phentolamine mesylate
Regitine

Class and Category
Chemical class: Imidazoline
Therapeutic class: Antihypertensive, diagnostic aid, vasodilator
Pregnancy category: Not rated

Indications and Dosages
➤ *To diagnose pheochromocytoma*
I.V. INJECTION
Adults. 2.5 mg as a single dose. After negative result, repeat test with 5-mg dose, as prescribed.
Children. 1 mg as a single dose. After negative result, repeat test with 0.1-mg/kg dose, as prescribed.
➤ *To manage hypertension before or during pheochromocytomectomy*
I.V. OR I.M. INJECTION
Adults. 5 mg 1 to 2 hr before surgery, repeated as needed and as prescribed. During surgery, 5 mg I.V., as ordered.
Children. 1 mg 1 to 2 hr before surgery, repeated as needed and as prescribed. During surgery, 1 mg I.V., as ordered.
➤ *To prevent dermal necrosis or sloughing after extravasation of I.V. norepinephrine*
I.V. INJECTION
Adults, children, and infants. 10 mg/L of I.V. fluid that contains norepinephrine at rate determined by patient response.
➤ *To treat dermal necrosis or sloughing after extravasation of I.V. norepinephrine*

INTRADERMAL INJECTION

Adults. 5 to 10 mg in 10 ml of normal saline solution infiltrated in affected area within 12 hr of extravasation.

Children. 0.1 to 0.2 mg/kg. *Maximum:* 10 mg.

Mechanism of Action

Blocks the actions of circulating epinephrine and norepinephrine by antagonizing $alpha_1$ and $alpha_2$ receptors. Phentolamine causes peripheral vasodilation through direct relaxation of vascular smooth muscle and alpha blockade. Positive inotropic and chronotropic effects increase cardiac output. A positive inotropic effect primarily raises blood pressure, but in larger doses, phentolamine causes peripheral vasodilation and can reduce blood pressure.

In patients with pheochromocytoma, phentolamine causes systolic and diastolic blood pressures to fall dramatically. In those without pheochromocytoma, it causes blood pressure to fall or rise slightly or remain the same.

Contraindications

Angina, hypersensitivity to phentolamine or its components, MI

Interactions

DRUGS

antihypertensives: Additive hypotensive effect
dopamine: Antagonized vasopressor activity of dopamine
epinephrine, methoxamine, norepinephrine, phenylephrine: Inhibited alpha adrenergic effects of these drugs
metaraminol: Possibly decreased vasopressor effect of metaraminol

ACTIVITIES

alcohol use: Additive vasodilation, increased risk of hypotension and tachycardia

Adverse Reactions

CNS: Dizziness
CV: Angina; arrhythmias, including tachycardia; hypotension
EENT: Nasal congestion
GI: Diarrhea, nausea, vomiting
GU: Ejaculation disorders, priapism
MS: Muscle weakness
SKIN: Flushing

Nursing Considerations

- Reconstitute each 5-mg vial of phentolamine with 1 ml of sterile water for injection.
- Use reconstituted solution immediately; don't store unused portion.
- Dilute 5 to 10 mg of reconstituted solution in 500 ml of D_5W. Inspect drug for particles and discoloration before administering.
- When diagnosing pheochromocytoma, hold nonessential drugs, as ordered, for at least 24 hours (preferably 48 to 72) before test.
- Before giving I.V. test dose for pheochromocytoma, place patient in supine position and assess baseline blood pressure with readings every 10 minutes for at least 30 minutes.
- In pheochromocytoma, expect excessive hypotension after patient receives drug.
- Take safety precautions according to facility policy if patient experiences dizziness.

PATIENT TEACHING

- Instruct patient to move slowly after phentolamine administration to minimize dizziness and avoid falls.

phenylephrine hydrochloride

Alconefrin Nasal Drops 12, Alconefrin Nasal Drops 25, Alconefrin Nasal Drops 50, Alconefrin Nasal Spray 25, Doktors, Duration, Neo-Synephrine, Neo-Synephrine Nasal Drops, Neo-Synephrine Nasal Jelly, Neo-Synephrine Nasal Spray, Neo-Synephrine Pediatric Nasal Drops, Nostril Spray Pump, Nostril Spray Pump Mild, Rhinall, Rhinall-10 Children's Flavored Nose Drops, Vicks Sinex

Class and Category

Chemical class: Sympathomimetic amine
Therapeutic class: Antiarrhythmic, decongestant, vasoconstrictor, vasopressor
Pregnancy category: C (parenteral), Not rated (nasal)

Indications and Dosages

➤ *To manage mild to moderate hypotension*

I.V. INJECTION

Adults. *Initial:* 0.1 to 0.5 mg. *Usual:* 0.2 mg, repeated no more than every 10 to 15 min.

I.M. OR SUBCUTANEOUS INJECTION

Adults. *Initial:* 1 to 5 mg. *Usual:* 2 to 5 mg (range, 1 to 10 mg), repeated no more than every 10 to 15 min, as prescribed.

➤ *To treat severe hypotension or shock*

I.V. INFUSION

Adults. *Initial:* 100 to 180 mcg/min (0.1 to 0.18 mg/min) until blood pressure is stable. *Maintenance:* 40 to 60 mcg/min (0.04 to 0.06 mg/min). Infusion concentration and flow rate adjusted as prescribed, based on patient response.

➤ *To prevent hypotension during spinal anesthesia*

I.M. OR SUBCUTANEOUS INJECTION

Adults. 2 to 3 mg 3 or 4 min before injection of spinal anesthetic.

Children. 0.5 to 1 mg for each 11.3 kg (25 lb).

➤ *To treat hypotension during spinal anesthesia*

I.V. INJECTION

Adults. *Initial:* 0.2 mg, increased by no more than 0.2 mg, as prescribed. *Maximum:* 0.5 mg/dose.

Children. 0.5 to 1 mg for each 11.3 kg (25 lb).

➤ *To treat paroxysmal supraventricular tachycardia*

I.V. INJECTION

Adults. *Initial:* Up to 0.5 mg by rapid injection; later doses increased 0.1 to 0.2 mg higher than preceding dose, as prescribed. *Maximum:* 1 mg/dose.

➤ *To treat sinus, nasal, and eustachian tube congestion*

NASAL JELLY OR SOLUTION

Adults and children age 12 and over. 2 or 3 drops or sprays of 0.25% or 0.5% solution every 4 hr, p.r.n., or small quantity of 0.5% nasal jelly in each nostril every 3 to 4 hr, p.r.n. A 1% solution may be used for severe congestion.

Children ages 6 to 12. 2 or 3 drops or sprays of 0.25% solution in each nostril every 4 hr, p.r.n.

Children ages 2 to 6. 2 or 3 drops or sprays of 0.125% or 0.16% solution in each nostril every 4 hr, p.r.n.

Incompatibilities

Don't combine nasal form with alkalies, butacaine, ferrous salts, metals, or oxidizing agents.

Contraindications

Hypersensitivity to bisulfites, phenylephrine, or their components; severe coronary artery disease or hypertension; use within 14 days of MAO inhibitor; ventricular tachycardia

Route	Onset	Peak	Duration
I.V.	Immediately	Unknown	15 to 20 min
I.M.	10 to 15 min	Unknown	30 min to 2 hr
SubQ	10 to 15 min	Unknown	50 min to 1 hr
Nasal	Unknown	Unknown	30 min to 4 hr

Mechanism of Action

Directly stimulates alpha-adrenergic receptors and inhibits the intracellular enzyme adenyl cyclase, which then inhibits production of cAMP. Inhibition of cAMP causes arterial and venous constriction and increases peripheral vascular resistance and systolic blood pressure. With greater-than-therapeutic doses, phenylephrine directly stimulates beta-adrenergic receptors in the myocardium, which increases activity of adenyl cyclase and produces positive inotropic and chronotropic effect. Intranasal use directly stimulates alpha-adrenergic receptors on the nasal mucosa, constricting local vessels and decreasing blood flow and mucosal edema.

Interactions

DRUGS

alpha blockers, haloperidol, loxapine, phenothiazines, thioxanthenes: Possibly decreased vasoconstrictor effect of phenylephrine; decreased decongestant effect of nasal phenylephrine (with phenothiazines)

antihypertensives, diuretics: Possibly decreased antihypertensive effects

atropine: Possibly enhanced vasopressor effect of phenylephrine

beta blockers: Decreased therapeutic effects of both drugs

bretylium: Possibly potentiated vasopressor effect and arrhythmias

doxapram: Increased vasopressor effect of both drugs

ergot alkaloids: Possibly cerebral blood vessel rupture, increased vasopressor effect, peripheral vascular ischemia, and gangrene (with ergotamine)

guanadrel, guanethidine: Increased vasopressor effect of phenylephrine, increased risk of severe hypertension and arrhythmias
hydrocarbon inhalation anesthetics: Increased risk of serious arrhythmias
MAO inhibitors: Increased and prolonged cardiac stimulation, increased vasopressor effect, increased risk of severe cardiovascular and cerebrovascular effects, hyperpyrexia, vomiting
maprotiline, tricyclic antidepressants: Increased risk of severe cardiovascular effects (including arrhythmias, hyperpyrexia, severe hypertension); possibly increased or decreased sensitivity to I.V. phenylephrine
mecamylamine, methyldopa: Decreased hypotensive effects of these drugs, increased vasopressor effect of phenylephrine
nitrates: Possibly decreased vasopressor effect of phenylephrine and decreased antianginal effect of nitrates
oxytocin: Possibly severe, persistent hypertension
phenoxybenzamine: Decreased vasoconstrictor effect of phenylephrine, possibly hypotension and tachycardia
theophylline: Possibly enhanced toxicity (including cardiotoxicity); decreased blood theophylline level (with nasal phenylephrine)
thyroid hormones: Increased cardiovascular effects of both drugs
urinary acidifiers: Possibly increased elimination and decreased therapeutic effects (with nasal phenylephrine)
urinary alkalizers: Possibly decreased elimination and toxic effects (with nasal phenylephrine)

Adverse Reactions

CNS: Dizziness, headache, insomnia, nervousness, paresthesia, restlessness, sleep disturbance (nasal), tremor, weakness
CV: Angina, bradycardia, hypertension, hypotension, palpitations, peripheral vasoconstriction that may lead to necrosis or gangrene, tachycardia, ventricular arrhythmias
EENT: Burning, dry, or stinging nasal mucosa; rebound congestion; and rhinitis (nasal forms)
GI: Nausea, vomiting
RESP: Dyspnea
SKIN: Extravasation with tissue necrosis and sloughing, pallor
Other: Allergic reaction

Nursing Considerations

• Don't dilute phenylephrine for I.M. or subcutaneous use.
• To reduce the risk of tissue extravasation, don't inject subcutaneous drug intradermally.
• For I.V. use, dilute with D_5W or sodium chloride for injection and prepare as prescribed—usually 10 mg/500 ml.
• After nasal application, rinse spray bottle tip or nasal dropper with hot water and dry with clean tissue. Wipe tip of nasal jelly tube with clean tissue.
• To prevent transmission of infection, don't use nasal form on more than one patient.
• Assess for signs and symptoms of angina, arrhythmias, and hypertension because phenylephrine may increase myocardial oxygen demand and the risk of proarrhythmias and blood pressure changes.
• **WARNING** If patient has thyroid disease, watch for increased sensitivity to catecholamines and possible thyrotoxicity or cardiotoxicity.
• **WARNING** Be aware that extravasation may cause tissue necrosis, gangrene, and other reactions around injection site. Expect to use phentolamine if extravasation occurs.

PATIENT TEACHING
• If patient uses nasal form, explain that excessive use may cause rebound congestion. Urge her not to exceed recommended dosage and to use for only 3 to 5 days.
• Teach patient who uses nasal form how to care for spray bottle, dropper, or tube.
• Advise patient to avoid potentially hazardous activities until drug's CNS effects are known.

P

phenytoin

Dilantin-30 (CAN), Dilantin-125, Dilantin Infatabs

phenytoin sodium

Dilantin, Dilantin Kapseals, Phenytex

Class and Category

Chemical class: Hydantoin derivative
Therapeutic class: Anticonvulsant
Pregnancy category: C

Indications and Dosages

➤ *To treat tonic-clonic, simple, or complex partial seizures in patients who have had no prior treatment*

CHEWABLE TABLETS, ORAL SUSPENSION (PHENYTOIN)

Adults and adolescents. *Initial:* 125 mg suspension or 100 to 125 mg tablet t.i.d., adjusted every 7 to 10 days as needed and tolerated.

Children. *Initial:* 5 mg/kg daily in divided doses b.i.d. or t.i.d., adjusted as needed and tolerated. *Maintenance:* 4 to 8 mg/kg daily in divided doses b.i.d. or t.i.d. *Maximum:* 300 mg daily.

EXTENDED CAPSULES (PHENYTOIN SODIUM)

Adults and adolescents. *Initial:* 100 mg t.i.d., adjusted every 7 to 10 days as needed and tolerated. *Maintenance:* Once seizures are controlled, adjusted dosage given daily if needed and tolerated.

DOSAGE ADJUSTMENT For hospitalized patients without hepatic or renal disease, oral loading dose of 400 mg followed in 2 hr by 300 mg and then in 2 more hr by another 300 mg for a total of 1 g.

Children. *Initial:* 5 mg/kg daily in divided doses b.i.d. or t.i.d., adjusted as needed and tolerated. *Maintenance:* 4 to 8 mg/kg daily in divided doses b.i.d. or t.i.d. *Maximum:* 300 mg daily.

PROMPT CAPSULES (PHENYTOIN SODIUM)

Adults and adolescents. 100 mg t.i.d., adjusted every 7 to 10 days as needed and tolerated.

Children. *Initial:* 5 mg/kg daily in divided doses b.i.d. or t.i.d., adjusted as needed and tolerated. *Maintenance:* 4 to 8 mg/kg daily in divided doses b.i.d. or t.i.d. *Maximum:* 300 mg daily.

➤ *To treat status epilepticus*

I.V. INJECTION (PHENYTOIN SODIUM)

Adults and adolescents. *Initial:* 15 to 20 mg/kg by slow push in 50 ml sodium chloride injection at no more than 50 mg/min. *Maintenance:* Beginning within 12 to 24 hr of initial dose, 5 mg/kg daily P.O. in divided doses b.i.d. to q.i.d., or 100 mg I.V. every 6 to 8 hr.

Children. 15 to 20 mg/kg at no more than 1 mg/kg/min. *Maximum:* 50 mg/min.

DOSAGE ADJUSTMENT For elderly or very ill patients and those with CV or hepatic disease, dosage reduced to 25 mg/min, as prescribed, or possibly as low as 5 to 10 mg/min to reduce the risk of adverse reactions.

➤ *To prevent or treat seizures during neurosurgery*

I.V. INJECTION (PHENYTOIN SODIUM)

Adults. 100 to 200 mg every 4 hr at no more than 50 mg/min during or immediately after neurosurgery.

Mechanism of Action

Limits the spread of seizure activity and the start of new seizures by regulating voltage-dependent sodium and calcium channels in neurons, inhibiting calcium movement across neuronal membranes, and enhancing sodium-potassium ATP activity in neurons and glial cells. These actions all help stabilize the neurons.

Incompatibilities

Don't mix phenytoin in same syringe with any other drugs or with any I.V. solutions other than sodium chloride for injection because precipitate will form.

Contraindications

Adams-Stokes syndrome, hypersensitivity to phenytoin or its components, SA block, second- or third-degree heart block, sinus bradycardia

Interactions

DRUGS

acetaminophen: Possibly hepatotoxicity, decreased acetaminophen effects

activated charcoal, antacids, calcium salts, enteral feedings, sucralfate: Decreased absorption of oral phenytoin

allopurinol, benzodiazepines, chloramphenicol, cimetidine, disulfiram, fluconazole, isoniazid, itraconazole, methylphenidate, metronidazole, miconazole, omeprazole, phenacemide, ranitidine, sulfonamides, trazodone, trimethoprim: Decreased metabolism and increased effects of phenytoin

amiodarone, ticlopidine: Possibly increased blood phenytoin level

antifungals (azole): Increased blood phenytoin level, decreased blood antifungal level

antineoplastics, nitrofurantoin, pyridoxine: Decreased phenytoin effects

barbiturates: Variable effects on blood phenytoin level

bupropion, clozapine, loxapine, MAO inhibitors, maprotiline, molindone, phenothiazines, pimozide, thioxanthenes, tricyclic antidepressants: Decreased seizure threshold, de-

creased anticonvulsant effect of phenytoin
calcium channel blockers: Increased metabolism and decreased effects of these drugs, possibly increased blood phenytoin level
carbamazepine: Decreased blood level and effects of carbamazepine, possibly phenytoin toxicity
carbonic anhydrase inhibitors: Increased risk of osteopenia from phenytoin
chlordiazepoxide, diazepam: Possibly increased blood phenytoin level, decreased effects of these drugs
clonazepam: Possibly decreased blood level and effects of clonazepam, possibly phenytoin toxicity
corticosteroids, cyclosporine, dicumarol, digoxin, disopyramide, doxycycline, estrogens, furosemide, lamotrigine, levodopa, methadone, metyrapone, mexiletine, oral contraceptives, quinidine, sirolimus, tacrolimus, theophylline: Increased metabolism and decreased effects of these drugs
dopamine: Increased risk of severe hypotension and bradycardia (with I.V. phenytoin)
fluoxetine: Increased blood phenytoin level and risk of phenytoin toxicity
folic acid, leucovorin: Decreased blood phenytoin level, increased risk of seizures
haloperidol: Decreased effects of haloperidol, decreased anticonvulsant effect of phenytoin
halothane anesthetics: Increased risk of hepatotoxicity and phenytoin toxicity
ifosfamide: Decreased phenytoin effects, possibly increased toxicity
influenza virus vaccine: Possibly decreased phenytoin effects
insulin, oral antidiabetic drugs: Possibly hyperglycemia, increased blood phenytoin level (with tolbutamide)
levonorgestrel, mebendazole, streptozocin, sulfonylureas: Decreased effects of these drugs
lidocaine, propranolol (possibly other beta blockers): Increased cardiac depressant effects (with I.V. phenytoin), possibly decreased blood level and increased adverse effects of phenytoin
lithium: Increased risk of lithium toxicity, increased risk of neurologic symptoms with normal blood lithium level
meperidine: Increased metabolism and decreased effects of meperidine, possibly meperidine toxicity
methadone: Possibly increased metabolism of

methadone and withdrawal symptoms
neuromuscular blockers: Shorter duration of action and decreased effects of neuromuscular blockers
oral anticoagulants: Decreased metabolism and increased effects of phenytoin; early increase and then decrease in anticoagulation
paroxetine: Decreased bioavailability of both drugs
phenylbutazone, salicylates: Increased phenytoin effects, possibly phenytoin toxicity
primidone: Increased primidone effects, possibly primidone toxicity
rifampin: Increased hepatic metabolism of phenytoin
valproic acid: Possibly decreased phenytoin metabolism, resulting in increased phenytoin effects; possibly decreased blood valproic acid level
vitamin D: Possibly decreased vitamin D effects, resulting in rickets or osteomalacia (with long-term use of phenytoin)

ACTIVITIES
alcohol use: Additive CNS depression, increased phenytoin clearance

Adverse Reactions

CNS: Ataxia, confusion, depression, dizziness, drowsiness, excitement, fever, headache, involuntary motor activity, lethargy, nervousness, peripheral neuropathy, restlessness, slurred speech, tremor, weakness
CV: Cardiac arrest, hypotension, vasculitis
EENT: Amblyopia, conjunctivitis, diplopia, earache, epistaxis, eye pain, gingival hyperplasia, hearing loss, loss of taste, nystagmus, pharyngitis, photophobia, rhinitis, sinusitis, taste perversion, tinnitus
ENDO: Gynecomastia, hyperglycemia
GI: Abdominal pain, anorexia, constipation, diarrhea, epigastric pain, hepatic dysfunction, hepatic necrosis, hepatitis, nausea, vomiting
GU: Glycosuria, priapism, renal failure
HEME: Acute intermittent porphyria (exacerbation), agranulocytosis, anemia, eosinophilia, leukopenia, pancytopenia, thrombocytopenia
MS: Arthralgia, arthropathy, bone fractures, muscle twitching, osteomalacia, polymyositis
RESP: Apnea, asthma, bronchitis, cough, dyspnea, hypoxia, increased sputum production, pneumonia, pneumothorax, pulmonary fibrosis

P

SKIN: Exfoliative dermatitis, jaundice, maculopapular or morbilliform rash, purpuric dermatitis, Stevens-Johnson syndrome, toxic epidermal necrolysis, unusual hair growth, urticaria

Other: Facial feature enlargement, injection site pain, lupus-like symptoms, lymphadenopathy, polyarteritis, weight gain or loss

Nursing Considerations

•**WARNING** Patients of Asian ancestry who have the genetic allelic variant HLA-B 1502 develop serious and sometimes fatal dermatologic reactions ten times more often than people without this variant when given carbamazepine, another antiepileptic drug. Because early data suggest a similar effect with phenytoin, this drug shouldn't be used as a substitute for carbamazepine in these patients.

Be aware that preferred administration routes for phenytoin are oral and I.V. injection. With I.M. administration, phenytoin has a variable absorption rate.

•If patient has difficulty swallowing, open prompt (rapid-release) capsules and mix contents with food or fluid.

•Shake oral suspension before measuring dose, and use a calibrated measuring device.

•To minimize GI distress, give phenytoin with or just after meals.

•Inspect I.V. form for particles and discoloration before administering.

•**WARNING** Avoid rapid I.V. injection because it may cause cardiac arrest, CNS depression, or severe hypotension.

•To decrease vein irritation, follow I.V. injection with flush of sodium chloride for injection through same I.V. catheter.

•Continuously monitor ECG tracings and blood pressure when administering I.V. phenytoin.

•Frequently assess I.V. site for signs of extravasation because drug can cause tissue necrosis.

•If patient has an NG tube in place, minimize drug absorption by polyvinyl chloride tubing by diluting suspension threefold with sodium chloride for injection, D₅W, or sterile water. After administration, flush tube with at least 20 ml of diluent.

•Separate oral phenytoin administration by at least 2 hours from antacids and calcium salts.

•Expect continuous enteral feedings to disrupt phenytoin absorption and, possibly, reduce blood phenytoin level. Discontinue tube feedings 1 to 2 hours before and after phenytoin administration, as prescribed. Anticipate giving increased phenytoin doses to compensate for reduced bioavailability during continuous tube feedings.

•Monitor blood phenytoin level. Therapeutic level ranges from 10 to 20 mcg/L.

•**WARNING** Monitor patient's hematologic status during therapy because phenytoin can cause blood dyscrasias. A patient with a history of agranulocytosis, leukopenia, or pancytopenia may have an increased risk of infection because phenytoin can cause myelosuppression.

•Anticipate that drug may worsen intermittent porphyria.

•Frequently monitor blood glucose level of patient with diabetes mellitus because drug can stimulate glucagon secretion and impair insulin secretion, either of which can raise blood glucose level.

•Monitor thyroid hormone levels in patient receiving thyroid replacement therapy because phenytoin may decrease circulating thyroid hormone levels and increase thyroid-stimulating hormone level.

•Be aware that long-term phenytoin therapy may increase patient's requirements for folic acid or vitamin D supplements. However, keep in mind that a diet high in folic acid may decrease seizure control.

PATIENT TEACHING

•Instruct patient to crush or thoroughly chew phenytoin chewable tablets before swallowing or to shake oral solution well before using.

•Advise patient to take drug exactly as prescribed and not to change brands or dosage or stop taking drug unless instructed by prescriber.

•Instruct patient to avoid taking antacids or calcium products within 2 hours of phenytoin.

•Urge patient to avoid alcohol during therapy.

•Caution patient to avoid potentially hazardous activities until drug's CNS effects are known.

•Inform patient with diabetes mellitus about the increased risk of hyperglycemia and the possible need for increased antidiabetic drug dosage during therapy. Advise her to monitor her blood glucose level frequently.

• Stress the importance of good oral hygiene, and encourage patient to inform her dentist that she's taking phenytoin.
• Encourage patient to obtain medical identification that indicates her diagnosis and drug therapy.

physostigmine salicylate

Antilirium

Class and Category
Chemical class: Salicylic acid derivative
Therapeutic class: Anticholinergic antidote, cholinesterase inhibitor
Pregnancy category: Not rated

Indications and Dosages
➤ *To counteract toxic anticholinergic effects (anticholinergic syndrome)*
I.V. OR I.M. INJECTION
Adults and adolescents. 0.5 to 2 mg at no more than 1 mg/min; then 1 to 4 mg, repeated every 20 to 30 min as needed and as prescribed.
Children. 0.02 mg/kg I.V., at no more than 0.5 mg/min, repeated every 5 to 10 min as prescribed. *Maximum:* 2 mg/dose.

Route	Onset	Peak	Duration
I.V.	3 to 8 min	5 min	30 to 60 min
I.M.	3 to 8 min	20 to 30 min	30 to 60 min

Mechanism of Action
Inhibits the destruction of acetylcholine by acetylcholinesterase. This action increases the concentration of acetylcholine at cholinergic transmission sites and prolongs and exaggerates the effects of acetylcholine that are blocked by toxic doses of anticholinergics.

Contraindications
Asthma; cardiovascular disease; diabetes mellitus; gangrene; GI or GU obstruction; hypersensitivity to physostigmine, sulfites, or their components

Interactions
DRUGS
choline esters: Enhanced effects of carbachol and bethanechol with concurrent use of physostigmine, enhanced effects of acetylcholine and methacholine with prior use of physostigmine
succinylcholine: Prolonged neuromuscular paralysis

Adverse Reactions
CNS: CNS stimulation, fatigue, hallucinations, restlessness, seizures (with too-rapid I.V. administration), weakness
CV: Bradycardia (with too-rapid I.V. administration), irregular heartbeat, palpitations
EENT: Increased salivation, lacrimation, miosis
GI: Abdominal pain, diarrhea, nausea, vomiting
GU: Urinary urgency
MS: Muscle twitching
RESP: Bronchospasm, chest tightness, dyspnea (with too-rapid I.V. administration), increased bronchial secretions, wheezing
SKIN: Diaphoresis

Nursing Considerations
• Use physostigmine cautiously in patients with bradycardia, epilepsy, or Parkinson's disease.
• Avoid rapid I.V. delivery, which may lead to bradycardia, respiratory distress, or seizures.
• Frequently monitor pulse and respiratory rates, blood pressure, and neurologic status.
• Monitor ECG tracing during I.V. use.
• Closely monitor patient with asthma for asthma attack because physostigmine may precipitate attack by causing bronchoconstriction.
• Watch for seizures in patient with a history of seizures because physostigmine can induce seizures by causing CNS stimulation.
• **WARNING** Be alert for life-threatening cholinergic crisis, which may indicate physostigmine overdose and may include confusion, diaphoresis, hypotension, miosis, muscle weakness, nausea, paralysis (including respiratory paralysis), salivation, seizures, sinus bradycardia, and vomiting. If you detect such signs, prepare to give atropine (the antidote) and use resuscitation equipment. Keep in mind that atropine counteracts only muscarinic cholinergic effects; paralytic effects may continue.
PATIENT TEACHING
• Reassure patient that vital signs will be monitored often to help prevent or detect adverse reactions.

•Instruct patient to notify prescriber immediately about evidence of cholinergic crisis.

pindolol

NovoPindol (CAN), SynPindol (CAN), Visken

Class and Category

Chemical class: Nonselective beta blocker
Therapeutic class: Antihypertensive
Pregnancy category: B

Indications and Dosages

➤ *To manage hypertension*

TABLETS

Adults. *Initial:* 5 mg b.i.d., increased by 10 mg daily every 3 to 4 wk, as prescribed. *Maintenance:* 10 to 30 mg daily. *Maximum:* 60 mg daily (U.S.), 45 mg daily (Canada).

Route	Onset	Peak	Duration
P.O.	Unknown	1 to 2 hr	Up to 24 hr

Mechanism of Action

Blocks sympathetic stimulation of beta$_1$ receptors in the heart and beta$_2$ receptors in vascular and bronchial smooth muscle by competing with adrenergic neurotransmitters, such as catecholamines. Pindolol's negative chronotropic effects slow the resting heart rate and reduce exercise-induced tachycardia. Its negative inotropic effects reduce cardiac output, myocardial contractility, systolic and diastolic blood pressure, and myocardial oxygen consumption during stress or exercise. Among beta blockers, pindolol has the most intrinsic sympathomimetic activity and nonselective antagonism.

Contraindications

Advanced AV block; asthma; bronchospasm; cardiogenic shock; heart failure; hepatic disease; hypersensitivity to pindolol, other beta blockers, or their components; hypotension (with systolic pressure less than 100 mm Hg); sinus bradycardia

Interactions

DRUGS

allergy extracts or immunotherapy, iodinated contrast media: Increased risk of systemic reaction or anaphylaxis

aluminum salts, barbiturates, calcium salts, certain penicillins, cholestyramine, colestipol, NSAIDs, rifampin, salicylates, sulfinpyrazone: Decreased blood level and effects of pindolol

antihypertensives: Additive hypotensive effect

beta blockers, digoxin: Increased risk of bradycardia

calcium channel blockers, quinidine: Possibly increased effects of both drugs, symptomatic bradycardia (with diltiazem or verapamil), excessive hypertension or heart failure (with nifedipine)

cimetidine: Increased blood pindolol level

epinephrine: Possibly hypertension followed by bradycardia

ergotamine: Possibly severe peripheral vasoconstriction with pain and cyanosis

estrogens: Decreased antihypertensive effect

fentanyl, fentanyl derivatives: Risk of bradycardia after anesthesia induction

insulin, oral antidiabetic drugs: Masked symptoms of hypoglycemia, increased risk of hyperglycemia

lidocaine: Increased risk of lidocaine toxicity

MAO inhibitors: Possibly hypertension

neuromuscular blockers: Possibly increased or prolonged neuromuscular blockade

phenothiazines: Increased blood levels of both drugs

phenytoin: Possibly increased cardiac depressant effects

prazosin, reserpine: Increased risk of orthostatic hypotension, bradycardia (with reserpine)

quinolones: Possibly increased bioavailability of pindolol

xanthines: Possibly decreased effects of both drugs, decreased xanthine clearance

Adverse Reactions

CNS: Anxiety, confusion, depression, dizziness, fatigue, fever, hallucinations, hypothermia, insomnia, memory loss, paresthesia, peripheral neuropathy, stroke, syncope, weakness

CV: Arrhythmias (including AV block and bradycardia), chest pain, decreased peripheral circulation, heart failure, hyperlipidemia, hypotension, MI, orthostatic hypotension, peripheral edema and ischemia, thrombosis of renal or mesenteric artery

EENT: Pharyngitis

ENDO: Hyperglycemia, hypoglycemia
GI: Colitis (ischemic), constipation, diarrhea, elevated liver function test results, gastritis, nausea, pancreatitis, vomiting
GU: Cystitis, decreased libido, renal colic, renal failure, urinary frequency, urine retention, UTI
HEME: Agranulocytosis, bleeding, eosinophilia, leukopenia, nonthrombocytopenic purpura, thrombocytopenia, thrombocytopenic purpura, unusual bleeding or bruising
MS: Arthralgia, back pain
RESP: Bronchospasm, pulmonary edema, pulmonary emboli
SKIN: Acne; alopecia; crusted, red, or scaly skin; diaphoresis; eczema; exfoliative dermatitis; hyperpigmentation; pruritus; purpura; rash
Other: Angioedema, positive ANA titer

Nursing Considerations

• Monitor blood pressure and pulse rate frequently, especially at start of pindolol therapy. Also monitor fluid intake and output and daily weight, and assess for signs of heart failure, such as dyspnea, edema, fatigue, and jugular vein distention.
• Be aware that drug shouldn't be stopped abruptly because MI, myocardial ischemia, severe hypertension, or ventricular arrhythmias may result.
• Expect to discontinue drug up to 2 days before surgery, as prescribed, to reduce the risk of heart failure.
• Assess distal circulation and peripheral pulses in patient with Raynaud's phenomenon or other peripheral vascular disorder because drug can worsen these conditions.
• Be aware that pindolol can mask tachycardia from hyperthyroidism and that abrupt withdrawal can cause thyroid storm. Drug also may potentiate diplopia and muscle weakness in patient with myasthenia gravis; decrease blood glucose level, prolong or mask symptoms of hypoglycemia, and promote hyperglycemia in patient with diabetes mellitus; and worsen psoriasis.

PATIENT TEACHING
• Instruct patient to weigh herself daily during pindolol therapy and to notify prescriber if she gains more than 2 lb (0.9 kg) in 1 day or 5 lb (2.3 kg) in 1 week.
• Caution patient not to stop drug abruptly.

• Advise patient to rise slowly from a seated or lying position to minimize effects of orthostatic hypotension.
• Advise patient to avoid potentially hazardous activities until drug's CNS effects are known.
• Instruct patient to contact prescriber about bleeding or bruising, cough at night, depression, dizziness, edema, rash, shortness of breath, slow pulse rate, or sore throat.
• Advise diabetic patient to monitor her blood glucose level more often during pindolol therapy because drug may mask symptoms of hypoglycemia.
• Inform patient with psoriasis that drug may aggravate this condition.

pioglitazone hydrochloride

Actos

Class and Category

Chemical class: Thiazolidinedione
Therapeutic class: Antidiabetic
Pregnancy category: C

Indications and Dosages

➤ *To achieve glucose control in type 2 diabetes mellitus as monotherapy or in combination with insulin, metformin, or a sulfonylurea*

TABLETS
Adults. *Initial:* 15 or 30 mg daily. *Maximum:* 45 mg daily.
DOSAGE ADJUSTMENT For patients taking insulin, insulin dosage decreased by 10% to 25%, as prescribed, once glucose level reaches 100 mg/dl or less. If hypoglycemia occurs, dosage of any concurrent antidiabetic is reduced, as prescribed.

Contraindications

Diabetic ketoacidosis, hypersensitivity to pioglitazone or its components, New York Heart Association (NYHA) Class III or IV heart falure, severe hepatic dysfunction, type 1 diabetes mellitus

Interactions

DRUGS
gemfibrozil, rifampin: Possibly altered glucose control
ketoconazole: Possibly decreased metabolism

of pioglitazone
oral contraceptives: Possibly decreased effectiveness of oral contraceptives

Mechanism of Action
Decreases insulin resistance by enhancing the sensitivity of insulin-dependent tissues, such as adipose tissue, skeletal muscle, and the liver, and reduces glucose output from the liver. Drug activates peroxisome proliferator-activated receptor-gamma (PPARγ) receptors, which modulate transcription of insulin-responsive genes involved in glucose control and lipid metabolism. In this way, pioglitazone reduces hyperglycemia, hyperinsulinemia, and hypertriglyceridemia in patients with type 2 diabetes mellitus and insulin resistance. However, to work effectively, pioglitazone needs endogenous insulin. Unlike sulfonylureas, it doesn't increase pancreatic insulin secretion.

Adverse Reactions
CNS: Headache
CV: Congestive heart failure, edema
EENT: Blurred vision, decreased visual acuity, macular edema, pharyngitis, sinusitis, tooth disorders
HEME: Decreased hemoglobin level and hematocrit
MS: Fractures, myalgia
RESP: Upper respiratory tract infection
Other: Weight gain

Nursing Considerations
•Be aware that pioglitazone isn't recommended for patients with symptopmatic heart failure.
•Be prepared to monitor liver function test results before therapy begins, every 2 months during first year, and annually thereafter, as ordered, because drug is extensively metabolized in the liver. Expect to stop drug if jaundice develops or ALT values exceed 2½ times normal.
• WARNING Monitor patient for signs and symptoms of congestive heart failure—such as shortness of breath, rapid weight gain, or edema—because pioglitazone can cause fluid retention that may lead to or worsen heart failure. Notify prescriber immediately of any

deterioration in the patient's cardiac status, and expect to discontinue the drug, as ordered.
•Assess for signs and symptoms of hypoglycemia, especially if patient is also taking another antidiabetic drug.
•Monitor fasting glucose level, as ordered, to evaluate effectiveness of therapy.
•Monitor glycosylated hemoglobin level to assess drug's long-term effectiveness.
PATIENT TEACHING
•Stress the need for patient to continue exercise program, diet control, and weight management during pioglitazone therapy.
•Advise patient to notify prescriber immediately if she experiences shortness of breath, fluid retention, or sudden weight gain because drug may need to be discontinued.
•Urge patient to report vision changes promptly and expect to have an eye examination by an ophthalmologist regardless of when the last examination occurred.
•Instruct patient to keep appointments for liver function tests, as ordered, typically every 2 months during first year of therapy and annually thereafter.
•Inform female patient who uses oral contraceptives that drug decreases their effectiveness; suggest that she use another method of contraception while taking pioglitazone.
•Also inform female patient that she may be at risk for fractures during pioglitazone therapy, and urge her to take safety precautions to prevent falls and other injuries.

piperacillin sodium
Pipracil

Class and Category
Chemical class: Piperazine derivative of ampicillin, acylureidopenicillin
Therapeutic class: Antibiotic
Pregnancy category: B

Indications and Dosages
➤ *To treat moderate to severe bacterial infections, including bone and joint infections, gynecologic infections, intra-abdominal infections, lower respiratory tract infections, septicemia, and skin and soft-tissue infections, caused by susceptible strains of* Acinetobacter *species,* anaerobic cocci, Bacteroides *species,* En-

terobacter *species,* Escherichia coli, Haemophilus influenzae, Klebsiella *species,* Proteus *species,* Pseudomonas aeruginosa, *and* Serratia *species*

I.V. INFUSION

Adults and adolescents. 12 to 18 g daily or 200 to 300 mg/kg daily in divided doses every 4 to 6 hr. *Maximum:* 24 g daily.

➤ *To treat bacterial meningitis*

I.V. INFUSION

Adults and adolescents. 4 g every 4 hr or 75 mg/kg every 6 hr. *Maximum:* 24 g daily.

➤ *To treat uncomplicated UTI and community-acquired pneumonia caused by susceptible organisms, including* E. coli, Klebsiella *species, and* Serratia *species*

I.V. INFUSION, I.M. INJECTION

Adults. 6 to 8 g daily or 100 to 125 mg/kg daily in divided doses every 6 to 12 hr.

➤ *To treat complicated UTI caused by susceptible organisms, including* Acinetobacter *species,* Klebsiella *species, and* Serratia *species*

I.V. INFUSION

Adults. 8 to 16 g daily or 125 to 200 mg/kg daily in divided doses every 6 to 8 hr.

➤ *To treat uncomplicated gonorrhea caused by susceptible strains of* Neisseria gonorrhoeae

I.M. INJECTION

Adults. 2 g as a single dose 30 min after 1-g dose of probenecid P.O.

➤ *To provide surgical prophylaxis in intra-abdominal procedures, including GI and biliary surgery*

I.V. INFUSION

Adults. 2 g 20 to 30 min before anesthesia, 2 g during surgery, and 2 g every 6 hr for 24 hr after surgery.

➤ *To provide surgical prophylaxis in abdominal hysterectomy*

I.V. INFUSION

Adults. 2 g 20 to 30 min before anesthesia, 2 g just after surgery, and 2 g 6 hr later.

➤ *To provide surgical prophylaxis in vaginal hysterectomy*

I.V. INFUSION

Adults. 2 g 20 to 30 min before anesthesia, then 2 g 6 and 12 hr after initial dose.

➤ *To provide surgical prophylaxis in cesarean section*

I.V. INFUSION

Adults. 2 g after cord is clamped, then 2 g 4 and 8 hr after initial dose.

Mechanism of Action

Binds to specific penicillin-binding proteins and inhibits the third and final stage of bacterial cell wall synthesis by interfering with an autolysin inhibitor. Uninhibited autolytic enzymes destroy the cell wall and result in cell lysis.

Incompatibilities

Don't mix piperacillin sodium in same container with aminoglycosides because of chemical incompatibility (depending on concentrations, diluents, pH, and temperature). Don't mix with solutions that contain only sodium bicarbonate because of chemical instability.

Contraindications

Hypersensitivity to cephalosporins, penicillins, or their components

Interactions

DRUGS

aminoglycosides: Additive or synergistic effects against some bacteria, possibly mutual inactivation

anti-inflammatory drugs (including aspirin and NSAIDs), heparin, oral anticoagulants, platelet aggregation inhibitors, sulfinpyrazone, thrombolytics: Increased risk of bleeding

hepatotoxic drugs (including labetalol and rifampin): Increased risk of hepatotoxicity

methotrexate: Increased blood methotrexate level and risk of toxicity

probenecid: Increased blood piperacillin level and risk of toxicity

vecuronium: Possibly prolonged perioperative neuromuscular blockade of vecuronium

Adverse Reactions

CNS: Dizziness, fever, hallucinations, headache, lethargy, seizures, stroke

CV: Cardiac arrest, hypotension, palpitations, tachycardia, vasodilation, vasovagal reactions

EENT: Oral candidiasis, pharyngitis

GI: Diarrhea, epigastric distress, intestinal necrosis, nausea, pseudomembranous colitis, vomiting

P

GU: Hematuria, impotence, nephritis, neurogenic bladder, priapism, proteinuria, renal failure, vaginal candidiasis
HEME: Agranulocytosis, eosinophilia, hemolytic anemia, leukopenia, neutropenia, pancytopenia, prolonged bleeding time, thrombocytopenia
MS: Arthralgia
RESP: Dyspnea, pulmonary embolism, pulmonary hypertension
SKIN: Exfoliative dermatitis, mottling, rash, toxic epidermal necrolysis, urticaria
Other: Anaphylaxis; facial edema; hypokalemia; hyponatremia; injection site pain, phlebitis, and skin ulcer; superinfection

Nursing Considerations
•Obtain blood, sputum, or other samples for culture and sensitivity testing, as ordered, before giving piperacillin. Expect to begin piperacillin therapy before results are available.
•Be aware that sunlight may darken piperacillin powder for dilution but won't alter drug potency.
•For initial dilution for I.V. infusion, reconstitute each gram of drug with at least 5 ml of sterile water for injection, sodium chloride for injection, D_5W, dextrose 5% in normal saline solution, or bacteriostatic water that contains parabens or benzyl alcohol. Shake solution vigorously after adding diluent to help drug dissolve, and inspect for particles and discoloration before giving.
•For further dilution, use sodium chloride for injection, D_5W, dextrose 5% in normal saline solution, lactated Ringer's solution, or dextran 6% in normal saline solution. Solutions diluted with lactated Ringer's solution should be given within 2 hours.
•For intermittent infusion, infuse appropriate dose over 20 to 30 minutes.
•Give aminoglycosides 1 hour before or after piperacillin; use a separate site, I.V. bag, and tubing.
•For I.M. injection, reconstitute each gram of piperacillin with at least 2 ml of an appropriate diluent listed above.
•Don't give more than 2 g I.M. at any one site. Use deltoid area cautiously and only if well developed to avoid injuring the radial nerve.
•Watch for bleeding or excessive bruising because drug can decrease platelet aggrega-

tion, especially in patients with renal failure. If bleeding occurs, notify prescriber and expect to stop piperacillin.
•Monitor CBC regularly, as ordered, to detect hematologic abnormalities, such as leukopenia and neutropenia.
•Monitor serum potassium level to detect hypokalemia from urinary potassium loss.
•Check for diarrhea during and after therapy because it may indicate pseudomembranous colitis caused by *Clostridium difficile.* If diarrhea occurs, notify prescriber and expect to withhold piperacillin and treat with fluids, electrolytes, protein, and an antibiotic effective against *C. difficile.*
•Watch closely for hypersensitivity reactions, especially if patient has cystic fibrosis. Notify prescriber, and expect to stop drug.

PATIENT TEACHING
•Advise patient to consult prescriber before using OTC drugs during piperacillin therapy because of the risk of interactions.
•Inform patient that increased bruising may occur if she takes anti-inflammatory drugs during piperacillin therapy.
•Advise patient to notify prescriber about signs of superinfection, such as white patches on tongue or in mouth.
•Urge patient to tell prescriber about diarrhea that's severe or lasts longer than 3 days. Remind patient that watery or bloody stools can occur 2 or more months after antibiotic therapy and can be serious, requiring prompt treatment.
•Instruct patient to complete full course of therapy, even if symptoms subside.

pirbuterol acetate

Maxair, Maxair Autohaler

Class and Category
Chemical class: Sympathomimetic amine
Therapeutic class: Bronchodilator
Pregnancy category: C

Indications and Dosages
➤ *To prevent or treat bronchospasm caused by COPD, to treat bronchospasm caused by asthma*

ORAL INHALATION
Adults and adolescents. 1 or 2 inhalations (200 to 400 mcg) every 4 to 6 hr. *Maximum:* 12 inhalations (2.4 mg) daily.

Route	Onset	Peak	Duration
Oral inhalation	In 5 min	In 30 to 90 min	3 to 6 hr

Mechanism of Action

Attaches to beta$_2$ receptors on bronchial cell membranes, which stimulates the intracellular enzyme adenyl cyclase to convert adenosine triphosphate (ATP) to cAMP. The increased intracellular level of cAMP relaxes bronchial smooth-muscle cells and inhibits histamine release. Pirbuterol also stabilizes mast cells and inhibits the release of histamine.

Contraindications

Hypersensitivity to pirbuterol or its components, tachycardia

Interactions
DRUGS

beta-adrenergic bronchodilators: Additive effects
beta blockers (ophthalmic): Possibly decreased pirbuterol effects, increased risk of bronchospasm
beta blockers (systemic): Decreased effects of both drugs, increased risk of bronchospasm
MAO inhibitors, tricyclic antidepressants: Potentiated cardiovascular effects

Adverse Reactions

CNS: Anxiety, confusion, depression, dizziness, headache, nervousness, tiredness, tremor
CV: Arrhythmias (including PVCs and tachycardia), chest pain, ECG changes (including flattening of T waves, prolonged QT interval, and ST-segment depression), hypotension, palpitations
EENT: Dry mouth
GI: Abdominal cramps, diarrhea, nausea, vomiting
RESP: Bronchospasm, cough
SKIN: Alopecia, rash, urticaria
Other: Facial edema, hypokalemia

Nursing Considerations

• For patient with a cardiovascular disorder, such as arrhythmias, hypertension, or ischemic cardiac disease, monitor blood pressure and heart rate and rhythm to detect significant changes after pirbuterol use.
• Be aware that elderly patients have a greater risk of adverse reactions than younger adults.
• **WARNING** Stop giving drug and notify prescriber immediately if patient has paradoxical bronchospasm, a life-threatening adverse reaction.
PATIENT TEACHING
• Teach patient how to use an inhaler and spacer correctly, and urge her to keep the inhaler readily available at all times.
• Recommend the use of an autohaler if patient has trouble coordinating inhalations with a regular inhaler.
• Advise patient to clean the inhaler's mouthpiece at least once daily.
• Caution patient against overusing drug because doing so may increase adverse reactions.
• Teach patient how to use a peak flow meter and how to determine her personal best reading.
• **WARNING** Advise patient to notify prescriber if symptoms worsen, if bronchospasm occurs more frequently, if she needs to use the inhaler more often, or if the inhaler becomes less effective.

piroxicam

Apo-Piroxicam (CAN), Feldene, Novo-Pirocam (CAN), Nu-Pirox (CAN), PMS-Piroxicam (CAN)

Class and Category

Chemical class: Oxicam derivative
Therapeutic class: Anti-inflammatory, antirheumatic
Pregnancy category: Not rated

Indications and Dosages

➤ *To treat acute and chronic osteoarthritis and rheumatoid arthritis*
CAPSULES
Adults. *Initial:* 20 mg once daily or 10 mg b.i.d.

Route	Onset	Peak	Duration
P.O.	Unknown	Several days to 1 wk*	Unknown

Contraindications

Angioedema, asthma, bronchospasm, nasal

---

* With severe inflammation, 2 wk or more.

P

polyps, rhinitis, or urticaria induced by aspirin, iodides, or other NSAIDs; hypersensitivity to piroxicam or its components

Mechanism of Action

Blocks the activity of cyclooxygenase, the enzyme needed for prostaglandin synthesis. Prostaglandins, important mediators of the inflammatory response, cause local vasodilation with swelling and pain. By blocking cyclooxygenase activity and inhibiting prostaglandins, this NSAID reduces inflammatory symptoms and pain.

Interactions

DRUGS

acetaminophen: Possibly increased adverse renal effects with long-term use of both drugs
antihypertensives: Possibly decreased or reversed effects of antihypertensives
aspirin, other NSAIDs: Increased risk of bleeding and adverse GI effects, possibly increased blood piroxicam level
cefamandole, cefoperazone, cefotetan: Increased risk of hypoprothrombinemia and bleeding
colchicine: Increased risk of GI bleeding, hemorrhage, and ulcers
corticosteroids, potassium supplements: Increased risk of adverse GI effects
cyclosporine: Increased risk of nephrotoxicity from both drugs, increased blood cyclosporine level
diuretics: Decreased antihypertensive, diuretic, and natriuretic effects of diuretics
gold compounds, nephrotoxic drugs: Increased risk of adverse renal effects
heparin, oral anticoagulants, thrombolytics: Increased anticoagulant effects, increased risk of hemorrhage
insulin, oral antidiabetic drugs: Possibly increased hypoglycemic effect of these drugs
lithium: Possibly increased blood lithium level and toxicity
methotrexate: Decreased methotrexate clearance and increased risk of methotrexate toxicity
platelet aggregation inhibitors: Increased risk of bleeding and GI ulceration or hemorrhage
plicamycin, valproic acid: Increased risk of hypoprothrombinemia and GI bleeding, hemorrhage, and ulceration
probenecid: Possibly increased blood level, effectiveness, and risk of toxicity of piroxicam

ACTIVITIES

alcohol use: Increased risk of adverse GI effects

Adverse Reactions

CNS: Anxiety, aseptic meningitis, asthenia, cerebral hemorrhage, confusion, depression, dizziness, dream disturbances, drowsiness, fever, headache, insomnia, ischemic stroke, malaise, nervousness, paresthesia, somnolence, syncope, transient ischemic attack, tremor, vertigo
CV: Deep vein thrombosis, edema, heart failure, hypertension, MI, peripheral edema, tachycardia
EENT: Blurred vision, dry mouth, epistaxis, glossitis, stomatitis, tinnitus
ENDO: Hypoglycemia
GI: Abdominal pain; anorexia; constipation; diarrhea; elevated liver function test results; esophagitis; flatulence; gastritis; GI bleeding, perforation, or ulceration; heartburn; hematemesis; hepatitis; indigestion; jaundice; liver failure; melena; nausea; vomiting
GU: Acute renal failure, cystitis, dysuria, elevated serum creatinine level, hematuria, interstitial nephritis, nephrotic syndrome, oliguria, polyuria, proteinuria, renal failure or insufficiency
HEME: Agranulocytosis, anemia, aplastic anemia, coagulation abnormalities, eosinophilia, leukopenia, pancytopenia, thrombocytopenia
RESP: Asthma, dyspnea
SKIN: Alopecia, diaphoresis, ecchymosis, erythema, erythema multiforme, exfoliative dermatitis, photosensitivity, pruritus, purpura, rash, Stevens-Johnson syndrome, toxic epidermal necrolysis, urticaria
Other: Anaphylaxis, angioedema, flulike symptoms, hyperkalemia, infection, sepsis, weight loss or gain

Nursing Considerations

• Administer piroxicam with food to decrease GI upset.
• Use piroxicam with extreme caution in patients with a history of ulcer disease or GI bleeding because NSAIDs such as piroxicam increase the risk of GI bleeding and ulceration. Expect to use piroxicam for the short-

est time possible in these patients.
•Be aware that serious GI tract ulceration, bleeding, and perforation may occur without warning symptoms. Elderly patients are at greater risk. To minimize risk, give drug with food. If GI distress occurs, withhold drug and notify prescriber immediately.
•Use piroxicam cautiously in patients with hypertension, and monitor blood pressure closely throughout therapy. Drug may cause hypertension or worsen it.
•**WARNING** Monitor patient closely for thrombotic events, including MI and stroke, because NSAIDs increase the risk.
•**WARNING** If patient has bone marrow suppression or is receiving antineoplastic drug therapy, monitor laboratory results (including WBC count), and watch for evidence of infection because anti-inflammatory and antipyretic actions of piroxicam may mask signs and symptoms, such as fever and pain.
•Especially if patient is elderly or taking drug long-term, watch for less common but serious adverse GI reactions, including anorexia, constipation, diverticulitis, dysphagia, esophagitis, gastritis, gastroenteritis, gastroesophageal reflux disease, hemorrhoids, hiatal hernia, melena, stomatitis, and vomiting.
•Monitor liver function test results because, in rare cases, elevated levels may progress to severe hepatic reactions, including fatal hepatitis, liver necrosis, and hepatic failure.
•Monitor BUN and serum creatinine levels in patients with heart failure, impaired renal function, or hepatic dysfunction; those taking diuretics or ACE inhibitors; and elderly patients because drug may cause renal failure.
•Monitor CBC for decreased hemoglobin and hematocrit because drug may worsen anemia.
•Assess patient's skin routinely for rash or other signs of hypersensitivity reaction because piroxicam and other NSAIDs may cause serious skin reactions without warning, even in patients with no history of NSAID hypersensitivity. Stop drug at first sign of reaction, and notify prescriber.
•**WARNING** Be aware that drug may cause premature closure of ductus arteriosus in growing fetus during third trimester of pregnancy. Be prepared to suggest referral for high-risk pregnancy.
PATIENT TEACHING
•Advise patient to take piroxicam with

meals to minimize GI distress. Also direct her to take drug with a full glass of water and to remain upright for 30 minutes afterward to decrease the risk of drug lodging in esophagus and causing irritation.
•Instruct patient to swallow capsules whole and not to crush, break, chew, or open them.
•Advise patient to avoid alcohol, aspirin, and other NSAIDs, unless prescribed, while taking piroxicam.
•Caution patient to avoid hazardous activities until drug's CNS effects are known.
•If patient also takes an anticoagulant, advise her to watch for and immediately report bleeding problems, such as bloody or tarry stools and bloody vomitus.
•If patient also takes insulin or an oral antidiabetic, advise her to closely monitor her blood glucose level to prevent hypoglycemia. Encourage her to carry candy or other simple sugars to treat mild hypoglycemia. Advise her to notify prescriber if hypoglycemic episodes are frequent or severe.
•Explain that piroxicam may increase the risk of serious adverse cardiovascular reactions; urge patient to seek immediate medical attention if signs or symptoms arise, such as chest pain, shortness of breath, weakness, and slurring of speech.
•Tell patient that piroxicam may increase the risk of serious adverse GI reactions; stress the need to seek immediate medical attention for such signs and symptoms as epigastric or abdominal pain, indigestion, black or tarry stools, or vomiting blood or material that looks like coffee grounds.
•Alert patient to the possibility of rare but serious skin reactions. Urge her to seek immediate medical attention for rash, blisters, itching, fever, or other indications of hypersensitivity.
•Instruct female patient to consult prescriber if she becomes pregnant because drug may cause premature closure of ductus arteriosus in growing fetus.

polymyxin B sulfate

Aerosporin

Class and Category

Chemical class: Bacillus polymyxa derivative
Therapeutic class: Antibiotic
Pregnancy category: Not rated

P

Indications and Dosages

➤ *To treat infections resistant to less toxic drugs, such as bacteremia, septicemia, and UTI caused by susceptible organisms, including* Enterobacter aerogenes, Escherichia coli, Haemophilus influenzae, *and* Klebsiella pneumoniae

I.V. INFUSION

Adults and children age 2 and over. 15,000 to 25,000 units/kg daily in divided doses every 12 hr or as a continuous infusion. *Maximum:* 2 million units daily.

Infants and children under age 2. Up to 40,000 units/kg daily in divided doses every 12 hr or as a continuous infusion.

I.M. INJECTION

Adults and children age 2 and over. 25,000 to 30,000 units/kg daily in divided doses every 4 to 6 hr. *Maximum:* 2 million units daily.

Infants and children under age 2. Up to 40,000 units/kg daily in divided doses every 4 to 6 hr.

DOSAGE ADJUSTMENT Dosage reduced by 50% for patients with creatinine clearance of 5 to 20 ml/min/1.73 m^2; by 85% for patients with creatinine clearance of less than 5 ml/min/ 1.73 m^2.

➤ *To prevent bacteriuria and bacteremia in patients with an indwelling catheter*

BLADDER IRRIGATION

Adults and children age 2 and over. Combination of 200,000 units (20 mg) of polymyxin B sulfate and 57 mg of neomycin sulfate added to 1,000 ml of normal saline solution daily as a continuous bladder irrigation for up to 10 days; rate adjusted as prescribed, based on patient's urine output.

➤ *To treat meningitis caused by susceptible strains of* Pseudomonas aeruginosa *or* H. influenzae

INTRATHECAL INJECTION

Adults and children age 2 and over. 50,000 units daily for 3 to 4 days, then 50,000 units every other day for at least 2 wk after CSF cultures are negative and glucose content is normal.

Infants and children under age 2. 20,000 units daily for 3 to 4 days, then 25,000 units every other day for at least 2 wk after CSF cultures are negative and glucose content is normal.

Mechanism of Action

Binds to cell membrane phospholipids in gram-negative bacteria, increasing the permeability of the cell membrane. Polymyxin B also acts as a cationic detergent, altering the osmotic barrier of the membrane and causing essential intracellular metabolites to leak out. Both actions lead to cell death.

Incompatibilities

Don't mix polymyxin B sulfate with amphotericin B, calcium salts, chloramphenicol, chlorothiazide, heparin sodium, magnesium salts, nitrofurantoin, penicillins, prednisolone, and tetracyclines. They're incompatible.

Contraindications

Hypersensitivity to polymyxin B or its components

Interactions

DRUGS

general anesthetics, neuromuscular blockers, skeletal muscle relaxants: Increased or prolonged skeletal muscle relaxation, possibly respiratory paralysis

nephrotoxic and neurotoxic drugs (such as aminoglycosides, amphotericin B, colistin, sodium citrate, streptomycin, tobramycin, and vancomycin): Increased risk of nephrotoxicity and neurotoxicity

Adverse Reactions

CNS: Ataxia, confusion, dizziness, drowsiness, fever, giddiness, headache, increased leukocyte and protein levels in CSF, neurotoxicity, paresthesia (circumoral or peripheral), slurred speech

CV: Thrombophlebitis

EENT: Blurred vision, nystagmus

GU: Albuminuria, azotemia, cylindruria, decreased urine output, hematuria, nephrotoxicity

HEME: Eosinophilia

RESP: Respiratory muscle paralysis

SKIN: Rash, urticaria

Other: Anaphylaxis, drug-induced fever, facial flushing, injection site pain, stiff neck (with intrathecal injection), superinfection

Nursing Considerations

•Be aware that patients receiving polymyxin B sulfate are hospitalized to allow appropriate supervision.

•Obtain blood, urine, or other samples for culture and sensitivity tests, as ordered, before giving drug. Expect to begin polymyxin B therapy before results are known. Keep in mind that baseline renal function tests should have been performed before administration. Check these test results, if available, and notify prescriber of abnormalities.

•For I.M. injection, reconstitute sterile powder with 2 ml of sterile water for injection or sodium chloride for injection.

•Be aware that I.M. route isn't usually recommended (especially for infants and children) because it can cause severe pain at injection site.

•For I.V. infusion, dissolve polymyxin B in 300 to 500 ml of D₅W and infuse over 60 to 90 minutes.

•For intrathecal route, add 10 ml of sodium chloride for injection to vial of polymyxin B.

•Inspect for particles and discoloration before giving drug.

•During therapy, monitor renal function, including BUN and serum creatinine levels, especially in patients with a history of renal insufficiency.

•**WARNING** Be aware that declining urine output and rising BUN level suggest nephrotoxicity, which also is characterized by albuminuria, azotemia, cylindruria, excessive excretion of electrolytes, hematuria, leukocyturia, and rising blood drug level. Notify prescriber immediately if you detect any of these signs.

•**WARNING** Notify prescriber immediately if patient experiences blurred vision, circumoral or peripheral paresthesia, confusion, dizziness, drowsiness, facial flushing, giddiness, myasthenia, nystagmus, or slurred speech. These may be signs of neurotoxicity, a serious adverse reaction that may lead to respiratory arrest or paralysis if untreated.

•Assess for signs of superinfection, such as mouth sores, severe diarrhea, and white patches on tongue or in mouth, especially in debilitated or elderly patients.

•Monitor fluid intake and output and provide adequate fluids to reduce the risk of nephrotoxicity.

PATIENT TEACHING

•Encourage patient to maintain adequate fluid intake during polymyxin B therapy.

•Instruct patient to notify prescriber immediately about diarrhea, mouth sores, or vaginitis, which may be early signs of superinfection.

posaconazole

Noxafil

Class and Category

Chemical class: Triazole
Therapeutic class: Antifungal
Pregnancy category: C

Indications and Dosages

➤ *To prevent invasive aspergillus and candida infections in patients at high risk because of severe immunocompromise from such conditions as graft-versus-host disease with hematopoietic stem-cell transplant or hematologic malignancies with prolonged neutropenia from chemotherapy*

ORAL SUSPENSION

Adults. 200 mg (5 ml) t.i.d. until recovery from neutropenia or immunosuppression.

➤ *To treat oropharyngeal candidiasis*

ORAL SUSPENSION

Adults. *Initial:* 100 mg (2.5 ml) b.i.d. on first day, followed by 100 mg (2.5 ml) once daily for 13 days.

➤ *To treat oropharyngeal candidiasis refractory to itraconazole and or fluconazole*

ORAL SUSPENSION

Adults. 400 mg (10 ml) b.i.d. until underlying condition improves.

Route	Onset	Peak	Duration
P.O.	Unknown	3 to 5 hr	Unknown

Mechanism of Action

Blocks synthesis of ergosterol, an essential component of the fungal cell membrane, by inhibiting 14 alpha-demethylase, an enzyme needed for conversion of lanosterol to ergosterol. Lack of ergosterol increases cellular permeability, and cell contents leak.

Contraindications

Concurrent therapy with sirolimus; hypersensitivity to posaconazole, its components, or other azole antifungals; use with ergot alkaloids or CYP3A4 substrates such as astemizole, cisapride, halofantrine, pimozide, quinidine, and terfenadine

Interactions

DRUGS

astemizole, cisapride, halofantrine, pimozide, quinidine, terfenadine: Increased risk of QT-interval prolongation and torsades de pointes
atazanavir, calcium channel blockers, cyclosporine, midazolam, phenytoin, rifabutin, ritonavir, sirolimus, tacrolimus: Increased plasma levels of these drugs, with increased risk of adverse reactions
cimetidine, efavirenz, phenytoin, rifabutin: Possibly decreased plasma level of posaconazole
digoxin: Increased risk of digitalis toxicity
ergot alkaloids: Increased plasma ergot alkaloid level and increased risk of ergotism
HMG-CoA reductase inhibitors: Increased plasma statin level and increased risk of rhabdomyolysis
vinca alkaloids: Increased plasma vinca alkaloid level and increased risk of neurotoxicity

Adverse Reactions

CNS: Anxiety, asthenia, dizziness, fatigue, fever, headache, insomnia, rigors, tremor, weakness
CV: Edema, hypertension, hypotension, QT-interval prolongation, tachycardia
EENT: Blurred vision, epistaxis, herpes simplex, mucositis, pharyngitis, taste perversion
ENDO: Hyperglycemia, hypocalcemia
GI: Abdominal pain, anorexia, bilirubinemia, constipation, diarrhea, dyspepsia, elevated liver enzyme levels, hepatomegaly, jaundice, nausea, vomiting
GU: Acute renal failure, elevated blood creatinine level, vaginal hemorrhage
HEME: Anemia, neutropenia, thrombocytopenia
MS: Arthralgia, back or musculoskeletal pain
RESP: Coughing, dyspnea, pneumonia, upper respiratory tract infection
SKIN: Diaphoresis, petechiae, pruritus, rash
Other: Bacteremia, cytomegalovirus infection, dehydration, hypokalemia, hypomagnesemia, weight loss

Nursing Considerations

•Use cautiously in patients who have had a hypersensitivity reaction to other azoles because of risk for cross-sensitivity.
•Use cautiously in patients with renal or hepatic dysfunction.
•Use cautiously in patients with potentially proarrhythmic conditions because posaconazole may prolong QT interval.
•Obtain baseline assessment of liver function and then check it periodically throughout therapy. If elevations occur or patient develops evidence of abnormal liver function, notify prescriber.

PATIENT TEACHING

•Advise patient to use the measuring spoon supplied by manufacturer and to rinse it with water after each use.
•Instruct patient to take posaconazole with a full meal or liquid nutritional supplement to increase drug absorption.
•Tell patient to notify prescriber if severe diarrhea or vomiting develops because these conditions may interfere with drug effectiveness.

potassium acetate

(contains 2 or 4 mEq of elemental potassium per 1 ml of injection)

potassium bicarbonate

(contains 6.5 mEq of elemental potassium per tablet, 20 or 25 mEq of elemental potassium per effervescent tablet for oral solution)
K+Care ET, K-Electrolyte, K-Ide, Klor-Con/EF, K-Lyte, K-Vescent

potassium bicarbonate and potassium chloride

(contains 20 mEq of elemental potassium per 2.8-g granule packet; 20, 25, or 50 mEq of elemental potassium per effervescent tablet for oral solution)
Klorvess Effervescent Granules, K-Lyte/Cl, K-Lyte/Cl 50, Neo-K (CAN), Potassium Sandoz (CAN)

potassium bicarbonate and potassium citrate

(contains 25 or 50 mEq of elemental potassium per effervescent tablet for oral solution)
Effer-K, K-Lyte DS

potassium chloride

(contains 8 or 10 mEq of elemental potassium per E.R. capsule; 6.7, 8, 10, 12, or 20 mEq of elemental potassium per E.R. tablet; 10, 20, 30, or 40 mEq of elemental potassium per 15 ml of oral solution; 10, 15, 20, or 25 mEq of elemental potassium per packet for oral solution; 20 mEq of elemental potassium per packet for oral suspension; 0.1, 0.2, 0.3, 0.4, 1.5, 2, 3, or 10 mEq of elemental potassium per 1 ml of injection)
Apo-K (CAN), Cena-K, Gen-K, K-8, K-10 (CAN), K+ 10, Kalium Durules (CAN), Kaochlor 10%, Kaochlor S-F 10%, Kaon-Cl, Kato, Kay Ciel, K+ Care, KCL 5% (CAN), K-Dur, K-Ide, K-Lease, K-Long (CAN), K-Lor, Klor-Con 10, Klor-Con Powder, Klor-Con/25 Powder, Klorvess 10% Liquid, Klotrix, K-Lyte/Cl Powder, K-Med 900 (CAN), K-Norm, K-Sol, K-Tab, Micro-K, Micro-K 10, Potasalan, Roychlor 10% (CAN), Rum-K, Slow-K, Ten-K

potassium gluconate

(contains 20 mEq of elemental potassium per 15 ml of elixir; 2, 2.3, or 2.5 mEq of elemental potassium per tablet)
Glu-K, Kaon, Kaylixir, K-G Elixir, Potassium-Rougier (CAN)

potassium gluconate and potassium chloride

(contains 20 mEq of elemental potassium per 15 ml of oral solution; 20 mEq of elemental potassium per 5-g packet for oral solution)
Kolyum

potassium gluconate and potassium citrate

(contains 20 mEq of elemental potassium per 15 ml of oral solution)
Twin-K

trikates

(contains 15 mEq of elemental potassium per 5 ml of oral solution)
Tri-K

Class and Category
Chemical class: Electrolyte cation
Therapeutic class: Electrolyte replacement
Pregnancy category: C

Indications and Dosages

➤ *To prevent or treat hypokalemia in patients who can't ingest sufficient dietary potassium or who are losing potassium because of certain conditions (such as hepatic cirrhosis and prolonged vomiting) or drugs (such as potassium-wasting diuretics and certain antibiotics)*

EFFERVESCENT TABLETS (POTASSIUM BICARBONATE)
Adults and adolescents. 25 to 50 mEq/g once or twice daily, as needed and tolerated. *Maximum:* 100 mEq daily.

EFFERVESCENT TABLETS (POTASSIUM BICARBONATE AND POTASSIUM CHLORIDE)
Adults and adolescents. 20, 25, or 50 mEq once or twice daily, as needed and tolerated. *Maximum:* 100 mEq daily.

EFFERVESCENT TABLETS (POTASSIUM BICARBONATE AND POTASSIUM CITRATE)
Adults and adolescents. 25 or 50 mEq once or twice daily, as needed and tolerated. *Maximum:* 100 mEq daily.

ELIXIR (POTASSIUM GLUCONATE)
Adults and adolescents. 20 mEq b.i.d. to q.i.d., as needed and tolerated. *Maximum:* 100 mEq daily.
Children. 2 to 3 mEq/kg daily in divided doses.

E.R. CAPSULES (POTASSIUM CHLORIDE)
Adults and adolescents. 40 to 100 mEq daily in divided doses b.i.d. or t.i.d. for treatment; 16 to 24 mEq daily in divided doses b.i.d. or t.i.d. for prevention. *Maximum:* 100 mEq daily.

E.R. TABLETS (POTASSIUM CHLORIDE)
Adults and adolescents. 6.7 to 20 mEq t.i.d. *Maximum:* 100 mEq daily.

GRANULE PACKETS (POTASSIUM BICARBONATE AND POTASSIUM CHLORIDE)
Adults and adolescents. 20 mEq once or twice daily, as needed and tolerated. *Maximum:* 100 mEq daily.

GRANULES FOR ORAL SUSPENSION (POTASSIUM CHLORIDE)
Adults and adolescents. 20 mEq 1 to 5 times/day, as needed. *Maximum:* 100 mEq daily.

ORAL SOLUTION (POTASSIUM CHLORIDE)
Adults and adolescents. 20 mEq once daily to q.i.d., as needed and tolerated. *Maximum:* 100 mEq daily.
Children. 1 to 3 mEq/kg daily in divided doses.

ORAL SOLUTION (POTASSIUM GLUCONATE AND POTASSIUM CHLORIDE, POTASSIUM GLUCONATE AND POTASSIUM CITRATE)
Adults and adolescents. 20 mEq b.i.d. to

P

q.i.d., as needed and tolerated. *Maximum:* 100 mEq daily.
Children. 2 to 3 mEq/kg daily in divided doses.
POWDER PACKET FOR ORAL SOLUTION (POTASSIUM CHLORIDE)
Adults. 15 to 25 mEq b.i.d. to q.i.d., as needed and tolerated. *Maximum:* 100 mEq daily.
Children. 1 to 3 mEq/kg daily in divided doses, as needed and tolerated.
POWDER PACKET FOR ORAL SOLUTION (POTASSIUM GLUCONATE AND POTASSIUM CHLORIDE)
Adults and adolescents. 20 mEq b.i.d. to q.i.d., as needed and tolerated. *Maximum:* 100 mEq daily.
Children. 2 to 3 mEq/kg daily in divided doses.
ORAL TRIKATES SOLUTION (POTASSIUM ACETATE, POTASSIUM BICARBONATE, AND POTASSIUM CITRATE)
Adults and adolescents. 15 mEq t.i.d. to q.i.d., as needed and tolerated. *Maximum:* 100 mEq daily.
Children. 2 to 3 mEq/kg daily in divided doses.
TABLETS (POTASSIUM GLUCONATE)
Adults and adolescents. 5 to 10 mEq b.i.d. to q.i.d., as needed and tolerated. *Maximum:* 100 mEq daily.
I.V. INFUSION (POTASSIUM ACETATE AND POTASSIUM CHLORIDE)
Adults and adolescents with serum potassium level above 2.5 mEq/L. Up to 10 mEq/hr. Maximum: 200 mEq daily.
Adults and adolescents with serum potassium level below 2 mEq/L, ECG changes, or paralysis. Up to 20 mEq/hr. *Maximum:* 400 mEq daily.
Children. 3 mEq/kg daily.
DOSAGE ADJUSTMENT Dosage adjusted as prescribed based on patient's ECG patterns and serum potassium level.

Mechanism of Action
Acts as the major cation in intracellular fluid, activating many enzymatic reactions that are essential for physiologic processes, including nerve impulse transmission and cardiac and skeletal muscle contraction. Potassium also helps maintain electroneutrality in cells by controlling the exchange of intracellular and extracellular ions. It also helps maintain normal renal function and acid-base balance.

Incompatibilities
Don't mix potassium chloride for injection in same syringe with amino acid solutions, lipid solutions, or mannitol because these drugs may precipitate from solution. Administration with blood or blood products can cause lysis of infused RBCs.

Contraindications
Acute dehydration, Addison's disease (untreated), concurrent use of potassium-sparing diuretics, crush syndrome, heat cramps, hyperkalemia, hypersensitivity to potassium salts or their components, renal impairment with azotemia or oliguria, severe hemolytic anemia

Interactions
DRUGS
ACE inhibitors, beta blockers, blood products, cyclosporine, heparin, NSAIDs, potassium-containing drugs, potassium-sparing diuretics: Increased risk of hyperkalemia
amphotericin B, corticosteroids (glucocorticoids or mineralocorticoids), gentamicin, penicillins, polymyxin B: Possibly hypokalemia
anticholinergics, drugs with anticholinergic activity: Increased risk of GI ulceration, stricture, and perforation
calcium salts (parenteral): Possibly arrhythmias
digoxin: Increased risk of digitalis toxicity
insulin, laxatives, sodium bicarbonate: Decreased serum potassium level
sodium polystyrene sulfonate: Possibly decreased serum potassium level and fluid retention
thiazide diuretics: Possibly hyperkalemia when diuretic is discontinued
FOODS
low-salt milk, salt substitutes: Increased risk of hyperkalemia

Adverse Reactions
CNS: Confusion, paralysis, paresthesia, weakness
CV: Arrhythmias, ECG changes
EENT: Throat pain when swallowing
GI: Abdominal pain; bloody stools; diarrhea; flatulence; GI bleeding, perforation, or ulceration; intestinal obstruction; nausea; vomiting
RESP: Dyspnea
SKIN: Rash
Other: Hyperkalemia

Nursing Considerations
•Administer oral potassium with or immediately after meals.

•Mix potassium chloride for oral solution or potassium gluconate elixir in cold water, orange juice, tomato juice (if patient isn't sodium restricted), or apple juice, and stir for 1 full minute before administering.

•Mix potassium bicarbonate, potassium bicarbonate and potassium chloride, and potassium bicarbonate and potassium citrate effervescent tablets with cold water and allow to dissolve completely.

•Be aware that liquid form of oral potassium is prescribed for patients with delayed gastric emptying, esophageal compression, or intestinal obstruction or stricture to decrease the risk of tissue damage.

•**WARNING** Be aware that direct injection of a potassium concentrate may be immediately fatal. Dilute potassium concentrate for injection with an adequate volume of solution before I.V. use. Maximum concentration suggested is 40 mEq/L, although stronger concentrations (up to 80 mEq/L) may be used for severe hypokalemia. Inappropriate solutions or improper technique may cause extravasation, fever, hyperkalemia, hypervolemia, I.V. site infection, phlebitis, venospasm, and venous thrombosis.

•Infuse potassium slowly to avoid phlebitis and decrease the risk of adverse cardiac reactions. Keep in mind that different forms of potassium salts contain different amounts of elemental potassium per gram and that not all forms are dosage equivalent.

•Monitor serum potassium level before and during administration of I.V. potassium.

•**WARNING** Be aware that some forms of potassium contain tartrazine, which may cause an allergic reaction, such as asthma. Some forms may also contain aluminum, which may become toxic in a patient with impaired renal function.

•Regularly assess patient for signs of hypokalemia, such as arrhythmias, fatigue, and weakness, and for signs of hyperkalemia, such as arrhythmias, confusion, dyspnea, and paresthesia.

•Because adequate renal function is needed for potassium supplementation, monitor serum creatinine level and urine output during administration. Notify prescriber about signs of decreased renal function.

PATIENT TEACHING
•Inform patient that potassium is part of a normal diet and that most meats, seafoods, fruits, and vegetables contain sufficient potassium to meet the recommended daily intake. Also advise her not to exceed the recommended daily amount of potassium.

•Teach patient the correct way to take the prescribed potassium. This can vary from swallowing a tablet with a full glass of water to mixing certain preparations with one-half to a full glass of cold water or juice.

•Caution patient not to crush or chew E.R. forms unless instructed otherwise.

•Instruct patient to take drug with or right after food.

•Teach patient how to take her radial pulse, and advise her to notify prescriber about significant changes in heart rate or rhythm.

•Advise patient to watch stools for changes in color and consistency and to notify prescriber if they become black, tarry, or red.

•Inform patient that although she may see waxy form of E.R. tablet in stools, she has received all of the potassium.

•Urge patient to keep follow-up laboratory appointments as directed by prescriber to determine serum potassium level.

potassium iodide
(KI, SSKI)

Pima, Thyro-Block

Class and Category
Chemical class: Iodine
Therapeutic class: Antithyroid, radiation protectant
Pregnancy category: D

Indications and Dosages
➤ *To prepare for thyroidectomy*
ORAL SOLUTION
Adults and children. 50 to 250 mg t.i.d. for 10 to 14 days before surgery.

➤ *To manage thyrotoxic crisis*
ORAL SOLUTION
Adults. 50 to 250 mg t.i.d. or 500 mg every 4 hr.

➤ *To protect thyroid gland during radiation exposure*
ORAL SOLUTION, SYRUP, TABLETS
Adults and adolescents. 100 to 150 mg 24 hr before administration of or exposure to radioactive isotopes of iodine and daily for 3 to 10 days afterward. *Maximum:* 12 g daily.

P

Children age 1 and over. 130 mg daily for 10 days after administration of or exposure to radioactive isotopes of iodine.
Children under age 1. 65 mg daily for 10 days after administration of or exposure to radioactive isotopes of iodine.

Route	Onset	Peak	Duration
P.O.*	24 hr	10 to 15 days	Up to 6 wk

Mechanism of Action
Inhibits the release of thyroid hormone into the circulation, thus alleviating symptoms caused by excessive thyroid hormone stimulation. Potassium iodide also blocks thyroidal uptake of radioactive iodine isotopes that are released as a result of radiation exposure.

Contraindications
Acute bronchitis, Addison's disease, dehydration, heat cramps, hyperkalemia, hypersensitivity to iodides or their components, hyperthyroidism, iodism, renal impairment, tuberculosis

Interactions
DRUGS
antithyroid drugs, lithium: Increased risk of hypothyroidism and goiter
captopril, enalapril, lisinopril, potassium-sparing diuretics: Increased risk of hyperkalemia

Adverse Reactions
CNS: Confusion, fatigue, headache, heaviness or weakness in legs, paresthesia
CV: Irregular heartbeat
EENT: Burning in mouth or throat, increased salivation, metallic taste, sore teeth or gums
GI: Diarrhea, epigastric pain, indigestion, nausea, vomiting
HEME: Eosinophilia
MS: Arthralgia
SKIN: Acneiform lesions, urticaria
Other: Angioedema, lymphadenopathy

Nursing Considerations
•Be aware that potassium iodide shouldn't be given to patients with tuberculosis because drug may cause pulmonary irritation

---

* For antithyroid effects.

and increased secretions.
•**WARNING** Monitor serum potassium level regularly in patients with renal impairment because of the risk of hyperkalemia.
•Monitor thyroid function test results periodically to assess drug's effectiveness.
PATIENT TEACHING
•Advise patient taking potassium iodide oral solution or syrup to use a calibrated liquid-measuring device to ensure accurate doses.
•Urge patient to mix solution or syrup in a full glass (8 oz) of water, fruit juice, milk, or broth to improve taste and lessen GI reactions. Advise patient taking tablet form to dissolve each tablet in half a glass (4 oz) of water or milk before ingestion.
•If crystals form in solution, advise patient to place the closed container in warm water and gently shake to dissolve.
•Instruct patient to discard bottle and obtain a new one if solution turns brownish yellow.

potassium phosphates
K-Phos Original, Neutra-Phos-K

potassium and sodium phosphates
K-Phos M.F., K-Phos-Neutral, K-Phos No. 2, Neutra-Phos

sodium phosphates

Class and Category
Chemical class: Anion, soluble salts
Therapeutic class: Antiurolithic, electrolyte replenisher, urinary acidifier
Pregnancy category: C

Indications and Dosages
➤ *As adjunct to treat UTI, to prevent renal calculus formation*
MONOBASIC TABLETS (POTASSIUM PHOSPHATES)
Adults and adolescents. 1 g in 180 to 240 ml of water q.i.d., after meals and at bedtime.
MONOBASIC TABLETS (POTASSIUM AND SODIUM PHOSPHATES)
Adults and adolescents. 250 mg in 240 ml of water q.i.d., after meals and at bedtime. Dosage interval may be increased to every 2 hr if urine is difficult to acidify. *Maximum:* 2 g/24 hr.
➤ *To prevent or treat hypophosphatemia*

CAPSULES (POTASSIUM PHOSPHATES)
Adults and children age 4 and over. 1.45 g in 75 ml of water or juice q.i.d., after meals and at bedtime.
Children up to age 4. 200 mg in 60 ml of water or juice q.i.d., after meals and at bedtime.

CAPSULES (POTASSIUM AND SODIUM PHOSPHATES)
Adults and children age 4 and over. 1.25 g in 75 ml of water or juice q.i.d., after meals and at bedtime.
Children up to age 4. 200 mg in 60 ml of water or fruit juice q.i.d., after meals and at bedtime.

MONOBASIC TABLETS (POTASSIUM PHOSPHATES)
Adults and children age 4 and over. 1 g in 180 to 240 ml of water q.i.d., after meals and at bedtime.
Children up to age 4. 200 mg in 60 ml of water q.i.d., after meals and at bedtime.

MONOBASIC TABLETS (POTASSIUM AND SODIUM PHOSPHATES)
Adults and children age 4 and over. 250 mg in 240 ml of water q.i.d., after meals and at bedtime.
Children up to age 4. 200 mg in 60 ml of water q.i.d., after meals and at bedtime.

ORAL SOLUTION (POTASSIUM PHOSPHATES, POTASSIUM AND SODIUM PHOSPHATES)
Adults and children age 4 and over. 250 mg q.i.d., after meals and at bedtime.
Children up to age 4. 200 mg q.i.d., after meals and at bedtime.

TABLETS (POTASSIUM AND SODIUM PHOSPHATES)
Adults and children age 4 and over. 250 mg in a full glass of water q.i.d., after meals and at bedtime.
Children up to age 4. 200 mg in 60 ml of water q.i.d., after meals and at bedtime.

I.V. INFUSION (SODIUM PHOSPHATES)
Adults and adolescents. 10 to 15 mmol (310 to 465 mg) daily.
Children. 1.5 to 2 mmol (46.5 to 62 mg)/kg daily.

Mechanism of Action

Reverses symptoms of hypophosphatemia by replenishing the body's supply of phosphate; acidifies urine by causing hydrogen to be exchanged for sodium in the renal distal tubule; and inhibits formation of calcium renal calculi by preventing solidification of calcium oxalate.

Incompatibilities

Don't add phosphates to calcium- or magnesium-containing solutions because precipitate may form.

Contraindications

Hyperkalemia (potassium formulations only), hypernatremia (sodium formulations only), hyperphosphatemia, magnesium ammonium phosphate urolithiasis accompanied by infection, severe renal insufficiency, UTI caused by urea-splitting organisms

Interactions
DRUGS

ACE inhibitors, cyclosporine, heparin (long-term use), NSAIDs, potassium-containing drugs, potassium-sparing diuretics: Increased risk of hyperkalemia (potassium forms only)
aluminum- or magnesium-containing antacids: Possibly impaired phosphate absorption
anabolic steroids, androgens, corticosteroids, estrogens: Increased risk of edema (sodium formulations only)
calcium-containing drugs: Increased risk of calcium deposition in soft tissues
iron supplements: Decreased absorption of oral iron
phosphate-containing drugs, vitamin D: Increased risk of hyperphosphatemia
salicylates: Increased blood salicylate level
zinc supplements: Reduced zinc absorption
FOODS
low-salt milk, salt substitutes: Increased risk of hyperkalemia
oxalates (in spinach and rhubarb), phyates (in bran and whole grains): Decreased absorption of phosphate

Adverse Reactions

CNS: Anxiety, confusion, dizziness, fatigue, headache, paresthesia, seizures, tremor, weakness
CV: Arrhythmias, edema of legs, tachycardia
GI: Diarrhea, epigastric pain, nausea, thirst, vomiting
GU: Decreased urine output
MS: Muscle cramps or weakness
RESP: Dyspnea
Other: Hyperkalemia, hypernatremia, hyperphosphatemia, hypocalcemia, weight gain

Nursing Considerations

•Monitor serum phosphorus level, as appropriate, in patient who receives phosphates

and has a condition that may be associated with an elevated phosphorus level, such as chronic renal disease, hypoparathyroidism, and rhabdomyolysis; phosphates may further increase serum phosphorus level.
•Monitor serum calcium level, as appropriate, in patient who receives phosphates and has a condition that may be associated with a low calcium level, such as acute pancreatitis, chronic renal disease, hypoparathyroidism, osteomalacia, rhabdomyolysis, and rickets; phosphates may further decrease serum calcium level.
•Monitor serum potassium level, as appropriate, if patient who receives potassium phosphate has a condition linked to an elevated potassium level, such as acute dehydration, adrenal insufficiency, extensive tissue breakdown (as in severe burns), myotonia congenita, pancreatitis, rhabdomyolysis, and severe renal insufficiency; she may have an increased risk of hyperkalemia.
•Monitor serum sodium level in patient who receives sodium phosphates and has a condition that may be exacerbated by sodium excess, such as heart failure, hypernatremia, hypertension, peripheral or pulmonary edema, preeclampsia, renal impairment, and severe hepatic disease.
•Monitor urine pH, as ordered, to assess drug effectiveness when it's used to acidify urine.
•When administering sodium phosphates, monitor ECG tracing frequently during I.V. infusion to detect arrhythmias.

PATIENT TEACHING
•Instruct patient to take phosphates after meals to avoid GI upset and decrease laxative effect.
•Stress the importance of not swallowing capsules or tablets whole; instead, advise patient to soak tablets in water or fruit juice for 2 to 3 minutes to dissolve them.
•Suggest chilling the diluted drug to improve the flavor, but caution against freezing.
•Encourage increased intake of fluids (8 oz/hour, if not contraindicated) to prevent kidney stones.
•Urge patient to notify prescriber immediately about muscle weakness or cramps, unexplained weight gain, or shortness of breath.
•Instruct patient who needs an iron supplement to take it 1 to 2 hours after taking phosphates.

pralidoxime chloride
(2-PAM chloride, 2-pyridine aldoxime methochloride)
Protopam Chloride

Class and Category
Chemical class: Quaternary ammonium oxime
Therapeutic class: Anticholinesterase antidote
Pregnancy category: C

Indications and Dosages
➤ *As adjunct to reverse organophosphate pesticide toxicity*
I.V. INFUSION, I.M. OR SUBCUTANEOUS INJECTION
Adults. *Initial:* 1 to 2 g in 100 ml of normal saline solution infused over 15 to 30 min, given concurrently with atropine 2 to 6 mg every 5 to 60 min until muscarinic signs and symptoms disappear; may be repeated in 1 hr and then every 3 to 8 hr if muscle weakness persists. If I.V. route isn't feasible, administer I.M. or subcutaneously.
Children. *Initial:* 20 mg/kg in 100 ml of normal saline solution infused over 15 to 30 min, given concurrently with atropine (dosage individualized); may be repeated in 1 hr and then every 3 to 8 hr if muscle weakness persists. If I.V. route isn't feasible, administer I.M. or subcutaneously.

➤ *To treat anticholinesterase overdose secondary to myasthenic drugs (including ambenonium, neostigmine, and pyridostigmine)*
I.V. INJECTION
Adults. *Initial:* 1 to 2 g, followed by 250 mg every 5 min.

➤ *To treat exposure to nerve agents*
I.V. INJECTION
Adults. *Initial:* 1 atropine-containing autoinjector followed by 1 pralidoxime-containing autoinjector as soon as atropine's effects are evident; both injections repeated every 15 min for 2 additional doses if nerve agent symptoms persist.
DOSAGE ADJUSTMENT Dosage reduced for patients with renal insufficiency.

Contraindications
Hypersensitivity to pralidoxime chloride or its components

Mechanism of Action

Reverses muscle paralysis by removing the phosphoryl group from inhibited cholinesterase molecules at the neuromuscular junction of skeletal and respiratory muscles. Reactivation of cholinesterase restores body's ability to metabolize acetylcholine, which is inhibited by organophosphate pesticides, anticholinesterase overdose, or nerve agent poisoning.

Interactions
DRUGS

aminophylline, morphine, phenothiazines, reserpine, succinylcholine, theophylline: Increased symptoms of organophosphate poisoning

barbiturates: Potentiated barbiturate effects

Adverse Reactions

CNS: Dizziness, drowsiness, headache
CV: Increased systolic and diastolic blood pressure, tachycardia
EENT: Accommodation disturbances, blurred vision, diplopia
GI: Nausea, vomiting
MS: Muscle weakness
RESP: Hyperventilation
Other: Injection site pain

Nursing Considerations

• Be aware that pralidoxime must be given within 36 hours of toxicity to be effective.
• Use drug with extreme caution in patients with myasthenia gravis being treated for organophosphate poisoning because pralidoxime may precipitate myasthenic crisis.
• Reconstitute drug according to manufacturer's guidelines and administration route.
• For intermittent infusion, further dilute with normal saline solution to 100 ml and infuse over 15 to 30 minutes.
• Avoid too-rapid delivery, which may cause hypertension, laryngospasm, muscle spasms, neuromuscular blockade, and tachycardia. Also be sure to avoid intradermal injection.
• Closely monitor neuromuscular status during therapy.
• Monitor BUN and serum creatinine levels, as appropriate, in patients with renal insufficiency because drug is excreted in urine.
• When pralidoxime is administered with atropine, expect signs of atropination, such as dry mouth and nose, flushing, mydriasis, and tachycardia, to occur earlier than might be expected when atropine is given alone.

PATIENT TEACHING

• Inform patient receiving I.M. pralidoxime that she'll experience pain at the injection site for 40 to 60 minutes afterward.
• Reassure patient that she'll be closely monitored throughout therapy.

pramipexole dihydrochloride

Mirapex

Class and Category

Chemical class: Benzothiazolamine derivative
Therapeutic class: Antidyskinetic
Pregnancy category: C

Indications and Dosages

➤ *To treat Parkinson's disease, with or without concurrent levodopa therapy*
TABLETS

Adults. *Initial:* 0.125 mg t.i.d. for 1 wk, increased weekly thereafter as follows: for week 2, 0.25 mg t.i.d.; for week 3, 0.5 mg t.i.d.; for week 4, 0.75 mg t.i.d.; for week 5, 1 mg t.i.d.; for week 6, 1.25 mg t.i.d.; and for week 7, 1.5 mg t.i.d. *Maintenance:* 1.5 to 4.5 mg daily in divided doses t.i.d. *Maximum:* 4.5 mg daily.
DOSAGE ADJUSTMENT For patients with renal impairment, dosage reduced as follows: for creatinine clearance of 35 to 59 ml/min/1.73 m^2, initial dose of 0.125 mg b.i.d., maximum of 3 mg daily; for creatinine clearance of 15 to 34 ml/min/1.73 m^2, initial dose of 0.125 mg daily, maximum of 1.5 mg daily. Drug should not be given to patients with creatinine clearance of less than 15 ml/min/1.73 m^2.

➤ *To treat restless legs syndrome*
TABLETS

Adults. *Initial:* 0.125 mg once daily, 2 to 3 hours before bedtime, increased in 4 to 7 days to 0.25 mg once daily 2 to 3 hours before at bedtime as needed and further increased in 4 to 7 days to 0.5 mg once daily 2 to 3 hours before bedtime, as needed.
DOSAGE ADJUSTMENT For patients with moderate to severe renal impairment (creatinine clearance 20 to 60 ml/min/1.73 m^2) dosage interval for titration, if needed, increased to 14 days.

P

> **Mechanism of Action**
> May stimulate dopamine receptors in the brain, thereby easing symptoms of Parkinson's disease, which is thought to be caused by a dopamine deficiency.

Contraindications

Hypersensitivity to pramipexole or its components

Interactions

DRUGS

carbidopa, levodopa: Possibly increased peak blood levodopa level and potentiation of levodopa's dopaminergic adverse effects
diltiazem, quinidine, quinine, ranitidine, triamterene, verapamil: Decreased pramipexole clearance
haloperidol, metoclopramide, phenothiazines, thioxanthenes: Decreased pramipexole effectiveness

Adverse Reactions

CNS: Abnormal behavior, amnesia, anxiety, asthenia, confusion, dream disturbances, drowsiness, dyskinesia, dystonia, fatigue, fever, hallucinations, headache, insomnia, malaise, paranoia, restlessness, syncope
CV: Edema, orthostatic hypotension
EENT: Diplopia, dry mouth, rhinitis, vision changes
GI: Anorexia, constipation, dysphagia, nausea
GU: Altered libido, impotence, urinary frequency, urinary incontinence
MS: Arthralgia, myalgia, myasthenia
RESP: Pneumonia
SKIN: Diaphoresis, rash
Other: Eating disorders (binge or compulsive eating, hyperphagia), weight gain or loss

Nursing Considerations

•Use pramipexole cautiously in patients with hallucinations, hypotension, or retinal problems (such as macular degeneration) because drug may worsen these conditions.
•Also use cautiously in patients with renal impairment because pramipexole elimination may be decreased.
•Take safety precautions according to facility policy until drug's CNS effects are known.
•Avoid stopping pramipexole abruptly because doing so may cause a symptom complex resembling neuroleptic malignant syndrome, consisting of hyperpyrexia, muscle rigidity, altered level of consciousness, and autonomic instability.

PATIENT TEACHING

•Advise patient to take pramipexole with meals if nausea occurs.
•Caution patient about possible dizziness, drowsiness, or light-headedness, which may result from orthostatic hypotension. Advise her not to rise quickly from a lying or sitting position to minimize these effects.
•Instruct patient to notify prescriber immediately about vision problems or urinary frequency or incontinence.
•Inform patient that improvement in motor performance and activities of daily living may take 2 to 3 weeks.

pramlintide acetate

Symlin

Class and Category

Chemical class: Synthetic analogue of human amylin, a pancreatic beta cell hormone
Therapeutic class: Antidiabetic
Pregnancy category: C

Indications and Dosages

➤ *To achieve euglycemia in patients with type 1 diabetes who use mealtime insulin therapy but have not achieved desired glucose control*

SUBCUTANEOUS INJECTION

Adults. *Initial:* 15 mcg just before major meals with 50% reduced dosage of preprandial rapid-acting or short-acting insulin, including fixed-mix insulins such as 70/30. When nausea has abated at least 3 days, dosage increased in increments of 15 mcg. *Maintenance:* 30 to 60 mcg before major meals.
DOSAGE ADJUSTMENT Dosage decreased to 30 mcg if nausea occurs and persists at higher dosages.

➤ *To achieve euglycemia in patients with type 2 diabetes who use mealtime insulin, with or without a sulfonylurea and/or metformin, and have not achieved desire glucose control*

SUBCUTANEOUS INJECTION

Adults. *Initial:* 60 mcg immediately before major meals combined with dosage reduction of preprandial rapid-acting or short-acting insulin, including fixed-mix insulins such as 70/30, by 50%. When nausea has been absent for 3 to 7 days, dosage increased to 120 mcg before major meals.

DOSAGE ADJUSTMENT Dosage decreased to 60 mcg before major meals if nausea occurs and persists with 120-mcg dosage.

Route	Onset	Peak	Duration
SubQ	Unknown	19 to 21 min	3 hr

Mechanism of Action

Slows the rate at which food is released from the stomach to the small intestine, thus reducing the initial postprandial rise in serum glucose level. Pramlintide also suppresses glucagon secretion and promotes satiety, thus furthering weight loss, which also lowers serum glucose level.

Pramlintide is a synthetic analogue of amylin, a naturally occurring neuroendocrine hormone secreted with insulin by pancreatic beta cells. In diabetes, secretion of insulin and amylin is reduced or absent.

Contraindications

Gastroparesis, hypersensitivity to pramlintide, cresol or its components; hypoglycemia unawareness

Incompatibilities

Do not mix in same syringe as insulin because pharmacokinetic parameters of pramlintide become altered.

Interactions

DRUGS

drugs that alter GI motility (such as anticholinergics) or slow intestinal absorption of nutrients (such as alpha-glucosidase inhibitors): Altered effects of these drugs
oral drugs: Delayed absorption

Adverse Reactions

CNS: Dizziness, fatigue, headache
EENT: Blurred vision, pharyngitis
ENDO: Insulin-induced hypoglycemia
GI: Abdominal pain, anorexia, nausea, vomiting
MS: Arthralgia
RESP: Coughing

SKIN: Diaphoresis
Other: Hypersensitivity reactions; local injection site reaction, such as redness, swelling, or pruritus

Nursing Considerations

• Because of the risks involved with pramlintide therapy, insulin-using patients with type 1 or 2 diabetes must have failed to achieve adequate glycemic control despite individualized insulin management and must be receiving ongoing care under the guidance of the insulin prescriber and a diabetes educator before pramlintide is prescribed.

• Expect that certain patients won't be prescribed pramlintide because its risks may outweigh its benefits. These include patients with poor compliance to the current insulin regimen, poor compliance with monitoring blood glucose level, a glycosylated hemoglobin greater than 9%, recurrent severe hypoglycemia that required assistance during the past 6 months, hypoglycemia unawareness, gastroparesis, concurrent therapy with drugs that stimulate GI motility, and pediatric patients.

• Before pramlintide therapy starts, make sure patient's pre-meal insulin dosage has been reduced by 50%.

• Give drug immediately before major meals.

• Monitor patient's pre- and post-meal blood glucose levels regularly to determine effectiveness of pramlintide and insulin therapy and to detect hypoglycemia.

• For 3 hours after each dose of pramlintide, monitor patient closely for hypoglycemia, which may be severe, especially in patients with type 1 diabetes. Effects may include hunger, headache, sweating, tremor, irritability, and trouble concentrating. They may occur with a rapid decrease in blood glucose level regardless of glucose values.

• Although pramlintide doesn't cause hypoglycemia, it's use with insulin increases the risk of insulin-induced severe hypoglycemia, which can result in loss of consciousness, coma, or seizures. If hypoglycemia occurs, provide supportive care, including glucagon if prescribed, and notify prescriber. Expect insulin dosage accompanying pramlintide to be reduced.

• Keep in mind that early warning symptoms of hypoglycemia may be different or less severe if patient has had diabetes for a long

P

time; has diabetic nerve disease; takes a beta blocker, clonidine, guanethidine, or reserpine; or is under intensified diabetes control.
•Closely monitor patients who are taking oral antidiabetics, ACE inhibitors, disopyramide, fibrates, fluoxetine, MAO inhibitors, pentoxifylline, propoxyphene, salicylates, or sulfonamide antibiotics because of an increased risk of hypoglycemia.
•Expect pramlintide to be stopped if patient develops recurrent hypoglycemia that requires medical assistance, develops persistent nausea, or becomes noncompliant with therapy or follow-up visits.

PATIENT TEACHING
•Alert patient that insulin-induced hypoglycemia may occur within 3 hours of injecting pramlintide. Review signs and symptoms and appropriate treatment. Tell patient to notify prescriber if hypoglycemia occurs because insulin dosage will need to be reduced.
•Stress importance of monitoring blood glucose level often, especially before and after eating.
•Tell patient to inject drug subcutaneously immediately before major meals using an insulin syringe to draw up dose and using the same technique as with insulin administration, including rotating sites. Or, if patient has been prescribed the Symlin Pen injector, show her how to use it. Advise patient to inject drug into her abdomen or thigh and not to use her arm as an injection site because absorption may be too variable.
•Warn patient not to mix pramlintide and insulin together in the same syringe.
•Warn patient that nausea is common with pramlintide; urge her to notify prescriber because dosage may need to be decreased.
•Caution patient that if she misses a dose, she should skip the missed dose and continue with the next scheduled dose.
•Instruct patient to keep unopened pramlintide vials in the refrigerator; vials that have been opened may be kept in the refrigerator or at room temperature. Vials should be discarded 28 days after opening.
•Caution patient to avoid hazardous activities that require mental alertness until effects of pramlintide are known.
•Reassure patient that pramlintide won't alter her awareness of or her body's response to insulin-induced hypoglycemia.
•Alert patient that she'll need close follow-up care, at least weekly until a target dose of pramlintide has been reached, she's tolerating the drug well, and her blood glucose level is stable.
•Instruct female patients of childbearing age to notify prescriber about planned, suspected, or known pregnancy because drug therapy will need to be adjusted.
•Tell patient that local injection site reactions, such as redness, swelling or itching, may occur but that they usually resolve within a few weeks.

pravastatin sodium

Pravachol

Class and Category

Chemical class: Mevinic acid derivative
Therapeutic class: Antihyperlipidemic
Pregnancy category: X

Indications and Dosages

➤ *To prevent coronary and cardiovascular events in patients at risk, to treat hyperlipidemia*

TABLETS
Adults. *Initial:* 10 to 40 mg daily at bedtime, increased every 4 wk, as needed. *Maintenance:* 10 to 80 mg at bedtime.
DOSAGE ADJUSTMENT For patients with significant renal or hepatic impairment, those taking immunosuppressants, and elderly patients, initial dosage reduced to 10 mg daily at bedtime. For elderly patients and those taking immunosuppressants, maintenance dosage usually limited to 20 mg daily.

➤ *To treat pediatric heterozygous familial hypercholesterolemia*

TABLETS
Adolescents ages 14 to 18. 40 mg daily at bedtime.
Children ages 8 to 14. 20 mg daily at bedtime.

Mechanism of Action

Inhibits cholesterol synthesis in the liver by blocking the enzyme needed to convert hydroxymethylglutaryl-CoA (HMG-CoA) to mevalonate, an early precursor of cholesterol. When cholesterol synthesis is blocked, the liver also increases the breakdown of LDL cholesterol.

Contraindications
Active hepatic disease or unexplained, persistent elevated liver function test results; breastfeeding; hypersensitivity to pravastatin or its components; pregnancy

Interactions
DRUGS
cholestyramine, colestipol: Decreased pravastatin bioavailability
cyclosporine, erythromycin, gemfibrozil, immunosuppressants, niacin: Increased risk of rhabdomyolysis and acute renal failure
oral anticoagulants: Increased bleeding or prolonged PT

Adverse Reactions
CNS: Anxiety, depression, dizziness, fatigue, headache, nervousness, sleep disturbance
CV: Angina pectoris, chest pain
EENT: Blurred vision, diplopia, rhinitis
ENDO: Abnormal thyroid function
GI: Abdominal pain, constipation, diarrhea, elevated liver function test results, flatulence, heartburn, indigestion, nausea, pancreatitis, vomiting
GU: Dysuria, nocturia, urinary frequency
MS: Arthralgia, musculoskeletal cramps or pain, myalgia, myopathy, rhabdomyolysis
RESP: Cough, dyspnea, upper respiratory tract infection
SKIN: Rash
Other: Angioedema

Nursing Considerations
• Use pravastatin cautiously in patients with renal or hepatic impairment and in elderly patients.
• Monitor liver function test results before pravastatin therapy starts, before dosage increases, and periodically throughout therapy, as prescribed.
• Give drug 1 hour before or 4 hours after giving cholestyramine or colestipol.
• Report unexplained muscle aches or weakness and significant increases in CK level to prescriber because drug rarely causes rhabdomyolysis with acute renal failure caused by myoglobinuria. Expect to stop drug and provide supportive care.
• Monitor patient's BUN and serum creatinine levels periodically for abnormal elevations.
• Monitor blood lipoprotein level, as indicated, to evaluate response to therapy.

PATIENT TEACHING
• Instruct patient to take drug at bedtime, without regard to meals.
• Advise patient to notify prescriber immediately about muscle pain, tenderness, weakness, and other signs and symptoms of myopathy.
• Urge female patient of childbearing age to use a reliable method of contraception during pravastatin therapy and to notify prescriber at once if she becomes pregnant or thinks she may be pregnant.
• Instruct patient not to stop taking pravastatin without consulting prescriber, even when cholesterol level returns to normal.

prazosin hydrochloride
Minipress

Class and Category
Chemical class: Quinazoline derivative
Therapeutic class: Antihypertensive
Pregnancy category: C

Indications and Dosages
➤ *To manage hypertension*
CAPSULES
Adults. *Initial:* 1 mg b.i.d. or t.i.d. *Maintenance:* 6 to 15 mg daily in divided doses b.i.d. or t.i.d. *Maximum:* 40 mg daily.
Children. *Initial:* 50 to 400 mcg/kg daily in divided doses b.i.d. or t.i.d. *Maximum:* 7 mg/dose, 15 mg daily.
TABLETS
Adults. *Initial:* 0.5 mg b.i.d. or t.i.d. for at least 3 days, then increased to 1 mg b.i.d. or t.i.d., if tolerated, for an additional 3 days. Subsequent dosages adjusted gradually, as needed and tolerated. *Maintenance:* 6 to 15 mg daily in divided doses b.i.d. or t.i.d. *Maximum:* 40 mg daily.
Children. *Initial:* 50 to 400 mcg/kg daily in divided doses b.i.d. or t.i.d. *Maximum:* 7 mg/dose, 15 mg daily.
DOSAGE ADJUSTMENT For elderly patients and those with renal impairment, initial dosage possibly reduced to 1 mg once to twice daily.

Route	Onset	Peak	Duration
P.O.	0.5 to 1.5 hr	2 to 4 hr*	7 to 10 hr

* For a single dose; 3 to 4 wk for multiple doses.

> **Mechanism of Action**
> Selectively and competitively inhibits alpha$_1$-adrenergic receptors. This action promotes peripheral arterial and venous dilation and reduces peripheral vascular resistance, thereby lowering blood pressure.

Contraindications
Hypersensitivity to prazosin, other quinazolines, or their components

Interactions
DRUGS
antihypertensives, beta blockers, diuretics: Increased risk of hypotension and syncope
dopamine: Antagonized peripheral vasoconstrictive effect of dopamine (with high doses)
ephedrine: Decreased vasopressor response to ephedrine
epinephrine: Possibly severe hypotension and tachycardia
metaraminol: Decreased vasopressor effect of metaraminol
methoxamine, phenylephrine: Possibly decreased vasopressor effect and shortened duration of action of these drugs
NSAIDs, sympathomimetics: Decreased effectiveness of prazosin

Adverse Reactions
CNS: Dizziness, drowsiness, fatigue, headache, malaise, nervousness, syncope
CV: Edema, orthostatic hypotension, palpitations
EENT: Dry mouth
GI: Nausea
GU: Urinary frequency, urinary incontinence

Nursing Considerations
• Use prazosin cautiously in patients with renal impairment because of increased sensitivity to prazosin's effects; in those with angina pectoris because drug may induce or aggravate angina; in those with narcolepsy because prazosin may exacerbate cataplexy; and in elderly patients because they're at increased risk for drug-induced hypotension.
• Monitor blood pressure regularly to evaluate effectiveness of therapy.
PATIENT TEACHING
• Instruct patient who is beginning prazosin therapy to take drug at bedtime to minimize effects of first-dose hypotension.

• Stress need to take drug even if feeling well.
• Advise patient to avoid drinking alcohol, standing for long periods, and exercising in hot weather because these activities increase the risk of orthostatic hypotension.
• Suggest rising slowly from a lying or sitting position to minimize orthostatic hypotension.
• Urge patient to avoid potentially hazardous activities until drug's CNS effects are known.
• Advise patient to notify prescriber immediately about adverse reactions, especially dizziness and fainting.
• Instruct patient not to take any drugs, including OTC preparations, without consulting prescriber, to avoid serious interactions.

prednisolone
Cotolone, Delta-Cortef, Prelone

prednisolone acetate
Articulose-50, Flo-Pred, Key-Pred, Predacort 50, Predalone 50, Predate 50, Predcor-25, Predcor-50, Pred-Ject 50

prednisolone sodium phosphate
Orapred ODT, Pediapred

prednisolone tebutate
Nor-Pred T.B.A., Predalone T.B.A., Predate TBA, Predcor-TBA

Class and Category
Chemical class: Glucocorticoid
Therapeutic class: Anti-inflammatory, immunosuppressant
Pregnancy category: C

Indications and Dosages
➤ *To treat adrenal insufficiency and acute and chronic inflammatory and immunosuppressive disorders*
SYRUP, TABLETS (PREDNISOLONE); DISINTEGRATING TABLETS, ORAL SOLUTION (PREDNISOLONE SODIUM PHOSPHATE); ORAL SUSPENSION (PREDNISOLONE ACETATE)
Adults and adolescents. 5 to 60 mg daily or in divided doses. *Maximum:* 250 mg daily.
I.M. INJECTION (PREDNISOLONE ACETATE)
Adults and adolescents. 4 to 60 mg daily.
INTRA-ARTICULAR, INTRALESIONAL, OR SOFT-TISSUE INJECTION (PREDNISOLONE ACETATE, PREDNISOLONE TEBUTATE)

Adults and adolescents. 4 to 100 mg of prednisolone acetate, repeated as needed, or 4 to 40 mg of prednisolone tebutate, repeated every 1 to 3 wk, as needed.

➤ *To treat adrenocortical insufficiency in children*

SYRUP, TABLETS (PREDNISOLONE); DISINTEGRATING TABLETS, ORAL SOLUTION (PREDNISOLONE SODIUM PHOSPHATE); ORAL SUSPENSION (PREDNISOLONE ACETATE)
Children. 0.14 mg/kg daily in divided doses t.i.d.

I.M. INJECTION (PREDNISOLONE ACETATE)
Children. 0.14 mg/kg over a 24-hr period in divided doses t.i.d. every third day.

➤ *To treat acute exacerbations of multiple sclerosis*

SYRUP, TABLETS (PREDNISOLONE); DISINTEGRATING TABLETS, ORAL SOLUTION (PREDNISOLONE SODIUM PHOSPHATE); ORAL SUSPENSION (PREDNISOLONE ACETATE)
Adults. 200 mg daily for 1 wk, followed by 80 mg every other day for 1 mo.

Route	Onset	Peak	Duration
P.O. (prednisolone)	Unknown	1 to 2 hr	1.25 to 1.5 days
I.M. (prednisolone acetate)	Slow	Unknown	Unknown
Intra-articular, intralesional, soft-tissue injection (prednisolone tebutate)	1 to 2 days	Unknown	1 to 3 wk

Mechanism of Action

Binds to intracellular glucocorticoid receptors and suppresses inflammatory and immune responses by:
• inhibiting neutrophil and monocyte accumulation at inflammation site and suppressing their phagocytic and bactericidal activity
• stabilizing lysosomal membranes
• suppressing antigen response of macrophages and helper T cells
• inhibiting synthesis of inflammatory response mediators, such as cytokines, interleukins, and prostaglandins.

Contraindications

Hypersensitivity to prednisolone or its components, idiopathic thrombocytopenic purpura (I.M. form), systemic fungal infection

Interactions

DRUGS
acetaminophen: Possibly hepatotoxicity (with long-term use or high doses of acetaminophen)
acetazolamide: Possibly hypernatremia or edema
amphotericin B (parenteral): Possibly severe hypokalemia
anabolic steroids, androgens: Possibly edema and severe acne
anticholinergics: Increased intraocular pressure
asparaginase: Increased hyperglycemic effect of asparaginase, possibly neuropathy and disturbances in erythropoiesis
carbonic anhydrase inhibitors: Possibly hypocalcemia, hypokalemia, and osteoporosis
digoxin: Possibly arrhythmias and digitalis toxicity from hypokalemia
diuretics: Possibly decreased natriuretic and diuretic effects of diuretics, severe hypokalemia (with potassium-depleting diuretics)
ephedrine: Increased metabolic clearance of prednisolone
estrogens, oral contraceptives: Decreased clearance, increased elimination half-life, and increased therapeutic and toxic effects of prednisolone
folic acid: Increased folic acid requirements (with long-term prednisolone use)
heparin, oral anticoagulants, streptokinase, urokinase: Possibly decreased anticoagulant effect and increased risk of GI ulceration and bleeding
immunosuppressants: Increased risk of infection, lymphomas, and other lymphoproliferative disorders
isoniazid: Decreased blood isoniazid level
mexiletine: Possibly accelerated metabolism and decreased blood level of mexiletine
neuromuscular blockers: Increased neuromuscular blockade
NSAIDs: Increased risk of GI ulceration and bleeding, possibly added therapeutic effect when NSAIDs are used to treat arthritis
potassium supplements: Decreased effectiveness of both drugs
rifampin, other hepatic enzyme inducers: Decreased prednisolone effect

P

ritodrine: Increased risk of pulmonary edema in pregnant women
salicylates: Possibly decreased blood salicylate level, increased risk of GI ulceration and bleeding
sodium-containing drugs: Possibly edema and hypertension
somatrem, somatropin: Inhibited growth response to somatrem or somatropin
streptozocin: Increased risk of hyperglycemia
toxoids, vaccines: Possibly loss of antibody response, increased risk of neurologic complications
tricyclic antidepressants: Possibly exacerbated adverse psychiatric effects of prednisolone
troleandomycin: Increased therapeutic and toxic effects of prednisolone

FOODS
sodium-containing foods: Increased risk of edema and hypertension

ACTIVITIES
alcohol use: Increased risk of GI ulceration and bleeding

Adverse Reactions

CNS: Euphoria, headache, insomnia, nervousness, psychosis, restlessness, seizures, vertigo
CV: Edema, heart failure, hypertension
EENT: Cataracts, exophthalmos, glaucoma, increased ocular pressure
ENDO: Adrenal insufficiency, Cushing's syndrome, growth suppression in children, hyperglycemia
GI: Anorexia, GI bleeding and ulceration, increased appetite, indigestion, intestinal perforation, nausea, pancreatitis, vomiting
GU: Menstrual irregularities
MS: Avascular necrosis of joints, bone fractures, muscle atrophy or weakness, myalgia, osteoporosis, tendon rupture (local injection only)
SKIN: Acne; cutaneous or subcutaneous atrophy (with frequent repository injections); diaphoresis; ecchymosis; flushing; petechiae; striae; thin, fragile skin
Other: Delayed wound healing, hypernatremia, hypokalemia, injection site scarring, negative nitrogen balance

Nursing Considerations

•**WARNING** Avoid using prednisolone in patients with a history of active tuberculosis because drug can reactivate the disease.
•Give once-daily doses in the morning to mirror the body's normal cortisol secretion.

•Inspect injectable form for particulates and discoloration before administering.
•For I.M. injection, shake suspension well before withdrawing. Keep in mind that I.M. innjections are contraindicated in patients with idiopathic thrombocytopenic purpura.
•For intra-articular injection, attach a 20G to 24G needle to an empty syringe, using aseptic technique, so prescriber can remove a few drops of synovial fluid to confirm that needle is in the joint. The aspirating syringe is then exchanged with a prenisolone-filled syringe to inject drug into joint.
•Because prednisolone can produce many adverse reactions, assess patient regularly for evidence of such reactions, including heart failure and hypertension. Also monitor patient's intake, output, and daily weight.
•Monitor growth pattern in children because prednisolone may retard bone growth.
•Be aware that prolonged use may cause hypothalamic-pituitary-adrenal suppression.
•**WARNING** Withdraw drug gradually, as ordered, if therapy lasts longer than 2 weeks. Abrupt discontinuation may cause acute adrenal insufficiency or, possibly, death.
•Be aware that patient may be at risk for emotional instability or psychic disturbance while taking prednisolone, especially if predisposed to them or taking high doses.

PATIENT TEACHING
•Instruct patient to take oral prednisolone with food to decrease stomach upset and to take once-daily dose in the morning.
•Stress the importance of taking drug exactly as prescribed; taking too much increases the risk of serious adverse reactions.
•Instruct patient taking the orally disintegrating tablets to remove the tablet from the blister pack only when ready to take and to place tablet on the tongue. Warn her not to split, cut, or break tablets.
•Caution patient not to discontinue drug abruptly.
•Urge patient to avoid alcohol during therapy because of increased risk of GI ulcers and bleeding.
•Encourage patient to avoid potentially hazardous activities until drug's CNS effects are known.
•Advise patient to avoid people with contagious infections because drug has an immunosuppressant effect. Urge her to notify prescriber immediately about exposure to

measles or chickenpox.
• Caution against receiving vaccinations or other immunizations and coming in contact with people who have recently received the oral poliovirus vaccine.
• Teach patient about potential side effects of prednisolone therapy, including restlessness, mood swings, nervousness, and delayed wound healing.
• Instruct patient to notify prescriber immediately about joint pain, swelling, tarry stools, and visual disturbances. Also instruct her to report signs of infection or injury for up to 12 months after therapy.
• Advise patient to restrict joint use after intra-articular injection and to obtain activity guidelines from prescriber.
• Instruct diabetic patient to monitor her blood glucose level frequently because prednisolone may cause hyperglycemia.
• Advise patient to comply with follow-up visits to assess drug's effectiveness and detect adverse reactions.
• Urge patient to carry medical identification notifying others of prednisolone therapy.

prednisone

Apo-Prednisone (CAN), Deltasone Liquid Pred, Meticorten, Orasone 1, Orasone 5, Orasone 10, Prednicen-M, Prednicot, Prednisone Intensol, Sterapred, Sterapred DS, Winpred (CAN)

Class and Category
Chemical class: Glucocorticoid
Therapeutic class: Anti-inflammatory, immunosuppressant
Pregnancy category: Not rated

Indications and Dosages
➤ *To treat adrenal insufficiency and acute and chronic inflammatory and immunosuppressive disorders*
ORAL SOLUTION, SYRUP, TABLETS
Adults and adolescents. 5 to 60 mg daily as a single dose or in divided doses. *Maximum:* 250 mg daily.
➤ *To treat adrenogenital syndrome*
ORAL SOLUTION, SYRUP, TABLETS
Adults and adolescents. 5 to 10 mg daily.
Children. 5 mg/m² daily in divided doses b.i.d.

➤ *To treat acute exacerbations of multiple sclerosis*
ORAL SOLUTION, SYRUP, TABLETS
Adults. 200 mg daily for 1 wk, then 80 mg every other day for 1 mo. *Maximum:* 250 mg daily.
➤ *To treat nephrosis in children*
ORAL SOLUTION, SYRUP, TABLETS
Children age 10 and over. 20 mg q.i.d.
Children ages 4 to 10. 15 mg q.i.d.
Children ages 18 months to 4 years. 7.5 to 10 mg q.i.d.
➤ *To treat rheumatic carditis, leukemia, and tumors in children*
ORAL SOLUTION, SYRUP, TABLETS
Children. 0.5 mg/kg q.i.d. for 2 to 3 wk, then 0.375 mg/kg q.i.d. for 4 to 6 wk.
➤ *As adjunct to treat tuberculosis in children (with concurrent antitubercular therapy)*
ORAL SOLUTION, SYRUP, TABLETS
Children. 0.5 mg/kg q.i.d. for 2 mo.

Route	Onset	Peak	Duration
P.O.	Rapid	1 to 2 hr	1.25 to 1.5 days

Mechanism of Action
Binds to intracellular glucocorticoid receptors and suppresses inflammatory and immune responses by:
• inhibiting neutrophil and monocyte accumulation at inflammation site and suppressing their phagocytic and bactericidal activity
• stabilizing lysosomal membranes
• suppressing antigen response of macrophages and helper T cells
• inhibiting synthesis of inflammatory response mediators, such as cytokines, interleukins, and prostaglandins.

Contraindications
Hypersensitivity to prednisone or its components, systemic fungal infection

Interactions
DRUGS
acetaminophen: Possibly hepatotoxicity (with long-term use or high doses of acetaminophen)
acetazolamide sodium: Possibly hypernatremia or edema

amphotericin B (parenteral): Possibly severe hypokalemia

anabolic steroids, androgens: Possibly edema and severe acne

antacids: Decreased absorption of prednisone (with long-term use)

anticholinergics: Increased intraocular pressure

asparaginase: Increased hyperglycemic effect of asparaginase, possibly neuropathy and disturbances in erythropoiesis

carbonic anhydrase inhibitors: Possibly hypocalcemia, hypokalemia, and osteoporosis

digoxin: Possibly arrhythmias and digitalis toxicity from hypokalemia

diuretics: Possibly decreased natriuretic and diuretic effects of diuretics, severe hypokalemia (with potassium-depleting diuretics)

ephedrine: Increased metabolic clearance of prednisone

estrogens, oral contraceptives: Decreased clearance, increased elimination half-life, and increased therapeutic and toxic effects of prednisone

folic acid: Increased folic acid requirements (with long-term prednisone use)

heparin, oral anticoagulants, streptokinase, urokinase: Possibly decreased anticoagulant effect and increased risk of GI ulceration and bleeding

immunosuppressants: Increased risk of infection, lymphomas, and other lymphoproliferative disorders

isoniazid: Decreased blood isoniazid level

mexiletine: Possibly accelerated metabolism and decreased blood level of mexiletine

neuromuscular blockers: Increased neuromuscular blockade

NSAIDs: Increased risk of GI ulceration and bleeding, possibly added therapeutic effect when NSAIDs are used to treat arthritis

potassium supplements: Decreased effectiveness of both drugs

ritodrine: Increased risk of pulmonary edema in pregnant women

salicylates: Possibly decreased blood salicylate level, increased risk of GI ulceration and bleeding

sodium-containing drugs: Possibly edema and hypertension

somatrem, somatropin: Inhibited growth response to somatrem or somatropin

streptozocin: Increased risk of hyperglycemia

toxoids, vaccines: Possibly loss of antibody response, increased risk of neurologic complications

tricyclic antidepressants: Possibly exacerbated adverse psychiatric effects of prednisone

troleandomycin: Increased therapeutic and toxic effects of prednisone

FOODS

sodium-containing foods: Increased risk of edema and hypertension

ACTIVITIES

alcohol use: Increased risk of GI ulceration and bleeding

Adverse Reactions

CNS: Euphoria, headache, insomnia, nervousness, psychosis, restlessness, seizures, vertigo

CV: Edema, heart failure, hypertension

EENT: Cataracts, exophthalmos, glaucoma, increased ocular pressure

ENDO: Adrenal insufficiency, Cushing's syndrome, growth suppression in children, hyperglycemia

GI: Anorexia, GI bleeding and ulceration, increased appetite, indigestion, intestinal perforation, nausea, pancreatitis, vomiting

GU: Menstrual irregularities

MS: Avascular necrosis of joints, bone fractures, muscle atrophy or weakness, myalgia, osteoporosis

SKIN: Acne; diaphoresis; ecchymosis; flushing; petechiae; striae; thin, fragile skin

Other: Delayed wound healing, hypernatremia, hypokalemia, negative nitrogen balance

Nursing Considerations

•Administer once-daily doses of prednisone in the morning to match the body's normal cortisol secretion schedule.

•Because prednisone can produce many adverse reactions, assess regularly for signs and symptoms of such reactions as heart failure and hypertension. Also monitor fluid intake and output and daily weight.

•Monitor growth pattern in children because prednisone may retard bone growth.

•Be aware that prolonged use of prednisone may cause hypothalamic-pituitary-adrenal suppression.

•**WARNING** Withdraw prednisone gradually, as ordered, if therapy lasts longer than 2 weeks. Abrupt discontinuation may cause acute adrenal insufficiency and, possibly, death.

PATIENT TEACHING
• Instruct patient to take prednisone with food to decrease GI distress and to take once-daily dose in the morning.
• Stress the importance of taking drug exactly as prescribed; taking more than prescribed dosage increases the risk of serious adverse reactions.
• Caution patient not to discontinue drug abruptly.
• Urge patient to avoid alcohol during therapy because of the increased risk of GI ulcers and bleeding.
• Encourage patient to avoid hazardous activities until drug's CNS effects are known.
• Advise patient to avoid people with contagious infections because drug has an immunosuppressant effect. Urge her to notify prescriber immediately about possible exposure to measles or chickenpox.
• Caution against receiving vaccinations or other immunizations and coming in contact with people who have recently received the oral poliovirus vaccine.
• Instruct patient to notify prescriber immediately about joint pain, swelling, tarry stools, and visual disturbances. Also instruct her to report signs of infection or injury for up to 12 months after therapy.
• Instruct diabetic patient to monitor her blood glucose level frequently because prednisone may cause hyperglycemia.
• Advise patient to comply with follow-up visits to assess drug effectiveness and detect adverse reactions.
• Urge patient to carry medical identification to notify others of prednisone therapy.

pregabalin

Lyrica

Class and Category

Chemical class: Structural derivative of gamma-aminobutyric acid (GABA)
Therapeutic class: Analgesic, anticonvulsant
Pregnancy category: C

Indications and Dosages

➤ *To relieve neuropathic pain associated with diabetic peripheral neuropathy*
CAPSULES
Adults. *Initial:* 50 mg t.i.d., increased to 100 mg t.i.d. within 1 wk as needed.

➤ *To relieve postherpetic neuralgia; as adjunct therapy to manage partial onset seizures*
CAPSULES
Adults. *Initial:* 75 mg b.i.d. or 50 mg t.i.d., increased to 150 mg b.i.d. or 100 mg t.i.d. within 1 week as needed. Then increased to 300 mg b.i.d. or 200 mg t.i.d. in 2 to 4 weeks as needed.

➤ *To manage fibromyalgia*
CAPSULES
Adults. *Initial:* 75 mg b.i.d., increased to 150 mg b.i.d. in 1 wk, as needed, and then to 225 mg b.i.d. in 1 wk as needed. *Maximum:* 450 mg daily.

DOSAGE ADJUSTMENT If patient's creatinine clearance is 30 to 60 ml/min/1.73 m^2, daily dosage reduced by 50%. If creatinine clearance is 15 to 30 ml/min/1.73 m^2, daily dosage reduced by 75% and frequency reduced to once or twice daily. If creatinine clearance is less than 15 ml/min/1.73 m^2, daily dosage decreased to as low as 25 mg daily. If patient has hemodialysis, daily dosage is reduced and supplemental dose given immediately after every 4-hour hemodialysis session as follows: If reduced daily dosage is 25 mg daily, give supplemental dose of 25 to 50 mg. If reduced daily dosage is 25 to 50 mg daily, give supplemental dose of 50 to 75 mg. If reduced daily dosage is 75 mg, give supplemental dose of 100 to 150 mg.

Route	Onset	Peak	Duration
P.O.	Unknown	1.5 hr	Unknown

Contraindications

Hypersenstivity to pregabalin or its components

Interactions

DRUGS
ACE inhibitors: Increased risk of pregabalin-induced angioedema
CNS depressants: Additive CNS effects such as somnolence
lorazepam, oxycodone: Additive effects on cognitive and gross motor function
thiazolidinedione antidiabetics: Possibly increased risk of peripheral edema and weight gain

ACTIVITIES
alcohol use: Additive effects on cognitive and gross motor function

P

Mechanism of Action
Binds to the alpha$_2$-delta site, an auxiliary subunit of voltage calcium channels, in CNS tissue where it may reduce calcium-dependent release of several neurotransmitters, possibly by modulating calcium channel function. With fewer neurotransmitters present, pain sensation and seizure activity are reduced.

Adverse Reactions
CNS: Abnormal gait, amnesia, anxiety, asthenia, ataxia, balance disorder, confusion, depression, difficulty concentrating, dizziness, euphoria, extrapyramidal syndrome, fatigue, fever, headache, hypertonia, hypesthesia, incoordination, intracranial hypertension, myoclonus, nervousness, neuropathy, paresthesia, psychotic depression, schizophrenic reaction, somnolence, stupor, tremor, twitching, vertigo
CV: Chest pain, heart failure, peripheral edema, ventricular fibrillation
EENT: Amblyopia, blurred vision, conjunctivitis, decreased visual acuity, diplopia, dry mouth, nystagmus, otitis media, sinusitis, tinnitus, visual field defect
ENDO: Hypoglycemia
GI: Abdominal distention or pain, constipation, diarrhea, flatulence, gastroenteritis, gastrointestinal hemorrhage, increased appetite, nausea, vomiting
GU: Acute renal failure, anorgasmia; decreased libido; glomerulitis, impotence; nephritis; urinary frequency, incontinence, or retention
HEME: Decreased platelet count, leukopenia, thrombocytopenia
MS: Arthralgia, back pain, elevated creatine kinase levels, leg or muscle cramps, myalgia, myasthenia
RESP: Apnea, dyspnea
SKIN: Ecchymosis, exfoliative dermatitis, pruritus
Other: Anaphylaxis, angioedema, facial edema, hypersensitivity reaction, Stevens-Johnson syndrome, weight gain

Nursing Considerations
• Pregabalin therapy should not be stopped abruptly but gradually over a minimum of 1 week to decrease the risk of seizure activity and avoid unpleasant symptoms such as diarrhea, headache, insomnia, and nausea.
• If patient has evidence of hypersensitivity (red skin, urticaria, rash, dyspnea, facial swelling, wheezing), stop drug immediately, notify prescriber, and give supportive care.
• Monitor patient closely for adverse reactions. Notify prescriber if significant adverse reactions persist.

PATIENT TEACHING
• Warn patient not to stop taking pregabalin abruptly.
• Urge patient to avoid potentially hazardous activities until she knows how drug affects her.
• Instruct patient to notify prescriber if she experiences changes in vision or unexplained muscle pain, tenderness, or weakness, especially if these muscle symptoms are accompanied by malaise or fever.
• Alert patient that drug may cause edema and weight gain.
• If patient also takes a thiazolidinedione antidiabetic drug, tell her these effects may be intensified. If significant, tell patient to notify prescriber.
• Inform male patient who plans to father a child that drug could impair his fertility.
• Instruct diabetic patients to inspect their skin while taking pregabalin.

primidone
Apo-Primidone (CAN), Myidone, Mysoline, PMS Primidone (CAN), Sertan (CAN)

Class and Category
Chemical class: Prodrug of phenobarbital
Therapeutic class: Anticonvulsant
Pregnancy category: Not rated

Indications and Dosages
➤ *To manage generalized tonic-clonic seizures, nocturnal myoclonic seizures, complex partial seizures, and simple partial seizures caused by epilepsy*

CHEWABLE TABLETS, ORAL SUSPENSION, TABLETS
Adults and children age 8 and over. *Initial:* 100 or 125 mg at bedtime for first 3 days, then increased to 100 or 125 mg b.i.d. for next 3 days, followed by 100 or 125 mg t.i.d. for next 3 days. On 10th day, begin maintenance dosage as prescribed. *Maintenance:* 250 mg t.i.d. or q.i.d., adjusted as needed. *Maximum:* 2 g daily.

Children up to age 8. *Initial:* 50 mg at bedtime for first 3 days, then increased to 50 mg b.i.d. for next 3 days, followed by increase to 100 mg b.i.d. for next 3 days. On 10th day, begin maintenance dosage. *Maintenance:* 125 to 250 mg t.i.d., adjusted as needed.

> ## Mechanism of Action
> Prevents seizures by decreasing the excitability of neurons and increasing the motor cortex's threshold of electrical stimulation.

Contraindications
Hypersensitivity to primidone, phenobarbital, or their components; porphyria

Interactions
DRUGS
acetaminophen: Decreased acetaminophen effectiveness, increased risk of hepatotoxicity
adrenocorticoids, chloramphenicol, cyclosporine, dacarbazine, disopyramide, doxycycline, levothyroxine, metronidazole, mexiletine, oral anticoagulants, oral contraceptives (estrogen-containing), quinidine, tricyclic antidepressants: Decreased effectiveness of these drugs
amphetamines: Possibly delayed absorption of primidone
anticonvulsants: Possibly altered pattern of seizures
carbamazepine: Decreased effectiveness of primidone
carbonic anhydrase inhibitors: Increased risk of osteopenia
CNS depressants: Possibly enhanced CNS and respiratory depressant effects of both drugs
cyclophosphamide: Reduced half-life and increased leukopenic activity of cyclophosphamide
enflurane, halothane, methoxyflurane: Increased risk of hepatotoxicity; increased risk of nephrotoxicity (with methoxyflurane)
fenoprofen: Decreased elimination half-life of fenoprofen
folic acid: Increased folic acid requirements
griseofulvin: Decreased antifungal effects of griseofulvin
guanadrel, guanethidine: Possibly aggravated orthostatic hypotension
haloperidol, loxapine, maprotiline, molin-done, phenothiazines, thioxanthenes: Possibly lowered seizure threshold and increased CNS depression
leucovorin: Possibly decreased anticonvulsant effects of primidone (with large doses)
MAO inhibitors: Possibly prolonged effects of primidone and altered pattern of seizures
methylphenidate: Possibly increased blood primidone level, resulting in toxicity
phenobarbital: Increased sedative effects of either drug, possibly altered seizure pattern
phenylbutazone: Decreased primidone effectiveness, increased metabolism and decreased half-life of phenylbutazone
rifampin: Decreased blood primidone level
valproic acid: Increased blood primidone level, leading to increased CNS depression and neurotoxicity; decreased half-life of valproic acid and enhanced risk of hepatotoxicity
vitamin D: Decreased effects of vitamin D
xanthines: Increased metabolism and clearance of xanthines (except dyphylline)
ACTIVITIES
alcohol use: Possibly increased CNS and respiratory depressant effects of primidone

Adverse Reactions
CNS: Ataxia, confusion, dizziness, drowsiness, excitement, mental changes, mood changes, restlessness
EENT: Diplopia, nystagmus
GI: Anorexia, nausea, vomiting
GU: Impotence
RESP: Dyspnea
Other: Folic acid deficiency

Nursing Considerations
•Monitor blood levels of primidone and phenobarbital (its active metabolite), as ordered, to determine therapeutic level or detect toxic levels.
•Anticipate that drug may cause confusion, excitement, or mood changes in elderly patients and children.
•Assess for signs of folic acid deficiency: mental dysfunction, neuropathy, tiredness, and weakness.
PATIENT TEACHING
•Instruct patient to crush primidone tablets and mix with foods or fluids, as needed.
•Advise patient taking oral suspension to shake the bottle well and measure doses with a calibrated device.
•Suggest that patient take drug with meals

to minimize adverse GI reactions.
•Urge patient not to stop taking primidone abruptly because doing so can precipitate seizures.
•Caution patient about possible decreased alertness.
•Advise her to avoid potentially hazardous activities until drug's CNS effects are known.
•Urge patient to avoid consuming alcohol and other CNS depressants during primidone therapy.

probenecid

Benemid, Benuryl (CAN), Probalan

Class and Category
Chemical class: Sulfonamide derivative
Therapeutic class: Antibiotic adjunct, antigout, uricosuric
Pregnancy category: Not rated

Indications and Dosages
➤ *To treat chronic gouty arthritis and hyperuricemia due to chronic gout*
TABLETS
Adults and adolescents. *Initial:* 250 mg b.i.d. for 1 wk, then increased to maintenance dosage. *Maintenance:* 500 mg b.i.d.; if not effective or 24-hr uric acid excretion isn't greater than 700 mg, dosage increased by 500 mg/day every 4 wk, as needed and prescribed, up to a maximum of 3 g daily. If no acute attacks of gout occur over next 6 mo and serum uric acid level is within normal limits, dosage decreased, as prescribed, by 500 mg every 6 mo until lowest effective maintenance dose is reached. *Maximum:* 3 g daily.
DOSAGE ADJUSTMENT Dosage possibly increased for patients with mild renal dysfunction, except for elderly patients, who require a dosage reduction.
➤ *As adjunct to antibiotic therapy with penicillins and some cephalosporins*
TABLETS
Adults, adolescents age 14 and over, and children weighing more than 50 kg (110 lb). 500 mg q.i.d.; if given with I.V. or I.M. antibiotic, administer at least 30 min before antibiotic.
Children ages 2 to 14 weighing up to 50 kg. 25 mg/kg as a single dose, then 10 mg/kg q.i.d.; if given with I.V. or I.M. antibiotic, give at least 30 min before antibiotic.

➤ *As adjunct to treat sexually transmitted diseases*
TABLETS
Adults and adolescents. 1 g as a single dose administered together with appropriate antibiotic.
➤ *As adjunct to treat pediatric gonorrhea*
TABLETS
Postpubertal children and children weighing more than 45 kg (99 lb). 1 g as a single dose administered together with appropriate antibiotic.
➤ *As adjunct to treat neurosyphilis*
TABLETS
Adults and adolescents. 500 mg q.i.d. concurrently with 1 daily dose (2.4 million units) of penicillin G procaine for 10 to 14 days.

Route	Onset	Peak	Duration
P.O.	Unknown	30 min*	8 hr†

Mechanism of Action
Increases urinary excretion of uric acid and lowers serum uric acid level, which may prevent or resolve urate deposits, tophus formation, and joint changes. Eventually, the incidence of acute gout attacks decreases. Probenecid also inhibits renal excretion of penicillins and some cephalosporin antibiotics, thereby increasing their serum concentration and prolonging their duration of action.

Contraindications
Age less than 2 years, blood dyscrasias, hypersensitivity to probenecid or its components, renal calculi (urate)

Interactions
DRUGS
acyclovir: Decreased renal tubular secretion of acyclovir
allopurinol: Additive antihyperuricemic effects
aminosalicylate sodium, cephalosporins, ciprofloxacin, clofibrate, dapsone, ganciclovir,

---

* For renal clearance of uric acid; 2 hr for effect on blood antibiotic level.
† For effect on blood antibiotic level; unknown for renal clearance of uric acid.

imipenem, methotrexate, nitrofurantoin, norfloxacin, penicillins: Increased and possibly prolonged blood levels of these drugs, increased risk of toxicity
antineoplastics (rapidly cytolytic): Possibly uric acid nephropathy
diazoxide, mecamylamine, pyrazinamide: Increased risk of hyperuricemia, decreased probenecid effectiveness
dyphylline: Increased half-life of dyphylline
furosemide: Increased blood furosemide level
heparin: Increased and prolonged anticoagulant effect
indomethacin, ketoprofen, other NSAIDs: Possibly increased adverse effects
lorazepam, oxazepam, temazepam: Increased effects of these drugs and, possibly, excessive sedation
riboflavin: Decreased GI absorption of riboflavin
rifampin, sulfonamides: Increased blood levels of these drugs and, possibly, toxicity
salicylates: Decreased uricosuric effects of probenecid
sodium benzoate and sodium phenylacetate: Decreased renal elimination of these drugs
sulfonylureas: Increased sulfonylurea half-life
thiopental: Prolonged thiopental effect
zidovudine: Increased risk of zidovudine toxicity
ACTIVITIES
alcohol use: Increased risk of hyperuricemia, decreased probenecid effectiveness

Adverse Reactions
CNS: Dizziness, headache
EENT: Sore gums
GI: Anorexia, nausea, vomiting
GU: Hematuria, renal calculi (urate), renal colic, urinary frequency
MS: Costovertebral pain; joint pain, redness, and swelling
SKIN: Facial flushing, pruritus, rash, urticaria

Nursing Considerations
• Be aware that probenecid therapy shouldn't be started until acute gout attack has subsided. If acute gout attack begins during therapy, continue drug therapy as prescribed.
• Use drug cautiously in patients with peptic ulcer disease.
• Expect to give sodium bicarbonate (3 to

7.5 g daily) or potassium citrate (7.5 g daily), as prescribed, to keep urine alkaline and prevent renal calculus formation.
• Monitor CBC, serum uric acid level, and liver and renal function test results during therapy.
• Closely monitor patients receiving intermittent therapy because they're more likely to develop allergic reactions.
• Monitor blood glucose level frequently in diabetic patient who takes a sulfonylurea because of the risk of drug interactions.
PATIENT TEACHING
• Advise patient to take probenecid with meals to minimize GI distress.
• Encourage patient to increase fluid intake (up to 3 L daily, if not contraindicated) to help prevent renal calculus formation.
• Instruct patient to notify prescriber immediately if she experiences signs of an acute gout attack (joint pain, swelling, and redness) or of kidney stones (flank pain and blood in urine).
• Caution patient against taking salicylates while taking probenecid. Instead, advise her to use acetaminophen to treat mild pain or fever.

procainamide hydrochloride

Procan SR, Promine, Pronestyl, Pronestyl-SR

Class and Category
Chemical class: Ethyl benzamide monohydrochloride
Therapeutic class: Antiarrhythmic
Pregnancy category: C

Indications and Dosages
➤ *To treat life-threatening ventricular arrhythmias*
CAPSULES, TABLETS
Adults. 50 mg/kg daily in 8 divided doses (every 3 hr), adjusted as needed and tolerated. *Maximum:* 6 g daily (maintenance).
Children. 12.5 mg/kg q.i.d.
E.R. TABLETS
Adults. *Maintenance:* 50 mg/kg daily in divided doses q.i.d. (every 6 hr), adjusted as needed and tolerated. *Maximum:* 6 g daily (maintenance).
I.V. INFUSION OR INJECTION
Adults. *Initial:* 100 mg diluted in D_5W and

given at no more than 50 mg/min. Repeated every 5 min until arrhythmia is controlled or maximum total dose of 1 g is reached. Alternatively, 10 to 15 mg/kg I.V. bolus administered at a rate of 25 to 50 mg/min. *Maintenance:* 1 to 4 mg/min by continuous infusion.

I.M. INJECTION

Adults. 50 mg/kg daily in divided doses every 3 to 6 hr.

➤ *To treat ventricular extrasystoles and arrhythmias associated with anesthesia and surgery*

I.V. INFUSION OR INJECTION

Adults. *Initial:* 100 mg diluted in D_5W and administered at a rate not to exceed 50 mg/min. Dosage repeated every 5 min until arrhythmia is controlled or maximum total dose of 1 g is reached. Alternatively, 10 to 15 mg/kg I.V. bolus administered at a rate of 25 to 50 mg/min. *Maintenance:* 1 to 4 mg/min by continuous infusion.

I.M. INJECTION

Adults. 100 to 500 mg every 3 to 6 hr.

DOSAGE ADJUSTMENT For elderly patients or those with cardiac or hepatic insufficiency, dosage possibly reduced or dosing intervals increased. For patients with creatinine clearance less than 50 ml/min/1.73 m^2, initial dosage reduced to 1 to 2 mg/min.

Route	Onset	Peak	Duration
P.O.	Unknown	Unknown	60 to 90 min
P.O. (E.R.)	Unknown	60 to 90 min	Unknown
I.V.	Unknown	Immediate	Unknown
I.M.	10 to 30 min	15 to 60 min	Unknown

Mechanism of Action

Prolongs the recovery period after myocardial repolarization by inhibiting sodium influx through myocardial cell membranes. This action prolongs the refractory period, causing myocardial automaticity, excitability, and conduction velocity to decline.

Contraindications

Complete heart block, hypersensitivity to procainamide or its components, systemic lupus erythematosus, torsades de pointes

Interactions

DRUGS

antiarrhythmics: Additive cardiac effects
anticholinergics, antidyskinetics, antihistamines: Possibly intensified atropine-like adverse effects, increased risk of ileus
antihypertensives: Additive hypotensive effects
antimyasthenics: Possibly antagonized effect of antimyasthenic on skeletal muscle
bethanechol: Possibly antagonized cholinergic effect of bethanechol
bone marrow depressants: Possibly increased leukopenic or thrombocytopenic effects
bretylium: Possibly decreased inotropic effect of bretylium and enhanced hypotension
neuromuscular blockers: Possibly increased or prolonged neuromuscular blockade
pimozide: Possibly prolonged QT interval, leading to life-threatening arrhythmias

Adverse Reactions

CNS: Chills, disorientation, dizziness, lightheadedness
CV: Heart block (second-degree), hypotension, pericarditis, prolonged QT interval, tachycardia
EENT: Bitter taste
GI: Abdominal distress, anorexia, diarrhea, nausea, vomiting
HEME: Agranulocytosis, neutropenia, thrombocytopenia
MS: Arthralgia, myalgia
RESP: Pleural effusion
SKIN: Pruritus, rash
Other: Drug-induced fever

Nursing Considerations

•Place patient in a supine position before administering procainamide I.M. or I.V. to minimize hypotensive effects. Monitor blood pressure frequently and ECG tracings continuously during administration and for 30 minutes afterward.
•Inspect parenteral solution for particles and discoloration before giving drug; discard if particles are present or solution is darker than light amber.
•When possible, give drug by I.V. infusion or injection, as prescribed, rather than by I.M. injection.
•If drug is to be administered I.M. and patient's platelet count is below 50,000/mm^3, notify prescriber immediately because patient may develop bleeding, bruising, or hematomas from procainamide-induced bone

marrow suppression and thrombocytopenia. Expect to administer procainamide I.V.

•For I.V. injection, dilute procainamide with D₅W according to manufacturer's instructions before administration.

•For I.V. infusion, dilute 200 to 1,000 mg of procainamide to a concentration of 2 or 4 mg/ml using 50 to 500 ml of D₅W.

•Administer I.V. infusion with an infusion pump or other controlled-delivery device.

•Don't exceed 500 mg in 30 minutes by I.V. infusion or 50 mg/min by I.V. injection because heart block or cardiac arrest may occur.

•Anticipate that patient has reached maximum clinical response when ventricular tachycardia resolves, hypotension develops, or QRS complex is 50% wider than original width.

•Expect to administer first oral dose 3 to 4 hours after last I.V. dose.

PATIENT TEACHING

•Instruct patient to swallow E.R. procainamide tablets whole, without breaking, crushing, or chewing them.

•If patient has trouble swallowing, advise her to crush regular-release tablets or open capsules and mix contents with food or fluid.

•Instruct patient to take drug 1 hour before or 2 hours after meals with a full glass of water. Inform her that she may take procainamide with food if GI irritation develops.

•Urge patient to obtain needed dental work before therapy starts or after blood count returns to normal because drug can cause myelosuppression and increased risk of bleeding and infection. Encourage good oral hygiene during therapy, and urge patient to consult prescriber before having dental procedures.

•Advise patient to notify prescriber immediately about bruising, chills, diarrhea, fever, or rash.

prochlorperazine

Compazine, Stemetil (CAN)

prochlorperazine edisylate

Compazine

prochlorperazine maleate

Compazine Spansule, Nu-Prochlor (CAN), Stemetil (CAN)

Class and Category

Chemical class: Phenothiazine, piperazine
Therapeutic class: Antianxiety, antiemetic, antipsychotic
Pregnancy category: Not rated

Indications and Dosages

➤ *To control nausea and vomiting related to surgery*

I.V. INFUSION OR INJECTION (PROCHLORPERAZINE EDISYLATE)

Adults and adolescents. 5 to 10 mg at a rate not to exceed 5 mg/ml 15 to 30 min before anesthesia or during or after surgery, as needed. Dosage repeated once, if necessary. *Maximum:* 10 mg/dose, 40 mg daily.

I.M. INJECTION (PROCHLORPERAZINE EDISYLATE)

Adults and adolescents. 5 to 10 mg 1 to 2 hr before anesthesia or during or after surgery, as needed. Repeated once in 30 min, if needed. *Maximum:* 10 mg/dose, 40 mg daily.

➤ *To control severe nausea and vomiting*

E.R. CAPSULES (PROCHLORPERAZINE MALEATE)

Adults and adolescents. 15 to 30 mg daily in the morning, or 10 mg every 12 hr. *Maximum:* 40 mg daily.

ORAL SOLUTION (PROCHLORPERAZINE EDISYLATE)

Adults and adolescents. 5 to 10 mg t.i.d. or q.i.d. *Maximum:* 40 mg daily.

Children weighing 18 to 39 kg (40 to 86 lb). 2.5 mg t.i.d. or 5 mg b.i.d. *Maximum:* 15 mg daily.

Children weighing 14 to 18 kg (31 to 40 lb). 2.5 mg b.i.d. or t.i.d. *Maximum:* 10 mg daily.

Children weighing 9 to 14 kg (20 to 31 lb). 2.5 mg once or twice daily. *Maximum:* 7.5 mg daily.

TABLETS (PROCHLORPERAZINE MALEATE)

Adults and adolescents. 5 to 10 mg t.i.d. or q.i.d. *Maximum:* 40 mg daily.

I.V. INFUSION OR INJECTION (PROCHLORPERAZINE EDISYLATE)

Adults and adolescents. 2.5 to 10 mg at a rate not to exceed 5 mg/min. *Maximum:* 40 mg daily.

I.M. INJECTION (PROCHLORPERAZINE EDISYLATE)

Adults and adolescents. 5 to 10 mg every 3 to 4 hr, p.r.n. *Maximum:* 40 mg daily.

Children ages 2 to 12. 132 mcg/kg/dose to maximum of 10 mg on day 1, then increased as needed. *Maximum:* On day 1, 10 mg; thereafter, 25 mg daily for children ages 6 to 12, 20 mg daily for children ages 2 to 6.

P

Suppositories (prochlorperazine)
Adults and adolescents. 25 mg b.i.d.
Children weighing 18 to 39 kg. 2.5 mg t.i.d.
or 5 mg b.i.d. *Maximum:* 15 mg daily.
Children weighing 14 to 18 kg. 2.5 mg b.i.d.
or t.i.d. *Maximum:* 10 mg daily.
Children weighing 9 to 14 kg. 2.5 mg once or
twice daily. *Maximum:* 7.5 mg daily.

➤ *To manage psychotic disorders, such as
schizophrenia*

Oral solution (prochlorperazine edisylate)
Adults and adolescents. 5 to 10 mg t.i.d. or
q.i.d., increased gradually every 2 to 3 days,
as needed and tolerated. *Maximum:* 150 mg
daily.
Children ages 2 to 12. 2.5 mg b.i.d. or t.i.d.
Maximum: On day 1, 10 mg for all children;
thereafter, 25 mg daily for children ages 6 to
12, 20 mg daily for children ages 2 to 6.

Tablets (prochlorperazine maleate)
Adults and adolescents. 5 to 10 mg t.i.d. or
q.i.d., increased gradually every 2 to 3 days,
as needed and tolerated. *Maximum:* 150 mg
daily.

I.M. injection (prochlorperazine edisylate)
Adults and adolescents. *Initial:* 10 to 20 mg,
repeated every 2 to 4 hr, as prescribed, to
bring symptoms under control (usually 3 to
4 doses). *Maintenance:* 10 to 20 mg every
4 to 6 hr. *Maximum:* 200 mg daily.
Children ages 2 to 12. 132 mcg/kg/dose on
day 1, then increased as needed. *Maximum:*
On day 1, 10 mg for all children; thereafter,
25 mg daily for children ages 6 to 12, 20 mg/
day for children ages 2 to 6.

➤ *To treat anxiety short-term*

E.R. capsules (prochlorperazine maleate)
Adults and adolescents. 15 mg daily in the
morning, or 10 mg every 12 hr. *Maximum:*
20 mg/day for no longer than 12 wk.

**Oral solution, tablets (prochlorperazine
edisylate)**
Adults and adolescents. 5 mg t.i.d. or q.i.d.
Maximum: 20 mg daily for no longer than
12 wk.

**I.V. infusion or injection (prochlorperazine
edisylate)**
Adults and adolescents. 2.5 to 10 mg at no
more than 5 mg/min. *Maximum:* 40 mg daily.

I.M. injection (prochlorperazine edisylate)
Adults and adolescents. 5 to 10 mg every 3 to
4 hr, p.r.n.
DOSAGE ADJUSTMENT Initial dose usually reduced and subsequent dosage increased more

gradually for elderly, emaciated, and debilitated patients.

Route	Onset	Peak	Duration
P.O., I.V., I.M., P.R.	Up to several wk*	Up to 6 mo	Unknown

Mechanism of Action
Alleviates psychotic symptoms by blocking dopamine receptors, depressing the release of selected hormones, and producing
an alpha-adrenergic blocking effect in the
brain.
  Prochlorperazine also alleviates nausea
and vomiting by centrally blocking dopamine receptors in the medullary chemoreceptor trigger zone and by peripherally
blocking the vagus nerve in the GI tract.
  Anticholinergic effects and alpha-
adrenergic blockade reduce anxiety by decreasing arousal and filtering internal
stimuli to the brain stem reticular activating system.

Incompatibilities
Don't mix prochlorperazine in same syringe
with other drugs. A precipitate may form
when prochlorperazine edisylate is mixed in
same syringe with morphine sulfate.

Contraindications
Age less than 2 years, blood dyscrasias, bone
marrow depression, cerebral arteriosclerosis,
coma, coronary artery disease, hepatic dysfunction, hypersensitivity to phenothiazines,
myeloproliferative disorders, pediatric surgery, severe CNS depression, severe hypertension or hypotension, subcortical brain
damage, use of large quantities of CNS depressants, weight less than 9 kg (20 lb)

Interactions
Drugs
*aluminum- or magnesium-containing ant-
acids, antidiarrheals (adsorbent):* Possibly inhibited absorption of oral prochlorperazine
*amantadine, anticholinergics, antidyskinet-
ics, antihistamines:* Possibly intensified anticholinergic adverse effects, increased risk of
prochlorperazine-induced hyperpyretic effect

---

*For antipsychotic effects; unknown for
 other indications.

amphetamines: Decreased stimulant effect of amphetamines, decreased antipsychotic effect of prochlorperazine

anticonvulsants: Lowered seizure threshold

antithyroid drugs: Increased risk of agranulocytosis

apomorphine: Possibly decreased emetic response to apomorphine, additive CNS depression

appetite suppressants: Possibly antagonized anorectic effect of appetite suppressants (except for phenmetrazine)

astemizole, cisapride, disopyramide, erythromycin, pimozide, probucol, procainamide: Additive QT interval prolongation, increased risk of ventricular tachycardia

beta blockers: Increased risk of additive hypotensive effects, irreversible retinopathy, arrhythmias, and tardive dyskinesia

bromocriptine: Decreased effectiveness of bromocriptine

CNS depressants: Additive CNS depression

dopamine: Possibly antagonized peripheral vasoconstriction (with high doses of dopamine)

ephedrine, epinephrine: Decreased vasopressor effects of these drugs

hepatotoxic drugs: Increased incidence of hepatotoxicity

hypotension-producing drugs: Possibly severe hypotension with syncope

levodopa: Inhibited antidyskinetic effect of levodopa

lithium: Reduced absorption of oral prochlorperazine, increased excretion of lithium, increased extrapyramidal effects, possibly masking of early symptoms of lithium toxicity

MAO inhibitors, maprotiline, tricyclic antidepressants: Possibly prolonged and intensified anticholinergic and sedative effects, increased blood antidepressant levels, inhibited prochlorperazine metabolism, and increased risk of neuroleptic malignant syndrome

mephentermine: Possibly antagonized antipsychotic effect of prochlorperazine and vasopressor effect of mephentermine

metrizamide: Increased risk of seizures

opioid analgesics: Increased risk of CNS and respiratory depression, orthostatic hypotension, severe constipation, and urine retention

ototoxic drugs: Possibly masking of some symptoms of ototoxicity, such as dizziness, tinnitus, and vertigo

phenytoin: Possibly inhibited phenytoin metabolism and increased risk of phenytoin toxicity

thiazide diuretics: Possibly potentiated hyponatremia and water intoxication

ACTIVITIES

alcohol use: Additive CNS depression

Adverse Reactions

CNS: Akathisia, altered temperature regulation, dizziness, drowsiness, extrapyramidal reactions (such as dystonia, pseudoparkinsonism, tardive dyskinesia)

CV: Hypotension, orthostatic hypotension, tachycardia

EENT: Blurred vision, dry mouth, nasal congestion, ocular changes, pigmentary retinopathy

ENDO: Galactorrhea, gynecomastia

GI: Constipation, epigastric pain, nausea, vomiting

GU: Dysuria, ejaculation disorders, menstrual irregularities, urine retention

SKIN: Decreased sweating, photosensitivity, pruritus, rash

Other: Weight gain

Nursing Considerations

•Prochlorperazine shouldn't be used to treat dementia-related psychosis in the elderly because of an increased mortality risk.

•Avoid contact between skin and solution forms of prochlorperazine because contact dermatitis could result.

•Inject I.M. form slowly, deep into upper outer quadrant of buttocks. Keep patient supine for 30 minutes after injection to minimize hypotensive effects.

•Rotate I.M. injection sites to prevent irritation and sterile abscesses.

•Be aware that I.V. form may be administered undiluted as injection or diluted in isotonic solution as infusion (mesylate form requires dilution in at least 1 L). Both forms should be administered at a rate not to exceed 5 mg/minute.

•Protect prochlorperazine from light.

•Be aware that parenteral solution may develop a slight yellowing that won't affect potency. Don't use if discoloration is pronounced or precipitate is present.

•Expect antipsychotic effects to occur in 2 to 3 weeks, although the range is days to months.

•**WARNING** Monitor closely for numerous ad-

verse reactions that may be serious.
• Be aware that adverse reactions may occur for up to 12 weeks after discontinuation of E.R. capsules.

PATIENT TEACHING
• Instruct patient to take prochlorperazine with food or a full glass of milk or water to minimize GI distress.
• Advise patient to swallow E.R. capsules whole, not to crush or chew them.
• Instruct patient using a suppository to refrigerate it for 30 minutes or hold it under running cold water before removing the wrapper if it softens during storage.
• Teach patient the correct administration technique for suppository.
• Caution patient on long-term therapy not to stop taking prochlorperazine abruptly; doing so may lead to such adverse reactions as nausea, vomiting, and trembling.
• Urge patient to avoid alcohol and OTC drugs that may contain CNS depressants.
• Advise patient to rise slowly from lying and sitting positions to minimize effects of orthostatic hypotension.
• Urge patient to avoid hazardous activities because of the risk of drowsiness and impaired judgment and coordination.
• Instruct patient to avoid excessive sun exposure and to wear sunscreen outdoors.
• Urge patient to notify prescriber about involuntary movements and restlessness.
• Explain that adverse effects may occur for up to 12 weeks after stopping E.R. capsules.

progestins

hydroxyprogesterone caproate

Gesterol LA 250, Hy/Gestrone, Hylutin, Prodrox, Pro-Span

levonorgestrel

Norplant System

medrogestone

Colprone (CAN)

medroxyprogesterone acetate

Alti-MPA (CAN), Amen, Curretab, Cycrin, Depo-Provera, Gen-Medroxy (CAN), Novo-Medrone (CAN), Provera

megestrol acetate

Apo-Megestrol (CAN), Megace, Megace OS (CAN)

norethindrone

Aygestin, Norlutate (CAN)

norgestrel

Ovrette

progesterone

Crinone, Gesterol 50, PMS-Progesterone (CAN), Prometrium

Class and Category

Chemical class: Progesterone derivative, steroid hormone
Therapeutic class: Antianorectic, anticachectic, antineoplastic, ovarian hormone replacement
Pregnancy category: D (hydroxyprogesterone, megestrol [tablets], progesterone); X (levonorgestrel, medroxyprogesterone [parenteral], megestrol [parenteral and suspension], norethindrone, norgestrel); NR (medrogestone, medroxyprogesterone [tablets])

Indications and Dosages
➤ *To treat renal cancer*
I.M. INJECTION (MEDROXYPROGESTERONE)
Adults and adolescents. *Initial:* 400 mg to 1 g every wk until improvement and stabilization occur. *Maintenance:* 400 mg or more every mo.

➤ *To treat breast cancer*
TABLETS (MEGESTROL)
Adults and adolescents. 160 mg daily as single dose or in divided doses.

➤ *To treat endometrial cancer*
TABLETS (MEGESTROL)
Adult and adolescent women. 40 to 320 mg daily in divided doses.
I.M. INJECTION (MEDROXYPROGESTERONE)
Adults and adolescents. *Initial:* 400 mg to 1 g every wk until improvement and stabilization occur. *Maintenance:* 400 mg or more every mo.

➤ *To treat anorexia, cachexia, or significant weight loss in patients who have AIDS*
SUSPENSION (MEGESTROL)
Adults and adolescents. 800 mg daily for the first mo, and then 400 or 800 mg daily for the next 3 mo.

➤ *To treat endometriosis*

TABLETS (NORETHINDRONE ACETATE)

Adult and adolescent women. *Initial:* 5 mg daily for 2 wk, increased by 2.5 mg daily at 2-wk intervals to total dose of 15 mg daily. *Maintenance:* 15 mg daily for 6 to 9 mo unless temporarily discontinued because of breakthrough menstrual bleeding.

➤ *As adjunct to treat endometrial shedding in menopausal women*

TABLETS (MEDROGESTONE)

Adult and adolescent women. 5 to 10 mg daily on days 15 through 25 of menstrual cycle.

➤ *To treat secondary amenorrhea*

TABLETS (MEDROGESTONE)

Adult and adolescent women. 5 to 10 mg daily on days 15 through 25 of menstrual cycle.

TABLETS (MEDROXYPROGESTERONE)

Adult and adolescent women. 5 to 10 mg daily for 5 to 10 days, starting anytime during menstrual cycle.

TABLETS (NORETHINDRONE ACETATE)

Adult and adolescent women. 2.5 to 10 mg daily on days 5 through 25 of menstrual cycle. Alternatively, 2.5 to 10 mg daily for 5 to 10 days during last half of menstrual cycle.

CAPSULES (PROGESTERONE)

Adult and adolescent women. 400 mg daily in evening for 10 days.

I.M. INJECTION (HYDROXYPROGESTERONE)

Adult and adolescent women. 375 mg as one-time dose.

I.M. INJECTION (PROGESTERONE)

Adult and adolescent women. 5 to 10 mg daily for 6 to 10 days. Alternatively, 100 to 150 mg injected as single dose.

VAGINAL GEL (PROGESTERONE)

Adult and adolescent women. 45 mg (1 applicatorful of 4% vaginal gel) every other day for up to 6 doses. Dosage increased, as needed, to 90 mg (1 applicatorful of 8% vaginal gel) every other day for up to 6 doses.

➤ *To treat dysfunctional uterine bleeding*

TABLETS (MEDROGESTONE)

Adult and adolescent women. 5 to 10 mg daily on days 15 through 25 of menstrual cycle.

TABLETS (MEDROXYPROGESTERONE)

Adult and adolescent women. 5 to 10 mg daily for 5 to 10 days, starting on day 16 or 21 of menstrual cycle.

TABLETS (NORETHINDRONE ACETATE)

Adult and adolescent women. 2.5 to 10 mg daily on days 5 through 25 of menstrual cycle. Alternatively, 2.5 to 10 mg daily for 5 to 10 days during last half of menstrual cycle.

I.M. INJECTION (HYDROXYPROGESTERONE)

Adult and adolescent women. 375 mg as one-time dose.

I.M. INJECTION (PROGESTERONE)

Adult and adolescent women. 5 to 10 mg daily for 6 consecutive days.

➤ *To induce menses*

TABLETS (MEDROGESTONE)

Adult and adolescent women. 5 to 10 mg daily on days 15 through 25 of the menstrual cycle.

TABLETS (MEDROXYPROGESTERONE)

Adult and adolescent women. 10 mg daily for 10 days, starting on day 16 of menstrual cycle. Repeated for 2 or more cycles if bleeding is satisfactorily controlled.

I.M. INJECTION (HYDROXYPROGESTERONE)

Adult and adolescent women. 125 to 250 mg on day 10 of menstrual cycle, repeated every 7 days until suppression is no longer desired.

➤ *To prevent pregnancy (postcoital)*

TABLETS (LEVONORGESTREL)

Adult and adolescent women. 0.75 mg as soon as possible within 72 hr of intercourse. Second dose given 12 hr later.

➤ *To prevent pregnancy*

TABLETS (NORETHINDRONE)

Adult and adolescent women. 0.35 mg daily, starting on day 1 of menstrual cycle and continuing uninterrupted through the year, whether or not menstrual bleeding occurs.

TABLETS (NORGESTREL)

Adult and adolescent women. 0.075 mg daily starting on day 1 of menstrual cycle and continuing uninterrupted throughout the year, whether or not menstrual bleeding occurs.

I.M. INJECTION (MEDROXYPROGESTERONE)

Adult and adolescent women. 150 mg every 3 mo.

SUBDERMAL IMPLANT (LEVONORGESTREL)

Adult and adolescent women. One set of implants surgically inserted every 2 yr.

Contraindications

Active thromboembolic disorder; thrombophlebitis; significant hepatic disease; hyper-

P

Mechanism of Action

Progestins may diminish the response to endogenous hormones in tumor cells by decreasing the number of steroid hormone receptors, causing a direct cytotoxic or antiproliferative effect on cell cycle growth and increased terminal cell differentiation. At higher doses, some progestins decrease adrenal production of estradiol and androstenedione, which may decrease estrogen- or testosterone-sensitive tumors. Megestrol stimulates appetite and metabolic effects, which promotes weight gain. Progestins also bind to cytosolic receptors that are loosely bound in the cell nucleus, increasing protein synthesis and improving cachexia.

Progestins affect other hormones, especially estrogen, by reducing the availability or stability of the hormone receptor complex, shutting off estrogen-responsive genes, or causing a negative feedback mechanism that decreases the number of functioning estrogen receptors. These actions allow the menstrual cycle to function normally, alleviating amenorrhea and dysfunctional uterine bleeding and inducing menses. Progestins also act to transform a proliferative uterine endometrium into a more differentiated, secretory one, which is the basis for using medroxypro-gesterone to treat some types of amenorrhea. In a normal ovulatory cycle not resulting in pregnancy, the decline in pro-gesterone secretion caused by degeneration of the corpus luteum in the late luteal phase results in endometrial sloughing. A similar sloughing occurs after 5 to 10 days of medroxy-progesterone, provided that adequate estrogen-stimulated proliferation has occurred during the follicular phase.

Selected progestins also inhibit secretion of gonadotropins from the pituitary gland, which prevents ovulation, follicular maturation, thickening of cervical mucus to prevent sperm penetration, and creation of an atrophic endometrium, resulting in a contraceptive effect.

sensitivity to peanuts (progesterone); progestins, or their components; known or suspected breast cancer; pregnancy; undiagnosed genital, uterine, or urinary tract bleeding

Interactions
DRUGS
aminoglutethimide: Possibly decreased blood level of medroxyprogesterone
carbamazepine, phenobarbital, phenytoin, rifabutin, rifampin: Possibly decreased effectiveness of progestin
thyroid hormone: Decreased thyroid hormone effectiveness

Adverse Reactions
CNS: Altered or reduced coordination or speech, depression, dizziness, drowsiness, fatigue, headache, irritability, migraine, mood changes, nervousness, postmenopausal dementia, syncope, unusual tiredness or weakness
CV: Ankle or foot edema; hypotension; numbness or pain in chest, arm, or leg; thromboembolism
ENDO: Adrenal insufficiency or suppression, breast pain or tenderness, Cushing's syndrome, decreased T_3 resin uptake, delayed return of fertility in women, elevated thyroid-binding globulin, galactorrhea, hyperglycemia, vaginal spotting
EENT: Gingival bleeding, swelling, or tenderness; vision changes or loss
GI: Abdominal cramps or pain, diarrhea, nausea, vomiting
GU: Amenorrhea, breakthrough bleeding or metromenorrhagia, decreased libido, hypermenorrhea, ovarian enlargement or cysts
HEME: Clotting and bleeding abnormalities
MS: Back pain, decreased bone density, osteoporosis, osteoporotic fractures
RESP: Dyspnea
SKIN: Acne, alopecia, melasma, rash
Other: Anaphylaxis; facial fullness; hot flashes; injection or implantation site irritation, pain, or redness; weight gain

Nursing Considerations
• Use progestins cautiously in patients with risk factors for arterial vascular disease, such as hypertension, diabetes mellitus, tobacco use, hypercholesterolemia, obesity, systemic lupus erythematosus, or a family or personal history of venous thromboembolism. Progestins may worsen these conditions.
• Use progestins cautiously in patients who

have CNS disorders, such as seizures or depression, because progestins may worsen these conditions.

•Be aware that drug causes significant loss of bone mineral density in adolescence and early adulthood and isn't recommended for long-term contraception. If other contraceptive methods are inadequate, evaluate bone mineral density routinely, as ordered.

•Confirm that patient isn't pregnant before giving progestin as a contraceptive.

•Shake container vigorously for at least 1 minute before giving medroxyprogesterone acetate injection suspension or megestrol acetate oral suspension.

•Inject parenteral medroxyprogesterone slowy, over 5 to 7 seconds, into the deltoid muscle. Don't inject it into the gluteal muscle to lessen absorption problems that may occur when patient inadvertently sits on the injection site. Pat site lightly after injection; don't rub injection site.

•Be aware that cyclical use of progestins is based on a menstrual cycle of 28 days.

•WARNING Notify prescriber immediately if patient develops sudden vision loss, abnormal protrusion of eyeball, diplopia, papilledema, migraine, or other signs of thrombotic events. Expect to discontinue progestin if such signs occur.

•Monitor patient for adrenal suppression, especially with megestrol therapy. If suspected, notify prescriber.

PATIENT TEACHING

•Instruct woman to notify prescriber if uterine bleeding continues longer than 3 months or if menstruation is delayed by 45 days.

•Warn patient taking progestin for noncontraceptive purposes to use a contraceptive method to prevent pregnancy because drug may harm fetus.

•Advise female patient to contact prescriber immediately if she suspects pregnancy or misses a menstrual period.

•Stress the importance of using a second method of birth control when taking other drugs that could reduce the contraceptive effectiveness of progestins.

•Advise female patient who vomits shortly after taking the progestin-only oral contraceptive pill not to take another dose immediately thereafter but to wait until next scheduled dose before resuming therapy and to use an additional contraceptive method for 48 hours afterward.

•Caution female patient who vomits within 1 hour of taking progestin for emergency contraception to contact prescriber about whether to repeat dose.

•Teach female patient how to administer vaginal gel, if prescribed. Tell her to avoid using other vaginal products for 6 hours before and after administration to ensure the gel's complete absorption.

•Direct patient to alert all prescribers about progestin therapy because certain blood tests may be affected.

•Emphasize importance of good dental hygiene and regular dental checkups because elevated progestin blood level increases the growth of normal oral flora, which may lead to gum tenderness, bleeding, or swelling.

•Caution postmenopausal women about increased risk of dementia associated with progestin therapy.

promethazine hydrochloride

Anergan 25, Anergan 50, Antinaus 50, Histantil (CAN), Pentazine, Phenazine 25, Phenazine 50, Phencen-50, Phenergan, Phenergan Fortis, Phenergan Plain, Phenerzine, Phenoject-50, Pro-50, Promacot, Pro-Med 50, Promet, Prorex-25, Prorex-50, Prothazine, Shogan, V-Gan-25, V-Gan-50

Class and Category

Chemical class: Phenothiazine derivative
Therapeutic class: Antiemetic, antihistamine, antivertigo, sedative-hypnotic
Pregnancy category: C

Indications and Dosages

➤ *To prevent or treat motion sickness*
SYRUP, TABLETS
Adults and adolescents. 25 mg 30 to 60 min before travel and repeated 8 to 12 hr later, if needed. *Maximum:* 150 mg daily.
➤ *To treat vertigo*
SYRUP, TABLETS
Adults and adolescents. 25 mg b.i.d., p.r.n. *Maximum:* 150 mg daily.
Children age 2 and over. 0.5 mg/kg or 10 to 25 mg every 12 hr, p.r.n.
SUPPOSITORIES
Adults and adolescents. 25 mg b.i.d., p.r.n.

P

Maximum: 150 mg daily.

Children age 2 and over. 0.5 mg/kg or 12.5 to 25 mg every 12 hr.

➤ *To prevent or treat nausea and vomiting associated with certain types of anesthesia and surgery*

SYRUP, TABLETS

Adults and adolescents. *Initial:* 25 mg, then 10 to 25 mg every 4 to 6 hr, p.r.n. *Maximum:* 150 mg daily.

Children age 2 and over. 0.25 to 0.5 mg/kg or 10 to 25 mg every 4 to 6 hr, p.r.n.

I.V. OR I.M. INJECTION

Adults and adolescents. 12.5 to 25 mg every 4 hr, p.r.n. *Maximum:* 150 mg daily.

I.M. INJECTION

Children age 2 and over. 0.25 to 0.5 mg/kg or 12.5 to 25 mg every 4 to 6 hr, p.r.n.

SUPPOSITORIES

Adults and adolescents. *Initial:* 25 mg, then 12.5 to 25 mg every 4 to 6 hr, p.r.n. *Maximum:* 150 mg daily.

Children age 2 and over. 0.25 to 0.5 mg/kg or 12.5 to 25 mg every 4 to 6 hr.

➤ *To treat signs and symptoms of allergic response*

SYRUP, TABLETS

Adults and adolescents. 10 to 12.5 mg q.i.d. before meals and at bedtime, p.r.n. Alternatively, 25 mg at bedtime, p.r.n. *Maximum:* 150 mg daily.

Children age 2 and over. 0.125 mg/kg every 4 to 6 hr or 5 to 12.5 mg t.i.d., p.r.n. Alternatively, 0.5 mg/kg or 25 mg at bedtime, p.r.n.

I.V. INJECTION

Adults and adolescents. 25 mg, repeated within 2 hr, if needed.

I.M. INJECTION, SUPPOSITORIES

Adults and adolescents. 25 mg, repeated in 2 hr, p.r.n. *Maximum:* 150 mg daily.

Children age 2 and over. 0.125 mg/kg every 4 to 6 hr or 6.25 to 12.5 mg t.i.d., p.r.n. Alternatively, 0.5 mg/kg or 25 mg at bedtime, p.r.n.

➤ *To provide nighttime, preoperative, or postoperative sedation*

SYRUP, TABLETS

Adults and adolescents. 25 to 50 mg as a single dose. *Maximum:* 150 mg daily.

Children age 2 and over. 0.5 to 1 mg/kg or 10 to 25 mg as a single dose. Alternatively, for preoperative sedation, 1.1 mg/kg along with 1.1 mg/kg of meperidine and appropri-ate dose of an atropine-like drug.

I.V. INJECTION

Adults and adolescents. 25 to 50 mg as a single dose. Alternatively, for preoperative and postoperative sedation, 25 to 50 mg combined with appropriately reduced dosages of analgesics and anticholinergics.

I.M. INJECTION, SUPPOSITORIES

Adults and adolescents. 25 to 50 mg as a single dose. Alternatively, for preoperative and postoperative sedation, 25 to 50 mg combined with appropriately reduced dosages of analgesics and anticholinergics.

Children age 2 and over. 0.5 to 1 mg/kg or 12.5 to 25 mg as a single dose. Alternatively, for preoperative sedation, 1.1 mg/kg along with 1.1 mg/kg of meperidine and an appropriate dose of an atropine-like drug.

➤ *To relieve apprehension and promote sleep the night before surgery*

SYRUP, TABLETS, SUPPOSITORIES

Adults and adolescents. 50 mg along with 50 mg of meperidine and an appropriate dose of an atropine-like drug at bedtime on the night before surgery.

DOSAGE ADJUSTMENT Dosage usually decreased for elderly patients.

➤ *To provide obstetric sedation*

I.V. OR I.M. INJECTION

Adults and adolescents. 50 mg for early stages of labor, followed by 1 or 2 doses of 25 to 75 mg after labor is definitely established, repeated every 4 hr during normal labor.

Route	Onset	Peak	Duration
P.O.	15 to 60 min	Unknown	4 to 6 hr
I.V.	3 to 5 min	Unknown	4 to 6 hr
I.M., P.R.	20 min	Unknown	4 to 6 hr

Contraindications

Angle-closure glaucoma; benign prostatic hyperplasia; bladder neck obstruction; bone marrow depression; breastfeeding; children under age 2; coma; hypersensitivity or history of idiosyncratic reaction to promethazine, other phenothiazines, or their components; hypertensive crisis; lower respiratory tract disorders (including asthma) when used as an antihistamine; pyloroduodenal obstruction; stenosing peptic ulcer; use of large quantities of CNS depressants

Mechanism of Action

Competes with histamine for H$_1$-receptor sites, thereby antagonizing many histamine effects and reducing allergy signs and symptoms. Promethazine also prevents motion sickness, nausea, and vertigo by acting centrally on the medullary chemoreceptive trigger zone and by decreasing vestibular stimulation and labyrinthine function in the inner ear. In addition, it promotes sedation and relieves anxiety by blocking receptor sites within the CNS, directly reducing stimuli to the brain.

Interactions

DRUGS

amphetamines: Decreased stimulant effect of amphetamines
anticholinergics: Possibly intensified anticholinergic adverse effects
anticonvulsants: Lowered seizure threshold
appetite suppressants: Possibly antagonized anorectic effect of appetite suppressants
beta blockers: Increased risk of additive hypotensive effects, irreversible retinopathy, arrhythmias, and tardive dyskinesia
bromocriptine: Decreased effectiveness of bromocriptine
CNS depressants: Additive CNS depression
dopamine: Possibly antagonized peripheral vasoconstriction (with high doses of dopamine)
ephedrine, metaraminol, methoxamine: Decreased vasopressor response to these drugs
epinephrine: Blocked alpha-adrenergic effects of epinephrine, increased risk of hypotension
guanadrel, guanethidine: Decreased antihypertensive effects of these drugs
hepatotoxic drugs: Increased risk of hepatotoxicity
hypotension-producing drugs: Possibly severe hypotension with syncope
levodopa: Inhibited antidyskinetic effects of levodopa
MAO inhibitors: Possibly prolonged and intensified anticholinergic and CNS depressant effects of promethazine
metrizamide: Increased risk of seizures
ototoxic drugs: Possibly masking of some symptoms of ototoxicity, such as dizziness, tinnitus, and vertigo
quinidine: Additive cardiac effects

riboflavin: Increased riboflavin requirements

ACTIVITIES

alcohol use: Additive CNS depression

Adverse Reactions

CNS: Akathisia, CNS stimulation, confusion, dizziness, drowsiness, dystonia, euphoria, excitation, fatigue, hallucinations, hysteria, incoordination, insomnia, irritability, nervousness, neuroleptic malignant syndrome, paradoxical stimulation, pseudoparkinsonism, restlessness, sedation, seizures, syncope, tardive dyskinesia, tremor
CV: Bradycardia, hypertension, hypotension, tachycardia
EENT: Blurred vision; diplopia; dry mouth, nose, and throat; nasal congestion; tinnitus; vision changes
ENDO: Hyperglycemia
GI: Anorexia, cholestatic jaundice, ileus, nausea, rectal burning or stinging (suppository form), vomiting
GU: Dysuria
HEME: Agranulocytosis, leukopenia, thrombocytopenia, thrombocytopenic purpura
RESP: Apnea, respiratory depression, tenacious bronchial secretions
SKIN: Dermatitis, diaphoresis, jaundice, photosensitivity, rash, urticaria
Other: Angioedema, paradoxical reactions

Nursing Considerations

• Use promethazine cautiously in children and elderly patients because they may be more sensitive to drug effects and in patients with cardiovascular disease or hepatic dysfunction because of potential adverse effects.
• Also use drug cautiously in patients with asthma because of its anticholinergic effects and in patients with seizure disorders or those who use medication that may affect seizure threshold because drug may lower patient's seizure threshold.
• Inject I.M. form deep into large muscle mass and rotate sites.
• **WARNING** Avoid inadvertent intra-arterial injection of promethazine because it can cause arteriospasm; gangrene may develop from impaired circulation.
• Give I.V. injection at a rate not to exceed 25 mg/min; rapid I.V. administration may produce a transient fall in blood pressure.
• **WARNING** Monitor respiratory function because drug may suppress cough reflex and cause thickening of bronchial secretions, ag-

P

gravating such conditions as asthma and COPD, and, in rare cases, may depress respirations and induce apnea.

•Monitor patient's hematologic status as ordered because promethazine may cause bone marrow depression, especially when used with other known marrow-toxic agents. Assess patient for signs and symptoms of infection or bleeding.

•**WARNING** Monitor patient for evidence of neuroleptic malignant syndrome, such as fever, hypertension or hypotension, involuntary motor activity, mental changes, muscle rigidity, tachycardia, and tachypnea. Be prepared to provide supportive treatment and additional drug therapy, as prescribed.

•Be aware that patient shouldn't have intradermal allergen tests within 72 hours of receiving promethazine because drug may significantly alter flare response.

PATIENT TEACHING
•Tell patient to use a calibrated device to ensure accurate doses of promethazine syrup.

•Teach patient correct administration technique for suppository, if needed.

•Advise patient to avoid OTC drugs unless approved by prescriber.

•Instruct patient to notify prescriber immediately if she experiences involuntary movements and restlessness.

•Urge patient to avoid consuming alcohol and other CNS depressants while taking promethazine.

•Instruct patient to avoid potentially hazardous activities until drug's CNS effects are known.

•Suggest frequent rinsing and use of sugarless gum or hard candy to relieve dry mouth.

•Caution patient to avoid excessive sun exposure and to use sunscreen when outdoors.

propafenone hydrochloride

Rythmol

Class and Category

Chemical class: 3-Phenylpropriophenone
Therapeutic class: Class IC antiarrhythmic
Pregnancy category: C

Indications and Dosages

➤ *To treat life-threatening ventricular arrhythmias*

TABLETS
Adults. *Initial:* 150 mg every 8 hr; after 3 or 4 days, increased to 225 mg every 8 hr (U.S.) or 300 mg every 12 hr (Canada), if needed; after an additional 3 or 4 days, further increased to 300 mg every 8 hr, if needed. *Maximum:* 900 mg daily.

Mechanism of Action

Prolongs the recovery period after myocardial repolarization by inhibiting sodium influx through myocardial cell membranes. This action prolongs the refractory period, causing myocardial automaticity, excitability, and conduction velocity to decline.

Contraindications

Bronchospastic disorders, such as asthma; cardiogenic shock; electrolyte imbalances; heart failure (uncontrolled); hypersensitivity to propafenone or its components; severe hypotension; sinus bradycardia or AV conduction disturbances (in patient without artificial pacemaker)

Interactions

DRUGS
amiodarone: Possibly altered cardiac conduction and repolarization; possibly increased blood propafenone level
anesthetics (local): Increased risk of adverse CNS effects
antiarrhythmics, fluoxetine: Increased propafenone levels and risk of adverse CV effects
cimetidine, erythromycin, ketoconazole, paroxetine, ritonavir, saquinavir, sertraline: Possibly increased blood propafenone level
desipramine: Possibly increased blood level of desipramine or propafenone
digoxin: Increased risk of digitalis toxicity
haloperidol, imipramine, venlafaxine: Possibly increased blood levels of these drugs
metoprolol, propranolol: Increased blood level and half-life of these drugs
orlistat: Possibly decreased absorption of propafenone
quinidine: Inhibited propafenone metabolism
rifampin: Possibly decreased propafenone level
warfarin: Increased blood warfarin level and risk of bleeding

FOODS
grapefruit juice: Possibly increased blood propafenone level

Adverse Reactions
CNS: Dizziness, fatigue, headache
CV: Angina, AV block, bradycardia, heart failure, irregular heartbeat, tachycardia, ventricular arrhythmias
EENT: Altered taste, blurred vision, dry mouth
GI: Constipation, diarrhea, nausea, vomiting
SKIN: Rash

Nursing Considerations
•Assess patient for electrolyte imbalances, such as hyperkalemia, before beginning therapy with propafenone or any antiarrhythmic to reduce the risk of adverse cardiac reactions.
•Use propafenone cautiously in patients with heart failure or myocardial dysfunction because drug's beta-blocking activity may further depress myocardial contractility.
•Monitor ECG tracings, blood pressure, and pulse rate, particularly at the start of therapy and with dosage increases.

PATIENT TEACHING
•Instruct patient to take a missed dose if she remembers within 4 hours; otherwise, tell her to skip the missed dose and to resume the regular dosing schedule.
•Advise patient not to discontinue propafenone or change dosage without consulting prescriber.
•Urge patient to carry or wear medical identification indicating that she takes propafenone.
•Advise patient to avoid hazardous activities until drug's CNS effects are known.
•Urge patient to increase fluid intake and add fiber to diet if she becomes constipated.
•Inform patient that drug may cause an unusual taste in her mouth. Advise her to notify prescriber if taste interferes with compliance.

propantheline bromide

Pro-Banthine, Propanthel (CAN)

Class and Category
Chemical class: Quaternary amine
Therapeutic class: Anticholinergic
Pregnancy category: C

Indications and Dosages
➤ *As adjunct to treat peptic ulcer disease*
TABLETS
Adults. 15 mg t.i.d. before meals and 30 mg at bedtime, adjusted as needed and tolerated. *Maximum:* 120 mg daily.
Children. 0.375 mg/kg q.i.d., adjusted as needed and tolerated.
DOSAGE ADJUSTMENT For elderly patients with mild symptoms or patients of below-average weight, dosage possibly reduced to 7.5 mg t.i.d. or q.i.d.

Route	Onset	Peak	Duration
P.O.	Unknown	Unknown	6 hr

Mechanism of Action
Prevents the neurotransmitter acetylcholine from combining with receptors on the postganglionic parasympathetic nerve terminal, thereby reducing smooth-muscle spasms in the GI system, slowing GI motility, and inhibiting gastric acid secretion. All these effects help to heal peptic ulcers.

Contraindications
Adhesions between iris and lens, angle-closure glaucoma, hemorrhage accompanied by hemodynamic instability, hepatic dysfunction, hypersensitivity to propantheline or its components, ileus, myasthenia gravis, myocardial ischemia, obstructive GI or urinary disease, renal dysfunction, severe ulcerative colitis, tachycardia

Interactions
DRUGS
amantadine, other anticholinergics, tricyclic antidepressants: Additive anticholinergic effects
antacids, antidiarrheals (adsorbent): Possibly reduced absorption of propantheline
antimyasthenics: Possibly further reduction in intestinal motility
atenolol: Increased effects of atenolol
cyclopropane: Possibly ventricular arrhythmias
digoxin: Possibly digitalis toxicity
haloperidol: Decreased antipsychotic effect of haloperidol in schizophrenic patients
ketoconazole: Decreased ketoconazole absorption

P

metoclopramide: Possibly decreased metoclopramide effect on GI motility
opioid analgesics: Increased risk of severe constipation and urine retention
phenothiazines: Possibly decreased antipsychotic effects
potassium chloride: Possibly increased severity of potassium chloride–induced GI ulceration, stricture, or perforation
urinary alkalizers: Delayed urinary excretion of propantheline

Adverse Reactions

CNS: Dizziness, excitement, insomnia, nervousness, paradoxical CNS stimulation
CV: Palpitations, tachycardia
EENT: Blurred vision; dry mouth, nose, and throat
GI: Constipation, dysphagia, heartburn, ileus, nausea, vomiting
GU: Impotence, urinary hesitancy, urine retention
SKIN: Decreased sweating, dry skin, flushing

Nursing Considerations

•Don't administer propantheline within 1 hour of antacids or antidiarrheals.
•Monitor elderly patients closely because they may respond to usual drug dose with agitation, confusion, drowsiness, or excitement.
•WARNING Be aware that drug can interfere with sweating reflex, thereby increasing the risk of heatstroke.

PATIENT TEACHING

•Instruct patient to take propantheline 30 to 60 minutes before meals and at bedtime, as prescribed.
•Inform patient that drug may cause dizziness. Advise her not to perform potentially hazardous activities until drug's CNS effects are known.
•Encourage patient to increase her fluid and fiber intake to decrease constipation. Instruct her to report persistent constipation and urine retention.
•Advise patient to avoid excessive exposure to heat to reduce the risk of heat prostration and heatstroke, because propantheline decreases sweating.
•Suggest that patient relieve dry mouth with frequent rinsing and sugar-free hard candy or gum.

propofol
(disoprofol)

Diprivan

Class and Category

Chemical class: 2,6-diisopropylphenol derivative
Therapeutic class: Sedative-hypnotic
Pregnancy category: B

Indications and Dosages

➤ *To provide sedation for critically ill patients in intensive care*
I.V. INFUSION
Adults. 2.8 to 130 mcg/kg/min. *Usual:* 27 mcg/kg/min.
DOSAGE ADJUSTMENT For elderly, debilitated, or American Society of Anesthesiologists Physical Status (ASA-PS) III or IV patients, induction dose decreased and maintenance rate slower.

Route	Onset	Peak	Duration
I.V.	Within 40 sec	Unknown	3 to 5 min

Mechanism of Action

Decreases cerebral blood flow, cerebral metabolic oxygen consumption, and intracranial pressure and increases cerebrovascular resistance, which may play a role in propofol's hypnotic effects.

Incompatibilities

Don't mix propofol with other drugs before administration. Don't administer propofol through same I.V. line as blood or plasma products because globular component of emulsion will aggregate.

Contraindications

Hypersensitivity to propofol or its components, to eggs or egg products, or to soybeans or soy products

Interactions

DRUGS

CNS depressants: Additive CNS depressant, respiratory depressant, and hypotensive effects; possibly decreased emetic effects of opioids
droperidol: Possibly decreased control of nausea and vomiting

ACTIVITIES
alcohol use: Additive CNS depressant, respiratory depressant, and hypotensive effects

Adverse Reactions

CV: Bradycardia, hypotension
GI: Nausea, vomiting
MS: Involuntary muscle movements (transient)
RESP: Apnea
Other: Anaphylaxis, injection site burning, pain, or stinging

Nursing Considerations

- Use propofol cautiously in patients with cardiac disease, peripheral vascular disease, impaired cerebral circulation, or increased intracranial pressure because drug may aggravate these disorders.
- If ordered to dilute drug before administration, use only D_5W to yield a final concentration of 2 mg/ml or more.
- Consult prescriber about pretreating injection site with 1 ml of 1% lidocaine to minimize pain, burning, or stinging that may occur with propofol administration. However, be aware that lidocaine, if ordered, should not be added to propofol solution in quantities greater than 20 mg/200 mg propofol because the emulsion may become unstable. Giving drug through a larger vein in the forearm or antecubital fossa may also minimize injection site discomfort.
- Shake container well before using, administer drug promptly after opening, and use vial for a single patient. Use prefilled syringes within 6 hours of opening.
- Use a drop counter, syringe pump, or volumetric pump to safely control infusion rate. Don't infuse drug through filter with a pore size of less than 5 microns because doing so could cause emulsion to break down.
- Discard all unused portions of propofol solution as well as reservoirs, I.V. tubing, and solutions immediately after or within 12 hours of administration (6 hours if propofol was transferred from original container) to prevent bacterial growth in stagnant solution. Also, protect solution from light.
- Be aware that dosage must be tapered before stopping therapy. Stopping abruptly will cause rapid awakening, anxiety, agitation and resistance to mechanical ventilation.
- Expect patient to recover from sedation within 8 minutes.
- **WARNING** Monitor patient for propofol infusion syndrome, especially with prolonged high-dose infusions. It may cause severe metabolic acidosis, hyperkalemia, lipemia, rhabdomyolysis, hepatomegaly and cardiac and renal failure. Alert prescriber immediately and be prepared to provide emergency supportive care as ordered.

PATIENT TEACHING

- Urge patient and family to voice concerns and ask questions before administration.
- Reassure patient that she'll be closely monitored throughout drug administration and that her vital functions, including breathing, will be supported as needed.

propoxyphene hydrochloride

Cotanol-65, Darvon, PP-Cap

propoxyphene napsylate

Darvon-N

Class, Category, and Schedule

Chemical class: Synthetic opioid
Therapeutic class: Analgesic
Pregnancy category: Not rated
Controlled substance schedule: IV

Indications and Dosages

➤ *To relieve mild to moderate pain*

CAPSULES, ORAL SUSPENSION, TABLETS (PROPOXYPHENE NAPYSLATE)
Adults. 100 mg every 4 hr, p.r.n. *Maximum:* 600 mg daily.

CAPSULES, TABLETS (PROPOXYPHENE HYDROCHLORIDE)
Adults. 65 mg every 4 hr, p.r.n. *Maximum:* 390 mg daily.

Route	Onset	Peak	Duration
P.O.	15 to 60 min	2 hr	4 to 6 hr

Contraindications

Hypersensitivity to propoxyphene or its components (including acetaminophen and aspirin), respiratory depression, severe asthma, upper airway obstruction, use within 14 days of MAO inhibitor therapy

Interactions

DRUGS
amphetamines: Possibly fatal seizures (with

P

Mechanism of Action

Produces analgesia through a synergistic analgesic effect.

Propoxyphene strongly agonizes mu receptors, blocking the release of such inhibitory neurotransmitters as gamma-aminobutyric acid (GABA) and acetylcholine. It also mediates analgesia by changing pain perception at the spinal cord and higher CNS levels and by altering the emotional response to pain.

Acetaminophen acts centrally to increase the pain threshold by inhibiting cyclooxygenase, an enzyme involved in prostaglandin synthesis.

Aspirin possesses analgesic, anti-inflam-matory, antiplatelet, and antipyretic properties. It interferes with arachidonate metabolism as it acetylates proteins and inhibits prostaglandin synthesis by irreversibly inhibiting cyclooxygenase-2, one of two major enzymes that act on arachidonic acid. Aspirin also decreases the perception of pain.

Caffeine exhibits a direct stimulant effect at all levels of the CNS and cardiovascular system. It stimulates the medullary respiratory center, relaxes bronchial smooth muscle, stimulates gastric acid secretion, increases renal blood flow, and acts as a mild diuretic.

propoxyphene overdose)

anticholinergics: Increased risk of severe constipation and urine retention

antidiarrheals: Severe constipation, possibly increased CNS depression

antihypertensives: Possibly exaggerated antihypertensive response

buprenorphine: Possibly decreased propoxyphene effectiveness, increased respiratory depression

carbamazepine: Possibly carbamazepine toxicity

CNS depressants: Increased CNS and respiratory depression, hypotensive effects, and risk of habituation

hydroxyzine: Increased analgesic, CNS depressant, and hypotensive effects

MAO inhibitors: Severe, possibly fatal reactions, including hypertensive crisis

metoclopramide: Possibly antagonized effects of metoclopramide on GI motility

naloxone: Antagonized analgesic and CNS and respiratory depressant effects of propoxyphene

naltrexone: Risk of withdrawal symptoms in patients who are dependent on propoxyphene, possibly decreased analgesic effect of propoxyphene

neuromuscular blockers: Additive respiratory depressant effects

opioid analgesics: Additive CNS and respiratory depressant and hypotensive effects

warfarin: Increased anticoagulation effects

ACTIVITIES

alcohol use: Increased CNS and respiratory depression, hypotensive effects, and risk of habituation

nicotine chewing gum, other smoking deterrents, smoking cessation: Decreased effectiveness of propoxyphene

Adverse Reactions

CNS: Dizziness, drowsiness, fatigue, insomnia, light-headedness, malaise, nervousness, sedation, tremor

CV: Orthostatic hypotension, tachycardia

EENT: Blurred vision, diplopia, dry mouth, tinnitus

GI: Abdominal cramps, anorexia, constipation, nausea, vomiting

GU: Decreased urine output

MS: Muscle weakness

RESP: Dyspnea, respiratory depression, wheezing

SKIN: Flushing of face, pruritus, rash, urticaria

Other: Psychological dependence

Nursing Considerations

• Use propoxyphene cautiously in patients with hepatic or renal dysfunction because delayed elimination may occur. Monitor hepatic and renal function test results.

• WARNING Be aware that long-term, high-dose propoxyphene therapy may lead to psychological dependence in some patients. Assess for opioid and alcohol use, which increase the risk of drug abuse or dependence.

• Be aware drug is also available in combination products with aspirin or acetaminophen and caffeine.

• Be aware that abruptly discontinuing drug

can result in withdrawal symptoms.

PATIENT TEACHING

•Inform patient that she may take propoxyphene with food if she experiences GI distress.

•Instruct patient not to take more than the prescribed amount because drug may be addictive.

•Inform patient that drug may cause blurred vision, drowsiness, dizziness, and impaired judgment and coordination. Urge her to avoid potentially hazardous activities until drug's CNS effects are known.

•Instruct patient to avoid alcohol and other sedatives while taking drug.

•Advise smokers to inform prescriber if they attempt to stop smoking during propoxyphene therapy because increased drug dosage may be required for effective analgesia.

•Urge patient to notify prescriber immediately if pain isn't relieved or worsens.

propranolol hydrochloride

Apo-Propranolol (CAN), Detensol (CAN), Inderal, Inderal LA, Novopranol (CAN), pms Propranolol (CAN)

Class and Category

Chemical class: Beta-adrenergic blocker
Therapeutic class: Antianginal, antiarrhythmic, antihypertensive, anti-MI, antimigraine, antitremor, hypertrophic cardiomyopathy and pheochromocytoma therapy adjunct
Pregnancy category: C

Indications and Dosages

➤ *To manage hypertension*

E.R. TABLETS

Adults. *Initial:* 80 mg daily, increased gradually up to 160 mg daily *Maximum:* 640 mg daily.

ORAL SOLUTION, TABLETS

Adults. *Initial:* 40 mg b.i.d., increased gradually to 120 to 240 mg daily, as needed. *Maximum:* 640 mg daily.

Children. *Initial:* 0.5 to 1 mg/kg daily in divided doses b.i.d. to q.i.d., adjusted as needed. *Maintenance:* 2 to 4 mg/kg daily in divided doses b.i.d.

➤ *To treat chronic angina*

E.R. TABLETS

Adults. *Initial:* 80 mg daily, increased every 3 to 7 days, as prescribed. *Maximum:*

320 mg/day.

ORAL SOLUTION, TABLETS

Adults. 80 to 320 mg daily in divided doses b.i.d., t.i.d., or q.i.d.

➤ *To treat supraventricular arrhythmias and ventricular tachycardia*

ORAL SOLUTION, TABLETS

Adults. 10 to 30 mg t.i.d. or q.i.d., adjusted as needed.

I.V. INJECTION

Adults. 1 to 3 mg at a rate not to exceed 1 mg/min; repeated after 2 min and again after 4 hr, if needed.

Children. 0.01 to 0.1 mg/kg at a rate not to exceed 1 mg/min; repeated every 6 to 8 hr, as needed. *Maximum:* 1 mg/dose.

➤ *To control tremor*

ORAL SOLUTION, TABLETS

Adults. *Initial:* 40 mg b.i.d., adjusted as needed and prescribed. *Maximum:* 320 mg daily.

➤ *To prevent vascular migraine headaches*

E.R. TABLETS

Adults. *Initial:* 80 mg daily, increased gradually, as needed. *Maximum:* 240 mg daily.

ORAL SOLUTION, TABLETS

Adults. *Initial:* 20 mg q.i.d., increased gradually, as needed. *Maximum:* 240 mg daily.

➤ *As adjunct to treat hypertrophic cardiomyopathy*

ORAL SOLUTION, TABLETS

Adults. 20 to 40 mg t.i.d. or q.i.d., adjusted as needed.

➤ *As adjunct to manage pheochromocytoma*

ORAL SOLUTION, TABLETS

Adults. For operable tumors, 20 mg t.i.d. to 40 mg t.i.d. or q.i.d. for 3 days before surgery, concomitantly with an alpha blocker. For inoperable tumors, 30 to 160 mg daily in divided doses.

➤ *To prevent MI*

ORAL SOLUTION, TABLETS

Adults. 180 to 240 mg daily in divided doses.

DOSAGE ADJUSTMENT Dosage increased or decreased for elderly patients, depending on sensitivity to propranolol.

Contraindications

Asthma, cardiogenic shock, greater than first-degree AV block, heart failure (unless secondary to tachyarrhythmia that's respon-

P

sive to propranolol), hypersensitivity to propranolol or its components, sinus bradycardia

Route	Onset	Peak	Duration
P.O.	Unknown	1 to 1.5 hr*	Unknown

Mechanism of Action

Exerts the following effects through its beta-blocking actions:
• prevents arterial dilation and inhibits renin secretion, resulting in decreased blood pressure (in hypertension and pheochromocytoma) and relief of migraine headaches
• decreases the heart rate, which helps resolve tachyarrhythmias
• improves myocardial contractility, which helps ease the symptoms of hypertrophic cardiomyopathy
• decreases myocardial oxygen demand, which helps prevent angina pain and death of myocardial tissue.

In addition, peripheral beta-adrenergic blockade may play a role in propranolol's ability to alleviate tremor.

Interactions

DRUGS

ACE inhibitors: Increased risk of hypotension, especially in presence of acute MI
allergen immunotherapy, allergenic extracts for skin testing: Increased risk of serious systemic adverse reactions or anaphylaxis
amiodarone: Additive depressant effects on conduction, negative inotropic effects
anesthetics (hydrocarbon inhalation): Increased risk of myocardial depression and hypotension
beta blockers: Additive beta blockade effects
calcium channel blockers, clonidine, diazoxide, guanabenz, resperpine, other hypotension-producing drugs: Additive hypotensive effect and, possibly, other beta blockade effects
catecholamine-depleting drugs, such as reserpine: Increased risk of hypotension, bradycardia, vertigo, syncope, and orthostatic hypotension

cimetidine: Possibly interference with propranolol clearance
digitalis glycosides: Increased risk of bradycardia
diltiazem: Increased risk of bradycardia, hypotension, high-degree heart block, and heart failure
dobutamine, isoproterenol: Reversed effects of propranolol
doxazosin, terazosin: Increased risk of orthostatic hypotension
epinephrine: Increased risk of uncontrolled hypertension
estrogens: Decreased antihypertensive effect of propranolol
fentanyl, fentanyl derivatives: Possibly increased risk of initial bradycardia after induction doses of fentanyl or a derivative (with long-term propranolol use)
glucagon: Possibly blunted hyperglycemic response
insulin, oral antidiabetic drugs: Possibly impaired glucose control, masking of tachycardia in response to hypoglycemia
lidocaine: Decreased lidocaine clearance, increased risk of lidocaine toxicity
MAO inhibitors, tricyclic antidepressants: Increased risk of significant hypertension
neuroleptic drugs: Increased risk of hypotension and cardiac arrest
neuromuscular blockers: Possibly potentiated and prolonged action of these drugs
NSAIDs: Possibly decreased hypotensive effects
phenothiazines: Increased blood levels of both drugs
phenytoin: Additive cardiac depressant effects (with parenteral phenytoin)
prazosin: Increased risk of first-dose hypotension
propafenone: Increased blood level and half-life of propranolol
quinidine: Increased propranolol level, resulting in higher degrees of beta blockade and orthostatic hypotension
sympathomimetics, xanthines: Possibly mutual inhibition of therapeutic effects
thyroxine: Possibly decreased T_3 level
verapamil: Increased risk of bradycardia, heart failure, and cardiovascular collapse
warfarin: Increased risk of bleeding

ACTIVITIES

alcohol: Possibly increased plasma propranolol level

---

* For regular-release form; unknown for E.R. form.

nicotine chewing gum, smoking cessation, smoking deterrents: Increased therapeutic effects of propranolol

Adverse Reactions
CNS: Anxiety, depression, dizziness, drowsiness, fatigue, fever, insomnia, lethargy, nervousness, weakness
CV: AV conduction disorders, cold limbs, heart failure, hypotension, sinus bradycardia
EENT: Dry eyes, laryngospasm, nasal congestion, pharyngitis
GI: Abdominal pain, constipation, diarrhea, nausea, vomiting
GU: Impotence, peyronie's disease, sexual dysfunction
HEME: Agranulocytosis
MS: Muscle weakness
RESP: Bronchospasm, dyspnea, respiratory distress, wheezing
SKIN: Alopecia, erythema multiforme, erythematous rash, exfoliative dermatitis, psoriasiform rash, Stevens-Johnson syndrome, toxic epidermal necrolysis, urticaria
Other: Anaphylaxis, flulike symptoms, systemic lupuslike reaction

Nursing Considerations
• Use propranolol cautiously in patients with bronchospastic lung disease because it may induce an asthmatic attack.
• Monitor blood pressure, apical and radial pulses, fluid intake and output, daily weight, respiration, and circulation in extremities before and during propranolol therapy.
• Give I.V. injection at no more than 1 mg/minute.
• **WARNING** Monitor ECG continuously, as ordered, when giving I.V. injection. Have emergency drugs and equipment available in case of hypotension or cardiac arrest.
• Protect injection solution from light.
• Because drug's negative inotropic effect can depress cardiac output, monitor cardiac output in patients with heart failure, particularly those with severely compromised left ventricular dysfunction.
• Be aware that propranolol can mask tachycardia that occurs in hyperthyroidism and that abrupt withdrawal of drug in patients with hyperthyroidism or thyrotoxicosis can precipitate thyroid storm.
• Monitor diabetic patient receiving antidiabetic drugs because propranolol can prolong hypoglycemia or promote hyperglycemia.

Propranolol also can mask signs of hypoglycemia, especially tachycardia, palpitations, and tremor, but it doesn't suppress diaphoresis or hypertensive response to hypoglycemia.
• **WARNING** Be aware that abruptly stopping drug may cause myocardial ischemia, MI, ventricular arrhythmias, or severe hypertension, especially in patients with cardiac disease. Stopping abruptly also may cause a return of increased intraocular pressure. Dosage should be reduced gradually.

PATIENT TEACHING
• Instruct patient to take propranolol at the same time every day.
• Caution patient not to change dosage without consulting prescriber and not to stop taking drug abruptly.
• Advise patient to notify prescriber immediately if she experiences shortness of breath.
• Instruct diabetic patient to regularly monitor blood glucose level and urine for ketones.
• Advise patient to consult prescriber before taking OTC drugs, especially cold remedies.
• Urge patient to avoid hazardous activities until CNS effects of drug are known.
• Advise smoker to notify prescriber immediately if she stops smoking because smoking cessation may decrease drug metabolism, calling for dosage adjustments.
• Tell patient to notify prescriber if she is or could be pregnant because drug may need to be discontinued.

propylthiouracil (PTU)

Propyl-Thyracil (CAN)

Class and Category
Chemical class: Thiourea derivative
Therapeutic class: Antithyroid
Pregnancy category: D

Indications and Dosages
➤ *To treat hyperthyroidism*
TABLETS
Adults and adolescents. *Initial:* For mild to moderate hyperthyroidism, 300 to 900 mg daily in 1 to 4 divided doses until patient becomes euthyroid; for severe hyperthyroidism, 300 to 1,200 mg daily in 1 to 4 divided doses until patient becomes euthyroid. *Maintenance:* 50 to 600 mg daily in 1 to 4 divided doses.

P

Children age 10 and over. *Initial:* 50 to 300 mg daily in 1 to 4 divided doses. *Maintenance:* Adjusted based on response to initial dosage. **Children ages 6 to 10.** *Initial:* 50 to 150 mg/day in 1 to 4 divided doses. *Maintenance:* Adjusted based on response to initial dosage. **Neonates.** 10 mg/kg daily in divided doses.

➤ *As adjunct to treat thyrotoxic crisis*
TABLETS
Adults and adolescents. 200 to 400 mg every 4 hr on day 1 plus other measures. Dosage gradually decreased as crisis subsides.
DOSAGE ADJUSTMENT If creatinine clearance is 10 to 50 ml/min/1.73 m², recommended dosage reduced by 25%; if creatinine clearance is less than 10 ml/min/1.73 m², recommended dosage reduced by 50%.

Route	Onset	Peak	Duration
P.O.	Unknown	17 wk	Unknown

Mechanism of Action

Inhibits conversion of peripheral thyroxine to triiodothyronine by interfering with incorporation of iodide into thyroglobulin; drug remains iodinated and degraded in the thyroid gland. Diversion of oxidized iodine away from thyroglobulin diminishes thyroid hormone synthesis and levels of circulating thyroid hormone.

Contraindications

Breastfeeding, hypersensitivity to propylthiouracil or its components

Interactions
DRUGS
amiodarone, iodinated glycerol, iodine, potassium iodide: Decreased efficacy of propylthiouracil
digoxin: Risk of digitalis toxicity
oral anticoagulants: Possibly enhanced anticoagulant effect
sodium iodide 131 (radioactive iodine, ^{131}I): Decreased thyroid uptake of ^{131}I

Adverse Reactions
CNS: Dizziness, paresthesia, peripheral neuropathy
CV: Vasculitis
ENDO: Hypothyroidism
GI: Abdominal pain, nausea, vomiting
HEME: Agranulocytosis, leukopenia

MS: Arthralgia, joint redness or swelling
SKIN: Pruritus, rash, urticaria
Other: Lupuslike symptoms

Nursing Considerations
•Monitor CBC, PT, and liver and thyroid function test results in patients taking propylthiouracil. Elevated serum triiodothyronine (T_3) level may be the sole indicator of inadequate treatment.
•Expect to stop drug 3 to 4 days before ^{131}I treatment to prevent decreased thyroid uptake of ^{131}I; therapy may be resumed 3 to 5 days after radiation, if needed.
•Serum T_3 and thyroxine levels should decrease after about 3 weeks of therapy.
•Expect to decrease beta blocker or theophylline dosage once patient is euthyroid.
PATIENT TEACHING
•Instruct patient to take propylthiouracil with meals to decrease risk of adverse GI reactions.
•Urge patient to avoid dietary sources of iodine, such as iodized salt and shellfish.
•Tell patient to monitor her pulse rate and weight daily and to report increased heart rate and excessive weight loss to prescriber.
•Urge patient to report signs and symptoms of infection, such as fever and sore throat, or signs and symptoms that could reflect hepatic dysfunction, such as anorexia and right-upper-quadrant pain.
•Instruct patient to notify prescriber immediately if she becomes pregnant.
•Advise patient to report signs and symptoms of hypothyroidism, such as cold intolerance, depression, and increased fatigue.
•Tell patient to consult prescriber before using OTC cold remedies (some contain iodides).

protamine sulfate

Class and Category
Chemical class: Simple low-molecular-weight protein
Therapeutic class: Heparin antagonist
Pregnancy category: C

Indications and Dosages
➤ *To treat heparin toxicity or hemorrhage associated with heparin therapy*
I.V. INJECTION
Adults and children. 1 mg for each 100 units

of heparin to be neutralized, or as indicated by coagulation test results. *Maximum:* 100 mg (within 2-hr period).

Route	Onset	Peak	Duration
I.V.	5 min	Unknown	2 hr

Mechanism of Action
Neutralizes anticoagulant activity. A strong basic polypeptide, protamine combines with strongly acidic heparin complex to form an inactive stable salt, thereby neutralizing the anticoagulant activity of both drugs.

Incompatibilities
Don't mix protamine sulfate in same syringe with other drugs unless they're known to be compatible. Several cephalosporins, penicillins, and other antibiotics are incompatible.

Contraindications
Allergy to fish, hypersensitivity to protamine or its components

Interactions
DRUGS
heparin: Neutralized anticoagulant effect of both drugs

Adverse Reactions
CNS: Weakness
CV: Bradycardia, hypertension, hypotension, shock
GI: Nausea, vomiting
HEME: Unusual bleeding or bruising
RESP: Dyspnea, pulmonary edema (noncardiogenic), pulmonary hypertension
SKIN: Flushing, sensation of warmth
Other: Anaphylaxis

Nursing Considerations
•Expect to administer I.V. protamine undiluted. However, dilute drug if needed (for patients other than neonates) with 5 ml of bacteriostatic water for injection containing 0.9% benzyl alcohol. For neonates, reconstitute with preservative-free sterile water for injection.
•Inject drug slowly at a rate of 5 mg/minute; administer no more than 50 mg in 10 minutes or 100 mg in 2 hours.
•**WARNING** Be aware that rapid delivery may cause severe hypotension and anaphylaxis.
•Be prepared to obtain coagulation studies (APTT, activated clotting time) 5 to 15 minutes after administering drug and to repeat studies in 2 to 8 hours to assess for heparin-rebound hypotension, shock, and bleeding.
•Monitor vital signs, hemodynamic parameters, and fluid intake and output, and assess for flushing sensation.
•Have fluids—epinephrine 1:1,000, dobutamine, or dopamine—available for allergic or hypotensive reactions.
•Be aware that vasectomized males have an increased risk of hypersensitivity reaction because of possible accumulation of antiprotamine antibodies.
PATIENT TEACHING
•Instruct patient to report adverse reactions immediately.

protriptyline hydrochloride
Triptil (CAN), Vivactil

Class and Category
Chemical class: Dibenzocycloheptene derivative
Therapeutic class: Antidepressant
Pregnancy category: Not rated

Indications and Dosages
➤ *To treat depression*
TABLETS
Adults. *Initial:* 5 to 10 mg t.i.d. or q.i.d., increased every wk by 10 mg daily, as needed. *Maximum:* 60 mg daily.
Children age 12 and over. *Initial:* 5 mg t.i.d., increased as needed.
DOSAGE ADJUSTMENT For elderly patients, initial dosage limited to 5 mg t.i.d., then adjusted as needed.

Route	Onset	Peak	Duration
P.O.	2 to 3 wk	Unknown	Unknown

Mechanism of Action
May block the reuptake of norepinephrine and serotonin (and possibly other neurotransmitters) at neuronal membranes, thus enhancing their effects at postsynaptic receptors. These neurotransmitters may play a role in relieving symptoms of depression.

P

Contraindications

Acute recovery phase after MI, hypersensitivity to protriptyline or its components, use within 14 days of MAO inhibitor therapy

Interactions

DRUGS

amantadine, anticholinergics, antidyskinetics, antihistamines: Additive anticholinergic effects, potentiated effects of antihistamines or protriptyline, possibly impaired detoxification of atropine and related drugs
anticonvulsants: Possibly lowered seizure threshold and decreased anticonvulsant effectiveness; enhanced CNS depression
antithyroid drugs: Possibly agranulocytosis
barbiturates, carbamazepine: Decreased therapeutic effects of protriptyline
bupropion, clozapine, cyclobenzaprine, haloperidol, loxapine, maprotiline, molindone, phenothiazines, thioxanthenes: Prolonged and intensified anticholinergic and sedative effects, lowered seizure threshold, increased risk of neuroleptic malignant syndrome; increased blood protriptyline level and inhibited phenothiazine metabolism (with phenothiazine use)
cimetidine: Increased risk of protriptyline toxicity
clonidine, guanadrel, guanethidine: Decreased hypotensive effects; increased CNS depression (with clonidine use)
CNS depressants: Possibly serious potentiation of CNS and respiratory depression and hypotensive effect
disulfiram, ethchlorvynol: Possibly transient delirium; increased CNS depression (with ethchlorvynol use)
fluoxetine: Increased protriptyline level
MAO inhibitors: Increased risk of hyperpyretic crisis, severe seizures, and death
methylphenidate: Possibly antagonized effects of methylphenidate and increased blood protriptyline level
metrizamide: Increased risk of seizures
naphazoline, oxymetazoline, phenylephrine, xylometazoline: Possibly increased vasopressor effects of these drugs
oral anticoagulants: Possibly increased anticoagulant activity
pimozide, probucol: Possibly prolonged QT interval and ventricular tachycardia
sympathomimetics: Possibly potentiated cardiovascular effects, decreased vasopressor effects of ephedrine and mephentermine

thyroid hormones: Increased therapeutic and toxic effects of both drugs
ACTIVITIES
alcohol use: Possibly increased response to alcohol

Adverse Reactions

CNS: Agitation, ataxia, confusion, dizziness, drowsiness, exacerbation of psychosis, extrapyramidal reactions, fatigue, lack of coordination, paresthesia, peripheral neuropathy, suicidal ideation, tremor, weakness
CV: Arrhythmias, including heart block and tachycardia; hypertension; hypotension; MI; orthostatic hypotension; palpitations; stroke
EENT: Black tongue, blurred vision, dry mouth, increased intraocular pressure, lacrimation, stomatitis, tongue swelling
ENDO: Hyperglycemia, hypoglycemia
GI: Abdominal cramps, anorexia, constipation, diarrhea, epigastric discomfort, hepatic dysfunction, nausea, vomiting
GU: Impotence, libido changes, nocturia, urinary frequency and hesitancy, urine retention
SKIN: Diaphoresis, petechiae, photosensitivity, rash, urticaria
Other: Facial edema, weight gain or loss

Nursing Considerations

• Use protriptyline cautiously in patients with a history of seizures because drug can lower seizure threshold.
• Use cautiously in patients with a history of urine retention or increased intraocular pressure because of drug's autonomic activity.
• **WARNING** Avoid giving protriptyline with an MAO inhibitor. If patient is being switched from an MAO inhibitor to protriptyline, ensure that MAO inhibitor has been discontinued for 14 days before starting protriptyline.
• Watch patient closely (especially children, adolescents, and young adults) for suicidal tendencies, particularly when therapy starts or dosage changes, because depression may worsen temporarily during these times, possibly leading to suicidal ideation.
PATIENT TEACHING
• Inform patient that protriptyline therapy may take several weeks to reach full effect.
• Instruct patient to avoid hazardous activities until drug's CNS effects are known.
• Advise patient to change position slowly to minimize effects of orthostatic hypotension.
• Urge patient to avoid alcohol while taking drug.

•Suggest drinking water and using sugarless gum or hard candy to relieve dry mouth.
•Advise patient to avoid sunlight and tanning booths and to wear protective clothing, a hat, and sunscreen when outdoors.
•Instruct diabetic patient to check blood glucose level frequently during first few weeks of protriptyline therapy.
•Urge family or caregiver to watch patient for suicidal tendencies, especially when therapy starts or dosage changes and particularly if patient is a child, teenager, or young adult.

pyrazinamide

pms-Pyrazinamide (CAN), Tebrazid (CAN)

Class and Category
Chemical class: Pyrazine analogue of nicotinamide
Therapeutic class: Antitubercular
Pregnancy category: C

Indications and Dosages
➤ *As adjunct to treat tuberculosis, along with other antitubercular drugs*
TABLETS
Adults and children. 15 to 30 mg/kg daily; or, 50 to 70 mg/kg 2 or 3 times/wk. *Maximum:* For daily regimen, 2 g daily; for twice/wk regimen, 4 g daily; for 3-times/wk regimen, 3 g daily.
DOSAGE ADJUSTMENT For patients with HIV infection, 20 to 30 mg/kg daily for first 2 mo of therapy.

Contraindications
Acute gout, hypersensitivity to pyrazinamide or its components, severe hepatic damage

Interactions
DRUGS
allopurinol, colchicine, probenecid, sulfinpyrazone: Possibly increased blood uric acid level and decreased antigout efficacy
cyclosporine: Possibly decreased blood level and therapeutic effects of cyclosporine

Adverse Reactions
CNS: Fever
GI: Anorexia, hepatotoxicity, nausea, vomiting
GU: Dysuria
HEME: Porphyria
MS: Arthralgia, gout, myalgia
SKIN: Acne, photosensitivity, pruritus, rash, urticaria

Mechanism of Action
Inhibits growth of *Mycobacterium tuberculosis* by decreasing pH level; exhibits bactericidal or bacteriostatic action, depending on blood pyrazinamide level.

Nursing Considerations
•Review liver function test results before and every 2 to 4 weeks during therapy.
•Be aware that drug can affect the accuracy of certain urine ketone strip test results.
•Because drug is metabolized by liver, monitor for signs of hepatotoxicity, such as darkened urine, fever, jaundice, malaise, nausea, severe pain in feet or toes, and vomiting.
PATIENT TEACHING
•Explain the importance of complying with long-term pyrazinamide therapy.
•Tell diabetic patient about possible changes in ketone measurement during therapy.
•Instruct patient to report dark urine, fever, malaise, nausea, severe pain in feet or toes, vomiting, and yellowing of skin or eyes.
•Inform patient of need for regular blood tests and follow-up visits with prescriber.
•Urge patient to minimize exposure to sun and to wear protective clothing, hat, sunglasses, and sunscreen when outdoors.

pyridostigmine bromide

Mestinon, Mestinon-SR (CAN), Mestinon Timespans, Regonol (CAN)

Class and Category
Chemical class: Bromide dimethylcarbamate
Therapeutic class: Antimyasthenic
Pregnancy category: Not rated

Indications and Dosages
➤ *To treat symptoms of myasthenia gravis*
E.R. TABLETS
Adults and adolescents. 180 to 540 mg once or twice daily (at least 6 hr between doses).
SYRUP, TABLETS
Adults and adolescents. *Initial:* 30 to 60 mg every 3 to 4 hr, adjusted as needed. *Maintenance:* 60 mg to 1.5 g daily.
Children. 7 mg/kg daily in 5 or 6 divided doses.
I.V. OR I.M. INJECTION
Adults and adolescents. 2 mg every 2 to 3 hr.
I.M. INJECTION
Neonates of myasthenic mothers. 0.05 to

0.15 mg/kg every 4 to 6 hr.

➤ *To reverse the effects of neuromuscular blockers*

I.V. INJECTION

Adults and adolescents. 10 to 20 mg after 0.6 to 1.2 mg of I.V. atropine has been given.

DOSAGE ADJUSTMENT Dosage possibly reduced for patients with renal impairment.

Route	Onset	Peak	Duration
P.O.	30 to 45 min	1 to 2 hr	3 to 6 hr
P.O. (E.R.)	30 to 60 min	1 to 2 hr	6 to 12 hr
I.V.	2 to 5 min	Unknown	2 to 4 hr
I.M.	15 min	Unknown	2 to 4 hr

Mechanism of Action

Improves muscle strength compromised by myasthenia gravis or neuromuscular blockade by competing with acetylcholine for its binding site on acetylcholinesterase. This action potentiates the effects of acetylcholine on skeletal muscle and the GI tract. Inhibited destruction of acetylcholine allows freer transmission of nerve impulses across the neuromuscular junction.

Contraindications

Hypersensitivity to pyridostigmine or its components, mechanical obstruction of GI or urinary tract

Interactions

DRUGS

aminoglycosides (systemic), anesthetics (hydrocarbon inhalation), capreomycin, lidocaine (I.V.), lincomycins, polymyxins, quinine: Possibly antagonized effect of pyridostigmine on skeletal muscle; possibly decreased neuromuscular blocking activity of these drugs (with large doses of pyridostigmine)

anesthetics (local): Inhibited neuronal transmission, increased anesthesia effects

anticholinergics: Possibly masked pyridostigmine overdose; reduced intestinal motility

cholinesterase inhibitors: Increased risk of additive toxicity

edrophonium: Possibly worsening of status

guanadrel, guanethidine, mecamylamine, neuromuscular blockers, procainamide: Possibly prolonged phase I blocking effect or reversal of nondepolarization blockade

quinidine, trimethaphan: Possibly antagonized effects of pyridostigmine

Adverse Reactions

EENT: Increased salivation, lacrimation, miosis

GI: Abdominal cramps, diarrhea, increased peristalsis, nausea, vomiting

GU: Urinary frequency, incontinence, or urgency

MS: Fasciculations, muscle spasms or weakness

RESP: Increased tracheobronchial secretions

SKIN: Diaphoresis

Nursing Considerations

• Use pyridostigmine cautiously in patients with renal disease because drug is mainly excreted unchanged by kidneys. Monitor BUN and serum creatinine levels.

• **WARNING** Maintain a rigid dosing schedule because a missed or late dose can precipitate myasthenic crisis.

• Observe for cholinergic reactions when administering drug I.V. or I.M.

• **WARNING** Pyridostigmine overdose may obscure diagnosis of myasthenic crisis because main symptom in both is muscle weakness. Treat cholinergic crisis by stopping anticholinesterase, giving atropine as prescribed, and helping with endotracheal intubation and mechanical ventilation, if needed.

• Be aware that reversal of neuromuscular blockade usually occurs in 15 to 30 minutes. Be prepared to maintain patent airway and ventilation until normal voluntary respiration returns completely. Assess respiratory measurements and muscle tone with peripheral nerve stimulator device, as indicated.

PATIENT TEACHING

• Instruct patient to take pyridostigmine as directed and on schedule. Explain that a late or missed dose can precipitate a crisis. Suggest the use of a battery-operated alarm clock as a reminder.

• Tell patient to take drug with a full glass of water or with food or milk if GI distress occurs.

• Warn patient not to crush or chew E.R. tablets.

• Ask patient to record pyridostigmine dosage, times taken, and drug effects to help determine optimal dosage and schedule.

• Urge patient to carry medical identification describing her condition and drug regimen.

➤ ◄

Q·R·S

quazepam

Doral

Class, Category, and Schedule

Chemical class: Benzodiazepine
Therapeutic class: Sedative-hypnotic
Pregnancy category: X
Controlled substance schedule: IV

Indications and Dosages

➤ *To treat insomnia*

TABLETS

Adults. 15 mg at bedtime.

DOSAGE ADJUSTMENT In elderly and debilitated patients, dosage may be reduced to 7.5 mg at bedtime after 1 or 2 nights of therapy.

Mechanism of Action

May antagonize mu receptors at limbic, thalamic, and hypothalamic regions of the brain, blocking release of such inhibitory neurotransmitters as gamma-aminobutyric acid (GABA) and acetylcholine. Central receptors interact with GABA receptors, allowing for greater influx of chloride into the neuron, thereby suppressing neuronal excitability. GABA effects may inhibit spinal afferent pathways and block the cortical and limbic arousal that normally occurs when reticular pathways are stimulated. These effects result in various levels of CNS depression, including sleep.

Contraindications

Hypersensitivity to quazepam or its components, pregnancy, sleep apnea (known or suspected)

Interactions

DRUGS

addictive drugs: Possibly habituation
carbamazepine: Decreased blood quazepam level, possibly increased blood carbamazepine level
cimetidine, diltiazem, disulfiram, erythromycin, fluoxetine, fluvoxamine, isoniazid, itraconazole, ketoconazole, nefazodone, oral contraceptives, propoxyphene, ranitidine, verapamil: Possibly potentiated effects of quazepam
clozapine: Possibly syncope, with respiratory depression or arrest
CNS depressants, tricyclic antidepressants: Increased CNS depression
digoxin: Possibly increased blood digoxin level and risk of digitalis toxicity
levodopa: Possibly decreased therapeutic effects of levodopa
phenytoin: Increased risk of phenytoin toxicity
theophyllines: Possibly antagonized effects of quazepam
zidovudine: Increased risk of zidovudine toxicity

FOODS

grapefruit juice: Increased blood quazepam level

ACTIVITIES

alcohol use: Additive CNS depression
smoking: Possibly decreased effectiveness of quazepam

Adverse Reactions

CNS: Abnormal complex behaviors, such as sleep driving; amnesia (anterograde); anxiety; ataxia; confusion; depression; dizziness; drowsiness; euphoria; fatigue; headache; light-headedness; paresthesia; slurred speech; suicidal ideation; tremor; weakness
CV: Chest pain, palpitations, tachycardia
EENT: Blurred vision, dry mouth, hyperacusis, photophobia, throat tightness, worsening of glaucoma
GI: Abdominal cramps, constipation, diarrhea, heartburn, nausea, thirst, vomiting
GU: Renal dysfunction, urinary incontinence, urine retention
MS: Muscle spasms
RESP: Dyspnea, increased tracheobronchial secretions
Other: Anaphylaxis, angioedema

Nursing Considerations

•Use quazepam cautiously in patients with angle-closure glaucoma because of drug's anticholinergic effects; in patients with hepatic dysfunction because this condition may prolong quazepam's half-life; in patients with myasthenia gravis because drug may worsen condition; in patients with severe COPD because adverse effects of quazepam may compromise respiratory function; in patients with renal dysfunction because accumulation of metabolites may result in toxicity; and in elderly patients because of age-related decreases in hepatic, renal, and cardiac function.

•**WARNING** Monitor patient closely for signs and symptoms of hypersensitivity reactions, such as dyspnea, throat tightness, nausea, vomiting, and swelling. If present, discontinue quazepam immediately, notify prescriber, and provide supportive care.

•**WARNING** Notify prescriber if eye pain develops in patient with angle-closure glaucoma.

•**WARNING** Be aware that quazepam may intensify signs and symptoms of depression. Monitor patient closely for evidence of suicidal ideation, and institute suicide precautions, as needed.

PATIENT TEACHING

•Instruct patient to stop taking quazepam and seek emergency care if she has trouble breathing, throat tightness, nausea, vomiting, or abnormal swelling.

•Advise patient that drug may cause abnormal behaviors during sleep, such as driving a car, eating, talking on the phone, or having sex without any recall of the event. If family members notice any such behavior, or if patient sees evidence of such behavior upon awakening, prescriber should be notified.

•Urge patient to avoid consuming alcohol during quazepam therapy because sedation and risk of abnormal behaviors, such as sleep driving, may increase.

•Instruct patient not to discontinue drug abruptly after prolonged use (6 weeks or more).

•Instruct female patient of childbearing age to use effective contraception during therapy and to notify prescriber immediately of known or suspected pregnancy.

•Urge family or caregiver to watch patient closely for suicidal tendencies, especially when therapy starts or dosage changes.

quetiapine fumarate

Seroquel, Seroquel XR

Class and Category

Chemical class: Dibenzothiazepine derivative
Therapeutic class: Antipsychotic
Pregnancy category: C

Indications and Dosages

➤ *To treat schizophrenia*

TABLETS

Adults. *Initial:* 25 mg b.i.d. on day 1. Increased by 25 to 50 b.i.d. or t.i.d. on days 2 and 3. *Usual:* 300 to 400 mg daily by day 4, in divided doses b.i.d. or t.i.d. Increased every 2 days in increments of 25 to 50 mg b.i.d., as needed. *Maximum:* 800 mg daily.

E.R. TABLETS

Adults. *Initial:* 300 mg once daily in evening. Dosage increased daily in increments up to 300 mg, as needed. *Maximum:* 800 mg daily.

➤ *To manage psychotic disorders other than schizophrenia*

TABLETS

Adults. *Initial:* 25 mg b.i.d. on day 1. Dosage increased by 25 to 50 mg b.i.d. or t.i.d. on days 2 and 3. *Usual:* 300 to 400 mg daily by day 4, in divided doses b.i.d. or t.i.d. Dosage increased every 2 days in increments of 25 to 50 mg b.i.d., as needed. *Maximum:* 800 mg daily.

➤ *To treat depressive episodes in bipolar disorder*

TABLETS

Adults. *Initial:* On day one, 50 mg once at bedtime; day two, 100 mg once at bedtime; day three, 200 mg once at bedtime; day four, 300 mg once at bedtime. *Maintenance:* 300 mg once daily at bedtime.

E.R. TABLETS

Adults. *Initial:* 50 mg once daily in evening on day 1, followed by 100 mg once daily in evening on day 2, 200 mg once daily in evening on day 3, and 300 mg once daily in evening on day 4 and thereafter.

➤ *To treat acute manic episodes in bipolar I disorder*

TABLETS

Adults. 50 mg b.i.d., increased to 200 mg b.i.d on day 4 (in increments no greater than 100 mg daily) and then further increased to 400 mg b.i.d. on day 6 (in increments no greater than 200 mg daily), as needed.

➤ *To treat acute manic episodes in bipolar I disorder as monotherapy; as adjunct with lithium or divalproex to treat acute manic episodes in bipolar I disorder*

E.R. TABLETS

Adults. *Initial:* 300 mg once daily in evening on day 1, followed by 600 mg once daily in evening on day 2 and 200 to 400 mg b.i.d. on day 3 and thereafter. *Maintenance:* 200 to 400 mg b.i.d.

DOSAGE ADJUSTMENT For elderly patients and patients with hepatic impairment, initial dosage no higher than 50 mg once daily and increased in increments of 50 mg/day depending on response and tolerance.

Mechanism of Action
May produce antipsychotic effects by interfering with dopamine binding to dopamine type 2 (D_2)-receptor sites in the brain and by antagonizing serotonin 5-HT$_2$, dopamine type 1 (D_1), histamine H$_1$, and adrenergic alpha$_1$ and alpha$_2$ receptors.

Contraindications
Hypersensitivity to quetiapine or its components

Interactions
DRUGS
antihypertensives: Possibly enhanced antihypertensive effects of these drugs
cimetidine, erythromycin, fluconazole, itraconazole, ketoconazole: Decreased clearance and possibly increased effects of quetiapine
CNS depressants: Possibly increased CNS depression
lorazepam: Possibly increased effects of lorazepam
phenytoin, thioridazine: Increased clearance and possibly decreased effectiveness of quetiapine
ACTIVITIES
alcohol use: Possibly enhanced CNS depression

Adverse Reactions
CNS: Depression, dizziness, drowsiness, dystonia, extrapyramidal reactions, hypertonia, lethargy, restless leg syndrome, somnolence, suicidal ideation, tardive dyskinesia
CV: Cardiomyopathy, hypercholesterolemia, myocarditis, orthostatic hypotension, palpitations
EENT: Dry mouth, nasal congestion, pharyngitis, rhinitis
ENDO: Hyperglycemia, syndrome of inappropriate antidiuretic hormone secretion
GI: Anorexia, constipation, indigestion
HEME: Agranulocytosis, leukopenia, neutropenia
MS: Dysarthria, muscle weakness, rhabdomyolysis

RESP: Cough, dyspnea
SKIN: Diaphoresis, Stevens-Johnson syndrome
Other: Anaphylaxis, flulike symptoms, weight gain

Nursing Considerations
•**WARNING** Quetiapine shouldn't be used to treat elderly patients with dementia-related psychosis because drug increases the risk of death in these patients.
•Monitor patients (particularly children, adolescents, and young adults) closely for suicidal tendencies, especially when therapy starts or dosage changes, because depression may worsen temporarily during these times.
•**WARNING** Monitor patient taking quetiapine for predisposing factors for neuroleptic malignant syndrome, such as heat stress, physical exhaustion, dehydration, and organic brain disease. Neuroleptic malignant syndrome includes hyperpyrexia, muscle rigidity, altered mental status, and autonomic instability (which may include irregular pulse or blood pressure, tachycardia, diaphoresis, and arrhythmias).
•Monitor patient for signs of tardive dyskinesia, a potentially irreversible complication characterized by involuntary, dyskinetic movements of tongue, mouth, jaw, eyelids, or face. Notify prescriber if such signs develop because quetiapine therapy may need to be stopped.
•Monitor patient for orthostatic hypotension, especially during initial dosage titration period. Be prepared to correct underlying conditions, such as hypovolemia and dehydration, before starting quetiapine therapy, as prescribed.
•Monitor patient for prolonged abnormal muscle contractions, especially during the first few days of quetiapine therapy, in male patients, and in younger patients.
•Assess patient for hypothyroidism because drug can cause dose-dependent decreases in total and free thyroxine (T$_4$) levels.
•Monitor laboratory results during first 3 weeks of therapy for transient elevations in hepatic enzyme levels. Notify prescriber if they persist or worsen.
•Monitor patient's blood glucose and lipid levels routinely, as ordered, because drug increases the risk of hyperglycemia and hypercholesterolemia.

Q
R
S

• Check CBC often during the first few months of therapy, as ordered, in patients with a low white blood cell count or a history of drug-induced hematologic problems. If counts drop or patient develops a fever or other signs of infection, notify prescriber and expect to discontinue drug and provide supportive care.

PATIENT TEACHING
• Instruct patient to take quetiapine with food to reduce stomach upset.
• Advise patient not to stop taking quetiapine suddenly because doing so may exacerbate his symptoms.
• Inform patient that quetiapine therapy may cause dizziness or drowsiness. Advise him not to drive or perform other activities that require alertness until drug's full CNS effects are known.
• Instruct patient to rise slowly from a seated or lying position to reduce the risk of dizziness or fainting.
• Caution patient to avoid consuming alcoholic beverages because they can increase dizziness and drowsiness.
• Urge family or caregiver to watch patient closely for suicidal tendencies, especially when therapy starts or dosage changes and particularly if patient is a child, teenager, or young adult.
• Encourage patient on long-term therapy to have regular eye examinations so that cataracts can be detected.

quinapril hydrochloride

Accupril

Class and Catgeory

Chemical class: Ethylester of quinaprilat
Therapeutic class: Antihypertensive
Pregnancy category: C (first trimester), D (later trimesters)

Indications and Dosages

➤ *To treat hypertension*

TABLETS
Adults. *Initial:* 10 or 20 mg daily, adjusted every 2 wk based on clinical response. *Maintenance:* 20 to 80 mg daily or in divided doses b.i.d.
DOSAGE ADJUSTMENT Initial dosage reduced to 5 mg daily for patients who are dehydrated from previous diuretic therapy, those who are still receiving diuretic therapy, and those with creatinine clearance of 30 to 60 ml/min/1.73 m². Dosage reduced to 2.5 mg daily for patients with creatinine clearance of 10 to 30 ml/min/1.73 m².

Route	Onset	Peak	Duration
P.O.	In 1 hr	2 to 4 hr	Up to 24 hr

Mechanism of Action
Blocks conversion of angiotensin I to angiotensin II, leading to vasodilation, and reduces aldosterone secretion, which prevents water retention. Quinapril also reduces peripheral arterial resistance. These combined actions lead to a reduction in blood pressure.

Contraindications
History of angioedema related to previous treatment with ACE inhibitor, hypersensitivity to quinapril or its components

Interactions
DRUGS
allopurinol, bone marrow depressants, corticosteroids (systemic), procainamide: Increased risk of fatal neutropenia or agranulocytosis
CNS depressants, other hypotension-producing drugs: Additive hypotensive effects
cyclosporine, potassium preparations, potassium-sparing diuretics: Possibly hyperkalemia
lithium: Possibly increased blood lithium level and risk of toxicity
NSAIDs, sympathomimetics: Decreased antihypertensive effect of quinapril
tetracyclines: Reduced tetracycline absorption
FOODS
low-salt milk, salt substitutes: Increased risk of hyperkalemia
ACTIVITIES
alcohol use: Additive hypotensive effects

Adverse Reactions
CNS: Depression, dizziness, drowsiness, fatigue, fever, headache, insomnia, lightheadedness, malaise, paresthesia, sleep disturbance, syncope, vertigo
CV: Chest pain, hypotension, orthostatic hypotension, palpitations, tachycardia
EENT: Amblyopia, dry mouth, loss of taste,

pharyngitis
GI: Abdominal pain, constipation, diarrhea, indigestion, nausea, vomiting
GU: Impotence
MS: Arthralgia, back pain, myalgia
RESP: Cough, dyspnea
SKIN: Alopecia, diaphoresis, flushing, photosensitivity, pruritus, rash, urticaria
Other: Anaphylaxis, angioedema

Nursing Considerations

• Use quinapril cautiously in patients with renal impairment.
• **WARNING** Patients with heart failure, hyponatremia, or severe volume or salt depletion; those who've recently received intensive diuresis or an increase in diuretic dosage; and those undergoing dialysis may be at risk for excessive hypotension. Monitor blood pressure often for first 2 weeks of therapy and whenever quinapril or diuretic dosage increases. If excessive hypotension occurs, notify prescriber immediately, place patient in a supine position, and, if prescribed, infuse normal saline solution.
• **WARNING** Because of the risk of angioedema, be prepared to discontinue drug and administer emergency measures, including subcutaneous epinephrine 1:1,000 (0.3 to 0.5 ml), if swelling of tongue, glottis, or larynx causes airway obstruction.
• Monitor blood pressure often to assess drug's effectiveness.

PATIENT TEACHING
• Instruct patient to notify prescriber immediately and stop taking quinapril if he has swelling of the face, eyes, lips, or tongue or difficulty breathing.
• Explain that drug may cause dizziness and light-headedness, especially for first few days of therapy. Advise patient to avoid hazardous activities until drug's CNS effects are known and to notify prescriber if he faints.
• Inform woman of childbearing age of risks of taking quinapril during pregnancy, especially during the second and third trimesters. Caution her to use effective contraception and to notify prescriber immediately of known or suspected pregnancy.
• Advise patient having surgery or anesthesia to tell specialist that he takes quinapril.
• Instruct patient to consult prescriber before using potassium supplements or salt substitutes that contain potassium.

quinidine gluconate
Quinaglute Dura-tabs, Quinate (CAN), Quin-Release

quinidine polygalacturonate
Cardioquin

quinidine sulfate
Apo-Quinidine (CAN), Novoquinidin (CAN), Quinidex Extentabs

Class and Category
Chemical class: Dextrorotatory isomer of quinine
Therapeutic class: Class IA antiarrhythmic
Pregnancy category: C

Indications and Dosages
➤ *To prevent or treat cardiac arrhythmias, including established atrial fibrillation, atrial flutter, paroxysmal atrial fibrillation, paroxysmal atrial tachycardia, paroxysmal atrioventricular junctional rhythm, paroxysmal ventricular tachycardia not associated with complete heart block, and premature atrial and ventricular contractions*

E.R. TABLETS (QUINIDINE GLUCONATE)
Adults. 324 to 660 mg every 8 to 12 hr. *Maximum:* 1,944 mg daily.

E.R. TABLETS (QUINIDINE SULFATE)
Adults. 300 to 600 mg every 8 to 12 hr.

TABLETS (QUINIDINE GLUCONATE)
Adults. *Initial:* 325 mg every 2 to 3 hr for 5 to 8 doses, gradually increasing dosage as needed and prescribed. *Maintenance:* 325 to 488 mg t.i.d. or q.i.d.

TABLETS (QUINIDINE POLYGALACTURONATE)
Adults. *Initial:* 275 to 825 mg every 3 to 4 hr for 3 or 4 doses, then increased by 137.5 to 275 mg every 3rd or 4th dose until rhythm is restored or toxic effects occur. *Maintenance:* 275 mg b.i.d. or t.i.d.

TABLETS (QUINIDINE SULFATE)
Adults. *Initial:* For premature atrial and ventricular contractions, 200 to 300 mg t.i.d. or q.i.d.; for paroxysmal supraventricular tachycardia, 400 to 600 mg every 2 to 3 hr until terminated; for atrial flutter, individual titration after digitalization; for conversion of atrial fibrillation, 200 mg every 2 to 3 hr for 5 to 8 doses, followed by subsequent

Q
R
S

daily increases, as needed. *Maintenance:* 200 to 400 mg t.i.d. or q.i.d.
Children. 6 mg/kg 5 times daily.
I.V. INFUSION (QUINIDINE GLUCONATE)
Adults. 800 mg in 40 ml of D_5W at up to 0.25 mg/kg/min.
I.M. INJECTION (QUINIDINE SULFATE)
Adults. 190 to 380 mg every 2 to 4 hr. *Maximum:* 3 g daily.

Route	Onset	Peak	Duration
P.O.	Unknown	Unknown	6 to 8 hr
P.O. (E.R.)	Unknown	Unknown	12 hr

Mechanism of Action
Depresses excitability, conduction velocity, and contractility of the myocardium and increases the effective refractory period, thus suppressing arrhythmic activity in the atria, ventricles, and His-Purkinje system.

Contraindications
Digitalis toxicity; history of quinidine-induced thrombocytopenic purpura or torsades de pointes; hypersensitivity to quinidine, other cinchona derivatives, or their components; long-QT syndrome; myasthenia gravis; pacemaker-dependent conduction disturbances

Interactions
DRUGS
antiarrhythmics, phenothiazines, rauwolfia alkaloids: Additive cardiac effects
anticholinergics: Possibly intensified atropine-like adverse effects
antimyasthenics: Antagonized antimyasthenic effects on skeletal muscle
barbiturates, rifampin: Possibly accelerated elimination and decreased effectiveness of quinidine
cimetidine: Increased elimination half-life, possibly leading to quinidine toxicity
digoxin: Possibly digitalis toxicity
hepatic enzyme inducers: Possibly decreased blood quinidine level
neuromuscular blockers: Possibly potentiated neuromuscular blockade
oral anticoagulants: Additive hypoprothrombinemia, increased risk of bleeding
pimozide: Risk of arrhythmias

quinine: Increased risk of quinidine toxicity
urinary alkalizers (such as antacids, carbonic anhydrase inhibitors, citrates, sodium bicarbonate, thiazide diuretics): Increased renal tubular reabsorption of quinidine, possibly leading to quinidine toxicity
verapamil: Possibly AV block, bradycardia, pulmonary edema, significant hypotension, and ventricular tachycardia

Adverse Reactions
CNS: Anxiety, asthenia, ataxia, confusion, delirium, difficulty speaking, dizziness, drowsiness, extrapyramidal reactions, fever, headache, hypertonia, syncope, vertigo
CV: Complete heart block, orthostatic hypotension, palpitations, peripheral edema, prolonged QT interval, torsades de pointes, vasculitis, ventricular arrhythmias, widening QRS complex
EENT: Blurred vision, change in color perception, diplopia, dry mouth, hearing loss (high-frequency), pharyngitis, photophobia, rhinitis, tinnitus
GI: Abdominal pain, anorexia, constipation, diarrhea, indigestion, nausea, vomiting
HEME: Agranulocytosis, hemolytic anemia, leukopenia, neutropenia, thrombocytopenia, thrombocytopenic purpura
MS: Arthralgia, myalgia
RESP: Dyspnea
SKIN: Diaphoresis, eczema, exfoliative dermatitis, flushing, hyperpigmentation, photosensitivity, pruritus, psoriasis, purpura, rash, urticaria
Other: Angioedema, flulike symptoms, weight gain

Nursing Considerations
• Give I.M. form of quinidine undiluted.
• For intermittent I.V. infusion, dilute drug in 40 ml of D_5W and administer using an infusion pump at a rate of 0.25 mg/kg/min or less. Rapid administration may cause hypotension. Monitor ECG tracings and blood pressure throughout administration.
• Monitor therapeutic blood level of quinidine, as ordered.
• Monitor heart rate and rhythm closely because quinidine may cause serious adverse reactions and can be cardiotoxic, especially at dosages exceeding 2.4 g daily. Implement continuous cardiac monitoring, as ordered.
• Assess for early signs and symptoms of cinchonism, including blurred vision, change in

color perception, confusion, diplopia, headache, and tinnitus, which may indicate quinidine toxicity.

PATIENT TEACHING
• Advise patient to take quinidine at the same times every day and at evenly spaced intervals.
• Instruct patient to swallow E.R. tablets whole, with a full glass of water, preferably while sitting upright.
• Advise patient to take drug with food if GI upset occurs.
• Urge patient to inform prescriber immediately of blurred or double vision, change in color perception, confusion, diarrhea, fever, headache, loss of hearing, or tinnitus.

quinine sulfate

Class and Category
Chemical class: Cinchona alkaloid
Therapeutic class: Antimalarial
Pregnancy category: X

Indications and Dosages
➤ *As adjunct to treat chloroquine-resistant malaria caused by* Plasmodium falciparum

CAPSULES, TABLETS
Adults. 600 to 650 mg every 8 hr for at least 3 days with one of the following: 250 mg of tetracycline every 6 hr for 7 days; 1.5 g of sulfadoxine and 75 mg of pyrimethamine combined as a single dose; 900 mg of clindamycin every 8 hr for 3 days; or 100 mg of doxycycline every 12 hr for 7 days.
Children over age 8. 8.3 mg/kg every 8 hr for at least 3 days with one of the following: 5 mg/kg of tetracycline every 6 hr for 7 days; 6.7 to 13.3 mg/kg of clindamycin every 8 hr for 3 days; or 1.25 mg/kg of pyrimethamine and 25 mg/kg of sulfadoxine combined as a single dose.

Mechanism of Action
May disrupt function in malarial parasite by elevating intracellular pH in parasitic acid vesicles.

Contraindications
G6PD deficiency, history of quinine-induced blackwater fever or thrombocytopenic purpura, hypersensitivity to quinine or its components, optic neuritis, pregnancy, tinnitus

Interactions
DRUGS
acetazolamide, sodium bicarbonate: Increased risk of quinine toxicity
aluminum-containing antacids: Possibly delayed or decreased quinine absorption
antimyasthenics: Possibly antagonized antimyasthenic effect on skeletal muscle
astemizole, cisapride, halofantrine, mefloquine, pimozide, quinidine, terfenadine: Increased risk of prolonged QT interval
atorvastatin: Increased blood atorvastatin level; increased risk of myopathy or rhabdomyolysis
carbamazepine, phenobarbital, phenytoin: Possibly increased blood level of these drugs; possibly decreased blood quinine level
cimetidine: Possibly reduced quinine clearance
debrisoquine, desipramine, dextromethorphan, flecainide, metoprolol, paroxetine: Possibly increased bood levels of these drugs; increased risk of adverse reactions
digoxin: Increased blood digoxin level
erythromycin, ketoconazole, troleandomycin: Possibly increased blood quinine level
hemolytics, neurotoxic drugs, ototoxic drugs: Increased risk of toxicity of these drugs
hepatic enzyme inducers, rifampin: Possibly decreased blood quinine level
mefloquine: Increased risk of seizures
neuromuscular blockers: Potentiated neuromuscular blockade
oral anticoagulants: Possibly increased anticoagulant effects and risk of bleeding

Adverse Reactions
CNS: Headache
EENT: Blurred vision, hearing loss, tinnitus, vision changes
ENDO: Hypoglycemia
GI: Abdominal or epigastric pain, diarrhea, nausea, vomiting
HEME: Thrombocytopenia

Nursing Considerations
• Be aware that quinine shouldn't be used in patients with blackwater fever, which can follow chronic malaria, because they're at increased risk for anemia and hemolysis with renal failure.

Q
R
S

•Be aware that quinine shouldn't be given I.M. Doing so may cause bleeding, bruising, or hematomas because of quinine's effect on platelets.

•Monitor patient with type 2 diabetes mellitus for alterations in blood glucose level because quinine stimulates release of insulin and may promote hypoglycemia.

•Be aware that quinine can exacerbate optic neuritis or tinnitus. It may also exacerbate muscle weakness and cause dysphagia and respiratory distress in myasthenic patients.

•Assess for early signs and symptoms of cinchonism, including blurred vision, confusion, diplopia, fever, headache, loss of hearing, and tinnitus, which may indicate quinine toxicity.

PATIENT TEACHING

•Instruct patient not to crush or chew quinine tablets; they taste bitter and can irritate the mouth and throat.

•Advise patient to take drug with food or after meals to minimize GI irritation.

•Urge patient to notify prescriber immediately if he experiences blurred or double vision, confusion, fever, headache, loss of hearing, or tinnitus, which are indicators of quinine toxicity.

•Advise patient to avoid potentially hazardous activities until he knows how quinine will affect his vision.

rabeprazole sodium

AcipHex

Class and Category

Chemical class: Substituted benzimidazole
Therapeutic class: Antiulcer
Pregnancy category: B

Indications and Dosages

➤ *To provide short-term treatment of erosive esophagitis or ulcerative gastroesophageal reflux disease (GERD)*

DELAYED-RELEASE TABLETS

Adults. For mild to moderate disease, 20 mg daily for 4 to 8 wk; course may be repeated if healing has not occurred at the end of 8 wk. For severe reflux with ulceration or stricture formation, 40 mg daily for 4 to 8 wk.

➤ *To treat symptomatic GERD*

DELAYED-RELEASE TABLETS

Adults and adolescents age 12 and over. 20 mg daily for 4 wk. Course may be repeated if symptoms aren't completely resolved.

➤ *To provide maintenance treatment of erosive esophagitis or GERD*

DELAYED-RELEASE TABLETS

Adults. 20 mg daily.

➤ *To promote healing of duodenal ulcer, as adjunct to treat* Helicobacter pylori–*positive duodenal ulcer*

DELAYED-RELEASE TABLETS

Adults. 20 mg daily after breakfast for up to 4 wk for ulcer healing and 2 wk when used with antibiotic therapy for *H. pylori.*

➤ *As adjunct to reduce the risk of duodenal ulcer recurrence by eradicating* H. pylori

DELAYED-RELEASE TABLETS

Adults. 20 mg b.i.d with morning and evening meals in conjunction with amoxicillin 1000 mg b.i.d for 7 days and clarithromycin 500 mg b.i.d. for 7 days.

➤ *To treat hypersecretory conditions, such as Zollinger-Ellison syndrome*

DELAYED-RELEASE TABLETS

Adults. *Initial:* 60 mg daily; may be increased, if needed, to 100 mg daily or 60 mg b.i.d.

DOSAGE ADJUSTMENT Dosage reduction may be needed in severe hepatic dysfunction.

Mechanism of Action

Decreases gastric acid secretion by suppressing its release at the secretory surface of gastric parietal cells. Rabeprazole also increases gastric pH and decreases basal acid output, which helps to heal ulcerated areas. In gastric parietal cells, it's transformed to an active sulfonamide, which increases the clearance rate of *Helicobacter pylori.*

Contraindications

Hypersensitivity to rabeprazole, other substituted benzimidazoles (omeprazole, lansoprazole), or their components

Interactions

DRUGS

cyclosporine: Possibly inhibited cyclosporine metabolism

digoxin: Increased risk of digitalis toxicity
warfarin: Possibly increased PT, INR

Adverse Reactions

CNS: Coma, delirium, disorientation, dizziness, headache, malaise
GI: Abdominal pain, diarrhea, jaundice, nausea, vomiting
GU: Interstitial nephritis
HEME: Agranulocytosis, hemolytic anemia, leukopenia, pancytopenia, thrombocytopenia
MS: Rhabdomyolysis
RESP: Interstitial pneumonia
SKIN: Erythema multiforme, rash, Stevens-Johnson syndrome, toxic epidermal necrolysis
Other: Anaphylaxis, angioedema, hyperammonemia

Nursing Considerations

•Use rabeprazole cautiously in patients with hepatic dysfunction.
•Monitor serum gastrin level during long-term therapy, as ordered, to detect elevation.
•Closely monitor Japanese men receiving rabeprazole therapy for adverse reactions because they're more likely than other patients to have increased blood drug levels.

PATIENT TEACHING
•Instruct patient to swallow delayed-release rabeprazole tablets whole.
•Inform patients with hypersecretory conditions, such as Zollinger-Ellison syndrome, that treatment can last as long as 1 year.

raloxifene hydrochloride
(keoxifene hydrochloride)

Evista

Class and Category

Chemical: Benzothiophene derivative
Therapeutic: Osteoporosis prophylactic
Pregnancy category: X

Indications and Dosages

➤ *To prevent osteoporosis in postmenopausal women; to reduce risk of invasive breast cancer in postmenopausal women with osteoporosis; to reduce risk of invasive breast cancer in postmenopausal women at high risk*

TABLETS
Adults. 60 mg daily.

Mechanism of Action

Prevents osteoporosis by binding to estrogen receptors, which decreases bone resorption and increases bone mineral density in postmenopausal women.

Contraindications

History of thromboembolic disease, hypersensitivity to raloxifene or its components, pregnancy

Interactions

DRUGS
ampicillin, cholestyramine: Decreased raloxifene absorption
warfarin: Possibly decreased PT

Adverse Reactions

CNS: Depression, fever, insomnia, migraine, stroke
CV: Chest pain, hot flashes, peripheral edema, thromboembolism, thrombophlebitis
EENT: Laryngitis, pharyngitis, sinusitis
ENDO: Hot flashes
GI: Abdominal pain, cholelithiasis, flatulence, indigestion, nausea, vomiting
GU: Cystitis, infertility, leukorrhea, UTI, vaginitis
MS: Arthralgia, arthritis, leg cramps or spasms, myalgia
RESP: Cough, pneumonia, pulmonary embolism
SKIN: Diaphoresis, rash
Other: Flulike symptoms, weight gain

Nursing Considerations

•Use cautiously in patients who smoke or have a history of stroke, TIA, atrial fibrillation, or hypertension because raloxifene may increase the risk of stroke.
•Use cautiously in patients with renal impairment because effects of raloxifene on renal system are unknown.
•**WARNING** Monitor patient's limbs for impaired circulation and pain (possible thromboembolism).
•Expect prescriber to stop drug at least 72 hours before and during periods of prolonged immobilization. Resume raloxifene therapy as prescribed after patient is fully ambulatory.

PATIENT TEACHING
•Advise patient to avoid lengthy immobility

during travel while taking raloxifene because of the increased risk of thromboembolism.

•Instruct patient to report adverse reactions to prescriber immediately, especially leg pain or swelling, sudden chest pain, shortness of breath, coughing up blood, or a sudden change in vision.

•Stress the importance of compliance with long-term raloxifene therapy.

•Advise patient that postmenopausal women require an average of 1,500 mg of elemental calcium and 400 to 800 international units of vitamin D daily. Vitamin D requirement is increased in women over age 70, women with GI malabsorption syndromes, and women who are chronically ill or nursing home bound. Review dietary sources of calcium and vitamin D, and have patient discuss supplements with prescriber, as needed.

ramelteon

Rozerem

Class and Category

Chemical class: Melatonin receptor agonist
Therapeutic class: Hypnotic
Pregnancy category: C

Indications and Dosages

➤ *To treat insomnia in patients having difficulty falling asleep*

TABLETS

Adults. 8 mg 30 min before at bedtime.

Route	Onset	Peak	Duration
P.O.	Unknown	0.5 to 1.5 hr	Unknown

Mechanism of Action

Binds to melatonin receptors MT1 and MT2 in the suprachiasmatic nucleus (SCN) of the hypothalamus. The SCN regulates the sleep-wake cycle, and endogenous melatonin probably is involved in maintaining the circadian rhythm underlying that cycle.

Contraindications

Concurrent therapy with fluvoxamine, history of angioedema with previous ramelteon treatment, hypersensitivity to ramelteon or its components, severe hepatic dysfunction

Interactions

DRUGS

benzodiazepines, melatonin, other sedative-hypnotics: Possible additive sedative effects
fluconazole, fluvoxamine, ketoconazole: Increased plasma ramelteon levels
rifampin: Decreased ramelteon effectiveness

ACTIVITIES

alcohol use: Possibly additive CNS effect

Adverse Reactions

CNS: Agitation, amnesia, anxiety, bizarre behavior, complex behaviors such as sleep driving, depression, dizziness, fatigue, hallucinations, headache, insomnia exacerbation, mania, somnolence, suicidal ideation
EENT: Throat tightness
ENDO: Decreased testosterone level, increased prolactin level
GI: Diarrhea, dysgeusia, nausea, vomiting
MS: Arthralgia, myalgia
RESP: Dyspnea, upper respiratory tract infection
Other: Anaphylaxis, angioedema

Nursing Considerations

•Be aware that ramelteon therapy is not recommended for patients with severe sleep apnea or COPD because its effects have not been studied in these patient populations.

•Use cautiously in patients with mild to moderate hepatic dysfunction. Drug is contraindicated in severe hepatic dysfunction.

•Ramelteon is the first approved hypnotic not classified as a controlled substance.

•**WARNING** Monitor patient closely for hypersensitivity reactions such as dyspnea, throat tightness, nausea, vomiting, and swelling. If present, discontinue ramelteon immediately, notify prescriber, and provide supportive care.

•Watch patient closely for suicidal tendencies, particularly when therapy starts and dosage changes, because depression may worsen temporarily during these times, possibly leading to suicidal ideation.

PATIENT TEACHING

•Instruct patient not to take ramelteon with or immediately after a high-fat meal.

•Caution patient to avoid potentially hazardous activities after taking ramelteon; drug's intended effect is to decrease alertness.

•Advise patient that drug may cause abnormal behaviors during sleep, such as driving a

car, eating, talking on the phone, or having sex without any recall of the event. If family members notice any such behavior or patient sees evidence of such behavior upon awakening, prescriber should be notified.
•Advise limiting alcohol during therapy.
•Tell patient to notify prescriber if insomnia worsens or new signs or symptoms occur.
•Inform patient that drug may affect reproductive hormones; urge patient to report cessation of menses or galactorrhea (females) or decreased libido or problems with infertility.
•Urge family or caregiver to watch patient closely for suicidal tendencies, especially when therapy starts or dosage changes.

ramipril

Altace

Class and Category
Chemical class: Ethylester of ramiprilat
Therapeutic class: Antihypertensive
Pregnancy category: C (first trimester), D (later trimesters)

Indications and Dosages
➤ *To treat heart failure after MI*
CAPSULES
Adults. *Initial:* 1.25 to 2.5 mg b.i.d. *Maintenance:* 5 mg b.i.d.
➤ *To treat hypertension*
CAPSULES
Adults. *Initial:* 2.5 mg daily. *Maintenance:* 2.5 to 20 mg once daily or in divided doses b.i.d.
DOSAGE ADJUSTMENT Initial dosage reduced to 1.25 mg daily for patients dehydrated from diuretics, those receiving diuretics, and those with creatinine clearance less than 40 ml/min/1.73 m^2; dosage then slowly increased until blood pressure is under control or maximum daily dose of 5 mg is reached.

Route	Onset	Peak	Duration
P.O.	1 to 2 hr	4 to 6.5 hr	24 hr

Contraindications
Hypersensitivity to ramipril, its components, or any other ACE inhibitors

Interactions
DRUGS
*allopurinol, bone marrow depressants, corti-*costeroids (systemic), procainamide:* Increased risk of fatal neutropenia or agranulocytosis
CNS depressants, other hypotension-producing drugs: Additive hypotensive effect
cyclosporine, potassium preparations, potassium-sparing diuretics: Possibly hyperkalemia
insulin, oral antidiabetics: Increased risk of hypoglycemia
lithium: Increased risk of lithium toxicity
NSAIDs, sympathomimetics: Decreased antihypertensive effect of ramipril
tetracyclines: Reduced tetracycline absorption
FOODS
low-salt milk, salt substitutes: Increased risk of hyperkalemia
ACTIVITIES
alcohol use: Additive hypotensive effects

Mechanism of Action
Blocks conversion of angiotensin I to angiotensin II, causing vasodilation, and reduces aldosterone secretion, which prevents water retention. Ramipril also reduces peripheral arterial resistance. Combined, these actions reduce blood pressure.

Adverse Reactions
CNS: Depression, dizziness, drowsiness, fatigue, fever, headache, insomnia, lightheadedness, malaise, paresthesia, sleep disturbance, syncope, vertigo
CV: Chest pain, hypotension, orthostatic hypotension, palpitations, tachycardia
EENT: Amblyopia, dry mouth, loss of taste, pharyngitis
GI: Abdominal pain, constipation, diarrhea, elevated liver function test results, hepatic failure, hepatitis, nausea, vomiting
GU: Acute renal failure, elevated BUN and serum creatinine levels, impotence, oliguria, progressive azotemia
HEME: Agranulocytosis, anemia, bone marrow depression, pancytopenia
MS: Arthralgia, back pain, myalgia
RESP: Cough, dyspnea
SKIN: Alopecia, diaphoresis, flushing, jaundice, onycholysis, pemphigoid, photosensitivity, pruritus, rash, Stevens-Johnson syndrome, toxic epidermal necrolysis, urticaria
Other: Angioedema

Q
R
S

Nursing Considerations

•Use ramipril cautiously in patients with renal or hepatic impairment.

•**WARNING** Patients with dehydration, heart failure, or hyponatremia; those who've recently received intensive diuresis or an increase in diuretic dosage; and those having dialysis may risk excessive hypotension. Monitor such patients closely the first 2 weeks of therapy and whenever ramipril or diuretic dosage increases. If excessive hypotension occurs, notify prescriber immediately, place patient in a supine position, and, if prescribed, infuse normal saline solution.

•**WARNING** Because of the risk of angioedema, be prepared to stop drug and provide emergency measures, including subcutaneous epinephrine 1:1,000 (0.3 to 0.5 ml), if swelling of tongue, glottis, or larynx causes airway obstruction.

•Monitor blood pressure frequently during therapy to assess drug's effectiveness.

•Monitor patient's renal and hepatic function closely during therapy.

PATIENT TEACHING

•Advise patient to stop taking ramipril and inform prescriber immediately if she experiences swelling of the face, eyes, lips, or tongue or has difficulty breathing.

•Explain that drug may cause dizziness and light-headedness, especially during first few days of therapy. Instruct patient to notify prescriber immediately if she faints.

•Inform female patient of childbearing age of the risks of taking ramipril during pregnancy, especially during the second and third trimesters. Caution patient to use effective contraception and to report known or suspected pregnancy immediately.

•Urge patient to tell providers that she takes ramipril before having surgery or anesthesia.

•Tell patient to ask prescriber before using supplements or salt substitutes that contain potassium.

ranitidine hydrochloride

Apo-Ranitidine (CAN), Gen-Ranitidine (CAN), Novo-Ranitidine (CAN), Nu-Ranit (CAN), Zantac, Zantac EFFERdose Tablets, Zantac 150 GELdose, Zantac 300 GELdose

Class and Category

Chemical class: Aminoalkyl-substituted furan derivative

Therapeutic class: Antiulcer agent, gastric acid secretion inhibitor

Pregnancy category: B

Indications and Dosages

➤ *To prevent duodenal and gastric ulcers*

CAPSULES, EFFERVESCENT GRANULES, EFFERVESCENT TABLETS, SYRUP, TABLETS

Adults and adolescents. 150 mg at bedtime.

➤ *To provide short-term treatment of active duodenal and benign gastric ulcers*

CAPSULES, EFFERVESCENT GRANULES, EFFERVESCENT TABLETS, SYRUP, TABLETS

Adults and adolescents. 150 mg b.i.d. for gastric ulcers; 150 mg b.i.d. or 300 mg at bedtime for duodenal ulcers.

Children ages 1 month to 16 years. 2 to 4 mg/kg b.i.d. up to 300 mg daily. *Maintenance:* 2 to 4 mg/kg daily up to 150 mg daily.

CONTINUOUS I.V. INFUSION

Adults and adolescents. 6.25 mg/hr. *Maximum:* 400 mg daily.

INTERMITTENT I.V. INFUSION

Adults and adolescents. 50 mg diluted to total volume of 100 ml and infused over 15 to 20 min every 6 to 8 hr. *Maximum:* 400 mg daily.

Children. 2 to 4 mg/kg daily diluted to a suitable volume and infused over 15 to 20 min.

I.V. INJECTION

Adults and adolescents. 50 mg diluted to total volume of 20 ml and injected slowly over no less than 5 min every 6 to 8 hr. *Maximum:* 400 mg daily.

I.M. INJECTION

Adults and adolescents. 50 mg every 6 to 8 hr. *Maximum:* 400 mg daily.

➤ *To treat acute gastroesophageal reflux disease*

CAPSULES, EFFERVESCENT GRANULES, EFFERVESCENT TABLETS, SYRUP, TABLETS

Adults and adolescents. 150 mg b.i.d.

EFFERVESCENT TABLETS

Children ages 1 month to 16 years. 2.5 to 5 mg/kg b.i.d.

INTERMITTENT I.V. INFUSION

Children. 2 to 8 mg/kg diluted to suitable volume and infused over 15 to 20 min t.i.d.

➤ *To treat erosive esophagitis*

CAPSULES, EFFERVESCENT GRANULES, EFFERVESCENT TABLETS, SYRUP, TABLETS

Adults and adolescents. 150 mg q.i.d.

EFFERVESCENT TABLETS

Children ages 1 month to 16 years. 2.5 to 5 mg/kg b.i.d.

➤ *To treat hypersecretory GI conditions, such as Zollinger-Ellison syndrome, systemic mastocytosis, and multiple endocrine adenoma syndrome*

CAPSULES, EFFERVESCENT GRANULES, EFFERVESCENT TABLETS, SYRUP, TABLETS

Adults and adolescents. *Initial:* 150 mg b.i.d., adjusted as needed. *Maximum:* 6 g daily in divided doses.

CONTINUOUS I.V. INFUSION

Adults and adolescents. *Initial:* 1 mg/kg/hr, increased by 0.5 mg/kg/hr up to 2.5 mg/kg/hr. *Maximum:* 400 mg daily.

INTERMITTENT I.V. INFUSION

Adults. 50 mg diluted to total volume of 100 ml and infused over 15 to 20 min every 6 to 8 hr. *Maximum:* 400 mg daily.

I.V. INJECTION

Adults and adolescents. 50 mg diluted to total of 20 ml and injected slowly over at least 5 min every 6 to 8 hr. *Maximum:* 400 mg daily.

I.M. INJECTION

Adults. 50 mg every 6 to 8 hr.

➤ *To prevent acid indigestion, heartburn, and sour stomach caused by eating certain foods or drinking certain beverages*

TABLETS

Adults and adolescents. 75 mg 30 to 60 min before food or beverages expected to cause symptoms. *Maximum:* 150 mg daily over no more than 2 continuous wk.

➤ *To treat acid indigestion, heartburn, and sour stomach*

TABLETS

Adults and adolescents. 75 mg when symptoms start; repeated once within 24 hr, if needed.

DOSAGE ADJUSTMENT For patients whose creatinine clearance is less than 50 ml/min/1.73 m^2, 150 mg P.O. every 24 hr with dosage interval increased thereafter to every 12 hr, as needed. Or 50 mg I.V. every 18 to 24 hr with dosage interval increased to every 12 hr, as needed. Dosage reduction may also be necessary for patients with hepatic dysfunction.

Route	Onset	Peak	Duration
P.O., I.V., I.M.	Unknown	1 to 3 hr	13 hr

Mechanism of Action

Inhibits basal and nocturnal secretion of gastric acid and pepsin by competitively inhibiting the action of histamine at H$_2$ receptors on gastric parietal cells. This action reduces total volume of gastric juices and, thus, irritation of GI mucosa.

Contraindications

Acute porphyria, hypersensitivity to ranitidine or its components

Interactions

DRUGS

antacids: Decreased ranitidine absorption
bone marrow depressants: Increased risk of neutropenia or other blood dyscrasias
diazepam, itraconazole, ketoconazole, sucralfate: Decreased absorption of these drugs
glipizide, glyburide, metoprolol, midazolam, nifedipine, phenytoin, theophylline, warfarin: Increased effects of these drugs, possibly leading to toxic reactions

ACTIVITIES

alcohol use: Increased blood alcohol level (with oral ranitidine)

Adverse Reactions

CNS: Dizziness, drowsiness, fever, headache, insomnia
CV: Vasculitis
GI: Abdominal distress, constipation, diarrhea, nausea, vomiting
GU: Impotence
MS: Arthralgia, myalgia
RESP: Bronchospasm
SKIN: Alopecia, erythema multiforme, rash
Other: Anaphylaxis, angioedema

Nursing Considerations

• Be aware that ranitidine must be diluted for I.V. use if not using premixed solution. For I.V. injection, dilute to total of 20 ml with normal saline solution, D$_5$W, D$_{10}$W, lactated Ringer's solution, or 5% sodium bicarbonate. For I.V. infusion, dilute to total volume of 100 ml of same solutions.
• Give I.V. injection at no more than 4 ml/min, intermittent I.V. infusion at 5 to 7 ml/min, and continuous I.V. infusion at 6.25 mg/hr (except with hypersecretory conditions, when initial infusion rate is 1 mg/kg/hr, gradually increased after 4 hours, as needed, in increments of 0.5 mg/kg/hr).

• Don't add additives to premixed solution.
• Stop primary I.V. solution infusion during piggyback administration.

PATIENT TEACHING

• Tell patient to dissolve 150-mg effervescent tablets or granules in 6 to 8 oz water or 25-mg effervescent tablets in at least 5 ml water.
• Advise patient (or parent) to wait until effervescent tablet is completely dissolved before taking (or giving to child or infant).
• Caution patient not to chew effervescent tablets, swallow them whole, or let them dissolve on the tongue.
• Alert patients with phenylketonuria that effervescent tablets and granules contain phenylalanine.
• Tell patient that she may take drug with food.
• Tell patient to stop taking ranitidine and contact prescriber if she has trouble swallowing, vomits blood, or passes black or bloody stools.
• If needed, advise patient to take antacids, 2 hours before or after ranitidine; advise against taking other acid reducers with drug.
• If patient takes drug to prevent heartburn, tell her to contact prescriber about frequent chest pain or wheezing with heartburn; stomach pain; unexplained weight loss; nausea; vomiting; heartburn lasting more than 3 months; heartburn with light-headedness, dizziness, or sweating; chest or shoulder pain with shortness of breath, sweating, light-headedness, or pain spreading to arms, neck, or shoulders. These problems may be serious.
• Inform patient that healing of an ulcer may require 4 to 8 weeks of therapy.

ranolazine

Ranexa

Class and Category

Chemical class: Piperazineacetamide
Therapeutic class: Antianginal
Pregnancy category: C

Indications and Dosages

➤ *To treat chronic angina*

E.R. TABLETS

Adults. *Initial:* 500 mg b.i.d., increased to 1,000 mg b.i.d., as needed. *Maximum:* 1,000 mg b.i.d.

DOSAGE ADJUSTMENT For patients taking a moderate CYP3A inhibitor, such as diltiazem or verapamil, maximum dosage reduced to 500 mg b.i.d. For patients taking cyclosporine, dosage reduced according to clinical response

Route	Onset	Peak	Duration
P.O.	Unknown	2 to 5 hr	Unknown

Mechanism of Action

Exerts anti-ischemic and antianginal effects by an unknown mechanism not dependent on reductions in heart rate or blood pressure. Ranolazine inhibits cardiac late sodium current, but how this action inhibits angina symptoms is also unknown.

Contraindications

Hypersensitivity to ranolazine or its components, hepatic impairment, QT-interval prolongation, torsades de pointes, use of CYP3A inducers or strong inhibitors

Interactions

DRUGS

CYP3A inducers, such as carbamazepine, phenobarbital, phenytoin, rifabutin, rifampin, rifapentin, St. John's wort: Decreased blood ranolazine level and decreased effectiveness
CYP3A substrates, such as cyclosporine: Possibly increased cyclosporine level
CYP3A inhibitors, such as clarithromycin, diltiazem, indinavir, itraconazole, ketoconazole, nefazodone, nelfinavir, ritonavir, saquinavir, verapamil: Increased blood ranolazine level and increased risk of adverse reactions
digoxin: Increased blood digoxin level

Adverse Reactions

CNS: Asthenia, confusion, dizziness, headache, hypoesthesia, paresthesia, tremor, vertigo
CV: Bradycardia, hypotension, orthostatic hypotension, palpitations, peripheral edema, QT-interval prolongation
EENT: Blurred vision, dry mouth, tinnitus
GI: Abdominal pain, constipation, nausea, vomiting
GU: Elevated creatinine level, hematuria, renal failure

HEME: Eosinophilia, leukopenia, pancytopenia, thrombocytopenia
RESP: Dyspnea, pulmonary fibrosis
Other: Angioedema

Nursing Considerations
•Monitor patient's QT interval, as ordered, because ranolazine prolongs it in a dose-related manner.
•Assess effectiveness of ranolazine at preventing anginal pain.
•Monitor patient's serum creatinine, BUN, magnesium, potassium, and liver enzyme levels.

PATIENT TEACHING
•Instruct patient to take ranolazine exactly as prescribed.
•Inform patient that drug may be taken with or without food.
•Caution patient to swallow tablets whole and not to crush, break, or chew them.
•Advise patient to limit the amount of grapefruit and grapefruit juice consumed while taking this drug.
•Advise patient to notify prescriber if serious or persistent adverse reactions occur.

rasagiline

Azilect

Class and Category
Chemical class: Propargylamine
Therapeutic class: Irreversible MAO inhibitor
Pregnancy category: C

Indications and Dosages
➤ *To treat idiopathic Parkinson's disease as initial monotherapy in early-stage disease*

TABLETS
Adults. 1 mg once daily.

➤ *As adjunct with levodopa or levodopa and carbidopa in treatment of later-stage idiopathic Parkinson's disease*

TABLETS
Adults. 0.5 mg once daily increased to 1 mg once daily, as needed.

DOSAGE ADJUSTMENT For patients with mild hepatic failure, dosage shouldn't exceed 0.5 mg daily.

Route	Onset	Peak	Duration
P.O.	Unknown	1 hr	Unknown

Mechanism of Action
Inhibits metabolic degradation of catecholamines and serotonin in the CNS and peripheral tissues, increasing extracellular dopamine level in the striatum. The increased dopamine level helps control alterations in voluntary muscle movement (such as tremors and rigidity) in Parkinson's disease because dopamine, a neurotransmitter, is essential for normal motor function. By stimulating peripheral and central dopaminergic 2 (D_2) receptors on postsynaptic cells, dopamine inhibits firing of striatal neurons (such as cholineric neurons), improving motor function.

Contraindications
Acute MI; angina; cardiac arrhythmias; coronary artery disease; cerebrovascular disease; elective surgery that requires general anesthesia; hypersensitivity to rasagiline or its components; pheochromocytoma; moderate to severe hepatic impairment; stroke; use within 14 days of cyclobenzaprine, dextromethorphan, MAO inhibitors, meperidine, mirtazapine, tramadol, methadone, propoxyphene, St. John's wort, or sympathomimetic amines

Interactions
DRUGS
ciprofloxacin and other CYP1A2 inhibitors: Increased rasagiline plasma level
dextromethorphan: Increased risk of psychosis or bizarre behavior
levodopa, levodopa and carbidopa: Increased risk of dyskinesias
MAO inhibitors, sympathomimetics: Increased risk of hypertensive crisis
meperidine, methadone, propoxyphene, tramadol: Increased risk of life-threatening adverse reactions characterized by coma, severe hypertension or hypotension, severe respiratory depression, seizures, malignant hyperpyrexia, excitation, and peripheral vascular collapse
selective serotonin reuptake inhibitors, tetracyclic antidepressants, tricyclic antidepressants: Increased risk of severe CNS toxicity with hyperpyrexia, behavioral and mental status changes, diaphoresis, muscle rigidity, hypertension, syncope, and possible death

Q
R
S

Adverse Reactions

CNS: Abnormal dreams, amnesia, anxiety, asthenia, ataxia, cerebral ischemia, coma, confusion, depression, difficulty thinking, dizziness, dyskinesia, dystonia, fever, hallucinations, headache, malaise, manic depressive reaction, nightmares, paresthesia, seizures, somnolence, stroke, stupor, syncope, vertigo

CV: Angina, bundle branch heart block, chest pain, heart failure, MI, hypertensive crisis, postural hypotension, thrombophlebitis, ventricular tachycardia or fibrillation

EENT: Blurred vision, conjunctivitis, dry mouth, gingivitis, hemorrhage, laryngeal edema, retinal detachment or hemorrhage, rhinitis

GI: Abdominal pain, anorexia, constipation, diarrhea, dyspepsia, dysphagia, epistaxia, gastroenteritis, gastrointestinal hemorrhage, intestinal obstruction or perforation, liver function test abnormalities, nausea, vomiting

GU: Acute renal failure, albuminuria, decreased libido, hematuria, impotence, incontinence, priapism

HEME: Anemia, leukopenia, thrombocytopenia

MS: Arthralgia, arthritis, bone necrosis, bursitis, leg cramps, myasthenia, neck pain or stiffness, tenosynovitis

RESP: Apnea, asthma, cough, dyspnea, pleural effusion, pneumothorax, interstitial pneumonia

SKIN: Alopecia, carcinoma, diaphoresis, ecchymosis, exfoliative dermatitis, pruritus, ulcer, vesiculobullous rash

Other: Angioedema, flu syndrome, hypersensitivity reaction, hypocalcemia, weight loss

Nursing Considerations

•WARNING Notify prescriber immediately if patient has evidence of hypertensive crisis, such as blurred vision, chest pain, difficulty thinking, stupor or coma, seizures, severe headache, neck stiffness, nausea, vomiting, palpitations or signs and symptoms suggesting a stroke. Expect to stop drug immediately if these occur.

•Keep phentolamine readily available to treat hypertensive crisis. Give 5 mg by slow I.V. infusion, as prescribed, to reduce blood pressure without causing excessive hypotension. Use external cooling measures, as prescribed, to manage fever.

•Maintain tyramine restriction and avoid-ance of amine-containing medications for at least 2 weeks after stopping rasagiline because of the irreversible inhibition of MAO and the need for new MAO enzyme synthesis.

•Monitor patient receiving rasagline with levodopa for worsening of pre-existing dyskinesia. If it occurs, notify prescriber and expect levodopa dosage to be decreased.

PATIENT TEACHING

•WARNING Instruct patient to avoid the following foods, beverages, and drugs during rasagline therapy and for 2 weeks afterward: alcohol-free and reduced-alcohol beer and wine; appetite suppressants; beer; broad beans; cheese (except cottage and cream cheese); chocolate and caffeine in large quantities; dry sausage (including Genoa salami, hard salami, Lebanon bologna, and pepperoni); hay fever drugs; inhaled asthma drugs; liver; meat extract; OTC cold and cough preparations (including those containing dextromethorphan), nasal decongestants (tablets, drops, or sprays); pickled herring products that contain tryptophan; protein-rich foods that may have undergone protein changes by aging, fermenting, pickling, or smoking; sauerkraut; sinus drugs; weight-loss preparations; yeast extracts (including brewer's yeast in large quantities); yogurt; and wine.

•Advise patient to stop taking rasagline and to notify prescriber immediately if he develops blurred vision, chest pain, trouble thinking, stupor or coma, seizures, severe headache, stiff neck, nausea, vomiting, palpitations, or evidence of stroke.

•Suggest that patient change position slowly to minimize orthostatic hypotension.

•Alert patient that drug may cause hallucinations. If they occur, tell patient to notify prescriber promptly.

rasburicase

Elitek

Class and Category

Chemical class: Tetrameric protein
Therapeutic class: Uric acid reducer
Pregnancy category: C

Indications and Dosages

➤ *To manage plasma uric acid levels ini-*

tially in pediatric patients with leuke-mia, lymphoma, or solid tumor malig-nancies who receive anticancer therapy that elevates plasma uric acid

I.V. INFUSION
Children. 0.15 or 0.20 mg/kg infused over 30 min daily for 5 days.

Mechanism of Action
Converts uric acid into an inactive and soluble metabolite at the end of the purine catabolic pathway. This prevents plasma uric acid levels from rising due to tumor lysis from anticancer therapy.

Contraindications
Glucose-6-phosphatase dehydrogenase (G6PD) deficiency; history of anaphylaxis or hypersensitivity reactions, hemolytic reactions, or methemoglobinemia reactions; hypersensitivity to rasburicase or its components

Adverse Reactions
CNS: Anxiety, fever, headache, paresthesia, rigors, seizures
CV: Arrhythmia, cardiac failure or arrest, cerebrovascular disorder, chest pain, hemorrhage, hypotension, myocardial infarction, pulmonary edema, thrombophlebitis, thrombosis
EENT: Mucositis, retinal hemorrhage
ENDO: Hot flashes
GI: Abdominal pain, constipation, diarrhea, ileus, intestinal obstruction, nausea, vomiting
GU: Acute renal failure
HEME: Anemia, hemolysis, methemoglobinemia, neutropenia, pancytopenia
RESP: Cyanosis, dyspnea, pneumonia, pulmonary hypertension, respiratory distress
SKIN: Cellulitis, rash
Other: Anaphylaxis, dehydration, infection, sepsis

Nursing Considerations
•Be aware that children at high risk for G6PD, such as patients of African or Mediterranean ancestry, should be screened before administering rasburicase because severe hemolysis can occur.
•Expect to give only one course of therapy because of risk of severe allergic reactions.
•Reconstitute rasburicase using only diluent

provided. Add 1 ml of diluent to each vial needed, and mix by swirling very gently. Don't shake or invert vial.
•Inject reconstituted solution into an infusion bag containing the appropriate volume of 0.9% NaCl to obtain a final volume of 50 ml. Infuse over 30 minutes in a different line than for infusion of other drugs. If a separate line isn't possible, flush the line with at least 15 ml of normal saline solution before and after rasburicase infusion. Don't use filters.
•Store reconstituted solution at 2° to 8° C (36° to 46° F) for no longer than 24 hours. Protect drug from light.
•**WARNING** Monitor patient closely for severe hypersensitivity reactions, including anaphylaxis (chest pain, dyspnea, hypotension, urticaria), hemolysis (severe anxiety, pain, dyspnea), and methemoglobinemia (anxiety, hypoxemia, shortness of breath). If such a reaction occurs, discontinue rasburicase immediately, notify prescriber, and start emergency treatment. Rasburicase shouldn't be restarted after such a reaction occurs.
•Ensure that blood samples to measure uric acid levels are collected in chilled tubes containing heparin anticoagulant and are immediately placed in ice water until analysis is done (within 4 hours); blood samples left at room temperature will result in low uric acid levels because of enzyme degradation of uric acid at room temperature.
PATIENT TEACHING
•Inform child and parents that chemotherapy will start 4 to 24 hours after rasburicase.
•Stress the importance of reporting any adverse reaction immediately.

remifentanil hydrochloride
Ultiva

Class, Category, and Schedule
Chemical class: Fentanyl analogue
Therapeutic class: Anesthesia adjunct
Pregnancy category: C
Controlled substance schedule: II

Indications and Dosages
➤ *As adjunct to induce general anesthesia*
INTERMITTENT I.V. INFUSION
Adults and children age 2 and over. 0.5 to 1 mcg/kg plus inhalation or I.V. anesthetic.

➤ *To maintain general anesthesia*

INTERMITTENT I.V. INFUSION

Adults and children age 2 and over. 0.05 to 0.2 mcg/kg, followed by 0.5 to 1 mcg/kg every 2 to 5 min, as needed.

➤ *To continue analgesic effect in immediate postoperative period*

CONTINUOUS I.V. INFUSION

Adults and children age 2 and over. *Initial:* 0.1 mcg/kg/min, adjusted by 0.025 mcg/kg/min every 5 min, as prescribed, to balance level of analgesia and respiratory rate. *Maximum:* 0.2 mcg/kg/min.

➤ *To supplement local or regional anesthesia in a monitored anesthetic setting*

I.V. INFUSION

Adults and children age 2 and over. *With a benzodiazepine:* 0.05 mcg/kg/min, beginning 5 min before placement of local or regional block; after placement of block, decreased to 0.025 mcg/kg/min and then further adjusted every 5 min in increments of 0.025 mcg/kg/min, as needed. *Without a benzodiazepine:* 0.1 mcg/kg/min, starting 5 min before placement of local or regional block; after placement of block, decreased to 0.05 mcg/kg/min and then further adjusted every 5 min in increments of 0.025 mcg/kg/min, as needed.

I.V. INJECTION

Adults and children age 2 and over. *With a benzodiazepine:* 0.5 mcg/kg over 30 to 60 sec as a single dose 60 to 90 sec before local anesthetic is administered. *Without a benzodiazepine:* 1 mcg/kg administered over 30 to 60 sec as a single dose 60 to 90 sec before local anesthetic is administered.

DOSAGE ADJUSTMENT For elderly patients, starting dose possibly reduced by half. If patient is more than 30% over ideal body weight, starting dose based on ideal body weight.

Route	Onset	Peak	Duration
I.V.	1 min	1 to 2 min	5 to 10 min

Incompatibilities

Don't give remifentanil through same I.V. line as blood because nonspecific esterases in blood products may inactivate drug.

Contraindications

Epidural or intrathecal administration, hypersensitivity to fentanyl analogues

Interactions

DRUGS

anesthetics (barbiturate, inhalation), benzodiazepines, propofol: Possibly synergistic ef-

Mechanism of Action

Remifentanil decreases the transmission and perception of pain by stimulating mu-opioid receptors in neurons. This action decreases the activity of adenyl cyclase in neurons, which in turn decreases cAMP production. With less cAMP available, potassium (K⁺) is forced out of neurons, and calcium (Ca⁺⁺) is prevented from entering neurons. As a result, neuron excitability declines, and fewer neurotransmitters (such as substance P) leave the neurons, thereby decreasing pain transmission.

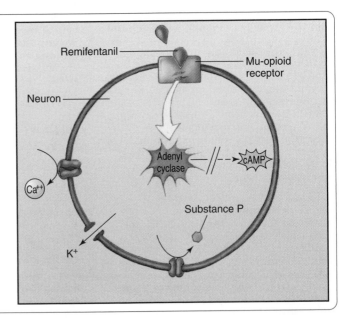

fects, increasing risk of hypotension and respiratory depression

atropine, glycopyrrolate: Possibly reversal of remifentanil-induced bradycardia

ephedrine, epinephrine, norepinephrine: Possibly reversal of remifentanil-induced hypotension

neuromuscular blockers: Prolonged remifentanil-induced skeletal muscle rigidity

opioid antagonists: Possibly reversal of remifentanil's effects

Adverse Reactions
CNS: Headache, shivering
CV: Asystole, bradycardia, hypotension
GI: Nausea, vomiting
MS: Skeletal muscle rigidity
RESP: Apnea, cough, dyspnea, respiratory depression, stridor, wheezing
Other: Anaphylaxis

Nursing Considerations
•Inject remifentanil into I.V. tubing at or as close as possible to venous cannula.
•Use infusion device to deliver continuous infusion.
•Monitor vital signs and oxygenation continuously during administration.
•Expect analgesic effects to dissipate rapidly when drug is discontinued. Expect to start adequate postoperative analgesia, as prescribed, before stopping drug.
•WARNING After stopping drug, clear I.V. tubing to prevent inadvertent later delivery.
•Monitor respiratory status continuously because of risk of respiratory depression from residual effects of other anesthetics for up to 30 minutes after infusion stops.

PATIENT TEACHING
•Explain expected drug effects to patient, and reassure her that she'll be monitored continuously during drug administration.

repaglinide

Prandin

Class and Category
Chemical class: Meglitinide
Therapeutic class: Antidiabetic
Pregnancy category: C

Indications and Dosages
➤ *To achieve glucose control in type 2 diabetes mellitus as monotherapy in pa-*

tients whose glycosylated hemoglobin (HbA₁c) level is less than 8%

TABLETS
Adults. *Initial:* 0.5 mg 15 to 30 min before meals b.i.d. Dosage doubled, as needed, every wk until adequate glucose response obtained. *Maintenance:* 0.5 to 4 mg/dose up to q.i.d. *Maximum:* 16 mg daily in divided doses of not more than 4 mg/dose.

➤ *To achieve glucose control in type 2 diabetes mellitus as monotherapy in patients whose HbA₁c is 8% or greater and in combination with metformin or thiazolidinedione (pioglitazone hydrochloride, rosiglitazone maleate) therapy*

TABLETS
Adults. *Initial:* 1 or 2 mg 15 to 30 min before meals b.i.d. Dosage doubled, as needed, every wk until adequate glucose response obtained. *Maintenance:* 1 to 4 mg/dose up to q.i.d. *Maximum:* 16 mg daily in divided doses of not more than 4 mg/dose.

DOSAGE ADJUSTMENT For patients with moderate to severe hepatic or renal impairment, increased time between dosage adjustments.

Mechanism of Action
Stimulates release of insulin from functioning pancreatic beta cells. In patients with type 2 diabetes mellitus, a shortage of these cells decreases blood insulin levels and causes glucose intolerance. By interacting with the adenosine triphosphatase (ATP)–potassium channel on the beta cell membrane, repaglinide prevents potassium from leaving the cell. This causes the beta cell to depolarize and the cell membrane's calcium channel to open. As a result, calcium moves into the cell and insulin moves out. The extent of insulin release is glucose dependent; the lower the glucose level, the less insulin is secreted from the cell.

Contraindications
Diabetic ketoacidosis, hypersensitivity to repaglinide or its components, severe hepatic or renal impairment, type 1 diabetes mellitus

Interactions
DRUGS
barbiturates, carbamazepine, rifampin, tro-

glitazone: Possibly increased repaglinide metabolism

beta blockers, chloramphenicol, clarithromycin, MAO inhibitors, NSAIDs, oral anticoagulants, probenecid, salicylates, sulfonamides: Enhanced hypoglycemic effects

calcium channel blockers, corticosteroids, diuretics, estrogens, isoniazid, niacin, oral contraceptives, phenothiazines, phenytoin, sympathomimetics, thyroid hormones: Possibly loss of glucose control

erythromycin, ketoconazole, miconazole: Possibly inhibited repaglinide metabolism

gemfibrozil: Increased blood repaglinide level, resulting in enhanced and prolonged blood glucose–lowering effects

NPH insulin: Possibly increased risk of angina

trimethoprim: Increased plasma repaglinide level

Adverse Reactions

CNS: Headache
CV: Angina
EENT: Rhinitis, sinusitis
ENDO: Hypoglycemia
GI: Diarrhea, elevated liver enzymes, hepatitis, nausea, pancreatitis
HEME: Hemolytic anemia, leukopenia, thrombocytopenia
MS: Arthralgia, back pain
RESP: Bronchitis, upper respiratory tract infection
SKIN: Alopecia, Stevens-Johnson syndrome
Other: Anaphylaxis

Nursing Considerations

•Be aware that repaglinide shouldn't be used with NPH insulin because the combination may increase the risk of angina.
•Expect to check HbA$_{1c}$ level every 3 months, as ordered, to assess patient's long-term control of blood glucose level.
•During times of increased stress, such as from infection, surgery, or trauma, monitor blood glucose level often and assess need for additional insulin.

PATIENT TEACHING

•Instruct patient to take repaglinide 15 to 30 minutes before meals and to skip dose whenever she skips a meal.
•Explain that repaglinide is an adjunct to diet in managing type 2 diabetes mellitus.
•Teach patient how to monitor her blood glucose level and when to notify prescriber

about changes.
•Review signs and symptoms of hyperglycemia and hypoglycemia with patient and family. Instruct patient to notify prescriber immediately if she experiences anxiety, confusion, dizziness, excessive sweating, headache, increased thirst, increased urination, or nausea.
•Advise patient to wear or carry identification indicating that she has diabetes. Encourage her to carry candy or other simple carbohydrates with her to treat mild episodes of hypoglycemia.
•Inform patient that her HbA$_{1c}$ level will be tested every 3 to 6 months until her blood glucose level is controlled.

reserpine

Novoreserpine (CAN), Reserfia (CAN), Serpalan, Serpasil (CAN)

Class and Category

Chemical class: Rauwolfia alkaloid
Therapeutic class: Antihypertensive
Pregnancy category: C

Indications and Dosages

➤ *To treat hypertension*

TABLETS

Adults. 0.1 to 0.25 mg daily.
Children. 0.005 to 0.02 mg/kg daily once daily or in divided doses b.i.d.

DOSAGE ADJUSTMENT Lower dosage possibly required for elderly or severely debilitated patients.

Route	Onset	Peak	Duration
P.O.	Days to 3 wk	3 to 6 wk	1 to 6 wk

Contraindications

Active peptic ulcer, electroconvulsive therapy, hypersensitivity to reserpine or its components, mental depression (current or history of), ulcerative colitis

Interactions

DRUGS

anticholinergics: Decreased effectiveness of anticholinergics
barbiturates: Increased CNS depression
beta blockers: Additive and, possibly, excessive beta-adrenergic blockade
bromocriptine: Possibly interference with

Mechanism of Action

Reserpine reduces blood pressure by decreasing norepinephrine stores in presynaptic sympathetic neurons.

Normally, when a nerve impulse activates a sympathetic neuron, the nerve ending releases norepinephrine, which stimulates alpha or beta receptors on target cell membranes, as shown below left. Stimulation of alpha receptors may produce vasoconstriction; stimulation of beta receptors may increase the heart rate and force of myocardial contraction, which raises cardiac output. Through a reuptake mechanism, some norepinephrine returns to the neuron and is stored in vesicles for reuse.

Reserpine displaces norepinephrine from vesicles in the nerve fiber, and MAO degrades the displaced norepinephrine, as shown below right. These actions reduce the amount of norepinephrine available to stimulate postsynaptic alpha and beta receptors, leading to a reduction in vasoconstriction, cardiac output, and blood pressure.

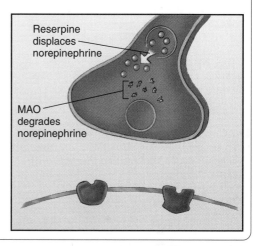

bromocriptine's effects
digoxin, procainamide, quinidine: Increased risk of arrhythmias
hypotension-producing drugs: Increased antihypertensive effect; increased risk of orthostatic hypotension or bradycardia (with guanadrel or guanethidine)
levodopa: Decreased levodopa effectiveness
MAO inhibitors: Increased risk of severe hypertension and hyperpyrexia, additive CNS depression
NSAIDs: Decreased antihypertensive effect
sympathomimetics: Increased vasopressor effects, decreased antihypertensive effect
ACTIVITIES
alcohol use: Increased CNS depression

Adverse Reactions

CNS: Anxiety, depression, dizziness, drowsiness, headache, nervousness, nightmares, sleep disturbance, syncope, weakness
CV: Arrhythmias, such as bradycardia; chest pain; peripheral edema
EENT: Conjunctival injection, dry mouth, epistaxis, glaucoma, hearing loss, nasal congestion, optic atrophy, uveitis
ENDO: Breast engorgement
GI: Abdominal cramps or pain, anorexia, diarrhea, increased gastric secretions, melena, nausea, vomiting
GU: Decreased libido, galactorrhea, gynecomastia, impotence
MS: Myalgia
RESP: Dyspnea
SKIN: Purpura
Other: Weight gain

Nursing Considerations

•If patient has a history of depression, use reserpine cautiously because it may cause depression masked as somatic complaints.
•Monitor blood pressure frequently during

Q
R
S

drug therapy.
•Alert anesthesiologist if patient is scheduled for surgery. Drug may cause circulatory instability even if withheld before procedure.
PATIENT TEACHING
•Instruct patient to take reserpine with food or milk to minimize stomach upset.
•Caution patient about possible drowsiness, and advise her to avoid potentially hazardous activities until drug's CNS effects are known.
•Explain the need for frequent appointments to monitor blood pressure and adjust dosage at start of therapy.

reteplase

Retavase

Class and Category

Chemical class: Recombinant plasminogen activator (r-PA)
Therapeutic class: Thrombolytic
Pregnancy category: C

Indications and Dosages

➤ *To improve ventricular function, prevent heart failure, and reduce mortality after acute MI*

I.V. INJECTION
Adults. 10 units over 2 min; repeated after 30 min.

Mechanism of Action

Converts plasminogen to plasmin, which works to break up fibrin clots that have formed in the coronary arteries. Elimination of the clots improves cardiac blood and oxygen flow to the area, thus improving ventricular function.

Incompatibilities

Don't add other drugs to reteplase injection solution or administer them through same I.V. line as reteplase.

Contraindications

Active internal bleeding, aneurysm, arteriovenous malformation, bleeding diathesis, brain tumor, history of stroke or other cerebrovascular disease, hypersensitivity to reteplase or its components, intracranial or intraspinal surgery or trauma during previous 2 months, severe uncontrolled hyperten-

sion (systolic 200 mm Hg or higher, diastolic 110 mm Hg or higher)

Interactions

DRUGS
antifibrinolytics (including aminocaproic acid, aprotinin, and tranexamic acid): Decreased effectiveness of reteplase
antineoplastics, antithymocyte globulin, certain cephalosporins (such as cefamandole, cefoperazone, and cefotetan), heparin, oral anticoagulants, platelet aggregation inhibitors (such as abciximab, aspirin, and dipyridamole), strontium-89 chloride, sulfinpyrazone, valproic acid: Increased risk of bleeding

Adverse Reactions

CNS: Intracranial hemorrhage
GI: GI bleeding, nausea, vomiting
HEME: Thrombocytopenia
RESP: Hemoptysis
SKIN: Bleeding from wounds, ecchymosis, hematoma, purpura
Other: Allergic reaction, injection site bleeding

Nursing Considerations

•Expect to start reteplase, as prescribed, as soon as possible after MI symptoms begin.
•Closely monitor patient with atrial fibrillation, severe hypertension, or other cardiac disease for signs and symptoms of cerebral embolism.
•To reconstitute, use diluent, syringe, needle, and dispensing pin provided. Withdraw 10 ml of preservative-free sterile water for injection. Remove and discard needle from syringe, and connect dispensing pin to syringe. Remove protective cap from spike end of dispensing pin, and insert spike into reteplase vial. Inject 10 ml of sterile water into the vial. With the spike still in the vial, swirl gently to dissolve the powder. Don't shake. Expect to see slight foaming. Let the vial stand for several minutes. When the bubbles dissipate, withdraw 10 ml of reconstituted solution into the syringe (about 0.7 ml may remain in the vial). Now detach the syringe from the dispensing pin and attach the 20G needle.
•Use the solution within 4 hours. Discard if it's discolored or contains particulates.
•Don't administer heparin and reteplase in the same solution. Instead, flush the heparin line with normal saline solution or D$_5$W be-

fore and after reteplase injection.
•Because fibrin is lysed during therapy, closely monitor all possible bleeding sites (catheter insertions, arterial and venous punctures, cutdowns, and needle punctures).
•Avoid I.M. injections, venipunctures, and nonessential handling of patient during therapy.
•If arterial puncture is needed, use an arm vessel that can be compressed, if possible. After sample is obtained, apply pressure for at least 30 minutes; then apply a pressure dressing. Check site often for bleeding.
•If bleeding occurs and can't be controlled by local pressure, notify prescriber immediately. Be prepared to stop concurrent anticoagulant therapy immediately and to discontinue second reteplase bolus, as prescribed.
•Anticipate that reperfusion arrhythmias, such as premature ventricular contractions or ventricular tachycardia, may follow coronary thrombolysis.

PATIENT TEACHING
•Advise patient to report adverse reactions immediately.

rifabutin

Mycobutin

Class and Category
Chemical class: Spiropiperidyl derivative
Therapeutic class: Antimycobacterial antibiotic
Pregnancy category: B

Indications and Dosages
➤ *To prevent disseminated* Mycobacterium avium *complex in patients with advanced HIV infection*

CAPSULES
Adults. 300 mg once daily or 150 mg b.i.d.

Contraindications
Hypersensitivity to rifabutin or rifamycins

Interactions
DRUGS
aminophylline, barbiturates, beta blockers, chloramphenicol, clofibrate, corticosteroids, cyclosporine, dapsone, diazepam, digoxin, disopyramide, estramustine, estrogens, ketoconazole, mexiletine, oral anticoagulants, oral antidiabetic drugs, oral contraceptives (containing estrogen), oxtriphylline, pheny-
toin, quinidine, theophylline, tocainide, verapamil (oral): Reduced therapeutic effects of these drugs
fluconazole: Increased blood rifabutin level
methadone: Possibly withdrawal symptoms
zidovudine: Decreased blood zidovudine level

Mechanism of Action
Suppresses RNA synthesis by inhibiting DNA-dependent RNA polymerase in a wide variety of bacteria, including *Mycobacterium avium.* Exhibits dose-dependent bactericidal or bacteriostatic action.

Adverse Reactions
CNS: Asthenia, fever, headache, insomnia
CV: Chest pain
EENT: Discolored saliva, tears, and sputum
GI: Abdominal pain, anorexia, diarrhea, discolored feces, elevated liver function test results, eructation, flatulence, indigestion, nausea, pseudomembranous colitis, vomiting
GU: Discolored urine
HEME: Neutropenia, thrombocytopenia
MS: Myalgia
SKIN: Discolored skin and sweat, rash

Nursing Considerations
•Monitor laboratory values during rifabutin therapy to detect neutropenia and thrombocytopenia.
•Expect drug to cause reddish orange to reddish brown discoloration of skin and body fluids.
•Be aware that drug may cause myelosuppression and increased risk of infection. Notify prescriber immediately if signs of infection, such as fever, develop.
•Monitor patient for diarrhea during therapy and for at least 2 months afterward; diarrhea may signal pseudomembranous colitis caused by *Clostridium difficile.* If diarrhea occurs, notify prescriber and expect to withhold rifabutin and treat with fluids, electrolytes, protein, and an antibiotic effective against *C. difficile.*

PATIENT TEACHING
•Advise patient to take rifabutin with food if GI distress develops.
•Encourage patient to have needed dental work done before rifabutin therapy starts to reduce the risk of bleeding or infection.

Q
R
S

•Explain that drug may turn urine, feces, saliva, sputum, sweat, tears, and skin reddish orange to reddish brown.
•Caution patient against wearing soft contact lenses during therapy because drug may permanently stain them.
•Advise patient to notify prescriber about signs of *Mycobacterium avium* complex (chills, fever, night sweats, weight loss), tuberculosis, myositis, or uveitis.
•Advise woman of childbearing age that rifabutin may decrease effectiveness of oral contraceptives; advise her to use a nonhormonal method of birth control.
•Urge patient to tell prescriber about diarrhea that's severe or prolonged. Remind patient that watery or bloody stools can occur 2 months or more after antibiotic therapy ends and can be serious, requiring prompt treatment.

rifampin
(rifampicin)

Rifadin, Rifadin IV, Rimactane, Rofact (CAN)

Class and Category

Chemical class: Semisynthetic antibiotic derivative of rifamycin
Therapeutic class: Antimycobacterial antitubercular
Pregnancy category: C

Indications and Dosages

➤ *As adjunct to treat tuberculosis caused by all strains of* Mycobacterium tuberculosis

CAPSULES, ORAL SUSPENSION, I.V. INFUSION

Adults. 10 mg/kg daily with other antitubercular drugs for 2 mo. *Maximum:* 600 mg daily.

Infants and children. 10 to 20 mg/kg daily in combination with other antitubercular drugs for 2 mo. *Maximum:* 600 mg daily.

➤ *To eliminate meningococci from nasopharynx of asymptomatic carriers of* Neisseria meningitidis

CAPSULES, ORAL SUSPENSION, I.V. INFUSION

Adults. 600 mg every 12 hr for 2 days (total of 4 doses).

Infants age 1 month and over and children. 10 mg/kg every 12 hr for 2 days (total of 4 doses). *Maximum:* 600 mg daily.

Infants under age 1 month. 5 mg/kg every 12 hr for 2 days (total of 4 doses). *Maximum:* 600 mg daily.

DOSAGE ADJUSTMENT For patients with hepatic impairment, maximum dosage of 8 mg/kg daily. For patients with creatinine clearance of 10 ml/min/1.73 m^2 or less, recommended dosage usually decreased by 50%.

Mechanism of Action

Inhibits bacterial and mycobacterial RNA synthesis by binding to DNA-dependent RNA polymerase, thereby blocking RNA transcription. Exhibits dose-dependent bactericidal or bacteriostatic action. Rifampin is highly effective against rapidly dividing bacilli in extracellular cavitary lesions, such as those found in the nasopharynx.

Incompatibilities

Don't administer rifampin in the same I.V. line as diltiazem.

Contraindications

Concurrent use of nonnucleoside reverse transcriptase inhibitors or protease inhibitors by patients with HIV, hypersensitivity to rifamycins

Interactions

DRUGS

aminophylline, oxtriphylline, theophylline: Increased metabolism and clearance of these theophylline preparations
anesthetics (hydrocarbon inhalation, except isoflurane), hepatotoxic drugs, isoniazid: Increased risk of hepatotoxicity
beta blockers, chloramphenicol, clofibrate, corticosteroids, cyclosporine, dapsone, digitalis glycosides, disopyramide, hexobarbital, itraconazole, ketoconazole, mexiletine, oral anticoagulants, oral antidiabetic drugs, phenytoin, propafenone, quinidine, tocainide, verapamil (oral): Increased metabolism, resulting in lower blood levels of these drugs
bone marrow depressants: Increased leukopenic or thrombocytopenic effects
clofazimine: Reduced absorption of rifampin, delaying its peak concentration and increasing its half-life
diazepam: Enhanced diazepam elimination, resulting in decreased drug effectiveness

estramustine, estrogens, oral contraceptives: Decreased estrogenic effects

methadone: Possibly impaired absorption of methadone, leading to withdrawal symptoms

probenecid: Increased blood level or prolonged duration of rifampin, increasing risk of toxicity

nonnucleoside reverse transcriptase inhibitors, protease inhibitors (indinavir, nelfinavir, ritonavir, saquinavir): Accelerated metabolism of these drugs (by patients with HIV), resulting in subtherapeutic levels; delayed metabolism of rifampin, increasing risk of toxicity

trimethoprim: Increased elimination and shortened elimination half-life of trimethoprim

vitamin D: Increased metabolism and decreased efficacy of vitamin D, leading to decreased serum calcium and phosphate levels and increased parathyroid hormone levels

ACTIVITIES
alcohol use: Increased risk of hepatotoxicity

Adverse Reactions

CNS: Chills, dizziness, drowsiness, fatigue, headache, paresthesia
EENT: Discolored saliva, tears, and sputum; mouth or tongue soreness; periorbital edema
GI: Abdominal cramps, anorexia, diarrhea, discolored feces, elevated liver function test results, epigastric discomfort, flatulence, heartburn, hepatitis, nausea, pseudomembranous colitis, vomiting
GU: Discolored urine
MS: Arthralgia, myalgia
SKIN: Discolored skin and sweat
Other: Facial edema, flulike symptoms

Nursing Considerations

•Obtain blood samples or other specimens for culture and sensitivity testing, as ordered, before giving rifampin and throughout therapy to monitor response to drug.
•Expect to monitor liver function test results before and every 2 to 4 weeks during therapy. Immediately report abnormalities.
•For I.V. infusion, reconstitute by adding 10 ml sterile water for injection to 600-mg vial of rifampin. Swirl gently to dissolve. Withdraw appropriate dose and add to 500 ml D₅W (preferred solution) or normal saline solution and infuse over 3 hours. Or, withdraw appropriate dose and add to 100 ml D₅W (preferred solution) or normal

saline solution and infuse over 30 minutes. Use reconstituted drug promptly because rifampin may precipitate out of D₅W solution after 4 hours. In normal saline solution, drug is stable up to 24 hours at room temperature.
•Be aware that patient receiving intermittent therapy (once or twice weekly) is at increased risk for adverse reactions.
•Expect drug to discolor skin and body fluids reddish orange to reddish brown.
•Be aware that rifampin can cause myelosuppression and increase risk of infection. Notify prescriber immediately if signs of infection, such as fever, develop.

PATIENT TEACHING
•Instruct patient to take rifampin 1 hour before or 2 hours after a meal with a full glass of water.
•Stress the need to take drug exactly as prescribed. Explain that interruptions can lead to increased adverse reactions.
•Explain that drug may turn urine, feces, saliva, sputum, sweat, tears, and skin reddish orange to reddish brown.
•Caution patient against wearing soft contact lenses during therapy because drug may permanently stain them.
•Advise patient who takes an oral contraceptive to use an additional form of birth control during rifampin therapy.
•Urge patient to notify prescriber about flulike symptoms, anorexia, darkened urine, fever, joint pain or swelling, malaise, nausea, vomiting, and yellowish skin or eyes, which may indicate hepatitis.
•Advise patient to avoid alcohol during rifampin therapy.
•Instruct patient to notify prescriber if no improvement occurs within 2 to 3 weeks.

riluzole
Rilutek

Class and Category

Chemical class: Benzothiazole
Therapeutic class: Amyotrophic lateral sclerosis treatment agent
Pregnancy category: C

Indications and Dosages

➤ *To treat amyotrophic lateral sclerosis*
TABLETS
Adults. 50 mg every 12 hr.

Mechanism of Action

Inhibits release of glutamic acid, an excitatory amino acid neurotransmitter, in the CNS, thus reducing its effects on target cells. Glutamic acid affects degeneration of neurons; reducing its level may help slow amyotrophic lateral sclerosis.

Contraindications

Hypersensitivity to riluzole or its components

Interactions

DRUGS
allopurinol, hepatotoxic drugs, methyldopa, sulfasalazine: Increased risk of hepatotoxicity
amitriptyline, phenacetin, quinolones, tacrine, theophylline: Delayed elimination of riluzole
omeprazole, rifampin: Increased riluzole clearance
FOODS
charbroiled foods: Increased riluzole elimination
ACTIVITIES
alcohol use: Increased risk of hepatotoxicity
smoking: Increased riluzole elimination

Adverse Reactions

CNS: Asthenia, dizziness, headache, insomnia, paresthesia (circumoral), somnolence, spasticity, vertigo
CV: Peripheral edema
EENT: Dry mouth, rhinitis, stomatitis
GI: Abdominal pain, anorexia, constipation, diarrhea, elevated liver function test results, flatulence, indigestion, nausea, vomiting
HEME: Neutropenia
MS: Back or muscle pain or stiffness
RESP: Dyspnea, increased cough, pneumonia
SKIN: Alopecia, eczema, pruritus

Nursing Considerations

• Use riluzole cautiously in patients with impaired hepatic or renal function.
• Also use cautiously in elderly patients, women, and Japanese patients because of increased risk of toxicity from decreased drug clearance.
• Monitor liver function test results before and during riluzole therapy.
PATIENT TEACHING
• Instruct patient to take riluzole regularly, every 12 hours, either 1 hour before or 2 hours after a meal, and at the same time each day.
• Instruct patient to store riluzole at room temperature, protected from bright light.
• Urge patient to minimize alcohol, smoking, and charred foods because they speed drug excretion.
• Tell patient to report fever.

risedronate sodium

Actonel

Class and Category

Chemical class: Pyridinyl bisphosphonate
Therapeutic class: Bone resorption inhibitor
Pregnancy category: C

Indications and Dosages

➤ *To treat Paget's disease of bone when serum alkaline phosphatase level is at least twice normal and patient is symptomatic or at risk for complications*
TABLETS
Adults. 30 mg daily for 2 mo. Repeated after 2 mo if relapse occurs or if serum alkaline phosphatase level fails to normalize.

➤ *To prevent or treat glucocorticoid-induced osteoporosis*
TABLETS
Adults. 5 mg daily. Or, for postmenopausal osteoporosis, 35 mg once/wk or 75 mg taken on 2 consecutive days once/mo.

➤ *To prevent or treat postmenopausal osteoporosis*
TABLETS
Adults. 5 mg daily. Alternatively, 35 mg once weekly, 75 mg taken on 2 consecutive days once a month, or 150 mg once a month

➤ *To treat osteoporosis in men*
TABLETS
Adults. 35 mg once/wk.

Route	Onset	Peak	Duration
P.O.	Unknown	3 mo	16 mo

Mechanism of Action

Hinders excessive bone remodeling characteristic of Paget's disease by binding to bone and reducing the rate at which osteoclasts are resorbed by bone.

Contraindications
Hypersensitivity to risedronate or its components, hypocalcemia

Interactions
DRUGS
aspirin, NSAIDs: Increased risk of GI irritation
calcium-containing preparations, including antacids: Impaired absorption of risedronate
FOODS
all foods: Decreased risedronate bioavailability

Adverse Reactions
CNS: Anxiety, asthenia, depression, dizziness, fatigue, headache, insomnia, sciatica, syncope, vertigo, weakness
CV: Chest pain, hypercholesterolemia, hypertension, peripheral edema, vasodilation
EENT: Amblyopia, cataract, dry eyes, nasopharyngitis, pharyngitis, rhinitis, sinusitis, tinnitus
GI: Abdominal pain, colitis, constipation, diarrhea, dyspepsia, dysphagia, eructation, esophagitis, esophageal or gastric ulcers, flatulence, gastritis, nausea, vomiting
GU: UTI
MS: Arthralgia; back, limb, neck, or shoulder pain; jaw osteonecrosis; leg cramps or spasms; myasthenia; myalgia; osteoarthritis
RESP: Bronchitis, cough, pneumonia, upper respiratory tract infection
SKIN: Bullous reaction, pruritus, rash
Other: Angioedema, flulike symptoms, hypersensitivity reaction, hypocalcemia

Nursing Considerations
•Give supplemental calcium and vitamin D, as prescribed, during risedronate therapy if patient's dietary intake is inadequate.
•Give calcium supplements and antacids at different time of day than risedronate administration to avoid impaired drug absorption and altered effectiveness.
•Watch for rare but possibly severe rash, bullous skin reactions, and angioedema.
PATIENT TEACHING
•Instruct patient to take risedronate at least 1 hour before first food or drink of day (except water) while in an upright position and with 6 to 8 oz of water. Caution against lying down for at least 30 minutes after taking drug to keep it from lodging in esophagus and causing irritation. Also instruct patient not to chew or suck on tablet because doing so may irritate mouth or throat.
•Advise patient to stop taking risedronate and to notify prescriber if GI symptoms appear or become worse.
•Alert patient that drugs in the same class as risedronate have caused severe bone, joint, or muscle pain. If such symptoms appear while taking risedronate, advise patient to contact prescriber.
•If patient takes 35 mg once weekly and misses a dose, tell her to take it the morning after she remembers and then to take the next dose on its usual day. If patient takes 75 mg on 2 consecutive days once monthly and she misses both doses with more than 7 days until the next scheduled dose, tell her to take the first missed dose on the morning after she remembers and the second dose the following day. If she misses only one of the two doses, tell her to take it the morning after she remembers and then resume her normal schedule. If patient takes 150 mg once monthly and misses a dose, urge her to contact prescriber for instructions. Caution patient not to take more than 150 mg within a 7-day period and not to take two tablets of any strength on the same day.
•Tell patient to take calcium supplements or antacids at different times than risedronate.
•Urge women of childbearing age to tell prescriber about planned, suspected, or known pregnancy because of risk to fetal skeleton.
•Tell patient to stop risedronate and contact prescriber about swelling or skin abnormalities.

risperidone
Risperdal, Risperdal Consta

Class and Category
Chemical class: Benzisoxazole derivative
Therapeutic class: Antipsychotic
Pregnancy category: C

Indications and Dosages
➤ *To manage psychotic disorders*
ORAL SOLUTION, ORALLY DISINTEGRATING TABLETS, TABLETS
Adults. 1 mg b.i.d. on day 1; 2 mg b.i.d. on day 2; 3 mg b.i.d. on day 3. Or, 2 mg daily on day one; 4 mg daily on day two; 6 mg daily on day 3. Then increased by 1 to 2 mg daily

at 1- to 2-wk intervals, as needed. *Maximum:* 16 mg daily.

Adolescents ages 13 to 17. *Initial:* 0.5 mg once daily, increased as needed every 24 hr in 0.5- to 1-mg increments. *Maximum:* 3 mg once daily.

I.M. INJECTION (RISPERDAL CONSTA)
Adults. *Initial:* 25 mg every 2 wk, increased as needed every 4 wk to 37.5 or 50 mg. *Maximum:* 50 mg every 2 wk.

➤ *To treat bipolar mania*
ORAL SOLUTION, ORALLY DISINTEGRATING TABLETS, TABLETS
Adults. *Initial:* 2 or 3 mg daily, increased as needed by 1 mg daily up to 6 mg. Maximum: 6 mg daily for no more than 3 wk.

Children and adolescents ages 10 to 17. *Initial:* 0.5 mg once daily, increased as needed every 24 hr in 0.5- to 1-mg increments. *Maximum:* 2.5 mg once daily.

DOSAGE ADJUSTMENT Initially 0.5 mg b.i.d. for elderly or debilitated patients, those with renal or hepatic impairment, and those at risk for hypotension. Increased by 0.5 mg b.i.d. every wk, as needed. Given daily after target dosage maintained for 2 or 3 days. Maximum for patients with severe hepatic dysfunction, 4 mg daily; for elderly patients, 3 mg daily. Initially 12.5 mg for patients receiving drug I.M. who have renal or hepatic impairment, take other drugs that increase risperidone blood level, or have a history of tolerating psychotropic drugs poorly. For adolescents and children with persistent somnolence, dose may be split and given twice daily.

Mechanism of Action

Selectively blocks serotonin and dopamine receptors in the mesocortical tract of the CNS to suppress psychotic symptoms.

Incompatibilities

Don't mix oral solution with cola or tea.

Contraindications

Hypersensitivity to risperidone or its components

Interactions

DRUGS
antihypertensives: Increased antihypertensive effects

bromocriptine, levodopa, pergolide: Possibly antagonized effects of these drugs
carbamazepine: Increased risperidone clearance with long-term concurrent use
clozapine: Decreased risperidone clearance with long-term concurrent use
CNS depressants: Additive CNS depression
fluoxetine, paroxetine: Increased plasma risperidone level

ACTIVITIES
alcohol use: Additive CNS depression

Adverse Reactions

CNS: Aggressiveness, agitation, akathisia, anxiety, asthenia, confusion, decreased concentration, dizziness, dream disturbances, drowsiness, dyskinesia, dystonia, fatigue, fever, headache, lassitude, memory loss, nervousness, neuroleptic malignant syndrome, parkinsonism, restlessness, seizures, somnolence, tremor
CV: Atrial fibrillation, chest pain, hypercholesterolemia, orthostatic hypotension, palpitations, QT-interval prolongation, tachycardia
EENT: Decreased or increased salivation, dry mouth, pharyngitis, retinal artery occlusion, rhinitis, sinusitis, vision changes
ENDO: Diabetic ketoacidosis (patients with diabetes), elevated prolactin level, galactorrhea, hyperglycemia, pituitary adenoma
GI: Abdominal pain, anorexia, constipation, diarrhea, indigestion, intestinal obstruction, nausea, vomiting
GU: Amenorrhea, decreased libido, dysmenorrhea, dysuria, hypermenorrhea, incontinence, increased appetite, polyuria, sexual dysfunction, UTI
MS: Arthralgia, back pain, myalgia
RESP: Cough, dyspnea, sleep apnea, upper respiratory tract infection
SKIN: Diaphoresis, dry skin, hyperpigmentation, photosensitivity, pruritus, rash, seborrhea
Other: Anaphylaxis, angioedema, injection site induration, pain, redness, or swelling; weight gain or loss

Nursing Considerations

•Use risperidone cautiously in debilitated patients, elderly patients, and patients with hepatic or renal dysfunction or hypotension because of their increased sensitivity to drug. Also use risperidone cautiously in patients with a history of seizures; although rare, seizures may occur in those with schizophrenia.

•**WARNING** Be aware that risperidone should not be used to treat elderly patients with dementia-related psychosis because it increases risk of death in these patients.

•Be aware that oral risperidone or another antipsychotic should be continued for 3 weeks after long-acting I.M. form of risperidone is first administered to provide an adequate therapeutic plasma level until risperidone release from injection site has begun. If the patient has never received oral risperidone, an oral trial should be prescribed before use of I.M. form to determine patient's tolerance of the drug.

•Remove I.M. form of risperidone from refrigerator and allow it to come to room temperature before reconstitution. Follow manufacturer's guidelines for reconstitution, using only the diluent supplied in the dose pack.

•Give I.M. form using only the needle supplied in the dose pack. Inject entire contents of syringe into the upper outer quadrant of gluteal area within 2 minutes of reconstitution. If drug can't be given right after reconstitution, shake the upright vial vigorously back and forth until particles are resuspended. Discard reconstituted drug if not used within 6 hours. Never administer I.M. form intravenously.

•Monitor for orthostatic hypotension, especially in patients with cardiac or cerebrovascular disease.

•**WARNING** Immediately notify prescriber and expect to stop giving risperidone if patient shows evidence of neuroleptic malignant syndrome (altered mental status, autonomic instability, hyperpyrexia, muscle rigidity), which can be fatal.

•Monitor patient's blood glucose and lipid levels as ordered because drug increases the risk of hyperglycemia and hypercholesterolemia.

PATIENT TEACHING

•Instruct patient to dilute risperidone oral solution with water, coffee, orange juice, or low-fat milk but not with cola or tea.

•Tell patient prescribed orally disintegrating tablets to break open the blister unit with dry hands by peeling the foil back to expose the tablet. Stress the importance of not pushing tablet through the foil because this could damage the tablet. Once patient has removed tablet, she should place immediately on her tongue, where it will dissolve within seconds. Tell patient not to chew orally disintegrating tablet or attempt to spit it out of her mouth.

•Urge patient to avoid alcohol because of its additive CNS effects.

•Caution diabetic patient to monitor blood glucose level closely because risperidone may increase it.

rivastigmine tartrate

Exelon, Exelon Patch

Class and Category

Chemical class: Carbamate derivative
Therapeutic class: Antidementia
Pregnancy category: B

Indications and Dosages

➤ *To treat mild to moderate Alzheimer's-type dementia*

CAPSULES, ORAL SOLUTION

Adults. *Initial:* 1.5 mg b.i.d. Dosage increased by 3 mg daily every 2 wk, as needed. *Maximum:* 12 mg daily.

TRANSDERMAL

Adults. *Initial:* 4.6 mg/24 hr. After 4 wk, increased to 9.5 mg/24 hr.

➤ *To treat mild to moderate dementia in Parkinson's disease*

CAPSULES, ORAL SOLUTION

Adults. *Initial:* 1.5 mg b.i.d. Dosage increased by 3 mg daily every 4 wk, as needed. *Maximum:* 12 mg daily.

TRANSDERMAL

Adults. *Initial:* 4.6 mg/24 hr. After 4 wk, increased to 9.5 mg/24 hr.

➤ *To convert patient from oral to transdermal rivastigmine therapy*

TRANSDERMAL

Adults. If total oral dosage was less than 6 mg daily, use 4.6 mg/24 hr, with first transdermal patch applied the day after the last oral dose. If total oral dosage was 6 to 12 mg daily, use 9.5 mg/24 hr, with first transdermal patch applied the day after the last oral dose.

DOSAGE ADJUSTMENT If patient develops adverse effects (such as nausea or vomiting) during oral therapy, treatment should be discontinued for several doses, as prescribed, restarted at lowest dose, and increased by

Q
R
S

3 mg daily every 2 wk, as needed. If patient develops adverse effects during transdermal therapy, treatment should be discontinnued for several days and restarted at same or next lower dose level.

Mechanism of Action

May slow the decline of cognitive function in patients with Alzheimer's disease by increasing acetylcholine concentration at cholinergic transmission sites. This action prolongs and exaggerates the effects of acetylcholine that are otherwise blocked by toxic levels of anticholinergics. The cognitive decline in these patients is partially related to cholinergic deficits along neuronal pathways projecting from the basal forebrain to the cerebral cortex and hippocampus that are involved in memory, attention, learning, and cognition.

Contraindications

Hypersensitivity to carbamate derivatives, rivastigmine, or their components

Interac0tions

DRUGS

anticholinergics: Possibly decreased effectiveness of anticholinergics
bethanechol, succinylcholine: Possibly synergistic effects

Adverse Reactions

CNS: Aggression, anxiety, asthenia, confusion, depression, dizziness, extrapyramidal movements, fatigue, fever, hallucinations, headache, insomnia, malaise, parkinsonism, seizures, somnolence, tremor
CV: Hypertension
EENT: Rhinitis
GI: Abdominal pain, anorexia, constipation, diarrhea, flatulence, indigestion, nausea, vomiting
GU: UTI
SKIN: Increased sweating, reaction at patch application site (pruritus, redness, swelling)
Other: Dehydration, flulike symptoms, weight loss

Nursing Considerations

•WARNING Be aware that rivastigmine should be started at lowest recommended dosage and adjusted to effective maintenance dosage because initial therapy at high dosage can cause serious adverse GI reactions, including anorexia, nausea, and weight loss. Also, higher than recommended starting dosage may cause severe vomiting and possibly esophageal rupture. If treatment is interrupted for longer than several days, expect to restart at lowest recommended dosage.

•Be aware that drug shouldn't be stopped abruptly because doing so may increase behavioral disturbances and precipitate a further decline in cognitive function.

•Monitor respiratory status of patients with pulmonary disease, including asthma, chronic bronchitis, and emphysema, because rivastigmine has a weak affinity for peripheral cholinesterase, which may increase bronchoconstriction and bronchial secretions.

•Monitor patient for adequate urine output because cholinomimetics, such as rivastigmine, may induce or exacerbate urinary tract or bladder obstruction.

•Monitor patients with Parkinson's disease for exaggerated parkinsonian symptoms, which may result from drug's increased cholinergic effects on CNS.

PATIENT TEACHING

•Explain to patient and family that rivastigmine can't cure Alzheimer's or Parkinson's disease but may slow the progressive deterioration of memory and improve patient's ability to perform activities of daily living.

•Teach patient and family how to administer oral solution, if prescribed, emphasizing need to use the oral dosing syringe provided. Explain that dose may be swallowed directly from the syringe or mixed into a small glass of water, cold fruit juice, or soda; stirred; and then drunk.

•Explain that oral drug should be taken with food to reduce adverse GI effects.

•For transdermal patch, instruct patient or caregiver to apply it to clean, dry, hairless, intact skin in a location, such as the back, that won't be rubbed by tight clothing and won't be affected by lotion, cream, or powder. Tell patient to remove the old patch before applying a new one and to use a new application site daily. Caution against using the same site within 14 days.

•To apply transdermal patch, tell patient to press patch firmly against skin until the edges stick well. Reassure patient that patch may be worn while swimming or bathing.

•Instruct a family member to supervise pa-

tient's use of rivastigmine.
•Urge caregiver to contact prescriber and to withhold drug if patient stops taking it for more than several days.

rizatriptan benzoate

Maxalt, Maxalt-MLT

Class and Category

Chemical class: Selective 5-hydroxytrypta-mine
Therapeutic class: Antimigraine
Pregnancy category: C

Indications and Dosages

➤ *To relieve acute migraine headache*
DISINTEGRATING TABLETS, TABLETS
Adults. 5 to 10 mg when migraine headache starts; repeated every 2 hr, p.r.n. *Maximum:* 30 mg daily.
DOSAGE ADJUSTMENT For patients taking propranolol, initial dosage reduced to 5 mg, then repeated every 2 hr, p.r.n., up to maximum of 15 mg daily.

Mechanism of Action

Binds to selective 5-hydroxytryptamine receptor sites on cerebral blood vessels, causing vessels to constrict. This may decrease the characteristic pulsing sensation and thus relieve the pain of migraine headaches. Rizatriptan also may relieve pain by inhibiting the release of proinflammatory neuropeptides and reducing transmission of trigeminal nerve impulses from sensory nerve endings during a migraine attack.

Contraindications

Basilar or hemiplegic migraine, hypersensitivity to rizatriptan or its components, ischemic coronary artery disease, uncontrolled hypertension, use within 14 days of MAO inhibitor therapy, use within 24 hours of other serotonin-receptor agonists or ergotamine-containing or ergot-type drugs

Interactions

DRUGS
ergot-containing drugs: Prolonged vasospastic reactions

MAO inhibitors, propranolol: Increased blood rizatriptan level
selective serotonin-reuptake inhibitors: Increased risk of weakness, hyperreflexia, and lack of coordination
serotonin-receptor agonists: Additive vasospastic effects

Adverse Reactions

CNS: Altered temperature sensation, anxiety, asthenia, ataxia, chills, confusion, depression, disorientation, dizziness, dream disturbances, drowsiness, euphoria, fatigue, hangover, headache, hypoesthesia, insomnia, mental impairment, nervousness, paresthesia, somnolence, tremor, vertigo
CV: Arrhythmias, such as bradycardia and tachycardia; chest pain; hot flashes; hypertension; palpitations
EENT: Blurred vision; burning eyes; dry eyes, mouth, and throat; earache; eye pain or irritation; lacrimation; nasal congestion and irritation; pharyngeal edema; pharyngitis; tinnitus; tongue swelling
GI: Abdominal distention, constipation, diarrhea, dysphagia, flatulence, heartburn, indigestion, nausea, thirst, vomiting
GU: Menstrual irregularities, polyuria, urinary frequency
MS: Arthralgia; dysarthria; muscle spasms, stiffness, or weakness; myalgia
RESP: Dyspnea, upper respiratory tract infection, wheezing
SKIN: Diaphoresis, flushing, pruritus, rash, urticaria
Other: Angioedema, dehydration, facial edema

Nursing Considerations

•Use rizatriptan cautiously in patients with renal or hepatic dysfunction because of impaired drug metabolism or excretion. Monitor patient's BUN and serum creatinine levels and liver function test results, as appropriate.
•Also use cautiously in patients with peripheral vascular disease because drug may cause vasospastic reactions, leading to vascular and colonic ischemia with abdominal pain and bloody diarrhea. Assess peripheral circulation and bowel sounds frequently during therapy.
•Assess patient's cardiovascular status and institute continuous ECG monitoring, as ordered, immediately after giving rizatriptan in

patients with cardiovascular risk factors because of possible asymptomatic cardiac ischemia.

•Monitor blood pressure regularly in patients with hypertension because rizatriptan may increase blood pressure.

PATIENT TEACHING

•Instruct patient taking rizatriptan disintegrating tablets to remove tablet from blister pack with dry hands just before taking, to place tablet on tongue, and to allow it to dissolve and be swallowed with saliva.

•Advise phenylketonuric patient not to use disintegrating tablet form because it contains phenylalanine.

•Instruct patient to seek emergency care immediately if cardiac symptoms, such as chest pain, occur after administration.

•Caution patient about possible adverse CNS reactions, and advise her to avoid potentially hazardous activities until drug's CNS effects are known.

romiplostim

Nplate

Class and Category

Chemical class: Fc-peptide fusion protein
Therapeutic class: Platelet production enhancer
Pregnancy category: C

Indications and Dosages

➤ *To treat thrombocytopenia in patients with chronic immune (idiopathic) thrombocytopenic purpura (ITP) who have had an insufficient response to corticosteroids, immunoglobulins, or splenectomy*

SUBCUTANEOUS INJECTION

Adults. *Initial:* 1 mcg/kg based on actual body weight, followed by weekly doses adjusted in increments of 1 mcg/kg to keep platelet count at or above 50×10^9/L. *Maximum:* 10 mcg/kg weekly.

DOSAGE ADJUSTMENT If platelet count is less than 50×10^9/L, dosage increased by 1 mcg/kg. If platelet count exceeds 200×10^9/L for 2 consecutive weeks, dosage reduced by 1 mcg/kg. If platelet count exceeds 400×10^9/L, dose held until count has fallen to less than 200×10^9/L and then resumed at a weekly dosage reduced by 1 mcg/kg.

Route	Onset	Peak	Duration
SubQ	Unknown	7 to 50 hr	Unknown

Mechanism of Action

Increases platelet production by binding and activating the thrombopoietin receptor in the same manner as endogenous thrombopoietin to prevent bleeding.

Contraindications

Hypersensitivity to romiplostim or its components

Adverse Reactions

CNS: Dizziness, headache, insomnia, paresthesia
CV: Thrombosis
GI: Abdominal pain, dyspepsia
HEME: Bone marrow reticulin deposition
MS: Arthralgia, extremity or shoulder pain, myalgia
Other: Antibody formation to romiplostim

Nursing Considerations

•Be aware that romiplostim can only be administered by prescribers or healthcare providers under their direction who are enrolled in the romiplostim NEXUS program.

•Know that romiplostim therapy is used to reduce the risk of bleeding and not as a therapy to normalize platelet counts.

•Be aware that romiplostim may increase patient's risk for hematologic malignancies.

•Obtain a CBC, including platelet count and peripheral blood smears, before starting therapy, weekly until dosage is stable, monthly throughout therapy, and for at least 2 weeks after stopping therapy, as ordered.

•Expect dosage to be adjusted based on weekly platelet count response.

•Reconstitute drug using only preservative-free sterile water for injection, adding 0.72 ml to 250-mcg vial or 1.2 ml to 500-mcg vial. Gently swirl and invert vial to dissolve powder, which normally occurs within 2 minutes. Don't shake or agitate vigorously. Protect reconstituted drug from light.

•To determine amount of reconstituted drug to administer, first identify patient's total dose in micrograms based on actual body weight. For example, a patient starting therapy at 1 mcg/kg who weighs 75 kg will receive 75 mcg. Then, divide ordered microgram dose by concentration of reconstituted drug solution (500 mcg/ml). For example, a 75-mcg dose divided by 500 mcg/ml will result in 0.15 ml of drug being administered. Discard any unused portion, and don't administer more than one dose from a vial because reconstituted drug can only be stored 24 hours, and drug is given only weekly.

• Administer drug using a syringe that contains 0.01-ml graduations to ensure accurate dosage because volume to be administered may be quite small.

• Be aware that drug may be administered with other ITP therapies, such as corticosteroids, danazol, azathioprine, I.V. immunoglobulin and anti-D immunoglobulin.

• Expect therapy to be discontinued after 4 weeks at maximum dosage if platelet count doesn't increase enough to prevent serious bleeding or if patient develops new or worsening abnormalities or cytopenias.

• Monitor patient closely for bleeding after drug has been discontinued because thromboyctopenia may occur at greater severity than when therapy was started.

PATIENT TEACHING

• Inform patient about increased risk of hematologic malignancies before starting romiplostim therapy.

• Stress importance of weekly blood tests to ensure accurate dosing and early detection of serious blood adverse reactions.

• Urge patient to take precautions to prevent bleeding and to avoid aspirin, NSAIDs, and other drugs that may increase bleeding risk.

• Instruct patient to seek emergency care immediately if unusual signs and symptoms occur that suggest a blood clot, such as shortness of breath, anxiety, change in skin color or mental status, or development of abnormal sensory or motor function.

• When therapy ends, warn patient to report any serious or prolonged bleeding episodes because additional therapy may be needed to control bleeding.

ropinirole hydrochloride

Requip

Class and Category

Chemical class: Non-ergot alkaloid dopamine agonist

Therapeutic class: Antidyskinetic
Pregnancy category: C

Indications and Dosages

➤ *To treat signs and symptoms of Parkinson's disease*

TABLETS

Adults. *Initial:* 0.25 mg t.i.d. Dosage titrated upward every wk according to the following schedule: 0.25 mg t.i.d. in wk 1; 0.5 mg t.i.d. in wk 2; 0.75 mg t.i.d. in wk 3; 1 mg t.i.d. in wk 4. After wk 4, dosage increased by 1.5 mg daily every wk up to 9 mg daily, then by 3 mg/day up to 24 mg daily. *Maximum:* 24 mg/day.

➤ *To treat moderate to severe primary restless legs syndrome*

TABLETS

Adults. *Initial:* 0.25 mg 1 to 3 hr before bedtime. Dosage increased after 2 days to 0.5 mg and then to 1 mg at the end of the first wk. If needed, dosage further increased in 0.5-mg increments every wk. *Maximum:* 4 mg daily.

Mechanism of Action

Directly stimulates postsynaptic dopamine type 2 (D_2) receptors within the brain and acts as an agonist at peripheral D_2 receptors. These actions inhibit the firing of striatal cholinergic neurons, thus helping to control alterations in voluntary muscle movement (such as tremors and rigidity) associated with Parkinson's disease.

Contraindications

Hypersensitivity to ropinirole or its components

Interactions

DRUGS

carbamazepine, cimetidine, ciprofloxacin, clarithromycin, diltiazem, enoxacin, erythromycin, fluvoxamine, mexiletine, norfloxacin, omeprazole, phenobarbital, phenytoin, rifampin, ritonavir, troleandomycin: Altered drug clearance and increased blood level of ropinirole

chlorprothixene, domperidone, droperidol, haloperidol, metoclopramide, phenothiazines, thiothixene: Possibly decreased effectiveness of ropinirole

CNS depressants: Additive effects

Q
R
S

ethinyl estradiol: Possibly reduced clearance of ropinirole

ACTIVITIES
alcohol use: Additive effects

Adverse Reactions
CNS: Asthenia, confusion, dizziness, falling asleep during activities of daily living, fatigue, hallucinations, headache, hypoesthesia, malaise, neuralgia, paresthesia, rigors, somnolence, syncope, transient ischemic attack, vertigo
CV: Acute coronary syndrome, angina, bradycardia, cardiac failure, chest pain, hypertension, MI, orthostatic hypotension, palpitations, peripheral edema, sick sinus syndrome, tachycardia
EENT: Abnormal vision, dry mouth, nasal congestion, nasopharyngitis, rhinitis, toothache
GI: Abdominal pain, constipation, diarrhea, dyspepsia, gastric hemorrhage, gastroenteritis, indigestion, intestinal obstruction, ischemic hepatitis, nausea, pancreatitis, vomiting
GU: Elevated BUN level, erectile dysfunction, UTI
HEME: Anemia
MS: Arthralgia; arthritis; exacerbation of restless leg syndrome in the early-morning hours; limb pain; muscle cramps, spasms, or stiffness; myalgia; neck pain; osteoarthritis; tendinitis
RESP: Asthma, bronchitis, cough, upper respiratory tract infection
SKIN: Diaphoresis, flushing, hot flashes, night sweats, rash
Other: Influenza, viral infection, weight loss

Nursing Considerations
•WARNING Expect to reassess patient for excessive sedation periodically during therapy. Excessive, acute drowsiness may arise as late as 1 year after starting therapy.
•When ropinirole is given as adjunct to levodopa, expect concurrent dosage of levodopa to be gradually decreased as tolerated.
•Expect to stop ropinirole gradually over 7 days, as follows: over first 4 days, reduce from t.i.d to b.i.d.; during last 3 days, reduce to once daily, followed by complete withdrawal of drug.
•WARNING Watch for altered mental status during drug withdrawal. Rapid dose reduction may lead to a symptom complex resembling neuroleptic malignant syndrome that

includes fever, muscle rigidity, altered level of consciousness, and autonomic instability.
•Watch for orthostatic hypotension, especially in patient with early Parkinson's disease. Orthostatic hypotension can occur more than 4 weeks after start of therapy or after a dosage reduction because ropinirole may impair systemic regulation of blood pressure.
•Monitor patient for hallucinations, especially if patient has Parkinson's disease, is elderly, or takes levodopa.
•Monitor patient for worsening of preexisting dyskinesia; ropinirole may potentiate dopaminergic adverse effects of levodopa.
•Avoid giving CNS depressants, sleep aids, and other CNS-interacting drugs during ropinirole therapy because they increase the risk of somnolence.

PATIENT TEACHING
•Inform patient with Parkinson's disease that ropinirole helps to improve muscle control and movement but doesn't cure Parkinson's disease.
•Encourage patient to take ropinirole with food to decrease risk of adverse GI effects.
•Caution patient to avoid hazardous activities until CNS effects of drug—including sedation—are known.
•If patient falls asleep during normal activities, advise her to notify prescriber.
•Urge patient to avoid consuming alcohol and other sedating drugs (such as sleep aids) during ropinirole therapy because they may increase the drug's CNS depressant effects.
•If patient has restless legs syndrome, explain that symptoms might appear in early morning during ropinirole therapy and could be worse or spread to other limbs. Urge patient to notify prescriber if this occurs.
•Instruct patient to change positions slowly to minimize effect on blood pressure.

rosiglitazone maleate

Avandia

Class and Category
Chemical class: Thiazolidinedione
Therapeutic class: Antidiabetic drug
Pregnancy category: C

Indications and Dosages
➤ *To achieve glucose control in type 2 diabetes mellitus as monotherapy or in*

combination with metformin
TABLETS
Adults. *Initial:* 4 mg once daily or 2 mg
b.i.d., increased to 8 mg once daily or 4 mg
b.i.d. if glucose control is inadequate after
12 wk. *Maximum:* 8 mg daily.
➤ *To achieve glucose control in type 2 dia-*
betes mellitus in combination with in-
sulin therapy
TABLETS
Adults. 4 mg daily with no change in insulin
dosage. Insulin dosage decreased by 10% to
25% if hypoglycemia occurs or fasting
plasma concentrations decrease to less than
100 mg/dl with combination therapy.

Mechanism of Action
Increases tissue sensitivity to insulin. This
peroxisome proliferator-activated receptor
agonist regulates the transcription of insulin-
responsive genes found in key target tissues, such as adipose tissue, skeletal muscle, and the liver. Enhanced tissue sensitivity to insulin lowers the blood glucose
level.

Contraindications
Hypersensitivity to rosiglitazone or its com-
ponents, New York Heart Association
(NYHA) class III or IV heart failure

Interactions
DRUGS
CYP2C8 inducers, such as rifampin: Possibly
decreased effects of rosiglitazone
CYP2C8 inhibitors, such as gemfibrozil: Pos-
sibly increased effects of rosiglitazone

Adverse Reactions
CNS: Fatigue, headache
CV: Angina, congestive heart failure, edema,
hypertension, myocardial ischemia or infarc-
tion
EENT: Blurred vision, decreased visual acu-
ity, macular edema, nasopharyngitis, sinusitis
ENDO: Hyperglycemia, hypoglycemia
GI: Diarrhea, elevated liver enzymes, hepato-
toxicity
HEME: Anemia
MS: Arthralgia, back pain, fracture (women)
RESP: Dyspnea, upper respiratory tract in-
fection
SKIN: Pruritus, rash, Stevens-Johnson syn-
drome, urticaria
Other: Anaphylaxis, angioedema, weight gain

Nursing Considerations
•Give rosiglitazone cautiously in patients
with edema, heart failure, or hepatic impairment because of potential adverse reactions.
•Be aware that drug isn't recommended for
patients with symptomatic heart failure.
•Evaluate patient's liver function before
starting drug and periodically throughout
therapy, as ordered. Notify prescriber about
abnormalities, such as nausea, vomiting, abdominal pain, fatigue, anorexia, and dark
urine. Drug may need to be stopped.
•**WARNING** Monitor patient for evidence of
congestive heart failure—such as shortness of
breath, rapid weight gain, or edema—because rosiglitazone can cause fluid retention
that may lead to or worsen heart failure. Notify prescriber immediately if the patient's
cardiac status deteriorates, and expect to
stop the drug, as ordered.
•Monitor fasting glucose and glycosylated
hemoglobin A_{1c} levels periodically, as ordered, to evaluate rosiglitazone effectiveness.
•Be aware that drug is effective only in the
presence of endogenous insulin.
PATIENT TEACHING
•Stress the need to follow an exercise program and a diet control program during
rosiglitazone therapy.
•Advise patient to notify prescriber immediately if she has shortness of breath, fluid retention, or sudden weight gain because drug
may need to be discontinued.
•Instruct patient to have liver function tests,
as prescribed, about every 2 months for first
year and then annually.
•Inform premenopausal, anovulatory patient
that drug may induce ovulation, increasing
risk of pregnancy.
•Urge women to take precautions against
falling; drug increases risk of fractures.

rosuvastatin calcium

Crestor

Class and Category
Chemical class: HMG-CoA reductase
inhibitor
Therapeutic class: Antihyperlipidemic
Pregnancy category: X

Indications and Dosages

➤ *To treat hyperlipidemia, mixed dyslipidemia, hypertriglyceridemia, and primary dysbetalipoproteinemia (Type III hyperlipoproteinemia); to slow the progression of atherosclerosis*

TABLETS

Adults with LDL-C level of 190 mg/dl or below. *Initial:* 10 mg daily, increased every 2 to 4 wk, as needed. *Maximum:* 40 mg daily.

Adults with LDL-C level greater than 190 mg/dl. *Initial:* 20 mg daily, increased every 2 to 4 wk, as needed. *Maximum:* 40 mg daily.

➤ *To treat homozygous familial hypercholesterolemia*

TABLETS

Adults. *Initial:* 20 mg daily, increased every 2 to 4 wk, as needed. *Maximum:* 40 mg daily.

DOSAGE ADJUSTMENT For patients taking cyclosporine, dosage shouldn't exceed 5 mg daily; for Asian patients, initial dosage should be limited to 5 mg daily; for patients taking gemfibrozil or combined lopinavir and ritonavir, 10 mg daily; for patients with severe renal impairment (creatinine clearance greater than 30 ml/min/1.73 m²) who are not undergoing hemodialysis, dosage should start at 5 mg daily but not exceed 10 mg daily; for patients taking niacin or fenofbrate, dosage reduction should be considered.

Route	Onset	Peak	Duration
P.O.	Unknown	3 to 5 hr	Unknown

Mechanism of Action

Cholesterol and triglycerides circulate in the blood as part of lipoprotein complexes. Rosuvastatin inhibits the enzyme 3-hydroxy-3-methylglutaryl-coenzyme A (HMG-CoA) reductase. This inhibition reduces lipid levels by increasing the number of hepatic low-density-lipoprotein (LDL) receptors on the cell surface to increase uptake and catabolism of LDL. It also inhibits hepatic synthesis of very-low-density lipoprotein (VLDL), which decreases the total number of VLDL and LDL particles.

Contraindications

Active liver disease, breast-feeding, hypersensitivity to rosuvastatin or its components, pregnancy, unexplained persistent elevations of serum transaminase levels

Interactions

DRUGS

antacids: Decreased blood rosuvastatin level if given within 2 hours of rosuvastatin

cyclosporine, gemfibrozil, lopinavir/ritonavir, niacin, other lipid-lowering drugs: Increased blood rosuvastatin level and risk of myopathy

oral contraceptives: Increased blood ethinyl estradiol and norgestrel levels

warfarin: Increased INR

Adverse Reactions

CNS: Asthenia, depression, dizziness, headache, hypertonia, insomnia, memory loss, paresthesia

CV: Chest pain, hypertension, peripheral edema

EENT: Pharyngitis, rhinitis, sinusitis

ENDO: Thyroid function abnormalities

GI: Abdominal pain, constipation, diarrhea, elevated liver function test results, gastroenteritis, hepatitis, jaundice, nausea, pancreatitis

GU: Acute renal failure, proteinuria, UTI

MS: Arthralgia, arthritis, back pain, myalgia, myopathy, rhabdomyolysis

RESP: Bronchitis, increased cough

SKIN: Rash, urticaria

Other: Angioedema, flulike symptoms, generalized pain, infection

Nursing Considerations

• Use rosuvastatin cautiously in patients who consume large quantities of alcohol or have a history of liver disease because drug is contraindicated in patients with active liver disease or unexplained persistent elevations of transaminase levels.

• Also use cautiously in patients with risk factors for myopathy, such as renal impairment, advanced age, and hypothyroidism.

• Obtain baseline liver function test results and expect to monitor them every 3 months for abnormal elevations. Notify prescriber if elevations occur. If ALT or AST levels increase to more than three times the normal range, expect dosage to be reduced or drug discontinued.

• Monitor serum lipoprotein levels, as ordered, to evaluate patient's response to therapy.

•Expect rosuvastatin to be temporarily withheld if patient develops any condition that may be related to myopathy or that predisposes her to renal failure, such as sepsis, hypotension, major surgery, trauma, uncontrolled seizures, or severe metabolic, endocrine, or electrolyte disorders.
•Notify prescriber if proteinuria or hematuria appears on patient's routine urinalysis because rosuvastatin dosage may need to be reduced.

PATIENT TEACHING
•Encourage patient to follow a low-fat, low-cholesterol diet.
•Tell patient to wait at least 2 hours after taking rosuvastatin before taking antacids.
•Instruct patient to notify prescriber immediately about muscle pain, tenderness, or weakness, especially if accompanied by malaise or fever.
•Tell woman of childbearing age about the need to use reliable contraceptive method while taking drug. Instruct her to notify prescriber at once if she suspects she may be pregnant.

rufinamide

Banzel

Class and Category
Chemical class: Triazole derivative
Therapeutic class: Anticonvulsant
Pregnancy category: C

Indications and Dosages
➤ *As adjunct treatment of seizures associated with Lennox-Gastaut syndrome*

TABLETS
Adults. *Initial:* 200 to 400 mg b.i.d., increased in daily increments of 200 to 400 mg b.i.d. every 2 days until reaching 1,600 mg b.i.d. *Maximum:* 1,600 mg b.i.d.
Children age 4 and over. *Initial:* 5 mg/kg b.i.d., increased in daily increments of 5 mg/kg b.i.d. every 2 days until reaching 22.5 mg/kg b.i.d. or 1600 mg b.i.d., whichever is less.
DOSAGE ADJUSTMENT For patients undergoing dialysis, dosage may need to be increased. For patients also receiving valproate, initial dosage reduced to less than 400 mg daily.

Route	Onset	Peak	Duration
P.O.	Unknown	4 to 6 hr	Unknown

Mechanism of Action
Unknown, although rufinamide is known to slow sodium channel recovery from inactivation after a prolonged prepulse and to limit repetitive firing of sodium-dependent action potentials in neurons in the brain. These actions may help to limit seizure activity.

Contraindications
Familial short-QT syndrome, hypersensitivity to rufinamide or its components

Interactions
DRUGS
contraceptives containing ethinyl estradiol and norethindrone: Decreased effectiveness of the oral contraceptive
phenytoin: Increased plasma phenytoin level and risk of adverse reactions
valproate: Increased plasma rufinamide level and risk of adverse reactions
ACTIVITIES
alcohol use: Increased CNS effects

Adverse Reactions
CNS: Aggression, anxiety, ataxia, attention disturbance, dizziness, fatigue, headache, hyperactivity, seizures, somnolence, status epilepticus, suicidal ideation, tremor, vertigo
CV: First-degree AV block, right bundle branch block
EENT: Sinusitis
ENDO: Blurred vision, diplopia, nasopharyngitis, nystagmus
GI: Abdominal pain, anorexia, constipation, dyspepsia, nausea, vomiting
GU: Dysuria, enuresis, hematuria, incontinence, nephrolithiasis, pollakiuria, polyuria
HEME: Anemia, leukopenia, lymphadenopathy, neutropenia, thrombocytopenia
MS: Back pain
RESP: Bronchitis
SKIN: Pruritus, rash
Other: Multi-organ hypersensitivity

Nursing Considerations
•Administer rufinamide with food because absorption is increased.
•Monitor patient's QT interval regularly, as ordered, because rufinamide may shorten the QT interval and possibly predispose patient to ventricular fibrillation if the interval falls

Q
R
S

below 300 msec.

•**WARNING** Watch closely for multi-organ hypersensitivity, especially if patient develops a rash. Although uncommon, it may cause serious adverse effects, such as urticaria, facial edema, fever, elevated eosinophils or liver enzymes, hematuria, stupor, lymphadenopathy and severe hepatitis, in addition to rash. Notify prescriber immediately if such changes appear, and expect to discontinue drug and provide supportive care.

•Watch closely for suicidal tendencies, especially when therapy starts and dosage changes and particularly in children and adolescents.

•When therapy is stopped, expect to taper dosage to minimize adverse effects rather than stopping drug abruptly.

PATIENT TEACHING
•Make sure patient receives medication guide describing drug use and possible suicidal tendencies.

•Instruct patient to take drug exactly as prescribed and to take each dose with food. If patient has trouble swallowing tablets, tell him they may be crushed.

•Inform woman that rufinamide decreases effectiveness of contraceptives containing ethinyl estradiol and norethindrone. Tell her to use a different contraceptive during therapy and to contact prescriber immediately if she thinks she's pregnant.

•Tell patient to report a rash accompanied by fever or other symptoms immediately.

•Warn family or caregiver to watch patient for suicidal tendencies, especially when therapy starts or dosage changes, and particularly if patient is a child or adolescent.

•Advise patient to avoid hazardous activities until drug's CNS effects are known.

•Caution patient not to stop taking drug abruptly. Explain that gradual tapering helps to avoid withdrawal symptoms.

•Explain that alcohol consumption may intensify drug effects.

salmeterol xinafoate

Serevent Diskus

Class and Category
Chemical class: Sympathomimetic amine
Therapeutic class: Bronchodilator
Pregnancy category: C

Indications and Dosages
➤ *To prevent asthma-induced bronchospasm*
ORAL INHALATION POWDER
Adults and children age 4 and over. 1 inhalation (50 mcg) every 12 hr.

➤ *To prevent COPD-induced bronchospasm*
ORAL INHALATION POWDER
Adults. 1 inhalation (50 mcg) every 12 hr.

➤ *To prevent exercise-induced bronchospasm*
ORAL INHALATION POWDER
Adults and children age 4 and over. 1 inhalation (50 mcg) at least 30 min before exercise.

Route	Onset	Peak	Duration
Inhalation	10 to 20 min	3 to 4 hr	12 hr

Mechanism of Action
Attaches to beta$_2$ receptors on bronchial cell membranes, stimulating the intracellular enzyme adenylate cyclase to convert adenosine triphosphate to cAMP. The resulting increase in the intracellular cAMP level relaxes bronchial smooth-muscle cells, stabilizes mast cells, and inhibits histamine release.

Contraindications
Hypersensitivity to salmeterol or its components

Interactions
DRUGS
atazanavir, clarithromycin, indinavir, itraconazole, ketoconazole, nefazodone, nelfinavir, ritonavir, saquinavir, telithromycin: Possibly increased risk of adverse cardiovascular effects
beta blockers: Mutual inhibition of therapeutic effects
loop or thiazide diuretics: Increased risk of hypokalemia and potentially life-threatening arrhythmias
MAO inhibitors, tricyclic antidepressants: Potentiated adverse vascular effects, such as hypertensive crisis

Adverse Reactions
CNS: Dizziness, fever, headache, nervous-

ness, paresthesia, tremor
CV: Palpitations, tachycardia
EENT: Dry mouth, nose, and throat; sinus problems
GI: Nausea
MS: Arthralgia
RESP: Cough, paradoxical bronchospasm
SKIN: Contact dermatitis, eczema, rash, urticaria
Other: Angioedema, generalized aches and pains

Nursing Considerations
•Be aware that salmeterol shouldn't be used to relieve bronchospasm quickly because of its prolonged onset of action and that patients already taking drug twice daily shouldn't take additional doses for exercise-induced bronchospasm.
•**WARNING** Be aware that a recent study suggests that asthma-related deaths may increase in asthmatics receiving salmeterol. Monitor this patient population closely throughout salmeterol therapy, and notify prescriber immediately of any changes in patient's respiratory status.
•Watch for arrhythmias and changes in blood pressure after use in patients with cardiovascular disorders, including ischemic cardiac disease, hypertension, and arrhythmias, because of drug's beta-adrenergic effects.
•Be aware that Serevent Diskus delivers full dose of salmeterol in only one inhalation.
•**WARNING** Stop salmeterol immediately and notify prescriber if patient develops paradoxical bronchospasm. Risk is greatest with first use of a new canister or vial used as an inhalant.
PATIENT TEACHING
•Advise patient who is using salmeterol to prevent asthma-induced bronchospasm to take doses 12 hours apart for optimum effect. Caution against using drug more than every 12 hours.
•Teach patient how to use the diskus by instructing him to slide the lever only once when preparing dose to avoid wasting doses. Advise him to exhale immediately before using the diskus and then to place mouthpiece to his lips and inhale through his mouth, not his nose. Then he should remove mouthpiece from his mouth, hold his breath for at least 10 seconds, and exhale slowly.
•Advise patient to rinse mouth with water after each dose to minimize dry mouth.
•Advise patient to discard diskus 6 weeks after removing it from overwrap or when dose indicator reads zero.
•Instruct patient to notify prescriber if he needs four or more oral inhalations of rapid-acting inhaled bronchodilator a day for 2 or more consecutive days, or if he uses more than one canister of rapid-acting bronchodilator in an 8-week period.
•Caution patient not to use other drugs to treat his underlying respiratory condition without consulting prescriber and to let all prescribers know that he takes salmeterol.

salsalate
(salicylsalicylic acid)

Amigesic, Anaflex 750, Argesic-SA, Disalcid, Marthritic, Mono-Gesic, Salflex, Salsitab

Class and Category
Chemical class: Salicylic acid ester
Therapeutic class: Analgesic, anti-inflammatory
Pregnancy category: C

Indications and Dosages
➤ *To relieve symptoms of rheumatoid arthritis and related rheumatic disorders*
CAPSULES
Adults and adolescents. *Initial:* 1 g t.i.d.; dosage then titrated, as needed.
TABLETS
Adults and adolescents. *Initial:* 0.5 to 1 g b.i.d. or t.i.d.; dosage then titrated, as needed.

Route	Onset	Peak	Duration
P.O.	Unknown	2 to 3 wk	Unknown

Mechanism of Action
Exerts peripherally induced analgesic and anti-inflammatory effects by blocking pain impulses and inhibiting prostaglandin synthesis.

Contraindications
Bleeding disorders; hypersensitivity to NSAIDs, salicylates, or their components

Interactions
DRUGS
acetaminophen: Increased risk of renal dys-

function with prolonged use of both drugs
anticoagulants, thrombolytics: Increased risk
and severity of GI bleeding
antiemetics: Masked symptoms of salicylate-
induced ototoxicity
bismuth subsalicylate: Increased risk of salicylate toxicity with large doses of salsalate
*cefamandole, cefoperazone, cefotetan, plate-
let aggregation inhibitors, plicamycin, valproic acid:* Possibly hypoprothrombinemia
corticosteroids: Possibly decreased blood salsalate level; additive therapeutic effects
when both drugs are used to treat arthritis
furosemide: Increased risk of ototoxicity and
salicylate toxicity
hydantoins: Possibly decreased hydantoin
metabolism, leading to toxicity
insulin, oral antidiabetic drugs: Potentiated
hypoglycemic effect
laxatives (cellulose-containing): Possibly reduced salsalate effectiveness due to impaired
absorption
methotrexate: Increased risk of methotrexate
toxicity
NSAIDs: Increased risk of adverse GI effects
ototoxic drugs, vancomycin: Increased risk of
ototoxicity
probenecid, sulfinpyrazone: Decreased uricosuric effects
topical salicylic acid, other salicylates: Increased risk of salicylate toxicity if significant quantities are absorbed
*urinary acidifiers (ammonium chloride,
ascorbic acid, potassium or sodium phosphates):* Decreased salicylate excretion, possibly leading to salicylate toxicity
*urinary alkalizers (antacids [long-term high-
dose use], carbonic anhydrase inhibitors, citrates, sodium bicarbonate):* Increased salicylate excretion, leading to reduced effectiveness and shortened half-life; increased risk
of salicylate toxicity with carbonic anhydrase inhibitor–induced metabolic acidosis
vitamin K: Increased vitamin K requirements
ACTIVITIES
alcohol use: Increased risk of GI bleeding

Adverse Reactions

CNS: CNS depression, confusion, dizziness,
drowsiness, fever, headache, lassitude
EENT: Hearing loss, tinnitus, vision changes
GI: Anorexia, diarrhea, epigastric discomfort, GI bleeding, heartburn, hepatotoxicity,
indigestion, nausea, thirst, vomiting

HEME: Hemolytic anemia, leukopenia, pro-
longed bleeding time, thrombocytopenia
SKIN: Diaphoresis, purpura, rash, urticaria
Other: Angioedema, Reye's syndrome

Nursing Considerations

•Avoid using salsalate in patients with hypoprothrombinemia or vitamin K deficiency
because drug's hypoprothrombinemic effect
may precipitate bleeding.
•Monitor hepatic and renal function, as appropriate, during long-term salsalate therapy.
•Assess for signs and symptoms of GI bleeding, such as abdominal pain or black, tarry
stools, especially in patient with peptic ulcer
disease.
•Assess for symptoms of ototoxicity, such as
ringing or roaring in ears.
PATIENT TEACHING
•Instruct patient to take salsalate with food
or a full glass of water and to remain upright for 1 hour after administration to prevent drug from lodging in esophagus and
causing irritation.
•Inform patient that therapeutic response
may not occur for 2 to 3 weeks.
•Urge patient to notify prescriber immediately of abdominal pain or black, tarry
stools; these symptoms may indicate GI
bleeding or drug toxicity.

sapropterin dihydrochloride

Kuvan

Class and Category

Chemical class: Synthetic tetrahydro-
biopterin salt
Therapeutic class: Phenylalanine reducer
Pregnancy category: C

Indications and Dosages

➤ *To reduce blood phenylalanine level in
patients with hyperphenylalaninemia
from tetrahydrobiopterin-responsive
phenylketonuria, with phenylalanine-
restricted diet*
TABLETS
Adults and children age 4 and over. *Initial:*
10 mg/kg daily with dosage increased or decreased after 1 wk based on response and
then periodically adjusted, as needed. Expect

to discontinue drug if levels fail to increase after 1 mo of therapy at 20 mg/kg/day. *Maintenance:* 5 to 20 mg/kg daily. *Maximum:* 20 mg/kg daily.

Mechanism of Action
As a synthetic form of tetrahydro-biopterin, the cofactor of the enzyme phenylalanine hydroxylase (PAH), sapropterin hydroxylates phenylalanine to form tyrosine. This improves the oxidative metabolism of phenylalanine, which decreases blood phenylalanine.

Contraindications
Hypersensitivity to sapropterin or its components

Interactions
DRUGS
folate metabolism inhibitors, such as methotrexate: Possibly decreased effectiveness of sapropterin
levodopa: Possibly increased risk of irritability, over stimulation or seizures
sildenafil, tadalafil, vardenafil: Possibly additive vasorelaxation effect leading to hypotension

Adverse Reactions
CNS: Agitation, dizziness, fever, headache, irritability, over stimulation, seizures
CV: MI, peripheral edema
EENT: Nasal congestion, pharyngolaryngeal pain, rhinorrhea
GI: Abdominal pain, diarrhea, elevated liver enzymes, gastrointestinal bleeding, nausea, vomiting
GU: Polyurina
HEME: Bleeding, neutropenia
MS: Arthralgia
RESP: Cough, respiratory failure, upper respiratory infection
SKIN: Rash

Nursing Considerations
• Use cautiously in patients with hepatic impairment because impaired phenylalanine metabolism may be linked to hepatic damage.
• Administer drug at the same time each day.
• Dissolve tablets in 4 to 8 ounces of water or apple juice, which may take a few minutes.

Stirring or crushing tablets will hasten process. Know that tablets may not dissolve completely. Administer solution within 15 minutes with food. If there are particles left in glass after administration, add more water or apple juice and have patient drink again to ensure a complete dose.
• Monitor patient's blood phenylalanine level regularly, as ordered.
• Expect drug to be discontinued if the patient's blood phenylalanine level does not decrease after one month with patient receiving maximum dosage.
• Continue to restrict dietary phenylalanine intake.

PATIENT TEACHING
• Tell patient to dissolve tablets in 4 to 8 ounces of water or apple juice, which may take a few minutes. Advise him to stir or crush tablets to hasten process and to drink solution within 15 minutes of dissolving. Alert him that tablets may not completely dissolve but that solution is alright to drink with particles floating in solution. After drinking solution, tell him to add more water or apple juice if any particles are clinging to glass and drink again.
• Stress to patient or caregiver importance of continuing dietary restriction of phenylalanine intake.
• Inform patient of continual need for periodic blood tests to determine drug effectiveness.
• Tell patient to a missed dose as soon as he remembers, unless it's almost time for the next dose. Warn patient not to take more than 1 dose per day.

scopolamine hydrobromide

scopolamine transdermal system

Transderm-Scōp, Transderm-V (CAN)

Class and Category
Chemical class: Belladonna alkaloid, tertiary amine
Therapeutic class: Anesthesia adjunct, anticholinergic, antiemetic, antispasmodic, antivertigo
Pregnancy category: C

Q
R
S

Indications and Dosages

➤ *To treat biliary tract disorders, enuresis, nausea and vomiting, and nocturia*

I.V., I.M., OR SUBCUTANEOUS INJECTION (HYDROBROMIDE)
Adults and adolescents. 300 to 600 mcg (0.3 to 0.6 mg) as a single dose.
Children. 6 mcg (0.006 mg)/kg as a single dose.

➤ *To prevent excessive salivation and respiratory tract secretions during anesthesia*

I.M. INJECTION (HYDROBROMIDE)
Adults and adolescents. 0.2 to 0.6 mg 30 to 60 min before induction of anesthesia.
Children ages 8 to 12. 0.3 mg 45 to 60 min before induction of anesthesia.
Children ages 3 to 8. 0.2 mg 45 to 60 min before induction of anesthesia.
Children ages 7 months to 3 years. 0.15 mg 45 to 60 min before induction of anesthesia.
Infants ages 4 to 7 months. 0.1 mg 45 to 60 min before induction of anesthesia.

➤ *As adjunct to anesthesia to induce sleep and calmness*

I.V., I.M., OR SUBCUTANEOUS INJECTION (HYDROBROMIDE)
Adults and adolescents. 0.6 mg t.i.d. or q.i.d.

➤ *As adjunct to anesthesia to induce amnesia*

I.V., I.M., OR SUBCUTANEOUS INJECTION (HYDROBROMIDE)
Adults and adolescents. 0.32 to 0.65 mg.

➤ *To prevent nausea, vomiting, and vertigo associated with motion sickness*

TRANSDERMAL SYSTEM
Adults and adolescents. 1 U.S. transdermal system (0.5 mg) applied behind ear for 3-day period, beginning at least 4 hr before antiemetic effect is required. Alternatively, 1 Canadian transdermal system (1 mg) applied behind ear for 3-day period, beginning at least 12 hr before antiemetic effect is required.

DOSAGE ADJUSTMENT Dosage reduction possible for elderly patients because of their increased sensitivity to scopolamine.

Contraindications

Angle-closure glaucoma; hemorrhage with hemodynamic instability; hepatic dysfunction; hypersensitivity to barbiturates, scopolamine, other belladonna alkaloids, or their components; ileus; intestinal atony; myasthenia gravis; myocardial ischemia; obstructive GI disease, such as pyloric stenosis; obstructive uropathy, as in prostatic hyperplasia; renal impairment; tachycardia; toxic megacolon; ulcerative colitis

Route	Onset	Peak	Duration
I.V., I.M., SubQ*	30 min	1 to 2 hr	4 to 6 hr
I.V.†	10 min	50 to 80 min	2 hr
I.M.‡	15 to 30 min	Unknown	4 hr
Transdermal	4 hr	Unknown	72 hr

Mechanism of Action

Competitively inhibits acetylcholine at autonomic postganglionic cholinergic receptors. Because the most sensitive receptors are in the salivary, bronchial, and sweat glands, this action reduces secretions from these glands. Scopolamine reduces GI smooth-muscle tone; decreases gastric secretions and GI motility; reduces bladder detrusor muscle tone; reduces nasal, oropharyngeal, and bronchial secretions; and decreases airway resistance by relaxing smooth muscles in the bronchi and bronchioles.

Scopolamine also blocks neural pathways in the inner ear to relieve motion sickness and depresses the cerebral cortex to produce sedation and hypnotic effects.

Interactions
DRUGS
adsorbent antidiarrheals, antacids: Decreased absorption and therapeutic effects of scopolamine
anticholinergics (other): Possibly intensified anticholinergic effects
antimyasthenics: Possibly reduced intestinal motility
CNS depressants: Possibly potentiated effects of either drug, resulting in additive sedation
cyclopropane: Increased risk of ventricular arrhythmias (with I.V. scopolamine)

---

* For inhibition of saliva.
† For amnesia.
‡ For antiemesis.

haloperidol: Decreased antipsychotic effect of haloperidol
ketoconazole: Decreased ketoconazole absorption
lorazepam (parenteral): Possibly hallucinations, irrational behavior, and sedation
metoclopramide: Possibly antagonized effect of metoclopramide on GI motility
opioid analgesics: Increased risk of severe constipation and ileus
potassium chloride: Possibly increased severity of potassium chloride–induced GI lesions
urinary alkalizers (antacids, carbonic anhydrase inhibitors, citrates, sodium bicarbonate): Delayed excretion of scopolamine, possibly leading to increased therapeutic and adverse effects
ACTIVITIES
alcohol use: Additive CNS effects

Adverse Reactions
CNS: Dizziness, drowsiness, euphoria, insomnia, memory loss, paradoxical stimulation
CV: Palpitations, tachycardia
EENT: Blurred vision; dry eyes, mouth, nose, and throat; mydriasis
GI: Constipation, dysphagia
GU: Urinary hesitancy, urine retention
SKIN: Decreased sweating, dry skin, flushing
Other: Injection site irritation or redness

Nursing Considerations
•For I.V. injection, dilute scopolamine with sterile water for injection.
•Assess for bladder distention and monitor urine output because drug's antimuscarinic effects can cause urine retention.
•Monitor for pain. In presence of pain, drug may act as a stimulant and produce delirium if used without morphine or meperidine.
•Monitor heart rate for transient tachycardia, which may occur with high doses of drug. Rate should return to normal within 30 minutes.

PATIENT TEACHING
•Instruct patient to apply scopolamine transdermal patch on hairless area behind ear and to wash hands thoroughly with soap and water before and after applying.
•Advise patient to avoid potentially hazardous activities until drug's CNS effects are known.
•Instruct patient to avoid alcohol while taking oral forms of scopolamine.

•If patient complains of dry eyes, suggest lubricating drops.

secobarbital sodium
Novosecobarb (CAN), Seconal

Class, Category, and Schedule
Chemical class: Barbiturate
Therapeutic class: Sedative-hypnotic
Pregnancy category: D
Controlled substance schedule: II

Indications and Dosages
➤ *To induce sedation before surgery*
CAPSULES
Adults. 200 to 300 mg 1 to 2 hr before surgery.
Children. 2 to 6 mg/kg 1 to 2 hr before surgery. *Maximum:* 100 mg.

➤ *To provide short-term treatment of insomnia*
CAPSULES
Adults. 100 mg at bedtime.

➤ *To relieve apprehension, daytime anxiety, and tension*
CAPSULES
Adults. 30 to 50 mg t.i.d. or q.i.d.
Children. 2 mg/kg t.i.d.
DOSAGE ADJUSTMENT Reduced dosage required for elderly or debilitated patients and those with renal or hepatic dysfunction.

Route	Onset	Peak	Duration
P.O.	10 to 15 min	15 to 30 min	1 to 4 hr

Mechanism of Action
Inhibits upward conduction of nerve impulses to the reticular formation of the brain, thereby disrupting impulse transmission to the cortex. This action depresses the CNS, producing drowsiness, hypnosis, and sedation.

Contraindications
History of barbiturate addiction; hypersensitivity to secobarbital, other barbiturates, or their components; nephritis; porphyria; severe hepatic or respiratory impairment

Interactions
DRUGS
acetaminophen, adrenocorticoids, beta block-

ers, chloramphenicol, cyclosporine, dacarbazine, digoxin, disopyramide, estrogens, metronidazole, oral anticoagulants, oral contraceptives, quinidine, thyroid hormones, tricyclic antidepressants: Decreased effectiveness of these drugs

addictive drugs: Increased risk of addiction

calcium channel blockers: Possibly excessive hypotension

carbamazepine, succinimide anticonvulsants: Decreased blood levels and increased elimination of these drugs

carbonic anhydrase inhibitors: Increased risk of osteopenia

CNS depressants: Increased CNS depressant effects

cyclophosphamide: Increased risk of leukopenic activity and reduced half-life of cyclophosphamide

divalproex sodium, valproic acid: Increased CNS depression and neurologic toxicity

doxycycline, fenoprofen: Increased elimination of these drugs

general anesthetics (enflurane, halothane, methoxyflurane): Increased risk of hepatotoxicity; increased risk of nephrotoxicity (with methoxyflurane)

griseofulvin: Decreased griseofulvin absorption

guanadrel, guanethidine: Possibly increased orthostatic hypotension

haloperidol: Possibly altered pattern or frequency of seizures, decreased blood haloperidol level

ketamine: Increased risk of hypotension or respiratory depression (when secobarbital is used as preanesthetic)

leucovorin (large doses): Decreased anticonvulsant effect of secobarbital

loxapine, phenothiazines, thioxanthenes: Possibly lowered seizure threshold

MAO inhibitors: Possibly prolonged CNS depressant effects of secobarbital

maprotiline: Increased CNS depressant effect; possibly lowered seizure threshold and decreased anticonvulsant effect with high doses of maprotiline

methylphenidate: Increased risk of barbiturate toxicity

mexiletine: Decreased blood mexiletine level

phenylbutazone: Decreased effectiveness of secobarbital

posterior pituitary hormones: Increased risk of arrhythmias and coronary insufficiency

primidone: Increased sedative effect of either drug, change in seizure pattern

vitamin D: Decreased vitamin D effects

xanthines (aminophylline, oxtriphylline, theophylline): Increased metabolism of xanthines (except dyphylline), decreased hypnotic effect of secobarbital

FOODS

caffeine: Increased caffeine metabolism, decreased hypnotic effect of secobarbital

ACTIVITIES

alcohol use: Increased CNS depression

Adverse Reactions

CNS: Anxiety, clumsiness, confusion, depression, dizziness, drowsiness, hangover, headache, insomnia, irritability, lethargy, nervousness, nightmares, paradoxical stimulation, syncope

CV: Hypotension

EENT: Laryngospasm

GI: Anorexia, constipation, nausea, vomiting

MS: Arthralgia, muscle weakness

RESP: Apnea, bronchospasm, respiratory depression

SKIN: Jaundice

Other: Drug dependence, weight loss

Nursing Considerations

•Be aware that prolonged use of secobarbital may lead to tolerance and physical and psychological dependence.

•**WARNING** To avoid withdrawal symptoms, expect to taper drug after long-term therapy. Withdrawal symptoms usually appear 8 to 12 hours after stopping drug and may include anxiety, insomnia, muscle twitching, nausea, orthostatic hypotension, vomiting, weakness, and weight loss. Severe symptoms may include delirium, hallucinations, and seizures. Generalized tonic-clonic seizures may occur within 16 hours or up to 5 days after last dose.

•Assess patient for signs and symptoms of barbiturate toxicity, including dyspnea, severe confusion, and severe drowsiness. Notify prescriber immediately if they appear because barbiturate toxicity may be life-threatening.

•Expect prescriber to provide patient with the least possible quantity of secobarbital to minimize the risk of acute or chronic overdosage. For patients who are depressed, suicidal, or drug-dependent or who have a history of drug abuse, institute precautions to

prevent drug hoarding and overdosage.
PATIENT TEACHING
•Instruct patient to take secobarbital exactly as prescribed because of the risk of addiction.
•Inform patient that taking drug with food may reduce adverse GI effects.
•Advise patient to avoid alcohol and caffeine and potentially hazardous activities during therapy.
•Inform patient about possible hangover effect.
•If patient takes an oral contraceptive, recommend using an additional form of birth control during therapy.
•Caution patient not to stop taking drug abruptly.
•Instruct patient to notify prescriber of bone pain, muscle weakness, or unexplained weight loss during therapy.

selegiline hydrochloride

Apo-Selegiline (CAN), Carbex, Eldepryl, Gen-Selegiline (CAN), Novo-Selegiline (CAN), Nu-Selegiline (CAN), SD Deprenyl (CAN), Selegiline-5 (CAN), Zelapar

selegiline transdermal system

Emsam

Class and Category

Chemical class: Phenethylamine derivative
Therapeutic class: Antidepressant (Emsam), antidyskinetic
Pregnancy category: C

Indications and Dosages

➤ *As adjunct to carbidopa-levodopa therapy to treat Parkinson's disease*
CAPSULES, TABLETS
Adults. 10 mg once daily, or 5 mg b.i.d. with breakfast and lunch.
DOSAGE ADJUSTMENT For patient with levodopa-induced adverse effects, 2.5 mg q.i.d.
➤ *As adjunct to carbidopa-levodopa therapy to treat Parkinson's disease in patients whose response to therapy has deteriorated*
ORALLY DISINTEGRATING TABLETS (ZELAPAR)
Adults. *Initial:* 1.25 mg once daily before

breakfast for at least 6 wk; then increased to 2.5 mg once daily, if needed.
➤ *To treat depression*
TRANSDERMAL SYSTEM (EMSAM)
Adults. *Initial:* 6 mg/24 hr with patch applied daily to upper torso, upper thigh, or outer surface of upper arm. Dosage increased every 2 wk in increments of 3 mg/24 hr, as needed. *Maximum:* 12 mg/24 hr.

Mechanism of Action
Reduces dopamine metabolism by noncompetitively inhibiting the brain enzyme monoamine oxidase type B. This increases the amount of dopamine available to relieve symptoms associated with parkinsonism. Selegiline's metabolites may also enhance dopamine transmission by inhibiting its reuptake at synapses.

Contraindications
Hypersensitivity to selegiline or its components; pheochromocytoma; use within 14 days of meperidine; use within 10 days of general anesthesia; use with carbamazepine, oxcarbazepine, selective serotonin reuptake inhibitors (fluoxetine, paroxetine, sertraline), dual serotonin and norephinephrine reuptake inhibitors (duloxetine, venlafaxine), tricyclic antidepressants (amitriptyline, bupropion, imipramine), analgesics (tramadol, propoxyphene), dextromethorphan; use with St. John's wort, mirtazapine, cyclobenzaprine, oral selegline, other MAO inhibitors, sympathomimetic amines (Emsam only)

Interactions
DRUGS
carbamazepine, oxcarbazepine: Increased blood selegiline level
fluoxetine, fluvoxamine, nefazodone, paroxetine, sertraline, venlafaxine: Increased risk of adverse reactions similar to those of serotonin syndrome (confusion, hypomania, restlessness, myoclonus), autonomic instability, delirium, muscle rigidity, and severe agitation
levodopa: Increased risk of confusion, dyskinesia, hallucinations, nausea, and orthostatic hypotension
meperidine, possibly other opioid agonists: Increased risk of diaphoresis, excitation, muscle rigidity, and severe hypertension

Q
R
S

sympathomimetics: Increased risk of severe hypertension
tricyclic antidepressants: Possibly serious CNS reactions, including decreased level of consciousness, hyperpyrexia, hypertension, muscle rigidity, seizures, and syncope
FOODS
caffeine: Increased risk of hypertension
foods that contain tyramine or other high-pressor amines: Increased risk of sudden and severe hypertension
ACTIVITIES
alcohol use: Increased risk of hypertension

Adverse Reactions

CNS: Anxiety, chills, confusion, dizziness, drowsiness, dyskinesia, euphoria, extrapyramidal reactions, fatigue, hallucinations, headache, insomnia, irritability, lethargy, memory loss, mood changes, nervousness, paresthesia, restlessness, suicidal ideation, syncope, tremor, weakness
CV: Arrhythmias, chest pain, hypertension, orthostatic hypotension, palpitations, peripheral edema
EENT: Altered taste, blepharospasm, blurred vision, burning lips or mouth, diplopia, dry mouth, pharyngitis, sinusitis, tinnitus
GI: Abdominal pain, anorexia, constipation, diarrhea, GI bleeding, heartburn, nausea, vomiting
GU: Dysuria, urinary hesitancy, urinary urgency, urine retention
MS: Arthralgia, back and leg pain, muscle fatigue and spasms, neck stiffness
RESP: Asthma
SKIN: Diaphoresis, photosensitivity, rash
Other: Application site reactions (Emsam)

Nursing Considerations

• Assess patient for mental status and mood changes because selegiline can worsen such conditions as dementia, severe psychosis, tardive dyskinesia, and tremor. Be especially alert for suicidal tendencies, particularly when therapy starts or dosage changes.
• Monitor patient who is also taking levodopa for levodopa-induced adverse reactions, including confusion, dyskinesia, hallucinations, nausea, and orthostatic hypotension.
• Monitor for decreased symptoms of Parkinson's disease to evaluate drug's effectiveness.
• Be aware that drug can reactivate gastric ulcers because it prevents breakdown of gastric histamine. Assess for related signs and

symptoms, such as abdominal pain.

PATIENT TEACHING
• Caution patient to take only prescribed amount because increased dosage may cause severe adverse reactions.
• Advise patient to avoid taking selegiline in the late afternoon or evening because it may interfere with sleep.
• For orally disintegrating tablets, tell patient to take it before breakfast without any liquid. Caution him not to push tablet through the foil on the blister pack but instead to peel back the foil with dry hands and gently remove the tablet. He should then immediately place the tablets on top of his tongue and let it disintegrate. Advise him not to drink or ingest any food for 5 minutes before and after taking the drug.
• If patient will use transdermal form, explain how and where to apply patch, stressing need to rotate sites. Tell patient to wash hands well after application and to dispose of removed patch immediately.
• Stress that only one patch may be worn at a time. If a patch falls off, tell patient to apply a new patch to a new site and to resume previous schedule.
• Urge patient to avoid tyramine-rich foods and beverages during and for 2 weeks after stopping selegiline therapy unless patient is prescribed the lowest dosage of transdermal system (6 mg per 24 hours), which doesn't require diet modification. Review which foods are considered tyramine-rich.
• Instruct patient to immediately report severe headache, neck stiffness, racing heart, palpitations, or other sudden or unusual symptoms.
• Caution patient to avoid exposing transdermal patch to sources of direct heat, such as heating pads, electric blankets, heat lamps, saunas, hot tubs, and prolonged sunlight exposure.
• Tell patient not to cut transdermal patch into smaller pieces.
• Urge caregiver to monitor patient closely for suicidal tendencies, especially when therapy starts or dosage changes.
• Urge patient to avoid potentially hazardous activities until drug's CNS effects are known.
• Advise patient to change positions slowly to minimize the effects of orthostatic hypotension.
• Suggest that patient elevate his legs when

sitting to reduce ankle swelling.
- Urge patient to avoid excessive sun exposure.
- Instruct patient to notify prescriber if symptoms develop that could indicate overdose, including muscle twitching and eye spasms.
- Urge patient to notify prescriber if dry mouth lasts longer than 2 weeks. Advise him to have routine dental checkups.

sertraline hydrochloride

Zoloft

Class and Category

Chemical class: Naphthylamine derivative
Therapeutic class: Antidepressant, antiobsessant, antipanic
Pregnancy category: C

Indications and Dosages

➤ *To treat major depression*
ORAL CONCENTRATE, TABLETS
Adults. *Initial:* 50 mg daily, increased after several wk in increments of 50 mg daily every wk, as needed. *Maximum:* 200 mg daily.

➤ *To treat obsessive-compulsive disorder*
ORAL CONCENTRATE, TABLETS
Adults and adolescents. *Initial:* 50 mg daily, increased after several wk in increments of 50 mg daily every wk, as needed. *Maximum:* 200 mg daily.
Children ages 6 to 12. *Initial:* 25 mg daily, increased every wk, as needed. *Maximum:* 200 mg daily.

➤ *To treat panic disorder, with or without agoraphobia; to treat posttraumatic stress disorder*
ORAL CONCENTRATE, TABLETS
Adults. *Initial:* 25 mg daily, increased to 50 mg daily after 1 wk; then increased by 50 mg daily every wk, as needed. *Maximum:* 200 mg daily.
DOSAGE ADJUSTMENT Initial dosage reduction recommended for elderly patients and those with hepatic impairment.

➤ *To treat premenstrual dysphoric disorder (PMDD)*
ORAL CONCENTRATE, TABLETS
Adult women. *Initial:* 50 mg daily in morning or evening throughout menstrual cycle;

or, 50 mg daily in morning or evening during luteal phase of menstrual cycle only. Dosage increased each menstrual cycle in 50-mg increments up to 150 mg daily, or each luteal phase up to 100 mg daily, as needed. Once 100-mg daily dosage established for luteal phase, each successive cycle requires a 50-mg titration step for 3 days at the beginning of each luteal phase. *Maximum:* 150 mg daily for dosing throughout menstrual cycle, or 100 mg daily for dosing during luteal phase only.

Route	Onset	Peak	Duration
P.O.	2 to 4 wk*	Unknown	Unknown

Mechanism of Action

Inhibits reuptake of the neurotransmitter serotonin by CNS neurons, thereby increasing the amount of serotonin available in nerve synapses. An elevated serotonin level may result in elevated mood and reduced depression. This action may also relieve symptoms of other psychiatric conditions attributed to serotonin deficiency.

Contraindications

Concurrent use of disulfiram (oral concentrate) or pimozide; hypersensitivity to sertraline or its components; use within 14 days of an MAO inhibitor

Interactions
DRUGS
aspirin, NSAIDs, warfarin: Increased anticoagulant activity and risk of bleeding
astemizole, terfenadine: Possibly increased blood levels of these drugs, leading to increased risk of arrhythmias
cimetidine: Increased sertraline half-life
MAO inhibitors: Possibly hyperpyretic episodes, hypertensive crisis, serotonin syndrome, and severe seizures
moclobemide, serotonergics: Increased risk of potentially fatal serotonin syndrome
serotonin and norepinephrine reuptake inhibitors: Increased risk of bleeding, especially GI bleeding
tolbutamide: Possibly hypoglycemia

---

* For antidepressant and antipanic effects; for antiobsessant effect, longer than 4 wk.

Q
R
S

tricyclic antidepressants: Possibly impaired metabolism of tricyclic antidepressants, resulting in increased risk of toxicity

Adverse Reactions

CNS: Aggressiveness, agitation, anxiety, dizziness, drowsiness, fatigue, fever, headache, hyperkinesia, insomnia, nervousness, neuroleptic malignant syndrome–like reaction, paresthesia, serotonin syndrome, suicidal ideation, tremor, weakness, yawning
CV: Palpitations
EENT: Dry mouth, epistaxis, sinusitis, vision changes
ENDO: Syndrome of inappropriate ADH secretion
GI: Abdominal cramps, anorexia, constipation, diarrhea, flatulence, increased appetite, indigestion, nausea, vomiting
GU: Anorgasmia, decreased libido, ejaculation disorders, impotence, urinary incontinence
SKIN: Diaphoresis, flushing, purpura, rash
Other: Weight loss

Nursing Considerations

•Monitor liver function test results and BUN and serum creatinine levels, as appropriate, in patients with hepatic or renal dysfunction.
•WARNING Monitor patient closely for evidence of serotonin syndrome, such as agitation, hallucinations, coma, tachycardia, labile blood pressure, hyperthermia, hyperreflexia, incoordination, nausea, vomiting, and diarrhea. Serotonin syndrome in its most severe form can resemble neuroleptic malignant syndrome, which includes hyperthermia, muscle rigidity, autonomic instability, possibly rapid changes in vital signs, and mental status changes. Notify prescriber immediately because serotonin syndrome reactions that resemble neuroleptic malignant syndrome may be life-threatening. Be prepared to provide supportive care.
•Monitor patient for hypo-osmolarity of serum and urine and for hyponatremia, which may indicate sertraline-induced syndrome of inappropriate ADH secretion.
•Be aware that effective antidepressant therapy can promote development of mania in predisposed people. If mania develops, notify prescriber immediately and expect to withhold sertraline.
•Watch closely for suicidal tendencies, espe-

cially when therapy starts and dosage changes and especially in children and adolescents.
•Monitor patient closely for evidence of GI bleeding, especially if patient takes a drug known to cause it, such as aspirin, an NSAID, a serotonin or norepinephrine reuptake inhibitor, or warfarin.
•When theray stops, expect to taper dosage to minimize adverse effects rather than stopping drug abruptly.

PATIENT TEACHING

•WARNING Tell patient that sertraline increases the risk of serotonin syndrome and reactions that resemble neuroleptic malignant syndrome, rare but serious complications, when taken with some other drugs. Teach patient to recognize signs and symptoms of serotonin syndrome and neuroleptic malignant syndrome, and advise him to notify prescriber immediately if they occur.
•Teach patient to dilute oral concentrate before taking it. Tell him to use supplied dropper to remove prescribed amount and mix it with 4 oz (½ cup) of water, ginger ale, lemon or lime soda, lemonade, or orange juice. Warn him not to mix oral concentrate with anything else. Explain that it's normal for mixture to be slightly hazy.
•Tell patient to take dose immediately after mixing it.
•If patient has latex sensitivity, advise him to use an alternate dispenser because the supplied dropper dispenser contains dry natural rubber.
•Advise patient to avoid potentially hazardous activities until drug's CNS effects are known.
•Warn family or caregiver to watch patient closely for evidence of suicidal thinking or behavior, especially when therapy starts or dosage changes, and especially if patient is a child or adolescent.
•Caution patient not to stop taking drug abruptly. Explain that gradual tapering helps to avoid withdrawal symptoms.
•Instruct female patients to notify prescriber if they are or could be pregnant and to discuss benefits and risks of continuing sertraline therapy throughout the pregnancy.
•Advise patient to consult prescriber before taking any OTC product, especially aspirin products or NSAIDs.

sevelamer hydrochloride
Renagel

sevelamer carbonate
Renvela

Class and Category
Chemical class: Polyallylamine-epichlorhydrin polymer
Therapeutic class: Antihyperphosphatemic
Pregnancy category: C

Indications and Dosages
➤ *To lower serum phosphate level during end-stage renal disease*
CAPSULES (RENAGEL)
Adults. 2 capsules (806 mg) t.i.d. if serum phosphorus level is 6 to 7.5 mg/dl; 3 capsules (1,209 mg) t.i.d. if serum phosphorus level is 7.6 to 8.9 mg/dl; or 4 capsules (1,612 mg) t.i.d. if serum phosphorus level is 9 mg/dl or more. Dosage increased or decreased gradually by 1 capsule (403 mg)/meal, as needed. *Maximum:* 30 capsules (12.1 g) daily.
TABLETS (RENVELA)
Adults. 1 tablet (800 mg) t.i.d. with meals if serum phosphorus level is 5.5 mg/dl to 7.5 mg/dl; or 2 tablets (1,600 mg) if serum phosphorus level is 7.5 mg/dl or greater. Dosage increased or decreased gradually by 1 tablet (800 mg)/meal at 2-wk intervals, as needed.
DOSAGE ADJUSTMENT For patients being switched from calcium acetate to sevelamer carbonate, 1 tablet of sevelamer (800 mg) can be substituted for every 1 tablet of calcium (667 mg) being taken.

Mechanism of Action
Inhibits phosphate absorption in the intestine by binding dietary phosphate, thereby lowering serum phosphorus level.

Contraindications
Fecal impaction, GI obstruction, hypersensitivity to sevelamer or its components, hypophosphatemia, ileus

Interactions
DRUGS
antiarrhythmics, anticonvulsants, digoxin, levothyroxine, liothyronine, quinolones, tetracyclines, theophylline, warfarin: Possibly altered absorption of these drugs
phosphate salts, phosphorus salts: Neutralized therapeutic effects of sevelamer
ciprofloxacin: Decreased ciprofloxacin effectiveness

Adverse Reactions
CNS: Headache, fever
CV: Hypertension, hypotension, thrombosis
EENT: Nasopharyngitis
GI: Abdominal pain, constipation (severe), diarrhea, fecal impaction, flatulence, ileus, indigestion, intestinal obstruction oir perforation, nausea, vomiting
RESP: Bronchitis, dyspnea, increased cough, upper respiratory tract infection
MS: Arthralgia, back or limb pain
SKIN: Pruritus, rash
Other: Infection

Nursing Considerations
•Give other drugs at least 1 hour before or 3 hours after sevelamer to prevent interaction.
•Be aware that severe hypophosphatemia may occur in patient with dysphagia, major GI tract surgery, or severe GI motility disorder (including severe constipation) because drug prevents phosphate absorption.
•Monitor blood pressure frequently.
•Monitor serum phosphorus level to determine drug's effectiveness; monitor other serum electrolyte levels, especially bicarbonate and chloride, to detect imbalances.
PATIENT TEACHING
•Tell patient to take drug with meals and to swallow capsules or tablets whole with water and not to open, break, or chew them.
•Caution patient to take other drugs 1 hour before or 3 hours after sevelamer.
•Review symptoms of thrombosis, and advise patient to report them immediately.
•Instruct patient to report severe or prolonged constipation to prescriber because additional treatment may be needed to prevent serious complications.

sibutramine hydrochloride monohydrate
Meridia

Class, Category, and Schedule
Chemical class: Cyclobutanemethanamine
Therapeutic class: Antiobesity

Q
R
S

Pregnancy category: C
Controlled substance schedule: IV

Indications and Dosages

➤ *As adjunct to calorie-controlled diet to manage obesity*

CAPSULES

Adults. *Initial:* 10 mg daily, increased to 15 mg daily after 4 wk if weight loss is inadequate. *Maximum:* 15 mg daily.

DOSAGE ADJUSTMENT Reduction to 5 mg daily may be needed if patient can't tolerate 10-mg dose.

Mechanism of Action

Inhibits central reuptake of dopamine, norepinephrine, and serotonin, thereby suppressing appetite and lowering food intake, leading to weight loss.

Contraindications

Anorexia nervosa, concomitant use of other centrally acting appetite suppressants, hypersensitivity to sibutramine or its components, use within 14 days of MAO inhibitor therapy

Interactions

DRUGS

certain decongestants and cough, cold, and allergy drugs; ephedrine; phenylpropanolamine; pseudoephedrine: Increased risk of elevated blood pressure or heart rate
certain opioid analgesics (dextromethorphan, fentanyl, meperidine, pentazocine), dihydroergotamine, lithium, MAO inhibitors, serotonergics, sumatriptan, tryptophan, zolmitriptan: Increased risk of serotonin syndrome
erythromycin, ketoconazole: Possibly decreased sibutramine clearance

Adverse Reactions

CNS: Anxiety, depression, dizziness, drowsiness, headache, insomnia, nervousness, paresthesia, somnolence
CV: Chest pain, edema, hypertension, palpitations, tachycardia
EENT: Dry mouth, earache, rhinitis, sinusitis, taste perversion
GI: Abdominal pain, anorexia, constipation, diarrhea, gastritis, increased appetite, indigestion, nausea, thirst, vomiting
GU: Dysmenorrhea, urine retention, UTI, vaginal candidiasis

HEME: Bleeding
MS: Arthralgia, back or neck pain, myalgia, tenosynovitis
SKIN: Acne, diaphoresis, ecchymosis, flushing, urticaria
Other: Anaphylaxis, angioedema, flulike symptoms

Nursing Considerations

• Administer sibutramine cautiously in patients with mild to moderate renal impairment, and expect to not use it in patients with severe renal impairment, including those with end-stage renal disease receiving hemodialysis.
• **WARNING** Use drug cautiously in patients with a history of substance abuse, and watch for signs of misuse.
• Measure blood pressure and pulse rate before and during sibutramine therapy.
• Because serotonin release from nerve terminals has been linked to cardiac valve dysfunction, assess for development of third heart sound.
• **WARNING** If patient takes drugs for migraine, notify prescriber immediately if evidence of serotonin syndrome develops: agitation, anxiety, ataxia, chills, confusion, diaphoresis, disorientation, dysarthria, emesis, excitement, hemiballismus, hyperreflexia, hyperthermia, hypomania, lack of coordination, loss of consciousness, mydriasis, myoclonus, restlessness, tachycardia, tremor, and weakness.
• Because drug decreases salivary flow, monitor patient for adverse dental effects.

PATIENT TEACHING

• Caution patient not to take sibutramine more often than prescribed.
• Teach patient how to measure his blood pressure and pulse rate during therapy.
• Explain that sibutramine is an adjunct to reduced-calorie diet, not a replacement for it.
• Advise patient to report unusual bleeding or bruising.
• Caution against taking OTC products that contain ephedrine because of the increased risk of hypertension.
• Urge patient to avoid potentially hazardous activities until drug's CNS effects are known.
• If patient reports dry mouth, suggest sugar-free hard candy or gum or a saliva substitute.

sildenafil citrate

Revatio, Viagra

Class and Category
Chemical class: Pyrazolopyrimidinone derivative
Therapeutic class: Antihypertensive (pulmonary arterial), anti-impotence
Pregnancy category: B

Indications and Dosages
➤ *To treat erectile dysfunction*
TABLETS
Adults. 50 mg daily, taken 1 hr before sexual activity; increased as prescribed, based on clinical response. *Maximum:* 100 mg daily.
DOSAGE ADJUSTMENT Initially 25 mg for elderly patients, those with hepatic cirrhosis or creatinine clearance less than 30 ml/min/ 1.73 m^2, and those taking potent cytochrome P-450 3A4 inhibitors or ritonavir. Dosage reduced to 25 mg if taken within 4 hr of an alpha blocker. *Maximum:* 25 mg/48 hr.

➤ *To treat pulmonary arterial hypertension in order to improve exercise ability in patients classified as group 1 by the World Health Organization*
TABLETS
Adults. 20 mg t.i.d.

Route	Onset	Peak	Duration
P.O.	In 30 min	Unknown	4 hr

Mechanism of Action
Enhances the effect of nitric oxide released in the penis by stimulation. Nitric oxide increases the cGMP level, relaxes smooth muscle, and increases blood flow to the corpus cavernosum, thus producing an erection.

Contraindications
Continuous or intermittent nitrate therapy, hypersensitivity to sildenafil or components

Interactions
DRUGS
barbiturates, bosentan, carabamazepine, efavirenza, nevirapine, phenytoin, rifabutin, rifampin: Altered plasma level of either drug
cimetidine, erythromycin, itraconazole, ketoconazole, mibefradil: Prolonged sildenafil effect

doxazosin and other alpha-blockers: Increased risk of symptomatic hypotension
nitrates: Profound hypotension
protease inhibitors: Increased sildenafil effect
rifampin: Decreased sildenafil effect
FOODS
high-fat meals: Drug absorption delayed by up to 60 minutes

Adverse Reactions
CNS: Cerebrovascular, intracerebral, or subarachnoid hemorrhage; dizziness; headache; migraine; seizures; syncope; transient global amnesia, transient ischemic attack
CV: Heart failure, hypertension, hypotension, myocardial infarction or ischemia, orthostatic hypotension, palpitations, sudden cardiac death, tachycardia, ventricular arrhythmias
EENT: Blurred vision; change in color perception; diplopia; epistaxis; hearing loss; increased intraocular pressure; nasal congestion; nonarteritic anterior ischemic optic neuropathy; ocular burning, pressure, redness or swelling; paramacular edema; photophobia; retinal vascular bleeding or disease; tinnitus, visual decrease or temporary vision loss; vitreous detachment
ENDO: Uncontrolled diabetes mellitus
GI: Diarrhea, indigestion
GU: Cystitis, dysuria, painful erection, priapism, UTI
MS: Arthralgia, back pain
RESP: Pulmonary hemorrhage, upper respiratory tract infection
SKIN: Flushing, photosensitivity

Nursing Considerations
•Use sildenafil cautiously in patients with renal or hepatic dysfunction, in elderly patients, and in men with penile abnormalities that may predispose them to priapism.
•Also use cautiously in patients with left ventricular outflow obstruction, such as aortic stenosis and idiopathic hypertrophic subaortic stenosis, and those with severely impaired autonomic control of blood pressure because these conditions increase patient's sensitivity to vasodilators such as sildenafil.
•Monitor patient's blood pressure and heart rate and rhythm before and often during therapy.
•Monitor vision, especially in patients who are over age 50; who have diabetes, hypertension, coronary artery disease, or hyper-

Q
R
S

lipidemia; or who smoke because sildenafil rarely may prompt nonarteritic anterior ischemic optic neuropathy that may lead to decreased vision or permanent vision loss.

PATIENT TEACHING

•Explain that sildenafil used to treat erectile dysfunction may be taken up to 4 hours before sexual activity but that taking it 1 hour beforehand provides most effective results.

•**WARNING** Warn patient not to take sildenafil if he also takes any form of organic nitrate, either continuously or intermittently, because profound hypotension and death could result. Also caution patient taking sildenafil for erectile dysfunction not to take more than 25 mg within 4 hours of an alpha blocker, such as doxazosin, because symptomatic orthostatic hypotension can occur.

•Tell patient to stop taking drug and contact prescriber if vision decreases suddenly in one or both eyes or if he has a loss of hearing, possibly with tinnitus and dizziness.

•Advise patient taking sildenafil for erectile dysfunction to seek sexual counseling to enhance the drug's effects.

•To avoid possible penile damage and permanent loss of erectile function, urge patient to notify prescriber immediately if erection is painful or lasts longer than 4 hours.

•Instruct diabetic patient to monitor his blood glucose level frequently because drug may affect glucose control.

silodosin

Rapaflo

Class and Category

Chemical class: Highly selective alpha-1 adrenergic receptor blocker
Therapeutic class: Benign prostatic antihyperplasia agent
Pregnancy category: B

Indications and Dosages

➤ *To treat symptomatic benign prostatic hyperplasia*

CAPSULES

Adult males. 8 mg daily. Maximum: 8 mg daily.

DOSAGE ADJUSTMENT For patients with moderate renal impairment (creatinine clearance between 30 and 50 ml/min), dosage reduced to 4 mg daily.

Mechanism of Action

Binds to postsynaptic alpha-1 adreno-receptors located in the prostate gland, bladder base and neck, and prostatic capsule and urethra. Blocking action at these adrenoreceptor sites causes relaxation of smooth muscle in the local area, which improves urine flow and reduces other benign prostatic hyperplasia symptoms.

Contraindications

Hypersensitivity to silodosin and its components, severe hepatic insufficiency (Child-Pugh score 10 or above), severe renal insufficiency (creatinine clearance less than 30 ml/min/1.73 m^2), use with strong CYP3A4 inhibitors such as clarithromycin, ketoconazole, itraconazole, and ritonavir

Interactions

DRUGS

alpha blockers: Possibly increased effects and risk of adverse reactions
antihypertensives: Increased risk of dizziness and orthostatic hypotension
cyclosporin, CYP3A4 inhibitors such as clarithromycin, diltiazem, erythromycin, itraconazole, ketoconazole, ritonavir: Possibly increased serum silodosin levels and risk of adverse reactions

Adverse Reactions

CNS: Asthenia, dizziness, headache, insomnia, syncope
CV: Orthostatic hypotension
EENT: Nasal congestion, nasopharyngitis, rhinorrhea, sinusitis
GI: Abdominal pain, diarrhea, elevated liver enzymes, impaired hepatic function, jaundice
GU: Elevated prostate specific antigen level, retrograde ejaculation
SKIN: Purpura, toxic skin eruption

Nursing Considerations

•Use cautiously in patients with mild renal impairment and mild and moderate hepatic impairment. Patients with moderate renal impairment need dosage adjustment.

•Monitor patient's blood pressure for reduction, especially if he takes an antihypertensive with silodosin.

PATIENT TEACHING

•Instruct patient to take drug with a meal.

•Advise patient to avoid hazardous activities until drug's CNS effects are known.
•Advise patient planning cataract surgery or other ocular procedure to tell ophthalmologist that he takes silodosin or has taken it in the past because of potential adverse reactions.

simvastatin

Zocor

Class and Category
Chemical class: Synthetically derived fermentation product of *Aspergillus terreus*
Therapeutic class: Antihyperlipidemic
Pregnancy category: X

Indications and Dosages
➤ *To treat hyperlipidemia*
TABLETS
Adults. *Initial:* 20 to 40 mg daily in the evening. Dosage adjusted at 4-wk intervals, as needed, to achieve target LDL-cholesterol level. *Maintenance:* 5 to 80 mg daily. *Maximum:* 80 mg daily.
➤ *To treat homozygous familial hypercholesterolemia*
TABLETS
Adults. 40 mg daily in the evening, or 80 mg/day in 3 divided doses—20 mg, 20 mg, and 40 mg (in the evening). Dosage adjusted every 4 wk, as needed, to achieve target LDL-cholesterol level. *Maintenance:* 5 to 40 mg/day. *Maximum:* 80 mg daily.
DOSAGE ADJUSTMENT Patients taking cyclosporine or who have severe renal insufficiency should initially receive 5 mg simvastatin daily and be increased as needed to no more than 10 mg daily. Maximum dosage of 10 mg daily should also not be exceeded in patients who are also taking fibrates or niacin.
➤ *To treat adolescent heterozygous familial hypercholesterolemia*
TABLETS
Children ages 10 to 17 at least 1 year postmenarche. *Initial:* 10 mg daily in the evening. Adjusted every 4 wk, as needed, to achieve target LDL-cholesterol level. *Maintenance:* 10 to 40 mg daily. *Maximum:* 40 mg daily.
DOSAGE ADJUSTMENT For patients who take cyclosporine, initial dosage reduced to 5 mg/day and maximum dosage reduced to 10 mg/

day. For elderly patients and those with renal impairment, initial dosage reduced to 5 mg daily. For patients who take danazol, fibric-acid derivative lipid-lowering drugs, such as gemfibrozil, or lipid-lowering doses of niacin (1 g daily or more), maximum dosage reduced to 10 mg daily. For patients who take amiodarone or verapamil, maximum dosage shouldn't exceed 20 mg daily.

Route	Onset	Peak	Duration
P.O.	2 wk	4 to 6 wk	Unknown

Mechanism of Action
Interferes with the hepatic enzyme hydroxymethylglutaryl-coenzyme A reductase. This action reduces the formation of mevalonic acid, a cholesterol precursor, thus interrupting the pathway necessary for cholesterol synthesis. When the cholesterol level declines in hepatic cells, LDLs are consumed, which in turn reduces the levels of circulating total cholesterol and serum triglycerides.

Contraindications
Active hepatic disease; breast-feeding; concurrent use with clarithromycin, erythromycin, more than 1 quart of grapefruit juice daily, HIV protease inhibitors, itraconazole, ketoconazole, nefazodone, or telithromycin; hypersensitivity to simvastatin or its components; pregnancy

Interactions
DRUGS
amiodarone, antiretroviral protease inhibitors (amprenavir, indinavir, nelfinavir, ritonavir, saquinavir), clarithromycin, cyclosporine, danazol, gemfibrozil and other fibrates, itraconazole, ketoconazole, erythromycin, nefazodone, niacin (1 g daily or more), telithromycin, verapamil: Increased risk of myopathy or rhabdomyolysis
azole antifungals, cyclosporine, gemfibrozil, immunosuppressants, macrolide antibiotics (including erythromycin), niacin, verapamil: Increased risk of acute renal failure
bile acid sequestrants, cholestyramine, colestipol: Decreased simvastatin bioavailability
digoxin: Possibly slight elevation in blood digoxin level
diltiazem, verapamil: Possibly increased

Q
R
S

blood simvastatin level, increased risk of myopathy
oral anticoagulants: Increased bleeding or prolonged PT
FOODS
grapefruit juice (1 or more quarts daily): Possibly increased blood simvastatin level

Adverse Reactions
CNS: Asthenia, dizziness, fatigue, headache
CV: Chest pain
EENT: Cataracts, rhinitis
GI: Abdominal pain, constipation, diarrhea, elevated liver function test results, flatulence, heartburn, hepatic failure, indigestion, nausea, pancreatitis, vomiting
MS: Myalgia, myopathy, rhabdomyolysis
RESP: Upper respiratory tract infection
SKIN: Eczema, pruritus, rash

Nursing Considerations
•Use simvastatin cautiously in elderly patients and those with renal or hepatic impairment.
•Give drug 1 hour before or 4 hours after giving bile acid sequestrant, cholestyramine, or colestipol.
•Expect to monitor liver function test results every 3 to 6 months for abnormal elevations.
•Monitor serum lipoprotein level, as ordered, to evaluate response to therapy.
PATIENT TEACHING
•Urge patient to take drug in the evening.
•Encourage patient to follow a low-fat, cholesterol-lowering diet.
•Urge patient to notify prescriber immediately about muscle pain, tenderness, or weakness and other symptoms of myopathy.
•Inform female patient of childbearing age of need to use reliable contraceptive method while taking drug. Instruct her to notify prescriber at once if she suspects pregnancy.
•Advise patient to avoid grapefruit juice to decrease risk of drug toxicity.

sirolimus
(rapamycin)

Rapamune

Class and Category
Chemical class: Macrocyclic lactone
Therapeutic class: Immunosuppressant
Pregnancy category: C

Indications and Dosages
➤ *To prevent rejection of kidney transplantation*
ORAL SOLUTION
Adults and adolescents over age 13 weighing 40 kg or more. *Initial:* 6-mg loading dose. *Maintenance:* 2 mg daily.
Adolescents over age 13 weighing less than 40 kg. *Initial:* 3-mg/m^2 loading dose. *Maintenance:* 1 mg/m^2 daily.
DOSAGE ADJUSTMENT Maintenance dosage reduced by one-third for patients with impaired hepatic function. Maintenance dosage increased by as much as 400% for patients discontinuing concomitant cyclosporine therapy in order to maintain blood sirolimus trough level of 12 to 24 nanograms/ml.

Contraindications
Hypersensitivity to sirolimus or its components, malignancy

Route	Onset	Peak	Duration
P.O.	Unknown	Unknown	Up to 6 mo after discontinuation

Mechanism of Action
Inhibits activation and proliferation of T lymphocytes and antibody production. Sirolimus also inhibits cell cycle progression from the G1 to the S phase, possibly by inhibiting a key regulatory kinase believed to suppress cytokine-driven T-cell proliferation.

Interactions
DRUGS
aminoglycosides, amphotericin B, cyclosporine: Possibly impaired renal function
bromocriptine, cimetidine, cisapride, clarithromycin, clotrimazole, cyclosporine, danazol, diltiazem, erythromycin, fluconazole, indinavir, itraconazole, ketoconazole, metoclopramide, nicardipine, ritonavir, troleandomycin, verapamil: Possibly increased blood sirolimus level and toxicity
calcineurin inhibitors, corticosteroids: Increased risk of deteriorating renal function, serum lipid abnormalities, and UTI
carbamazepine, phenobarbital, phenytoin, rifabutin, rifapentine, St. John's wort: Possibly

decreased blood sirolimus level
HMG-CoA reductase inhibitors: Increased
risk of rhabdomyolysis when administered
concurrently with sirolimus and cyclosporine
rifampin: Significantly increased sirolimus
clearance
vaccines (killed virus): Possibly decreased
immune response to vaccines
vaccines (live virus): Increased risk of con-
tracting disease from live virus
FOODS
grapefruit juice: Possibly decreased metabolism of sirolimus
high-fat diet: Reduced rate of sirolimus absorption

Adverse Reactions
CNS: Asthenia, fever, headache, insomnia,
tremor
CV: Atrial fibrillation, chest pain, hyperlipidemia, hypersensitivity vasculitis, hypertension, pericardial effusion, peripheral edema
ENDO: Hyperglycemia
GI: Abdominal pain, constipation, diarrhea,
elevated liver enzymes, hepatotoxicity, nausea, vomiting
GU: Azoospermia, elevated serum creatinine
level, nephrotic syndrome, proteinuria, UTI
HEME: Anemia, lymphoma, neutropenia,
pancytopenia, thrombocytopenia
MS: Arthralgia, low back or flank pain, joint
abnormality
RESP: Dyspnea on exertion, interstitial lung
disease, pleural effusion, pulmonary hemorrhage
SKIN: Acne, exfoliative dermatitis, rash
Other: Anaphylaxis; angioedema; delayed
wound healing; hypercholesterolemia; hypokalemia; hypophosphatemia; increased susceptibility to infection, including opportunistic infections such as tuberculosis; lymphedema; weight gain or loss

Nursing Considerations
• Use sirolimus cautiously in patients who
are receiving other drugs known to adversely
affect renal function, such as aminoglycosides and amphotericin B; together, they may
further decrease renal function.
• Monitor patients with existing or recent
(including recent exposure to) chickenpox
and patients with herpes zoster for worsening symptoms because they have an increased risk of developing severe generalized
disease while taking sirolimus.

• Mix oral sirolimus with at least 2 oz (60 ml)
of water or orange juice in a glass or plastic
container. Don't dilute drug in grapefruit
juice or any other liquid.
• Stir well and have patient drink solution
immediately. Then rinse glass with at least
4 oz (120 ml) of additional liquid, stir well,
and have patient drink that liquid to make
sure that all of drug is taken.
• Give initial dose as soon after transplantation as possible and daily dose 4 hours after
cyclosporine, as prescribed.
• Monitor whole blood sirolimus concentrations, as ordered, in patients receiving concentrated form of drug, patients weighing
less than 40 kg (88 lb), patients with hepatic
impairment, and those receiving potent
CYP3A4 inducers or inhibitors concurrently.
• Monitor serum creatinine level, as ordered,
in patients receiving sirolimus and cyclosporine because this combination may impair
renal function. Notify prescriber of any increases in serum creatinine level because
sirolimus or cyclosporine dosage may need to
be adjusted or drug discontinued.
• Monitor patient for urinary protein excretion, as ordered. If protein appears in urine,
sirolimus may be discontinued.
• Monitor patient for signs and symptoms of
infection and check CBC results, as ordered,
to detect sirolimus-induced blood dyscrasias
or changes in neutrophil count, which may
indicate infection.
• For patients with hyperlipidemia, be prepared to institute dietary changes, an exercise program, or a lipid-lowering drug regimen if blood cholesterol or triglyceride levels
increase because drug may aggravate hyperlipidemia.

PATIENT TEACHING
• Advise patient to take sirolimus consistently either with or without food (but not
food high in fat) to prevent changes in absorption rate.
• Instruct patient to take daily dose with at
least 2 oz (60 ml) of water or orange juice.
Caution him not to dilute drug in grapefruit
juice or any other liquid. Advise him to stir
mixture well and drink immediately, then to
add at least another 4 oz (120 ml) of liquid
to empty container, stir mixture again, and
drink that liquid to ensure that he has swallowed all of drug.
• Urge patient to avoid people with colds,

flu, or other infections because immunosuppression makes him more vulnerable.
•Instruct patient not to take live vaccines, such as measles, mumps, rubella, oral polio, bacille Calmette-Guérin, yellow fever, varicella, and TY21a typhoid, during sirolimus therapy.
•Advise patient to keep follow-up appointments for blood tests, as ordered.

sitagliptin

Januvia

Class and Category

Chemical class: Beta amino acid derivative
Therapeutic class: Antidiabetic
Pregnancy category: C

Indications and Dosages

➤ *To achieve control of glucose level in type 2 diabetes mellitus as monotherapy or with metformin or other thiazolidinediones*

TABLETS

Adults. 100 mg once daily.

DOSAGE ADJUSTMENT For patients with moderate renal insufficiency (creatinine clearance 30 to 50 ml/min/1.73 m^2), dosage reduced to 50 mg once daily; for patients with severe renal insufficiency (creatinine clearance less than 30 ml/min/1.73 m^2) or end-stage renal disease requiring hemodialysis or peritoneal dialysis, dosage reduced to 25 mg once daily.

Route	Onset	Peak	Duration
P.O.	Unknown	1 to 4 hr	Unknown

Mechanism of Action

Inhibits the dipeptidyl peptidase-4 enzyme to slow inactivation of incretin hormones. These hormones are released by the intestine throughout the day but increase in response to a meal. When blood glucose level is normal or increased, incretin hormones increase insulin synthesis and release from pancreatic beta cells. One type of incretin hormone, glucagon-like peptide (GLP-1) also lowers glucagon secretion from pancreatic alpha cells which reduces hepatic glucose production. These combined actions decrease blood glucose level in type 2 diabetes.

Contraindications

Diabetic ketoacidosis, hypersensitivity to sitagliptin or its components, type 1 diabetes

Interactions

DRUGS

ACE inhibitors, disopyramide, fibric acid derivatives, fluoxetine, sulfonylureas: Possibly increased hypoglycemic effects
beta blockers: Possibly prolonged hypoglycemia or promotion of hyperglycemia
digoxin: Slightly increased plasma digoxin level
estrogens, oral contraceptives, phenytoin, progestines, thiazide diuretics, triamterene: Possibly decreased hypoglycemic effects

Adverse Reactions

CNS: Headache
EENT: Nasopharyngitis
GI: Abdominal pain, diarrhea, elevated hepatic enzymes, nausea, vomiting
RESP: Upper respiratory tract infection
SKIN: Rash, Stevens-Johnson syndrome, urticaria
Other: Anaphylaxis, angioedema

Nursing Considerations

•Assess patient's renal function before starting sitagliptin therapy, as ordered, and periodically thereafter. In moderate to severe renal dysfunction, dosage will be reduced.
•Monitor patient for hypersensitivity reactions that, although uncommon, may be severe. If present, notify prescriber and expect sitagliptin to be discontinued.
•Monitor patient's blood glucose level, as ordered, to determine effectiveness of sitagliptin therapy.

PATIENT TEACHING

•Stress the need to follow an exercise program and a diet control program during sitagliptin therapy.
•Advise patient to notify prescriber immediately if she has trouble breathing, hives, rash, or swelling.
•Inform patient that periodic blood tests will be done to determine effectiveness of drug and assess kidney function.
•Teach patient how to monitor blood glucose level and when to report changes.
•Caution patient that taking other drugs in addition to sitagliptin to control his diabetes may lead to hypoglycemia. Review signs, symptoms, and appropriate prescribed treat-

ment with him.

•Instruct patient to contact prescriber if he develops other illnesses, such as infection, or experiences trauma or surgery because his diabetes medication may need adjustment.

•Advise patient to carry identification indicating that she has diabetes.

sodium bicarbonate

Arm and Hammer Pure Baking Soda, Bell/ans, Citrocarbonate, Soda Mint

Class and Category

Chemical class: Electrolyte
Therapeutic class: Antacid, electrolyte replenisher, systemic and urinary alkalizer
Pregnancy category: C

Indications and Dosages

➤ *To treat hyperacidity*
EFFERVESCENT POWDER

Adults and adolescents. 3.9 to 10 g in a glass of water after meals. *Maximum:* 19.5 g daily.

Children ages 6 to 12. 1 to 1.9 g in a glass of water after meals.

ORAL POWDER

Adults and adolescents. ½ tsp in a glass of water every 2 hr, p.r.n. *Maximum:* 4 tsp daily in patients up to age 60.

TABLETS

Adults and adolescents. 325 mg to 2 g daily to q.i.d., p.r.n. *Maximum:* 16 g daily.

Children ages 6 to 12. 520 mg, repeated once after 30 min, p.r.n.

➤ *To provide urinary alkalization*
ORAL POWDER

Adults and adolescents. 1 tsp in a glass of water every 4 hr. *Maximum:* 4 tsp daily in patients up to age 60.

TABLETS

Adults and adolescents. *Initial:* 4 g, then 1 to 2 g every 4 hr. *Maximum:* 16 g daily.

Children. 23 to 230 mg/kg daily, adjusted p.r.n.

I.V. INFUSION

Adults and children. 2 to 5 mEq/kg over 4 to 8 hr.

➤ *To treat metabolic acidosis during cardiac arrest*
I.V. INJECTION

Adults and children. *Initial:* 1 mEq/kg, followed by 0.5 mEq/kg every 10 min while arrest continues.

➤ *To treat less urgent forms of metabolic acidosis*
I.V. INFUSION

Adults and children. 2 to 5 mEq/kg over 4 to 8 hr.

DOSAGE ADJUSTMENT Dosage reduction possible for elderly patients because of age-related renal impairment.

Mechanism of Action

Increases plasma bicarbonate level, buffers excess hydrogen ions, and raises blood pH, thereby reversing metabolic acidosis. Sodium bicarbonate also increases the excretion of free bicarbonate ions in urine, raising urine pH; increased alkalinity of urine may help to dissolve uric acid calculi. In addition, it relieves symptoms of hyperacidity by neutralizing or buffering existing stomach acid, thereby increasing the pH of stomach contents.

Incompatibilities

Don't admix I.V. form of sodium bicarbonate in same solution or administer through same I.V. line as other drugs because precipitate may form.

Contraindications

Hypocalcemia in which alkalosis may lead to tetany; hypochloremic alkalosis secondary to vomiting, diuretics, or nasogastric suction; preexisting metabolic or respiratory alkalosis

Interactions

DRUGS

amphetamines, quinidine: Decreased urinary excretion of these drugs, possibly resulting in toxicity

anticholinergics: Decreased anticholinergic absorption and effectiveness

calcium-containing products: Increased risk of milk-alkali syndrome

chlorpropamide, lithium, salicylates, tetracyclines: Increased renal excretion and decreased absorption of these drugs

ciprofloxacin, norfloxacin, ofloxacin: Decreased solubility of these drugs, leading to crystalluria and nephrotoxicity

citrates: Increased risk of systemic alkalosis; increased risk of calcium calculus formation and hypernatremia in patients with history of uric acid calculi

Q
R
S

digoxin: Possibly elevated blood digoxin level

enteric-coated drugs: Increased risk of gastric or duodenal irritation from rapid removal of enteric coating

ephedrine: Increased ephedrine half-life and duration of action

H₂-receptor antagonists, iron supplements or preparations, ketoconazole: Decreased absorption of these drugs

mecamylamine: Decreased excretion and prolonged effect of mecamylamine

methenamine: Decreased methenamine effectiveness

mexiletine: Possibly mexiletine toxicity

potassium supplements: Decreased serum potassium level

sucralfate: Interference with binding of sucralfate to gastric mucosa

urinary acidifiers (ammonium chloride, ascorbic acid, potassium and sodium phosphates): Counteracted effects of urinary acidifiers

FOODS

dairy products: Increased risk of milk-alkali syndrome with prolonged use of sodium bicarbonate

Adverse Reactions

CNS: Mental or mood changes
CV: Irregular heartbeat, peripheral edema (with large doses), weak pulse
EENT: Dry mouth
GI: Abdominal cramps, thirst
MS: Muscle spasms, myalgia
SKIN: Extravasation with necrosis, tissue sloughing, or ulceration

Nursing Considerations

• Monitor sodium intake of patient taking sodium bicarbonate because effervescent powder contains 700.6 mg of sodium/3.9 g; oral powder contains 952 mg of sodium/tsp; and tablets contain 325 mg/3.9-mEq tablet, 520 mg/6.2-mEq tablet, and 650 mg/7.7-mEq tablet.
• For I.V. infusion, dilute drug with normal saline solution, D₅W, or other standard electrolyte solution before administration.
• Avoid rapid I.V. infusion, which can cause severe alkalosis. Be aware that during cardiac arrest, risk of death from acidosis may outweigh risks of rapid infusion.
• Monitor urine pH, as ordered, to determine drug's effectiveness as urine alkalizer.

• If patient receiving long-term sodium bicarbonate therapy is consuming a diet that includes calcium or milk, monitor her for milk-alkali syndrome, characterized by anorexia, confusion, headache, hypercalcemia, metabolic acidosis, nausea, renal insufficiency, and vomiting.
• Be aware that parenteral formulations are hypertonic and that increased sodium intake can produce edema and weight gain.
• Assess I.V. site frequently for signs and symptoms of extravasation. If this occurs, notify prescriber immediately and remove I.V. catheter. Elevate the limb, apply warm compresses, and expect prescriber to administer a local injection of hyaluronidase or lidocaine.

PATIENT TEACHING
• Advise patient not to take sodium bicarbonate with large amounts of dairy products or for longer than 2 weeks, unless directed by prescriber.
• Caution patient not to take more than the prescribed amount of drug to avoid adverse reactions.
• Direct patient not to take drug within 2 hours of other oral drugs.
• Advise patient to avoid taking other prescribed or OTC drugs without prescriber's approval because many drugs interact with sodium bicarbonate.

sodium ferric gluconate

(contains 62.5 mg of elemental iron per 5 ml)

Ferrlecit

Class and Category

Chemical class: Iron salt, mineral
Therapeutic class: Antianemic
Pregnancy category: B

Indications and Dosages

➤ *To treat iron deficiency anemia in patients receiving long-term hemodialysis and erythropoietin*

I.V. INFUSION OR INJECTION

Adults. 125 mg of elemental iron. *Usual:* Minimum cumulative dose of 1 g of elemental iron given over eight sequential dialysis treatment. Dosage repeated at lowest dosage necessary to maintain target levels of hemoglobin and hematocrit and acceptable limits of blood iron levels.

Mechanism of Action

Acts to replenish iron stores lost during hemodialysis as a result of increased blood loss or increased iron utilization from epoetin therapy. Iron is an essential component of hemoglobin, myoglobin, and several enzymes, including cytochromes, catalase, and peroxidase, and is needed for catecholamine metabolism and normal neutrophil function. Sodium ferric gluconate also normalizes RBC production by binding with hemoglobin or being stored as ferritin in reticuloendothelial cells of the liver, spleen, and bone marrow.

Incompatibilities

Don't mix sodium ferric gluconate with other drugs or parenteral nutrition solutions for I.V. infusion.

Contraindications

Anemia other than iron deficiency, hypersensitivity to iron salts or their components, iron overload

Interactions

DRUGS

oral iron preparations: Possibly reduced absorption of oral iron supplements

Adverse Reactions

CNS: Asthenia, dizziness, fatigue, fever, headache, hypertonia, nervousness, paresthesia, syncope
CV: Chest pain, generalized edema, hypertension, hypotension, tachycardia
EENT: Dry mouth
GI: Abdominal pain, diarrhea, nausea, vomiting
HEME: Hemorrhage
MS: Back pain, leg cramps
RESP: Cough, dyspnea, upper respiratory tract infection, wheezing
SKIN: Diaphoresis, pruritus
Other: Anaphylaxis, generalized pain, hyperkalemia, hypersensitivity, infusion or injection site reaction

Nursing Considerations

• To reconstitute sodium ferric gluconate for I.V. infusion, dilute prescribed dosage in 100 ml of normal saline solution immediately before infusion. Infuse over 1 hour. Discard any unused diluted solution.

• Inspect drug for particles and discoloration before administration and discard if present.
• Give undiluted drug by slow I.V. injection at up to 12.5 mg/min, not to exceed 125 mg per injection.
• Be aware that most patients need a minimum cumulative dose of 1 gram of elemental iron administered over eight sequential dialysis treatments.
• **WARNING** Assess patient for signs and symptoms of an allergic reaction, including chills, facial flushing, pruritus, and rash, and of a hypersensitivity reaction, including diaphoresis, dyspnea, nausea, severe lower back pain, vomiting, and wheezing. Discontinue drug and notify prescriber immediately if patient develops an allergic or hypersensitivity reaction, and be prepared to provide emergency interventions.
• **WARNING** Assess blood pressure frequently after drug administration because hypotension may occur and may be related to infusion rate or total cumulative dose. Avoid rapid infusion and be prepared to provide I.V. fluids for volume expansion.
• Expect to monitor blood hemoglobin level, hematocrit, serum ferritin level, and transferrin saturation, as ordered, before, during, and after sodium ferric gluconate therapy. Make sure serum iron level is tested 48 hours after last dose. To prevent iron toxicity, notify prescriber and expect to end therapy if blood iron level is normal or elevated.
• Assess patient for possible iron overload, characterized by bleeding in GI tract and lungs, decreased activity, pale conjunctivae, and sedation.

PATIENT TEACHING
• Warn patient not to take any oral iron preparations during sodium ferric gluconate therapy without first consulting prescriber.
• Inform patient that symptoms of iron deficiency may include decreased stamina, learning problems, shortness of breath, and fatigue.

sodium phenylbutyrate

Buphenyl

Class and Category

Chemical class: Phenylacetate prodrug
Therapeutic class: Antihyperammonemic
Pregnancy category: C

Indications and Dosages

➤ *As adjunct to treat urea cycle disorders in combination with low-protein diet*

POWDER, TABLETS

Adults and children weighing more than 20 kg (44 lb). 9.9 to 13 g/m² daily in 4 to 6 divided doses with meals.
Children weighing up to 20 kg. 450 to 600 mg/kg daily in 4 to 6 divided doses with meals.

Mechanism of Action

Provides alternate pathway for eliminating waste nitrogen by forming phenylacetate, an active metabolite that conjugates with glutamine to produce phenylacetylglutamine, which is excreted by the kidneys.

Contraindications

Acute hyperammonemia, hypersensitivity to sodium phenylbutyrate or its components

Interactions

DRUGS

corticosteroids: Increased serum ammonia level
haloperidol, valproate: Increased risk of hyperammonemia
probenecid: Decreased excretion of conjugated product of sodium phenylbutyrate

Adverse Reactions

CNS: Depression, disorientation, fatigue, headache, light-headedness, memory loss, syncope
CV: Arrhythmias
EENT: Hypoacusis, taste perversion
GI: Abdominal pain, anorexia, constipation, elevated liver function test results, gastritis, nausea, peptic ulcer, rectal bleeding, vomiting
GU: Amenorrhea, menstrual irregularities
HEME: Anemia, aplastic anemia, leukocytosis, leukopenia, thrombocytopenia
SKIN: Rash
Other: Body odor, hyperchloremia, hypoalbuminemia, hypophosphatemia, metabolic acidosis, metabolic alkalosis, weight gain

Nursing Considerations

• Mix powder form of sodium phenylbutyrate with food or liquid, but not with acidic beverages such as coffee and tea.
• Be aware that drug shouldn't be used to treat acute hyperammonemia, which is a medical emergency.
• Monitor patient with history of heart failure or severe renal failure for fluid retention because of drug's sodium content.

PATIENT TEACHING

• Instruct patient to take sodium phenylbutyrate with meals but not to mix it with acidic beverages such as coffee and tea.
• Advise patient to comply with follow-up laboratory tests, as prescribed.
• Urge patient to notify prescriber immediately about changes in body odor because they may signal metabolic imbalance.

sodium polystyrene sulfonate

Kayexalate, K-Exit (CAN), Kionex, PMS-Sodium Polystyrene Sulfonate (CAN), SPS Suspension

Class and Category

Chemical class: Sulfonated cation-exchange resin
Therapeutic class: Antihyperkalemic
Pregnancy category: C

Indications and Dosages

➤ *To treat hyperkalemia*

ORAL POWDER, SUSPENSION

Adults. 15 g (4 level tsp) once daily to q.i.d. *Maximum:* 40 g q.i.d.
Children. 1 g/kg/dose, as needed.

RECTAL POWDER, SUSPENSION

Adults. 25 to 100 g as retention enema, as needed.
Children. 1 g/kg/dose as retention enema, as needed.

Mechanism of Action

Releases sodium ions in exchange for other cations in intestines. Resin enters large intestine and releases sodium ions in exchange for hydrogen ions. As the resin moves through the intestines, hydrogen ions are then exchanged for potassium ions, which are in greater concentration. Bound resin leaves the body in feces, carrying potassium and other ions with it, thereby reducing serum potassium level.

Route	Onset	Peak	Duration
P.O.	2 to 12 hr	Unknown	Unknown

Contraindications

Hypersensitivity to sodium polystyrene sulfonate or its components, hypokalemia, obstructive bowel disease, reduced intestinal motility in neonates, oral administration in neonates

Interactions

DRUGS

antacids, laxatives: Increased risk of metabolic alkalosis

potassium-sparing diuretics, potassium supplements: Increased risk of fluid retention

Adverse Reactions

CV: Peripheral edema

GI: Abdominal cramps, anorexia, constipation, epigastric pain, fecal impaction, indigestion, nausea, vomiting

GU: Decreased urine output

Other: Hypernatremia, hypocalcemia, hypokalemia, weight gain

Nursing Considerations

• Use sodium polystyrene sulfonate cautiously in patients with heart failure, hypertension, or marked edema.

• Be aware that drug is available as powdered resin or as solution that contains sorbitol to facilitate movement of resin through intestines. As a result, patient may experience abdominal cramps, diarrhea, nausea, and vomiting.

• Because the drug doesn't take effect for several hours, be aware that it's inappropriate for treating acute, life-threatening hyperkalemia.

• If patient has hypokalemia or hypocalcemia, notify prescriber immediately and expect to withhold drug because it reduces potassium and calcium levels. Evidence of hypokalemia includes abdominal cramps, acidic urine, anorexia, drowsiness, ECG changes, hypotension, hypoventilation, muscle weakness, and tachycardia. Evidence of hypocalcemia includes abdominal pain, agitation, anxiety, ECG changes, hypotension, muscle twitching, psychosis, seizures, and tetany.

• To administer powdered resin as an oral suspension, mix powder in water, syrup (such as sorbitol), or food and give promptly.

If necessary, administer through gastric feeding tube.

• Precede rectal administration with a cleansing enema, as ordered.

• When giving rectally, suspend powdered resin in 100 ml of aqueous solution warmed to body temperature, in bag connected to soft, large (French 28) catheter. Have patient lie on his left side with his lower leg straight and upper leg flexed or with his knees to his chest. Gently insert the tube into the rectum and well into the sigmoid colon. The solution should flow into the colon by way of gravity and be retained for 30 to 60 minutes or longer, if possible. After patient is unable to retain the solution any longer, administer a non-sodium-containing cleansing enema, as prescribed.

• After administration, assess for constipation and fecal impaction.

PATIENT TEACHING

• Instruct patient not to mix oral form of sodium polystyrene sulfonate with foods and liquids high in potassium content, such as bananas and orange juice.

• If patient will self-administer rectal solution, teach the correct technique and body position. Remind him to let the solution flow into the colon by gravity and to retain it for at least 30 to 60 minutes, longer if possible.

• Advise patient to notify prescriber immediately about abdominal cramps, nausea, and vomiting.

sodium thiosalicylate

Rexolate, Tusal

Class and Category

Chemical class: Salicylic acid derivative
Therapeutic class: Analgesic, anti-inflammatory
Pregnancy category: Not rated

Indications and Dosages

➤ *To relieve symptoms of acute gout*

I.V. OR I.M. INJECTION

Adults. *Initial:* 100 mg every 3 to 4 hr for 2 days; then 100 mg daily.

➤ *To relieve pain from musculoskeletal conditions*

I.V. OR I.M. INJECTION

Adults. 50 to 100 mg daily or every other day.

Q
R
S

➤ *To relieve symptoms of osteoarthritis*
I.V. OR I.M. INJECTION
Adults. 100 mg 3 times/wk for several wk, then once/wk, usually up to a total dosage of 2.5 g. After 1 to 2 wk, another course of treatment may be given.
➤ *To treat rheumatic fever*
I.V. OR I.M. INJECTION
Adults. *Initial:* 100 to 150 mg every 4 to 8 hr for 3 days, then 100 mg b.i.d.

Mechanism of Action

Exerts peripherally induced analgesic and anti-inflammatory effects by blocking pain impulses and inhibiting prostaglandin synthesis.

Contraindications

GI bleeding; hemophilia; hemorrhage; hypersensitivity to sodium thiosalicylate, NSAIDs, or their components; Reye's syndrome

Interactions

DRUGS

ACE inhibitors, beta blockers: Decreased antihypertensive effect of these drugs
activated charcoal: Decreased sodium thiosalicylate absorption
antacids, urinary alkalizers: Increased excretion of sodium thiosalicylate, leading to reduced drug effectiveness and shortened half-life
carbonic anhydrase inhibitors (such as acetazolamide): Increased risk of salicylate toxicity; possibly displacement of acetazolamide from protein-binding sites, resulting in toxicity
corticosteroids: Possibly increased sodium thiosalicylate excretion
insulin, oral antidiabetic drugs: Altered glucose control (with large sodium thiosalicylate doses)
loop diuretics: Possibly decreased effectiveness of loop diuretics in patients with renal or hepatic impairment
methotrexate: Increased risk of methotrexate toxicity
nizatidine: Increased blood sodium thiosalicylate level
probenecid, sulfinpyrazone: Decreased uricosuric effects
spironolactone: Possibly inhibited diuretic effect of spironolactone

urinary acidifiers (including ammonium chloride, ascorbic acid, methionine): Decreased sodium thiosalicylate excretion, possibly leading to salicylate toxicity

ACTIVITIES

alcohol use: Increased risk of gastrointestinal ulceration

Adverse Reactions

GI: Anorexia, diarrhea, GI bleeding, heartburn, hepatotoxicity, indigestion, nausea, thirst, vomiting
HEME: Leukopenia, platelet dysfunction, prolonged bleeding time, thrombocytopenia
RESP: Bronchospasm
SKIN: Rash, urticaria
Other: Angioedema

Nursing Considerations

•Use drug cautiously in patients with asthma, chronic urticaria, or nasal polyps because these patients are more prone to hypersensitivity.
•Expect to monitor hepatic and renal function during long-term drug therapy.
•After repeated use or large doses, look for signs of salicylate toxicity: CNS depression, confusion, diaphoresis, diarrhea, difficulty hearing, dizziness, headache, hyperventilation, lassitude, tinnitus, and vomiting.
•Be aware that tinnitus usually means that the blood sodium thiosalicylate level has reached or exceeded the upper limit for therapeutic effects.

PATIENT TEACHING

•Instruct patient to notify prescriber immediately about bleeding or symptoms of salicylate toxicity.

solifenacin succinate

VESIcare

Class and Category

Chemical class: Muscarinic receptor antagonist
Therapeutic class: Bladder antispasmodic
Pregnancy category: C

Indications and Dosages

➤ *To treat overactive urinary bladder with symptoms of urge incontinence, urgency, and frequency*
TABLETS
Adults. 5 mg daily; if tolerated well, in-

creased to 10 mg daily.

DOSAGE ADJUSTMENT For patients with severe renal impairment or moderate hepatic impairment or patients taking ketoconazole or other potent CYP3A4 inhibitors, dosage limited to 5 mg daily.

Route	Onset	Peak	Duration
P.O.	Unknown	3 to 8 hr	Unknown

Mechanism of Action

Antagonizes the effect of acetylcholine on muscarinic receptors in detrusor muscle, decreasing the muscle spasms that cause inappropriate bladder emptying. This action increases bladder capacity and volume, which relieves the sensation of urgency and frequency and enhances bladder control.

Contraindications

Gastric retention, hypersensitivity to solifenacin or its components, uncontrolled angle-closure glaucoma, urine retention

Interactions

DRUGS

ketoconazole, other potent CYP3A4 inhibitors: Possibly decreased metabolism of solifenacin and increased risk of adverse effects

Adverse Reactions

CNS: Confusion, depression, dizziness, fatigue, hallucinations, headache
CV: Hypertension, prolonged QT interval, peripheral edema, torsades de pointes
EENT: Blurred vision, dry eyes or mouth, pharyngitis
GI: Abdominal pain, constipation, indigestion, nausea, vomiting
GU: UTI, uriney retention
RESP: Cough
RESP: Pruritus, rash, urticaria
Other: Angioedema, influenza

Nursing Considerations

•Use cautiously in patients with ulcerative colitis, intestinal atony, or myasthenia gravis because solifenacin may decrease GI motility; in patients with significant bladder outflow obstruction because solifenacin may cause urine retention; in patients with he-patic impairment because solifenacin is metabolized in the liver; and in patients with renal impairment because solifenacin excretion may be impaired.
•Monitor elderly patients, especially those age 75 and over, for adverse reactions because they're at increased risk for solifenacin-induced adverse reactions.

PATIENT TEACHING

•Instruct patient to take solifenacin with a full glass of water and to swallow the tablet whole.
•Caution patient to avoid exertion in a warm or hot environment because sweating may be delayed, which could increase body temperature and increase risk of heatstroke.
•Advise patient to avoid hazardous activities until drug's CNS effects are known.
•Inform patient that alcohol may cause drowsiness, and urge patient to limit or avoid alcoholic beverages while taking solifenacin.

somatropin

Accretropin, Genotropin, Humatrope, Norditropin, Nutropin, Nutropin AQ, Omnitrope, Saizen, Serostim, Tev-Tropin

Class and Category

Chemical class: Recombinant DNA product
Therapeutic class: Growth hormone
Pregnancy category: B (Serostim) or C (Genotropin, Humatrope, Norditropin, Nutropin, Nutropin AQ, Saizen)

Indications and Dosages

➤ *To treat growth failure caused by growth hormone deficiency*

SUBCUTANEOUS INJECTION (NUTROPIN, NUTROPIN AQ)
Adults. 0.3 mg (0.9 international units)/kg/wk.

SUBCUTANEOUS INJECTION (SAIZEN)
Adults. *Initial:* 0.005 mg/kg daily, increased after 4 wk by no more than 0.01 mg/kg daily, as needed.

I.M. OR SUBCUTANEOUS INJECTION (HUMATROPE, NUTROPIN, SAIZEN)
Children. 0.18 to 0.3 mg (0.54 to 0.9 international units)/kg/wk, divided into equal doses given daily or every other day over 6 to 7 days.

SUBCUTANEOUS INJECTION (NORDITROPIN)
Adults. *Initial:* 0.004 mg/kg daily, increased

Q
R
S

after 6 wk by no more than 0.016 mg/kg daily, as needed.

SUBCUTANEOUS INJECTION (GENOTROPIN, NORDITROPIN)
Children. 0.16 to 0.24 mg (0.48 to 0.72 international units)/kg/wk, divided into equal doses given daily over 6 to 7 days.

SUBCUTANEOUS INJECTION (TEV-TROPIN)
Children. Up to 0.1 mg/kg three times/wk.

SUBCUTANEOUS INJECTION (OMNITROPE)
Adults. *Initial:* 0.04 mg/kg/wk divided into 7 daily doses and increased at 4- to 8-wk intervals, as needed. *Maximum:* 0.08 mg/kg/wk. Alternatively, 0.15 to 0.30 mg/day.
Children. 0.16 to 0.24 mg/kg/wk divided into 6 to 7 daily doses.

SUBCUTANEOUS INJECTION (ACCRETROPIN)
Children. 0.18 to 0.3 mg/kg/wk divided into 6 to 7 daily doses.

➤ *To treat growth failure caused by chronic renal insufficiency*

SUBCUTANEOUS INJECTION (NUTROPIN, NUTROPIN AQ)
Children. Up to 0.35 mg (1.05 international units)/kg/wk, divided into equal doses given daily.

➤ *To treat growth failure caused by Turner's syndrome*

SUBCUTANEOUS INJECTION (NUTROPIN, NUTROPIN AQ)
Adults and children. Up to 0.375 mg (1.125 international units)/kg/wk, divided into equal doses given daily or every other day over 7 days.

SUBCUTANEOUS INJECTION (NORDITROPIN)
Adults and children. Up to 0.067 mg/kg/day.

SUBCUTANEOUS INJECTION (ACCRETROPIN)
Children. 0.36 mg/kg/wk divided into 6 to 7 daily doses.

➤ *To treat short stature or growth failure in children with short stature homeobox-containing gene (SHOX) deficiency whose epiphyses are not closed*

SUBCUTANEOUS INJECTION (HUMATROPE)
Children. 0.35 mg/kg weekly divided into equal daily doses.

➤ *To provide long-term treatment of growth failure in children born small for gestational age and no catch-up growth by age 2*

SUBCUTANEOUS INJECTION (GENOTROPIN)
Children. 0.48 mg/kg/wk, divided into equal doses and administered daily over 6 to 7 days.

SUBCUTANEOUS INJECTION (HUMATROPE)
Children. Up to 0.37 mg/kg/wk, divided into

equal doses and administered daily over 6 to 7 days.

SUBCUTANEOUS INJECTION (NORDITROPIN)
Children. Up to 0.067 mg/kg/day.

➤ *To treat growth factor failure due to Prader-Willi syndrome*

SUBCUTANEOUS INJECTION (GENOTROPIN)
Children. 0.24 mg/kg/wk.

➤ *To treat AIDS-related cachexia or weight loss*

SUBCUTANEOUS INJECTION (SEROSTIM)
Adults weighing more than 55 kg (121 lb). 6 mg at bedtime.
Adults weighing 45 to 55 kg (99 to 121 lb). 5 mg at bedtime.
Adults weighing 35 to 45 kg (77 to 99 lb). 4 mg at bedtime.
Adults weighing less than 35 kg. 0.1 mg/kg at bedtime.

DOSAGE ADJUSTMENT For patients at increased risk for adverse effects related to Serostim therapy, 0.1 mg/kg every other day. For elderly patients, regardless of type of somatropin prescribed, lower starting dose and smaller dosage titration recommended.

Route	Onset	Peak	Duration
I.M., SubQ	Unknown	Unknown	12 to 48 hr

Mechanism of Action
Increases production of somatomedins (or insulin-like growth factor) in the liver and other tissues, which mediates somatropin's anabolic and growth-promoting effects. The drug binds to specific receptors throughout the body, stimulating amino acid transport; DNA, RNA, and protein synthesis; cell proliferation; and growth of bone and soft tissue.

Somatropin also decreases insulin cell receptor sensitivity, thereby increasing blood glucose level; stimulates triglyceride hydrolysis in adipose tissue and hepatic glucose output; and aids bone growth by promoting a positive calcium balance and retention of sodium and potassium.

Contraindications
Active neoplasia; active proliferative or severe nonproliferative diabetic retinopathy; acute critical illness due to complications following open-heart surgery, abdominal sur-

gery, or multiple trauma; acute respiratory failure; cancer; closed epiphyses; hypersensitivity to somatropin, its components, or benzyl alcohol; Prader-Willi syndrome coupled with severe obesity, history of upper airway obstruction or sleep apnea, or severe respiratory impairment

Interactions
DRUGS
anabolic steroids, androgens, estrogens, thyroid hormones: Possibly accelerated epiphyseal closure
anticonvulsants, corticosteroids, cyclosporine, sex steroids: Possibly altered clearance of these drugs, increasing risk of adverse effects
corticosteroids, corticotropin: Inhibited growth response to somatropin; decreased response of corticosteroids or corticotropin
oral estrogens: Decreased somatropin effectiveness

Adverse Reactions
CNS: Depression, dizziness, fatigue, headache, hypoesthesia, insomnia, intracranial hypertension or tumor, paresthesia, weakness
CV: Chest pain, edema, hypertriglyceridemia
EENT: Otitis, papilledema, rhinitis, sinusitis, tonsillitis, vision changes, worsening of diabetic retinopathy
ENDO: Breast pain, edema, tenderness, or mass; gynecomastia; hyperglycemia; hypothyroidism
GI: Nausea, pancreatitis, vomiting
GU: UTI
HEME: Eosinophilia
MS: Arthralgia; back, bone, joint, or leg pain; carpal tunnel syndrome; myalgia; progression of existing scoliosis; slipped capital femoral epiphysis (children)
RESP: Upper respiratory tract infection
SKIN: Increased growth of nevi, rash
Other: Elevated serum alkaline phosphatase, inorganic phosphorus, and parathyroid hormone levels; flulike symptoms; injection site inflammation, lipoatrophy

Nursing Considerations
• Be aware that somatropin shouldn't be used in patients with malignancy and should be stopped if patient is diagnosed with malignancy. Cancer treatment must be completed with evidence of remission before somatropin can be started or restarted.

• Make sure patient with Prader-Willi syndrome has been evaluated for upper airway obstruction and sleep apnea before starting somatropin because of increased risk of respiratory arrest. Notify prescriber immediately and expect to stop drug if patient starts snoring, snoring increases, or other evidence of upper airway obstruction develops.
• Make sure patient has a funduscopic eye examination before starting and periodically throughout somatropin therapy to rule out papilledema.
• Use cautiously in elderly patients because they're more prone to adverse reactions to somatropin. Expect initial dosage to be lower and dosage adjustment more gradual to minimize adverse effects.
• Reconstitute somatropin according to package directions. (Nutropin AQ and forms available in cartridges, such as Norditropin NordiFlex, don't require reconstitution.) In general, swirl vial gently to dissolve contents rather than shaking it.
• Don't reconstitute with diluent that contains benzyl alcohol if drug will be given to neonate. Don't use diluent supplied for Humatrope for patients sensitive to Metacresol or glycerin; use sterile water for injection.
• Store Nutropin AQ vials and cartridges refrigerated in a dark place.
• Remember to rotate injection sites to avoid tissue atrophy at injection site.
• **WARNING** Although uncommon, intracranial hypertension is possible. Monitor patient for such signs and symptoms as headache, nausea, papilledema, vision changes, and vomiting, especially during first 8 weeks of therapy. If intrancranial hypertension occurs, notify prescriber, expect to discontinue drug, and provide supportive care, as needed.
• Because somatropin is a protein, monitor patient for local or systemic allergic reaction.
• Monitor patient's blood glucose level because somatropin may decrease insulin sensitivity, especially at higher does.
• Monitor patient's thyroid function and obtain periodic test results, as ordered, because untreated hypothyroidsm may interfere with somatropin, especially in children.
• Assess patient's skin regularly for changes that suggest skin malignancy.
PATIENT TEACHING
• Instruct diabetic patient who takes insulin to monitor blood glucose level frequently; so-

Q
R
S

matropin may induce insulin resistance.
•Inform parents of a child with Turner's syndrome about increased risk of ear infections.
•Advise family or cargiver to observe patient for limping, which may indicate a slipped epiphysis.
•Instruct patient or caregiver how to measure and administer drug at home using either pen device or vial, syringe, and needle.

sotalol hydrochloride

Betapace, Betapace AF, Sotacor (CAN)

Class and Category

Chemical class: Methanesulfonanilide
Therapeutic class: Class III antiarrhythmic
Pregnancy category: B

Indications and Dosages

➤ *To treat life-threatening ventricular arrhythmias*

TABLETS

Adults. *Initial:* 80 mg b.i.d. *Maintenance:* 160 to 320 mg daily in divided doses b.i.d. or t.i.d. *Maximum:* 640 mg daily.
DOSAGE ADJUSTMENT If creatinine clearance is 30 to 60 ml/min/1.73 m^2, dosage interval extended to every 24 hr; if creatinine clearance is less than 30 ml/min/1.73 m^2, dosage interval extended to every 36 to 48 hr, according to response; if creatinine clearance less than 10 ml/min/1.73 m^2, dosage adjusted as prescribed.

➤ *To maintain normal sinus rhythm in patients with highly symptomatic atrial fibrillation who are currently in sinus rhythm*

TABLETS

Adults. *Initial:* If creatinine clearance is 40 to 60 ml/min/1.73 m^2, give 80 mg daily; if creatinine clearance exceeds 60 ml/min/1.73 m^2, give 80 mg b.i.d. *Maintenance:* After at least 3 days (five or six doses given daily), if 80-mg dose is tolerated and QT interval less than 500 msec, dosage maintained and patient discharged. Or hospitalized patient monitored closely to determine maintenance dosage while increasing to 120 mg b.i.d. for 3 days (five or six doses if daily dosing). *Maximum:* 160 mg b.i.d. if creatinine clearance exceeds 60 ml/min/1.73 m^2.
DOSAGE ADJUSTMENT If 80-mg once or twice daily doesn't reduce frequency of atrial fib-

rillation relapses and is tolerated without excessive QT-interval prolongation (greater than 520 msec), dosage increased to 120 mg once or twice daily, depending on creatinine clearance. If 120-mg dose doesn't reduce frequency of early relapse and is tolerated using same criteria, dosage increased to 160 mg once or twice daily, depending on creatinine clearance.
DOSAGE ADJUSTMENT If QT interval is 520 msec or more, dosage reduced until it returns to less than 520 msec. If QT interval exceeds 520 msec with lowest maintenance dosage of 80 mg, drug stopped. If renal function deteriorates, daily dose reduced by half and given daily.

Route	Onset	Peak	Duration
P.O.	Unknown	2 to 3 hr	Unknown

Mechanism of Action

Combines class II and class III antiarrhythmic activity to increase sinus cycle length. This beta blocker decreases AV nodal conduction and increases AV nodal refractoriness. Suppression of SA node automaticity and AV node conductivity decreases atrial and ventricular ectopy.

Contraindications

Asthma, atrial arrhythmias (if baseline QT interval exceeds 450 msec or creatinine clearance is less than 40 ml/min/1.73 m^2), cardiogenic shock, congenital or acquired QT syndromes, COPD, heart failure (unless it results from tachyarrhythmia that's treatable by sotalol), hypersensitivity to sotalol or its components, second- or third-degree AV block without functioning pacemaker, sinus bradycardia

Interactions

DRUGS

allergen immunotherapy, allergenic extracts for skin testing: Increased risk of serious systemic adverse reaction or anaphylaxis
amiodarone: Additive depressant effect on conduction, negative inotropic effect
anesthetics (hydrocarbon inhalation): Increased risk of myocardial depression and hypotension
antacids: Altered sotalol effectiveness

astemizole, class I antiarrhythmics, phenothiazines, terfenadine, tricyclic antidepressants: Prolonged QT interval, life-threatening
torsades de pointes
beta blockers (other): Additive beta blockade
beta$_2$-receptor stimulants: Decreased effectiveness of these drugs
calcium channel blockers, clonidine, diazoxide, guanabenz, reserpine and other antihypertensives: Additive antihypertensive effect and, possibly, other beta-blocking effects
cimetidine: Possibly impaired sotalol clearance
glucagon: Possibly blunted hyperglycemic response
insulin, oral antidiabetic drugs: Impaired glucose control, increased risk of hyperglycemia
lidocaine: Decreased lidocaine clearance, increased risk of lidocaine toxicity
MAO inhibitors: Increased risk of significant
hypertension
neuromuscular blockers: Possibly potentiated
and prolonged neuromuscular blockade
phenothiazines: Increased blood levels of both
drugs
propafenone: Increased blood level and half-
life of sotalol
sympathomimetics, xanthines: Possibly mutual inhibition of therapeutic effects

Adverse Reactions

CNS: Anxiety, depression, dizziness, drowsi-
ness, fatigue, insomnia, lethargy, nervous-
ness, weakness
CV: AV conduction disorders, bradycardia,
heart failure, hypotension, peripheral vascu-
lar insufficiency
EENT: Nasal congestion
ENDO: Hyperglycemia, hypoglycemia
GI: Abdominal pain, constipation, diarrhea,
nausea, vomiting
GU: Sexual dysfunction
MS: Muscle weakness
RESP: Bronchospasm, dyspnea, wheezing

Nursing Considerations

•Expect to obtain baseline creatinine clearance and QT interval before starting sotalol.
•Monitor blood pressure, apical and radial
pulses, fluid intake and output, daily weight,
respiratory rate, and circulation in extremities before and during sotalol therapy.
•If prescriber is stopping amiodarone, be
aware that sotalol shouldn't be started until
QT interval has returned to baseline because

of possible adverse cardiac effects.
•Be aware that stopping sotalol abruptly
may cause life-threatening reactions.
•Monitor serum electrolyte levels because
drug can increase risk of torsades de pointes
in patients with electrolyte imbalances, especially hypokalemia or hypomagnesemia.
•Assess carefully if patient has diabetes mellitus or thyrotoxicosis because they may
mask hypoglycemia and hyperthyroidism.
PATIENT TEACHING
•Advise patient to notify prescriber immediately if he has difficulty breathing.
•Urge patient to consult prescriber before
taking OTC drugs, especially cold remedies,
which may decrease sotalol's effectiveness.
•Urge patient to avoid potentially hazardous
activities until drug's CNS effects are known.

sparfloxacin

Zagam

Class and Category

Chemical class: Fluoroquinolone
Therapeutic class: Antibiotic
Pregnancy category: C

Indications and Dosages

➤ *To treat community-acquired pneumonia
caused by* Chlamydia pneumoniae, Haemophilus influenzae, H. parainfluenzae,
Moraxella catarrhalis, Mycoplasma
pneumoniae, *or* Streptococcus pneumoniae *and acute bacterial exacerbations
of chronic bronchitis caused by* C. pneumoniae, Enterobacter cloacae, H. influenzae, H. parainfluenzae, Klebsiella
pneumoniae, M. catarrhalis, Staphylococcus aureus, *or* S. pneumoniae
TABLETS
Adults. 400 mg on day 1, followed by 200 mg/
day for 10 days.
DOSAGE ADJUSTMENT For patients with creatinine clearance less than 50 ml/min/1.73 m^2,
400 mg on day 1 and then dosing interval
extended to 200 mg every 48 hr for 9 days.

Contraindications

History of photosensitivity, hypersensitivity
to quinolone derivatives, job or lifestyle that
precludes compliance with measures to prevent phototoxicity, prolonged QTc interval or
use of drugs that can prolong QTc interval

Q
R
S

> **Mechanism of Action**
> Causes bacterial cells to die by inhibiting the enzyme DNA gyrase, which is responsible for unwinding and supercoiling bacterial DNA before it replicates.

Interactions

DRUGS

aluminum-, calcium-, or magnesium-containing antacids; ferrous sulfate; magnesium-containing laxatives; sucralfate; zinc: Decreased bioavailability of sparfloxacin
amiodarone, astemizole, bepridil, cisapride, class IA antiarrhythmics (disopyramide, quinidine, procainamide), class III antiarrhythmics (ibutilide, sotalol), erythromycin, pentamidine, phenothiazines, terfenadine, tricyclic antidepressants, other drugs that can prolong QTc interval: Possibly prolonged QTc interval and torsades de pointes

Adverse Reactions

CNS: Asthenia, cerebral thrombosis, dizziness, drowsiness, headache, insomnia, lightheadedness, nervousness, seizures, somnolence
CV: Cardiopulmonary arrest, embolism, prolonged QTc interval, torsades de pointes, vasodilation
EENT: Laryngeal edema, taste perversion
GI: Abdominal pain, diarrhea, hepatic necrosis or failure, hepatitis, intestinal perforation, nausea, pseudomembranous colitis, vomiting
GU: Acute renal failure, vaginal candidiasis
HEME: Agranulocytosis, hemolytic anemia, pancytopenia, thrombocytopenia
MS: Rhabdomyolysis, tendinitis, tendon rupture
RESP: Interstitial pneumonia, pulmonary edema
SKIN: Photosensitivity, pruritus, rash, Stevens-Johnson syndrome, toxic epidermal necrolysis
Other: Acidosis, anaphylaxis, angioedema, squamous cell carcinoma

Nursing Considerations

• Use sparfloxacin cautiously in patients with known or suspected CNS disorders because of risk of seizures. Institute seizure precautions according to facility policy.
• Monitor renal and liver function test re-

sults, as appropriate, during prolonged therapy.
• Measure QTc interval regularly because sparfloxacin has been found to increase QTc interval and risk of torsades de pointes.
• Severe diarrhea may indicate pseudomembranous colitis; give fluid, electrolyte, and protein replacement, as ordered.

PATIENT TEACHING

• Urge patient to avoid potentially hazardous activities until sparfloxacin's CNS effects are known.
• Advise patient to notify prescriber immediately about aching or throbbing tendon pain.
• Instruct patient to wait 4 hours after taking sparfloxacin before taking antacids that contain aluminum, calcium, or magnesium; laxatives that contain magnesium; or vitamins that contain iron or zinc.
• Caution patient to avoid exposure to sunlight, bright natural light, and other sources of ultraviolet light during therapy and for 5 days afterward. Urge him to wear sunscreen and protective clothing when outdoors.
• Urge patient to notify prescriber at first sign of photosensitivity reaction (blistering, burning or swelling sensation, itching, rash, redness).

spectinomycin hydrochloride

Trobicin

Class and Category

Chemical class: Aminocyclitol, aminoglycoside derivative
Therapeutic class: Antibiotic
Pregnancy category: Not rated

Indications and Dosages

➤ *To treat acute endocervical, rectal, and urethral gonorrhea caused by susceptible strains of* Neisseria gonorrhoeae

I.M. INJECTION

Adults and children weighing 45 kg (99 lb) or more. 2 g as a single dose, repeated as prescribed for adult if reinfection occurs or is strongly suspected. *Maximum:* 4 g for adults, 2 g for children.
Children weighing less than 45 kg (except infants). 40 mg/kg as a single dose.

Mechanism of Action
Binds to negatively charged sites on bacterial outer cell membrane, disrupting cell integrity, and binds to bacterial ribosomal subunits, inhibiting protein synthesis. Both actions lead to bacterial cell death.

Contraindications
Hypersensitivity to spectinomycin or its components

Adverse Reactions
CNS: Dizziness, insomnia
GI: Abdominal cramps, nausea, vomiting
Other: Injection site pain

Nursing Considerations
•To reconstitute spectinomycin, add 3.2 ml of bacteriostatic water for injection (with benzyl alcohol) to each 2-g vial or 6.2 ml of diluent to each 4-g vial. Shake vial vigorously before withdrawing dose.
•Administer I.M. injection deep into large muscle mass, preferably upper outer quadrant of gluteal muscle.

PATIENT TEACHING
•Tell patient he'll be tested for syphilis at the start of treatment and 3 months later because spectinomycin treatment may mask or delay syphilis symptoms.
•Explain risk factors for sexually transmitted diseases, and teach correct condom use.
•Advise patient to encourage sexual partner to be tested for gonorrhea.
•Instruct patient to notify prescriber if signs and symptoms persist after a few days.

spironolactone
Aldactone, Novospiroton (CAN)

Class and Category
Chemical class: Aldosterone antagonist
Therapeutic class: Aldosterone antagonist, antihypertensive, diagnostic aid for primary hyperaldosteronism, diuretic
Pregnancy category: Not rated

Indications and Dosages
➤ *To treat edema cause by heart failure, hepatic cirrhosis, or nephrotic syndrome*
TABLETS
Adults. *Initial:* 25 to 200 mg daily in divided doses b.i.d. to q.i.d. for at least 5 days. *Maintenance:* 75 to 400 mg daily in divided doses b.i.d. to q.i.d. *Maximum:* 400 mg daily.
Children. *Initial:* 1 to 3 mg/kg daily as a single dose or in divided doses b.i.d. to q.i.d. for at least 2 wk; adjusted, as needed, after 5 days. *Maximum:* 3 times initial dose.
➤ *To treat hypertension*
TABLETS
Adults. *Initial:* 50 to 100 mg daily as a single dose or in divided doses b.i.d. to q.i.d. for at least 2 wk; gradually adjusted every 2 wk, as needed, to control blood pressure, up to 200 mg daily. *Maximum:* 400 mg daily.
Children. *Initial:* 1 to 3 mg/kg daily as a single dose or in divided doses b.i.d. to q.i.d. for at least 2 wk; adjusted, as needed, after 5 days. *Maximum:* 3 times initial dose.
➤ *To aid in the diagnosis of primary hyperaldosteronism*
TABLETS
Adults. For long test, 400 mg daily in divided doses b.i.d. to q.i.d. for 3 to 4 wk; for short test, 400 mg daily in divided doses b.i.d. to q.i.d. for 4 days.
➤ *To treat primary hyperaldosteronism*
TABLETS
Adults. 100 to 400 mg daily in divided doses b.i.d. to q.i.d. before surgery. *Maximum:* 400 mg daily.
DOSAGE ADJUSTMENT Long-term maintenance dosage decreased for patients at risk for complications during surgery.
➤ *To substitute as therapy for diuretic-induced hypokalemia*
TABLETS
Adults. 25 to 100 mg daily as a single dose or in divided doses b.i.d. to q.i.d. *Maximum:* 400 mg daily.

Route	Onset	Peak	Duration
P.O.*	Unknown	2 to 3 days	2 to 3 days

Contraindications
Acute renal insufficiency, anuria, hyperkalemia, hypersensitivity to spironolactone or its components

Interactions
DRUGS
ACE inhibitors, cyclosporine, other potas-

* For diuretic effect; others unknown.

Mechanism of Action

Normally, aldosterone attaches to receptors on the walls of distal convoluted tubule cells, causing sodium (Na^+) and water (H_2O) reabsorption in the blood, as shown at left.

Spironolactone competes with aldosterone for these receptors, thereby preventing sodium and water reabsorption and causing their excretion through the distal convoluted tubules, as shown below right. Increased urinary excretion of sodium and water reduces blood volume and blood pressure.

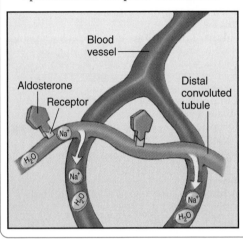
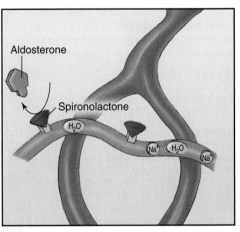

sium-sparing diuretics, potassium-containing drugs, potassium supplements: Increased risk of hyperkalemia
digoxin: Possibly increased half-life of digoxin
exchange resins (sodium cycle), such as sodium polystyrene sulfonate: Increased risk of hypokalemia and fluid retention
heparin, oral anticoagulants: Decreased anticoagulant effect of these drugs
hypotension-producing drugs: Possibly potentiated antihypertensive or diuretic effect of spironolactone
lithium: Possibly lithium toxicity
NSAIDs, sympathomimetics: Decreased antihypertensive effect of spironolactone

FOODS

low-salt milk, salt substitutes: Increased risk of hyperkalemia

Adverse Reactions

CNS: Dizziness, encephalopathy, fatigue, headache
EENT: Increased intraocular pressure, nasal congestion, tinnitus, vision changes
ENDO: Gynecomastia
GI: Abdominal pain, anorexia, constipation, diarrhea, flatulence, nausea, vomiting

GU: Impotence
HEME: Aplastic anemia, neutropenia
RESP: Cough, dyspnea
MS: Arthralgia, back and leg pain, muscle weakness, myalgia
Other: Hyperkalemia

Nursing Considerations

•Be aware that for children or patients who have trouble swallowing, pharmacist may crush spironolactone tablets, mix with a flavored syrup, and dispense as a suspension. It's stable for 1 month when refrigerated.
•In diagnosing primary aldosteronism, the test is considered positive if patient's serum potassium level rises when spironolactone is given and falls when it's discontinued.
•Expect to evaluate patient's serum potassium level 1 week after spiraonolactone therapy begins, after each dosage adjustment, monthly for the first 3 months, quarterly for 1 year, and then every 6 months thereafter or as ordered. Notify prescriber if level exceeds 5 mEq/L or patient's renal function deteriorates (serum creatinine level exceeding 4 mg/dl). If patient has severe heart failure, follow closely because hyperkalemia may be fatal in such patients.

- Evaluate spironolactone's effectiveness by assessing blood pressure and edema.
- Stop drug for several days, as prescribed, before patient undergoes adrenal vein catheterization to measure serum aldosterone level and plasma renin activity.

PATIENT TEACHING
- Instruct patient to take spironolactone with meals or milk.
- If patient can't swallow tablets, mention that pharmacist can crush and mix them with a flavored syrup as a suspension.
- Teach patient who takes spironolactone for hypertension how to measure his blood pressure. Urge him to monitor it regularly and report pressure greater than 140 mm Hg systolic or 90 mm Hg diastolic to prescriber.
- Caution patient that he may experience dizziness during spironolactone therapy if fluid balance is altered.

streptokinase

Kabikinase, Streptase

Class and Category
Chemical class: Purified beta-hemolytic *Streptococcus* filtrate
Therapeutic class: Thrombolytic
Pregnancy category: C

Indications and Dosages
➤ *To lyse coronary artery thrombi*
I.V. INFUSION
Adults. 1,500,000 international units within 60 min of event.
INTRACORONARY INFUSION
Adults. 20,000-international unit bolus, followed by 2,000 international units/min for 60 min for total dose of 140,000 international units.

➤ *To lyse acute arterial thromboembolism or thrombosis, acute pulmonary embolism, or deep vein thrombosis*
I.V. INFUSION
Adults. 250,000-international unit bolus over 30 min, followed by 100,000 international units/hr for 24 to 72 hr.

➤ *To clear occluded arteriovenous cannula*
I.V. INJECTION
Adults. 100,000 to 250,000 international units instilled slowly into each occluded lumen.

Route	Onset	Peak	Duration
I.V.	Immediate	20 to 120 min	4 hr

Mechanism of Action
Binds to fibrin in thrombus and converts trapped plasminogen to plasmin. Plasmin breaks down fibrin, fibrinogen, and other clotting factors, thereby dissolving the thrombus.

Incompatibilities
Don't mix streptokinase in the same syringe or give through the same I.V. line as other drugs.

Contraindications
Active internal bleeding, AV malformation or aneurysm, bleeding diathesis, history of stroke or intracranial or intraspinal surgery within the previous 2 months, hypersensitivity to streptokinase or its components, intracranial cancer, severe uncontrolled hypertension

Interactions
DRUGS
anticoagulants, enoxaparin, heparin, NSAIDs, platelet aggregation inhibitors: Increased risk of bleeding
antifibrinolytics: Antagonized effects of both drugs
antihypertensives: Increased risk of severe hypotension, especially when streptokinase is administered rapidly to treat coronary artery occlusion
cefamandole, cefoperazone, cefotetan, plicamycin, valproic acid: Possibly hypoprothrombinemia and increased risk of severe hemorrhage
corticosteroids, ethacrynic acid, salicylates: Possibly GI ulceration or bleeding

Adverse Reactions
CNS: Chills, fever
CV: Arrhythmias, hypotension
HEME: Unusual bleeding or bruising

Nursing Considerations
- Obtain hematocrit, platelet count, APTT, PT, and INR, as ordered, before giving streptokinase.
- To prevent foaming, don't shake drug dur-

Q
R
S

ing reconstitution.

•Check requently for bleeding at I.V. site and for blood in urine and stool. Perform neurologic assessment to detect intracranial bleeding.

•If serious spontaneous bleeding (not controlled by local pressure) occurs, stop streptokinase infusion immediately and notify prescriber.

•Monitor heart rate and rhythm by continuous ECG, as ordered.

•Treat fever with acetaminophen, as prescribed, rather than aspirin to reduce the risk of bleeding.

PATIENT TEACHING

•Explain to patient that he'll be on bed rest during streptokinase therapy.

•Inform patient that minor bleeding may occur at arterial puncture or surgical sites. Reassure him that appropriate care measures will be taken if bleeding occurs.

•Advise patient to wear or carry medical alert identification stating that he takes streptokinase.

•Inform patient that if he experiences chest pain within 12 months of therapy, he should notify health care providers that he has received streptokinase because repeated administration within 12 months may be ineffective.

streptomycin sulfate

Class and Category

Chemical class: Aminoglycoside
Therapeutic class: Antibiotic
Pregnancy category: D

Indications and Dosages

➤ *To treat gram-negative bacillary bacteremia, meningeal infections, pneumonia, systemic infections, and UTI caused by susceptible strains of* Aerobacter aerogenes, Brucella, Calymmatobacterium granulomatis, Enterococcus faecalis, Escherichia coli, Haemophilus ducreyi, H. influenzae, Klebsiella pneumoniae, *and* Proteus

I.M. INJECTION

Adults. 1 to 2 g daily in divided doses every 6 to 12 hr. *Maximum:* 2 g daily.

Children. 20 to 40 mg/kg daily in divided doses every 6 to 12 hr.

➤ *As adjunct to treat endocarditis caused by* Streptococcus viridans *or* E. faecalis

I.M. INJECTION

Adults. 1 g b.i.d. for 1 wk *(S. viridans)* or 2 wk *(E. faecalis)* with a penicillin. Then, 500 mg b.i.d. for 1 wk *(S. viridans)* or 4 wk *(E. faecalis).*

➤ *As adjunct to treat tuberculosis caused by* Mycobacterium tuberculosis

I.M. INJECTION

Adults. 1 g daily with other antibiotics; dosage reduced to 1 g 2 or 3 times/wk, as appropriate and prescribed. *Maximum:* 2 g daily.

Children. 20 mg/kg daily with other antibiotics. *Maximum:* 1 g daily.

DOSAGE ADJUSTMENT For elderly patients, dosage decreased to 500 to 750 mg daily in combination with other antibiotics.

➤ *To treat plague caused by* Yersinia pestis

I.M. INJECTION

Adults. 2 g daily in 2 equally divided doses for at least 10 days.

Children. 30 mg/kg daily in divided doses b.i.d. or t.i.d. for 10 days.

➤ *To treat tularemia caused by* Francisella tularensis

I.M. INJECTION

Adults. 1 to 2 g daily in divided doses for 7 to 14 days.

DOSAGE ADJUSTMENT If creatinine clearance is 50 to 80 ml/min/1.73 m^2, dosage reduced to 7.5 mg/kg I.M. every 24 hr; if 10 to 49 ml/min/1.73 m^2, 7.5 mg/kg I.M. every 24 to 72 hr; if less than 10 ml/min/1.73 m^2, 7.5 mg/kg I.M. every 72 to 96 hr.

Mechanism of Action

Binds to negatively charged sites on the bacteria's outer cell membrane, disrupting cell integrity. Streptomycin also binds to bacterial ribosomal subunits and inhibits protein synthesis. Both actions lead to bacterial cell death.

Incompatibilities

Don't mix streptomycin in same solution or administer through same I.V. line as other antibiotics.

Contraindications

Hypersensitivity to streptomycin or other aminoglycosides

Interactions

DRUGS

antimyasthenics: Possibly decreased effect of antimyasthenics on skeletal muscle

beta-lactam antibiotics: Inactivation of streptomycin

capreomycin, other aminoglycosides: Increased potential for ototoxicity, nephrotoxicity, and neuromuscular blockade

indomethacin (I.V.): Decreased renal clearance of streptomycin when given to premature neonates, possibly leading to aminoglycoside toxicity

methoxyflurane, polymyxins (parenteral): Increased risk of nephrotoxicity and neuromuscular blockade

nephrotoxic and ototoxic drugs: Increased risk of nephrotoxicity and ototoxicity

neuromuscular blockers: Increased neuromuscular blockade

Adverse Reactions

CNS: Clumsiness, dizziness, neurotoxicity, paresthesia, peripheral neuropathy, seizures, unsteadiness, vertigo

EENT: Hearing loss, sensation of fullness in ears, tinnitus, vision loss

GI: Anorexia, nausea, thirst, vomiting

GU: Decreased or increased urine output, nephrotoxicity

MS: Muscle twitching

SKIN: Erythema, pruritus, rash, urticaria

Nursing Considerations

• Use streptomycin cautiously in patients with renal impairment. In severely uremic patients, single dose can produce high blood level of drug for several days; cumulative effects may produce ototoxicity.

• Expect prescriber to order baseline renal function studies and to assess cranial nerve VIII function (responsible for hearing) at start of streptomycin therapy to allow for later comparisons.

• Monitor serum peak and trough levels, as ordered, to ensure adequate but not toxic drug level.

• Be aware that streptomycin should be given only by I.M. injection.

• To reconstitute streptomycin, add between 4.2 and 4.5 ml of sodium chloride for injection or sterile water for injection to each 1-g vial to provide a concentration of 200 mg/ml, or add between 3.2 and 3.5 ml of diluent to each 5-g vial to provide a concentration of 250 mg/ml. Alternatively, add 6.5 ml of diluent to each 5-g vial to provide a concentration of 500 mg/ml.

• Don't give more than 500 mg/ml.

• Rotate injection sites to prevent sterile abscess formation.

PATIENT TEACHING

• Advise patient to refrigerate streptomycin solution at 36° to 46° F (2° to 8° C).

• Inform patient that treatment for tuberculosis lasts at least 1 year.

• Urge patient to notify prescriber if he has fullness or ringing in ears, hearing loss, or vertigo.

sucralfate

Apo-sucralfate (CAN), Carafate, Sulcrate (CAN), Sulcrate Suspension Plus (CAN)

Class and Category

Chemical class: Disulfated disaccharide, aluminum salt

Therapeutic class: Antiulcer

Pregnancy category: B

Indications and Dosages

➤ *To prevent duodenal ulcer*

TABLETS

Adults and adolescents. 1 g b.i.d.

➤ *To treat active duodenal ulcer*

ORAL SUSPENSION

Adults and adolescents. 1 g q.i.d. 1 hr before meals and at bedtime for 4 to 8 wk, possibly less. Or, 2 g b.i.d. on empty stomach on waking and at bedtime for 4 to 8 wk, possibly less.

TABLETS

Adults and adolescents. 1 g q.i.d. 1 hr before meals and at bedtime for 4 to 8 wk, possibly less.

Q
R
S

Mechanism of Action

May react with hydrochloric acid in the stomach to form a complex that buffers acid. The complex adheres electrostatically to proteins on the ulcer's surface and creates a protective barrier at the ulcer site. Sucralfate also inhibits back-diffusion of hydrogen ions and adsorbs pepsin and bile acids, actions that promote healing of an existing duodenal ulcer and prevent ulcer formation.

Interactions
DRUGS
aluminum-containing drugs (such as antacids, antidiarrheals, buffered aspirin with aluminum, and vaginal douches): Possibly aluminum toxicity in patients with renal failure
antacids: Possibly interference with binding of sucralfate to GI mucosa
cimetidine, ciprofloxacin, digoxin, norfloxacin, ofloxacin, phenytoin, ranitidine, tetracycline, theophylline: Decreased bioavailability of these drugs

Adverse Reactions
CNS: Dizziness, drowsiness, light-headedness
EENT: Dry mouth
GI: Constipation, diarrhea, indigestion, nausea, vomiting
MS: Back pain
SKIN: Pruritus, rash, urticaria

Nursing Considerations
•Use sucralfate cautiously in patients with chronic renal failure because of increased risk of aluminum toxicity.
•Administer drug to patient when he has an empty stomach.
PATIENT TEACHING
•Instruct patient to take sucralfate on an empty stomach at least 1 hour before meals and at bedtime.
•Advise patient not to take antacids within 30 minutes of sucralfate.
•Caution patient to check with prescriber before taking another drug within 2 hours of sucralfate.

sulfadiazine

Class and Category
Chemical class: Sulfonamide
Therapeutic class: Antibiotic, antiprotozoal
Pregnancy category: C

Indications and Dosages
➤ *To treat asymptomatic carriers of meningitis*
TABLETS
Adults and adolescents. 1 g every 12 hr for 2 days.
Children ages 1 to 12. 500 mg every 12 hr for 2 days.
Children ages 2 to 12 months. 500 mg daily for 2 days.

➤ *To prevent recurrent rheumatic fever*
TABLETS
Adults and adolescents. 500 mg daily (for patients weighing less than 30 kg [66 lb]) to 1 g daily (for patients weighing 30 kg or more).
➤ *To treat inclusive nocardiosis*
TABLETS
Adults and adolescents. 4 to 8 g daily for at least 6 wk.
➤ *As adjunct to treat toxoplasmosis in patients with AIDS*
TABLETS
Adults and adolescents. 1 to 2 g every 6 hr, with 50 to 100 mg daily of pyrimethamine and 10 to 25 mg daily of leucovorin.
Children age 2 months and over. 50 mg/kg b.i.d. for 12 mo, together with 2 mg/kg daily of pyrimethamine for 2 days, then 1 mg/kg/day of pyrimethamine for 2 to 6 mo, then 1 mg/kg daily of pyrimethamine 3 times/wk for remainder of 12 mo; in addition, 5 mg of leucovorin given 3 times/wk for 12 mo. *Maximum:* 6 g daily.
➤ *To treat toxoplasmosis in pregnant women after week 16 of gestation*
TABLETS
Adults. 1 g every 6 hr, together with 25 mg daily of pyrimethamine and 5 to 15 mg daily of leucovorin.

Mechanism of Action
Inhibits para-aminobenzoic acid, a bacterial enzyme responsible for synthesizing folic acid, which susceptible bacteria require for growth. By inactivating bacteria, sulfadiazine prevents or alleviates infection.

Contraindications
Breastfeeding; hypersensitivity to sulfadiazine, its components, or other chemically related drugs, such as sulfonamides; pregnancy at term

Interactions
DRUGS
bone marrow depressants: Increased risk of leukopenic or thrombocytopenic effects
cyclosporine: Decreased blood cyclosporine level, increased risk of nephrotoxicity
estrogen-containing oral contraceptives: In-

creased risk of breakthrough bleeding and pregnancy
hemolytics: Increased risk of adverse effects
hepatotoxic drugs: Increased risk of hepatotoxicity
hydantoins, oral anticoagulants, oral antidiabetic drugs: Increased or prolonged effects of these drugs, possibly toxicity
indomethacin, probenecid, salicylates: Increased blood level of free sulfadiazine caused by displacement from plasma protein-binding sites
methotrexate: Increased risk of leukopenic or thrombocytopenic effects of methotrexate
phenylbutazone, sulfinpyrazone: Increased blood sulfadiazine level
uricosuric drugs: Potentiated uricosuric action

Adverse Reactions
CNS: Dizziness, fatigue, fever, headache, lethargy, weakness
EENT: Pharyngitis
GI: Anorexia, diarrhea, dysphagia, nausea, vomiting
GU: Crystalluria
HEME: Agranulocytosis, aplastic anemia, hemolytic anemia, leukopenia, thrombocytopenia, unusual bleeding or bruising
MS: Arthralgia, myalgia
SKIN: Blisters, erythema, jaundice, pallor, photosensitivity, pruritus, rash
Other: Drug-induced fever

Nursing Considerations
•Use sulfadiazine cautiously in patients with blood dyscrasias or megaloblastic anemia from folate deficiency because drug may cause blood dyscrasias; in those with G6PD deficiency because hemolysis may occur; in those with hepatic or renal impairment because of increased risk of toxicity; and in those with porphyria because drug may precipitate an acute attack.
•Obtain blood sample for CBC and body tissue or fluid specimen for culture and sensitivity tests, as ordered, before giving drug. Expect first dose to be given before results are available.
•WARNING Monitor patient for drug-induced fever, which may develop 7 to 10 days after starting sulfadiazine therapy. Signs and symptoms may include abdominal pain, anorexia, ataxia, depression, diarrhea, headache, insomnia, nausea, peripheral neuropa-

thy, tinnitus, and vomiting.
•Monitor fluid intake and output during therapy. Altered fluid balance may increase risk of crystalluria.
•Frequently monitor blood glucose level and assess for signs and symptoms of hypoglycemia in patients who take an oral antidiabetic drug. Be prepared to respond if hypoglycemia develops.
PATIENT TEACHING
•Instruct patient to take sulfadiazine exactly as prescribed and to complete the full course even if he feels better.
•Advise patient to take drug with a full glass of water and to drink plenty of fluids during therapy.
•Urge patient to notify prescriber if urine turns reddish brown; this may indicate crystalluria.
•Inform patient about possible dizziness, and urge him to avoid potentially hazardous activities until drug's CNS effects are known.
•Advise patient to avoid prolonged exposure to sunlight and to wear sunscreen and protective clothing when outdoors.
•Urge patient who takes oral contraceptives to use an additional method of birth control during therapy.
•Advise patient who takes an oral antidiabetic drug to check his blood glucose level frequently because of the increased risk of hypoglycemia during therapy.

sulfamethizole
Thiosulfil Forte

Class and Category
Chemical class: Sulfonamide
Therapeutic class: Antibiotic
Pregnancy category: C

Indications and Dosages
➤ *To treat cystitis and other UTIs caused by* Enterobacter *species,* Escherichia coli, Klebsiella *species,* Proteus mirabilis, P. vulgaris, *or* Staphylococcus aureus
TABLETS
Adults. 0.5 to 1 g every 6 to 8 hr.
Children age 2 months and over. 7.5 to 11.25 mg/kg every 6 hr.
DOSAGE ADJUSTMENT Dosage usually reduced for patients with impaired renal function.

Mechanism of Action

Inhibits para-aminobenzoic acid, a bacterial enzyme responsible for synthesizing folic acid, which susceptible bacteria require for growth. By inactivating bacteria, sulfamethizole prevents or alleviates infection.

Contraindications

Breastfeeding; hypersensitivity to sulfamethizole, its components, or other chemically related drugs, such as sulfonamides; pregnancy at term

Interactions

DRUGS

bone marrow depressants: Increased risk of leukopenic or thrombocytopenic effects
cyclosporine: Decreased blood cyclosporine level, increased risk of nephrotoxicity
estrogen-containing oral contraceptives: Increased risk of breakthrough bleeding and pregnancy
hemolytics: Increased risk of adverse effects
hepatotoxic drugs: Increased risk of hepatotoxicity
hydantoins, oral anticoagulants, oral antidiabetic drugs: Increased or prolonged effects of these drugs, possibly toxicity
indomethacin, probenecid, salicylates: Increased blood level of free sulfamethizole caused by displacement from plasma protein-binding sites
methotrexate: Increased risk of leukopenic or thrombocytopenic effects of methotrexate
phenylbutazone, sulfinpyrazone: Increased blood sulfamethizole level
uricosuric drugs: Potentiated uricosuric action

Adverse Reactions

CNS: Dizziness, fatigue, fever, headache, lethargy, weakness
EENT: Pharyngitis
GI: Anorexia, diarrhea, dysphagia, nausea, vomiting
GU: Crystalluria
HEME: Agranulocytosis, aplastic anemia, hemolytic anemia, leukopenia, thrombocytopenia, unusual bleeding or bruising
MS: Arthralgia, myalgia
SKIN: Blisters, erythema, jaundice, pallor, photosensitivity, pruritus, rash
Other: Drug-induced fever

Nursing Considerations

• Use sulfamethizole cautiously in patients with blood dyscrasias or megaloblastic anemia from folate deficiency because drug may cause blood dyscrasias; in those with G6PD deficiency because hemolysis may occur; in those with hepatic or renal impairment because of increased risk of toxicity; and in those with porphyria because drug may precipitate an acute attack.
• Obtain blood sample for CBC and body tissue or fluid specimen for culture and sensitivity tests, as ordered, before giving drug. Expect first dose to be given before results are available.
• **WARNING** Monitor patient for drug-induced fever, which may develop 7 to 10 days after he starts taking sulfamethizole. Signs and symptoms include abdominal pain, anorexia, ataxia, depression, diarrhea, headache, insomnia, nausea, peripheral neuropathy, tinnitus, and vomiting.
• Monitor fluid intake and output during therapy. Altered fluid balance may increase risk of crystalluria.
• Frequently monitor blood glucose level and assess for signs and symptoms of hypoglycemia in patients who take an oral antidiabetic drug. Be prepared to respond if hypoglycemia develops.

PATIENT TEACHING

• Instruct patient to take sulfamethizole exactly as prescribed and to complete the full course even if he feels better.
• Advise patient to take drug with a full glass of water and to drink plenty of fluids during therapy.
• Urge patient to notify prescriber if urine turns reddish brown; this may indicate crystalluria.
• Inform patient about possible dizziness, and urge him to avoid potentially hazardous activities until sulfamethizole's CNS effects are known.
• Advise patient to avoid prolonged exposure to sunlight and to wear sunscreen and protective clothing when outdoors.
• Urge patient who takes oral contraceptives to use an additional method of birth control during therapy.
• Advise patient who takes an oral antidiabetic drug to check his blood glucose level frequently because of the increased risk of hypoglycemia during therapy.

sulfamethoxazole

Apo-Sulfamethoxazole (CAN), Gantanol, Urobak

Class and Category
Chemical class: Sulfonamide
Therapeutic class: Antibiotic, antiprotozoal
Pregnancy category: C

Indications and Dosages
➤ *To treat chlamydial conjunctivitis; malaria (as adjunct to quinine sulfate and pyrimethamine); toxoplasmosis (as adjunct to pyrimethamine); and UTI, including pyelonephritis and cystitis, caused by susceptible organisms*

TABLETS
Adults. *Initial:* 2 g, followed by 1 g every 8 to 12 hr.
Children age 2 months and over. *Initial:* 50 to 60 mg/kg, then 25 to 30 mg/kg every 12 hr. *Maximum:* 2 g for initial dose, 75 mg/kg daily for subsequent doses.
DOSAGE ADJUSTMENT Dosage reduction usually needed for patients with impaired renal function.

➤ *To treat uncomplicated urethritis, cervicitis, and proctitis caused by* Chlamydia trachomatis

TABLETS
Adults. 1 g every 12 hr for 10 days.
DOSAGE ADJUSTMENT For patients with creatinine clearance of 10 to 30 ml/min/1.73 m^2, recommended dose reduced by 50% or dosing interval extended; for creatinine clearance of less than 10 ml/min/1.73 m^2, recommended dose reduced by 75% or dosing interval extended, as prescribed.

Mechanism of Action
Inhibits para-aminobenzoic acid, a bacterial enzyme responsible for synthesizing folic acid, which susceptible bacteria require for growth. By inactivating bacteria, sulfamethoxazole prevents or alleviates infection.

Contraindications
Breastfeeding; hypersensitivity to sulfamethoxazole, its components, or other chemically related drugs, such as sulfonamides; pregnancy at term

Interactions
DRUGS
bone marrow depressants: Increased risk of leukopenic or thrombocytopenic effects
cyclosporine: Decreased blood cyclosporine level, increased risk of nephrotoxicity
estrogen-containing oral contraceptives: Increased risk of breakthrough bleeding and pregnancy
hemolytics: Increased risk of adverse effects
hepatotoxic drugs: Increased risk of hepatotoxicity
hydantoins, oral anticoagulants, oral antidiabetic drugs: Increased or prolonged effects of these drugs, possibly toxicity
indomethacin, probenecid, salicylates: Increased blood level of free sulfamethoxazole caused by displacement from plasma protein-binding sites
methotrexate: Increased risk of leukopenic or thrombocytopenic effects of methotrexate
phenylbutazone, sulfinpyrazone: Increased blood sulfamethoxazole level
uricosuric drugs: Potentiated uricosuric action

Adverse Reactions
CNS: Dizziness, fatigue, fever, headache, lethargy, weakness
EENT: Pharyngitis
GI: Anorexia, diarrhea, dysphagia, nausea, vomiting
GU: Crystalluria
HEME: Agranulocytosis, aplastic anemia, hemolytic anemia, leukopenia, thrombocytopenia, unusual bleeding or bruising
MS: Arthralgia, myalgia
SKIN: Blisters, erythema, jaundice, pallor, photosensitivity, pruritus, rash
Other: Drug-induced fever

Nursing Considerations
•Use sulfamethoxazole cautiously in patients with blood dyscrasias or megaloblastic anemia from folate deficiency because drug may cause blood dyscrasias; in those with G6PD deficiency because hemolysis may occur; in those with hepatic or renal impairment because of increased risk of toxicity; and in those with porphyria because drug may precipitate an acute attack.
•Obtain blood sample for CBC and body tissue or fluid specimen for culture and sensitivity tests, as ordered, before giving drug. Expect first dose to be given before results are available.

Q
R
S

•**WARNING** Monitor patient for drug-induced fever, which may develop 7 to 10 days after he starts taking sulfamethoxazole. Signs and symptoms include abdominal pain, anorexia, ataxia, depression, diarrhea, headache, insomnia, nausea, peripheral neuropathy, tinnitus, and vomiting.

•Monitor fluid intake and output during therapy. Altered fluid balance may increase risk of crystalluria.

•Frequently monitor blood glucose level and assess for signs and symptoms of hypoglycemia in patients who take an oral antidiabetic drug. Be prepared to respond if hypoglycemia develops.

PATIENT TEACHING

•Instruct patient to take sulfamethoxazole exactly as prescribed and to complete the full course even if he feels better.

•Advise patient to take drug with a full glass of water and to drink plenty of fluids during therapy.

•Urge patient to notify prescriber if urine turns reddish brown; this may indicate crystalluria.

•Inform patient about possible dizziness, and urge him to avoid potentially hazardous activities until drug's CNS effects are known.

•Advise patient to avoid prolonged exposure to sunlight and to wear sunscreen and protective clothing when outdoors.

•Urge patient who takes oral contraceptives to use an additional method of birth control during therapy.

•Advise patient who takes an oral antidiabetic drug to check his blood glucose level frequently because of increased risk of hypoglycemia during therapy.

sulfasalazine

Alti-Sulfasalazine (CAN), Azulfidine, Azulfidine EN-Tabs, PMS-Sulfasalazine (CAN), PMS-Sulfasalazine E.C. (CAN), Salazopyrin EN-Tabs (CAN), S.A.S.-500 (CAN), S.A.S. Enteric-500 (CAN)

Class and Category

Chemical class: Salicylate, sulfonamide
Therapeutic class: Anti-inflammatory, antirheumatic, immunomodulator
Pregnancy category: B

Indications and Dosages

➤ *To treat inflammatory bowel diseases,* *such as ulcerative colitis, and to maintain or prolong remission*

DELAYED-RELEASE TABLETS, TABLETS

Adults and adolescents. *Initial:* 500 to 1,000 mg every 6 to 8 hr. Or 500 mg every 6 to 12 hr to decrease adverse GI reactions. *Maintenance:* 500 mg every 6 hr.
Children over age 6. *Initial:* 6.7 to 10 mg/kg every 4 hr, 10 to 15 mg/kg every 6 hr, or 13.3 to 20 mg/kg every 8 hr. *Maintenance:* 7.5 mg/kg every 6 hr.

➤ *To treat rheumatoid arthritis*

DELAYED-RELEASE TABLETS, TABLETS

Adults. *Initial:* 500 to 1,000 mg daily during wk 1, increased by 500 mg daily every wk, as needed, up to 2,000 mg daily in divided doses. If no response after 12 wk, increased to 3,000 mg daily. *Maintenance:* 1,000 mg every 12 hr. *Maximum:* 3,000 mg daily.

➤ *To treat juvenile rheumatoid arthritis in patients who have not responded to salicylates or other NSAIDs*

DELAYED-RELEASE TABLETS

Children ages 6 to 16. 30 to 50 mg/kg daily in divided doses b.i.d. *Maximum:* 2 g daily.

Mechanism of Action

As a prodrug of sulfapyridine and 5-aminosalicylic acid (mesalamine), delivers more sulfapyridine and mesalamine to the colon than either metabolite could provide alone. Sulfapyridine provides antibacterial action along the intestinal wall; mesalamine inhibits cyclooxygenase, thereby decreasing the production of arachidonic acid metabolites and reducing colonic inflammation.

Contraindications

Hypersensitivity to salicylates, sulfasalazine, sulfonamides, chemically related drugs, or their components; intestinal or urinary obstruction; porphyria

Interactions

DRUGS

bone marrow depressants: Increased leukopenic and thrombocytopenic effects of both drugs
digoxin: Possibly inhibited absorption and decreased blood level of digoxin
folic acid (vitamin B₉): Decreased folic acid absorption

hepatotoxic drugs: Increased risk of hepatotoxicity
hydantoins, oral anticoagulants, oral antidiabetic drugs: Increased, prolonged, or toxic effects of these drugs
methotrexate, phenylbutazone, sulfinpyrazone: Possibly potentiated effects of these drugs

Adverse Reactions
CNS: Ataxia, chills, depression, fatigue, fever, Guillain-Barré syndrome, headache, insomnia, meningitis, peripheral neuropathy, seizures, vertigo, weakness
EENT: Hearing loss, orange-yellow tears, pharyngitis, tinnitus
GI: Abdominal pain, anorexia, diarrhea, hepatitis, indigestion, nausea, pancreatitis, ulcerative colitis exacerbation, vomiting
GU: Crystalluria, decreased ejaculatory volume, male infertility, nephritis, nephrotic syndrome, orange-yellow urine, toxic nephrosis
HEME: Agranulocytosis, aplastic anemia, Heinz body or hemolytic anemia, leukopenia, neutropenia, thrombocytopenia, unusual bleeding or bruising
MS: Arthralgia
RESP: Idiopathic pulmonary fibrosis, lymphocytic interstitial pneumonitis
SKIN: Cyanosis, jaundice, photosensitivity, pruritus, purpura, rash, Stevens-Johnson syndrome, toxic epidermal necrolysis, urticaria

Nursing Considerations
•Monitor CBC, liver function test results, and BUN and serum creatinine levels before and periodically during prolonged sulfasalazine therapy.
•Be aware that sulfasalazine doses over 4 g or a blood level over 50 mcg/ml increases the risk of adverse and toxic reactions.
•Monitor fluid intake and output and urine color, pH, and consistency. Acidic urine may require alkalization to prevent crystalluria.
PATIENT TEACHING
•Instruct patient to take sulfasalazine with meals, milk, or an antacid to decrease GI distress, and to swallow tablets whole.
•Advise patient to prevent crystalluria by taking drug with a full glass of water and drinking at least 64 oz of fluid per day.
•Instruct patient and family to administer drug around the clock.

•Inform patient that symptom relief may take 2 to 5 days for ulcerative colitis and 4 to 12 weeks for rheumatoid arthritis.
•Alert patient that drug may turn urine and skin orange-yellow.
•Advise contact lens wearer to consider wearing glasses during therapy because drug can permanently stain contact lenses yellow.
•Instruct patient to avoid prolonged sun exposure and to wear protective clothing and sunscreen when outdoors.
•Advise patient to brush with a soft-bristled toothbrush and to use dental floss and toothpicks gently because leukopenic and thrombocytopenic drug effects increase the risk of infections and gingival bleeding.
•Urge patient to return for laboratory tests and follow-up visits to monitor drug's effect.

sulfinpyrazone

Anturane, Apo-Sulfinpyrazone (CAN), Novopyrazone (CAN)

Class and Category
Chemical class: Pyrazalone derivative
Therapeutic class: Antigout, uricosuric
Pregnancy category: Not rated

Indications and Dosages
➤ *To treat chronic or intermittent gouty arthritis*
CAPSULES, TABLETS
Adults. *Initial:* 100 to 200 mg b.i.d., increased by 200 mg daily every 2 to 4 days, if needed. *Maintenance:* 100 to 200 mg b.i.d. *Maximum:* 400 mg b.i.d. during wk 1; then 200 to 400 mg b.i.d. until serum urate level is controlled.

Route	Onset	Peak	Duration
P.O.	Unknown	Unknown	4 to 10 hr

Mechanism of Action
Inhibits renal tubular reabsorption of uric acid, thereby increasing uric acid excretion and decreasing serum urate level. Decreased serum urate level prevents urate deposition, tophus formation, and chronic joint changes. It also helps resolve existing urate deposits and eventually reduces the number of gouty arthritis attacks.

Contraindications

Active peptic ulcer disease, blood dyscrasias, hypersensitivity to sulfinpyrazone or its components, symptoms of GI inflammation or ulceration

Interactions

DRUGS

acetaminophen: Increased risk of hepatotoxicity, decreased acetaminophen effects
aminosalicylate sodium: Increased blood level and prolonged duration of this drug, possibly leading to toxicity
antineoplastics: Increased risk of uric acid nephropathy
bismuth subsalicylate and other salicylates: Decreased sulfinpyrazone effects
cefamandole, cefoperazone, cefotetan, moxalactam, plicamycin, valproic acid: Possibly hypoprothrombinemia, increased risk of severe hemorrhage
diazoxide, mecamylamine, pyrazinamide: Possibly increased serum uric acid level
hydantoins: Increased blood hydantoin level, possibly leading to hydantoin toxicity
niacin: Possibly decreased uricosuric effect of sulfinpyrazone
nitrofurantoin: Decreased nitrofurantoin effectiveness, possibly nitrofurantoin toxicity
NSAIDs, oral anticoagulants, platelet aggregation inhibitors, thrombolytics: Increased risk of bleeding
oral antidiabetic drugs: Increased risk of hypoglycemia
probenecid: Increased sulfinpyrazone effects
theophylline: Possibly decreased blood theophylline level
verapamil: Increased clearance and decreased bioavailability of verapamil

ACTIVITIES

alcohol use: Possibly increased serum uric acid level

Adverse Reactions

CNS: Dizziness
EENT: Tinnitus
GI: Abdominal pain, epigastric discomfort, GI bleeding, indigestion, nausea, vomiting
GU: Dysuria, flank pain, hematuria, renal calculi, renal colic, renal failure
HEME: Agranulocytosis, anemia, aplastic anemia, leukopenia, thrombocytopenia
MS: Arthralgia, gouty arthritis (acute attack)
RESP: Bronchospasm, dyspnea, wheezing
SKIN: Erythema, rash

Nursing Considerations

•Expect to start with full maintenance dose, as ordered, for patient being switched to sulfinpyrazone from another uricosuric.
•Monitor serum uric acid level periodically, as ordered, to evaluate drug effectiveness.
•Assess for signs of acute gouty arthritis, especially during first few months of sulfinpyrazone therapy.

PATIENT TEACHING

•Instruct patient to take sulfinpyrazone with food, milk, or an antacid to prevent GI distress.
•Stress the importance of taking drug every day, even when feeling better, to prevent acute gouty arthritis attacks.
•Inform patient that acute gouty arthritis may worsen during initial therapy but should improve as treatment continues. Explain that he may not experience drug's full therapeutic effect for 6 months.
•If an acute gouty arthritis attack occurs, advise patient to seek additional treatment but to continue taking sulfinpyrazone, as prescribed, to help prevent exacerbation.
•Advise patient to drink at least 80 oz of fluids per day to decrease the risk of renal calculus formation.
•Instruct patient to consult prescriber before taking OTC products that contain aspirin or acetaminophen.
•Advise patient to avoid alcohol while taking sulfinpyrazone.
•Encourage patient to return for ordered follow-up laboratory tests to check for blood dyscrasias.

sulfisoxazole

Apo-Sulfisoxazole (CAN), Gantrisin, Novo-Soxazole (CAN), Sulfizole (CAN)

sulfisoxazole acetyl

Gantrisin

Class and Category

Chemical class: Sulfonamide
Therapeutic class: Antibiotic, antiprotozoal
Pregnancy category: C

Indications and Dosages

➤ *To treat nocardiosis; plague; malaria (as adjunct to quinine sulfate and pyrimethamine); and UTI, including pyelo-*

nephritis and cystitis, caused by susceptible organisms
ORAL SUSPENSION, ORAL SYRUP, TABLETS
Adults and adolescents. *Initial:* 2 to 4 g daily in divided doses. *Maintenance:* 4 to 8 g daily in divided doses every 4 to 6 hr. *Maximum:* 8 g daily.
Children over age 2 months. *Initial:* 75 mg/kg, followed by 120 to 150 mg/kg daily in divided doses every 4 to 6 hr. *Maximum:* 6 g daily.
➤ *To treat uncomplicated cystitis in women*
ORAL SUSPENSION, ORAL SYRUP, TABLETS
Adults. 2 g as a single dose.
➤ *To treat acute or recurrent otitis media in combination with erythromycin in penicillin-allergic patients*
ORAL SUSPENSION, ORAL SYRUP, TABLETS
Children. 150 mg of sulfisoxazole/kg daily and 50 mg of erythromycin/kg daily in divided doses q.i.d.
➤ *To treat lymphogranuloma venereum*
ORAL SUSPENSION, ORAL SYRUP, TABLETS
Adults. 500 mg every 6 hr for 21 days.
➤ *To treat uncomplicated urethritis, cervicitis, or proctitis caused by* Chlamydia trachomatis
ORAL SUSPENSION, ORAL SYRUP, TABLETS
Adults. 500 mg every 6 hr.
DOSAGE ADJUSTMENT For patients with renal impairment, dosing interval changed to every 8 to 24 hr, as prescribed.

Mechanism of Action
Inhibits para-aminobenzoic acid, a bacterial enzyme responsible for synthesizing folic acid, which susceptible bacteria require for growth. By inactivating bacteria, sulfisoxazole prevents or alleviates infection.

Contraindications
Breastfeeding; hypersensitivity to sulfisoxazole, other chemically related drugs, such as sulfonamides, or their components; pregnancy at term

Interactions
DRUGS
bone marrow depressants, methotrexate: Increased risk of leukopenia or thrombocytopenia
cyclosporine: Increased risk of nephrotoxicity
diuretics: Increased incidence of thrombocytopenic purpura
hemolytics (such as doxapram and methyldopa): Increased risk of toxic reaction
hepatotoxic drugs (such as amiodarone): Increased risk of hepatotoxicity
hydantoins, oral anticoagulants, oral antidiabetic drugs: Increased or prolonged effects of these drugs, possibly toxicity
indomethacin, probenecid, salicylates: Increased blood sulfisoxazole level
oral contraceptives: Increased risk of breakthrough bleeding with long-term sulfisoxazole use
phenylbutazone, sulfinpyrazone: Risk of increased blood sulfisoxazole level
thiopental: Increased anesthetic effect of thiopental
tolbutamide: Prolonged half-life of tolbutamide
uricosurics: Potentiated uricosuric action

Adverse Reactions
CNS: Dizziness, fatigue, fever, headache, lethargy, weakness
EENT: Pharyngitis
GI: Anorexia, diarrhea, dysphagia, nausea, vomiting
GU: Crystalluria
HEME: Agranulocytosis, aplastic anemia, hemolytic anemia, leukopenia, thrombocytopenia, unusual bleeding or bruising
MS: Arthralgia, myalgia
SKIN: Blisters, erythema, jaundice, pallor, photosensitivity, pruritus, rash
Other: Drug-induced fever

Nursing Considerations
•Use sulfisoxazole cautiously in patients with blood dyscrasias or megaloblastic anemia from folate deficiency because drug may cause blood dyscrasias; in those with G6PD deficiency because hemolysis may occur; in those with hepatic or renal impairment because of increased risk of toxicity; and in those with porphyria because drug may precipitate an acute attack.
•Obtain blood sample for CBC and tissue or fluid specimen for culture and sensitivity testing, as ordered, before beginning sulfisoxazole therapy. Expect to give first dose before results are available.
•**WARNING** Expect prescriber to discontinue

sulfisoxazole if patient exhibits signs of blood dyscrasias, including fever, jaundice, maculopapular or other rash, pallor, pharyngitis, or purpura.

•Monitor CBC often, as appropriate, during treatment for signs of adverse reactions.

•Closely monitor patients with AIDS, who are at increased risk for adverse reactions.

•**WARNING** Monitor patient for drug-induced fever, which may develop 7 to 10 days after he starts taking sulfisoxazole. Signs and symptoms include abdominal pain, anorexia, ataxia, depression, diarrhea, headache, insomnia, nausea, peripheral neuropathy, tinnitus, and vomiting.

•Monitor fluid intake and output. Unless contraindicated, provide sufficient fluids to maintain a daily urine output of at least 1,200 ml.

•For otitis media caused by *Haemophilus influenzae*, expect to give drug with erythromycin, as prescribed.

•Frequently monitor blood glucose level and assess for signs of hypoglycemia in patients who take oral antidiabetic drugs.

PATIENT TEACHING

•Instruct patient to take sulfisoxazole exactly as prescribed and to complete the full course of therapy even if he feels better.

•Advise patient to take drug with a full glass of water.

•Inform patient that tablet may be chewed or crushed and mixed with liquid to ease swallowing.

•Advise patient to shake oral suspension well before use and to measure oral suspension or syrup dose with calibrated device to ensure accuracy.

•Inform patient that oral suspension or syrup form of drug may be stored at room temperature.

•Advise patient to drink 2 to 3 L of fluid daily to maintain hydration, unless contraindicated.

•Caution patient to avoid potentially hazardous activities until drug's CNS effects are known.

•Instruct patient who takes an oral antidiabetic drug to monitor her blood glucose level frequently because of the risk of hypoglycemia.

•Advise patient to avoid prolonged exposure to sunlight and to use sunscreen and wear protective clothing when outdoors.

sulindac

Apo-Sulin (CAN), Clinoril, Novo-Sundac (CAN)

Class and Category
Chemical class: Pyrroleacetic acid derivative
Therapeutic class: Antigout, anti-inflammatory, antirheumatic
Pregnancy category: Not rated

Indications and Dosages
➤ *To decrease pain and inflammation in ankylosing spondylitis, acute attacks of gout or pseudogout, bursitis, moderately painful arthralgia, osteoarthritis, rheumatoid arthritis, and tendinitis*

TABLETS

Adults and adolescents over age 14. *Initial:* 150 to 200 mg b.i.d., adjusted based on patient's response. *Maximum:* 200 mg b.i.d.

➤ *To relieve symptoms of acute gouty arthritis, acute subacromial bursitis, and supraspinatus tendinitis*

TABLETS

Adults and adolescents over age 14. 200 mg b.i.d. for 7 to 14 days; decreased to lowest effective dosage after satisfactory response occurs.

DOSAGE ADJUSTMENT For elderly patients, dosage reduced to 50% of usual adult dosage, if needed.

Route	Onset	Peak	Duration
P.O.	In 1 wk*	2 to 3 wk*	Unknown

Mechanism of Action
May block the activity of cyclooxygenase, an enzyme needed to synthesize prostaglandins, which mediate the inflammatory response and cause local vasodilation, swelling, and pain. By blocking cyclooxygenase and inhibiting prostaglandins, this NSAID reduces inflammatory symptoms and pain.

Contraindications
Angioedema, asthma, bronchospasm, nasal polyps, rhinitis, or urticaria induced by aspirin, iodides, or other NSAIDs

---

* For antirheumatic effects; unknown for antigout or anti-inflammatory effects.

Interactions

DRUGS

acetaminophen, cyclosporine, gold compounds, nephrotoxic drugs: Increased risk of adverse renal effects

antacids: Decreased blood level and effects of sulindac

antihypertensives: Risk of decreased antihypertensive effect

aspirin, salicylates: Decreased sulindac effects, increased risk of GI hemorrhage

bone marrow depressants: Increased risk of leukopenia and thrombocytopenia

cefamandole, cefoperazone, cefotetan, colchicine, oral anticoagulants, plicamycin, thrombolytics, valproic acid: Increased risk of bleeding

cimetidine, ranitidine: Increased bioavailability of both drugs

digoxin: Increased blood digoxin level and risk of digitalis toxicity

dimethyl sulfoxide (DMSO): Decreased sulindac effectiveness, possibly peripheral neuropathy with topical application of DMSO

diuretics: Possibly decreased loop diuretic effects and increased thiazide diuretic effects

glucocorticoids, other NSAIDs, potassium supplements: Increased risk of adverse GI effects

hydantoins: Increased blood hydantoin level and risk of phenytoin toxicity

insulin, oral antidiabetic drugs: Increased risk of hypoglycemia

lithium: Possibly increased blood level and toxic effects of lithium

methotrexate: Decreased methotrexate excretion, possibly leading to toxicity

platelet aggregation inhibitors: Increased risk of bleeding, additive effects of these drugs

probenecid: Increased blood level and adverse and toxic effects of sulindac

ACTIVITIES

alcohol use: Increased risk of adverse GI effects, including GI bleeding

Adverse Reactions

CNS: Aseptic meningitis, cerebral hemorrhage, chills, drowsiness, fever, headache, ischemic stroke, malaise, nervousness, transient ischemic attack

CV: Deep vein thrombosis, edema, heart failure, hypertension, MI, palpitations, peripheral edema

EENT: Tinnitus

ENDO: Hypoglycemia

GI: Abdominal cramps or pain, anorexia, constipation, diarrhea, esophageal irritation, flatulence, gastritis, gastrointestinal bleeding or ulceration, hepatic failure, hepatitis, hepatotoxicity, indigestion, jaundice, liver failure, nausea, perforation of stomach or intestines, vomiting

GU: Acute renal failure, decreased urine output, interstitial nephritis, nephrotic syndrome, polyuria, proteinuria

HEME: Agranulocytosis, aplastic anemia, leukopenia, pancytopenia

RESP: Pulmonary edema, wheezing

SKIN: Diaphoresis, erythema multiforme, exfoliative dermatitis, maculopapular rash, pruritus, purpura, Stevens-Johnson syndrome, toxic epidermal necrolysis

Other: Anaphylaxis, angioedema, facial edema

Nursing Considerations

•Use sulindac with extreme caution in patients with a history of ulcer disease or GI bleeding because NSAIDs such as sulindac increase the risk of GI bleeding and ulceration. Expect to use sulindac for the shortest time possible in these patients.

•Be aware that serious GI tract ulceration, bleeding, and perforation may occur without warning symptoms. Elderly patients are at greater risk. To minimize risk, give drug with food. If GI distress occurs, withhold drug and notify prescriber immediately.

•Use sulindac cautiously in patients with hypertension, and monitor blood pressure closely throughout therapy. Drug may cause hypertension or worsen it.

•**WARNING** Monitor patient closely for thrombotic events, including MI and stroke, because NSAIDs increase the risk.

•If patient has systemic lupus erythematosus and mixed connective tissue disease, monitor him closely because sulindac increases the risk of aseptic meningitis.

•**WARNING** If patient has bone marrow suppression or is receiving antineoplastic drug therapy, monitor laboratory results (including WBC count), and watch for evidence of infection because anti-inflammatory and antipyretic actions of sulindac may mask signs and symptoms, such as fever and pain.

•Especially if patient is elderly or taking

sulindac long-term, watch for less common but serious adverse GI reactions, including anorexia, constipation, diverticulitis, dysphagia, esophagitis, gastritis, gastroenteritis, gastroesophageal reflux disease, hemorrhoids, hiatal hernia, melena, stomatitis, and vomiting.
•Monitor liver function test results because, in rare cases, elevated levels may progress to severe hepatic reactions, including fatal hepatitis, liver necrosis, and hepatic failure.
•Watch BUN and serum creatinine levels in elderly patients; those with heart failure, impaired renal function, or hepatic dysfunction; and those taking diuretics or ACE inhibitors; because drug may cause renal failure.
•Monitor CBC for decreased hemoglobin and hematocrit because drug may worsen anemia.
•Assess patient's skin routinely for rash or other signs of hypersensitivity reaction because sulindac and other NSAIDs may cause serious skin reactions without warning, even in patients with no history of NSAID hypersensitivity. Stop drug at first sign of reaction, and notify prescriber.
•**WARNING** Monitor patient for adventitious breath sounds and dyspnea; sulindac may cause fluid retention, which may precipitate heart failure in susceptible patients.
•Expect patient to undergo audiometric examinations before and periodically during prolonged therapy, as ordered.
PATIENT TEACHING
•Instruct patient to take sulindac exactly as prescribed. Explain that higher doses don't increase effectiveness and may increase risk of adverse reactions.
•Advise patient to crush tablet and mix with food, if needed, to aid in swallowing.
•Instruct patient to take drug with or immediately after meals to decrease GI distress, to take with a full glass of water, and to remain upright for 20 to 30 minutes after administration to prevent drug from lodging in esophagus and causing esophageal irritation.
•Urge patient to notify prescriber immediately of chills, fever, rash, or sweating, which may indicate hypersensitivity.
•Advise patient to consult prescriber before using acetaminophen, alcohol, aspirin, other NSAIDs, or any OTC drugs during sulindac therapy.
•Caution patient to avoid hazardous activi-

ties until drug's CNS effects are known.
•Explain the need for periodic physical examinations and laboratory tests during prolonged therapy to monitor drug effectiveness.
•Inform patient that sulindac may increase the risk of serious adverse cardiovascular reactions; urge patient to seek immediate medical attention if signs or symptoms arise, such as chest pain, shortness of breath, weakness, and slurring of speech.
•Tell patient that sulindac also may increase the risk of serious adverse GI reactions; stress the need to seek immediate medical attention for such signs and symptoms as epigastric or abdominal pain, indigestion, black or tarry stools, or vomiting blood or material that looks like coffee grounds.
•Alert patient to the possibility of rare but serious skin reactions. Urge him to seek immediate medical attention for rash, blisters, itching, fever, or other indications of hypersensitivity.

sumatriptan succinate
Imitrex

Class and Category
Chemical class: Serotonin 5-HT$_1$-receptor agonist
Therapeutic class: Antimigraine
Pregnancy category: C

Indications and Dosages
➤ *To relieve acute migraine attacks, with or without aura, or cluster headaches*
TABLETS
Adults. 25 to 100 mg as a single dose as soon as possible after onset of symptoms, repeated every 2 hr, as needed and prescribed. *Maximum:* 300 mg daily.
DOSAGE ADJUSTMENT For patients with hepatic dysfunction, 50 mg is maximum single dose.
SUBCUTANEOUS INJECTION
Adults. *Initial:* 6 mg, repeated after 1 or 2 hr, if needed. *Maximum:* 2 (6-mg) injections/24 hr. If migraine symptoms return after initial subcutaneous injection, 50 mg P.O. every 2 hr up to 200 mg daily.
NASAL SPRAY
Adults. 1 or 2 sprays (5 or 10 mg) into one nostril as a single dose or 1 spray (20 mg) into

one nostril as a single dose. One additional dose may be taken if another attack occurs after at least 2 hr. *Maximum:* 40 mg daily.

Route	Onset	Peak	Duration
P.O.	In 30 min	2 to 4 hr	Up to 24 hr
SubQ	In 10 min	1 to 2 hr	Up to 24 hr
Nasal	In 15 min	Unknown	Up to 24 hr

Mechanism of Action
May stimulate 5-HT$_1$ receptors, causing selective vasoconstriction of inflamed and dilated cranial blood vessels in carotid circulation, thus decreasing carotid arterial blood flow and relieving acute migraines.

Contraindications
Basilar or hemiplegic migraine, cardiovascular disease, concurrent use of ergotamine-containing drugs, hypersensitivity to sumatriptan or its components, ischemic heart disease, Prinzmetal's angina, use within 14 days of MAO inhibitor therapy, use within 24 hours of another serotonin 5-HT$_1$-receptor agonist

Interactions
DRUGS
antidepressants, lithium: Increased risk of serious adverse effects
ergotamine-containing drugs: Possibly additive or prolonged vasoconstrictive effects
fluoxetine, fluvoxamine, paroxetine, sertraline: Possibly incoordination, hyperreflexia, and weakness
MAO inhibitors: Risk of decreased sumatriptan clearance, increased risk of serious adverse effects

Adverse Reactions
CNS: Anxiety, atypical sensations, dizziness, drowsiness, fatigue, fever, headache, malaise, sedation, seizures, vertigo, weakness
CV: Arrhythmias; chest heaviness, pain, pressure, or tightness; coronary artery vasospasm; ECG changes; hypertension; hypotension; palpitations
EENT: Abnormal vision; nasal burning (P.O., subcutaneous); jaw or mouth discomfort; nasal irritation (nasal); nose or throat discomfort; photophobia (P.O., subcutaneous);

taste perversion (nasal); tongue numbness or soreness
GI: Abdominal discomfort, dysphagia
MS: Jaw discomfort, muscle cramps, myalgia, neck pain or stiffness
SKIN: Dermatitis, diaphoresis, erythema, flushing, pallor, photosensitivity (P.O., subcutaneous), pruritus, rash, urticaria
Other: Injection site burning, pain, and redness

Nursing Considerations
•Be aware that sumatriptan shouldn't be given to elderly patients because they're more likely to have decreased hepatic function, coronary artery disease (CAD), and more pronounced blood pressure increases.
•Assess patient for chest pain, and monitor blood pressure in patients with CAD before and for at least 1 hour after sumatriptan administration.
•Don't give sumatriptan within 24 hours of another 5-HT$_1$-receptor agonist, such as naratriptan, rizatriptan, or zolmitriptan.
•After nasal administration, rinse tip of bottle with hot water (don't suction water into bottle) and dry with a clean tissue. Replace cap after cleaning.
•Inspect injection solution for particles and discoloration before administering. Discard solution if you detect these changes.
•Be aware that drug shouldn't be administered I.V. because this may precipitate coronary artery vasospasm.
•Assess patients with risk factors for CAD for arrhythmias, chest pain, and other signs of heart disease.
•For patients with seizure disorder, institute seizure precautions according to facility policy because sumatriptan may lower seizure threshold.

PATIENT TEACHING
•Advise patient to use sumatriptan as soon as possible after the onset of migraine symptoms.
•Urge patient to contact prescriber and avoid taking sumatriptan if headache symptoms aren't typical.
•Remind patient not to exceed prescribed daily dosage.
•Advise patient to swallow tablets whole and drink fluids to disguise unpleasant taste.
•Show patient suitable sites for subcutaneous injection, and teach him how to load, administer, and discard autoinjector.

Q
R
S

•Instruct patient to administer no more than two subcutaneous doses in 24 hours and not to take a second dose if first dose doesn't provide significant relief.

•Inform patient that he may experience burning, pain, and redness for 10 to 30 minutes after subcutaneous injection. Suggest that he apply ice to relieve pain and redness.

•Teach patient how to use nasal form correctly.

•To avoid cross-contamination, advise patient not to use the same nasal container for more than one person.

•Encourage patient to lie down in a dark, quiet room after taking drug to help relieve migraine.

•Instruct patient to seek emergency care for chest, jaw, or neck tightness after drug use because drug may cause coronary artery vasospasm; subsequent doses may require ECG monitoring.

•Urge patient to report palpitations or rash to prescriber.

•Advise patient to avoid potentially hazardous activities until drug's CNS effects are known.

•Alert patient with seizure disorder that drug may lower seizure threshold.

•Encourage yearly ophthalmologic examinations for patients who require prolonged drug therapy.

T

tacrine hydrochloride
(tetrahydroaminoacridine, THA)

Cognex

Class and Category
Chemical class: Monoamine acridine
Therapeutic class: Dementia treatment
Pregnancy category: C

Indications and Dosages
➤ *To treat mild to moderate Alzheimer's-type dementia*
CAPSULES
Adults. *Initial:* 10 mg q.i.d. for 4 wk, increased to 20 mg q.i.d. and adjusted every 4 wk as prescribed. *Maximum:* 160 mg daily in 4 divided doses.

Contraindications
Hypersensitivity to tacrine, other acridine derivatives, or their components; jaundice from previous tacrine use; serum bilirubin level that exceeds 3 mg/dl

Interactions
DRUGS
anticholinergics: Decreased effects of both drugs
cholinergics, other cholinesterase inhibitors: Increased effects of these drugs and tacrine, possibly leading to toxicity
cimetidine: Increased blood tacrine level, possibly leading to toxicity
neuromuscular blockers: Prolonged or exaggerated muscle relaxation
NSAIDs: Increased gastric acid secretion, possibly GI irritation and bleeding
theophylline: Increased blood theophylline

Mechanism of Action
Tacrine may relieve dementia in Alzheimer's disease by increasing acetylcholine level in the CNS. In Alzheimer's disease, some cholinergic neurons lose their ability to function, which decreases the acetylcholine level. The remaining functioning cholinergic neurons release acetylcholine, but it's enzymatically broken down by cholinesterases into acetic acid and choline, as shown below left. Without acetylcholine

to activate muscarinic (M) and nicotinic (N) receptors on postsynaptic cell membranes, nerve transmission and excitability decrease.

Tacrine binds with and inhibits cholinesterases, making more intact acetylcholine available in cholinergic synapses, as shown below right. This prolongs and enhances acetylcholine's effects, which increases nerve transmission and reduces symptoms of dementia.

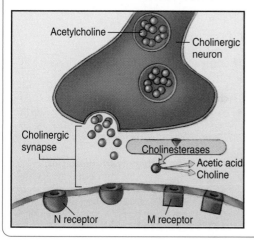

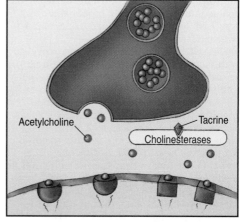

T

level, possibly leading to toxicity

FOODS

all foods: Reduced tacrine bioavailability

ACTIVITIES

smoking: Possibly decreased tacrine effectiveness

Adverse Reactions

CNS: Agitation, anxiety, asthenia, ataxia, confusion, depression, dizziness, fatigue, hallucinations, headache, hostility, insomnia, seizures, somnolence, syncope, tremor

CV: Arrhythmias, chest pain, conduction disturbances, hypertension, hypotension, palpitations, peripheral edema, sick sinus syndrome

EENT: Rhinitis

GI: Abdominal pain, anorexia, constipation, diarrhea, elevated liver function test results, flatulence, indigestion, nausea, vomiting

GU: Bladder obstruction, urinary frequency and incontinence, UTI

MS: Back pain, muscle stiffness, myalgia

RESP: Asthma, cough, upper respiratory tract infection, wheezing

SKIN: Flushing, jaundice, purpura, rash

Other: Weight loss

Nursing Considerations

•Monitor patients with asthma for wheezing and increased mucus production because drug may increase bronchoconstriction and bronchial secretions.

•Expect to monitor hepatic enzyme levels (specifically ALT), as ordered, every other week from at least week 4 to week 16 of tacrine therapy.

•If patient has elevated serum ALT level, monitor for signs and symptoms of hepatitis, such as jaundice and right-upper-quadrant pain. ALT level should return to normal 4 to 6 weeks after therapy stops.

•Once ALT level returns to normal, expect to begin tacrine again (starting at 10 mg q.i.d.) as prescribed, and check hepatic enzyme levels weekly for 16 weeks, monthly for 2 months, and every 3 months thereafter, as ordered.

•Monitor patient for bradyarrhythmias, conduction disturbances, and sick sinus syndrome because tacrine may have a vagotonic effect on the heart rate.

•**WARNING** Be aware that tacrine's cholinergic effects may exacerbate seizures or parkinsonian symptoms.

•Monitor patient's urine output and assess for abdominal distention and abnormal bowel sounds because drug's cholinergic effects may exacerbate conditions involving urinary tract or GI obstruction or ileus.

•Be aware that patients with peptic ulcer disease and those receiving NSAIDs are at increased risk for developing diarrhea, nausea, and vomiting because tacrine increases gastric acid secretion.

•Assess patient for increased symptoms because drug becomes less effective as Alzheimer's disease progresses and the number of intact cholinergic neurons declines.

PATIENT TEACHING

•Instruct patient to take tacrine on an empty stomach, and advise caregiver to make sure that drug is swallowed.

•If patient experiences GI distress, suggest taking drug with meals. Mention that drug's effects may be delayed.

•Urge patient to seek assistance when walking and changing position until drug's effects are known. Instruct her to avoid potentially hazardous activities during this period.

•Advise patient not to smoke because it decreases drug's effectiveness.

•Caution patient not to stop taking drug abruptly. Doing so may impair cognitive ability.

•Inform caregiver that drug becomes less effective as Alzheimer's disease progresses.

•Urge caregiver to make sure patient returns regularly for follow-up visits and laboratory tests to monitor drug effectiveness.

tacrolimus

Prograf

Class and Category

Chemical class: Macrolide
Therapeutic class: Immunosuppressant
Pregnancy category: C

Indications and Dosages

➤ *To prevent organ rejection in patients undergoing allogeneic liver, kidney, or heart transplantation*

CAPSULES

Adults having kidney transplantation.
0.2 mg/kg/day given in two equally divided doses every 12 hr beginning only after renal function has recovered (serum creatinine level of 4 mg/dl or less).

DOSAGE ADJUSTMENT Black patients may

need higher doses after kidney transplantation.

Adults having liver transplantation. 0.10 to 0.15 mg/kg/day given in two equally divided doses every 12 hr. Administer 6 hr after transplantation.

Adults having heart transplantation. 0.075 mg/kg/day given in two equally divided doses every 12 hr. Administer 6 hr after transplantation.

Children having liver transplantation. 0.15 to 0.20 mg/kg/day given in two equally divided doses every 12 hr. Administer 6 hr after transplantation.

I.V. INFUSION

Adults having kidney or liver transplantation. 0.03 to 0.05 mg/kg/day as a continuous infusion beginning no sooner than 6 hr after transplantation.

Adults having heart transplantation. 0.0187 to 0.025 mg/kg/day as a continuous infusion beginning no sooner than 6 hr after transplantation.

Children having liver transplantation. 0.03 to 0.05 mg/kg/day as a continuous infusion beginning no sooner than 6 hr after transplantation.

DOSAGE ADJUSTMENT Therapy delayed up to 48 hours or longer in patients with postoperative oliguria. For patients with hepatic or renal impairment, dosage kept at lower end of range with possible need for further reduction.

Incompatibilities

Don't store diluted drug in PVC containers because of increased instability of tacrolimus and possible extraction of phthalates. Don't mix or co-infused tacrolimus with solutions of pH 9 or greater, such as with acyclovir or ganciclovir, because of chemical instability of tacrolimus in alkaline media.

Contraindications

Breast-feeding, hypersensitivity to tacrolimus or its components, hypersensitivity to polyoxyl 60 hydrogenated castor oil (parenteral form), ocular exposure

Interactions

DRUGS

aminoglycosides, amphotericin B, cisplatin, cyclosporine, other nephrotoxic drugs such as sirolimus: Increased risk of renal impairment

bromocriptine, chloramphenicol, cimetidine, cisapride, clarithromycin, clotrimazole, cyclosporine, danazol, diltiazem, erythromycin, ethinyl estradiol, fluconazole, ganciclovir, itraconazole, ketoconazole, lansoprazole, magnesium-aluminum-hydroxide, metoclopramide, methylprednisolone, nefazodone, nicardipine, nifedipine, nelfinavir, omeprazole, protease inhibitors, ritonavir, troleandomycin, verapamil, voriconazole: Possibly increased blood tacrolimus level

carbamazepine, caspofungin, phenobarbital, phenytoin, rifabutin, rifampin, sirolimus, St. John's wort: Possibly decreased blood tacrolimus level

phenytoin: Possibly increased blood phenytoin level

vaccines (live or killed): Possibly suppressed immune response and increased adverse effects of vaccine

FOODS

grapefruit juice: Possibly increased blood tacrolimus trough levels in liver transplant patients

high-fat foods: Decreased absorption of oral tacrolimus

Mechanism of Action

Inhibits T-lymphocyte activation, possibly by binding to an intracellular protein, FKBP-12. This binding results in formation of a complex of tacrolimus-FKBP-12, calcium, calmodulin, and calcineurin, which inhibits phosphatase activity of calcineurin. This inhibition may prevent dephosphorylation and translocation of nuclear factor of activated T-cells, a nuclear component thought to initiate gene transcription for the formation of lymphokines. The result is inhibition of T-lymphocyte activation, which produces immunosuppression.

Adverse Reactions

CNS: Asthenia, fever, dizziness, headache, insomnia, jittery feeling, leukoencephalopathy, mental changes, paresthesia, posterior reversible encephalopathy syndrome, progressive multifocal leukoencephalopathy, seizures, stroke, syncope, tremor

CV: Atrial and ventricular arrhythmias, cardiac arrest, chest pain, hypercholesterolemia,

T

hyperlipemia, hypertension, hypertriglyceridemia, myocardial hypertrophy or ischemia, MI, pericardial effusion, peripheral edema, QT-interval prolongation, torsades de pointes, venous thrombosis
EENT: Blindness, cortical blindness, deafness, hearing loss, photophobia
ENDO: Cushingoid features, diabetes mellitus, hot flashes, hyperglycemia
GI: Abdominal pain, anorexia, ascites, bile duct stenosis, colitis, constipation, diarrhea, dyspepsia, enterocolitis, gastric ulcer, gastroenteritis, gastroesophageal reflux disease, hepatic impairment or toxicity, impaired gastric emptying, nausea, pancreatitis, veno-occlusive liver disease, vomiting
GU: Acute renal failure, elevated creatinine and BUN levels, hemorrhagic cystitis, hemolytic-uremic syndrome, micturition abnormality, oliguria, renal impairment, UTI
HEME: Anemia, decreased platelet count, disseminated intravascular coagulation, leukocytosis, neutropenia, pancytopenia, thrombocytopenia
MS: Arthralgia, back pain
RESP: Acute respiratory distress syndrome, atelectasis, bronchitis, cough increase, dyspnea, interstitial lung disease, lung infiltration, pleural effusion, respiratory distress or failure
SKIN: Flushing, malignancy, pruritus, rash, Stevens-Johnson syndrome, toxic epidermal necrolysis
OTHER: Anaphylaxis, cytomegalovirus infection, hyperkalemia, hypokalemia, hypomagnesemia, hypophosphatemia, impaired wound healing, lymphoproliferative or malignant disorders, multi-organ failure, opportunistic infections, primary graft dysfunction, weight loss

Nursing Considerations
•Don't start tacrolimus therapy within 24 hours of cyclosporine, and vice versa. If tacrolimus or cyclosporine blood levels are elevated beyond 24 hours of either drug being discontinued, the other drug should not be started until elevation is resolved.
•Be aware that I.V. tacrolimus therapy should only be given if patient can't tolerate oral tacrolimus. Patient should be switched to oral therapy as soon as possible.
•Expect to give drug with adrenal corticosteroid therapy.

•Dilute intravenous drug with normal saline solution or 5% dextrose to 0.004 to 0.02 mg/ml following manufacturer guidelines. Once diluted, drug should be stored in glass or polyethylene containers (not PVC, because of decreased stability and possible extraction of phthalates). Discard after 24 hours if not used.
•When converting patient from parenteral to oral therapy after heart transplantation, expect to give oral form 8 to 12 hours after infusion is discontinued.
•Be aware that children having liver transplantation usually need higher doses of tacrolimus than adults.
•**WARNING** Closely monitor patient for anaphylaxis at least during first 30 minutes of I.V. administration. Make sure emergency equipment and drugs, such as aqueous solution of epinephrine and oxygen, are immediately available.
•Monitor patient's blood tacrolimus trough levels regularly, as ordered. Higher trough levels increase risk of toxicity.
•Monitor blood pressure, especially in patients with history of hypertension, because drug can worsen this condition.
•Monitor results of liver and renal function tests, as ordered, to detect signs of decreased function.
•Tacrolimus may increase serum cholesterol, lipid, and triglyceride levels.
•Monitor patient's blood glucose level closely because tacrolimus may cause post-transplant diabetes mellitus with the need for insulin therapy, especially in black and Hispanic patients.
•Monitor patient's serum potassium level, as ordered, because drug can alter it.
•Watch for evidence neurotoxicity, especially in patients receiving high doses of drug. Evidence of encephalopathy includes headache, impaired consciousness, loss of motor function, psychiatric disturbance, seizures, and tremors.
PATIENT TEACHING
•Advise patient to take oral doses 12 hours apart at same time each day.
•Instruct patient to take capsules on an empty stomach.
•Tell patient to avoid consuming grapefruit juice while taking tacrolimus.
•Advise patient not to stop taking drug without consulting prescriber.

•Instruct patient not to receive virus vaccines during therapy. Urge him to avoid people who have received such vaccines or to wear a protective mask when he's around them.

•Caution patient to avoid having contact with people who have infections during therapy because tacrolimus causes immunosuppression.

•Stress importance of having repeated laboratory tests while taking tacrolimus, and urge compliance.

•Inform patient that tacrolimus therapy may result in insulin-dependent diabetes. Tell him to report frequent urination or an increase in thirst, hunger, or fatigue.

•Instruct patient to limit exposure to direct sunlight and to wear protective clothing and use sunscreen when exposure can't be avoided.

tadalafil

Cialis

Class and Category

Chemical class: Phosphodiesterase inhibitor
Therapeutic class: Anti-impotence
Pregnancy category: B

Indications and Dosages

➤ *To treat erectile dysfunction*

TABLETS

Adults. *Initial:* 10 mg daily taken 1 hr before sexual activity; dosage decreased to 5 mg or increased to 20 mg, as prescribed, based on clinical response. *Maximum:* 20 mg daily. Alternatively, 2.5 mg once daily, increased to 5 mg once daily, if needed.

DOSAGE ADJUSTMENT For patients taking potent CYP3A4 inhibitors such as itraconazole, ketoconazole, or ritonavir, dosage shouldn't exceed 10 mg every 72 hr. For patients with moderate to severe renal insufficiency who take drug on an as-needed basis, dosage shouldn't exceed 5 mg daily. For patients with mild to moderate hepatic impairment who take drug on an as-needed basis, dosage shouldn't exceed 10 mg daily. For patients who take drug once daily, no dosage adjustment is needed with mild to moderate hepatic or renal impairment; once daily dosing not recommended for use with severe hepatic or renal impairment.

Route	Onset	Peak	Duration
P.O.	Unknown	30 min to 6 hr	Unknown

Mechanism of Action

Enhances the effect of nitric oxide released in the penis during sexual stimulation. Nitric oxide activates the enzyme guanylate cyclase, which causes increased levels of cGMP in the corpus cavernosum. This leads to increased blood flow to the penis, thus producing an erection.

Contraindications

Continuous or intermittent nitrate therapy, hypersensitivity to tadalafil or its components, retinitis pigmentosa

Interactions

DRUGS

carbamazepine, phenytoin, phenobarbitol: Possibly decreased tadalafil effects
doxazosin, tamsulosin and other alpha blockers: Increased risk of symptomatic hypotension
erythromycin, itraconazole, ketoconazole, ritonavir: Prolonged tadalafil effects
nitrates: Profound hypotension
protease inhibitors (other than ritonavir): Possibly prolonged tadalafil effects
rifampin: Decreased tadalafil effects

FOODS

grapefruit juice: Possibly prolonged tadalafil effects

ACTIVITIES

alcohol use: Potentiated blood pressure lowering effects

Adverse Reactions

CNS: Asthenia, dizziness, fatigue, headache, hypesthesia, insomnia, migraine, paresthesia, seizures, somnolence, stroke, syncope, transient global amnesia, vertigo

CV: Angina pectoris, chest pain, hypotension, hypertension, MI, postural hypotension, palpitations, sudden cardiac death, tachycardia

EENT: Blurred vision, changes in color vision, conjunctivitis, dry mouth, epistaxis, eyelid swelling, eye pain, hearing loss, increased lacrimation, nasal congestion, nasopharyngitis, nonarteritic anterior ishcemic optic neuropathy, pharyngitis, retinal artery

T

or vein occlusion, visual field defects
GI: Abnormal liver function studies, diarrhea, dysphagia, dyspepsia, esophagitis, gastroesophageal reflux, gastritis, increased gamma-glutamyl transpeptidase levels, nausea, upper abdominal pain, vomiting
GU: Priapism, spontaneous penile erection, UTI
MS: Arthralgia, back or neck pain, extremity pain, myalgia
RESP: Bronchitis, cough, dyspnea, upper respiratory tract infection
SKIN: Diaphoresis, exfoliative dermatitis, flushing, pruritus, rash, Stevens-Johnson syndrome, urticaria
Other: Facial edema, flulike symptoms, hypersensitivity reactions

Nursing Considerations
•Know that patients with hereditary degenerative retinal disorders, including retinitis pigmentosa, should not receive tadalafil because of the risk of serious ophthalmic adverse reactions.
•Patients with severe hepatic impairment should not receive tadalafil because its effects in these patients are unknown.
•Use tadalafil cautiously in patients with left ventricular outflow obstruction, such as aortic stenosis and idiopathic hypertrophic subaortic stenosis, and those with severely impaired autonomic control of blood pressure because these conditions increase sensitivity to vasodilators such as tadalafil.
•Use tadalafil cautiously in patients with conditions that may predispose them to priapism, such as sickle cell anemia, multiple myeloma, leukemia, or penile deformities (such as angulation, cavernosal fibrosis, or Peyronie's disease).
•Monitor blood pressure and heart rate and rhythm before and during therapy.
PATIENT TEACHING
•Explain that tadalafil should be taken 1 hour before sexual activity to provide the most effective results unless patient has chosen to take a smaller dose daily. If patient takes drug daily, remind him to take it at about the same time every day regardless of timing of sexual activity.
•**WARNING** Tell patient not to take tadalafil if he takes any form of organic nitrate, either continuously or intermittently, because profound hypotension and death could result. Tell him to seek immediate medical attention

if he has a sudden loss of vision or hearing.
•Advise patient to seek sexual counseling to enhance drug's effects.
•To avoid possible penile damage and permanent loss of erectile function, urge patient to notify prescriber immediately if erection is painful or lasts longer than 4 hours.
•Advise patient to limit alcohol consumption while taking tadalafil.

tamoxifen citrate
Apo-Tamox (CAN), Gen-Tamoxifen (CAN), Nolvadex, Novo-Tamoxifen (CAN), Tamofen (CAN), Tamone (CAN)

Class and Category
Chemical class: Triphenylethylene derivative
Therapeutic class: Nonsteroidal antiestrogen agent, partial estrogen agonist
Pregnancy category: D

Indications and Dosages
➤ *To treat metastatic breast cancer in men and women; to treat node-negative breast cancer in women, or node-positive breast cancer in postmenopausal women, after total or segmental mastectomy, axillary dissection, and breast irradiation*
TABLETS
Adults. 20 to 40 mg daily. Dosages greater than 20 mg administered b.i.d.
➤ *To reduce the risk of invasive breast cancer in women with ductal carcinoma in situ (DCIS) after surgery and radiation, to reduce the risk of breast cancer in women at high risk*
TABLETS
Adults. 20 mg daily for 5 yr.

Mechanism of Action
May block the effects of estrogen on breast tissue by competing with estrogen for estrogen-receptor binding sites. Estrogen may stimulate the growth of cancer cells.

Contraindications
Hypersensitivity to tamoxifen or its components; women at high risk for breast cancer and women with DCIS and a history of deep

vein thrombosis or pulmonary embolus or who need coumarin-type anticoagulant therapy; use with anastrozole therapy

Interactions
DRUGS
bromocriptine: Possibly increased blood tamoxifen level
estrogens: Possibly altered therapeutic effect of tamoxifen
warfarin and other coumarin-type anticoagulants: Increased anticoagulant effect of these drugs

Adverse Reactions
CNS: Confusion, depression, dizziness, fatigue, headache, light-headedness, somnolence, stroke, weakness
CV: Edema, hyperlipidemia, thrombosis
EENT: Keratopathy, ocular toxicity (including cataracts), optic neuritis, retinopathy
GI: Elevated liver function test results, hepatotoxicity, nausea, vomiting
GU: Endometrial cancer, endometrial hyperplasia, endometrial polyps, genital itching, menstrual irregularities, ovarian cysts, uterine malignancies, vaginal discharge (females); impotence, decreased libido (males)
HEME: Anemia, leukopenia, thrombocytopenia
MS: Transient bone or tumor pain
RESP: Pulmonary embolism
SKIN: Bullous pemphigoid, dry skin, erythema multiforme, rash, Stevens-Johnson syndrome, thinning hair
Other: Angioedema, hot flashes, hypercalcemia, weight gain

Nursing Considerations
•**WARNING** Ensure that patient has been informed of serious or potentially life-threatening adverse effects associated with tamoxifen before therapy begins. Be aware that women with ductal carcinoma in situ or those at high risk for breast cancer are more likely to develop uterine cancer, stroke, or pulmonary emboli than others receiving tamoxifen.
•If patient is premenopausal, begin drug therapy in the middle of menstruation; if patient's menstrual cycles are irregular, verify that she has had a negative pregnancy test before therapy starts.
•Expect patient to undergo an ophthalmic examination before and periodically during tamoxifen therapy. Also expect to monitor patient for adverse ocular reactions, such as cataracts.
•Assess patient for signs and symptoms of thromboembolic events, such as shortness of breath, leg pain, and change in mental status.
•Periodically monitor platelet and WBC count, cholesterol and triglyceride levels, and liver function test results, as ordered.
•Monitor blood calcium level and assess patient for signs and symptoms of hypercalcemia, such as nausea, vomiting, and thirst; tamoxifen may cause hypercalcemia in breast cancer patients with bone metastasis within a few weeks of starting treatment.
•Store tamoxifen in a closed, light-resistant container at room temperature.
PATIENT TEACHING
•Advise patient to swallow tamoxifen tablet whole with water.
•Instruct premenopausal patient to use a nonhormonal form of contraception, such as a condom or diaphragm, during tamoxifen therapy. Emphasize that she shouldn't become pregnant while taking drug and for 2 months afterward. Advise her to notify prescriber at once if she becomes pregnant during therapy.
•Inform patient of the most common side effects—hot flashes, vaginal discharge, and irregular menses.
•Urge patient to immediately notify prescriber if she notices a rash, itching, difficulty breathing, or facial swelling, which may signify a hypersensitivity reaction.
•Advise patient to notify prescriber if she experiences leg pain or calf swelling, which may indicate a blood clot.
•Instruct patient to report signs of hepatotoxicity, such as tiredness, nausea, yellow skin, and flulike symptoms.
•Advise patient to have regular gynecologic checkups and to report abnormal symptoms, including abdominal or pelvic pain, new breast lumps, and unusual vaginal discharge or bleeding.
•Urge patients taking tamoxifen for prophylaxis to obtain regular mammograms because drug doesn't prevent all cancers.
•Stress the importance of taking tamoxifen regularly. Urge patient to consult prescriber if adverse reactions, such as nausea and vomiting, are interfering with dosage schedule. These symptoms may be a sign of hypercalcemia.

T

•Inform women who wish to breastfeed that tamoxifen my appear in breast milk and cause serious adverse effects in the infant.

tamsulosin hydrochloride

Flomax

Class and Category

Chemical class: Sulfamoylphenethylamine derivative
Therapeutic class: Benign prostatic hyperplasia (BPH) treatment
Pregnancy category: B

Indications and Dosages

➤ *To treat BPH*

CAPSULES

Adults. *Initial:* 0.4 mg daily 30 min p.c. for 2 to 4 wk, increased to 0.8 mg daily if no response to initial dosage. *Maximum:* 0.8 mg daily.

Mechanism of Action

Blocks alpha$_1$-adrenergic receptors in the prostate. This action inhibits smooth-muscle contraction in the prostate, prostatic capsule, prostatic urethra, and bladder neck, which improves the rate of urine flow and reduces the symptoms of BPH.

Contraindications

Hypersensitivity to tamsulosin, quinazolines, or their components

Interactions

DRUGS

alpha blockers: Additive effects of both drugs
cimetidine: Risk of decreased tamsulosin clearance
CYP2D6 inhibitors (such as fluoxetine), CYP3A4 inhibitors (such as ketoconazole): Possibly increased plasma tamsulosin level

Adverse Reactions

CNS: Asthenia, dizziness, drowsiness, headache, insomnia, syncope, vertigo
CV: Chest pain, orthostatic hypotension
EENT: Amblyopia, diplopia, intraoperative floppy iris syndrome, pharyngitis, rhinitis
GI: Diarrhea, nausea
GU: Decreased libido, ejaculation disorders, priapism

MS: Back pain
RESP: Respiratory impairment
SKIN: Pruritus, rash, urticaria
Other: Angioedema

Nursing Considerations

•Be aware that prostate cancer should be ruled out before tamsulosin therapy begins.
•Give drug about 30 minutes after the same meal each day.
•If patient takes drug on an empty stomach, monitor his blood pressure because of the increased risk of orthostatic hypotension.
•If patient doesn't take drug for several days, resume therapy at 0.4 mg/dose, as prescribed.

PATIENT TEACHING

•Instruct patient not to open, crush, or chew tamsulosin capsules and to take drug about 30 minutes after the same meal each day.
•Instruct patient to notify prescriber if he misses several days of therapy, and caution him against restarting drug at previous dosage.
•Advise patient to avoid potentially hazardous activities until drug's CNS effects are known. Mention the need for caution if dosage is increased.
•Advise patient to change position slowly, especially after initial dose and each dosage increase, to minimize effects of orthostatic hypotension.

telithromycin

Ketek

Class and Category

Chemical class: Semisynthetic ketolide
Therapeutic class: Antibiotic
Pregnancy category: C

Indications and Dosages

➤ *To treat mild to moderate community-acquired pneumonia caused by* Streptococcus pneumoniae, Haemophilus influenzae, Moraxella catarrhalis, Chlamydophila pneumoniae, *or* Mycoplasma pneumoniae

TABLETS

Adults. 800 mg daily P.O. for 7 to 10 days.

Route	Onset	Peak	Duration
P.O.	Unknown	1 hr	Unknown

Mechanism of Action

Binds to domains II and V of the 50S ribosomal subunit in many aerobic, anaerobic, gram-positive, and gram-negative bacteria of the respiratory tract. Telithromycin may also inhibit the assembly of nascent ribosomal units. These actions inhibit RNA-dependent protein synthesis in bacterial cells, causing them to die.

Contraindications

Cisapride or pimozide therapy; history of hepatitis or jaundice associated with use of telithromycin or any macrolide antibiotic; hypersensitivity to telithromycin, macrolide antibiotics, or their components; myasthenia gravis

Interactions

DRUGS

atorvastatin, lovastatin, midazolam, pimozide, simvastatin: Possibly increased blood levels of these drugs
cisapride, dofetilide, procainamide, quinidine: Increased risk of prolonged QT interval
itraconazole, ketoconazole: Increased blood level of telithromycin
oral anticoagulants: Possibly potentiated effects of oral anticoagulants
rifampin: Decreased blood level of telithromycin
sotalol: Decreased sotalol absorption
theophylline: Increased risk of adverse GI reactions

Adverse Reactions

CNS: Dizziness, fatigue, headache, insomnia, somnolence, transient loss of consciousness, vertigo
CV: Atrial arrhythmias, prolonged QT interval, torsades de pointes
EENT: Blurred vision, difficulty focusing eyes, diplopia, dry mouth, glossitis, oral candidiasis, stomatitis
GI: Abdominal distention or pain, anorexia, constipation, diarrhea, elevated liver function test results, flatulence, fulminant hepatitis, gastroenteritis, gastritis, hepatic failure or necrosis, hepatitis, nausea, pseudomembranous colitis, taste perversion, vomiting
GU: Vaginal candidiasis, vaginitis, vaginosis (fungal)
HEME: Increased platelet count

MS: Exacerbated myasthenia gravis, muscle cramps
RESP: Acute respiratory failure
SKIN: Diaphoresis, rash
Other: Angioedema, anaphylaxis

Nursing Considerations

•Be aware that telithromycin therapy should not be used in patients who have congenital prolonged QT interval or ongoing proarrhythmic conditions (such as uncorrected hypokalemia or hypomagnesemia, or serious bradycardia) or in those receiving concurrent therapy with class IA or class III antiarrhythmics because telithromycin increases the risk of QT prolongation, which may lead to ventricular arrhythmias, including torsades de pointes.
•Before administering the first telithromycin dose, expect to obtain respiratory specimens for culture and sensitivity testing.
•Monitor patient closely for diarrhea, which may indicate pseudomembranous colitis. If it occurs, notify prescriber and expect to withhold drug and give fluids, electrolytes, protein, and an antibiotic effective against *Clostridium difficile*.
•**WARNING** Monitor patient's liver studies for abnormalities, and assess patient for evidence of liver dysfunction such as fatigue, malaise, anorexia, nausea, jaundice, acholic stools, and liver tenderness, because telithromycin may cause potentially life-threatening acute hepatic failure and severe liver damage.

PATIENT TEACHING

•Stress need to take drug for prescribed duration even if patient feels better before prescription is finished.
•Caution patient to avoid hazardous activities until drug's CNS and visual effects are known. Explain that telithromycin can cause trouble focusing eyes, especially for first 30 minutes after a dose.
•Instruct patient to notify prescriber if visual disturbances occur, and tell her to avoid quick changes in viewing near and distant objects.
•Tell patient to alert prescriber if she faints because drug may alter heart rhythm.
•Caution patient to notify prescriber immediately about fatigue, malaise, anorexia, nausea, abdominal tenderness, yellow skin, or changes in stool appearance.

telmisartan

Micardis

Class and Category

Chemical class: Nonpeptide angiotensin II antagonist
Therapeutic class: Antihypertensive
Pregnancy category: C (first trimester), D (later trimesters)

Indications and Dosages

➤ *To manage hypertension, alone or with other antihypertensives*

TABLETS

Adults. *Initial:* 40 mg daily. *Maintenance:* 20 to 80 mg daily. *Maximum:* 80 mg daily.

Route	Onset	Peak	Duration
P.O.	Unknown	In 4 wk	Unknown

Mechanism of Action

Blocks angiotensin II from binding to receptor sites in many tissues, including vascular smooth muscle and adrenal glands. This action inhibits the vasoconstrictive and aldosterone-secreting effects of angiotensin II, which reduces blood pressure.

Contraindications

Hypersensitivity to telmisartan or its components

Interactions

DRUGS

digoxin: Increased peak blood digoxin level and risk of digitalis toxicity
diuretics, other antihypertensives: Enhanced hypotensive effect

Adverse Reactions

CNS: Asthenia, dizziness, fatigue, headache, syncope, weakness
CV: Atrial fibrillation, bradycardia, chest pain, congestive heart failure, hypertension, hypotension, MI, orthostatic hypotension, peripheral edema
EENT: Pharyngitis, sinusitis
GI: Abdominal pain, diarrhea, indigestion, nausea, vomiting
GU: Acute renal failure, erectile dysfunction, renal dysfunction, UTI
HEME: Anemia, eosinophilia, thrombocytopenia
MS: Back pain, leg or muscle cramps, myalgia
RESP: ACE cough, upper respiratory tract infection
SKIN: Diaphoresis, erythema, urticaria
Other: Angioedema, elevated uric acid level, flulike symptoms, hyperkalemia, hypovolemia

Nursing Considerations

•Administer telmisartan cautiously to patients with dehydration or hyponatremia.
•Expect prescriber to add a diuretic to regimen if patient's blood pressure isn't well controlled by telmisartan.
•Be prepared to treat symptomatic hypotension by placing patient in supine position and giving normal saline solution, as ordered.
•Monitor BUN and serum creatinine levels and urine output in patients with impaired renal function because they're at increased risk for oliguria, progressive azotemia, and possibly acute renal failure.
•Monitor liver function test results, as appropriate, and assess for signs of drug toxicity in patients with severe hepatic disease because they're at increased risk for toxicity from increased drug accumulation.
•Avoid using telmisartan in pregnant women during second and third trimesters because drug can increase the risk of fetal harm.

PATIENT TEACHING

•Advise patient to avoid hazardous activities until telmisartan's CNS effects are known.
•Instruct patient to change position slowly to minimize effects of orthostatic hypotension.
•Urge patient to immediately report diarrhea, dizziness, severe nausea, or vomiting.
•Instruct patient to consult prescriber before taking any new drug.
•Advise patient to drink adequate fluids during hot weather and when exercising.
•Advise female patients of childbearing age to notify presciber immediately about known or suspected pregnancy.

temazepam

Apo-Temazepam (CAN), Novo-Temazepam (CAN), Restoril

Class, Category, and Schedule

Chemical class: Benzodiazepine
Therapeutic class: Sedative-hypnotic

Pregnancy category: X
Controlled substance schedule: IV

Indications and Dosages

➤ *To provide short-term management of insomnia*

CAPSULES

Adults. 7.5 to 30 mg 30 min before at bedtime. *Maximum:* 30 mg daily.

DOSAGE ADJUSTMENT For elderly or debilitated patients, 7.5 mg 30 min before bedtime. *Maximum:* 15 mg daily.

Mechanism of Action

May potentiate the effects of gamma-aminobutyric acid (GABA) and other inhibitory neurotransmitters by binding to specific benzodiazepine receptor sites in the limbic and cortical areas of the CNS. By binding to these receptor sites, temazepam increases GABA's inhibitory effects and blocks cortical and limbic arousal.

Contraindications

Hypersensitivity to temazepam, other benzodiazepines, or their components; pregnancy

Interactions

DRUGS

antihistamines (such as brompheniramine, carbinoxamine, chlorpheniramine, clemastine, cyproheptadine, diphenhydramine, trimeprazine), anxiolytics, barbiturates, general anesthetics, opioid analgesics, phenothiazines, promethazine, sedative-hypnotics, tramadol, tricyclic antidepressants: Increased sedation or respiratory depression
clozapine: Risk of respiratory depression or arrest
digoxin: Increased risk of elevated blood digoxin level and digitalis toxicity
flumazenil: Increased risk of withdrawal symptoms
levodopa: Possibly decreased levodopa effects
oral contraceptives: Decreased response to temazepam
phenytoin: Possibly phenytoin toxicity
probenecid: Increased response to temazepam
zidovudine: Possibly zidovudine toxicity

ACTIVITIES

alcohol use: Increased CNS depression and risk of apnea
smoking: Increased temazepam clearance

Adverse Reactions

CNS: Aggressiveness, anxiety (in daytime), ataxia, complex behaviors (such as sleep driving), confusion, decreased concentration, depression, dizziness, drowsiness, euphoria, fatigue, headache, insomnia, nightmares, slurred speech, suicidal ideation, syncope, talkativeness, tremor, vertigo, wakefulness during last third of night
CV: Palpitations, tachycardia
EENT: Abnormal or blurred vision, increased salivation, throat tightness
GI: Abdominal pain, constipation, diarrhea, hepatic dysfunction, nausea, thirst, vomiting
GU: Decreased libido
HEME: Agranulocytosis, anemia, leukopenia, neutropenia, thrombocytopenia
MS: Muscle spasm or weakness
RESP: Dyspnea, increased bronchial secretions
SKIN: Diaphoresis, flushing, jaundice, pruritus, rash
Other: Anaphylaxis, angioedema, physical and psychological dependence

Nursing Considerations

• Use temazepam cautiously in patients with a history of depression or suicidal thoughts.
• **WARNING** Monitor patient closely for evidence of hypersensitivity reaction, such as dyspnea, throat tightness, nausea, vomiting, and swelling. If present, discontinue temazepam immediately, notify prescriber, and provide supportive care.
• Watch patient closely for suicidal tendencies, particularly when therapy starts and dosage changes, because depression may worsen temporarily during these times and could lead to suicidal ideation.
• **WARNING** Monitor patient for evidence of physical and psychological dependence during therapy.
• Implement safety precautions, according to facility policy, especially in elderly patients, because they're more sensitive to drug's CNS effects.
• Assess patients with respiratory depression, severe COPD, or sleep apnea for signs of ventilatory failure.
• Be aware that temazepam can aggravate acute intermittent porphyria, myasthenia gravis, and severe renal impairment.
• Be aware that temazepam may cause worsening psychosis or deterioration of cognition

T

or coordination in patients with late-stage Parkinson's disease.
•Be aware that drug shouldn't be discontinued abruptly, even after only 1 to 2 weeks of therapy, because doing so may cause seizures or withdrawal symptoms, such as insomnia, irritability, and nervousness.

PATIENT TEACHING
•Instruct patient to take temazepam exactly as prescribed and not to stop or change dosage without consulting prescriber.
•Explain the risks associated with abrupt cessation, including abdominal cramps, acute sense of hearing, confusion, depression, nausea, numbness, perceptual disturbances, photophobia, sweating, tachycardia, tingling, trembling, and vomiting.
•Advise patient to avoid consuming alcohol because it increases drug's sedative effects and the risk of such abnormal behaviors as sleep driving.
•Caution patient about possible drowsiness. Advise her to avoid hazardous activities until drug's CNS effects are known.
•Urge patient to notify prescriber immediately about excessive drowsiness, nausea, and known or suspected pregnancy.
• Instruct patient to stop taking temazepam and seek emergency care if she experiences difficulty breathing, throat tightness, nausea, vomiting, or abnormally swelling.
•Advise patient that drug may cause abnormal behaviors during sleep, such as driving a car, eating, talking on the phone, or having sex without any recall of the event. If family notices any such behavior or patient sees evidence of such behavior upon awakening, the prescriber should be notified.
•Urge family or caregiver to watch patient closely for suicidal tendencies, especially when therapy starts or dosage changes.

tenecteplase

TNKase

Class and Category
Chemical class: Purified glycoprotein
Therapeutic class: Thrombolytic
Pregnancy category: C

Indications and Dosages
➤ *To reduce mortality associated with acute MI*

I.V. INJECTION
Adults. Single bolus administered over 5 sec in individualized dosage based on patient's weight, as follows: 30 mg (6 ml) for patients weighing less than 60 kg; 35 mg (7 ml) for patients weighing 60 to 69 kg; 40 mg (8 ml) for patients weighing 70 to 79 kg; 45 mg (9 ml) for patients weighing 80 to 89 kg; 50 mg (10 ml) for patients weighing 90 kg or more. *Maximum:* 50 mg total dose.

Mechanism of Action
Binds to fibrin and converts plasminogen to plasmin. Plasmin breaks down fibrin, fibrinogen, and other clotting factors, resulting in dissolution of a coronary artery thrombus.

Incompatibilities
Don't administer tenecteplase through an I.V. line containing dextrose because precipitation may occur.

Contraindications
Active internal bleeding, aneurysm, arteriovenous malformation, bleeding disorders, brain tumor, history of cerebrovascular accident, hypersensitivity to tenecteplase or its components, intracranial or intraspinal surgery or trauma within past 2 months, severe uncontrolled hypertension

Interactions
DRUGS
abciximab, aspirin, clopidogrel, dipyridamole, heparin, oral anticoagulants, ticlopidine: Possibly increased risk of bleeding

Adverse Reactions
CNS: Intracranial hemorrhage
EENT: Epistaxis, gingival bleeding, pharyngeal bleeding
GI: GI and retroperitoneal bleeding
GU: Genitourinary bleeding, prolonged or heavy menstrual bleeding
HEME: Hematoma
RESP: Hemoptysis
SKIN: Bleeding at puncture sites, surgical incision sites, or venous cutdown sites

Nursing Considerations
•**WARNING** Reconstitute tenecteplase for injection immediately before use because drug

contains no antibacterial preservatives. If reconstituted drug isn't used immediately, refrigerate vial at 36° to 46° F (2° to 8° C). Discard solution if not used within 8 hours.
•To reconstitute and administer drug, use supplied 10-ml syringe with dual cannula device. Withdraw 10 ml of supplied (preservative-free) sterile water for injection into syringe, and inject entire contents into vial containing tenecteplase dry powder, directing stream of diluent into powder. Gently swirl—don't shake—vial until contents are completely dissolved. If slight foaming occurs during reconstitution, allow drug to stand undisturbed for a few minutes to allow large bubbles to dissipate. Then withdraw prescribed dose of tenecteplase from reconstituted drug in vial, using supplied syringe. Make sure that reconstituted preparation is a colorless to pale yellow transparent solution. Discard any unused solution.
•Give drug as a single I.V. bolus over 5 seconds. Although supplied syringe is intended for use with needleless I.V. systems, be aware that it is also compatible with a conventional needle. Follow manufacturer's directions for use with each system. Flush any dextrose-containing I.V. lines with saline solution before and after administering tenecteplase.
•**WARNING** Monitor for signs and symptoms of GI bleeding, including bloody or black, tarry stools; bloody or coffee-ground vomitus; and severe stomach pain. Notify prescriber immediately if any of these signs or symptoms develops.
•Assess tenecteplase injection site for signs and symptoms of hematoma, including deep, dark purple bruises under skin and itching, pain, redness, or swelling. Also monitor patient for superficial bleeding, delayed bleeding at puncture sites, and bleeding from surgical incisions.
•Assess for signs and symptoms of intracranial bleeding (such as decreased level of consciousness), retroperitoneal bleeding (such as abdominal pain or swelling and back pain), genitourinary bleeding (such as hematuria), or respiratory tract bleeding (such as hemoptysis). Notify prescriber immediately if patient develops any of these signs or symptoms.
•If serious bleeding (not controllable by local pressure) occurs, expect to discontinue concomitant heparin or oral antiplatelet therapy immediately.

•If possible, avoid I.M. injections and nonessential handling of patient for first few hours after drug administration.
•If arterial puncture becomes necessary during first few hours after tenecteplase administration, expect to use an upper extremity that's accessible to manual compression. Apply pressure for at least 30 minutes after procedure, use a pressure dressing, and frequently monitor puncture site for signs of bleeding.

PATIENT TEACHING
•Advise patient to immediately report any bleeding, including from nose or gums.
•Instruct patient to limit physical activity during tenecteplase administration to reduce the risk of injury or bleeding.

terazosin hydrochloride

Hytrin

Class and Category
Chemical class: Quinazoline derivative
Therapeutic class: Antihypertensive, benign prostatic hyperplasia (BPH) treatment
Pregnancy category: C

Indications and Dosages
➤ *To manage hypertension*
CAPSULES
Adults. *Initial:* 1 mg at bedtime. *Maintenance:* 1 to 5 mg daily as a single dose or in divided doses every 12 hr. *Maximum:* 20 mg daily.

➤ *To treat symptomatic BPH*
CAPSULES
Adults. *Initial:* 1 mg at bedtime, increased in increments to 2 mg, 5 mg, and then 10 mg, as prescribed, based on symptom improvement and urine flow rate. *Maintenance:* 5 to 10 mg daily as a single dose or in divided doses every 12 hr. *Maximum:* 20 mg daily.

Route	Onset	Peak	Duration
P.O.	15 min	2 to 3 hr	24 hr

Contraindications
Hypersensitivity to terazosin, other quinazolines, or their components

Interactions
DRUGS
clonidine: Possibly decreased clonidine effects

diuretics, other antihypertensives: Additive hypotensive effect

dopamine: Risk of decreased terazosin effects and antagonized vasoconstrictive effect of dopamine (in high doses)

epinephrine: Risk of decreased terazosin effects, possibly severe hypotension and tachycardia

indomethacin, other NSAIDS: Altered terazosin effects related to sodium and fluid retention

methoxamine, phenylephrine: Decreased vasopressor effects, and shortened duration of action of these drugs

sympathomimetics: Decreased terazosin effects

Mechanism of Action
Blocks postsynaptic alpha$_1$-adrenergic receptors in many tissues, including vascular smooth muscle, the bladder neck, and the prostate. This action promotes vasodilation, which reduces blood pressure and improves urine flow.

Adverse Reactions
CNS: Asthenia, dizziness, headache, lethargy, nervousness, paresthesia, somnolence, syncope, vertigo
CV: Chest pain, hypotension, orthostatic hypotension, palpitations, peripheral edema, sinus tachycardia
EENT: Blurred vision, dry mouth, intraoperative floppy iris syndrome, nasal congestion, sinusitis
GI: Constipation, diarrhea, nausea, vomiting
MS: Arthralgia, back pain
Other: Flulike symptoms, weight gain

Nursing Considerations
•Be aware that prostate cancer should be ruled out before giving terazosin for BPH.
•Expect prescriber to reduce terazosin dosage if a diuretic or another antihypertensive is added to patient's regimen.
•Monitor blood pressure 2 to 3 hours after initial dose because of possible first-dose hypotension and again after 24 hours to evaluate patient's response.
•If patient requires administration by feeding tube, place capsule in 60 ml of warm tap water. Stir until capsule shell dissolves and liquid contents are released into water (5 to 10 minutes).
•Be aware that elderly patients may have exaggerated hypotension and other adverse reactions.

PATIENT TEACHING
•Instruct patient to take terazosin at the same time each night.
•Explain possible first-dose hypotension. Advise patient to change position and rise slowly to prevent syncope early in therapy. Suggest sitting or lying down if dizziness or light-headedness occurs.
•Advise patient to avoid potentially hazardous activities until drug's CNS effects are known.
•Instruct patient to notify prescriber if she misses several doses in a row; caution her against resuming therapy at previous dose.
•Inform patient that drug may take 2 to 6 weeks to improve urinary hesitancy.
•Advise patient to avoid alcohol use, prolonged standing, and excessive exercise or exposure to hot weather because these activities can worsen orthostatic hypotension.
•Stress the importance of regular follow-up visits with prescriber to evaluate patient's response to drug.

terbinafine hydrochloride
Lamisil

Class and Category
Chemical class: Allylamine derivative
Therapeutic class: Antifungal
Pregnancy category: B

Indications and Dosages
➤ *To treat onychomycosis of fingernails and toenails*
TABLETS
Adults and adolescents. 125 mg b.i.d. or 250 mg daily for 6 to 12 wk.
DOSAGE ADJUSTMENT For patients with stable chronic hepatic dysfunction or renal dysfunction (creatinine clearance less than 50 ml/min/1.73 m^2 or serum creatinine greater than 3.4 mg/dl), dosage reduced by 50%.

Contraindications
Hypersensitivity to terbinafine or its components

Mechanism of Action
Inhibits the conversion of squalene monooxygenase to squalene epoxidase, a key enzyme in fungal biosynthesis. The resulting squalene accumulation weakens cell membranes and creates a deficiency of ergosterol, the fungal membrane component necessary for normal fungal growth.

Interactions
DRUGS
beta blockers, MAO inhibitors (type B), selective serotonin reuptake inhibitors, tricyclic antidepressants: Possibly increased blood levels of these drugs
cimetidine, other hepatic enzyme inhibitors: Significantly decreased terbinafine clearance, possibly increased adverse reactions
hepatotoxic drugs: Increased risk of hepatotoxicity
rifampin: Increased clearance and decreased effectiveness of terbinafine
FOODS
caffeine: Decreased caffeine clearance
ACTIVITIES
alcohol use: Increased risk of severe hepatitis

Adverse Reactions
CNS: Headache
EENT: Taste perversion
GI: Abdominal pain, anorexia, diarrhea, elevated liver function test results, flatulence, hepatic failure, indigestion, nausea, vomiting
SKIN: Cutaneous lupus erythematosus, pruritus, rash, urticaria
OTHER: Angioedema, systemic lupus erythematosus

Nursing Considerations
•Because terbinafine has been linked to serious adverse hepatic effects, expect to send nail specimens for laboratory testing to confirm onychomycosis before starting therapy.
•Be aware that drug shouldn't be given to patients with chronic or active hepatic disease or renal impairment.
•Monitor patient for hepatic failure (anorexia, dark urine, fatigue, jaundice, nausea, pale stools, right upper abdominal pain, and vomiting). Expect to stop drug and obtain liver function tests if these problems develop.

PATIENT TEACHING
•Instruct patient to space doses evenly if taking terbinafine more than once a day.
•Stress the need to complete the full course of therapy to prevent relapse of infection.
•Discourage use of alcohol during therapy.
•Tell patient to contact prescriber if onychomycosis doesn't improve in a few weeks.

terbutaline sulfate
Brethaire, Brethine, Bricanyl, Bricanyl Turbuhaler (CAN)

Class and Category
Chemical class: Sympathomimetic amine
Therapeutic class: Bronchodilator
Pregnancy category: B

Indications and Dosages
➤ *To prevent or reverse bronchospasm from asthma, bronchitis, or emphysema*
TABLETS (BRETHINE, BRICANYL)
Adults and adolescents age 15 and over. 2.5 to 5 mg t.i.d. at 6-hr intervals while awake. *Maximum:* 15 mg daily.
Children ages 12 to 15. 2.5 mg t.i.d. at 6-hr intervals while awake. *Maximum:* 7.5 mg daily.
Children ages 6 to 11. 50 to 75 mcg/kg t.i.d. at 6-hr intervals while awake. *Maximum:* 150 mcg/kg/dose or 5 mg daily.
SUBCUTANEOUS INJECTION (BRICANYL)
Adults and children age 12 and over. *Initial:* 0.25 mg, repeated in 15 to 30 min as prescribed. *Maximum:* 0.5 mg/4-hr period.
Children ages 6 to 12. 5 to 10 mcg (0.005 to 0.01 mg)/kg every 15 to 20 min, up to 3 doses. *Maximum:* 400 mcg (0.4 mg)/dose.
INHALATION AEROSOL (BRETHAIRE)
Adults and children. 2 inhalations (400 mcg) every 4 to 6 hr, as needed and as prescribed.
INHALATION AEROSOL (BRICANYL TURBUHALER)
Adults and children. 1 inhalation (500 mcg), repeated after 5 min, as needed and as prescribed. *Maximum:* 6 inhalations daily.

Route	Onset	Peak	Duration
P.O.	30 to 90 min	2 to 3 hr	4 to 8 hr
SubQ	15 to 30 min	30 to 60 min	1.5 to 4 hr
Inhalation	In 5 min	30 to 90 min	3 to 6 hr

T

Mechanism of Action

Stimulates beta$_2$-adrenergic receptors in the lungs, which is believed to increase production of cAMP. The increased cAMP level relaxes bronchial smooth muscles, thereby increasing bronchial airflow and relieving bronchospasm.

Contraindications

Hypersensitivity to terbutaline, other sympathomimetic amines, or their components

Interactions

DRUGS

antihypertensives, diuretics: Decreased antihypertensive effect

beta blockers: Mutual inhibition of therapeutic effects, increased risk of bronchospasm

CNS stimulants: Additive CNS stimulation, possibly resulting in adverse effects

digoxin: Increased risk of arrhythmias, possibly digitalis toxicity

halogenated anesthetics: Possibly ventricular arrhythmias

MAO inhibitors: Possibly potentiated action of terbutaline; headache, hyperpyrexia, hypertension, possible hypertensive crisis

maprotiline, tricyclic antidepressants: Possibly potentiated action of terbutaline

nitrates: Decreased effectiveness of nitrates

ritodrine: Increased effects of either drug and potential for adverse effects

sympathomimetics: Increased CNS stimulation and risk of adverse cardiovascular effects, including prolonged QT interval

thyroid hormones: Increased effects of either drug, risk of coronary insufficiency in patients with coronary artery disease

xanthines (theophylline): Increased CNS stimulation and other additive toxic effects

FOODS

caffeine: Increased CNS stimulation and other additive toxic effects

Adverse Reactions

CNS: Anxiety, dizziness, drowsiness, headache, insomnia, light-headedness, nervousness, restlessness, tremor, weakness

CV: Chest pain, irregular heartbeat, palpitations, tachycardia

EENT: Dry mouth, taste perversion

ENDO: Hyperglycemia

GI: Heartburn, nausea, vomiting

MS: Muscle spasms

RESP: Dyspnea

SKIN: Diaphoresis, flushing, rash

Nursing Considerations

• Use terbutaline cautiously in patients with cardiovascular disease because drug can adversely affect cardiovascular function. Monitor patient's heart rate and rhythm and blood pressure, and assess for chest pain.

• For subcutaneous use, inject into lateral deltoid area.

• Assess patient's respiratory rate, depth, and quality; oxygen saturation; and activity tolerance at regular intervals because continuous use of beta$_2$-agonists for 12 months or longer accelerates the decline in pulmonary function.

PATIENT TEACHING

• Teach patient how to use terbutaline aerosol inhaler or give subcutaneous injection, as needed.

• Instruct patient not to increase dose or frequency without consulting prescriber.

• Urge patient to seek immediate medical attention if symptoms worsen.

• Inform patient that she may experience transient nervousness or tremors during terbutaline therapy.

teriparatide

Forteo

Class and Category

Chemical class: Recombinant human parathyroid hormone (PTH)

Therapeutic class: Bone growth and density regulator

Pregnancy category: C

Indications and Dosages

➤ *To treat osteoporosis in postmenopausal women and primary or hypogonadal osteoporosis in men at high risk for fracture*

SUBCUTANEOUS INJECTION

Adults. 20 mcg daily for up to 2 yr.

Route	Onset	Peak	Duration
SubQ	2 hr	4 to 6 hr	16 to 24 hr

Contraindications

Hypersensitivity to teriparatide or its components

Interactions

DRUGS

digitalis glycosides: Possibly increased risk of digitalis toxicity

Adverse Reactions

CNS: Asthenia, depression, dizziness, headache, insomnia, paresthesia, syncope, vertigo
CV: Angina pectoris, chest pain, hypertension, transient orthostatic hypotension
EENT: Pharyngitis, rhinitis, taste perversion, tooth disorder
ENDO: Transient hypoparathyroidism
GI: Constipation, diarrhea, indigestion, vomiting
MS: Arthralgia, muscle cramps or spasms in back or leg, neck pain
RESP: Cough, dyspnea, pneumonia
SKIN: Diaphoresis, pruritus, rash, urticaria
Other: Angioedema, generalized pain, injection site reactions (erythema, localized bruising, minor bleeding, pain, pruritus, swelling), transient hypercalcemia or hypocalcemia

Nursing Considerations

•**WARNING** Be aware that teriparatide shouldn't be used to treat patients at risk for osteosarcoma (such as those with Paget's disease or a metabolic bone disease other than osteoporosis), unexplained elevations of alkaline phosphatase, open epiphyses, or prior skeletal radiation or malignancy.
•**WARNING** Be aware that patients with hypercalcemia shouldn't receive teriparatide because drug may worsen hypercalcemia.
•Use drug cautiously in patients with active or recent urolithiasis because drug could worsen this condition.
•Monitor patient closely for allergic reac-

Mechanism of Action

Teriparatide, which contains recombinant PTH, stimulates new bone growth and increases bone density. In a patient with osteoporosis, bone density and mass are diminished by an imbalance between bone destruction and formation. Normally, osteoclasts break down and resorb bone, leaving behind a cavity in a section of bone. Then bone-building cells, called osteoblasts, line the walls of the cavity and stimulate new bone formation. PTH stimulates these actions by attaching to receptors on osteoclasts and osteoblasts, as shown below.

Teriparatide binds to cell-surface receptors on osteoblasts and preferentially stimulates osteoblastic over osteoclastic activity. Also, the drug increases the amount of circulating calcium available for bone formation by increasing the intestinal absorption of calcium and phosphate, thus enhancing the rate of calcium resorption from bone, increasing the reabsorption of calcium, and inhibiting the reabsorption of phosphate in the kidneys. These actions stimulate new bone formation and increase bone density to reduce osteoporotic bone changes.

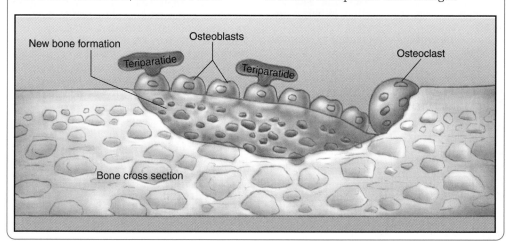

New bone formation
Osteoblasts
Teriparatide
Teriparatide
Osteoclast
Bone cross section

T

tions because teriparatide is a peptide agent.
•Monitor patient's blood calcium level, and
notify prescriber of any elevation; in persistent hypercalcemia, the drug may need to be
stopped.
•Monitor patient's blood pressure during the
first several doses of drug therapy because of
a risk of transient orthostatic hypotension. If
this occurs, place patient in a reclining position and alert prescriber.

PATIENT TEACHING
•Teach patient how to administer teriparatide by subcutaneous injection and how to
properly use the delivery pen device and dispose of needles. Advise her not to share pen
device with others.
•Inform patient that each delivery pen can
be used for up to 28 days after the first injection but then should be discarded even if
it still contains solution.
•Instruct patient to store the delivery pen in
the refrigerator and to recap it when not in
use to protect it from damage and light.
•Tell patient that delivery pen may be used
immediately after removal from refrigerator
and should be put back in refrigerator as
soon as the injection is given.
•Instruct patient to inject drug into thigh or
abdominal wall and to rotate injection sites.
•Caution patient to administer drug in a
room where she can immediately sit or lie
down if light-headedness or palpitations
occur. Advise her to notify prescriber if these
symptoms persist or worsen.
•Instruct patient to notify prescriber of persistent symptoms of hypercalcemia, such as
nausea, vomiting, constipation, lethargy, and
muscle weakness.
•Caution patient about potential developing
osteosarcoma.

tetracycline hydrochloride

Achromycin, Achromycin V, Apo-Tetra (CAN),
Novo-Tetra (CAN), Nu-Tetra (CAN), Panmycin,
Robitet, Sumycin, Tetracap, Tetracyn, Tetracyn 500

Class and Category

Chemical class: Chlortetracycline derivative
Therapeutic class: Antibiotic
Pregnancy category: D

Indications and Dosages

➤ *To treat actinomycosis caused by susceptible organisms*
CAPSULES, ORAL SUSPENSION, TABLETS
Adults and adolescents. 250 to 500 mg every
6 hr or 500 to 1,000 mg every 12 hr. *Maximum:*
4 g daily.
Children age 8 and over. 6.25 to 12.5 mg/kg
every 6 hr or 12.5 to 25 mg/kg every 12 hr.

➤ *To treat acne vulgaris*
CAPSULES, ORAL SUSPENSION, TABLETS
Adults and adolescents. *Initial:* 500 to
2,000 mg daily in divided doses until improvement occurs (usually in 3 wk); then
dosage reduced gradually. *Maintenance:*
125 to 1,000 mg daily. *Maximum:* 4 g daily.

➤ *To treat brucellosis caused by susceptible organisms*
CAPSULES, ORAL SUSPENSION, TABLETS
Adults and adolescents. 500 mg every 6 hr
for 3 wk, given with 1 g of streptomycin I.M.
every 12 hr in week 1 and daily in week 2.
Maximum: 4 g daily.
Children ages 8 to 12. 6.25 to 12.5 mg/kg
every 6 hr, or 12.5 to 25 mg/kg every 12 hr.

➤ *To treat gonorrhea caused by* Neisseria
gonorrhoeae
CAPSULES, ORAL SUSPENSION, TABLETS
Adults and adolescents. 1,500 mg, then
500 mg every 6 hr for 5 days. *Maximum:* 4 g
daily.

➤ *To treat syphilis caused by* Treponema
pallidum
CAPSULES, ORAL SUSPENSION, TABLETS
Adults and adolescents. 500 mg every 6 hr
for 15 days (for early syphilis) or 30 days
(for late syphilis). *Maximum:* 4 g daily.
Children ages 9 to 12. 6.25 to 12.5 mg/kg
every 6 hr, or 12.5 to 25 mg/kg every 12 hr.

➤ *To treat uncomplicated endocervical,
rectal, or urethral infections caused by*
Chlamydia trachomatis
CAPSULES, ORAL SUSPENSION, TABLETS
Adults and adolescents. 500 mg q.i.d. for at
least 7 days. *Maximum:* 4 g daily.
DOSAGE ADJUSTMENT For patients with renal
impairment, dosage possibly reduced because
of extended half-life.

Contraindications

Hypersensitivity to tetracycline or its components

Mechanism of Action
Exerts a bacteriostatic effect against a wide variety of gram-positive and gram-negative organisms by passing through the bacterial lipid bilayer, where it binds reversibly to 30S ribosomal subunits. Bound tetracycline blocks the binding of aminoacyl transfer RNA to messenger RNA, thus inhibiting bacterial protein synthesis.

Interactions
DRUGS
aluminum-, calcium-, or magnesium-containing antacids; iron supplements (oral); magnesium-containing laxatives; magnesium salicylate; multivitamins (containing manganese or zinc salts); sodium bicarbonate: Possibly impaired absorption of oral tetracycline and formation of nonabsorbable complexes
cholestyramine, colestipol: Possibly impaired absorption of oral tetracycline
digoxin: Possibly increased digoxin level
methoxyflurane: Possibly nephrotoxicity
oral contraceptives (containing estrogen): Possibly reduced contraceptive reliability and increased risk of breakthrough bleeding (with long-term tetracycline use)
penicillins: Possibly decreased bactericidal effect of penicillins
vitamin A: Possibly benign intracranial hypertension
FOODS
dairy products and other foods: Possibly impaired absorption of oral tetracycline

Adverse Reactions
CNS: Dizziness, light-headedness, unsteadiness
EENT: Darkened or discolored tongue, enamel hypoplasia, oral candidiasis, tooth discoloration (in children)
GI: Abdominal pain, diarrhea, hepatotoxicity, nausea, rectal candidiasis, vomiting
GU: Vaginal candidiasis
SKIN: Photosensitivity

Nursing Considerations
• Avoid giving tetracycline to children under age 8 because drug may cause permanent brown or yellow tooth discoloration and enamel hypoplasia.
• Be aware that tooth discoloration and enamel hypoplasia may occur in breastfeeding infants, along with inhibition of linear skeletal growth, oral and vaginal candidiasis, and photosensitivity.
• To reduce the risk of esophageal irritation or ulceration, avoid bedtime dosing of tetracycline for patient with esophageal obstruction or compression.
• Assess for photosensitivity, which can develop within a few minutes or up to several hours after exposure to sunlight or other ultraviolet (UV) light. Effects may last for 1 to 2 days after discontinuation of drug.
• Be aware that citric acid in tetracycline preparations may accelerate drug deterioration and that using outdated drug may cause Fanconi's syndrome, characterized by multiple defects in renal tubular function. Symptoms include acidosis, bicarbonate wasting, glycosuria, hypokalemia, osteomalacia, and phosphaturia.

PATIENT TEACHING
• Instruct patient to take oral tetracycline at least 1 hour before meals or 2 hours after meals because dairy products and some foods may interfere with absorption.
• Advise patient to take each dose with a full glass of water while in an upright position to avoid esophageal or GI irritation.
• Instruct patient taking oral suspension to shake container well before measuring dose and to use a calibrated measuring device.
• Advise patient to avoid taking other drugs, including OTC antacids and other preparations, within 3 hours of oral tetracycline.
• Urge patient to complete entire course of tetracycline therapy even if she feels better.
• Caution her to avoid direct sunlight or UV light and to wear sunscreen when outdoors.
• Advise women who use oral contraceptives containing estrogen to use another method of contraception while taking tetracycline because contraceptives may be less effective.
• Stress the need to discard outdated tetracycline because of the risk of toxic effects.
• Encourage patient to take safety precautions if she experiences dizziness or other adverse CNS reactions.

thalidomide
Thalomid

Class and Category
Chemical class: Glutamic-acid derivative
Therapeutic class: Anti-inflammatory,

T

immuno-modulator
Pregnancy category: X

Indications and Dosages

➤ *To treat acute cutaneous erythema no-*
dosum leprosum
CAPSULES
Adults and adolescents. 100 to 400 mg daily
at bedtime or at least 1 hr after the evening
meal. *Usual:* 200 mg.
DOSAGE ADJUSTMENT For patients weighing
less than 50 kg (110 lb), dosage started at
100 mg.
➤ *To prevent or suppress recurrence of cu-*
taneous erythema nodosum leprosum
CAPSULES
Adults and adolescents. Minimum dosage
necessary to control reaction; dosage tapered
every 3 to 6 mo in increments of 50 mg every
2 to 4 wk, as prescribed.

Mechanism of Action
Suppresses the production of tumor necrosis factor-alpha, which reduces neutrophils and CD4 T cells in erythema nodosum leprosum lesions, thus preventing or
controlling symptoms.

Contraindications
Hypersensitivity to thalidomide or its components; men, regardless of history of vasectomy, who refuse to wear latex condom during intercourse with women of childbearing
age; pregnancy; women of childbearing age
who aren't using two reliable contraceptive
methods or aren't abstaining from heterosex-
ual intercourse

Interactions
DRUGS
antihistamines, anxiolytics, barbiturates,
chlorpromazine, CNS depressants, hypnotics,
opioid analgesics, reserpine, sedatives: Increased CNS depression
chloramphenicol, cisplatin, dapsone, didano-
sine, ethambutol, ethionamide, hydralazine,
isoniazid, lithium, metronidazole, nitrofuran-
toin, nitrous oxide, other drugs associated
with peripheral neuropathy, phenytoin,
stavudine, vincristine, zalcitabine: Increased
risk of peripheral neuropathy
ACTIVITIES
alcohol use: Increased CNS depression

Adverse Reactions
CNS: Agitation, anxiety, asthenia, chills,
confusion, depression, dizziness, drowsiness,
fatigue, fever, headache, insomnia, lethargy,
loss of consciousness, malaise, mood changes,
nervousness, paresthesia, peripheral neuropathy, seizures, somnolence, status epilepticus, stupor, syncope, tremor, vertigo
CV: Arrhythmias, bradycardia, embolism, hyperlipidemia, hypertension, orthostatic hypotension, peripheral edema, tachycardia,
thrombosis
EENT: Dry mouth, oral candidiasis, pharyngitis, rhinitis, sinusitis, tooth pain
ENDO: Hypothyroidism
GI: Abdominal pain, anorexia, constipation,
diarrhea, elevated liver function test results,
flatulence, hepatic dysfunction, increased appetite, intestinal perforation, nausea, vomiting
GU: Albuminuria, elevated creatinine level,
hematuria, impotence
HEME: Anemia, decreased platelets count,
leukopenia, neutropenia, prolonged PT
MS: Arthralgia, back or bone pain, muscle
weakness, myalgia, neck pain or rigidity
RESP: Cough, dyspnea, pleural effusion, pulmonary embolism
SKIN: Acne, dermatitis, diaphoresis, dryness,
erythema multiforme, photosensitivity, pruritus, rash
Other: Facial edema, hypercalcemia, hyperkalemia, hypocalcemia, hypokalemia, hyponatremia, increased alkaline phosphatase
level, lymphadenopathy, pain (generalized),
tumor lysis syndrome, weight loss or gain

Nursing Considerations
•Be aware that all patients receiving thalidomide must complete an informed consent
form and participate in a confidential monitoring registry. Thalidomide may be obtained
only through physicians and pharmacies registered in the System for Thalidomide Education and Prescribing Safety (STEPS) Program, a comprehensive safety program designed to prevent fetal exposure to thalidomide. Thalidomide may be dispensed only in
original packaging and in no more than a
28-day supply. Prescriptions older than
7 days may not be filled.
•Be aware that female patients of childbearing age must use two contraceptive methods
during therapy. Pregnancy testing must be

performed 24 hours before starting thalidomide, weekly during first month of therapy,
then monthly thereafter in women with regular menstrual cycles or every 2 weeks in
women with irregular menstrual cycles.
•**WARNING** Be aware that thalidomide
shouldn't be given to pregnant patient. A
single dose may cause severe birth defects or
fetal death.
•Assess patient's medication history for use
of carbamazepine, griseofulvin, HIV-protease
inhibitors, modafinil, penicillins, phenytoin,
rifabutin, rifampin, and the herbal remedy
St. John's wort. These products can decrease
the effectiveness of hormonal contraceptives
during thalidomide therapy.
•**WARNING** Monitor patient closely for evidence of a venous thromboembolic event
(shortness of breath, chest pain, or arm or
leg swelling). Notify prescriber immediately
and expect to assist with diagnostic studies
to confirm suspicions and provide treatment,
as ordered.
•To minimize sedative effect, give thalidomide in divided doses t.i.d. or q.i.d., as prescribed, with larger dose in the evening.
•Assess for early signs of peripheral neuropathy (muscle cramps, numbness and tingling
in toes and fingers, pain or superficial sensory loss in feet or hands) in patients receiving long-term thalidomide therapy. Early detection and drug discontinuation, as prescribed, prevents further damage and increases the chance for reversal.
•Expect to stop thalidomide if absolute neutrophil count is less than 750/mm³. Routine
monitoring of WBC count is recommended
every other week for first 3 months of treatment in HIV-positive and other immunosuppressed patients and monthly in immunocompetent patients.
PATIENT TEACHING
•Instruct patient to have thalidomide prescription filled promptly because prescriptions more than 7 days old may not be filled.
•Urge patient to take drug exactly as prescribed.
•Inform female patient that drug will harm
a fetus, and stress the need to avoid pregnancy. Tell her that pregnancy tests will be
done before and frequently during therapy.
•Instruct female patient to abstain from sexual intercourse or to use two reliable methods of birth control simultaneously, starting

4 weeks before drug therapy and continuing
for up to 4 weeks after therapy has been
completed. One contraceptive method must
be highly effective, such as an intrauterine
device, oral contraceptive, or tubal ligation;
the other may be a cervical cap, diaphragm,
or latex condom.
•**WARNING** Inform male patient, even one who
has had a vasectomy, that he must use barrier contraception (latex condom) when having sexual intercourse with a woman of
childbearing age.
•Caution patient to avoid hazardous activities until drug's CNS effects are known.
•Suggest changing positions slowly to minimize effects of orthostatic hypotension.
•Instruct patient to immediately report signs
of peripheral neuropathy, including numbness, pain, or tingling in feet and hands.
•Inform HIV-positive patient of the need for
viral-load testing after first and third
months of therapy and then every 3 months.
•Urge patient to avoid using alcohol and do-
nating blood or sperm during therapy.

theophylline

Aerolate, Aerolate III, Aerolate Jr., Aerolate
Sr., Apo-Theo LA (CAN), Asmalix, Elixophyl-
lin, Lanophyllin, PMS Theophylline (CAN),
Pulmophylline (CAN), Quibron-T Dividose,
Quibron-T/SR Dividose, Respbid, Slo-Bid
Gyrocaps, Slo-Phyllin, Theo-24, Theo-SR
(CAN), Theobid Duracaps, Theochron, Theo-
clear, Theoclear LA, Theo-Dur, Theolair,
Theolair-SR, Theovent Long-Acting, T-Phyl,
Truxophyllin, Uni-Dur, Uniphyl

Class and Category
Chemical class: Xanthine derivative
Therapeutic class: Bronchodilator
Pregnancy category: C

Indications and Dosages
➤ *As loading dose to treat reversible air-
way obstruction in patients not cur-
rently receiving theophylline*
CAPSULES, ELIXIR, ORAL SOLUTION, SYRUP, TABLETS
Adults and children. 5 mg/kg as a single
dose.
I.V. INFUSION
Adults and children. 5 mg/kg infused over
20 to 30 min.

➤ *As partial loading dose to treat revers-*

ible airway obstruction in patients currently receiving theophylline

CAPSULES, ELIXIR, ORAL SOLUTION, SYRUP, TABLETS, I.V. INFUSION

Adults and children. Individualized dosage based on blood theophylline level, as prescribed. Loading dose based on principle that 0.5 mg/kg of theophylline will produce a 1-mcg/ml increase in blood theophylline level.

➤ *To provide maintenance treatment of reversible airway obstruction associated with asthma or COPD*

CAPSULES, TABLETS

Adults and children weighing more than 45 kg (99 lb). *Initial:* 300 mg daily in equally divided doses every 6 to 8 hr; after 3 days, if tolerated, increased to 400 mg daily in divided doses every 6 to 8 hr; after 3 more days, if tolerated, increased to 600 mg daily in divided doses every 6 to 8 hr. Dosages above 600 mg daily are based on blood theophylline level and clinical response.

Children age 1 and over weighing 45 kg or less. *Initial:* 12 to 14 mg/kg daily up to maximum of 300 mg daily in equally divided doses every 4 to 6 hr; after 3 days, if tolerated, increased to 16 mg/kg up to maximum of 400 mg daily in equally divided doses every 4 to 6 hr; after 3 more days, if tolerated, 20 mg/kg daily up to maximum of 600 mg daily in equally divided doses every 4 to 6 hr. Dosages above 600 mg daily are based on blood theophylline level and clinical response.

ELIXIR

Adults. *Initial:* 300 mg daily in equally divided doses every 6 to 8 hr; after 3 days, if tolerated, increased to 400 mg daily in divided doses every 6 to 8 hr; after 3 more days, if tolerated, increased to 600 mg daily in divided doses every 6 to 8 hr. Dosages above 600 mg daily are based on blood theophylline level and clinical response.

E.R. CAPSULES OR TABLETS

Adults and children weighing 45 kg or more. *Initial:* 300 mg daily in equally divided doses every 8 to 12 hr; after 3 days, if tolerated, increased to 400 mg daily in divided doses every 8 to 12 hr; after 3 more days, if tolerated, increased to 600 mg daily in divided doses every 8 to 12 hr. Dosages above 600 mg daily are based on blood theophylline level and clinical response.

Children age 1 and over weighing less than 45 kg. *Initial:* 12 to 14 mg/kg daily up to maximum of 300 mg daily in equally divided doses every 8 to 12 hr; after 3 days, if tolerated, increased to 16 mg/kg up to maximum of 400 mg daily in equally divided doses every 8 to 12 hr; after 3 more days, if tolerated, dosage increased to 20 mg/kg daily up to maximum of 600 mg daily in equally divided doses every 8 to 12 hr. Dosages above 600 mg daily are based on blood theophylline level and clinical response.

ORAL SOLUTION, SYRUP

Adults and children weighing more than 45 kg. *Initial:* 300 mg daily in equally divided doses every 6 to 8 hr; after 3 days, if tolerated, increased to 400 mg daily in divided doses every 6 to 8 hr; after 3 more days, if tolerated, increased to 600 mg daily in divided doses every 6 to 8 hr. Dosages above 600 mg daily are based on blood theophylline level and clinical response.

Children age 1 and over weighing 45 kg or less. *Initial:* 12 to 14 mg/kg daily up to maximum of 300 mg daily in equally divided doses every 4 to 6 hr; after 3 days, if tolerated, increased to 16 mg/kg up to a maximum of 400 mg daily in equally divided doses every 4 to 6 hr; after 3 more days, if tolerated, dosage increased to 20 mg/kg daily up to maximum of 600 mg daily in equally divided doses every 4 to 6 hr. Dosages above 600 mg daily are based on blood theophylline level and clinical response.

Full-term infants ages 26 to 52 weeks. Dosage individualized in mg/kg daily, as prescribed, and administered in equally divided doses every 6 hr.

Full-term infants up to age 26 weeks. Dosage individualized in mg/kg daily, as prescribed, and administered in equally divided doses every 8 hr.

Premature infants age 24 days and over. 1.5 mg/kg every 12 hr.

Premature infants under age 24 days. 1 mg/kg every 12 hr.

I.V. INFUSION

Adults and adolescents age 16 and over. 0.4 mg/kg/hr for nonsmokers, 0.7 mg/kg/hr for smokers.

DOSAGE ADJUSTMENT For elderly patients and adults with cardiac decompensation, cor pulmonale, or hepatic impairment, I.V. dosage reduced to 0.2 mg/kg/hr.

Children ages 9 to 16. 0.7 mg/kg/hr.
Children ages 1 to 9. 0.8 mg/kg/hr.
Full-term infants up to age 1. Dosage individualized in mg/kg daily as prescribed.

Mechanism of Action

Inhibits phosphodiesterase enzymes, causing bronchodilation. Normally, these enzymes inactivate cAMP and cGMP, which are responsible for bronchial smooth-muscle relaxation. Theophylline also may cause calcium translocation, antagonize prostaglandins and adenosine receptors, stimulate catecholamines, and inhibit cGMP metabolism.

Incompatibilities

Don't mix parenteral theophylline solution with any additives. Don't infuse theophylline through same I.V. line as Hetastarch (Hespan), a colloidal plasma volume expander, which is incompatible with theophylline.

Contraindications

Hypersensitivity to theophylline or its components, peptic ulcer disease, uncontrolled seizure disorder

Interactions

DRUGS
adenosine: Decreased adenosine effectiveness
allopurinol, cimetidine, ciprofloxacin, clarithromycin, disulfiram, enoxacin, erythromycin, fluvoxamine, interferon alpha (human recombinant), methotrexate, mexiletine, pentoxifylline, propafenone, propranolol, tacrine, thiabendazole, ticlopidine, troleandomycin, verapamil: Increased blood theophylline level and risk of toxicity
aminoglutethimide, carbamazepine, isoproterenol (I.V.), moricizine, oral contraceptives (containing estrogen), phenobarbital, phenytoin, rifampin: Decreased blood theophylline level and possibly drug effectiveness
benzodiazepines: Possibly reversal of benzodiazepine sedation
beta blockers: Possibly decreased bronchodilator effect of theophylline
ephedrine: Increased adverse effects, including insomnia, nausea, and nervousness
halothane anesthetics: Increased risk of ventricular arrhythmias
ketamine: Lowered seizure threshold

lithium: Decreased lithium effectiveness
neuromuscular blockers: Possibly antagonized neuromuscular blockade
sucralfate: Decreased absorption of oral theophylline
FOODS
high-carbohydrate, low-protein diet: Possibly decreased theophylline elimination
low-carbohydrate, high-protein diet; daily intake of charbroiled beef: Possibly increased theophylline elimination
ACTIVITIES
alcohol use: Increased blood theophylline level and risk of toxicity
smoking: Increased drug clearance, decreased drug effectiveness

Adverse Reactions

CNS: Agitation, anxiety (I.V. form), behavioral changes, confusion, disorientation, headache, insomnia, nervousness, seizures, tremor
CV: Hypotension, tachycardia, ventricular arrhythmias
ENDO: Hyperglycemia
GI: Abdominal pain, diarrhea, heartburn, nausea, vomiting
GU: Increased urine output
Other: Hypercalcemia

Nursing Considerations

• Be aware that ideal body weight is used to calculate theophylline dosages because drug doesn't bind well in body fat.
• Be aware that E.R. capsules and tablets shouldn't be used for oral loading doses.
• Infuse theophylline loading dose, bolus, or intermittent infusion at a rate that doesn't exceed 25 mg/min.
• Administer continuous theophylline infusion with rate-controlled infusion device.
• Monitor blood theophylline level, as ordered, to gauge therapeutic level and detect toxicity.
• Frequently assess heart rate and rhythm because theophylline can exacerbate existing arrhythmias.
• Be especially alert for signs of toxicity in patient with acute pulmonary edema, hypothyroidism, influenza vaccination, prolonged fever, sepsis with multiple organ failure, shock, or viral pulmonary infection because of decreased drug clearance.
• Monitor blood theophylline level in patients with uncorrected acidemia because they have

T

an increased risk of toxicity.
•Expect patient with cystic fibrosis or hyperthyroidism to have increased theophylline clearance and decreased drug effectiveness. Monitor blood theophylline level, as ordered.
•Suspect toxicity if patient experiences vomiting, and be prepared to obtain blood theophylline level.

PATIENT TEACHING
•Instruct patient to swallow theophylline tablets whole and not to chew or crush them, unless scored for breaking.
•Explain that patient may open capsules and mix contents with soft food but that she shouldn't chew or crush granules.
•Instruct patient to take drug with a full glass of water on an empty stomach (30 to 60 minutes before meals or 2 hours after meals). However, suggest that she take drug with food or antacids if GI distress occurs.
•Encourage patient to take drug at the same times every day.
•Advise patient to notify prescriber if she develops a fever, makes a significant dietary change, or starts or stops smoking or taking other drugs because these factors may alter blood theophylline level.
•Tell female patient to notify prescriber if she is or cold be pregnant.

thiethylperazine maleate

Torecan

Class and Category

Chemical class: Piperazine phenothiazine
Therapeutic class: Antiemetic
Pregnancy category: Not rated

Indications and Dosages

➤ *To treat nausea and vomiting*
TABLETS, I.M. INJECTION, SUPPOSITORIES
Adults and adolescents. 10 mg once daily to t.i.d. *Maximum:* 30 mg daily.

Route	Onset	Peak	Duration
P.O.	30 to 60 min	Unknown	4 hr

Mechanism of Action
Relieves nausea and vomiting by centrally blocking dopamine receptors in the medullary chemoreceptor trigger zone.

Contraindications

Breastfeeding; coma; hypersensitivity to thiethylperazine, sulfites, tartrazine dye, or their components; jaundice; severe CNS depression

Interactions

DRUGS
aluminum- or magnesium-containing antacids, antidiarrheals (adsorbent): Decreased absorption of thiethylperazine
anticonvulsants (including barbiturates): Lowered seizure threshold
antihistamines, tricyclic antidepressants: Additive CNS and GI effects, including ileus and severe constipation
antihypertensives: Enhanced hypotensive effect of both drugs
antimuscarinics (including antiparkinsonian drugs, MAO inhibitors, meperidine, and phenothiazines): Additive GI effects, including ileus and severe constipation
appetite suppressants: Decreased anorectic effect
barbiturates, benzodiazepines, CNS depressants, general anesthetics, opioid analgesics: Additive CNS effects
beta blockers: Increased blood levels of both drugs; additive hypotensive effects; possibly arrhythmias, irreversible retinopathy, and tardive dyskinesia
bromocriptine: Possibly decreased effectiveness of bromocriptine
hepatotoxic drugs: Increased risk of hepatotoxicity
levodopa: Decreased effectiveness of levodopa
lithium: Possibly acute encephalopathy
methoxsalen, porfimer: Possibly increased photosensitivity
metrizamide: Increased risk of seizures
ototoxic drugs: Possibly masked symptoms of ototoxicity (dizziness, tinnitus, and vertigo)
phenytoin: Increased risk of phenytoin toxicity
quinidine: Possibly adverse cardiac effects
riboflavin: Increased requirements for riboflavin
sympathomimetics: Reduced vasopressor response and duration of action of sympathomimetics
tramadol: Additive CNS effects, increased risk of seizures

ACTIVITIES
alcohol use: Additive CNS effects

Adverse Reactions

CNS: Confusion, dizziness, EEG abnormalities, extrapyramidal reactions (dystonia, pseudoparkinsonism), sedation
CV: ECG changes, hypotension, orthostatic hypotension, tachycardia
EENT: Blurred vision, dry mouth
ENDO: Gynecomastia
GI: Constipation, increased appetite
GU: Darkened urine, ejaculation disorders, menstrual irregularities, urine retention
HEME: Agranulocytosis, leukopenia (transient)
SKIN: Contact dermatitis, photosensitivity
Other: Weight gain

Nursing Considerations

• Avoid using thiethylperazine in patients with neurologic impairment because drug can disrupt central temperature regulation.
• Avoid inadvertent I.V. administration of thiethylperazine; injection is for I.M. administration only.
• Keep patient in recumbent position for 30 to 60 minutes after I.M. injection to minimize the risk of hypotension.
• Be aware that parenteral preparations contain sulfites and that tablets contain tartrazine dye.
• Moisten suppository with water or water-soluble lubricant before insertion. If suppository has softened excessively, chill for 30 minutes or run under cold water before removing wrapper.
• Avoid skin contact with drug to prevent contact dermatitis.
• Because thiethylperazine may cause reactions from anticholinergic effects and adrenergic blockade, assess for blurred vision, constipation, dry mouth, impotence, urine retention (from cholinergic activity) and priapism (from alpha-adrenergic blockade).
• During prolonged therapy, assess for visual disturbances because drug may cause corneal keratopathy and retinal discoloration (pigmentary retinopathy).
• **WARNING** Be aware that thiethylperazine may cause neuroleptic malignant syndrome, a rare but extremely serious reaction characterized by cardiovascular instability, decreased level of consciousness, extrapyramidal effects, and hyperpyrexia.
• Monitor CBC with differential, as ordered, because drug may worsen existing blood dyscrasias, such as agranulocytosis, neutro-

penia, and thrombocytopenia, in patients with bone marrow suppression. Be aware that drug may worsen angle-closure glaucoma, encephalopathy, organic or traumatic brain damage, or tardive dyskinesia.
• When possible, avoid combining thiethylperazine with CNS depressants because these drugs may potentiate thiethylperazine's effects.
• Monitor patient with cardiac disease for exaggerated cardiovascular reactions.
• Implement seizure precautions and monitor for seizures in patients with known seizure disorder because drug may lower seizure threshold.
• Implement safety precautions, according to facility policy, for elderly patients. They may be especially sensitive to drug's sedative and extrapyramidal effects.
• Be prepared to discontinue drug 48 hours before myelography and to resume drug 24 to 48 hours afterward to minimize the risk of seizures.
• Be aware that photosensitivity may turn patient's skin yellow-brown, gray, or purple because of hyperpigmentation.
• Be aware that drug shouldn't be given to pregnant patient because it may cause jaundice and extrapyramidal symptoms in her neonate.

PATIENT TEACHING
• Instruct patient to stay recumbent for 1 hour after taking thiethylperazine to minimize effects of orthostatic hypotension.
• Advise patient to notify prescriber immediately about adverse CNS reactions, decreased urine output, or vision changes.
• Urge patient to avoid alcohol use and potentially hazardous activities during therapy.
• Encourage patient to avoid excessive sun exposure and to use sunscreen when she's outdoors.
• Advise patient on long-term therapy to have periodic eye examinations to detect possible eye disorders.

thiopental sodium

Pentothal

Class, Category, and Schedule

Chemical class: Barbiturate
Therapeutic class: Anticonvulsant, sedative-hypnotic

Pregnancy category: C
Controlled substance: Schedule III

Indications and Dosages

➤ *To control seizures from anesthesia or other causes*

I.V. INJECTION

Adults. *Initial:* 75 to 125 mg (3 to 5 ml of 2.5% solution) as soon as possible after onset of seizure. *Maximum:* 250 mg given over 10 min.

➤ *To facilitate narcoanalysis*

I.V. INFUSION OR INJECTION

Adults. Dosage individualized based on patient's age, condition, sex, and weight; injected at 100 mg/min (4 ml/min of 2.5% solution) with patient counting backwards from 100. Expect to discontinue injection once patient becomes confused with her counting but is still awake. Or, use 0.2% concentration in D_5W for injection and infuse at 50 ml/min.

➤ *To treat cerebral hypertension*

I.V. INFUSION OR INJECTION

Adults. 1.5 to 3.5 mg/kg, repeated as needed, to reduce elevated intracranial pressure (ICP).

Route	Onset	Peak	Duration
I.V.	10 to 40 sec	Unknown	10 to 30 min

Mechanism of Action

Depresses the CNS and may inhibit the ascending transmission of impulses in the reticular formation. Thiopental possibly enhances or mimics the inhibitory action of gamma-aminobutyric acid, thereby having an anticonvulsant effect and producing sedation and hypnosis. Thiopental may reduce ICP by increasing cerebral vascular resistance, which decreases cerebral blood flow and volume.

Incompatibilities

Don't mix thiopental with acidic I.V. drugs or solutions, succinylcholine, or tubocurarine.

Contraindications

History of porphyria; hypersensitivity to thiopental, its components, or other barbiturates

Interactions

DRUGS

clonidine, CNS depressants, guanabenz, mag- *nesium sulfate, methyldopa, metyrosine, pargyline, rauwolfia alkaloids:* Additive CNS depressant effects
diazoxide, diuretics, guanadrel, guanethidine, mecamylamine, trimethaphan: Possibly additive hypotensive effect
ketamine: Increased risk of hypotension or respiratory depression; possibly countered hypnotic effect of thiopental
phenothiazines: Possibly increased CNS depression or excitation, increased hypotensive effect

ACTIVITIES

alcohol use: Additive CNS depressant effects

Adverse Reactions

CNS: Agitation, anxiety, seizures
CV: Bradycardia, hypotension, shock, tachycardia, thrombophlebitis
GI: Hiccups
RESP: Apnea, bronchospasm, cough, laryngospasm, respiratory depression, wheezing
SKIN: Hives, itching, rash, redness
Other: Angioedema

Nursing Considerations

•Before administering thiopental, expect to premedicate patient with an anticholinergic, such as atropine or glycopyrrolate, to minimize secretions.
•Be prepared to administer a test dose of 25 to 75 mg (1 to 3 ml of 2.5% solution) to determine tolerance or sensitivity. Expect to observe patient for at least 1 minute after administering test dose.
•Dilute drug with a compatible I.V. solution before administering, such as D_5W for injection, normal saline solution for injection, or sterile water for injection. Be aware that sterile water for injection shouldn't be used to prepare 0.2% or 0.4% solution because it would result in a hypotonic solution and cause hemolysis.
•To prepare 0.2% solution, dilute 1 g of thiopental with 500 ml of compatible diluent to produce a final concentration of 2 mg/ml.
•To prepare 0.4% solution, dilute 1 g thiopental with 250 ml compatible diluent or 2 g thiopental with 500 ml compatible diluent to produce a final concentration of 4 mg/ml.
•To prepare 2.5% solution, dilute 1 g of thiopental with 40 ml of compatible diluent or 5 g of thiopental with 200 ml of compatible diluent to produce a final concentration of 25 mg/ml.

•Inspect solution for particles before administration. Use solution within 24 hours of reconstitution, and discard unused portion after 24 hours.
•Monitor blood and tissue oxygenation and vital signs during I.V. administration. Keep emergency equipment and drugs nearby in case respiratory depression occurs.
•If patient has a history of CV disease or hypotension, monitor her for CV depressant effects, such as bradycardia, hypotension, or shock.
•In patient with a history of seizures, institute seizure precautions according to facility protocol.
•Monitor respiratory rate, rhythm, and quality for signs of respiratory depression in debilitated patient or one with a history of respiratory disease.
•Monitor neurologic status every hour, or as ordered, in patient with increased ICP.

PATIENT TEACHING
•Explain the need for frequent hemodynamic monitoring.
•Advise patient to use caution when driving or performing tasks that require alertness for at least 24 hours after receiving thiopental.
•Instruct patient not to consume alcohol or other CNS depressants for at least 24 hours after thiopental administration (unless prescribed) because they increase the effects of thiopental.
•Instruct patient to report persistent drowsiness, rash, severe dizziness, or skin lesions to prescriber.

thioridazine

Mellaril (CAN), Mellaril-S, Novo-Ridazine (CAN)

thioridazine hydrochloride

Apo-Thioridazine (CAN), Mellaril, Mellaril Concentrate, Novo-Ridazine (CAN), PMS Thioridazine

Class and Category
Chemical class: Piperidine phenothiazine
Therapeutic class: Antipsychotic drug
Pregnancy category: Not rated

Indications and Dosages
➤ *To treat schizophrenia in patients un-*

responsive to other antipsychotic drugs

ORAL SOLUTION, ORAL SUSPENSION, TABLETS
Adults and adolescents. *Initial:* 50 to 100 mg t.i.d., gradually increased, as needed and tolerated. *Maintenance:* 200 to 800 mg daily in two to four divided doses. *Maximum:* 800 mg daily.
Children ages 2 to 12. *Initial:* 0.5 mg/kg daily in divided doses, gradually increased, as needed and tolerated. *Maximum:* 3 mg/kg daily.

Route	Onset	Peak	Duration
P.O.	Up to several wk	6 wk to 6 mo	Unknown

Mechanism of Action
Depresses areas of the brain that control activity and aggression, including the cerebral cortex, hypothalamus, and limbic system by blocking postsynaptic dopamine$_2$ (D$_2$) receptors. Drug may relieve anxiety by indirectly reducing arousal and increasing filtration of internal stimuli to the brain stem reticular activating system.

Contraindications
Coma; concurrent use of drugs that inhibit the metabolism of thioridazine, such as fluoxetine, fluvoxamine, paroxetine, pindolol, and propranolol; concurrent use of drugs that prolong the QT interval; concurrent use of high doses of a CNS depressant; history of arrhythmias; hypersensitivity to thioridazine, other phenothiazines, or their components; prolonged QT interval; reduced cytochrome P450 2D6 activity; severe CNS depression; severe hypertensive or hypotensive cardiac disease

Interactions
DRUGS
amantadine, antihistamines, antimuscarinics, clozapine, cyclobenzaprine, diphenoxylate, disopyramide, maprotilene: Additive anticholinergic effects
amiodarone, bepridil, cisapride, disopyramide, erythromycin, flecainide, grepafloxacin, ibutilide, pimozide, probucol, procaina-

mide, quinidine, sotalol, sparfloxacin, tocainide: Possibly prolonged QT interval

amphetamine, chlorpromazine, dextroamphetamine: Possibly decreased effects of these drugs and thioridazine

antacids, antidiarrheals (adsorbent), kaolin, rifabutin, rifampin, rifapentine: Reduced bioavailability of thioridazine

anxiolytics, benzodiazepines, clonidine, dronabinol, guanabenz, guanfacine, opioid analgesics, phenothiazines, sedative-hypnotics: Possibly increased CNS effects or hypotension

barbiturates, fosphenytoin, phenytoin, valproic acid: Increased CNS depression, lowered seizure threshold

bromocriptine: Possibly decreased effectiveness of bromocriptine

carbamazepine: Possibly decreased blood thioridazine level

charcoal: Reduced thioridazine absorption

dopamine, droperidol, haloperidol, metoclopramide, metyrosine: Possibly increased adverse CNS effects

ephedrine, epinephrine, norepinephrine, phenylephrine: Possibly severe hypotension, MI, or tachycardia

fluoxetine, fluvoxamine, other cytochrome P450 2D6 inhibitors, paroxetine, pindolol: Inhibited metabolism of thioridazine, leading to elevated blood thioridazine level

general anesthetics: Possibly potentiated CNS depression

guanadrel, guanethidine, methyldopa: Inhibited hypotensive effect of these drugs

levodopa, pergolide, pramipexole, ropinirole: Possibly inhibited antiparkinsonian response

lithium (high doses): Risk of encephalopathic syndrome (characterized by confusion, elevated liver function test results and fasting blood glucose level, extrapyramidal symptoms, fever, lethargy, leukocytosis, and weakness)

MAO inhibitors: Possibly exaggerated extrapyramidal reactions

methoxsalen, oral contraceptives, porfimer, sulfonamides, sulfonylureas, tetracyclines, thiazide diuretics, vitamin A analogues: Possibly increased photosensitivity

propranolol: Increased blood propranolol and thioridazine levels, increased CNS effects, hypotension

tramadol: Increased blood tramadol level, possibly increased risk of seizures

trazodone: Possibly additive hypotension
ACTIVITIES
alcohol use: Additive CNS effects

Adverse Reactions

CNS: Akathisia, altered temperature regulation, depression, dizziness, drowsiness, extrapyramidal reactions (dystonia, laryngospasm, motor restlessness, pseudoparkinsonism), headache, insomnia

CV: ECG changes, hypertension, hypotension, prolonged QT interval, torsades de pointes, ventricular tachycardia

EENT: Blurred vision, change in color perception, dry mouth, impaired night vision, mydriasis, photophobia

ENDO: Breast engorgement, galactorrhea

GI: Constipation, ileus, nausea

GU: Amenorrhea, decreased libido, ejaculation disorders, impotence, menstrual irregularities, priapism, urine retention

HEME: Agranulocytosis, anemia, aplastic anemia, eosinophilia, leukocytosis, leukopenia, pancytopenia, thrombocytopenia

SKIN: Hyperpigmentation, jaundice, photosensitivity

Other: Weight gain

Nursing Considerations

•**WARNING** Expect to give thioridazine only if patient has failed to respond to therapy with at least two other antipsychotic drugs because it may prolong the QT interval and has been associated with torsades de pointes and sudden death.

•**WARNING** Thioridazine shouldn't be used to treat elderly patients with dementia-related psychosis because drug increases the risk of death in these patients.

•Obtain baseline and serial ECG tracings and serum potassium levels, as ordered. Notify prescriber if QT interval is greater than 500 msec or if potassium level is abnormal, and expect to discontinue drug immediately.

•Frequently monitor blood pressure and assess for chest pain in patients with heart disease because thioridazine has caused hypotension and has precipitated angina on occasion. Also monitor urine output in patients with benign prostatic hyperplasia because drug can worsen urine retention.

•Be aware that high doses and large dosage changes in patient with a seizure disorder may lower seizure threshold. Institute seizure precautions, as appropriate, according to facility policy.

•Administer drug with food, milk, or a full glass of water to minimize GI distress.

•Measure oral suspension using calibrated measuring device. Dilute with 60 to 120 ml of fruit juice, distilled water, or acidified tap water immediately before administration.

•Don't give thioridazine oral suspension with carbamazepine oral suspension; a rubbery orange precipitate may form in stool.

•To prevent contact dermatitis, don't let oral solution come in contact with skin.

•Administer antacid or adsorbent antidiarrheal at least 1 hour before or 2 hours after thioridazine.

•**WARNING** Be aware that thioridazine can cause neuroleptic malignant syndrome—most commonly in males. Signs and symptoms include altered level of consciousness, altered mental status, autonomic instability (diaphoresis, hypotension or hypertension, sinus tachycardia), hyperthermia, and severe extrapyramidal dysfunction. Acute renal failure, increased serum creatine phosphokinase level, and leukocytosis also have occurred. Notify prescriber immediately if such symptoms develop, and be prepared to discontinue therapy.

•Be aware that drug shouldn't be discontinued abruptly. Sudden withdrawal of thioridazine may produce transient dizziness, nausea, tremor, and vomiting.

•Assess for eye pain because drug's anticholinergic effects can worsen angle-closure glaucoma.

•Promptly investigate and report blurred vision, defective color perception, or impaired night vision because of the risk of pigmentary retinopathy.

•Expect prescriber to discontinue thioridazine and order CBC if patient experiences signs of infection. Also expect drug therapy to be stopped 48 hours before myelography and resumed 24 to 48 hours afterward.

•Monitor patient for signs and symptoms of tardive dyskinesia—such as uncontrollable movements of the arms, face, or legs—even after treatment stops. Notify prescriber if they develop.

PATIENT TEACHING

•Instruct patient to take thioridazine exactly as prescribed and not to stop taking drug without consulting prescriber because of the risk of withdrawal symptoms.

•Instruct patient to notify prescriber immediately if she develops unusual symptoms, such as dizziness, palpitations, and syncope, because they may indicate the presence of torsades de pointes.

•Advise patient not to take drug within 2 hours of an antacid.

•Caution patient to avoid alcohol use, which increases thioridazine's sedative effects, and to avoid hazardous activities if drowsiness occurs.

•Urge patient to notify prescriber immediately if she experiences blurred vision, defective color perception, difficulty with nighttime vision, excessive drowsiness, nausea, sore throat, or other signs of infection. Treatment may be discontinued.

•Advise female patient to use effective contraception while taking drug because its fetal effects are unknown. Instruct her to inform prescriber immediately of known or suspected pregnancy.

•Because drug may alter temperature regulation, encourage patient to avoid exposure to extreme temperatures during therapy.

•Advise patient to wear protective dark glasses to minimize the effects of adverse vision reactions.

•If patient requires long-term therapy, explain the risk of tardive dyskinesia, and urge her to notify prescriber immediately if she develops uncontrollable movements of her arms, face, or legs.

•Instruct patient to tell other prescribers that she's taking thioridazine before she takes any new drug.

thiothixene

Navane

thiothixene hydrochloride

Navane, Thiothixene HCl Intensol

Class and Category

Chemical class: Thioxanthene derivative
Therapeutic class: Antipsychotic
Pregnancy category: Not rated

Indications and Dosages

➤ *To treat psychotic disorders, such as acute psychosis, psychotic depression, and schizophrenia*

CAPSULES (THIOTHIXENE), ORAL SOLUTION (THIOTHIXENE HYDROCHLORIDE)

Adults and children age 12 and over. *Initial:* 2 mg t.i.d. (for mild conditions) or 5 mg b.i.d. (for more severe conditions), increased every wk, as needed. *Usual:* 10 to 40 mg daily in divided doses. *Maximum:* 60 mg daily (for severe conditions).

DOSAGE ADJUSTMENT For elderly patients, lowest effective dosage used for maintenance therapy; maximum dosage limited to 30 mg/day. For some patients, one daily dose possibly used for maintenance therapy.

I.M. INJECTION (THIOTHIXENE HYDROCHLORIDE)

Adults. *Initial:* 4 mg b.i.d. to q.i.d. *Optimal:* 4 mg every 6 to 12 hr. *Usual:* 16 to 20 mg daily in divided doses. *Maximum:* 30 mg daily.

Mechanism of Action

Increases dopamine turnover by blocking postsynaptic dopamine receptors in the mesolimbic system. Eventually, dopamine neurotransmission decreases, resulting in antipsychotic effects.

Contraindications

Blood dyscrasias, coma, hypersensitivity to thiothixene or its components, Parkinson's disease, severe CNS depression, shock, use of quinidine

Interactions

DRUGS

amphetamines: Decreased effectiveness of either drug

antacids, antidiarrheals (adsorbent): Possibly reduced bioavailability of thiothixene

antihistamines, tricyclic antidepressants: Additive anticholinergic effects, causing severe constipation, ileus, or increased intraocular pressure

bromocriptine: Possibly increased serum prolactin level and decreased effectiveness of bromocriptine

carbamazepine: Possibly decreased blood thiothixene level

dopamine: Decreased vasoconstrictive effect of dopamine (in high doses)

ephedrine, phenylephrine: Possibly reduced vasopressor response

epinephrine: Possibly epinephrine reversal, leading to severe hypotension, tachycardia, and possibly MI

erythromycin: Increased adverse effects of thiothixene

general anesthetics, opioid analgesics, tramadol: Additive CNS effects, increased risk of seizures

guanadrel, guanethidine: Possibly decreased antihypertensive effect of these drugs

hypotensive drugs: Possibly excessive hypotension

levodopa: Possibly reduced effectiveness of levodopa

lithium: Possibly encephalopathic syndrome (with a blood level that exceeds 12 mEq/L)

MAO inhibitors: Possibly exaggerated extrapyramidal reactions

metaraminol, methoxamine, norepinephrine: Possibly reduced vasopressor response

pergolide: Possibly reduced effectiveness of pergolide

propranolol: Possibly seizures and increased hypotension

quinidine: Additive orthostatic hypotension, possibly prolonged QT interval

ACTIVITIES

alcohol use: Additive CNS effects, increased risk of seizures

smoking: Possibly decreased blood thiothixene level

Adverse Reactions

CNS: Agitation, akathisia, drowsiness, dystonia, fatigue, insomnia, light-headedness, neuroleptic malignant syndrome, paradoxical exacerbation of psychotic disorder, restlessness, seizures, syncope, tardive dyskinesia, weakness

CV: ECG changes, edema, hypotension, peripheral edema, tachycardia

EENT: Blurred vision, dry mouth, increased salivation, miosis, mydriasis, nasal congestion, retinopathy

ENDO: Breast engorgement, galactorrhea, hyperglycemia, hypoglycemia

GI: Anorexia, constipation, diarrhea, elevated liver function test results, ileus, increased appetite, nausea, vomiting

GU: Amenorrhea, glycosuria, impotence, priapism

HEME: Agranulocytosis, anemia, eosino-

philia, hemolytic anemia, leukocytosis, leukopenia, pancytopenia, thrombocytopenia
SKIN: Contact dermatitis, decreased sweating, photosensitivity, pruritus, rash
Other: Hyperuricemia, weight gain

Nursing Considerations

•**WARNING** Thiothixene shouldn't be used to treat elderly patients with dementia-related psychosis because drug increases the risk of death in these patients.
•Administer thiothixene capsules with food or milk if needed to minimize GI distress.
•Don't give drug within 1 hr of an antacid.
•Dilute oral solution with 60 to 120 ml of fruit or tomato juice, milk, soup, water, or a carbonated beverage. Measure dose and administer using a calibrated measuring device. Avoid spilling solution on skin because drug may cause contact dermatitis.
•Avoid inadvertent I.V. delivery of thiothixene. It's intended for I.M. use.
•Be aware that I.M. administration usually is reserved for acute, severe agitation or for patients who can't take oral preparations.
•Maintain patient in recumbent position for 30 minutes after I.M. injection to minimize orthostatic hypotension.
•Assess patient for early signs of potentially irreversible tardive dyskinesia, a syndrome of involuntary rhythmic movements of the face, jaw, mouth, or tongue.
•**WARNING** Be aware that drug can precipitate neuroleptic malignant syndrome, a serious condition characterized by altered mental status, arrhythmias, diaphoresis, hyperpyrexia, muscle rigidity, and tachycardia, especially in patients with hyperthyroidism or thyrotoxicosis. Symptoms may be severe enough to cause life-threatening respiratory depression.
•Monitor patient's serum calcium level because hypocalcemia may lead to dystonic reactions.
•Keep in mind that hypotension from thiothixene may precipitate angina in patients with known cardiac disease.
•**WARNING** Be aware that drug-induced adverse CNS reactions may mimic or suppress neurologic evidence of CNS disorders, such as brain tumor, encephalitis, encephalopathy, meningitis, Reye's syndrome, and tetanus.
•Monitor for extrapyramidal symptoms—particularly dystonias—in children with acute illnesses, including CNS infections, de-hydration, gastroenteritis, measles, or varicella-zoster infections.
•Observe for signs of adverse hematologic reactions, such as sore throat and other symptoms of infection. If they occur, be prepared to obtain CBC, as ordered, and discontinue thiothixene, as prescribed.
•Implement seizure precautions in patients with a history of seizures or EEG abnormalities because thiothixene can lower the seizure threshold.
•Assess patient for eye pain because thiothixene's anticholinergic effects may worsen angle-closure glaucoma. Assess patient with benign prostatic hyperplasia for urine retention.

PATIENT TEACHING
•Fully inform patient facing long-term thiothixene therapy about risk of developing tardive dyskinesia.
•Advise patient to avoid exposure to sunlight or ultraviolet light, and to apply sunscreen when outdoors.
•Urge patient to avoid smoking or to begin a smoking cessation program while taking thiothixene.
•Encourage patient to avoid extreme temperature changes during drug therapy to prevent hyperthermia or hypothermia caused by decreased sweating.
•Instruct patient to immediately report sore throat or other signs of infection.

thyroid USP

Armour Thyroid, Thyrar, Thyroid Strong, Westhroid

Class and Category

Chemical class: Porcine thyroid gland hormone
Therapeutic class: Thyroid hormone replacement
Pregnancy category: A

Indications and Dosages

➤ *To treat hypothyroidism without myxedema*

TABLETS
Adults and children. *Initial:* 60 mg daily, increased by 30 mg daily every mo p.r.n. *Maintenance:* 60 to 120 mg daily.

➤ *To treat hypothyroidism or myxedema in patients with cardiovascular disease*

T

TABLETS

Adults. *Initial:* 15 mg daily; daily dosage doubled every 2 wk, as indicated to achieve desired response, up to 180 mg daily. *Maintenance:* 60 to 180 mg daily.

➤ *To treat congenital hypothyroidism (cretinism) or severe hypothyroidism in children and infants*

TABLETS

Children and infants. *Initial:* 15 mg daily; daily dosage doubled every 2 wk, as indicated to achieve desired response, up to 180 mg daily. If desired response isn't achieved, dosage further increased by 30 to 60 mg daily. *Maintenance:* Individualized.

Mechanism of Action

Stimulates growth and maturation of tissues, increases energy expenditure, and affects all enzyme actions through several mechanisms. Thyroid hormone:
• regulates cell differentiation and proliferation
• aids in myelination of nerves and development of axonal and dendritic processes in the nervous system
• enhances protein and carbohydrate metabolism by promoting metabolic processes that increase gluconeogenesis and protein synthesis and facilitate the mobilization of glycogen stores.

Contraindications

Acute MI not associated with hypothyroidism, hypersensitivity to thyroid USP or its components, obesity treatment, untreated thyrotoxicosis

Interactions

DRUGS

barbiturates, carbamazepine, phenytoin, rifampin: Possibly increased catabolism of thyroid hormone
cholestyramine, colestipol: Decreased effectiveness of thyroid hormone
corticosteroids: Decreased metabolism of corticosteroids
estrogens: Possibly increased circulating concentrations of thyroxine-binding globulin, decreased effectiveness of thyroid hormone
insulin, oral antidiabetic drugs: Possibly altered blood glucose control

ketamine: Risk of marked hypertension and tachycardia
oral anticoagulants: Altered anticoagulant effect
sympathomimetics: Increased adverse cardiovascular effects
tricyclic antidepressants: Increased therapeutic and toxic effects of both drugs

FOODS

all foods: Possibly altered absorption of thyroid hormone

Adverse Reactions

CNS: Headache, insomnia, nervousness, tremor
CV: Angina; arrhythmias, including atrial fibrillation and sinus tachycardia; palpitations
ENDO: Hyperthyroidism
GI: Diarrhea, vomiting
GU: Menstrual irregularities
SKIN: Alopecia, diaphoresis
Other: Heat intolerance, weight loss

Nursing Considerations

• Avoid giving oral thyroid hormone with food because it may alter drug absorption.
• Don't give thyroid hormone within 5 hours of cholestyramine or colestipol. Giving them together can reduce hormone absorption.
• **WARNING** Be aware that thyroid hormone therapy can unmask or worsen adrenal insufficiency, precipitate adrenal crisis in patients with uncontrolled adrenal insufficiency, and increase the risk of arrhythmias in patients with coronary artery disease.
• Monitor blood glucose level often because thyroid hormone therapy can unmask or exacerbate symptoms of other endocrine disorders and also may alter antidiabetic drug dosage requirements in patients with diabetes mellitus. Be aware that withdrawal of thyroid hormone can precipitate a hypoglycemic response in susceptible patients.

PATIENT TEACHING

• Tell patient to take thyroid hormone on an empty stomach at the same time each day.
• Advise her to inform prescriber immediately and seek medical attention if she experiences chest pain, nervousness, or sweating.
• Instruct patient who uses cholestyramine or colestipol not to take these drugs within 5 hours of thyroid dose.
• Inform patient that full effects may not be evident for 1 to 3 weeks.

•Instruct patient with diabetes mellitus to monitor blood glucose level frequently.

thyrotropin
(thyroid-stimulating hormone, TSH)

Thytropar

thyrotropin alfa

Thyrogen

Class and Category
Chemical class: Recombinant glycoprotein of human TSH
Therapeutic class: Diagnostic aid
Pregnancy category: C

Indications and Dosages

➤ *To provide diagnostic follow-up of patients with well-differentiated thyroid carcinoma*

I.M. INJECTION (THYROTROPIN ALFA)
Adults and adolescents age 16 and over. 0.9 mg every 24 hr for 2 doses or every 72 hr for 3 doses. Scanning or serum thyroglobulin testing performed 72 hr after last injection.

➤ *To provide differential diagnosis of subclinical hypothyroidism or low thyroid reserve*

I.M. OR SUBCUTANEOUS INJECTION (THYROTROPIN)
Adults and adolescents age 16 and over. 10 international units daily for 1 to 3 days, followed by radioactive iodine study 24 hr after last injection. No response indicates thyroid failure; substantial response indicates pituitary failure.

➤ *To determine thyroid status in patients receiving thyroid hormone, to differentiate between primary and secondary hypothyroidism*

I.M. OR SUBCUTANEOUS INJECTION (THYROTROPIN)
Adults and adolescents age 16 and over. 10 international units daily for 1 to 3 days.

➤ *To aid in diagnosing thyroid carcinoma remnant after surgery*

I.M. OR SUBCUTANEOUS INJECTION (THYROTROPIN)
Adults and adolescents age 16 and over. 10 international units daily for 3 to 7 days.

➤ *As adjunct for radioiodine ablation of thyroid tissue remnants in patients who have undergone a near-total or total thyroidectomy for well-differentiated thyroid cancer and who have no evidence of metastatic thyroid cancer*

I.M. INJECTION (THYROTROPIN ALPHA)
Adults. 0.9 mg, followed by a second 0.9 mg 24 hours later, followed by radioiodine administration 24 hours later.

Mechanism of Action
Stimulates production of thyroglobulin by active thyroid tissue and enhances uptake of iodine, synthesis of thyroid precursor hormones (monoiodotyrosine, diiodotyrosine, and levothyroxine), and release of triiodothyronine (T_3) and thyroxine (T_4) from the thyroid gland into systemic circulation. Thyrotropin also binds with thyroid cancer tissue and stimulates iodine uptake in radioactive iodine imaging to detect cancer cells in euthyroid patients after near-total or total thyroidectomy.

Contraindications
Coronary thrombosis, hypersensitivity to thyrotropin or its components, uncorrected adrenal insufficiency

Adverse Reactions
CNS: Asthenia, fever, headache, paresthesia
ENDO: Hyperthyroidism
GI: Nausea, vomiting
RESP: Respiratory distress
SKIN: Rash, urticaria
Other: Flulike symptoms; sudden, rapid, painful enlargement of locally recurring papillary carcinoma

Nursing Considerations
•**WARNING** Be aware that thyrotropin can unmask or worsen adrenal insufficiency, precipitate adrenal crisis in patients with uncontrolled adrenal insufficiency, and increase the risk of arrhythmias in patients with coronary artery disease.
•Reconstitute thyrotropin solution with manufacturer-provided diluent, which contains no preservatives.
•Administer I.M. injections to the buttocks.
•**WARNING** Avoid inadvertent I.V. or intradermal injection of thyrotropin. I.V. administration may result in severe reactions, including diaphoresis, hypotension, nausea, tachycardia, and vomiting. Intradermal injection may

T

damage tissue at injection site.
•Monitor patient closely, especially during first 24 hours after drug administration, because patients have died (rarely) during this time.
•Check for chest pain and increased heart rate, especially in patients with cardiac or coronary artery disease, including angina, hypertension, and recent acute MI, and in patients with residual thyroid tissue. Drug may increase serum thyroid hormone level.

PATIENT TEACHING
•Advise patient to continue taking any thyroid hormone replacement while receiving injections of thyrotropin alfa unless otherwise directed by prescriber.
•If patient is scheduled for radioactive iodine test, tell her to follow a low-iodine diet.
•Inform patient that testing may take 5 to 12 days to complete.

tiagabine hydrochloride

Gabitril

Class and Category

Chemical class: Nipecotic acid derivative
Therapeutic class: Anticonvulsant
Pregnancy category: C

Indications and Dosages

➤ *As adjunct to treat partial seizures*

TABLETS
Adults. *Initial:* 4 mg daily; increased by 4 mg/wk up to 16 mg daily, then dosage increased by 4 to 8 mg every wk until desired response occurs. *Usual:* 32 to 56 mg daily. *Maximum:* 56 mg daily in 2 to 4 divided doses.
Children ages 12 to 18. *Initial:* 4 mg daily for 1 wk, then increased by 4 to 8 mg/wk until desired response occurs. *Maximum:* 32 mg daily in 2 to 4 divided doses.
DOSAGE ADJUSTMENT For patients with impaired hepatic function, dosage individualized and reduced, or interval extended if needed, because of reduced drug clearance.

Contraindications

Hypersensitivity to tiagabine or its components

Interactions

DRUGS
benzodiazepines, CNS depressants: Possibly additive CNS depression
carbamazepine, phenobarbital, phenytoin: Possibly decreased tiagabine effectiveness

ACTIVITIES
alcohol use: Possibly additive CNS depression

Mechanism of Action

Appears to inhibit neuronal and glial uptake of gamma-aminobutyric acid (GABA), the major inhibitory neurotransmitter in the CNS. Tiagabine makes more GABA available in the CNS to open chloride channels in postsynaptic membranes, thereby leading to membrane hyperpolarization and preventing transmission of nerve impulses.

Adverse Reactions

CNS: Amnesia, anxiety, asthenia, ataxia, confusion, depression, dizziness, drowsiness, EEG abnormalities, hostility, impaired cognition, insomnia, light-headedness, paresthesia, seizures, status epilepticus, tremor, weakness
EENT: Pharyngitis, stomatitis
GI: Abdominal pain, diarrhea, increased appetite, nausea, vomiting
GU: UTI
MS: Dysarthria
SKIN: Ecchymosis, rash

Nursing Considerations

•Give tiagabine with food.
•**WARNING** Expect to taper dosage gradually, as prescribed, because stopping drug abruptly may increase seizure frequency.
•Take seizure precautions because tiagabine has caused seizures and status epilepticus in patients with no history of seizures.

PATIENT TEACHING
•Instruct patient to take tiagabine with food.
•Advise patient to avoid potentially hazardous activities until drug's CNS effects are known. Also urge her to avoid alcohol during therapy.
•Caution patient who takes CNS depressants that drug may increase depressant effect.
•Instruct patient not to stop taking tiagabine abruptly. Explain that prescriber usually tapers dosage over 4 weeks to reduce the risk of withdrawal seizures.

ticarcillin disodium

Ticar

Class and Category

Chemical class: Penicillin
Therapeutic class: Antibiotic
Pregnancy category: B

Indications and Dosages

➤ *To treat moderate to severe infections, such as bacteremia, diabetic foot ulcers, empyema, intra-abdominal infections, lower respiratory tract infections (including pneumonia), lung abscess, peritonitis, pulmonary infections due to complications of cystic fibrosis (including bronchiectasis and pneumonia), septicemia, and skin and soft-tissue infections (including cellulitis) caused by susceptible organisms*

I.V. INFUSION

Adults and children. 200 to 300 mg/kg daily in divided doses every 4 to 6 hr. *Usual:* 3 g every 4 hr or 4 g every 6 hr.

➤ *To treat uncomplicated UTI*

I.V. INFUSION, I.M. INJECTION

Adults and children weighing 40 kg (88 lb) or more. 1 g every 6 hr.

Children over age 1 month and weighing less than 40 kg. 50 to 100 mg/kg daily in divided doses every 6 to 8 hr.

➤ *To treat complicated UTI*

I.V. INFUSION

Adults and children. 150 to 200 mg/kg in equally divided doses every 4 to 6 hr. *Usual:* 3 g every 6 hr.

DOSAGE ADJUSTMENT For patients with creatinine clearance of 30 to 60 ml/min/1.73 m², 2 g I.V. every 4 hr; with creatinine clearance of 10 to 30 ml/min/1.73 m², 2 g I.V. every 8 hr; with creatinine clearance of less than 10 ml/min/1.73 m², 2 g I.V. every 12 hr or 1 g I.M. every 6 hr.

Incompatibilities

Don't administer ticarcillin through the same I.V. line as amikacin, gentamicin, or tobramycin. Don't give within 1 hr of aminoglycosides.

Contraindications

Hypersensitivity to ticarcillin, penicillins, or their components

Mechanism of Action

Inhibits bacterial cell wall synthesis by binding to specific penicillin-binding proteins inside the bacterial cell wall. Ultimately, this leads to cell wall lysis and death.

Interactions

DRUGS

aminoglycosides: Additive or synergistic activity against some bacteria, possibly mutual inactivation
anticoagulants: Possibly interference with platelet aggregation, prolonged PT
methotrexate: Prolonged blood methotrexate level, increased risk of methotrexate toxicity
probenecid: Prolonged blood ticarcillin level

Adverse Reactions

CV: Thrombophlebitis, vasculitis
GI: Elevated liver function test results, nausea, pseudomembranous colitis, vomiting
GU: Proteinuria
HEME: Anemia, eosinophilia, hemorrhage, leukopenia, neutropenia, prolonged bleeding time, thrombocytopenia
SKIN: Erythema nodosum, exfoliative dermatitis, pruritus, rash, toxic epidermal necrolysis, urticaria
Other: Anaphylaxis, hypernatremia, hypokalemia, injection site pain, superinfection

Nursing Considerations

•Obtain body fluid or tissue samples for culture and sensitivity testing, as ordered. Review test results, if possible, before giving first dose of ticarcillin.
•Don't inject more than 2 g of drug at any one I.M. injection site.
•Reconstitute each gram of ticarcillin with 4 ml of compatible diluent. Further dilute reconstituted I.V. solution to 10 to 100 mg/ml with compatible I.V. solution. To minimize vein irritation, don't exceed concentration of 100 mg/ml. Concentrations of 50 mg/ml or greater are preferred. Infuse appropriate I.V. dose over 30 to 120 minutes.
•Check for local injection site reaction, including thrombophlebitis, during therapy.
•Be aware that ticarcillin may worsen symptoms in patients with a history of GI disease or colitis.
•For patients with renal impairment, take

T

seizure precautions, according to facility policy, because of increased risk of seizures.
•Monitor patient closely for diarrhea, which may indicate pseudomembranous colitis caused by *Clostridium difficile.* If diarrhea occurs, notify prescriber and expect to withhold ticarcillin and treat with fluids, electrolytes, protein, and an antibiotic effective against *C. difficile.*
•Also look for signs of superinfection, such as oral candidiasis and rash in breastfeeding infant.
•Monitor serum electrolyte levels for hypernatremia due to drug's high sodium content and for hypokalemia due to increased urinary potassium loss.
•**WARNING** Monitor patient's platelet count, PT, and APTT because ticarcillin may increase bleeding time and, in rare cases, may induce thrombocytopenia.
PATIENT TEACHING
•Stress need to take full course of ticarcillin exactly as prescribed, even if feeling better.
•Urge patient to report past allergies to penicillins and to notify prescriber immediately about adverse reactions, including fever.
•Advise patient to decrease sodium intake to reduce the risk of electrolyte imbalance.
•Instruct patient to report diarrhea that's severe or prolonged. Remind patient that watery or bloody stools can occur 2 or more months after antibiotic therapy and can be serious, requiring prompt treatment.

ticlopidine hydrochloride

Ticlid

Class and Category
Chemical class: Thienopyridine derivative
Therapeutic class: Antithrombotic, platelet aggregation inhibitor
Pregnancy category: B

Indications and Dosages
➤ *To reduce the risk of initial thrombotic stroke in patients who have experienced transient ischemic attack, to reduce the risk of recurrent stroke in patients who have previously experienced thrombotic stroke*
TABLETS
Adults. 250 mg b.i.d.

➤ *As adjunct to reduce the risk of subacute stent thrombosis after successful coronary stent implantation*
TABLETS
Adults. 250 mg b.i.d with antiplatelet doses of aspirin for up to 30 days after successful stent implantation.

Route	Onset	Peak	Duration
P.O.	2 to 4 days	8 to 11 days	1 to 2 wk

Contraindications
Coagulopathy, GI bleeding, hematologic disorders related to hematopoiesis (including history of thrombotic thrombocytopenic purpura, neutropenia, and thrombocytopenia), hemophilia, hypersensitivity to ticlopidine or its components, intracranial bleeding, retinal bleeding, severe hepatic disease

Interactions
DRUGS
aluminum- and magnesium-containing antacids: Possibly decreased peak blood ticlopidine level
antineoplastics, antithymocyte globulin, heparin, NSAIDs, oral anticoagulants, platelet aggregation inhibitors, salicylates, strontium-89 chloride, thrombolytics: Increased risk of bleeding
cimetidine: Reduced clearance of ticlopidine, increased risk of adverse reactions
cyclosporine, digoxin: Decreased blood level and possibly reduced effects of these drugs
porfimer: Decreased effectiveness of porfimer photodynamic therapy
xanthines (aminophylline, oxytriphylline, theophylline): Decreased theophylline clearance, increased risk of toxicity

Adverse Reactions
CNS: Dizziness
CV: Hypercholesterolemia, vasculitis
EENT: Tinnitus
GI: Abdominal pain, anorexia, diarrhea, elevated liver function test results, flatulence, indigestion, nausea, vomiting
HEME: Agranulocytosis, aplastic anemia, hemolysis, hemolytic anemia, neutropenia, pancytopenia, thrombocytopenia, thrombotic thrombocytopenia, thrombotic thrombocytopenic purpura
SKIN: Pruritus, purpura, rash
Other: Hyponatremia, serum sicknesslike reaction

Mechanism of Action

Normally, platelets don't adhere to blood vessel walls. However, when a thrombotic stroke or other disorder damages blood vessel walls, platelets are activated and adhere within seconds. Once activated, platelets release adenosine diphosphate (ADP). This causes fibrinogen to bind to glycoprotein IIb/IIIa (GP IIb/IIIa) receptors on the surface of activated platelets and connect with other activated platelets. Then a thrombus forms.

Ticlopidine inhibits the release of ADP from activated platelets, which prevents fibrinogen from binding to GP IIb/IIIa receptors on the surface of activated platelets, as shown below. This action prevents platelets from aggregating to form a thrombus, which prevents thrombosis of an implanted stent or recurrence of stroke.

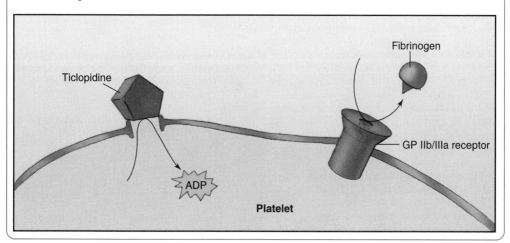

Nursing Considerations

• Give ticlopidine with food to maximize GI absorption and minimize any GI distress.
• Avoid I.M. injections of other drugs because excessive bleeding, bruising, or hematoma may occur.
• During first 3 months of therapy, monitor CBC every 2 weeks, as ordered (more frequently in patients with depressed neutrophil count).
• Be aware that ticlopidine therapy typically is used for patients with stroke or an increased risk of stroke who can't tolerate aspirin because of the risk of neutropenia or agranulocytosis.
• **WARNING** Be aware that ticlopidine therapy irreversibly affects platelet aggregation. Expect prescriber to discontinue drug 10 to 14 days before surgical procedures to prevent uncontrolled bleeding.
• Monitor serum cholesterol level during first month of ticlopidine therapy for expected increase. Hypercholesterolemia may persist for duration of treatment.

PATIENT TEACHING

• Urge patient to take ticlopidine with food.
• Inform patient that she may be at increased risk for infection because drug may decrease WBC or platelet count, especially in first 3 months of therapy.
• Advise patient to notify prescriber immediately if she has chills, fever, or sore throat.
• Urge patient to keep scheduled appointments for blood tests to detect abnormalities.
• Instruct patient to apply prolonged pressure to injured areas because bleeding may take longer than usual to stop. Urge her to immediately report to prescriber any unusual bleeding or bruising.

tigecycline

Tygacil

Class and Category

Chemical class: Glycylcycline

T

Therapeutic class: Antibiotic
Pregnancy category: D

Indications and Dosages

➤ *To treat complicated skin and skin structure infections caused by* Escherichia coli, Enterococcus faecalis *(vancomycin-susceptible isolates only),* Staphylococcus aureus *(methicillin-susceptible and -resistant isolates),* Streptococcus agalactiae, Streptococcus anginosus *group (includes* S. anginosus, S. intermedius, *and* S. constellatus*),* Streptococcus pyogenes, *and* Bacteroides fragilis; *to treat complicated intra-abdominal infections caused by* Citrobacter freundii, Enterobacter cloacae, Escherichia coli, Klebsiella oxytoca, Klebsiella pneumoniae, Enterococcus faecalis *(vancomycin-suseptible isolates only),* Staphylococcus aureus *(methicillin-susceptible isolates only),* Streptococcus anginosus *group (includes* S. anginosus, S. intermedius, *and* S. constellatus*),* Bacteroides fragilis, Bacteroides thetaiotaomicron, Bacteroides uniformis, Bacteroides vulgatus, Clostridium perfringens, *and* Peptostreptococcus micros; *to treat community-acquired bacterial pneumonia caused by* Streptococcus pneumoniae *(penicillin-susceptible isolates), including cases with concurrent bacteremia,* Haemophilus influenzae *(beta-lactamase negative isolates), and* Legionella pneumophila

I.V. INFUSION

Adults. *Initial:* 100 mg infused over 30 to 60 min followed by 50 mg infused over 30 to 60 min every 12 hr for 5 to 14 days for complicated skin and skin structure infections and intra-abdominal infections (7 to 14 days for community-acquired bacterial pneumonia).

DOSAGE ADJUSTMENT For patients with severe hepatic impairment, initial dosage of 100 mg should be followed by a reduced maintenance dosage of 25 mg every 12 hr.

Incompatibilities

Don't give amphotericin B, chlorpromazine, methylprednisolone, or voriconazole simultaneously through the same Y-site.

Mechanism of Action

Inhibits protein translation in bacteria by binding to the 30S ribosomal subunit, which prevents binding of amino-acyl tRNA molecules to the ribosome complex, thus interfering with protein synthesis. Through this bacteriostatic action, bacteria are weakened.

Contraindications

Hypersensitivity to tigecycline or its components

Adverse Reactions

CNS: Asthenia, chills, dizziness, fever, headache, insomnia, somnolence
CV: Bradycardia, hypertension, hypotension, peripheral edema, phlebitis, septic shock, tachycardia, thrombophlebitis, vasodilation
EENT: Dry mouth, taste perversion
ENDO: Hyperglycemia, hypoglycemia
GI: Abdominal pain, acute pancreatitis, anorexia, constipation, diarrhea, dyspepsia, elevated liver enzyme levels, jaundice, nausea, pancreatitis, pseudomembranous colitis, vomiting
GU: Elevated BUN and creatinine levels, vaginal candidiasis
HEME: Anemia, leukocytosis, thrombocythemia
MS: Back pain
RESP: Increased cough, dyspnea
SKIN: Diaphoresis, photosensitivity, pruritus, rash
Other: Hypersensitivity reaction, hypocalcemia; hypokalemia; hyponatremia; hypoproteinemia; injection site reaction, such as edema, phlebitis, inflammation, and pain

Nursing Considerations

•Obtain body tissue and fluid samples for culture and sensitivity tests as ordered before giving first dose of tigecycline. Expect to begin drug therapy before test results are known.

•Avoid giving tigecycline to children under age 8 because drug may cause permanent brown or yellow tooth discoloration and enamel hypoplasia.

•Use tigecycline cautiously in patients hypersensitive to tetracycline antibiotics because glycylcycline antibiotics are structurally similar to tetracyclines.

•Also use cautiously in patients with complicated intra-abdominal infections secondary to intestinal perforation because of the risk of septic shock.
•Determine whether female patients could be pregnant before starting tigecycline therapy because the drug may cause harm to fetus.
•Reconstitute each vial of tigecycline with 5.3 ml of 0.9% sodium chloride injection or 5% dextrose injection to achieve a concentration of 10 mg/ml. Note that the color will be yellow to orange. If not, the solution should be discarded. Immediately withdraw reconstituted solution from the vial and add to a 100-ml I.V. bag for infusion. Drug may be stored in the I.V. bag at room temperature for up to 6 hours or refrigerated up to 24 hours before use.
•If I.V. line is used to infuse other drugs, flush the line with either 0.9% sodium chloride injection or 5% dextrose injection before and after tigecycline infusion.
•Infuse tigecycline over 30 to 60 minutes.
•Monitor patient closely for diarrhea, which may indicate pseudomembranous colitis, which is known to occur with many antibiotics. If diarrhea occurs during therapy, notify prescriber and expect to withhold drug. Expect to treat psuedomembranous colitis, if confirmed, with fluids, electrolytes, protein, and an antibiotic effective against *Clostridium difficile*.
•Monitor patient for adverse reactions, keeping in mind the similarity between tigecycline and tetracycline.
•Assess patient for superinfection, such as vaginal candidiasis, that may result from overgrowth of nonsusceptible organisms, including fungi. If signs of infection are present, notify prescriber and provide supportive care, as prescribed.

PATIENT TEACHING
•Instruct patient to report adverse reactions, especially hypersensitivity reactions, such as a rash or itching, as well as diarrhea.
•Tell patient to report discomfort at the infusion site because the site may need to be changed.
•Urge patient to report diarrhea that's severe or prolonged. Remind patient that watery or bloody stools can occur 2 or more months after antibiotic therapy and can be serious, requiring prompt treatment.

tiludronate disodium
(contains 200 mg of tiludronic acid per tablet)
Skelid

Class and Category
Chemical class: Aminobiphosphonate
Therapeutic class: Bone resorption inhibitor
Pregnancy category: C

Indications and Dosages
➤ *To treat Paget's disease in patients with serum alkaline phosphatase levels at least twice the upper limit of normal, who are symptomatic or at risk for future complications of the disease*
TABLETS
Adults. *Initial:* 400 mg of tiludronic acid daily 2 hr a.c. or p.c. for 3 mo. *Maximum:* 400 mg of tiludronic acid daily.

Mechanism of Action
Reduces the activity of cells that cause bone loss and increases bone mass. Tiludronate may act by inhibiting osteoclast activity on newly formed bone resorption surfaces. This activity reduces the number of sites at which bone is remodeled. When bone formation exceeds bone resorption at these remodeling sites, bone mass increases. Tiludronate may also inhibit bone destruction by binding to hydroxyapatite crystals, which give bone its rigidity.

Contraindications
Creatinine clearance less than 30 ml/min/1.73 m², esophageal abnormalities that delay esophageal emptying, hypersensitivity to tiludronate or its components

Interactions
DRUGS
aluminum- or magnesium-containing antacids, mineral supplements (such as calcium, iron), salicylates, salicylate-containing compounds: Decreased absorption of tiludronate
indomethacin: Possibly increased bioavailability of tiludronate
FOODS
all foods and beverages (except plain water): Decreased absorption of tiludronate

Adverse Reactions
CNS: Dizziness, headache

CV: Chest pain, edema
EENT: Cataracts, conjunctivitis, glaucoma, pharyngitis, rhinitis
GI: Diarrhea, esophageal irritation and ulceration, flatulence, indigestion, nausea, vomiting
MS: Arthralgia, back pain, myalgia, osteonecrosis of jaw
RESP: Cough, upper respiratory tract infection
SKIN: Rash
Other: Flulike symptoms

Nursing Considerations
•Be prepared to monitor serum calcium levels before, during, and after tiludronate therapy because drug may exacerbate such conditions as hyperparathyroidism, hypocalcemia, and vitamin D deficiency. Ensure adequate dietary intake of calcium and vitamin D during and after treatment. If hypocalcemia occurs, expect to administer a calcium supplement, as prescribed.
•WARNING Be aware that tiludronate may irritate upper GI mucosa, causing such adverse reactions as esophageal ulcer. To help minimize these reactions, have patient take drug with full glass of plain water and remain upright for at least 30 minutes.

PATIENT TEACHING
•Instruct patient to take drug with 6 to 8 oz of plain water on an empty stomach (at least 2 hours before or after beverages, food, other drugs, or mineral supplements, including mineral water) because food and beverages may severely reduce drug's effect. Also, advise her to remain upright for at least 30 minutes after taking drug.
•Advise patient not to chew or suck on tablet to reduce the risk of esophageal irritation.
•Instruct patient to notify prescriber immediately if she develops signs or symptoms of esophageal irritation, such as trouble swallowing or worsening heartburn; these may indicate a serious esophageal disorder.
•Caution patient not to take salicylate-containing drugs, such as aspirin, during tiludronate therapy.

timolol maleate

Apo-Timol (CAN), Blocadren, Novo-Timol (CAN)

Class and Category
Chemical class: Beta blocker
Therapeutic class: Antihypertensive, MI prophylactic, vascular headache prophylactic
Pregnancy category: C

Indications and Dosages
➤ *To manage hypertension*
TABLETS
Adults. *Initial:* 10 mg b.i.d., increased every wk as prescribed. *Maintenance:* 20 to 40 mg daily in divided doses. *Maximum:* 60 mg daily.
➤ *To provide long-term prophylaxis after MI*
TABLETS
Adults. 10 mg b.i.d., beginning 1 to 4 wk after MI and continuing for at least 2 yr.
➤ *To prevent migraine headache*
TABLETS
Adults. *Initial:* 10 mg b.i.d. *Maintenance:* 20 mg daily in divided doses. *Maximum:* 30 mg daily; discontinued after 8 wk, as prescribed, if maximum dose is ineffective.

Route	Onset	Peak	Duration
P.O.	30 min	1 to 2 hr	4 to 8 hr

Mechanism of Action
Selectively blocks alpha$_1$ and beta$_2$ receptors in vascular smooth muscle and beta$_1$ receptors in the heart. This reduces peripheral vascular resistance and blood pressure and relieves migraine headaches. Timolol's potent beta blockade prevents the reflex tachycardia that typically occurs with most alpha blockers, and decreases cardiac excitability, cardiac output, and myocardial oxygen demand, thus preventing MI.

Contraindications
Acute bronchospasm; asthma; cardiogenic shock; children; COPD (severe); heart failure; hypersensitivity to timolol, other beta blockers, or their components; second- or third-degree AV block; severe sinus bradycardia

Interactions
DRUGS
allergen immunotherapy, allergenic extracts for skin testing: Increased risk of serious systemic adverse reactions or anaphylaxis
amiodarone: Additive depressant effect on cardiac conduction, negative inotropic effect

anesthetics (hydrocarbon inhalation): Increased risk of myocardial depression and hypotension
beta blockers: Additive beta blockade effects
calcium channel blockers, clonidine, diazoxide, guanabenz, reserpine, other hypotension-producing drugs: Additive hypotensive effect and, possibly, other beta blockade effects
cimetidine: Possibly interference with timolol clearance
estrogens: Decreased antihypertensive effect of timolol
fentanyl, fentanyl derivatives: Possibly increased risk of initial bradycardia after induction doses of fentanyl or derivative (with long-term timolol use)
glucagon: Possibly blunted hyperglycemic response
insulin, oral antidiabetic drugs: Possibly masking of tachycardia in response to hypoglycemia, impaired glucose control
lidocaine: Decreased lidocaine clearance, increased risk of lidocaine toxicity
MAO inhibitors: Increased risk of significant hypertension
neuromuscular blockers: Possibly potentiated and prolonged action of these drugs
NSAIDs: Possibly decreased hypotensive effect
phenothiazines: Increased blood levels of both drugs
phenytoin (parenteral): Additive cardiac depressant effect
sympathomimetics, xanthines: Possibly mutual inhibition of therapeutic effects

Adverse Reactions

CNS: Asthenia, decreased concentration, depression, dizziness, fatigue, fever, hallucinations, headache, insomnia, nervousness, nightmares, paresthesia, stroke, syncope, vertigo
CV: Angina, arrhythmias, bradycardia, cardiac arrest, chest pain, edema, palpitations, Raynaud's phenomenon, vasodilation
EENT: Diplopia, dry eyes, eye irritation, ptosis, tinnitus, vision changes
ENDO: Hyperglycemia, hypoglycemia
GI: Abdominal pain, diarrhea, hepatomegaly, indigestion, nausea, vomiting
GU: Decreased libido, impotence
MS: Arthralgia, decreased tolerance to exercise, extremity pain, muscle weakness
RESP: Bronchospasm, cough, crackles, dyspnea
SKIN: Alopecia, diaphoresis, hyperpigmenta-

tion, pruritus, purpura, rash
Other: Anaphylaxis, weight loss

Nursing Considerations

• **WARNING** Be aware that timolol may mask evidence of acute hypoglycemia in diabetic patient. It also may mask certain signs of hyperthyroidism, such as tachycardia.
• Be aware that timolol may prolong hypoglycemia by interfering with glycogenolysis or may promote hyperglycemia by decreasing tissue sensitivity to insulin.
• Monitor blood pressure and cardiac output, as appropriate, for patient with a history of systolic heart failure or left ventricular dysfunction because timolol's negative inotropic effect can depress cardiac output.
• **WARNING** Timolol shouldn't be discontinued abruptly because this may produce MI, myocardial ischemia, severe hypertension, or ventricular arrhythmias, particularly in patient with known cardiovascular disease.
• Expect varied drug effectiveness in elderly patients; they may be less sensitive to drug's antihypertensive effect or more sensitive because of reduced drug clearance.
• Monitor for impaired circulation in elderly patients with age-related peripheral vascular disease or patients with Raynaud's phenomenon. Such patients may experience exacerbated symptoms from increased alpha stimulation. Elderly patients also are at increased risk for beta blocker–induced hypothermia.
• If timolol worsens skin condition, such as psoriasis, notify prescriber.

PATIENT TEACHING
• Instruct patient taking timolol to inform prescriber of chest pain, fainting, light-headedness, or shortness of breath, which may indicate the need for dosage change.
• Caution patient not to stop taking drug abruptly. Timolol dosage must be tapered gradually under prescriber's supervision.
• Instruct patient with diabetes to monitor blood glucose level often during therapy.
• Warn patient with psoriasis about possible flare-ups of skin condition.

tinidazole

Tindamax

Class and Category

Chemical class: Synthetic nitroimidazole
Therapeutic class: Antiprotozoal

Pregnancy category: C

Indications and Dosages

➤ *To treat trichomoniasis caused by* Trichomonas vaginalis

TABLETS

Adults. 2 g one time with food.

➤ *To treat giardiasis caused by* Giardia duodenalis (G. lamblia)

TABLETS

Adults. 2 g one time with food.

Children age 4 and over. 50 mg/kg (up to 2 g) one time with food.

➤ *To treat intestinal amebiasis caused by* Entamoeba histolytica

TABLETS

Adults. 2 g daily for 3 days with food.

Children age 4 and over. 50 mg/kg (up to 2 g) daily for 3 days with food.

➤ *To treat amebic liver abscess caused by* Entamoeba histolytica

TABLETS

Adults. 2 g daily for 3 to 5 days with food.

Children age 4 and over. 50 mg/kg (up to 2 g) daily for 3 to 5 days with food.

DOSAGE ADJUSTMENT For patients receiving hemodialysis, an additional dose equivalent to one-half the dose prescribed should be given after the dialysis treatment on the days dialysis is performed.

Mechanism of Action

Undergoes intracellular chemical reduction during anaerobic metabolism. After tinidazole is reduced, it damages DNA's helical structure and breaks its strands, which inhibits bacterial nucleic acid synthesis and causes cell death.

Contraindications

Breastfeeding, hypersensitivity to tinidazole or its components, treatment of trichomoniasis during first trimester of pregnancy

Interactions

DRUGS

cholestyramine: Possibly decreased bioavailability of tinidazole

cimetidine, ketoconazole: Possibly delayed elimination and increased blood level of tinidazole

cyclosporine, tacrolimus: Possibly increased serum cyclosporine and tacrolimus levels

disulfiram: Possibly combined toxicity, resulting in confusion and psychosis

fluorouracil: Possibly decreased fluorouracil clearance

lithium: Possibly increased serum lithium levels

oral anticoagulants: Possibly increased anticoagulant effect

oxytetracycline: Possibly diminished effect of tinidazole

phenobarbital, phenytoin, rifampin: Possibly increased metabolism and decreased blood level of tinidazole

ACTIVITIES

alcohol use: Possibly disulfiram-like effects

Adverse Reactions

CNS: Ataxia, dizziness, coma, confusion, depression, drowsiness, fatigue, fever, headache, insomnia, malaise, peripheral neuropathy, seizures, vertigo, weakness

CV: Palpitations

EENT: Dry mouth, excessive salivation, furry tongue, metallic or bitter taste, oral candidiasis, pharyngitis, stomatitis, tongue discoloration

GI: Abdominal cramps, anorexia, constipation, diarrhea, epigastric discomfort, flatulence, hepatic abnormalities, indigestion, nausea, thirst, vomiting

GU: Darkened urine, dysuria, increased vaginal discharge, menorrhagia, UTI, vaginal candidiasis or odor, vulvo-vaginal discomfort

HEME: Reversible thrombocytopenia, transient leukopenia or neutropenia

MS: Arthralgia, arthritis, myalgia, pelvic pain

RESP: Bronchospasm, dyspnea, upper respiratory tract infection

SKIN: Diaphoresis, erythema multiforme, flushing, pruritus, rash, Stevens-Johnson syndrome, urticaria

Other: Angioedema

Nursing Considerations

• Use tinidazole cautiously in patients with CNS disease or blood dyscrasias because tinidazole's adverse effects may worsen these disorders. Also use cautiously in patients with hepatic impairment because a chemically related drug has reduced elimination.

• Take seizure precautions. If a seizure or other abnormal neurological symptoms occur, notify prescriber and expect to stop drug.

•Treat a patient diagnosed with trichomoniasis and her sexual partner with the same dose of tinidazole and at the same time, as ordered, because trichomoniasis is a sexually transmitted disease.

•Monitor patient's total WBC count and differential if retreatment with tinidazole is needed because adverse hematological reactions may occur with repeated tinidazole use.

PATIENT TEACHING

•Tell patient to take tinidazole with food to minimize gastric discomfort.

•Instruct patient unable to swallow tablets to crush tinidazole and mix in artificial cherry syrup and then take with food.

•Advise patient to avoid alcohol while taking tinidazole and for 3 days afterward because alcohol can cause intense flushing.

•Tell patient to alert prescriber before taking tinidazole if she thinks or knows she is pregnant because tinidazole crosses the placental barrier during the first trimester and its effects on the fetus are unknown.

•Instruct breastfeeding patient not to breastfeed during therapy and for 3 days after taking last dose.

tinzaparin sodium

Innohep

Class and Category

Chemical class: Low–molecular-weight heparin
Therapeutic class: Anticoagulant, antithrombotic
Pregnancy category: B

Indications and Dosages

➤ *As adjunct to treat pulmonary thromboembolism and acute symptomatic deep vein thrombosis*

SUBCUTANEOUS INJECTION

Adults. 175 anti-Xa international units/kg daily for at least 6 days. *Maximum:* 18,000 to 21,000 anti-Xa international units daily.

Route	Onset	Peak	Duration
SubQ	2 to 3 hr	4 to 6 hr	24 hr

Contraindications

Active major bleeding; heparin-induced thrombocytopenia (current or past); hypersensitivity to tinzaparin or its components, other low–molecular-weight heparins, sulfites, benzyl alcohol, or pork products

Interactions

DRUGS

alteplase, anistreplase, aspirin, dextran, dipyridamole, NSAIDs, oral anticoagulants, streptokinase, sulfinpyrazone, urokinase: Possibly increased risk of bleeding

Mechanism of Action

Potentiates the action of antithrombin III, a coagulation inhibitor. By binding with antithrombin III, tinzaparin rapidly binds with and inactivates clotting factors (primarily fibrin and factor Xa). Without thrombin, fibrinogen can't convert to fibrin and clots can't form.

Adverse Reactions

CNS: Confusion, dizziness, headache, insomnia, intracranial hemorrhage, paralysis
CV: Angina, hypertension, hypotension, tachycardia
EENT: Epistaxis, gingival bleeding, pharyngeal bleeding
GI: Constipation, elevated liver function test results, GI and retroperitoneal bleeding, hematemesis, nausea, vomiting
GU: Hematuria, genitourinary bleeding, prolonged or heavy menstrual bleeding, UTI
HEME: Anemia, thrombocytopenia, unusual bruising
MS: Back pain
RESP: Dyspnea, hemoptysis, pulmonary embolism
SKIN: Bleeding at puncture sites, surgical incision sites, or venous cutdown sites; rash
Other: Injection site hematoma, including itching, pain, redness, and swelling

Nursing Considerations

•Expect warfarin therapy to begin within 1 to 3 days of tinzaparin use.

•Monitor patient's international normalized ratio (INR). Expect therapy to continue until INR reaches 2.0 for 2 consecutive days.

•WARNING Monitor patient for signs and symptoms of GI bleeding, including bloody or black, tarry stools; bloody or coffee-ground vomitus; and severe stomach pain. Notify prescriber immediately if patient develops any of these signs or symptoms.

T

•Assess tinzaparin injection site for signs and symptoms of hematoma, including deep, dark purple bruises under skin and itching, pain, redness, or swelling.
•Assess patient for evidence of intracranial bleeding (such as decreased level of consciousness), retroperitoneal bleeding (such as abdominal pain or swelling and back pain), genitourinary bleeding (such as hematuria), or respiratory tract bleeding (such as hemoptysis). Notify prescriber immediately about any of these signs or symptoms.
•If serious bleeding (not controllable by local pressure) occurs, expect to discontinue any concomitant warfarin or antiplatelet drugs immediately.
•Expect to treat bleeding by administering 1 mg of protamine sulfate 1% solution I.V. per 100 anti-Xa international units of tinzaparin, as prescribed.
•If possible, avoid giving patient I.M. injections while she's receiving tinzaparin. If arterial puncture becomes necessary during tinzaparin therapy, expect to apply pressure after procedure and to monitor puncture site frequently for signs of bleeding.
•Monitor patient's laboratory tests for elevated liver enzyme levels. If significant elevations persist or worsen, notify prescriber immediately.

PATIENT TEACHING
•Advise patient who is receiving tinzaparin to immediately report any bleeding, including from nose or gums.
•Instruct patient to limit physical activity during tinzaparin administration to reduce the risk of injury or bleeding.
•Urge female patient to notify prescriber if she is or could be pregnant.

tiopronin

Thiola

Class and Category
Chemical class: Thiol compound
Therapeutic class: Antiurolithic
Pregnancy category: C

Indications and Dosages
➤ *To prevent the formation of urinary cystine calculi*
TABLETS
Adults. 800 mg daily in 3 divided doses.

Children over age 9. 15 mg/kg in 3 divided doses.
DOSAGE ADJUSTMENT For patients with a history of hypersensitivity to penicillamine, therapy initiated at a reduced dosage; later dosage adjusted as prescribed, according to urine cystine level.

Route	Onset	Peak	Duration
P.O.	Rapid	Unknown	8 to 10 hr

Mechanism of Action
Inhibits the formation of urinary cystine calculi by undergoing thiol-disulfide exchange with cystine (cystine-cystine disulfide) to form a water-soluble compound, tiopronin-cystine disulfide.

Contraindications
History of agranulocytosis, aplastic anemia, or thrombocytopenia; hypersensitivity to tiopronin or its components

Interactions
DRUGS
bone marrow depressants: Increased risk of adverse hematologic effects
hepatotoxic drugs: Increased risk of hepatotoxic effects
nephrotoxic drugs: Increased risk of nephrotoxic effects

Adverse Reactions
CNS: Chills, fever
CV: Peripheral edema
EENT: Laryngeal edema, stomatitis
GU: Hematuria, proteinuria
HEME: Anemia, eosinophilia, leukopenia, thrombocytopenia
MS: Arthralgia
SKIN: Ecchymosis, jaundice, pruritus, rash, urticaria

Nursing Considerations
•Watch for drug fever, which may occur during first month of tiopronin therapy.
•Be aware that drug may be stopped temporarily, then restarted at lower dose.
•Expect to monitor urine cystine level so dosage can be adjusted to keep cystine level below 250 g/ml.

PATIENT TEACHING
•Instruct patient to take tiopronin on an

empty stomach, 1 hour before or 2 hours after meals, for faster drug absorption.
• Advise patient to drink at least 3 L of fluid daily to maintain a urine output of at least 2 L daily during therapy.
• Encourage the patient to maintain a diet low in methionine, which is an essential amino acid that is found in eggs, cheese, fish, and milk.

tiotropium bromide

Spiriva HandiHaler

Class and Category

Chemical class: Nonane bromide monohydrate
Therapeutic class: Anticholingeric, bronchodilator
Pregnancy category: C

Indications and Dosages

➤ *To prevent bronchospasm associated with COPD, including chronic bronchitis and emphysema*

AEROSOL CAPSULES

Adults. 18 mcg (1 capsule) inhaled daily using HandiHaler inhalation device

Mechanism of Action

Prevents acetylcholine from attaching to muscarinic receptors on membranes of smooth-muscle cells. By blocking acetylcholine's effects in the bronchi and bronchioles, tiotropium relaxes smooth muscles and causes bronchodilation.

Contraindications

Hypersensitivity to atropine or its derivatives, including ipratropium, tiotropium, or their components

Interactions

DRUGS

anticholinergics: Possibly increased anticholinergic effects

Adverse Reactions

CNS: Depression, difficulty speaking, dizziness, paresthesia, stroke
CV: Angina, atrial fibrillation, chest pain, hypercholesterolemia, palpitations, peripheral edema, supraventricular tachycardia, tachycardia
EENT: Applicaiton site irritation (glossitis, mouth ulceration, pharyngolaryngeal pain), blurred vision, cataract, dry mouth, epistaxis, eye pain, glaucoma, hoarseness, laryngitis, oral candidiasis, pharyngitis, rhinitis, sinusitis, stomatitis, throat irritation, visual halos
ENDO: Hyperglycemia
GI: Abdominal pain, constipation, dysphagia, gastroesophageal reflux, indigestion, intestinal obstruction, ileus, vomiting
GU: Urinary difficulty, urine retention, UTI
MS: Arthritis, leg or skeletal pain, myalgia
RESP: Cough, paradoxical bronchospasm, upper respiratory tract infection
SKIN: Pruritus, rash, urticaria
Other: Allergic reaction, angioedema, flulike symptoms, infection, moniliasis

Nursing Considerations

• Use tiotropium cautiously in patients with angle-closure glaucoma, benign prostatic hyperplasia, or bladder neck obstruction.
• Monitor patient closely after giving first dose of tiotropium for immediate hypersensitivity reactions, including angioedema and paradoxical bronchospasm. If any reactions occur, notify prescriber and expect to stop tiotropium.
• Monitor patient's renal function, as ordered, especially in patients with moderate to severe renal impairment, because tiotropium is excreted mainly by the kidneys.
• Monitor patient's pulmonary function, as ordered, to evaluate the effectiveness of tiotropium.

PATIENT TEACHING

• Caution patient not to use tiotropium to treat acute bronchospasm.
• Instruct the patient on the proper use of the HandiHaler inhalation device. Tell patient to place the capsule into the center chamber of the inhalation device and then to press and release the button on the side of the inhalation device to pierce the capsule. Then have the patient exhale completely, close her lips around the mouthpiece, inhale slowly and deeply, and hold her breath for as long as is comfortable.
• Alert patient that the HandiHaler device should not be used for taking any other drug and that tiotropium must be taken only using the device and never swallowed.

T

•Tell patient not to expose capsules to air until ready for use. To remove a capsule from the blister pack, tell patient to open the foil only as far as the stop line to avoid exposing the rest of the capsules in the blister pack to air. Instruct patient to discard capsules if they are inadvertently exposed to air and won't be used immediately.

•Advise patient to keep powder out of her eyes because it may irritate them or blur her vision.

•Instruct patient to rinse her mouth after each treatment to help minimize throat dryness and irritation.

•Advise patient to tell prescriber about decreased response to tiotropium as well as difficulty urinating, eye pain, palpitations, and vision changes.

tirofiban hydrochloride

Aggrastat

Class and Category
Chemical class: Tyrosine derivative
Therapeutic class: Platelet aggregation inhibitor
Pregnancy category: B

Indications and Dosages
➤ *To treat acute coronary syndrome*
I.V. INFUSION
Adults. 0.4 mcg/kg/min for 30 min, followed by 0.1 mcg/kg/min.
DOSAGE ADJUSTMENT For patients with creatinine clearance of less than 30 ml/min/1.73 m², infusion rate reduced by one-half.

Route	Onset	Peak	Duration
I.V.	Immediate	30 min	4 to 8 hr

Mechanism of Action
Binds to glycoprotein IIb/IIIa receptor sites on the surface of activated platelets. Circulating fibrinogen can bind to these receptor sites and link platelets together, forming a clot that eventually blocks a coronary artery. By binding to receptor sites, tirofiban prevents the normal binding of fibrinogen and other factors and inhibits platelet aggregation.

Incompatibilities
Don't infuse tirofiban in same I.V. line with any drug other than atropine sulfate, dobutamine, dopamine, epinephrine hydrochloride, furosemide, heparin, lidocaine, midazolam hydrochloride, morphine sulfate, nitroglycerin, potassium chloride, propranolol hydrochloride, or famotidine (Pepcid injection).

Contraindications
Acute pericarditis; arteriovenous malformation; coagulopathy; stroke that occurred within previous 30 days or a history of hemorrhagic stroke; GI or GU bleeding; hemophilia; history of thrombocytopenia after tirofiban use; hypersensitivity to tirofiban or its components; intracranial aneurysm or mass, intracranial bleeding, retinal bleeding, aortic dissection, or any evidence of active abnormal bleeding within previous 30 days; major surgery or trauma within previous 6 weeks; severe uncontrolled hypertension (systolic blood pressure above 180 mm Hg, diastolic blood pressure above 110 mm Hg)

Interactions
DRUGS
antineoplastics, antithymocyte globulin, NSAIDs, oral anticoagulants, platelet aggregation inhibitors, strontium-89 chloride, thrombolytics: Increased risk of bleeding
levothyroxine, omeprazole: Increased rate of tirofiban clearance
porfimer: Decreased effectiveness of porfimer photodynamic therapy
salicylates: Increased risk of bleeding, possibly hypoprothrombinemia

Adverse Reactions
CNS: Chills, dizziness, fever, headache, intracranial hemorrhage
CV: Edema, hemopericardium, peripheral edema, sinus bradycardia
GI: Hematemesis, nausea, retroperitoneal bleeding, vomiting
GU: Hematuria, pelvic pain
HEME: Severe thrombocytopenia with chills, fever, and possibly fatal bleeding complications
RESP: Pulmonary hemorrhage
SKIN: Diaphoresis, rash, urticaria
Other: Allergic reaction, anaphylaxis, infusion site bleeding

Nursing Considerations
•**WARNING** Dilute 50-ml vial of tirofiban before use; don't dilute 500-ml container because it holds premixed solution ready for

I.V. infusion. Don't use solution unless it's clear and the seal is intact.

• If prescribed, give tirofiban with heparin for 48 to 108 hours. Expect to continue infusion throughout angiography and for 12 to 24 hours after angioplasty or atherectomy.

• **WARNING** If patient is also receiving a heparin infusion, expect to monitor APTT before treatment, 6 hours after heparin infusion starts, and regularly thereafter. Expect to adjust heparin dosage to maintain APTT at about two times the control. Notify prescriber immediately if patient develops an abnormally high APTT. Also, assess patient for signs and symptoms of abnormal bleeding and report them to prescriber immediately because potentially life-threatening bleeding may occur.

• After cardiac catheterization or percutaneous transluminal coronary angioplasty, keep patient on bed rest with head of bed elevated. Ensure hemostasis of percutaneous site for at least 4 hours before discharge. Minimize invasive procedures, including epidural procedures, to reduce the risk of bleeding.

• Monitor patient's platelet count, hemoglobin level, and hematocrit, as ordered. Expect to discontinue tirofiban if platelet count is less than 90,000/mm³. Expect to give a platelet transfusion, as prescribed, if platelet count falls below 50,000/mm³.

PATIENT TEACHING

• Advise patient to immediately report any bleeding, bruising, headache, pain, or swelling during I.V. infusion of tirofiban.

tizanidine hydrochloride

Zanaflex

Class and Category

Chemical class: Imidazoline
Therapeutic class: Antispasmodic
Pregnancy category: C

Indications and Dosages

➤ *To manage acute and intermittent increases of muscle tone with spasticity*

TABLETS

Adults. 4 mg every 6 to 8 hr, p.r.n., increased gradually by 2 to 4 mg/dose, as needed and as prescribed. *Maximum:* 36 mg daily or 3 doses daily.

Route	Onset	Peak	Duration
P.O.	Unknown	1 to 2 hr	3 to 6 hr

Mechanism of Action

Reduces spasticity by decreasing the release of excitatory amino acids. This alpha₂-adrenergic agonist's action increases presynaptic inhibition of spinal motor neurons, with the greatest effects on polysynaptic pathways.

Contraindications

Hypersensitivity to tizanidine or its components, use with ciprofloxacin or fluvoxamine

Interactions

DRUGS

acetaminophen: Delayed peak effects of acetaminophen

alpha₂-adrenergic agonists: Possibly significant hypotension

antihypertensives: Additive hypotensive effects

CYP1A2 inhibitors (such as acyclovir, amiodarone, cimetidine, famotidine, mexiletine, propafenone, ticlopidine, verapamil, zileuton), fluroquinolones (including ciprofloxacin, fluvoxamine): Possibly increased plasma tizanidine level; increased risk of hypotension and sedation

oral contraceptives: Decreased tizanidine clearance

rofecoxib: Possibly increased adverse reactions

ACTIVITIES

alcohol use: Increased adverse effects of tizanidine, additive CNS depression

Adverse Reactions

CNS: Anxiety, delusions, drowsiness, dyskinesia, fatigue, fever, hallucinations, slurred speech

CV: Orthostatic hypotension

EENT: Dry mouth, pharyngitis, rhinitis

GI: Abdominal pain, anorexia, constipation, diarrhea, dyspepsia, elevated liver function test results, hepatic failure, hepatomegaly, nausea, vomiting

GU: Urinary frequency, UTI

MS: Back pain, muscle weakness, myasthenia

SKIN: Diaphoresis, jaundice, rash, ulceration

Nursing Considerations

• Be aware that extreme caution is required

if tizanidine is prescribed for a patient with hepatic impairment because the drug is extensively metabolized in the liver.
•Monitor hepatic and renal function for first 6 months and periodically thereafter.
•Expect prolonged drug use to inhibit saliva.
•Be aware that tizanidine should be stopped slowly to prevent withdrawal and rebound hypertension, tachycardia, and hypertonia.

PATIENT TEACHING
•Caution patient not to stop taking tizanidine suddenly to prevent adverse effects.
•Advise patient to change positions slowly to minimize effects of orthostatic hypotension.
•Urge patient to avoid alcohol during drug therapy because of its additive CNS effects.
•Tell patient to notify prescriber or a dentist if dry mouth lasts longer than 2 weeks.
•Instruct patient to inform all prescribers and pharmacists about any drug he starts or stops taking.

tobramycin sulfate

Tobi

Class and Category
Chemical class: Aminoglycoside
Therapeutic class: Antibiotic
Pregnancy category: D

Indications and Dosages
➤ *To treat bacteremia; bone and joint, gynecologic, intra-abdominal, lower respiratory tract, skin and soft-tissue, and urinary tract infections; endocarditis; meningitis; neonatal sepsis; pyelonephritis; and septicemia caused by susceptible strains of* Acinetobacter *species,* Aeromonas *species,* Citrobacter *species,* Enterobacter *species,* Escherichia coli, Haemophilus influenzae *(beta lactamase–negative and –positive),* Klebsiella *species,* Morganella morganii, Proteus mirabilis, Proteus vulgaris, Providencia rettgeri, Pseudomonas aeruginosa, Salmonella *species,* Serratia *species,* Shigella *species,* Staphylococcus aureus, *and* Staphylococcus epidermidis; *to treat febrile neutropenia*

I.V. INFUSION, I.M. INJECTION
Adults. 3 to 6 mg/kg daily in divided doses every 8 to 12 hr.

Children over age 5. 2 to 2.5 mg/kg every 8 hr.
Children under age 5. 2.5 mg/kg every 8 to 16 hr.
Neonates over age 7 days weighing more than 2 kg (4.4 lb). 2.5 mg/kg every 8 hr.
Neonates over age 7 days weighing 1.2 to 2 kg (2.6 to 4.4 lb). 2.5 mg/kg every 8 to 12 hr.
Neonates age 7 days and under weighing 2 kg or more. 2.5 mg/kg every 12 hr.
Neonates age 7 days and under weighing 1.2 to 2 kg. 2.5 mg/kg every 12 to 18 hr.
Preterm neonates weighing 1 to 1.2 kg (2.2 to 2.6 lb). 2.5 mg/kg every 18 to 24 hr.
Preterm neonates weighing less than 1 kg. 3.5 mg/kg every 24 hr.

➤ *To treat pulmonary infection caused by* P. aeruginosa *in patients with cystic fibrosis*
I.V. INFUSION
Adults and children. 2.5 to 3.3 mg/kg every 8 hr; dosage adjusted to achieve peak blood drug level of 8 to 12 mcg/ml and trough blood drug level below 2 mcg/ml.

INHALATION
Adults and children over age 6. 1 ampule (300 mg) b.i.d. in alternating periods of 28 days on and 28 days off.

➤ *To treat meningitis caused by susceptible organisms*
INTRATHECAL INJECTION
Adults. 4 to 8 mg daily with parenteral therapy.
Children. 1 to 2 mg daily with parenteral therapy.

➤ *To treat systemic infection*
INTRAPERITONEAL INFUSION
Adults and children. 1.5 to 2 mg/kg.

➤ *To treat dialysis-associated peritonitis in patients with end-stage renal disease*
INTRAPERITONEAL INFUSION
Adults and children. 4 to 8 mg/L in each dialysate exchange bag, increased, as prescribed, to 6 to 8 mg/L in documented *Pseudomonas* infection or to 20 mg/L administered in one exchange bag daily.
DOSAGE ADJUSTMENT For patients with renal impairment, dosage possibly reduced.

Incompatibilities
Don't mix tobramycin in same solution with parenteral aminoglycosides or beta-lactam antibiotics because mutual inactivation may result. Don't dilute or mix inhalation solution in nebulizer with dornase alfa.

Mechanism of Action

Inhibits bacterial protein synthesis by binding irreversibly to one of two aminoglycoside-binding sites on the 30S ribosomal subunit, resulting in bacteriostatic effects. Bactericidal effects may stem from tobramycin's ability to accumulate within cells so that the intracellular drug level exceeds the extracellular level.

Contraindications

Concurrent cidofovir therapy; hypersensitivity to tobramycin, aminoglycosides, sodium bisulfite, or their components

Interactions

DRUGS

acyclovir, aminoglycosides, amphotericin B, carboplatin, cisplatin, NSAIDs, vancomycin: Additive nephrotoxicity
carbenicillin, ticarcillin: Possibly inactivation of tobramycin
dimenhydrinate: Possibly masking of symptoms of ototoxicity
ethacrynic acid, furosemide: Additive ototoxicity
general anesthetics, neuromuscular blockers: Possibly exaggerated neuromuscular blockade

Adverse Reactions

CNS: Confusion, dizziness, headache, lethargy, neurotoxicity, vertigo
EENT: Hearing loss, tinnitus
GI: Diarrhea, elevated liver function test results, nausea, vomiting
GU: Elevated BUN and serum creatinine levels, nephrotoxicity, oliguria, proteinuria, renal failure
HEME: Anemia, leukocytosis, leukopenia, neutropenia, thrombocytopenia
SKIN: Exfoliative dermatitis, pruritus, rash, urticaria
Other: Hypocalcemia, hypokalemia, hypomagnesemia, hyponatremia, injection site pain

Nursing Considerations

•Obtain fluid and tissue samples for culture and sensitivity testing before and during tobramycin therapy, as ordered. Review results, if available, before therapy starts.
•After reconstituting with 30 ml of sterile or bacteriostatic water for injection, dilute further with normal saline solution or D_5W.

•Give each I.V. dose over 20 to 60 minutes.
•**WARNING** Don't infuse tobramycin over less than 20 minutes to avoid neuromuscular blockade and excessive peak drug level.
•Don't expose ampules for inhalation solution to intense light. Refrigerate them at 36° to 46° F (2° to 8° C).
•Because drug can cause bilateral and irreversible hearing loss, assess for early signs of cochlear and vestibular ototoxicity, including high-frequency hearing loss and vertigo.
•Monitor serum calcium, magnesium, potassium, and sodium levels to detect electrolyte imbalances.
•**WARNING** Be alert for allergic reactions, including anaphylaxis, because some forms of drug contain sodium bisulfite.
•Stop tobramycin therapy 7 days before starting cidofovir therapy, as prescribed.
•Watch for signs of nephrotoxicity, such as elevated BUN and serum creatinine levels.
•Expect dehydration to increase the risk of nephrotoxicity.
•**WARNING** Monitor patient with myasthenia gravis or parkinsonism for increased muscle weakness because of tobramycin's potential curare-like effect.

PATIENT TEACHING

•For inhaled tobramycin, instruct patient to inhale over 10 to 15 minutes, using a handheld nebulizer with a compressor.
•Teach patient how to use nebulizer while sitting or standing upright and to breathe normally through its mouthpiece. Nose clips may help patient breathe through her mouth.
•Instruct patient to disinfect her nebulizer every other treatment day by boiling the nebulizer parts (except tubing) for a full 10 minutes and then drying the parts on a clean, lint-free cloth.
•Urge patient to immediately report high-frequency hearing loss and vertigo.
•Instruct female patient to notify prescriber immediately about known or suspected pregnancy because drug poses danger to fetus.

tocainide hydrochloride

Tonocard

Class and Category

Chemical class: Lidocaine analogue
Therapeutic class: Class IB antiarrhythmic
Pregnancy category: C

Indications and Dosages

➤ *To treat life-threatening, sustained ventricular tachycardia*

TABLETS

Adults. *Initial:* 400 mg every 8 hr. *Maintenance:* 1.2 to 1.8 g daily in divided doses every 8 hr.

DOSAGE ADJUSTMENT Dosage possibly reduced by 25% if creatinine clearance is 10 to 30 ml/min/1.73 m^2 and by 50% if creatinine clearance is less than 10 ml/min/1.73 m^2.

Route	Onset	Peak	Duration
P.O.	Unknown	0.5 to 2 hr	8 hr

Mechanism of Action

Combines with fast sodium channels in myocardial cell membranes, which inhibits sodium influx into cells and decreases ventricular depolarization, automaticity, and excitability during diastole.

Contraindications

Hypersensitivity to tocainide or its components, second- or third-degree AV block without ventricular pacemaker

Interactions

DRUGS

antiarrhythmics: Possibly additive cardiac effects, additive toxicity

beta blockers: Increased cardiac index, left ventricular pressures, and pulmonary artery wedge pressures

cimetidine: Possibly decreased blood tocainide level

rifampin: Accelerated hepatic metabolism of tocainide, reduced tocainide effectiveness

Adverse Reactions

CNS: Agitation, anxiety, ataxia, coma, confusion, depression, dizziness, fatigue, hallucinations, headache, mood changes, nervousness, paresthesia, psychosis, seizures, sleep disturbance, syncope, tremor, vertigo

CV: AV conduction disorders, bradycardia, chest pain, heart failure, hypertension, hypotension, palpitations, prolonged QT interval, PVCs, tachycardia, ventricular fibrillation

EENT: Blurred vision, vision changes

GI: Anorexia, diarrhea, nausea, vomiting

HEME: Agranulocytosis, anemia, aplastic anemia, bone marrow depression, hemolysis, leukopenia, neutropenia, thrombocytopenia

RESP: Pulmonary edema, fibrosis, and hypersensitivity (pneumonitis); respiratory arrest

SKIN: Diaphoresis, exfoliative dermatitis, pruritus, rash, skin lesions, urticaria

Nursing Considerations

•Monitor CBC with differential weekly during first 3 months of tocainide treatment and routinely thereafter to detect blood dyscrasias. Although rare, agranulocytosis, anemia, aplastic anemia, bone marrow depression, hemolysis, leukopenia, neutropenia, or thrombocytopenia may be fatal. Expect findings to normalize about 1 month after therapy stops.

•Maintain continuous cardiac monitoring or obtain periodic ECG tracings, as ordered, to assess drug effectiveness.

•Watch for tremor, a possible sign of maximum dosing.

•Assess patient for additive adverse cardiac effects, especially if tocainide is used with another antiarrhythmic.

•Be aware that tocainide is secreted in breast milk and has the potential to cause serious adverse reactions in breastfeeding infants.

PATIENT TEACHING

•Inform patient that electrophysiologic studies may be performed before tocainide therapy starts.

•Tell patient to notify prescriber about tremor because dosage may need adjustment.

•Explain that chest X-rays may be needed if adverse pulmonary reactions occur.

•Inform patient that ambulatory monitoring may be needed to verify antiarrhythmic response.

•Stress the need to keep all scheduled appointments for follow-up blood tests.

tolazamide

Tolinase

Class and Category

Chemical class: First-generation sulfonylurea
Therapeutic class: Antidiabetic
Pregnancy category: C

Indications and Dosages

➤ *As adjunct to treat type 2 diabetes mel-*

litus that's uncontrolled by diet and exercise

TABLETS

Adults. *Initial:* 100 mg daily with breakfast if fasting blood glucose level is less than 200 mg/dl; 250 mg daily if fasting blood glucose level is more than 200 mg/dl. Dose adjusted every wk by 100 to 250 mg, if needed. Doses greater than 500 mg daily are divided and given every 12 hr. *Maximum:* 1,000 mg daily.

DOSAGE ADJUSTMENT If patient takes more than 40 units daily of insulin, initial dosage increased to 250 mg daily and insulin dosage decreased by 50%.

Route	Onset	Peak	Duration
P.O.	Unknown	3 to 4 hr	10 to 20 hr

Mechanism of Action

Stimulates insulin release from beta cells in the pancreas. Tolazamide also increases peripheral tissue sensitivity to insulin either by enhancing insulin binding to cellular receptors or by increasing the number of insulin receptors.

Contraindications

Diabetic coma; diabetic ketoacidosis; hypersensitivity to tolazamide, sulfonylureas, or their components; pregnancy; sole therapy for type 1 diabetes mellitus

Interactions

DRUGS

ACE inhibitors, anabolic steroids, androgens, azole antifungals, bromocriptine, chloramphenicol, clofibrate, disopyramide, guanethidine, H_2-receptor antagonists, insulin, magnesium salts, MAO inhibitors, methyldopa, octreotide, oxyphenbutazone, phenylbutazone, probenecid, quinidine, salicylates, sulfonamides, tetracycline, theophylline, tricyclic antidepressants, urinary acidifiers: Increased risk of hypoglycemia

asparaginase, calcium channel blockers, cholestyramine, clonidine, corticosteroids, danazol, diazoxide, estrogen, glucagon, hydantoins, isoniazid, lithium, morphine, nicotinic acid, oral contraceptives, phenothiazines, rifabutin, rifampin, sympathomimetics, thiazide diuretics, thyroid drugs, urinary alkalizers: Increased risk of hyperglycemia

beta blockers: Possibly hyperglycemia or masking of signs and symptoms of hypoglycemia

digoxin: Increased risk of digitalis toxicity

pentamidine: Initial hypoglycemia and then hyperglycemia if beta cell damage occurs

ACTIVITIES

alcohol use: Altered blood glucose control (usually hypoglycemia), possibly disulfiram-like reaction

Adverse Reactions

CNS: Dizziness, fatigue, headache, malaise, paresthesia, vertigo

ENDO: Hypoglycemia

GI: Anorexia, cholestasis, heartburn, nausea, vomiting

HEME: Agranulocytosis, aplastic anemia, hemolysis, hemolytic anemia, leukopenia, thrombocytopenia

MS: Muscle weakness

SKIN: Erythema, photosensitivity, pruritus, rash, urticaria

Nursing Considerations

•When switching an insulin-treated patient with type 2 diabetes, expect to start tolazamide at 100 mg daily if patient takes less than 20 units daily of insulin, or 250 mg daily if patient takes 20 to 40 units daily of insulin.

•Anticipate that patient receiving tolazamide may need temporary insulin treatment during periods of physiologic stress, such as fever, surgery, systemic infection, and trauma.

•For patient over age 65, expect to start tolazamide at 100 mg daily.

•Assess elderly patients for signs of hypoglycemia because they're more susceptible to drug's hypoglycemic effect. Anticipate that hypoglycemia may be more difficult to detect.

•Assess patient with thyroid disease for altered blood glucose control because thyroid hormone increases GI absorption of glucose.

•Expect prescriber to stop tolazamide 2 weeks before pregnant patient delivers her neonate to minimize the risk of prolonged hypoglycemia in neonate.

PATIENT TEACHING

•Advise patient to avoid alcohol while taking tolazamide.

•Teach patient and family members how to monitor blood glucose level and how to rec-

T

ognize signs of hypoglycemia and hyperglycemia.

•Instruct patient to treat mild hypoglycemia with fruit juice or other simple sugars.

tolbutamide

Apo-Tolbutamide (CAN), Novo-Butamide (CAN), Orinase

Class and Category

Chemical class: First-generation sulfonylurea
Therapeutic class: Antidiabetic
Pregnancy category: C

Indications and Dosages

➤ *As adjunct to treat type 2 diabetes mellitus that's uncontrolled by diet and exercise*

TABLETS

Adults. *Initial:* 1 to 2 g daily in divided doses b.i.d. or t.i.d. *Maintenance:* 0.25 to 2 g daily. *Maximum:* 3 g daily.

Route	Onset	Peak	Duration
P.O.	Unknown	3 to 4 hr	6 to 12 hr

Mechanism of Action

Stimulates insulin release from beta cells in the pancreas. Tolbutamide also increases peripheral tissue sensitivity to insulin either by enhancing insulin binding to cellular receptors or by increasing the number of insulin receptors.

Contraindications

Diabetes complicated by pregnancy; diabetic coma; diabetic ketoacidosis; hypersensitivity to tolbutamide, sulfonylureas, or their components; sole therapy for type 1 diabetes mellitus

Interactions

DRUGS

ACE inhibitors, anabolic steroids, androgens, azole antifungals, bromocriptine, chloramphenicol, clofibrate, disopyramide, guanethidine, H_2-receptor antagonists, insulin, magnesium salts, MAO inhibitors, methyldopa, octreotide, oxyphenbutazone, phenylbutazone, probenecid, quinidine, salicylates, sulfonamides, tetracycline, theophylline, tricyclic antidepressants, urinary acidifiers: Increased risk of hypoglycemia
asparaginase, calcium channel blockers, cholestyramine, clonidine, corticosteroids, danazol, diazoxide, estrogen, glucagon, hydantoins, isoniazid, lithium, morphine, nicotinic acid, oral contraceptives, phenothiazines, rifabutin, rifampin, sympathomimetics, thiazide diuretics, thyroid drugs, urinary alkalizers: Increased risk of hyperglycemia
beta blockers: Possibly hyperglycemia or masking of signs and symptoms of hypoglycemia
digoxin: Increased risk of digitalis toxicity
pentamidine: Initial hypoglycemia and then hyperglycemia if beta cell damage occurs

ACTIVITIES

alcohol use: Altered blood glucose control (usually hypoglycemia), possibly disulfiramlike reaction

Adverse Reactions

CNS: Dizziness, fatigue, headache, malaise, paresthesia, vertigo
ENDO: Hypoglycemia
GI: Anorexia, cholestasis, heartburn, nausea, vomiting
HEME: Agranulocytosis, aplastic anemia, hemolysis, hemolytic anemia, leukopenia, thrombocytopenia
MS: Muscle weakness
SKIN: Erythema, photosensitivity, pruritus, rash, urticaria

Nursing Considerations

•If patient takes 20 units or less of insulin daily, expect a possible transfer from insulin to tolbutamide. If patient takes more than 20 units of insulin daily, expect to reduce insulin dosage as tolbutamide therapy starts.
•Anticipate that patient receiving tolbutamide may need temporary insulin treatment during periods of physiologic stress, such as fever, surgery, systemic infection, or trauma.
•Assess elderly patients for signs of hypoglycemia because they're more susceptible to drug's hypoglycemic effect. Anticipate that hypoglycemia may be more difficult to detect.
•Assess patient with thyroid disease for altered blood glucose control because thyroid hormone increases GI absorption of glucose.
•Expect prescriber to stop tolbutamide 2 weeks before pregnant patient delivers her neonate to minimize the risk of prolonged hypoglycemia in neonate.

PATIENT TEACHING
• Advise patient to avoid alcohol while taking tolbutamide.
• Teach patient and family members how to monitor blood glucose level and recognize signs of hypoglycemia and hyperglycemia.
• Instruct patient to treat mild hypoglycemia with fruit juice or other simple sugars.

tolcapone

Tasmar

Class and Category

Chemical class: Nitrobenzophenone
Therapeutic class: Antidyskinetic
Pregnancy category: C

Indications and Dosages

➤ *As adjunct (with levodopa and carbidopa) to treat Parkinson's disease*

TABLETS

Adults. *Initial:* 100 mg t.i.d. *Maximum:* 200 mg t.i.d.

Mechanism of Action

Prolongs plasma half-life of levodopa by inhibiting catechol-*O*-methyltransferase (COMT), an enzyme responsible for metabolizing catecholamines—including dopa, dopamine, epinephrine, norepinephrine, and their hydroxylated metabolites. COMT inhibition decreases the metabolizing enzyme for levodopa, which yields a more sustained plasma levodopa level, making more available for diffusion into the CNS to be converted to dopamine.

Contraindications

Confusion, hyperpyrexia, or rhabdomyolysis with previous use of tolcapone; hepatic dysfunction; hypersensitivity to tolcapone or its components

Interactions

DRUGS

desipramine: Possibly increased frequency of adverse effects
levodopa: Increased levodopa bioavailability, with increased risk of orthostatic hypotension and syncope
MAO inhibitors: Possibly inhibited catecholamine metabolism

Adverse Reactions

CNS: Confusion, dizziness, drowsiness, dyskinesia, fatigue, fever, hallucinations, headache, lethargy, loss of balance
CV: Chest pain, orthostatic hypotension
EENT: Dry mouth
GI: Abdominal pain, acute fulminant liver failure, anorexia, cholestasis, constipation, diarrhea, elevated liver function test results, vomiting
GU: Bright yellow urine, hematuria
MS: Muscle cramps, rhabdomyolysis
RESP: Dyspnea, upper respiratory tract infection
SKIN: Diaphoresis, jaundice

Nursing Considerations

• Ensure that patient has had the risks of tolcapone therapy explained fully to him and has signed the acknowledgement form before starting therapy.
• Use cautiously in patient with severe dyskinesia or dystonia because drug is known to cause rhabdomyolysis.
• Monitor liver function test results, as ordered, during tolcapone therapy to detect hepatic impairment. Expect to discontinue drug if patient's liver enzymes exceed twice the upper limit of normal or if patient has any signs or symptoms of liver dysfunction, such as persistent nausea, fatigue, lethargy, anorexia, jaundice, dark urine, pruritus, or right upper quadrant tenderness.
• Assess patient for hallucinations, especially in patient over age 75.
• Anticipate that drug may precipitate or exaggerate preexisting dyskinesia.
• Expect tolcapone to be discontinued if no improvement occurs after 3 weeks of drug therapy.

PATIENT TEACHING

• Inform patient that urine may turn bright yellow during tolcapone therapy.
• Advise patient to avoid hazardous activities until drug's CNS effects are known.
• Urge patient to notify prescriber immediately about darkened urine, decreased appetite, fatigue, jaundice, lethargy, and right-sided abdominal pain.
• Caution patient not to stop taking drug abruptly. Explain that prescriber will supervise tapering of drug dosage.
• Urge patient to have regular follow-up appointments and laboratory tests.

T

tolmetin

Novo-Tolmetin (CAN), Tolectin DS, Tolectin 200, Tolectin 400 (CAN), Tolectin 600

Class and Category

Chemical class: Pyrroleacetic acid derivative
Therapeutic class: Anti-inflammatory
Pregnancy category: C (first trimester), Not rated (later trimesters)

Indications and Dosages

➤ *To relieve moderate pain from rheumatoid arthritis and osteoarthritis*

CAPSULES, TABLETS

Adults. *Initial:* 400 mg t.i.d. *Maintenance:* 600 to 1,800 mg daily in divided doses t.i.d. or q.i.d. *Maximum:* 2,000 mg daily for rheumatoid arthritis, 1,600 mg daily for osteoarthritis.

➤ *To treat juvenile rheumatoid arthritis*

CAPSULES, TABLETS

Children over age 2. *Initial:* 20 mg/kg daily in divided doses t.i.d. or q.i.d. *Maintenance:* 15 to 30 mg/kg daily in divided doses. *Maximum:* 30 mg/kg daily.

Route	Onset	Peak	Duration
P.O.	Unknown	1 to 2 wk	Unknown

Mechanism of Action

Blocks cyclooxygenase, the enzyme needed to synthesize prostaglandins, which mediate the inflammatory response and cause local vasodilation, swelling, and pain. Prostaglandins also promote pain transmission from the periphery to the spinal cord. By blocking cyclooxygenase and inhibiting prostaglandins, tolmetin reduces inflammatory symptoms and relieves pain.

Contraindications

Angioedema, asthma, bronchospasm, nasal polyps, rhinitis, or urticaria caused by aspirin, iodides, or other NSAIDs

Interactions

DRUGS

ACE inhibitors, beta blockers: Decreased effectiveness of these drugs, possibly reduced renal function
alendronate, corticosteroids, other NSAIDs,
salicylates: Possibly adverse GI effects
anticoagulants, platelet aggregation inhibitors, thrombolytics: Additive inhibition of platelet aggregation; prolonged bleeding time
antineoplastics, antithymocyte globulin, strontium-89 chloride: Increased risk of bleeding
cidofovir: Possibly nephrotoxicity
cyclosporine: Potentiated cyclosporine nephrotoxicity
digoxin: Increased blood digoxin level
lithium: Possibly lithium toxicity
methotrexate: Increased or prolonged blood methotrexate level

ACTIVITIES

alcohol use: Increased risk of adverse GI effects

Adverse Reactions

CNS: Aseptic meningitis, cerebral hemorrhage, ischemic stroke, depression, dizziness, drowsiness, fatigue, headache, transient ischemic attack, weakness
CV: Chest pain, deep vein thrombosis, edema, hypertension, MI, peripheral edema
EENT: Tinnitus
ENDO: Hypoglycemia
GI: Abdominal pain; constipation; diarrhea; elevated liver function test results; flatulence; gastritis; GI bleeding, perforation, or ulceration; hepatitis; indigestion; jaundice; liver failure; nausea; peptic ulcer disease; vomiting
GU: Acute renal failure, dysuria, elevated BUN level, hematuria, interstitial nephritis, nephrotic syndrome, nephrotoxicity, proteinuria, UTI
HEME: Agranulocytosis, aplastic anemia, hemolytic anemia, leukopenia, pancytopenia, prolonged bleeding time
SKIN: Erythema multiforme, exfoliative dermatitis, maculopapular rash, Stevens-Johnson syndrome, toxic epidermal necrolysis, urticaria
Other: Anaphylaxis, angioedema, weight gain or loss

Nursing Considerations

• Give tolmetin with food or milk to reduce adverse GI reactions.
• Assess patient for improvement within 7 days and progressive improvement over several successive weeks.
• Use tolmetin with extreme caution in pa-

tients with a history of ulcer disease or GI bleeding because NSAIDs such as tolmetin increase the risk of GI bleeding and ulceration. Expect to use tolmetin for the shortest time possible in these patients.

•Be aware that serious GI tract ulceration, bleeding, and perforation may occur without warning symptoms. Elderly patients are at greater risk. To minimize risk, give drug with food. If GI distress occurs, withhold drug and notify prescriber immediately.

•Use tolmetin cautiously in patients with hypertension, and monitor blood pressure closely throughout therapy. Drug may cause hypertension or worsen it.

•WARNING Monitor patient closely for thrombotic events, including MI and stroke, because NSAIDs increase the risk.

•WARNING If patient has bone marrow suppression or is receiving antineoplastic drug therapy, monitor laboratory results (including WBC count), and watch for evidence of infection because anti-inflammatory and antipyretic actions of tolmetin may mask signs and symptoms, such as fever and pain.

•Especially if patient is elderly or taking tolmetin long-term, watch for less common but serious adverse GI reactions, including anorexia, constipation, diverticulitis, dysphagia, esophagitis, gastritis, gastroenteritis, gastroesophageal reflux disease, hemorrhoids, hiatal hernia, melena, stomatitis, and vomiting.

•Monitor liver function test results because, in rare cases, elevated levels may progress to severe hepatic reactions, including fatal hepatitis, liver necrosis, and hepatic failure.

•Monitor BUN and serum creatinine levels in patients with heart failure, impaired renal function, or hepatic dysfunction; those taking diuretics or ACE inhibitors; and elderly patients because drug may cause renal failure.

•Monitor CBC for decreased hemoglobin and hematocrit because drug may worsen anemia.

•Assess patient's skin routinely for rash or other signs of hypersensitivity reaction because tolmetin and other NSAIDs may cause serious skin reactions without warning, even in patients with no history of NSAID hypersensitivity. Stop drug at first sign of reaction, and notify prescriber.

•Assess invasive sites or wounds for bleeding and bruising from drug's effects on platelets.

PATIENT TEACHING
•Tell patient to take drug with food or milk.
•Urge patient to limit sodium intake because drug may cause fluid retention.
•Tell patient to avoid alcohol during therapy.
•Teach patient how to perform proper oral hygiene, and advise her to have needed dental work done before tolmetin therapy starts because of the increased risk of bleeding.
•Explain that tolmetin may increase the risk of serious adverse cardiovascular reactions; urge patient to seek immediate medical attention if signs or symptoms arise, such as chest pain, shortness of breath, weakness, and slurring of speech.
•Tell patient that tolmetin also may increase the risk of serious adverse GI reactions; stress the need to seek immediate medical attention for such signs and symptoms as epigastric or abdominal pain, indigestion, black or tarry stools, or vomiting blood or material that looks like coffee grounds.
•Alert patient to the possibility of rare but serious skin reactions. Urge her to seek immediate medical attention for rash, blisters, itching, fever, or other indications of hypersensitivity.

tolterodine tartrate
Detrol, Detrol LA

Class and Category
Chemical class: Prodrug of 5-hydroxymethyl-tolterodine
Therapeutic class: Antispasmodic
Pregnancy category: C

Indications and Dosages
➤ *To treat overactive bladder*
TABLETS
Adults. 2 mg b.i.d. Reduced to 1 mg b.i.d. based on patient response and tolerance.
DOSAGE ADJUSTMENT Dosage reduced to 1 mg b.i.d. for patients with significant hepatic or renal dysfunction and for patients who are also receiving cytochrome P-450 3A4 inhibitors, such as clarithromycin, erythromycin, and the antifungals itraconazole, ketoconazole, and miconazole.
E.R. TABLETS
Adults. 4 mg daily. Reduced to 2 mg daily based on individual response and tolerance.

T

Mechanism of Action

Exerts antimuscarinic (atropine-like) and potent direct antispasmodic (papaverine-like) actions on smooth muscle in the bladder, which decreases detrusor muscle contractions. This helps reduce urinary frequency and urgency as well as urge-related incontinence.

Contraindications

Gastric retention, hypersensitivity to tolterodine tartrate or its components, uncontrolled angle-closure glaucoma, urine retention

Interactions

DRUGS

clarithromycin, erythromycin, itraconazole, ketoconazole, miconazole: Possibly increased blood tolterodine level
class IA antiarrhythmics (such as quinidine, procainamide) or class III antiarrhythmics (such as amiodarone, sotalol): Possibly increased risk of prolonged QT interval
fluoxetine: Possibly decreased tolterodine metabolism

Adverse Reactions

CNS: Confusion, disorientation, dizziness, fatigue, hallucinations, headache, memory impairment, somnolence, worsening of dementia
CV: Chest pain, edema, hypertension, palpitations, QT interval prolongation, tachycardia
EENT: Abnormal vision, dry eyes, dry mouth
GI: Abdominal pain, constipation, diarrhea, flatulence, indigestion, nausea
GU: Dysuria, urine retention, UTI
Other: Anaphylaxis, angioedema, flulike symptoms

Nursing Considerations

• Use cautiously in patients with decreased GI motility, myasthenia gravis, or narrow-angle glaucoma because tolterodine could make these conditions worse.
• **WARNING** Monitor patients with a history of bladder outflow obstruction for decreased urine output or bladder distention because tolterodine poses a risk of urine retention.
• Monitor patients with a history of GI obstructive disorders, such as pyloric stenosis, for abdominal distention or bloating because of increased risk of gastric retention.
• Be aware that drug's antimuscarinic effects may produce blurred vision, dizziness, and drowsiness. If these occur, institute fall precautions according to institution policy.

PATIENT TEACHING

• Instruct patient taking tolterodine to immediately report to prescriber difficulty urinating or infrequent urination.
• Advise patient not to drive or perform activities that require high level of alertness until drug's CNS and vision effects are known. Instruct her to notify prescriber if dizziness or blurred vision persists.
• Encourage patient to use sugarless candy, gum, or ice to relieve dry mouth. Advise her to notify prescriber or dentist if dry mouth persists or worsens over 2 weeks.

topiramate

Topamax

Class and Category

Chemical class: Sulfamate-substituted monosaccharide
Therapeutic class: Anticonvulsant
Pregnancy category: C

Indications and Dosages

➤ *To treat partial-onset or primary generalized tonic-clonic seizures*

CAPSULES

Adults and chidren age 10 and over. *Initial:* 25 mg b.i.d. in morning and evening. Increased by 50 mg daily every wk. *Maintenance:* 200 mg b.i.d. in morning and evening.

➤ *As adjunct to treat partial seizures and primary generalized tonic-clonic seizures*

CAPSULES, TABLETS

Adults and adolescents age 17 and over. *Initial:* 25 to 50 mg daily in divided doses b.i.d. for 1 wk. Increased by 25 to 50 mg daily every wk. *Maintenance:* 200 to 400 mg daily in divided doses b.i.d. *Maximum:* 1,600 mg daily.
Children ages 2 to 16. *Initial:* 25 mg or less at bedtime for 1 wk. Increased every 1 to 2 wk by 1 to 3 mg/kg daily in divided doses every 12 hr, as prescribed. *Usual:* 5 to 9 mg/kg daily in divided doses every 12 hr.

➤ *As adjunct to treat seizures associated with Lennox-Gastaut syndrome*

CAPSULES, TABLETS
Children ages 2 to 16. 25 mg at bedtime for
1 wk. Increased every 1 to 2 wk by 1 to
3 mg/kg daily in divided doses every 12 hr,
as prescribed. *Usual:* 5 to 9 mg/kg daily in
divided doses every 12 hr.

➤ *To prevent migraine headache*
CAPSULES, TABLETS
Adults. *Initial:* 25 mg daily in evening for
1 wk; then 25 mg b.i.d. for 1 wk; then 25 mg
in morning and 50 mg in evening for 1 wk.
Maintenance: 50 mg b.i.d.
DOSAGE ADJUSTMENT For patients with moderate to severe renal impairment, dosage possibly reduced by 50%.

Mechanism of Action
May block the spread of seizures by reducing the length and frequency of excitatory
transmission. Topiramate increases the
availability of the inhibitory neurotransmitter gamma-aminobutyric acid by
blocking voltage-sensitive sodium channels. This action promotes the movement
of chloride ions into neurons.

Contraindications
Hypersensitivity to topiramate or its components

Interactions
DRUGS
*antihistamines, barbiturates, benzodiaze-
pines, CNS depressants, opioid analgesics,
skeletal muscle relaxants, tricyclic antidepressants:* Additive CNS depression
carbamazepine: Decreased blood topiramate
level
carbonic anhydrase inhibitors: Increased risk
of renal calculus formation
digoxin: Possibly decreased blood digoxin
level
ethinyl estradiol: Increased risk of breakthrough bleeding
oral contraceptives: Increased risk of breakthrough bleeding, decreased contraceptive
efficacy
phenobarbital: Altered blood phenobarbital
level
phenytoin: Decreased blood level of topiramate
probenecid: Possibly blocked renal tubular
reabsorption of topiramate and decreased

blood topiramate level
valproic acid: Decreased blood levels of both
drugs
ACTIVITIES
alcohol use: Additive CNS depression

Adverse Reactions
CNS: Agitation, anxiety, asthenia, ataxia,
confusion, decreased concentration, depression, dizziness, fatigue, fever, hallucinations,
headache, hyperthermia, hypoesthesia, insomnia, irritability, memory loss, mood
changes, nervousness, paresthesia, psychomotor slowing, psychosis, slurred speech,
somnolence, suicidal ideology, syncope,
tremor
CV: Cardiac arrest, chest pain, hot flashes,
hypertension, hypotension, palpitations, vasodilation
EENT: Diplopia, dry mouth, gingivitis, hearing loss, nystagmus, pharyngitis, rhinitis,
secondary angle-closure glaucoma with acute
myopia, sinusitis, taste perversion, tinnitus,
tongue edema, vision changes
ENDO: Breast pain, hyperglycemia
GI: Abdominal pain, anorexia, constipation,
diarrhea, flatulence, gastroenteritis, gastroesophageal reflux, hepatic failure, hepatitis,
indigestion, nausea, pancreatitis, vomiting
GU: Cystitis, decreased libido, dysmenorrhea, dysuria, frequent urination, impotence,
menstrual irregularities, renal calculi, renal
tubular acidosis, UTI, vaginitis
HEME: Anemia, leukopenia
MS: Arthralgia, back pain, leg cramps or
pain, muscle weakness
RESP: Bronchitis, cough, dyspnea, pulmonary embolism, upper respiratory tract infection
SKIN: Acne, alopecia, decreased sweating,
erythema multiforme, pemphigus, pruritus,
rash, Stevens-Johnson syndrome, toxic epidermal necrolysis
Other: Dehydration, metabolic acidosis,
weight gain or loss

Nursing Considerations
•Obtain baseline serum bicarbonate level before topiramate therapy and monitor periodically throughout therapy, as ordered.
•Give capsule with water and have patient
swallow it whole. If needed, open capsules
and empty contents onto a spoonful of soft
food. Discard unused portion.
•Never store food sprinkled with drug for

T

use at a later time.

•**WARNING** Anticipate an increase in seizures if therapy stops abruptly. Take seizure precautions, as appropriate.

•If patient reports ocular pain or decreased visual acuity, notify prescriber immediately; topiramate may cause increased intraocular pressure and secondary angle-closure glaucoma. Expect to stop drug immediately.

•If patient has a history of renal calculi, assess for signs of recurrence.

PATIENT TEACHING

•Instruct patient to swallow topiramate tablets whole.

•Urge patient to avoid potentially hazardous activities until drug's CNS effects are known.

•Advise patient to watch for decreased sweating and significantly increased body temperature, especially during hot weather, and to notify prescriber immediately if they occur.

•Tell patient to maintain adequate fluid intake to minimize the risk of developing kidney stones.

•Advise female patient of possible breakthrough bleeding. If she takes an oral contraceptive, encourage her to use another form of contraception during therapy.

torsemide

Demadex

Class and Category

Chemical class: Anilinopyridine sulfonylurea derivative
Therapeutic class: Antihypertensive, diuretic
Pregnancy category: B

Indications and Dosages

➤ *To treat edema in heart failure*

TABLETS, I.V. INJECTION

Adults. *Initial:* 10 to 20 mg daily, adjusted by doubling, as prescribed, to achieve desired effect. *Maximum:* 200 mg daily.

➤ *To treat edema in chronic renal failure*

TABLETS, I.V. INJECTION

Adults. *Initial:* 20 mg daily, adjusted by doubling, as prescribed, to achieve desired effect. *Maximum:* 200 mg daily.

➤ *To treat ascites, alone or with amiloride or spironolactone*

TABLETS, I.V. INJECTION

Adults. *Initial:* 5 to 10 mg daily. *Maximum:* 40 mg daily.

➤ *To manage hypertension*

TABLETS

Adults. *Initial:* 5 mg daily, increased to 10 mg daily after 4 to 6 wk, as prescribed, if response is inadequate. *Maximum:* 10 mg daily.

Route	Onset	Peak	Duration
P.O.	1 hr	1 to 2 hr	6 to 8 hr
I.V.	10 min	1 hr	6 to 8 hr

Mechanism of Action

Blocks active sodium and chloride reabsorption in the ascending loop of Henle by promoting rapid excretion of water, sodium, and chloride. Torsemide also increases the production of renal prostaglandins, increasing the plasma renin level and renal vasodilation. As a result, blood pressure falls, reducing preload and afterload.

Contraindications

Hypersensitivity to torsemide, sulfonamides, or their components

Interactions

DRUGS

ACE inhibitors, antihypertensives: Additive hypotension

amiloride, spironolactone, triamterene: Possibly counteracted torsemide-induced hypokalemia

amphotericin B: Increased risk of nephrotoxicity and severe, prolonged hypokalemia or hypomagnesemia

cisplatin: Increased risk of significant hypokalemia or hypomagnesemia, possibly permanent ototoxicity

cortisone, fluorocortisone, hydrocortisone: Increased risk of sodium retention and hypokalemia

digoxin: Increased risk of arrhythmias and digitalis toxicity due to hypokalemia or hypomagnesemia

indomethacin: Possibly decreased diuretic and antihypertensive effects of torsemide and increased risk of renal failure

lithium: Possibly lithium toxicity

metolazone, thiazide diuretics: Increased risk of severe fluid and electrolyte loss

neuromuscular blockers: Possibly increased

neuromuscular blockade due to hypokalemia
probenecid: Possibly decreased diuretic effect
of torsemide
quinidine and other ototoxic drugs: Increased
risk of ototoxicity
salicylates: Increased risk of salicylate toxicity
ACTIVITIES
alcohol use: Additive diuresis and, possibly,
dehydration

Adverse Reactions
CNS: Dizziness, drowsiness, fatigue, headache, insomnia, lethargy, nervousness, restlessness, weakness
CV: Chest pain, ECG abnormalities, edema, hypotension, tachycardia
EENT: Dry mouth, hearing loss, ototoxicity, pharyngitis, rhinitis, tinnitus
GI: Constipation, diarrhea, indigestion, nausea, thirst, vomiting
GU: Azotemia (prerenal), oliguria, urinary frequency
MS: Muscle spasms, myalgia
RESP: Cough
Other: Hypochloremia, hypokalemia, hypomagnesemia, hyponatremia, hypovolemia

Nursing Considerations
•Inject I.V. torsemide slowly over 2 minutes. Flush I.V. line with normal saline solution before and afterward.
•Don't exceed 200 mg in a single I.V. dose of torsemide.
•Monitor serum electrolyte levels and fluid intake and output to detect hypovolemia.
•**WARNING** Expect torsemide-induced electrolyte imbalances, such as hypokalemia and hypomagnesemia, to increase the risk of toxicity and fatal arrhythmias in a patient who takes a digitalis glycoside. Hypokalemia also potentiates the neuromuscular blockade effects of nondepolarizing neuromuscular blockers.
PATIENT TEACHING
•Advise patient to change position slowly to minimize the effects of orthostatic hypotension.
•Instruct patient to notify prescriber at once about drowsiness, dry mouth, hearing changes, lethargy, muscle pain, nausea, restlessness, thirst, vomiting, or weakness.
•Advise diabetic patient to monitor her blood glucose level often because drug may raise it.

tramadol hydrochloride
Ultram, Ultram ER

Class and Category
Chemical class: Cyclohexanol
Therapeutic class: Analgesic
Pregnancy category: C

Indications and Dosages
➤ *To relieve moderate to moderately severe pain*
TABLETS
Adults and adolescents over age 16. 50 to 100 mg every 4 to 6 hr, p.r.n. *Maximum:* 400 mg daily.
DOSAGE ADJUSTMENT If patient has hepatic impairment, dosage reduced to 50 mg every 12 hr. If patient is age 75 or over, maximum dosage reduced to 300 mg daily. If creatinine clearance is 30 ml/min/1.73 m² or less, interval increased to every 12 hr and maximum dosage limited to 200 mg daily.
E.R. TABLETS
Adults. 100 mg once daily, increased in 100-mg increments once daily every 5 days, as needed. *Maximum:* 300 mg once daily.

Route	Onset	Peak	Duration
P.O.	1 hr	2 to 3 hr	7 to 14 hr

Mechanism of Action
Binds with mu receptors and inhibits the reuptake of norepinephrine and serotonin, which may account for tramadol's analgesic effect.

Contraindications
Alcohol intoxication; excessive use of central-acting analgesics, hypnotics, opioids, or other psychotropic drugs; hypersensitivity to tramadol or its components; use within 14 days of MAO inhibitor therapy

Interactions
DRUGS
alpha blockers, CYP2D6 and CYP3A4 inhibitors (amitriptyline, erythromycin, fluoxetine, paroxetine, quinidine), linezolid, lithium, MAO inhibitors, St. John's wort, selective serotonin and norepinephrine reuptake inhibitors, tricyclic antidepressants, triptans: Increased risk of serotonin syndrome

T

amiodarone, cimetidine, clomipramine, desipramine, fluphenazine, haloperidol, propafenone, quinidine, ritonavir, thioridazine: Decreased analgesia, increased adverse effects of tramadol

amitriptyline, amphetamines, antipsychotics, bupropion, cyclobenzaprine, dextroamphetamine, erythromycin, fluoxetine, ketoconazole, paroxetine, quinidine, MAO inhibitors, naloxone, tricyclic antidepressants: Increased risk of seizures

barbiturates, benzodiazepines, opioid analgesics, sedative-hypnotics, tranquilizers: Additive CNS depression

carbamazepine: Increased tramadol metabolism

general anesthetics: Increased CNS and respiratory depression

phenothiazines, rifampin: Additive CNS depression, increased risk of seizures

warfarin: Possibly increased INR

ACTIVITIES

alcohol use: Additive CNS depression

Adverse Reactions

CNS: Agitation, anxiety, asthenia, depression, dizziness, emotional lability, euphoria, fatigue, fever, hallucinations, headache, hypertonia, hypoesthesia, insomnia, lethargy, nervousness, paresthesia, restlessness, rigors, seizures, serotonin syndrome, somnolence, tremor, vertigo, weakness

CV: Chest pain, orthostatic hypotension, vasodilation

EENT: Blurred vision, dry mouth, nasal or sinus congestion, sore throat, vision changes

ENDO: Hot flashes

GI: Abdominal pain, anorexia, constipation, diarrhea, indigestion, nausea, vomiting

GU: Urinary frequency, urine retention

MS: Arthralgia; back, limb, or neck pain

RESP: Cough, dyspnea

SKIN: Diaphoresis, dermatitis, flushing, pruritus, rash

Other: Flulike illness, physical and psychological dependence

Nursing Considerations

• Be aware that tramadol shouldn't be given to patients with a history of anaphylactoid reactions to codeine or other opioids.

• **WARNING** Monitor patient closely for evidence of serotonin syndrome, such as agitation, hallucinations, coma, tachycardia, labile blood pressure, hyperthermia, hyperreflexia, incoordination, nausea, vomiting, or diarrhea. Notify prescriber immediately because serotonin syndrome may be life-threatening. Be prepared to discontinue drug and provide supportive care.

• Because tramadol may lead to physical and psychological dependence, assess patient for evidence of dependence or abuse. Avoid giving drug to patients with a history of dependence on other opioids.

• Avoid giving tramadol to patients with acute abdominal conditions because it may mask evidence and disrupt assessment of the abdomen.

• After patient receives first tramadol dose, watch for allergic reactions, including angioedema, bronchospasm, pruritus, Stevens-Johnson syndrome, toxic epidermal necrolysis, and urticaria. Also watch for signs and symptoms of anaphylaxis, such as dyspnea and hypotension.

• If patient has respiratory depression, assess respiratory status often, and expect to give a nonopioid analgesic—not tramadol.

• If patient develops respiratory depression, expect to give naloxone. Watch for seizures because naloxone may increase this risk. Take seizure precautions.

• Assess respiratory status often if patient has increased intracranial pressure or head injury because of possible increased carbon dioxide retention and CSF pressure, either of which may cause respiratory depression. Also, be aware that tramadol may constrict pupils, obscuring evidence of intracranial complications.

• **WARNING** Watch for seizures in patients with epilepsy, a history of seizures, or an increased risk of seizures, such as those with head injury, metabolic disorders, alcohol or drug withdrawal, or CNS infection.

• Expect to taper tramadol rather than stopping it abruptly to avoid such acute withdrawal symptoms as anxiety, diarrhea, insomnia, nausea, pain, panic attacks, paresthesias, piloerection, rigors, sweating, tremor, and upper respiratory symptoms.

PATIENT TEACHING

• Urge patient to follow prescribed dose limits and dosing intervals to prevent respiratory depression and seizures.

• Instruct patient prescribed extended-release form to swallow tablet whole and not to chew, crush, or split tablet.

•Caution patient not to stop tramadol abruptly.
•Instruct patient to avoid hazardous activities until drug's CNS effects are known.
•Advise patient to avoid alcohol while taking tramadol.
•Urge patient to notify prescriber about known, suspected, or intended pregnancy.

trandolapril

Mavik

Class and Category

Chemical class: ACE inhibitor (non-sulfhydryl-containing)
Therapeutic class: Antihypertensive, vasodilator
Pregnancy category: C (first trimester), D (later trimesters)

Indications and Dosages

➤ *To manage hypertension*

TABLETS

Adults. *Initial:* 1 mg daily, increased every wk based on clinical response. Dosage may be given in two daily doses if antihypertensive effect diminishes before 24 hr. *Usual:* 2 to 4 mg daily. *Maximum:* 8 mg daily.

DOSAGE ADJUSTMENT Initial dosage increased to 2 mg daily for blacks with hypertension. Initial dosage reduced to 0.5 mg for patients also receiving a diuretic, those with a creatinine clearance of less than or equal to 30 ml/min/1.73 m², and those with cirrhosis.

➤ *To treat heart failure after MI*

TABLETS

Adults. *Initial:* 1 mg daily. *Usual:* 4 mg or more daily. *Maximum:* 8 mg daily.

Route	Onset	Peak	Duration
P.O.	2 hr	8 hr	24 hr

Contraindications

History of angioedema related to previous treatment with ACE inhibitor, hypersensitivity to trandolapril or its components

Interactions

DRUGS

allopurinol, bone marrow depressants (such as methotrexate), corticosteroids (systemic), cytostatic drugs, procainamide: Increased risk of potentially fatal neutropenia or agranulocytosis
antacids: Decreased blood trandolapril level
cyclosporine, potassium-containing drugs, potassium-sparing diuretics, potassium supplements: Increased risk of hyperkalemia
diuretics, other antihypertensives: Increased hypotensive effects
lithium: Increased blood lithium level and risk of lithium toxicity
NSAIDs, sympathomimetics: Possibly reduced antihypertensive effects

FOODS

high-potassium diet, low-sodium milk, potassium-containing salt substitutes: Increased risk of hyperkalemia

ACTIVITIES

alcohol use: Possibly increased hypotensive effect

Mechanism of Action

Reduces blood pressure by inhibiting the conversion of angiotensin I to angiotensin II. Angiotensin II is a potent vasoconstrictor that stimulates the renal cortex to secrete aldosterone. Decreased release of aldosterone reduces sodium and water retention and increases their excretion, thereby reducing blood pressure. Trandolapril may also inhibit renal and vascular production of angiotensin II.

Adverse Reactions

CNS: Dizziness, fatigue, fever, headache
CV: Hypotension, orthostatic hypotension
EENT: Loss of taste
GI: Diarrhea, nausea
GU: Decreased libido, impotence
MS: Myalgia
RESP: Cough, dyspnea, upper respiratory tract infection
SKIN: Pruritus, rash
Other: Angioedema

Nursing Considerations

•**WARNING** Closely monitor blood pressure during first 2 weeks of therapy and whenever dosage is adjusted, especially in patients with heart failure, hyponatremia, or severe volume or sodium loss. If excessive hypotension occurs, notify prescriber immediately, place patient in supine position, and infuse I.V. normal saline solution, as prescribed.

T

•**WARNING** Be alert for signs and symptoms of angioedema. If swelling of tongue, glottis, or larynx causes airway obstruction, notify prescriber and be prepared to discontinue drug and administer emergency measures, including subcutaneous epinephrine 1:1,000 (0.3 to 0.5 ml).

•Continue to monitor patient's blood pressure to assess drug's long-term effectiveness.

PATIENT TEACHING

•Instruct patient to notify prescriber immediately and stop taking trandolapril if she experiences swelling of face, eyes, lips, or tongue or has difficulty breathing.

•Explain that drug may cause dizziness and light-headedness, especially during first few days of therapy. Advise patient to avoid driving and other potentially hazardous activities until drug's CNS effects are known and to notify prescriber immediately if she faints.

•Inform female patient of childbearing age about risks of taking trandolapril during pregnancy, especially during second and third trimesters. Urge her to use effective contraceptive method and to notify prescriber immediately if she becomes or thinks she might be pregnant.

•Advise patient planning to undergo surgery or anesthesia to inform specialist that she's taking trandolapril.

•Instruct patient to consult prescriber before using potassium supplements or salt substitutes containing potassium.

•Inform patient about possible loss of taste, which may result in weight loss. Reassure her that loss of taste is usually reversed after 2 to 3 months.

tranylcypromine sulfate

Parnate

Class and Category

Chemical class: Nonhydrazine derivative
Therapeutic class: Antidepressant
Pregnancy category: Not rated

Indications and Dosages

➤ *To treat major depressive episodes without melancholia*

TABLETS

Adults and adolescents over age 16. 30 mg/day in divided doses. After first 2 wk, increased by 10 mg every 1 to 2 wk, as prescribed. *Maintenance:* 10 to 40 mg daily. *Maximum:* 60 mg daily.

DOSAGE ADJUSTMENT For elderly patients, initial dosage possibly reduced to 2.5 to 5 mg daily and increased by 2.5 to 5 mg every 3 to 4 days, as prescribed; maximum dosage 45 mg daily. Alternative therapies should be carefully considered for patients over age 60.

Route	Onset	Peak	Duration
P.O.	7 to 10 days	4 to 8 wk	10 days

Mechanism of Action

Reversibly binds to MAO, reducing its activity and resulting in increased levels of neurotransmitters, including dopamine, epinephrine, and norepinephrine. This regulation of CNS neurotransmitters helps ease depression.

Contraindications

Cardiovascular disease; cerebrovascular disease; heart failure; hepatic disease; history of headaches; hypersensitivity to tranylcypromine or its components; hypertension; pheochromocytoma; severe renal impairment; use of anesthetics, antihypertensives, bupropion, buspirone, carbamazepine, CNS depressants, cyclobenzaprine, dextromethorphan, meperidine, other MAO inhibitors, selective serotonin-reuptake inhibitors, sympathomimetics, or tricyclic antidepressants

Interactions

DRUGS

amoxapine, bupropion, maprotiline, selective serotonin-reuptake inhibitors, trazodone, tricyclic antidepressants: Increased risk of severe hypertensive crisis, increased anticholinergic effects
anticonvulsants: Additive CNS depression
antihistamines: Possibly prolonged anticholinergic and CNS depressant effects
antipsychotics: Additive anticholinergic, hypotensive, and sedative effects
beta blockers: Possibly worsened bradycardia
bromocriptine: Increased blood prolactin level and interference with bromocriptine effects
buspirone: Increased blood pressure
dextroamphetamine, isometheptene, local anesthetics, naphazoline, oxymetazoline, psy-

chostimulants, sympathomimetics, tetrahydrozoline, xylometazoline: Increased risk of severe hypertensive reaction
dextromethorphan, tryptophan: Increased risk of serotonin syndrome
diuretics: Additive hypotensive effects
doxapram: Increased vasopressor effects
furazolidone, procarbazine, selegiline: Increased risk of severe hyperpyretic or hypertensive crisis, seizures, or death
guanadrel, guanethidine: Increased risk of moderate to severe hypertension
insulin, oral antidiabetic drugs: Possibly prolonged hypoglycemic response
levodopa: Increased vasopressor effects, hypertension, adverse cardiovascular effects
meperidine: Increased risk of coma, diaphoresis, excitation, hypertension, rigidity, severe respiratory depression, shock, and, possibly, death
methyldopa: Increased risk of hallucinations
metrizamide, tramadol: Increased risk of seizures
succinylcholine: Possibly prolonged succinylcholine effects

FOODS
aged cheese; avocadoes; bananas; fava or broad beans; cured sausage (bologna, pepperoni, salami, and summer sausage) or other meat; overripe fruit; pickled fish, meats, or poultry; protein extract; smoked fish, meats, or poultry; soy sauce; yeast extract; and other foods high in pressor amines, such as tyramine: Increased risk of sudden, severe hypertension
caffeine-containing beverages and foods: Increased risk of severe hypertensive crisis and dangerous arrhythmias

ACTIVITIES
alcohol-containing products that also may contain tyramine, such as beer (including reduced-alcohol and alcohol-free beer), wine (red and white), sherry, hard liquor, liqueurs: Increased risk of hypertensive crisis

Adverse Reactions

CNS: Anxiety, chills, dizziness, drowsiness, fever, headache, insomnia, intracranial hemorrhage, paresthesia, restlessness, suicidal ideation, tremor, weakness
CV: Bradycardia, chest pain, edema, hypertensive crisis, orthostatic hypotension, palpitations, tachycardia

EENT: Blurred vision, dry mouth, mydriasis, photophobia, tinnitus
GI: Abdominal pain, anorexia, constipation, diarrhea, nausea, vomiting
GU: Ejaculation disorders, impotence, urine retention
HEME: Agranulocytosis, anemia, leukopenia, thrombocytopenia
MS: Muscle spasms, myoclonus, neck stiffness
SKIN: Clammy skin, diaphoresis

Nursing Considerations
•Monitor patient's blood pressure during tranylcypromine therapy to detect hypertensive crisis and to decrease the risk of orthostatic hypotension.
•**WARNING** Notify prescriber immediately if patient has signs of hypertensive crisis, such as chest pain, headache, neck stiffness, and palpitations. Expect to stop drug right away.
•Anticipate that therapeutic response may not occur for up to 4 weeks.
•Expect drug to aggravate symptoms of Parkinson's disease, including muscle spasms, myoclonic movement, and tremor.
•Keep dietary restrictions in place for at least 2 weeks after stopping tranylcypromine because of the slow recovery from drug's enzyme-inhibiting effects.
•Expect to stop tranylcypromine 10 days before elective surgery, as prescribed, to avoid hypotension.
•Be aware that abrupt cessation of drug can precipitate original symptoms.
•Check diabetic patient's blood glucose level often to detect possible loss of control.
•Anticipate that coadministration with a selective serotonin reuptake inhibitor may cause confusion, seizures, severe hypertension, and other, less severe symptoms.
•Monitor severely depressed patients, including children and teens, for suicidal tendencies. Take safety measures, and notify prescriber immediately.
•Assess patient for sudden insomnia. If it develops, notify prescriber and be prepared to administer drug early in the day.

PATIENT TEACHING
•Instruct patient to avoid foods that contain cheese and that are high in tyramine, such as anchovies, avocadoes, bananas, beer, canned figs, caviar, Chianti wine, chocolate, dried fruit, fava beans, liqueurs, meat tenderizers, overripe fruit, pickled herring, raspberries,

T

sauerkraut, sherry, sour cream, soy sauce, yeast extract, and yogurt while taking tranylcypromine.
• Urge patient to continue dietary restrictions for at least 2 weeks after tranylcypromine therapy stops.
• Advise patient to notify prescriber immediately about chest pain, dizziness, headache, nausea, neck stiffness, palpitations, rapid heart rate, sweating, and vomiting.
• Urge patient to avoid alcohol and excessive caffeine intake during therapy.
• Encourage patient to change positions slowly to minimize effects of orthostatic hypotension.
• Advise patient to avoid hazardous activities until drug's CNS effects are known.
• Caution patient not to take any other prescribed or OTC drugs without consulting prescriber.
• Caution patient not to stop tranylcypromine abruptly to avoid recurrence of original symptoms.
• Instruct female patient to use effective contraception during tranylcypromine therapy to prevent fetal abnormalities. Urge her to notify prescriber immediately about known or suspected pregnancy.
• **WARNING** Urge parents to watch their child or adolescent closely for abnormal thinking or behavior or increased aggression or hostility. Stress importance of notifying prescriber about unusual changes.

trazodone hydrochloride

Trazon, Trialodine

Class and Category
Chemical class: Triazolopyridine derivative
Therapeutic class: Antidepressant, anxiolytic
Pregnancy category: C

Indications and Dosages
➤ *To treat major depression, with or without generalized anxiety*
TABLETS
Adults. *Initial:* 150 mg daily in divided doses, increased by 50 mg daily every 3 to 4 days, p.r.n., as prescribed. *Maximum:* 400 mg daily for outpatients, 600 mg daily for inpatients.
Children ages 6 to 18. *Initial:* 1.5 to 2 mg/kg daily in divided doses, increased every 3 to

4 days, p.r.n., as prescribed. *Maximum:* 6 mg/kg daily in divided doses.

Route	Onset	Peak	Duration
P.O.	1 to 2 wk	Unknown	Unknown

Mechanism of Action
Blocks serotonin reuptake along the presynaptic neuronal membrane, causing an antidepressant effect. Trazodone exerts an alpha-adrenergic blocking action and produces modest histamine blockade, causing a sedative effect. It also inhibits the vasopressor response to norepinephrine, which reduces blood pressure.

Contraindications
Hypersensitivity to trazodone or its components, recovery from acute MI

Interactions
DRUGS
anticonvulsants: Decreased seizure threshold
antihypertensives: Increased risk of excessive hypotension
anxiolytics, brompheniramine, carbinoxamine, chlorpheniramine, clemastine, dimenhydrinate, diphenhydramine, doxylamine, general anesthetics, methdilazine, opioid analgesics, phenothiazines, sedative-hypnotics, skeletal muscle relaxants: Increased CNS depression, increased risk of respiratory depression and hypotension
barbiturates: Decreased seizure threshold and barbiturate effects, increased drowsiness
buspirone, selective serotonin-reuptake inhibitors, tricyclic antidepressants: Possibly excessive serotonergic stimulation
carbamazepine: Decreased trazodone level
clonidine: Interference with clonidine's antihypertensive effect
digoxin: Possibly increased blood digoxin level and risk of digitalis toxicity
erythromycin, indinavir, itraconazole, ketoconazole, nefazodone, protease inhibitors, ritonavir: Possibly increased blood trazodone level with increased risk of adverse effects
MAO inhibitors: Increased serotonin effects
warfarin: Decreased anticoagulation response
ACTIVITIES
alcohol use: Increased CNS depression, risk of respiratory depression and hypotension

Adverse Reactions
CNS: Dizziness, drowsiness, fatigue, headache, light-headedness, nervousness, suicidal ideation, syncope, tremor
CV: Arrhythmias, hypotension, orthostatic hypotension, palpitations
EENT: Blurred vision, dry mouth
GI: Constipation, indigestion, nausea, vomiting
GU: Anorgasmia, ejaculation disorders, increased libido, priapism
SKIN: Pruritus, rash

Nursing Considerations
•Give trazodone shortly after the patient has a meal or light snack to reduce nausea.
•Give larger portion of daily dose at bedtime if drowsiness occurs.
•Because trazadone's mechanism of action is similar to that of selective serotonin reuptake inhibitors, expect high doses (6 to 8 mg/kg) to increase blood serotonin level and low doses (0.05 to 1 mg/kg) to decrease blood serotonin level.
•Expect most patients who respond to trazodone to do so by the end of the second week of therapy.
•Closely monitor depressed patients, including children and teens, for suicidal thoughts and tendencies. Notify prescriber if they occur, and take suicide precautions according to facility policy.
•Be aware that adverse CNS reactions usually improve after patient completes a few weeks of therapy.
•**WARNING** Be aware that trazodone therapy may increase the risk of priapism.

PATIENT TEACHING
•Urge patient to avoid taking trazodone on an empty stomach because doing so may increase the risk of dizziness or light-headedness.
•Caution patient to avoid potentially hazardous activities during therapy.
•Advise patient not to fast during trazodone therapy because of possible adverse CNS reactions.
•Instruct male patient to notify prescriber immediately about priapism.
•**WARNING** Urge parents to watch their child or adolescent closely for abnormal thinking or behavior or increased aggression or hostility. Stress importance of notifying prescriber about unusual changes.

treprostinil sodium
Remodulin

Class and Category
Chemical class: Prostaglandin, tricyclic benzidene analog
Therapeutic class: Vasodilator
Pregnancy category: B

Indications and Dosages
➤ *To treat pulmonary artery hypertension in patients who have New York Heart Association Class II to IV symptoms in order to diminish exercise-induced symptoms*

I.V. INFUSION, SUBCUTANEOUS INFUSION
Adults. *Initial:* 1.25 nanograms/kg/min. *Maintenance:* Infusion rate increased in increments of no more than 1.25 nanograms/kg/min each wk for first 4 wk, and in increments of no more than 2.5 nanograms/kg/min each wk thereafter, as needed. *Maximum:* 40 nanograms/kg/min.
DOSAGE ADJUSTMENT If initial dosage isn't tolerated or if patient has mild to moderate hepatic insufficiency, decrease to 0.625 nanogram/kg/min (using ideal body weight).

Mechanism of Action
Acts directly on pulmonary and systemic arterial vascular beds to produce vasodilation. Vasodilatory effects reduce right and left ventricular afterload and increase cardiac output and stroke volume. These effects improve symptoms of pulmonary hypertension, such as dyspnea, and enable patients with pulmonary hypertension to walk farther with less discomfort.

Contraindications
Hypersensitivity to treprostinil, its components, or structurally related compounds

Interactions
DRUGS
anticoagulants: Increased risk of bleeding
antihypertensives, diuretics, other vasodilators: Increased risk of hypotension

Adverse Reactions
CNS: Anxiety, dizziness, fatigue, headache, restlessness

CV: Chest pain, edema, hypotension, right ventricular heart failure, vasodilatation
EENT: Jaw pain
GI: Diarrhea, nausea, vomiting
HEME: Thrombocytopenia
RESP: Dyspnea
MS: Bone or jaw pain
SKIN: Cellulitis, pallor, pruritus, rash
Other: Infusion site pain or reaction (erythema, hematoma, induration, pain, paresthesia, rash, swelling, thrombophlebitis)

Nursing Considerations

• Use treprostinil cautiously in patients with hepatic or renal impairment.
• Assess patient's ability to care for an I.V. or subcutaneous catheter and to use an infusion pump. Discuss findings with prescriber before starting treprostinil therapy.
• Be aware that drug shouldn't be diluted when given subcutaneously.
• When drug will be given I.V., dilute with sterile water for injection or normal saline solution according to instructions provided. Watch for blood-borne infections and sepsis in patients receiving drug through an indwelling central venous catheter, which increases the risk.
• Calculate infusion rate using the formula provided in the package insert, or refer to charts in package insert to find infusion delivery rate for prescribed dosage and administration route.
• **WARNING** Don't abruptly stop treprostinil infusion or make sudden large reductions in dose because symptoms of pulmonary hypertension may worsen.
• Assess patient often for drug effectiveness and for adverse reactions. Know that the goal of dosage adjustments is to find a dose that will improve symptoms of pulmonary hypertension, such as dyspnea and fatigue, while minimizing adverse effects, such as headache, nausea, vomiting, restlessness, anxiety, and infusion site pain or reaction.
• Monitor patients with mild to moderate hepatic insufficiency closely for adverse reactions, especially after dosage increases, because treprostinil is metabolized mainly by the liver.
• Be aware that patient must be discharged with a backup infusion pump. It should be adjustable to about 0.002 ml/hr and have alarms that indicate occlusion/no delivery, low battery, programming error, and motor malfunction. Also, the pump should have a delivery accuracy of ±6% or better, be positive-pressure driven, and have a reservoir made of polyvinyl chloride, polypropylene, or glass. Make sure patient has additional I.V. or subcutaneous infusion sets to prevent potential interruptions in drug delivery.

PATIENT TEACHING
• Explain to patient that treprostinil is infused continuously through an I.V. or subcutaneous catheter via an infusion pump.
• Teach patient to operate and maintain the I.V. or subcutaneous infusion pump and to recognize the drug's adverse effects.
• To reduce the risk of infection, caution patient to always use aseptic technique when preparing and giving drug.
• Tell patient that a vial of drug shouldn't be used beyond 14 days after opening and that once the drug is placed in the pump's reservoir, it shouldn't be used after 72 hours.
• Instruct patient to store treprostinil vials at room temperature (about 25° C [77° F]).
• Inform patient that drug will be needed for prolonged periods, possibly years. Stress the importance of not stopping drug abruptly or making sudden large reductions in dosage without consulting prescriber because symptoms could worsen.
• Make sure patient understands that treprostinil use doesn't preclude the subsequent use of an alternative I.V. prostacyclin therapy such as epoprostenol.
• Make sure patient has emergency contact information for problems or questions about giving treprostinil at home.

triamcinolone

Aristocort, Aristopak, Atolone, Kenacort, Nasacort AQ

triamcinolone acetonide

AllerNaze, Azmacort, Cenocort A-40, Cinonide-40, Kenaject-40, Kenalog-10, Kenalog-40, Ken-Jec-40, Nasacort, Nasacort HFA, Robalog, Tac-3, Triam-A, Triamonide, Tri-Kort, Trilog

triamcinolone diacetate

Acetocot, Amcort, Aristocort, Aristocort Forte, Articulose-LA, Cenocort Forte,

Cinalone 40, Clinacort, Kenacort Diacetate, Tilone, Tramacort-D, Triam-Forte, Triamolone 40, Tristoject

triamcinolone hexacetonide

Aristospan

Class and Category

Chemical class: Synthetic glucocorticoid
Therapeutic class: Anti-inflammatory, immunosuppressant
Pregnancy category: C (nasal and oral inhalation), Not rated (oral and parenteral)

Indications and Dosages

➤ *To prevent bronchospasm or provide long-term corticosteroid treatment to control asthma*

ORAL INHALATION (TRIAMCINOLONE ACETONIDE)

Adults and children age 12 and over. *Initial:* 2 metered sprays (200 mcg) t.i.d. or q.i.d. *Maintenance:* Individualized dosage given b.i.d. *Maximum:* 16 metered sprays daily in divided doses.
Children ages 6 to 11. 2 to 4 metered sprays (200 to 400 mcg) b.i.d. to q.i.d. *Maximum:* 12 metered sprays daily.

➤ *To treat acute rheumatic carditis, berylliosis, and Hodgkin's disease; as adjunct to treat fulminating or disseminated pulmonary tuberculosis (with appropriate antituberculosis therapy)*

SYRUP (TRIAMCINOLONE DIACETATE), TABLETS (TRIAMCINOLONE)

Adults and children age 12 and over. *Initial:* 4 to 48 mg daily as a single dose or in divided doses. Some patients may require an initial dose of 60 mg.
Children under age 12. 0.42 to 1.7 mg/kg daily as a single dose or in divided doses.

I.M. INJECTION (TRIAMCINOLONE ACETONIDE)

Adults and children age 12 and over. 40 to 80 mg every 4 wk, as needed.
Children ages 6 to 11. 40 mg every 4 wk, as needed, or 30 to 200 mcg/kg every 1 to 7 days.

I.M. INJECTION (TRIAMCINOLONE DIACETATE)

Adults and children age 12 and over. 40 mg every wk, or 4 to 7 times the daily P.O. dose as a single injection every 4 days to every 4 wk.
Children ages 6 to 11. 40 mg/wk.

➤ *To relieve inflammation caused by acute gouty arthritis, acute nonspecific tenosynovitis, acute or subacute bursitis, epicondylitis, osteoarthritis, posttraumatic osteoarthritis, rheumatoid arthritis, and synovitis*

SYRUP (TRIAMCINOLONE DIACETATE)

Adults and children age 12 and over. 4 to 48 mg daily as a single dose or in divided doses, adjusted, as prescribed, to lowest effective dose based on clinical response.

TABLETS (TRIAMCINOLONE)

Adults and children age 12 and over. 8 to 16 mg daily in divided doses t.i.d. or q.i.d., adjusted, as prescribed, to lowest effective dose based on clinical response.

SYRUP (TRIAMCINOLONE DIACETATE), TABLETS (TRIAMCINOLONE)

Children ages 6 to 11. 0.42 to 1.7 mg/kg daily as a single dose or in divided doses, adjusted based on clinical response.

I.M. INJECTION (TRIAMCINOLONE ACETONIDE)

Adults and children age 12 and over. 40 to 80 mg every 4 wk.
Children ages 6 to 11. 40 mg every 4 wk.

I.M. INJECTION (TRIAMCINOLONE DIACETATE)

Adults and children age 6 and over. 40 mg every wk as single injection, repeated every 4 wk if needed.

INTRA-ARTICULAR OR INTRABURSAL INJECTION (TRIAMCINOLONE ACETONIDE)

Adults and children age 6 and over. 2.5 to 15 mg, as needed.

INTRA-ARTICULAR OR INTRASYNOVIAL INJECTION (TRIAMCINOLONE DIACETATE)

Adults. 5 to 40 mg, repeated as prescribed every 1 to 8 wk, as needed.

INTRA-ARTICULAR INJECTION (TRIAMCINOLONE HEXACETONIDE)

Adults. 2 to 20 mg, repeated as prescribed every 3 to 4 wk, as needed.

➤ *To treat primary (Addison's disease) or secondary adrenocortical insufficiency*

SYRUP (TRIAMCINOLONE DIACETATE)

Adults and children age 12 and over. 4 to 12 mg daily as a single dose or in divided doses.

SYRUP (TRIAMCINOLONE DIACETATE), TABLETS (TRIAMCINOLONE)

Children ages 6 to 11. 0.12 mg (base)/kg daily as a single dose or in divided doses.

➤ *To treat inflammatory dermatoses*

T

TABLETS (TRIAMCINOLONE)
Adults and children age 12 and over. 8 to 16 mg daily. *Usual:* 1 to 2 mg daily.

➤ *To treat disseminated lupus erythematosus*
TABLETS (TRIAMCINOLONE)
Adults and children age 12 and over. 20 to 30 mg daily. *Usual:* 3 to 30 mg daily.

➤ *To treat nephrotic syndrome*
TABLETS (TRIAMCINOLONE)
Adults and children age 12 and over. 16 to 20 mg daily.

➤ *To relieve symptoms of perennial and seasonal allergic rhinitis*
TABLETS (TRIAMCINOLONE)
Adults and children age 12 and over. 8 to 12 mg daily. *Usual:* 2 to 6 mg daily.
Children ages 6 to 11. 0.42 to 1.7 mg/kg daily as a single dose or in divided doses.

NASAL INHALATION (NASACORT)
Adults and children age 12 and over. *Initial:* 220 mcg daily in 2 sprays (55 mcg each)/nostril. *Maintenance:* 110 mcg daily in 1 spray (55 mcg)/nostril. *Maximum:* 440 mcg (8 sprays daily).

NASAL INHALATION (NASACORT AQ)
Adults and children age 12 and over. *Initial:* 110 mcg daily in 2 sprays (55 mcg each)/nostril. *Maintenance:* 55 mcg daily in 1 spray/nostril. *Maximum:* 220 mcg or 4 sprays daily.
Children ages 6 to 11. 110 mcg daily in 1 spray (55 mcg each)/nostril. *Maximum:* 220 mcg or 4 sprays daily.
Children ages 2 to 5. 110 mcg daily in 1 spray (55 mcg)/nostril. *Maximum:* 100 mcg or 2 sprays daily.

NASAL INHALATION (NASACORT HFA)
Adults and children age 12 and over. *Initial:* 220 mcg daily in 2 sprays (55 mcg each)/nostril. May be increased to 440 mcg daily in 4 sprays/nostril, as needed.
Children ages 6 to 11. 220 mcg daily in 2 sprays (55 mcg each)/nostril.

NASAL INHALATION (ALLERNAZE)
Adults and children age 12 and over. *Initial:* 200 mcg daily in 2 sprays (50 mcg each)/nostril. *Maximum:* 400 mcg daily in 4 sprays (50 mcg each)/nostril or divided into 2 daily doses.

➤ *To treat chronic idiopathic thrombocytopenic purpura*
TABLETS (TRIAMCINOLONE)
Adults and children age 12 and over. 0.8 mg/kg daily.

Route	Onset	Peak	Duration
P.O. (tablets)	Unknown	1 to 2 hr	2.25 days
I.M. (acetonide)	24 to 48 hr	Unknown	1 to 6 wk
I.M. (diacetate)	Slow	Unknown	4 days to 4 wk
Inhalation	12 hr	3 to 4 hr	Unknown
Intra-articular, intrabursal (acetonide)	Unknown	Unknown	Several wk
Intra-articular, intrasynovial (diacetate)	Unknown	Unknown	1 to 8 wk

Mechanism of Action
Inhibits the release of prostaglandins and leukotrienes, thus reducing immediate and late-phase allergic responses in chronic asthma. Triamcinolone also:
• decreases peribronchial edema and mucus secretion by inhibiting the binding of allergens to immunoglobulin E antibodies on the surface of mast cells, thereby inactivating the release of chemotactic substances
• decreases inflammation by interfering with leukocyte adhesion to capillary walls
• inhibits the release of leukocytic acid hydrolases, preventing macrophage accumulation at the infection site
• inhibits histamine and kinin release, preventing the formation of scar tissue.

Incompatibilities
Don't mix triamcinolone hexacetonide with parenteral local anesthetics because precipitation can occur.

Contraindications
Acute status asthmaticus (inhalation form), hypersensitivity to triamcinolone or its components, live-virus vaccine therapy, systemic fungal infection

Interactions
DRUGS
amphotericin B, ethacrynic acid, furosemide, thiazide diuretics: Increased potassium-wasting effect, severe hypokalemia

aspirin: Increased blood salicylate level, increased risk of salicylate toxicity
barbiturates, carbamazepine, phenytoin, rifampin: Increased triamcinolone metabolism
cholinesterase inhibitors: Increased risk of severe muscle weakness in patients with myasthenia gravis
digitalis glycosides: Increased risk of arrhythmias and digitalis toxicity
estrogens: Increased triamcinolone effects
insulin, oral antidiabetic drugs: Increased blood glucose level
isoproterenol: Increased risk of cardiotoxicity
live-virus vaccines: Decreased antibody response, increased risk of neurologic complications
neuromuscular blockers: Increased risk of hypokalemia and enhanced neuromuscular blockade
NSAIDs: Increased risk of adverse GI effects
toxoids: Decreased resistance to toxoids

Adverse Reactions

CNS: Dizziness, emotional lability, exacerbated psychosis, fatigue, headache, insomnia, restlessness, seizures, vertigo
CV: Edema, heart failure, hypertension
EENT: Altered sense of smell or taste, cataracts, dry mouth, epistaxis (nasal form), glaucoma, hoarseness, nasal congestion, nasal irritation (inhalation form), nasal septal perforation (nasal form), oropharyngeal candidiasis, pharyngitis, posterior subcapsular cataracts, rhinorrhea, secondary ocular infection, sinusitis, sneezing
ENDO: Cushing's syndrome, diabetes mellitus, growth retardation (children)
GI: Abdominal pain, constipation, diarrhea, dyspepsia, esophageal ulceration, gastritis, nausea, vomiting
GU: Cystitis, renal disease, UTI, vaginitis
MS: Bone mineral density loss, bursitis, muscle wasting or weakness, myalgia, osteoporosis, tenosynovitis
RESP: Asthma, bronchitis, bronchospasm (inhalation form), chest congestion, dyspnea, increased cough
SKIN: Ecchymosis, petechiae (parenteral form), photosensitivity, pruritus, rash, striae, urticaria
Other: Anaphylaxis; angioedema; facial edema; flu syndrome; herpes infection; impaired wound healing; injection site atrophy, induration, pain, soreness, and sterile abscess; weight gain

Nursing Considerations

•Triamcinolone should be administered with extreme caution, if at all, in patients who have active or quiescent tuberculosis infection of the respiratory tract, untreated fungal or bacterial infection, systemic viral or parasitic infection, or ocular herpes simplex because this drug can make these infections worse.
•Give oral form of triamcinolone with meals to minimize GI distress.
•Use calibrated device to measure liquid doses.
•If necessary, crush tablets and mix with food or fluids.
•Shake I.M. suspension thoroughly before drawing it into syringe.
•Be aware that specialized training may be needed to administer parenteral triamcinolone.
•Don't administer parenteral forms of triamcinolone I.V.
•Be aware that triamcinolone may reactivate tuberculosis in patients who have a history of it.
•Monitor patients, especially infants, closely for gasping syndrome because parenteral triamcinolone contains benzyl alcohol. Exposure to high doses may result in toxicity evidenced by life-threatening hypotension and metabolic acidosis.
•**WARNING** Assess patient for signs and symptoms of adrenal insufficiency (fatigue, hypotension, lassitude, nausea, vomiting, and weakness) during times of stress, such as infection, surgery, or trauma. Notify prescriber immediately if you detect these signs and symptoms because adrenal insufficiency may be life-threatening.
•Be aware that, although rare, bone mineral density loss and osteoporosis may occur, which may increase risk of fractures, especially in patients on prolonged triamcinolone therapy.

Patient Teaching
•Caution patient not to adjust triamcinolone dosage without consulting prescriber.
•Teach patient how to administer nasal aerosols properly, using manufacturer's instructions, to avoid nasal irritation.
•Instruct patient to dispose of aerosol canister after 240 uses (100 uses for Nasacort HFA) because dosage may not be correct after that time.

•Teach patient how to use nasal spray, including how to prime spray pump bottle before use. Caution patient to not to get nasal spray in eyes. If this occurs, patient should rinse his eyes well with water.

•Inform patient that maximum benefit of triamcinolone therapy may not occur for up to 2 weeks.

•Advise patient to notify prescriber immediately if asthma fails to respond to inhaled drug because additional systemic therapy may be needed.

•Caution patient to avoid exposure to people who have chickenpox or measles throughout triamcinolone therapy and for 12 months afterward.

•Advise patient to have periodic eye examinations during long-term therapy because triamcinolone can cause glaucoma or ocular nerve damage.

triamterene

Dyrenium

Class and Category

Chemical class: Pterdine derivative
Therapeutic class: Diuretic
Pregnancy category: B

Indications and Dosages

➤ *To treat edema in cirrhosis, heart failure, and nephrotic syndrome*

CAPSULES

Adults. *Initial:* 25 to 100 mg daily. *Maximum:* 300 mg daily.

Route	Onset	Peak	Duration
P.O.	2 to 4 hr	1 to several days	7 to 9 hr

Mechanism of Action

Inhibits sodium reabsorption in distal convoluted tubules and cortical collecting ducts, causing sodium and water loss and enhancing potassium retention.

Contraindications

Anuria, diabetic nephropathy or renal disease linked to renal insufficiency, hyperkalemia (potassium level of 5.5 mEq/L or more), hypersensitivity to triamterene or its components, severe hepatic dysfunction

Interactions

DRUGS

ACE inhibitors, amiloride, angiotensin-II receptor antagonists, cyclosporine, heparin, potassium-containing drugs, potassium salts, potassium supplements, spironolactone: Increased risk of hyperkalemia

amantadine: Decreased amantadine clearance, possibly amantadine toxicity

antihypertensives: Increased antihypertensive effect

diuretics: Increased diuretic effect

folic acid: Possibly antagonized action of folic acid

indomethacin: Increased risk of renal impairment

lithium: Increased risk of lithium toxicity

NSAIDs: Decreased diuretic effect of triamterene, increased risk of hyperkalemia

oral antidiabetic drugs: Altered blood glucose control

Adverse Reactions

CNS: Dizziness, fatigue, headache, weakness
EENT: Dry mouth
ENDO: Hyperglycemia, hypoglycemia
GI: Diarrhea, nausea, vomiting
GU: Azotemia, elevated BUN and serum creatinine levels, renal calculi
SKIN: Jaundice, photosensitivity, rash

Nursing Considerations

•Be aware that triamterene shouldn't be given to patient with creatinine clearance below 10 ml/min/1.73 m^2 because this condition increases the risk of drug-induced hyperkalemia.

•Monitor serum potassium level during therapy, especially in patient with renal impairment or diabetes mellitus. Also monitor patient's BUN and serum creatinine levels to assess renal function and prevent hyperkalemia.

•Monitor patient for irregular heartbeat, which is usually the first sign of hyperkalemia.

•If you suspect hyperkalemia, obtain an ECG tracing, as ordered. A widened QRS complex or an arrhythmia requires prompt additional therapy.

•Monitor laboratory test results and watch for signs of metabolic or respiratory acidosis, which may occur suddenly in patient with

cardiac disease or uncontrolled diabetes mellitus.
•Monitor patient's serum uric acid and sodium levels, as ordered, because triamterene may reduce uric acid clearance and increase the risk of gout and hyperuricemia. This drug also may worsen preexisting hyponatremia.
•Monitor CBC with differential because drug may increase the risk of megaloblastic anemia in patient with folic acid deficiency.

PATIENT TEACHING
•Advise patient to take triamterene with food or milk.
•Instruct patient to avoid exposure to excessive heat or sunlight to prevent dehydration and, possibly, photosensitivity.
•Explain to patient with a history of gout that drug may increase the risk of an attack.
•Advise patient to notify prescriber about ineffective diuresis and unexplained weight gain during therapy.

triazolam

Alti-Triazolam (CAN), Apo-Triazo (CAN), Gen Triazolam (CAN), Halcion, Novo-Triolam (CAN)

Class, Category, and Schedule
Chemical class: Benzodiazepine
Therapeutic class: Sedative-hypnotic
Pregnancy category: X
Controlled substance schedule: IV

Indications and Dosages
➤ *To provide short-term management of insomnia*
TABLETS
Adults. 0.125 to 0.25 mg at bedtime. *Maximum:* 0.5 mg daily (for patients with inadequate response to usual dose).
DOSAGE ADJUSTMENT For elderly or debilitated patients, initial dosage reduced to 0.125 mg at bedtime and maximum dosage limited to 0.25 mg daily.

Route	Onset	Peak	Duration
P.O.	15 to 30 min	Unknown	Unknown

Contraindications
Hypersensitivity to triazolam or its components; itraconazole, ketoconazole, or nefazodone therapy; pregnancy

Mechanism of Action
Potentiates the effects of the inhibitory neurotransmitter gamma-aminobutyric acid, which increases the inhibition of the ascending reticular activating system and produces varying levels of CNS depression, including sedation, hypnosis, skeletal muscle relaxation, anticonvulsant activity, and coma.

Interactions
DRUGS
anxiolytics, barbiturates, brompheniramine, carbinoxamine, cetirizine, chlorpheniramine, clemastine, cyproheptadine, dimenhydrinate, diphenhydramine, doxylamine, general anesthetics, methdilazine, opioid analgesics, sedative-hypnotics, phenothiazines, promethazine, tramadol, tricyclic antidepressants, trimeprazine: Increased sedation, respiratory depression
cimetidine, diltiazem, disulfiram, erythromycin, probenecid, verapamil: Increased sedation
fluconazole: Increased blood triazolam level and effects
flumazenil: Increased risk of withdrawal symptoms
itraconazole, ketoconazole, nefazodone: Delayed triazolam elimination
oral contraceptives: Increased blood triazolam level
FOODS
grapefruit juice: Increased blood triazolam level and sedation
ACTIVITIES
alcohol use: Increased sedation, respiratory depression

Adverse Reactions
CNS: Anxiety, ataxia, complex behaviors (such as sleep driving), confusion, depression, dizziness, drowsiness, fatigue, headache, insomnia, nightmares, syncope, talkativeness, tremor, vertigo
EENT: Throat tightness
GI: Nausea, vomiting
RESP: Dyspnea
Other: Anaphylaxis, angioedema, physical and psychological dependence

Nursing Considerations
•Be aware that triazolam shouldn't be dis-

T

continued abruptly, even after only 1 to 2 weeks of therapy. Doing so can cause withdrawal symptoms, including abdominal cramps, confusion, depression, diaphoresis, hyperacusis, insomnia, irritability, nausea, nervousness, paresthesia, perceptual disturbances, photophobia, tachycardia, tremor, and vomiting.

•**WARNING** Assess patient for signs of physical and psychological dependence, and notify prescriber if they occur.

•Monitor patient's respiratory rate and depth and ABG results, as appropriate, because drug may worsen ventilatory failure in patient with pulmonary disease, such as severe COPD, respiratory depression, or sleep apnea. Use drug cautiously in patients with acute intermittent porphyria, myasthenia gravis, and severe renal impairment because it may aggravate these conditions.

•Take safety precautions for elderly patients because triazolam may impair cognitive and motor function and increase the risk for falls.

•Use drug cautiously in patients with advanced Parkinson's disease because it may worsen cognition, coordination, and psychosis.

•**WARNING** Monitor patient closely for hypersensitivity reactions such as dyspnea, throat tightness, nausea, vomiting, and swelling. If present, stop triazolam immediately, notify prescriber, and provide supportive care.

PATIENT TEACHING

•Instruct patient to take triazolam exactly as prescribed and not to stop taking it abruptly because of the risk of having withdrawal symptoms.

•Instruct patient to stop taking triazolam and seek emergency care if she has trouble breathing, throat tightness, nausea, vomiting, or abnormal swelling.

•Advise patient that drug may cause abnormal behaviors during sleep, such as driving a car, eating, talking on the phone, or having sex without any recall of the event. If family notices any such behavior or patient sees evidence of such behavior upon awakening, the prescriber should be notified.

•Caution patient about possible drowsiness during therapy.

•Urge patient to avoid alcohol consumption because it increases drug's sedative effects and risk of abnormal behaviors, such as sleep driving.

•Advise patient to notify prescriber about excessive drowsiness, known or suspected pregnancy, and nausea.

trifluoperazine hydrochloride

Apo-Trifluoperazine (CAN), PMS-Trifluoperazine (CAN)

Class and Category

Chemical class: Piperazine phenothiazine
Therapeutic class: Antianxiety, antipsychotic
Pregnancy category: Not rated

Indications and Dosages

➤ *To treat psychotic disorders*

SYRUP, TABLETS

Adults and adolescents. *Initial:* 2 to 5 mg b.i.d., increased gradually, as needed. *Maintenance:* 15 to 20 mg daily. *Maximum:* 40 mg daily.

Children age 6 and over. *Initial:* 1 mg daily or in divided doses b.i.d., increased gradually, as needed.

I.M. INJECTION

Adults and adolescents. 1 to 2 mg every 4 to 6 hr, as needed. *Maximum:* 10 mg daily.

Children age 6 and over. 1 mg daily or in divided doses b.i.d., as needed.

➤ *To relieve anxiety*

SYRUP, TABLETS, I.M. INJECTION

Adults and adolescents. *Initial:* 1 to 2 mg daily, increased gradually, as needed. *Maximum:* 6 mg daily for 12 wk.

Mechanism of Action

Blocks postsynaptic dopamine receptors, increasing dopamine turnover and decreasing dopamine neurotransmission. This action may depress the areas of the brain that control activity and aggression, including the cerebral cortex, hypothalamus, and limbic system. Trifluoperazine may relieve anxiety by indirectly reducing arousal and increasing the filtering of internal stimuli to the reticular activating system.

Contraindications

Blood dyscrasias; bone marrow depression; cerebral arteriosclerosis; coma; coronary artery disease; hepatic dysfunction; hypersensitivity to trifluoperazine, other phenothiazines, or their components; myeloproliferative disorders; severe hypertension or hypotension; significant CNS depression; subcortical brain damage; use of high doses of CNS depressants

Interactions

DRUGS

adsorbent antidiarrheals, aluminum- and magnesium-containing antacids: Possibly inhibited absorption of oral trifluoperazine

amantadine, anticholinergics, antidyskinetics, antihistamines: Possibly intensified adverse anticholinergic effects, increased risk of trifluoperazine-induced hyperpyrexia

amphetamines: Decreased stimulant effect of amphetamines, decreased antipsychotic effect of trifluoperazine

anticonvulsants: Lowered seizure threshold

antithyroid drugs: Increased risk of agranulocytosis

apomorphine: Possibly decreased emetic response to apomorphine, additive CNS depression

appetite suppressants: Decreased effects of appetite suppressants

astemizole, cisapride, disopyramide, erythromycin, pimozide, probucol, procainamide, quinidine: Prolonged QT interval, increased risk of ventricular tachycardia

beta blockers: Increased blood levels of both drugs, possibly leading to additive hypotensive effect, arrhythmias, irreversible retinopathy, and tardive dyskinesia

bromocriptine: Impaired therapeutic effects of bromocriptine

CNS depressants: Additive CNS depression

ephedrine, metaraminol: Decreased vasopressor response to ephedrine

epinephrine: Blocked alpha-adrenergic effects of epinephrine

extrapyramidal reaction–causing drugs (droperidol, haloperidol, metoclopramide, metyrosine, risperidone): Increased severity and frequency of extrapyramidal reactions

hepatotoxic drugs: Increased risk of hepatotoxicity

hypotension-producing drugs: Possibly severe hypotension with syncope

levodopa: Decreased antidyskinetic effect of levodopa

lithium: Reduced absorption of oral trifluoperazine, possibly encephalopathy and additive extrapyramidal effects

MAO inhibitors, maprotiline, tricyclic antidepressants: Possibly prolonged and intensified sedative and anticholinergic effects, increased blood level of antidepressants, impaired trifluoperazine metabolism, increased risk of neuroleptic malignant syndrome

mephentermine: Decreased antipsychotic effect of trifluoperazine and vasopressor effect of mephentermine

methoxamine, phenylephrine: Decreased vasopressor effect and shortened duration of action of these drugs

metrizamide: Increased risk of seizures

opioid analgesics: Increased risk of CNS and respiratory depression, orthostatic hypotension, severe constipation, and urine retention

ototoxic drugs: Possibly masking of some symptoms of ototoxicity, such as dizziness, tinnitus, and vertigo

phenytoin: Lowered seizure threshold; inhibited phenytoin metabolism, possibly leading to phenytoin toxicity

photosensitizing drugs: Possibly additive photosensitivity and intraocular photochemical damage to choroid, lens, or retina

thiazide diuretics: Possibly hyponatremia and water intoxication

ACTIVITIES

alcohol use: Increased CNS and respiratory depression, increased hypotensive effect

Adverse Reactions

CNS: Akathisia, altered temperature regulation, dizziness, drowsiness, extrapyramidal reactions (dystonia, pseudoparkinsonism, tardive dyskinesia)

CV: Hypotension, orthostatic hypotension, tachycardia

EENT: Blurred vision, dry mouth, nasal congestion, ocular changes (deposits of fine particles in cornea and lens), pigmentary retinopathy

ENDO: Galactorrhea, gynecomastia

GI: Constipation, epigastric pain, nausea, vomiting

GU: Ejaculation disorders, menstrual irregularities, urine retention

SKIN: Contact dermatitis, decreased sweating, photosensitivity, pruritus, rash

Other: Injection site irritation and sterile abscess, weight gain

Nursing Considerations

•**WARNING** Trifluoperazine shouldn't be used to treat elderly patients with dementia-related psychosis because drug increases the risk of death in these patients

•Use trifluoperazine cautiously in patients with glaucoma because of drug's anticholinergic effect.

•Before administration, observe parenteral solution, which may turn slightly yellow without altering its potency. Don't use solution if discoloration is pronounced or precipitate is present.

•For I.M. administration, inject drug slowly and deep into upper outer quadrant of the buttocks. Keep patient in a supine position for 30 minutes after injection to minimize hypotensive effect.

•Rotate I.M. injection sites to avoid irritation and sterile abscesses.

•**WARNING** Watch closely for tardive dyskinesia, which may continue after treatment stops. Signs include uncontrolled movements of arms, body, cheeks, jaw, legs, mouth, or tongue. Notify prescriber if such signs occur.

•Closely monitor elderly patients and severely ill or dehydrated children. They're at increased risk for certain adverse CNS reactions.

•To prevent contact dermatitis, avoid skin contact with oral or injection solution.

PATIENT TEACHING

•Instruct patient to take trifluoperazine exactly as prescribed and not to stop taking drug abruptly or without consulting prescriber.

•Advise patient to take drug with food or a full glass of milk or water to minimize adverse GI reactions.

•Urge patient to consult prescriber before using other drugs because of possible interactions.

•Instruct patient to notify prescriber immediately if she experiences difficulty swallowing or speaking and her tongue protrudes from her mouth.

•Caution patient to avoid alcohol during therapy.

•Advise patient to avoid potentially hazardous activities until drug's CNS effects are known.

•Instruct patient to change position slowly to minimize effects of orthostatic hypotension.

•Urge patient to avoid exposure to the sun and extreme heat because drug may cause photosensitivity and interfere with thermoregulation. Encourage her to wear sunscreen when outdoors.

triflupromazine

Vesprin

Class and Category

Chemical class: Phenothiazine
Therapeutic class: Antiemetic, antipsychotic
Pregnancy category: Not rated

Indications and Dosages

➤ *To treat psychotic disorders*

I.M. INJECTION

Adults and adolescents. 60 mg, as needed. *Maximum:* 150 mg daily.

Children age 30 months and over. 0.2 to 0.25 mg/kg, as needed. *Maximum:* 10 mg daily.

➤ *To treat nausea and vomiting*

I.V. INJECTION

Adults. 1 mg, p.r.n. *Maximum:* 3 mg daily.

I.M. INJECTION

Adults and adolescents. 5 to 15 mg every 4 hr. *Maximum:* 60 mg daily.

Children age 30 months and over. 0.2 to 0.25 mg/kg, p.r.n. *Maximum:* 10 mg daily.

Mechanism of Action

Blocks postsynaptic dopamine receptors, increasing dopamine turnover and decreasing dopamine neurotransmission. This action may depress the areas of the brain that control activity and aggression, including the cerebral cortex, hypothalamus, and limbic system. Triflupromazine also prevents nausea and vomiting by inhibiting or blocking dopamine receptors in the medullary chemoreceptor trigger zone and, peripherally, by blocking the vagus nerve in the GI tract.

Contraindications

Blood dyscrasias, bone marrow depression,

cerebral arteriosclerosis, coma or severe CNS depression, concurrent use of large amount of CNS depressants, coronary artery disease, hepatic dysfunction, hypersensitivity to phenothiazines, severe hypertension or hypotension, subcortical brain damage

Interactions

DRUGS

amantadine, anticholinergics, antidyskinetics, antihistamines: Possibly intensified adverse anticholinergic effects and increased risk of triflupromazine-induced hyperpyrexia

amphetamines: Decreased stimulant effect of amphetamines, decreased antipsychotic effect of triflupromazine

anticonvulsants: Lowered seizure threshold

antithyroid drugs: Increased risk of agranulocytosis

apomorphine: Possibly decreased emetic response to apomorphine, additive CNS depression

appetite suppressants: Decreased anorectic effect of appetite suppressants

astemizole, cisapride, disopyramide, erythromycin, pimozide, probucol, procainamide, quinidine: Prolonged QT interval, increased risk of ventricular tachycardia

beta blockers: Increased blood levels of both drugs, possibly leading to additive hypotensive effect, arrhythmias, irreversible retinopathy, and tardive dyskinesia

bromocriptine: Impaired therapeutic effects of bromocriptine

CNS depressants: Additive CNS depressant effects

ephedrine: Decreased vasopressor response to ephedrine

epinephrine: Blocked alpha-adrenergic effects of epinephrine

extrapyramidal reaction–causing drugs (droperidol, haloperidol, metoclopramide, metyrosine, risperidone): Increased severity and frequency of extrapyramidal reactions

hepatotoxic drugs: Increased risk of hepatotoxicity

hypotension-producing drugs: Possibly severe hypotension with syncope

levodopa: Decreased antidyskinetic effect of levodopa

lithium: Possibly encephalopathy and additive extrapyramidal effects

MAO inhibitors, maprotiline, tricyclic anti-

depressants: Increased CNS depression, impaired triflupromazine metabolism, increased risk of neuroleptic malignant syndrome

mephentermine: Possibly antagonized antipsychotic effect of triflupromazine and vasopressor effect of mephentermine

metaraminol: Decreased vasopressor effect of metaraminol

methoxamine, phenylephrine: Decreased vasopressor effect and shortened duration of action of these drugs

metrizamide: Increased risk of seizures

opioid analgesics: Increased risk of CNS and respiratory depression, orthostatic hypotension, severe constipation, and urine retention

ototoxic drugs: Possibly masking of symptoms of ototoxicity, such as dizziness, tinnitus, and vertigo

phenytoin: Lowered seizure threshold; inhibited phenytoin metabolism, possibly leading to phenytoin toxicity

photosensitizing drugs: Possibly additive photosensitivity and intraocular photochemical damage to choroid, lens, or retina

thiazide diuretics: Possibly hyponatremia and water intoxication

ACTIVITIES

alcohol use: Increased CNS and respiratory depression, increased hypotensive effect

Adverse Reactions

CNS: Akathisia, altered temperature regulation, dizziness, drowsiness, extrapyramidal reactions (dystonia, pseudoparkinsonism, tardive dyskinesia)

CV: Hypotension, orthostatic hypotension, tachycardia

EENT: Blurred vision, dry mouth, nasal congestion, ocular changes (deposits of fine particles in cornea and lens), pigmentary retinopathy

ENDO: Galactorrhea, gynecomastia

GI: Constipation, epigastric pain, nausea, vomiting

GU: Ejaculation disorders, menstrual irregularities, urine retention

SKIN: Decreased sweating, photosensitivity, pruritus, rash

Other: Injection site irritation and sterile abscess, weight gain

Nursing Considerations

•Use triflupromazine cautiously in patients with glaucoma because of drug's anticholin-

ergic effects.
•Before administration, observe parenteral solution, which may turn slightly yellow without altering potency. Don't use solution if discoloration is pronounced or precipitate is present.
•Don't let solution come in contact with your skin because contact dermatitis may occur.
•For I.M. administration, slowly inject triflupromazine deep into upper outer quadrant of buttocks. Keep patient supine for 30 minutes afterward to minimize hypotensive effect.
•Rotate I.M. injection sites to avoid irritation and sterile abscesses.
•WARNING Watch closely for tardive dyskinesia, which may continue after treatment stops. Signs include uncontrolled movements of arms, body, cheeks, jaw, legs, mouth, or tongue. Notify prescriber if such signs occur.
•Closely monitor elderly patients and severely ill or dehydrated children. They're at increased risk for certain adverse CNS reactions.

PATIENT TEACHING
•Instruct patient to change position slowly to minimize effects of orthostatic hypotension.
•Urge patient to avoid potentially hazardous activities until triflupromazine's CNS effects are known.
•Instruct patient to notify prescriber immediately if she experiences difficulty swallowing or speaking and her tongue protrudes from her mouth.
•Caution patient to avoid alcohol during therapy.
•Urge patient to avoid exposure to the sun and extreme heat because drug may cause photosensitivity and interfere with thermoregulation. Encourage her to wear sunscreen when outdoors.

trihexyphenidyl hydrochloride

Apo-Trihex (CAN), Artane, PMS Trihexyphenidyl (CAN), Trihexane, Trihexy

Class and Category
Chemical class: Tertiary amine

Therapeutic class: Antidyskinetic
Pregnancy category: C

Indications and Dosages
➤ *To treat parkinsonism*
ELIXIR, TABLETS
Adults. *Initial:* 1 to 2 mg on day 1, divided into 3 equal doses and given with meals. Total daily dose increased by 2 mg every 3 to 5 days until desired response or maximum dose is reached. *Maximum:* 15 mg daily.
E.R. CAPSULES
Adults. 5 mg after breakfast; additional 5 mg 12 hr later, if needed. *Maximum:* 15 mg daily.
➤ *To treat drug-induced extrapyramidal symptoms*
TABLETS
Adults. 1 mg daily, increased to 5 to 15 mg/day, as prescribed, to control symptoms.

Route	Onset	Peak	Duration
P.O.	1 hr	Unknown	6 to 12 hr

Mechanism of Action
Blocks acetylcholine's action at cholinergic receptor sites, which restores normal dopamine and acetylcholine balance in the brain, relaxing muscle movement and decreasing drooling, rigidity, and tremor. Drug also may inhibit reuptake and storage of dopamine, prolonging its action.

Contraindications
Achalasia, bladder neck or prostatic obstruction, narrow-angle glaucoma, hypersensitivity to trihexyphenidyl or its components, megacolon, myasthenia gravis, pyloric or duodenal obstruction, stenosing peptic ulcer

Interactions
DRUGS
amantadine, anticholinergics, MAO inhibitors, tricyclic antidepressants: Increased anticholinergic effects
antidiarrheals (adsorbent): Possibly decreased therapeutic effects of trihexyphenidyl
chlorpromazine: Decreased blood chlorpro-

mazine level
CNS depressants: Increased sedative effect
levodopa: Increased efficacy of levodopa
ACTIVITIES
alcohol use: Increased sedation

Adverse Reactions
CNS: Confusion, dizziness, drowsiness, nervousness
EENT: Blurred vision; dry eyes, mouth, nose, or throat; mydriasis
GI: Constipation, nausea, vomiting
GU: Dysuria, urine retention
SKIN: Decreased sweating

Nursing Considerations
•Use trihexyphenidyl cautiously in patients with cardiovascular, hepatic, or renal disorders. Patients with cardiovascular disorders, such as atherosclerosis, hypertension, and ischemic heart disease, are at risk for tachycardia and coronary ischemia from drug's positive chronotropic effects. Hepatic and renal dysfunction increase the risk of adverse reactions.
•Before therapy begins, assess patient's muscle rigidity and tremor to establish a baseline. During therapy, reassess patient to detect improvement in these signs and evaluate drug effectiveness.
•Obtain patient's intraocular pressure before and periodically during trihexyphenidyl therapy, as ordered, because drug can precipitate incipient glaucoma.

PATIENT TEACHING
•Instruct patient to take trihexyphenidyl after meals.
•Teach patient not to break or chew E.R. capsules.
•Instruct patient to use calibrated device to measure elixir.
•Advise patient to avoid potentially hazardous activities until drug's CNS effects are known.
•Advise patient with dry eyes or increased contact lens awareness to use lubricating drops or stop wearing contact lenses during drug therapy.
•Caution patient being treated for parkinsonism not to stop taking trihexyphenidyl suddenly because doing so may worsen symptoms.
•Advise patient to maintain adequate hydration and avoid exercising during hot weather because trihexyphenidyl increases the risk of heatstroke.

trimethobenzamide hydrochloride

Benzacot, Tebamide, Tigan, Tribenzagan, Trimazide

Class and Category
Chemical class: Ethanolamine derivative
Therapeutic class: Antiemetic
Pregnancy category: Not rated

Indications and Dosages
➤ *To treat nausea and vomiting*
CAPSULES
Adults and adolescents. 250 mg every 6 to 8 hr, p.r.n.
Children weighing 15 to 45 kg (33 to 99 lb). 100 to 200 mg every 6 to 8 hr, p.r.n.
I.M. INJECTION
Adults and adolescents. 200 mg every 6 to 8 hr, p.r.n.
DOSAGE ADJUSTMENT For patient with renal impairment, dosage decreased or dose interval lengthened.

Mechanism of Action
Prevents or stops nausea and vomiting by blocking dopamine receptors and emetic impulses at the chemoreceptor trigger zone in the brain.

Contraindications
Children (I.M.); hypersensitivity to trimethobenzamide, benzocaine, or any of their components

Interactions
DRUGS
apomorphine: Decreased emetic response to apomorphine, increased CNS effects
barbiturates, belladonna alkaloids, phenothiazines: Increased risk of coma, extrapyramidal reactions, opisthotonos, and seizures
CNS depressants: Possibly enhanced effects of both drugs
ototoxic drugs: Possibly masked signs of ototoxicity

Adverse Reactions

CNS: Dizziness, drowsiness, headache
EENT: Blurred vision
GI: Diarrhea
MS: Muscle cramps
Other: Injection site burning, irritation, pain, redness, or swelling

Nursing Considerations

• Use trimethobenzamide cautiously in patients who are dehydrated and those with an electrolyte imbalance, encephalitis, encephalopathy, gastroenteritis, or high fever.
• Be aware that trimethobenzamide shouldn't be used in children who have viral illnesses because they're at increased risk for Reye's syndrome, characterized by abrupt onset of irrational behavior; lethargy; persistent, severe vomiting; progressive encephalopathy leading to coma, seizures, and possibly death.
• To minimize injection site irritation, inject trimethobenzamide deep into a large muscle mass using the Z-track technique, which blocks solution from escaping along the injection route.

PATIENT TEACHING
• Inform patient that trimethobenzamide may cause blurred vision, dizziness, and drowsiness. Advise her to avoid potentially hazardous activities until drug's CNS effects are known.
• Inform patient's parents or caregivers that trimethobenzamide may cause Reye's syndrome, and urge them to notify prescriber immediately if they notice decreased level of consciousness, irrational behavior, lethargy, or severe vomiting.

trimethoprim

Proloprim, Trimpex

Class and Category

Chemical class: Dihydrofolic acid analogue
Therapeutic class: Antibiotic
Pregnancy category: C

Indications and Dosages

➤ *To treat UTI caused by* Enterobacter species, Escherichia coli, Klebsiella pneumoniae, Proteus mirabilis, *or coagulase-negative staphylococci, including* Staphylococcus saprophyticus

TABLETS
Adults and children age 12 and over. 100 mg every 12 hr or 200 mg daily for 10 days.
DOSAGE ADJUSTMENT For patients with creatinine clearance of 15 to 30 ml/min/1.73 m², dosage usually reduced by 50%.

Mechanism of Action

Inhibits formation of tetrahydrofolic acid, the metabolically active form of folic acid, in susceptible bacteria. This depletes folate, an essential component of bacterial development, thereby disrupting production of bacterial nucleic acid and protein.

Contraindications

Hypersensitivity to trimethoprim or its components, megaloblastic anemia from folate deficiency, severe renal impairment (creatinine clearance less than 15 ml/min/1.73 m²)

Interactions

DRUGS
bone marrow depressants: Increased risk of leukopenia, thrombocytopenia
cyclosporine: Increased risk of nephrotoxicity
dapsone: Increased blood levels and risk of adverse effects (especially methemoglobinemia) of both drugs
folate antagonists: Increased risk of megaloblastic anemia
phenytoin: Decreased phenytoin metabolism, increased risk of phenytoin toxicity
procainamide: Increased blood levels of procainamide and its metabolite, *N*-acetylprocainamide
rifampin: Increased elimination and decreased effectiveness of trimethoprim
warfarin: Increased anticoagulant activity of warfarin

Adverse Reactions

CNS: Fever, headache
EENT: Glossitis
GI: Abdominal pain, anorexia, diarrhea, elevated liver function test results, epigastric pain, nausea, vomiting
GU: Elevated BUN and serum creatinine levels
HEME: Leukopenia, megaloblastic anemia,

methemoglobinemia, neutropenia, thrombocytopenia

SKIN: Exfoliative dermatitis, pruritus, rash

Nursing Considerations
•Obtain urine specimen, as ordered, before trimethoprim therapy starts.
•Give drug on an empty stomach to enhance absorption.
•Evaluate patient's test values for folic acid deficiency and signs of bone marrow depression.
•Monitor serum potassium level and renal function studies, as ordered, in patients with decreased renal function because these patients are at increased risk for hyperkalemia and toxic reactions when receiving trimethoprim.

PATIENT TEACHING
•Instruct patient to complete entire course of trimethoprim therapy, as prescribed, even if she feels better beforehand.
•Advise patient to take drug with food or milk if GI distress occurs.
•Instruct patient to notify prescriber if she experiences rash, severe fatigue, sore throat, or unusual bleeding or bruising.

trimipramine maleate
Apo-Trimip (CAN), Novo-Tripramine (CAN), Rhotrimine (CAN), Surmontil

Class and Category
Chemical class: Dibenzazepine derivative
Therapeutic class: Antidepressant
Pregnancy category: C

Indications and Dosages
➤ *To treat depression*
CAPSULES
Adults in inpatient settings. *Initial:* 100 mg daily in divided doses, increased gradually in a few days to 200 mg daily. *Maximum:* 300 mg daily in 2 to 3 wk.
Adolescents in inpatient settings. *Initial:* 50 mg daily in divided doses, increased as needed. *Maximum:* 100 mg daily.
Adults in outpatient settings. *Initial:* 75 mg/day in divided doses, increased gradually up to 150 mg daily, as needed. *Maintenance:* 50 to 150 mg daily. *Maximum:* 200 mg daily.
Adolescents in outpatient settings. *Initial:* 50 mg daily in divided doses, increased as needed. *Maximum:* 100 mg daily.

DOSAGE ADJUSTMENT For elderly patients, initial dosage reduced to 50 mg daily in divided doses, and maximum dosage limited to 100 mg daily.

Route	Onset	Peak	Duration
P.O.	2 to 3 wk	Unknown	Unknown

Mechanism of Action
Inhibits the reuptake of norepinephrine at presynaptic neurons, thus increasing its concentration in synapses. This action may elevate mood and relieve depression.

Contraindications
Hypersensitivity to trimipramine, other dibenzazepine tricyclic antidepressants, or their components; recovery period after an MI; use within 14 days of an MAO inhibitor or other tricyclic antidepressant

Interactions
DRUGS
amantadine, anticholinergics, antidyskinetics, antihistamines: Increased anticholinergic effects (confusion, hallucinations, nightmares)
anticonvulsants: Increased CNS depression, lowered seizure threshold (high trimipramine doses), decreased anticonvulsant effect
antithyroid drugs: Risk of agranulocytosis
barbiturates, carbamazepine: Decreased blood level and effects of trimipramine
bupropion, clozapine, cyclobenzaprine, haloperidol, loxapine, maprotiline, molindone, phenothiazines, thioxanthenes: Increased and prolonged sedative and anticholinergic effects of both drugs, increased risk of seizures
cimetidine: Decreased trimipramine metabolism, possibly leading to trimipramine toxicity
clonidine: Decreased hypotensive effect and increased CNS depressant effect of clonidine
CNS depressants: Increased hypotension and CNS and respiratory depression
disulfiram, ethchlorvynol: Transient delirium, risk of CNS depression (ethchlorvynol)
fluoxetine: Increased trimipramine level
guanadrel, guanethidine: Decreased hypoten-

sive effect
MAO inhibitors: Increased risk of death, hyperpyrexia, hypertensive crisis, severe seizures
methylphenidate: Decreased methylphenidate effects, increased blood trimipramine level
metrizamide: Increased risk of seizures
naphazoline (ophthalmic), oxymetazoline (nasal or ophthalmic), phenylephrine (nasal or ophthalmic), xylometazoline (nasal): Increased vasopressor effect of these drugs
oral anticoagulants: Increased anticoagulation
phenothiazines: Increased blood trimipramine level, decreased phenothiazine metabolism
pimozide, probucol: Increased risk of arrhythmias, possibly prolonged QT interval
sympathomimetics: Increased risk of arrhythmias, hyperpyrexia, severe hypertension
thyroid hormones: Increased therapeutic and toxic effects of both drugs

ACTIVITIES
alcohol use: Increased hypotension and CNS and respiratory depression

Adverse Reactions
CNS: Anxiety, ataxia, confusion, delirium, dizziness, drowsiness, excitement, extrapyramidal reactions, hallucinations, headache, insomnia, nervousness, nightmares, parkinsonism, seizures, stroke, suicidal ideation, tremor
CV: Arrhythmias, orthostatic hypotension
EENT: Blurred vision, dry mouth, increased intraocular pressure, taste perversion, tinnitus, tongue swelling
ENDO: Gynecomastia, syndrome of inappropriate ADH secretion
GI: Constipation, diarrhea, heartburn, ileus, increased appetite, nausea, vomiting
GU: Sexual dysfunction, testicular swelling, urine retention
HEME: Agranulocytosis, bone marrow depression
RESP: Wheezing
SKIN: Alopecia, diaphoresis, jaundice, photosensitivity, pruritus, rash, urticaria
Other: Facial edema, weight gain

Nursing Considerations
•Watch patient closely for suicidal tendencies, especially when therapy starts or dos-

age changes and particularly if patient is a child, teenager, or young adult.
•Expect to gradually reduce trimipramine dosage, as prescribed, before electroconvulsive therapy.
PATIENT TEACHING
•Instruct patient to take the last trimipramine dose early in the evening to avoid insomnia.
•Advise patient to avoid potentially hazardous activities until drug's CNS effects are known.
•Encourage patient to change positions slowly to minimize effects of orthostatic hypotension.
•Urge patient to avoid alcohol during therapy.
•Advise patient to avoid exposure to excessive sunlight and to wear sunscreen when she's outdoors.
•Instruct patient to notify prescriber about the development of unusual bruising and signs of infection.
•Suggest that patient use sugarless gum or hard candy to relieve dry mouth.
•**WARNING** Urge parents to watch their child or adolescent closely for abnormal behavior, increased aggression or hostility, or suicidal tendencies, especially when therapy starts or dosage is adjusted. Stress need to notify prescriber about changes.

tromethamine

Tham

Class and Category
Chemical class: Organic amine
Therapeutic class: Alkalinizer
Pregnancy category: C

Indications and Dosages
➤ *To treat metabolic acidosis associated with cardiac arrest*
I.V. INFUSION
Adults and children. 3.6 to 10.8 g (111 to 333 ml) of 0.3 M solution.
I.V. INJECTION
Adults and children. If chest is opened, 2 to 6 g injected directly into open ventricular cavity.

➤ *To treat metabolic acidosis during cardiac bypass surgery*

I.V. INFUSION
Adults and children. 9 ml (2.7 mEq or 0.32 g) of 0.3 M solution/kg as a single dose. *Usual:* 500 ml (150 mEq or 18 g) infused over 1 hr. *Maximum:* 500 mg/kg over 1 hr.

Mechanism of Action
Combines with hydrogen ions and their associated acid anions, including lactic, pyruvic, and carbonic acid, to form salts that are excreted in urine. Tromethamine exerts additional alkalinizing effects by acting as an osmotic diuretic, promoting the excretion of alkaline urine that contains increased amounts of carbon dioxide and electrolytes.

Contraindications
Anuria, chronic respiratory acidosis, hypersensitivity to tromethamine or its components, uremia

Interactions
DRUGS
amphetamines, quinidine, other pH-dependent drugs: Altered excretion of these drugs

Adverse Reactions
CNS: Fever
CV: Vasospasm
ENDO: Hypoglycemia
GI: Hepatic necrosis (hemorrhagic)
RESP: Respiratory depression
Other: Hypervolemia; infusion site infection, phlebitis, or venous thrombosis; metabolic alkalosis

Nursing Considerations
•Evaluate blood pH, blood glucose, and serum bicarbonate and electrolyte levels, and partial pressure of arterial carbon dioxide before, during, and after tromethamine therapy, as ordered.
•Be aware that, except in life-threatening situations, tromethamine therapy is limited to no more than 1 day because of the risk of alkalosis.
•WARNING Be aware that exceeding the recommended dosage can cause alkalosis, respiratory depression, and reduced carbon dioxide level.

•Expect I.V. tromethamine administration to increase the risk of hypervolemia and pulmonary edema.
•Assess the infusion site often for infiltration, which may cause inflammation, necrosis, thrombosis, tissue sloughing, and vasospasm.
•Be aware that patients with renal failure have an increased risk of developing hyperkalemia. For such patients, be prepared to monitor ECG continuously and assess serum potassium level frequently.
•Monitor patient's blood glucose level often during and after therapy because rapid delivery can cause hypoglycemia for several hours.
PATIENT TEACHING
•Inform family members that patient's vital signs and laboratory test results will be measured frequently to monitor her progress.

trospium chloride
Sanctura, Sanctura XR

Class and Category
Chemical class: Quaternary ammonium compound
Therapeutic class: Bladder antispasmodic
Pregnancy category: C

Indications and Dosages
➤ *To treat overactive bladder with symptoms of urge urinary incontinence, urgency, and urinary frequency*
TABLETS
Adults. 20 mg b.i.d. 1 hour before meals or on empty stomach.
DOSAGE ADJUSTMENT For patients with severe renal insufficiency (creatinine clearance less than 30 ml/min/1.73 m^2) and patients age 75 or over, dosage reduced to 20 mg daily at bedtime.
E.R. TABLETS
Adults. 60 mg daily in the morning, 1 hour before a meal or on empty stomach.

Route	Onset	Peak	Duration
P.O.	Unknown	5 to 6 hr	Unknown

Contraindications
Gastric retention, hypersensitivity to trospium or its components, uncontrolled angle-closure glaucoma, urine retention

T

Mechanism of Action

Antagonizes the effect of acetylcholine on muscarinic receptors in the bladder. Trospium's parasympatholytic action reduces the tonus of smooth muscle in the bladder. These actions increase maximum cystometric bladder capacity and volume with the first detrusor contraction, which relieves the sensation of urgency and frequency and enhances bladder control.

Interactions

DRUGS
anticholinergics: Increased frequency or severity of adverse effects; possibly reduced absorption of trospium
digoxin, metformin, morphine, pancuronium, procainamide: Possibly increased plasma concentration of trospium, digoxin, metformin, morphine, pancuronium, procainamide

ACTIVITIES
alcohol use: Possibly increased drowsiness

Adverse Reactions

CNS: Dizziness, drowsiness, fatigue, headache, light-headedness
CV: Palpitations, tachycardia
EENT: Blurred vision; dry eyes, mouth, or throat
GI: Abdominal distention or pain, constipation, flatulence, indigestion, vomiting
GU: Urine retention
SKIN: Decreased sweating, dry skin, flushing, rash
Other: Angioedema

Nursing Considerations

• Use trospium cautiously in patients with ulcerative colitis, intestinal atony, or myasthenia gravis because drug may decrease GI motility; patients with significant bladder outflow obstruction because drug may cause urine retention; patients with hepatic impairment because drug's effects on the liver are unknown; and patients with renal impairment because drug excretion may be impaired.
• Monitor elderly patients carefully, especially those age 75 or over, for adverse reactions because elderly patients have an in-creased risk of trospium-induced adverse reactions.

PATIENT TEACHING
• Instruct patient to take trospium on an empty stomach or at least 1 hour before eating because food delays trospium's absorption.
• Caution patient to avoid performing activities in a warm or hot environment because sweating may be delayed, which could cause a sudden increase in body temperature and heatstroke.
• Advise patient to avoid potentially hazardous activities until drug's CNS effects are known.
• Inform patient that alcohol may increase the risk of drowsiness; urge patient to limit or abstain from alcoholic beverages while taking trospium.

tubocurarine chloride

Class and Category

Chemical class: Isoquinoline derivative
Therapeutic class: Anticonvulsant
Pregnancy category: C

Indications and Dosages

➤ *To manage muscle contractions of seizures associated with electroshock therapy*
I.V. INJECTION
Adults. 157 mcg/kg (0.157 mg/kg) over 30 to 90 sec, given just before electroshock therapy. Expect initial dose to be 3 mg less than calculated total dose.

➤ *To produce skeletal muscle paralysis during anesthesia*
I.V. OR I.M. INJECTION
Adults. *Initial:* 6 to 9 mg. *Maintenance:* 3 to 4.5 mg in 3 to 5 min. if needed. For prolonged procedures, 3-mg supplemental doses given.
Infants and children. 500 mcg/kg I.V.
Neonates. *Initial:* 250 to 500 mcg/kg I.V. *Maintenance:* One-fifth to one-sixth of initial dose if needed.

➤ *To facilitate endotracheal intubation and aid controlled respiration during mechanical ventilation*

Mechanism of Action

Tubocurarine reduces the intensity of skeletal muscle contractions caused by electrically induced seizures. Normally, when a nerve impulse arrives at a somatic motor nerve terminal, it triggers acetylcholine (ACh) stored in synaptic vesicles to be released into the neuromuscular junction. The released ACh binds with nicotinic receptors embedded in the skeletal muscle motor endplate, as shown below left, triggering muscle cell depolarization and contraction.

Tubocurarine is a nondepolarizing neuromuscular blocker that acts as a competitive antagonist of ACh. By binding to the nicotinic receptors, as shown below right, it prevents transmission of the action potential at the neuromuscular junction, thereby sustaining skeletal muscle relaxation and eliminating the peripheral muscular manifestations of seizures. The drug has no effect on the CNS processes involved with seizures because it doesn't cross the blood-brain barrier.

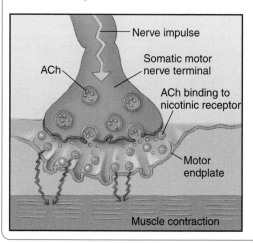

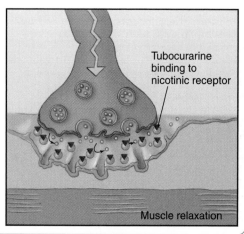

I.V. INJECTION
Adults. *Initial:* 16.5 mcg/kg. *Maintenance:* Dosage individualized based on patient response.

➤ *To aid in the diagnosis of myasthenia gravis*

I.V. INJECTION
Adults. 4 to 33 mcg/kg. After 2 to 3 min, 1.5 mg of neostigmine is given I.V. to terminate the test.

Route	Onset	Peak	Duration
I.V.	1 min	2 to 5 min	20 to 40 min

Incompatibilities

Don't mix tubocurarine with barbiturates, such as methohexital or thiopental, because a precipitate may form.

Contraindications

Hypersensitivity to tubocurarine or its components, patients in whom histamine release may be dangerous

Interactions
DRUGS
alfentanil, fentanyl, sufentanil: Prevented or reversed muscle rigidity from these drugs
aminoglycosides, anesthetics, capreomycin, citrate-anticoagulated blood, clindamycin, lidocaine (I.V.), lincomycin, polymyxins, procaine (I.V.), trimethaphan: Additive neuromuscular blocking effects
beta blockers, calcium salts: Prolonged and enhanced effects of tubocurarine
magnesium salts, procainamide, quinidine: Enhanced blockade effects
opioid analgesics: Additive histamine release

T

effects, additive respiratory depressant effects, worsened bradycardia and hypotension

Adverse Reactions
CV: Arrhythmias, bradycardia, edema, hypotension, shock, tachycardia
RESP: Bronchospasm
SKIN: Erythema, flushing, itching, rash
Other: Anaphylaxis

Nursing Considerations
•If patient has a history of CV disease or is hypotensive, monitor her for further decrease in blood pressure.
•Monitor patient for bronchospasm and hypotension because tubocurarine may cause increased histamine release.
•Keep emergency equipment and drugs readily available in case respiratory depression occurs.
PATIENT TEACHING
•Explain the need for frequent hemodynamic monitoring.

U·V·W

urea
(carbamide)

Ureaphil

Class and Category
Chemical class: Carbonic acid diamide salt
Therapeutic class: Antiglaucoma, diuretic
Pregnancy category: C

Indications and Dosages
➤ *To reduce cerebral edema and intracranial pressure*

I.V. INFUSION

Adults and children age 2 and over. 500 mg to 1.5 g/kg as 30% solution in D_5W, $D_{10}W$, or 10% invert sugar solution infused over 30 min to 2 hr at 4 or 6 ml/min, according to manufacturer's instructions. *Maximum:* 2 g/kg daily.
Children under age 2. 100 mg to 1.5 g/kg as 30% solution in D_5W, $D_{10}W$, or 10% invert sugar solution infused over 30 min to 2 hr at 4 or 6 ml/min, according to manufacturer's instructions.

➤ *To treat malignant or secondary glaucoma*

I.V. INFUSION

Adults. 500 mg to 1.5 g/kg as 30% solution in D_5W, $D_{10}W$, or 10% invert sugar solution infused over 30 min to 2 hr at 4 or 6 ml/min, according to manufacturer's instructions. *Maximum:* 2 g/kg daily.
DOSAGE ADJUSTMENT Dosage reduced or drug withheld for patients with renal impairment if BUN level rises to 75 mg/dl or more or if diuresis fails to occur within 2 hr after administration.

Route	Onset	Peak	Duration
I.V.	10 min	1 to 2 hr	3 to 10 hr*

Contraindications
Active intracranial bleeding, hepatic failure, hypersensitivity to urea or its components, renal impairment, severe dehydration

---

* For diuresis; 5 to 6 hr for reduced intraocular pressure.

Mechanism of Action
Elevates blood plasma osmolality, creating an osmotic effect that increases the movement of water from the brain, CSF, and anterior portion of the eyes into interstitial fluid and plasma. This action reduces cerebral edema, intracranial pressure, CSF volume, and intraocular pressure. Large doses inhibit the reabsorption of water and solutes in the renal tubules and induce diuresis by affecting the osmotic pressure gradient of the glomerular filtrate.

Interactions
DRUGS
carbonic anhydrase inhibitors, other diuretics: Additive diuretic and intraocular pressure–reducing effects
lithium: Increased renal excretion of lithium

Adverse Reactions
CNS: Agitation, confusion, fever, headache, hyperthermia, nervousness, subarachnoid hemorrhage, subdural hematoma, syncope
CV: Tachycardia
EENT: Dry mouth, intraocular hemorrhage
GI: Nausea, thirst, vomiting
GU: Elevated BUN level
HEME: Hemolysis
SKIN: Blemishes, extravasation with tissue necrosis and sloughing
Other: Dehydration, hypokalemia, hyponatremia, infusion site phlebitis or thrombosis

Nursing Considerations
•For maximum reduction of intracranial or intraocular pressure, expect to give urea 60 minutes before ocular or intracranial surgery.
•Don't mix urea with invert sugar solution if patient has fructose intolerance from aldolase deficiency.
•Avoid infusing drug into leg veins to reduce risk of phlebitis and thrombosis.
•Discard unused portion of drug after 24 hours.
•Be aware that rapid administration may cause hemolysis, increased capillary bleeding, and, in patients with glaucoma, intraocular hemorrhage.
•Maintain adequate hydration to minimize adverse reactions. Assess for signs of dehydration, including dry mucous membranes or tenting.
•Monitor BUN and serum electrolyte levels as well as fluid intake and output during

U V W

urea therapy because prolonged use can cause diuresis.

PATIENT TEACHING
•Instruct patient to notify prescriber immediately about difficulty breathing or shortness of breath because drug can cause transient increases in circulatory volume, leading to circulatory overload, exacerbations of heart failure, or pulmonary edema.
•Tell patient to expect increased urine output.
•Encourage patient to remain on bed rest during therapy.

urokinase

Abbokinase, Abbokinase Open-Cath

Class and Category

Chemical class: Renal enzymatic protein
Therapeutic class: Thrombolytic
Pregnancy category: B

Indications and Dosages

➤ *To treat acute coronary artery thrombosis*

INTRACORONARY INFUSION
Adults. 6,000 international units/min until artery is maximally opened (up to 2 hr may be required). *Usual:* 500,000 international units.

➤ *To treat acute pulmonary thromboembolism including massive events*

I.V. INFUSION
Adults. *Initial:* 4,400 international units/kg over 10 min, followed by 4,400 international units/kg/hr for 12 hr.

➤ *To clear I.V. catheter occlusion*

INSTILLATION
Adults and children. 5,000 international units/ml instilled into occluded line.

Route	Onset	Peak	Duration
I.V.	Unknown	20 min to 2 hr	4 hr
Intra-coronary	Unknown	Unknown	4 hr

Incompatibilities

Don't administer I.V. urokinase through the same I.V. line as other drugs or add other drugs to urokinase solution.

Contraindications

Arteriovenous malformation, bleeding disorder, CVA during previous 2 months, hypersensitivity to urokinase or its components, internal bleeding, intracranial aneurysm, intracranial or intraspinal surgery during previous 2 months, intracranial tumor, recent cardiopulmonary resuscitation, recent trauma, severe uncontrolled hypertension (systolic blood pressure of 200 mm Hg or higher, or diastolic blood pressure of 110 mm Hg or higher)

Mechanism of Action

Indirectly promotes conversion of plasminogen to plasmin, an enzyme that breaks down fibrin clots, fibrinogen, and other plasma proteins, including procoagulant factors V and VIII.

Interactions

DRUGS
antifibrinolytics (aminocaproic acid, aprotinin): Mutual antagonism
antihypertensives: Increased risk of severe hypotension
cefamandole, cefoperazone, cefotetan, plicamycin, valproic acid: Increased risk of hypoprothrombinemia and severe hemorrhage
corticosteroids, ethacrynic acid, salicylates (nonacetylated): Increased risk of GI ulceration and bleeding
enoxaparin, heparin, NSAIDs, oral anticoagulants, platelet-aggregation inhibitors: Increased risk of hemorrhage
thiotepa: Increased therapeutic effects of thiotepa

Adverse Reactions

CNS: Chills, CVA, fever, headache
CV: Arrhythmias, including tachycardia; chest pain; cholesterol embolization, hypertension; hypotension
EENT: Orolingual edema
GI: Nausea, vomiting
HEME: Unusual bleeding
MS: Back pain, myalgia
RESP: Bronchospasm, dyspnea, hypoxemia, wheezing
SKIN: Cyanosis, ecchymosis, flushing, pruritus, rash, urticaria
Other: Anaphylaxis, infusion site reactions, metabolic acidosis

Nursing Considerations

•To prevent foaming, don't shake urokinase

when reconstituting. Consult with pharmacist about giving drug through 0.45-micron or smaller cellulose membrane filter.
•Assess baseline hematocrit, platelet count, thrombin time, APTT, PT, and INR as ordered.
•Monitor heart rate and rhythm by continuous ECG during therapy, especially during rapid lysis of coronary thrombi, because arrhythmias can occur with reperfusion.
•Monitor blood pressure for hypotension. If hypotension occurs, notify prescriber and expect to reduce infusion rate.
•Check for bleeding at puncture sites and in urine and stool. Check for intracranial bleeding by performing frequent neurologic assessments.
•After arterial puncture is performed, apply pressure for at least 30 minutes and then apply pressure dressing. Check frequently for bleeding during therapy.
•To prevent bleeding and associated complications, avoid venipunctures; use an external blood pressure cuff to measure blood pressure; give acetaminophen (not aspirin), as prescribed, for fever; and handle patient as little as possible.
•WARNING If serious bleeding begins and can't be controlled with local pressure, stop infusion immediately and notify prescriber.
PATIENT TEACHING
•Instruct patient to remain on bed rest during urokinase therapy.
•Inform patient that minor bleeding may occur at wounds or puncture sites.

ursodiol
(ursodeoxycholic acid)
Actigall, Urso Forte, URSO 250, Ursofalk (CAN)

Class and Category
Chemical class: Naturally occurring bile acid
Therapeutic class: Bile salt replenisher, chole-litholytic
Pregnancy category: B

Indications and Dosages
➤ *To prevent gallstone formation in obese patients during rapid weight loss*
CAPSULES
Adults and adolescents. 300 mg b.i.d. Alternatively, 8 to 10 mg/kg daily in divided doses

b.i.d or t.i.d.
➤ *To dissolve gallstones*
CAPSULES
Adults and adolescents. 8 to 10 mg/kg daily in divided doses b.i.d. or t.i.d.
➤ *To treat primary biliary cirrhosis*
TABLETS
Adults. 13 to 15 mg/kg daily in two to four divided doses.

Mechanism of Action
Suppresses hepatic synthesis, biliary secretion, and intestinal reabsorption of cholesterol. Prolonged use promotes dissolution of gallstones.

Contraindications
Acute cholangiitis; gallstone complications (such as biliary GI fistula; biliary obstruction; calcified, radiopaque, or radiotranslucent bile-pigment gallstones; cholecystitis; pancreatitis); hypersensitivity to ursodiol, other bile acids, or their components

Interactions
DRUGS
aluminum-containing antacids, cholestyramine, colestipol: Decreased absorption and therapeutic effects of ursodiol
clofibrate, estrogens, neomycin, oral contraceptives, progestins: Interference with ursodiol's therapeutic effects; increased risk of gallstone formation
FOODS
any foods: Increased dissolution of drug

Adverse Reactions
CNS: Anxiety, asthenia, depression, fatigue, headache, sleep disturbance
CV: Chest pain, hypertension, peripheral edema
ENDO: Hyperglycemia
EENT: Metallic taste, rhinitis, stomatitis
GI: Abdominal pain, cholecystitis, constipation, diarrhea, esophagitis, flatulence, indigestion, nausea, peptic ulcer, vomiting
GU: Elevated CK level
HEME: Leukopenia
MS: Arthralgia, back pain, myalgia
RESP: Cough
SKIN: Alopecia, diaphoresis, dry skin, pruritus, rash, urticaria

U
V
W

Nursing Considerations
•Administer ursodiol with food to increase drug dissolution.
•Administer aluminum-containing antacids, cholestyramine, and colestipol at least 1 hour before or 4 hours after ursodiol because they may decrease drug's effects.
•Expect drug to be discontinued if gallstones haven't partially dissolved after 12 months of therapy.
•Be aware that if patient inadvertently takes too much ursodiol, diarrhea will most likely result and most likely warrant systemic treatment.

PATIENT TEACHING
•Instruct patient to take ursodiol with meals.
•Advise patient to take aluminum-containing antacids at least 1 hour before or 4 hours after taking ursodiol to avoid impaired absorption.
•Urge patient to notify prescriber immediately if signs of acute cholecystitis develop, such as acute right-upper-quadrant abdominal pain.
•Inform patient that he may need to take ursodiol for a prolonged period before gallstones dissolve.
•Advise diabetic patient to monitor blood glucose levels while taking ursodiol because drug may alter blood glucose control.

valproic acid
Alti-Valproic (CAN), Depakene, Depakote ER, Deproic (CAN), Dom-Proic (CAN), Med-Valproic (CAN), Novo-Valproic (CAN), Nu-Valproic (CAN), PMS-Valproic Acid (CAN), Stavzor

valproate sodium
Depacon

divalproex sodium
Depakote, Depakote Sprinkle, Epival (CAN)

Class and Category
Chemical class: Carboxylic acid derivative
Therapeutic class: Anticonvulsant
Pregnancy category: D

Indications and Dosages
➤ *To treat simple or complex absence seizures, complex partial seizures, myo-*clonic seizures, and generalized tonic-clonic seizures as monotherapy

CAPSULES, DELAYED-RELEASE SPRINKLE CAPSULES, DELAYED-RELEASE TABLETS, SYRUP, I.V. INFUSION (VALPROIC ACID, VALPROATE SODIUM, DIVALPROEX SODIUM)

Adults and adolescents. *Initial:* 10 to 15 mg/kg/day in divided doses b.i.d. or t.i.d., increased by 5 to 10 mg/kg daily every wk, as needed and as prescribed. *Maximum:* 60 mg/kg daily.
Children. *Initial:* 15 to 45 mg/kg daily in divided doses b.i.d. or t.i.d., increased by 5 to 10 mg/kg/day every wk, as needed and as prescribed.

➤ *As adjunct to treat simple or complex absence seizures, complex partial seizures, myoclonic seizures, and generalized tonic-clonic seizures*

CAPSULES, DELAYED-RELEASE SPRINKLE CAPSULES, DELAYED-RELEASE TABLETS, SYRUP, I.V. INFUSION (VALPROIC ACID, VALPROATE SODIUM, DIVALPROEX SODIUM)

Adults and adolescents. 10 to 30 mg/kg daily in divided doses, increased by 5 to 10 mg/kg daily every wk, as needed and as prescribed.
Children. 30 to 100 mg/kg daily in divided doses, as prescribed.

DOSAGE ADJUSTMENT For adults being converted from immediate-release divalproex tablets to delayed-release tablets, dosage increased to 8% to 20% more than total daily dose of immediate-release tablets and given once daily.

➤ *To treat acute manic phase of bipolar disorder*

DELAYED-RELEASE TABLETS (DIVALPROEX SODIUM), DELAYED-RELEASE CAPSULES (STAVZOR)

Adults. *Initial:* 750 mg daily in divided doses. *Maximum:* 60 mg/kg daily.

➤ *To prevent migraine headache*

TABLETS, TABLETS (DIVALPROEX SODIUM), DELAYED-RELEASE CAPSULES (STAVZOR)

Adults. 250 mg every 12 hr, increased p.r.n. *Maximum:* 1 g daily.

DELAYED-RELEASE TABLETS (DIVALPROEX SODIUM)

Adults. 500 mg daily, increased, as needed and prescribed, up to 1 g daily. *Maximum:* 1 g daily.

Contraindications
Hepatic dysfunction; hypersensitivity to valproic acid, valproate sodium, divalproex sodium, or their components; urea cycle disorders

Mechanism of Action

May decrease seizure activity by blocking the reuptake of gamma-aminobutyric acid (GABA), the most common inhibitory neurotransmitter in the brain. GABA is known to suppress the rapid firing of neurons by inhibiting voltage-sensitive sodium channels.

Interactions

DRUGS

aspirin, heparin, NSAIDs, oral anticoagulants, thrombolytics: Increased inhibition of platelet aggregation and risk of bleeding
barbiturates, primidone: Increased blood levels of both drugs, additive CNS effects
carbamazepine: Possibly decreased valproic acid effectiveness
carbapenem antibiotics (ertapenem, imipenem, meropenem): Reduced serum valproic acid level, causing loss of seizure control
cholestyramine: Decreased bioavailability of valproic acid
clonazepam: Increased risk of absence seizures
CNS depressants: Increased CNS depression
diazepam: Inhibited diazepam metabolism
ethosuximide: Unpredictable blood ethosuximide level
felbamate: Impaired valproic acid metabolism and increased blood drug level
haloperidol, loxapine, MAO inhibitors, maprotiline, phenothiazines, thioxanthenes, tricyclic antidepressants: Increased CNS depression, lowered seizure threshold
lamotrigine: Decreased lamotrigine clearance
mefloquine: Decreased blood levels of valproic acid, divalproex, and valproate sodium; increased risk of seizures
phenytoin: Increased risk of phenytoin toxicity, loss of seizure control

ACTIVITIES

alcohol use: Additive CNS depression

Adverse Reactions

CNS: Agitation, ataxia, confusion, depression, dizziness, drowsiness, euphoria, hallucinations, headache, hyperesthesia, hypothermia, lack of coordination, lethargy, loss of seizure control, paresthesia, psychosis, sedation, suicidal ideation, tremor, vertigo, weakness
EENT: Diplopia, nystagmus, pharyngitis, spots before eyes

ENDO: Galactorrhea, hyperglycemia
GI: Abdominal pain, anorexia, constipation, diarrhea, elevated liver function test results, hepatotoxicity, increased appetite, indigestion, nausea, pancreatitis, vomiting
GU: Menstrual irregularities
HEME: Eosinophilia, hematoma, leukopenia, prolonged bleeding time, thrombocytopenia
MS: Dysarthria
SKIN: Alopecia, diaphoresis, erythema multiforme, jaundice, petechiae, photosensitivity, pruritus, rash, Stevens-Johnson syndrome
Other: Facial edema, hyperammonemia, injection site pain, weight gain or loss

Nursing Considerations

•Give oral valproic acid or divalproex with food to minimize GI irritation, if necessary.
•Administer drug at least 2 hours before or 6 hours after cholestyramine.
•Don't mix syrup with carbonated beverages; doing so may produce an unpleasant-tasting mixture and irritate the mouth and throat.
•Don't break or allow patient to chew delayed-release tablets.
•As needed, sprinkle contents of delayed-release sprinkle capsules on small amount of semisolid food just before administration. Instruct patient not to chew contents of delayed-release sprinkle capsules.
•For I.V. administration, dilute prescribed dose with at least 50 ml of compatible diluent and infuse over 60 minutes.
•Be aware that patient should be switched from I.V. to P.O. form of valproic acid as soon as possible.
•Be aware that patient with hypoalbuminemia or another protein-binding deficiency is at increased risk for valproic acid toxicity.
•Assess for signs and symptoms of decreased hepatic function, including anorexia, facial edema, jaundice, lethargy, loss of seizure control, malaise, vomiting, and weakness.
•Monitor liver function test results, as ordered. Assess for signs and symptoms of hepatotoxicity during first 6 months of treatment, especially in children under age 2. Notify prescriber immediately if you suspect hepatotoxicity.
•Monitor platelet count, as ordered, for signs of thrombocytopenia, and notify prescriber if they appear.
•WARNING Be aware that hyperammonemia may occur even if patient's liver function test results are normal. Monitor ammonia levels,

U
V
W

as ordered. If patient develops unexplained lethargy, vomiting, or changes in mental status with an increase in ammonia level; if asymptomatic ammonia elevations are detected and persist; or if patient develops hypothermia even without hyperammonemia, expect valproic acid to be discontinued.

•Watch patient closely for suicidal tendencies, particularly when therapy starts and dosage changes, because depression may worsen temporarily during these times, possibly leading to suicidal ideation.

•Monitor patient's drug level, as ordered, especially early in therapy and if patient takes other drugs because interactions can alter the blood level.

•Drug may alter urine ketone test and thyroid function tests.

PATIENT TEACHING

•Instruct patient to swallow capsules whole to prevent irritation to mouth and throat. However, delayed-release sprinkle capsules may be opened and contents mixed with food for easier swallowing. Instruct patient not to chew contents of delayed-release sprinkle capsules.

•Advise patient to avoid potentially hazardous activities during therapy because drug may affect mental and motor performance.

•Urge patient to avoid alcohol during therapy.

•Urge female patient to notify prescriber immediately about suspected or known pregnancy.

•Advise patient to notify prescriber if tremor develops during therapy; occurrence of tremor may be dose-related.

•Urge family or caregiver to watch patient closely for suicidal tendencies, especially when therapy starts or dosage changes.

valsartan

Diovan

Class and Category

Chemical class: Nonpeptide tetrazole derivative
Therapeutic class: Antihypertensive
Pregnancy category: C (first trimester), D (later trimesters)

Indications and Dosages

➤ *To manage hypertension, alone or with other antihypertensives*

CAPSULES

Adults. *Initial:* 80 or 160 mg daily, increased as needed and prescribed. *Maximum:* 320 mg/day.

Children ages 6 to 16. 1.3 mg/kg (up to 40 mg total) once daily, increased as needed and prescribed. *Maximum:* 2.7 mg/kg (up to 160 mg) daily.

➤ *To treat New York Heart Association (NYHA) class II to IV heart failure*

CAPSULES

Adults. *Initial:* 40 mg b.i.d., increased to 80 mg b.i.d. and then 160 mg b.i.d., as needed and prescribed. *Maximum:* 320 mg daily.

➤ *To reduce cardiovascular mortality in stable patients with left ventricular failure or dysfunction following an MI*

CAPSULES

Adults. *Initial:* 20 mg b.i.d. starting as early as 12 hr after MI, increased to 40 mg b.i.d. within 7 days, followed by subsequent adjustments to 160 mg b.i.d., as tolerated. *Maintenance:* 160 mg b.i.d.

DOSAGE ADJUSTMENT If patient develops symptomatic hypotension or renal dysfunction, dosage decreased.

Route	Onset	Peak	Duration
P.O.	2 hr	6 hr	24 hr

Mechanism of Action

Blocks the hormone angiotensin II from binding to the receptor sites in vascular smooth muscle, adrenal glands, and other tissues. This action inhibits angiotensin II's vasoconstrictive and aldosterone-secreting effects, thereby reducing blood pressure.

Contraindications

Hypersensitivity to valsartan or its components

Interactions

DRUGS

antihypertensives, diuretics: Additive hypotensive effect
potassium salts, potassium-sparing diuretics: Possibly hyperkalemia

FOODS

potassium-containing salt substitutes: Possibly hyperkalemia

Adverse Reactions

CNS: Dizziness, fatigue, headache, insomnia
CV: Edema, hypotension
EENT: Pharyngitis, rhinitis, sinusitis
GI: Abdominal pain, diarrhea, elevated liver enzymes, hepatitis, indigestion, nausea, vomiting
GU: Increased blood creatinine level
HEME: Thrombocytopenia
MS: Arthralgia, back pain, rhabdomyolysis
RESP: Cough, upper respiratory tract infection
SKIN: Alopecia, rash
Other: Angioedema, hyperkalemia, viral infection

Nursing Considerations

•Be aware that valsartan shouldn't be given to patients who have hypovolemia or are taking a diuretic because of the increased risk of severe hypotension from volume depletion.
•Check patient's blood pressure often during therapy.
•Be aware that maximal blood pressure reduction typically occurs after 4 weeks.
•Monitor serum potassium level because drug may elevate potassium level by blocking aldosterone secretion.

PATIENT TEACHING

•Instruct patient to take valsartan exactly as prescribed at the same time each day to maintain therapeutic effect.
•Advise patient to avoid hazardous activities until drug's CNS effects are known.
•Advise patient to avoid using potassium-containing salt substitutes without consulting prescriber.
•Instruct female patient of childbearing age to use reliable birth control during therapy and to notify prescriber immediately about known or suspected pregnancy because valsartan will need to be discontinued.
•Urge patient to keep follow-up appointments with prescriber to monitor progress.

vancomycin hydrochloride

Vancocin

Class and Category

Chemical class: Tricyclic glycopeptide derivative

Therapeutic class: Antibiotic
Pregnancy category: B (oral), C (parenteral)

Indications and Dosages

➤ *To treat pseudomembranous colitis caused by* Clostridium difficile *and enterocolitis caused by staphylococci*

CAPSULES, ORAL SOLUTION

Adults and adolescents. 125 to 500 mg every 6 hr for 7 to 10 days. *Maximum:* 2 g daily.
Children. 10 mg/kg (up to 125 mg) every 6 hr for 7 to 10 days. *Maximum:* 2 g daily.

➤ *To treat bacterial endocarditis caused by methicillin-resistant* Staphylococcus aureus

I.V. INFUSION

Adults. 30 mg/kg daily in equally divided doses b.i.d. for 4 to 6 wk. *Maximum:* 2 g daily.

➤ *As adjunct to treat bacterial endocarditis caused by methicillin-resistant* S. aureus *in patients with prosthetic heart valve*

I.V. INFUSION

Adults. 30 mg/kg daily in equally divided doses b.i.d. to q.i.d. for 6 wk or longer in conjunction with rifampin and gentamicin. *Maximum:* 2 g daily.

➤ *To treat bacterial endocarditis caused by* Streptococcus bovis *or* Streptococcus viridans

I.V. INFUSION

Adults. 30 mg/kg daily in equally divided doses b.i.d. for 4 wk. *Maximum:* 2 g daily.

➤ *As adjunct to treat bacterial endocarditis caused by enterococci*

I.V. INFUSION

Adults. 30 mg/kg daily in equally divided doses b.i.d. for 4 to 6 wk in conjunction with gentamicin. *Maximum:* 2 g daily.

➤ *To treat bacterial septicemia, bone and joint infections, pneumonia, and skin and soft-tissue infections caused by staphylococcus, including methicillin-resistant strains, and life-threatening infections*

I.V. INFUSION

Adults and children age 12 and over. 500 mg every 6 hr or 1 g every 12 hr infused over at least 60 min. *Maximum:* 4 g daily.
Children ages 1 month to 12 years. 10 mg/kg every 6 hr or 20 mg/kg every 12 hr infused

U
V
W

over at least 60 min.

Neonates ages 1 week to 1 month. *Initial:* 15 mg/kg followed by 10 mg/kg every 8 hr infused over at least 60 min.

Neonates under age 1 week. *Initial:* 15 mg/kg followed by 10 mg/kg every 12 hr infused over at least 60 min.

Mechanism of Action

Inhibits bacterial RNA and cell wall synthesis; alters permeability of bacterial membranes, causing cell wall lysis and cell death.

Incompatibilities

Don't give I.V. vancomycin through the same I.V. line as other drugs. Don't add it to albumin-containing solutions, alkaline solutions, aminophylline, amobarbital sodium, aztreonam, cefepime, ceftazidime, chloramphenicol sodium succinate, chlorothiazide sodium, dexamethasone sodium phosphate, foscarnet sodium, heparin sodium, methicillin sodium, penicillin G, pentobarbital sodium, phenobarbital sodium, pipera-cillin sodium and tazobactam sodium, secobarbital sodium, and sodium bicarbonate. Vancomycin may precipitate with heavy metals.

Contraindications

Hypersensitivity to vancomycin or its components, hypersensitivity to corn or corn products when vancomycin is given with dextrose solutions

Interactions
DRUGS

aminoglycosides (amikacin, gentamicin, tobramycin), amphotericin B, bacitracin (parenteral), bumetanide, capreomycin, carmustine, cidofovir, cisplatin, cyclosporine, ethacrynic acid, furosemide, paromomycin, pentamidine (parenteral), polymyxins, salicylates (parenteral), streptozocin: Additive nephrotoxicity or ototoxicity

antihistamines, buclizine, cyclizine, meclizine, phenothiazines, thioxanthenes, trimethobenzamide: Masked symptoms of ototoxicity

cholestyramine, colestipol: Decreased antibacterial activity of oral vancomycin

dexamethasone: Decreased penetration of vancomycin into CSF

nephrotoxic drugs: Increased risk of nephrotoxicity

Adverse Reactions

CNS: Chills, dizziness, vertigo
CV: Hypotension
EENT: Ototoxicity
GI: Nausea, pseudomembranous colitis
GU: Nephrotoxicity
HEME: Eosinophilia, neutropenia
RESP: Dyspnea, wheezing
SKIN: Exfoliative dermatitis; extravasation with pain, tenderness, thrombophlebitis, and tissue necrosis; pruritus; rash; toxic epidermal necrolysis; urticaria
Other: Anaphylaxis, drug-induced fever, injection site inflammation, superinfection

Nursing Considerations

•To reconstitute 500-mg vial of vancomycin for I.V. use, add 10 ml of sterile water for injection; further dilute with at least 100 ml of compatible I.V. solution. For 1-g vial of dry, sterile powder, add 20 ml of sterile water for injection; further dilute with at least 200 ml of compatible I.V. solution.

•**WARNING** Infuse over at least 1 hour. Rapid administration may cause hypotension or transient "red man syndrome," characterized by chills; fainting; fever; flushing of face, neck, upper arms, and torso; hypotension; nausea; tachycardia; and vomiting.

•Monitor blood vancomycin levels, as ordered; be aware that therapeutic levels are 10 to 15 mcg/ml trough and 30 to 40 mcg/ml peak.

•Monitor serum vancomycin concentration in patients with renal impairment or colitis because significant increases in blood drug level have occurred in such patients taking multiple oral doses of vancomycin.

•If patient has an inflammatory intestinal disorder, assess him often for adverse reactions because vancomycin absorption may be increased in these conditions.

•Check CBC results and serum creatinine and BUN levels during therapy, especially if patient has renal impairment or takes an aminoglycoside.

•Observe I.V. infusion site for signs and symptoms of extravasation, including necrosis, pain, tenderness, and thrombophlebitis. If extravasation occurs, discontinue infusion immediately and notify prescriber.

• Assess hearing during therapy. Transient or permanent ototoxicity may occur if patient receives an excessive amount of drug, has an underlying hearing loss, or receives concurrent aminoglycosides.

• Monitor patient closely for diarrhea because it may indicate pseudomembranous colitis aused by *Clostridium difficile,* a risk with many antibiotics. If diarrhea occurs during therapy, notify prescriber and expect to withhold drug. If confirmed, treat with fluids, electrolytes, protein, and an antibiotic effective against *C. difficile.*

PATIENT TEACHING

• Instruct patient to use a calibrated measuring device to accurately measure doses of oral solution.

• Advise patient to notify prescriber if no improvement occurs after a few days.

• Instruct patient to complete full course of vancomycin, as prescribed.

• Instruct patient to notify prescriber if she develops severe or persistent diarrhea.

• Instruct patient to keep follow-up appointments during and after treatment.

vardenafil hydrochloride

Levitra

Class and Category

Chemical class: Type 5 phosphodiesterase inhibitor
Therapeutic class: Anti-impotence agent
Pregnancy category: B

Indications and Dosages

➤ *To treat erectile dysfunction*

TABLETS

Adults. 10 mg taken 1 hr before sexual activity; increased to 20 mg or decreased to 5 mg, as needed. *Maximum:* 20 mg and taken only once daily regardless of dosage used.

DOSAGE ADJUSTMENT If patient takes ritonavir, dosage of vardenfil shouldn't exceed 2.5 mg in 72 hr. If patient takes indinavir, saquinavir, atazanavir, clarithromycin, ketoconazole 400 mg daily, itraconazole 400 mg daily, or another potent CYP3A4 inhibitor, dosage or vardenafil shouldn't exceed 2.5 mg in 24 hr. If patient takes ketoconazole 200 mg and itraconazole 200 mg daily, dosage of vardenafil shouldn't exceed 5 mg in 24 hr.

Route	Onset	Peak	Duration
P.O.	30 min	30 min to 2 hr	4 to 5 hr

Mechanism of Action

Enhances effect of nitric oxide (released in the penis by sexual stimulation) and inhibits phosphodiesterase type 5, which increases cGMP level, relaxes smooth muscle, and increases blood flow into the corpus cavernosum, producing an erection.

Contraindications

Concurrent administration of alpha blockers, concomitant continuous or intermittent nitrate therapy, hypersensitivity to vardenafil or its components

Interactions

DRUGS

alpha blockers, nitrates: Profound hypotension
atazanavir, clarithromycin, erythromycin, indinavir, itraconazole, ketoconazole, ritonavir, saquinavir: Increased vardenafil effects
class IA (procainamide, quinidine) and class III (amiodarone, sotalol) antiarrhythmics: Possibly increased QT-interval prolongation
indinavir, ritonavir: Reduced blood levels of indinavir and ritonavir

FOODS

grapefruit juice: Possibly increased vardenafil effect

Adverse Reactions

CNS: Dizziness, headache, seizures, transient global amnesia
CV: Hypotension
EENT: Decreased vision, hearing loss, nonarteritic anterior ischemic optic neuropathy, rhinitis, sinusitis, tinnitus
GI: Indigestion, nausea
MS: Back pain
SKIN: Flushing
Other: Flulike symptoms, increased creatine kinase level

Nursing Considerations

• Be aware that vardenafil shouldn't be used by men taking class IA (procainamide, quinidine) or class III (amiodarone, sotalol) antiarrhythmics or by men who have congenital QT-interval prolongation because drug may potentiate QT-interval prolongation.

• Use vardenafil cautiously in men with renal or hepatic dysfunction, in elderly men, and in men with penile abnormalities that may predispose them to priapism.

• Also use cautiously in patients with left ventricular outflow obstruction, such as aortic stenosis, and those with severely impaired autonomic control of blood pressure because these conditions increase patient's sensitivity to vasodilators, such as vardenafil.

• Monitor blood pressure and heart rate before and after giving drug, especially if patient takes an alpha blocker, because of increased risk of symptomatic hypotension.

• Monitor patient's vision, especially if he is over age 50; has diabetes, hypertension, coronary artery disease, or hyperlipidemia; or smokes, because vardenafil rarely leads to nonarteritic ischemic optic neuropathy and decreased vision, possibly permanent.

• Monitor patient's hearing. Sudden decrease or loss, possibly with tinnitus and dizziness, may occur with vardenafil use. Report such changes immediately, and expect drug to be discontinued.

PATIENT TEACHING

• For best results, tell patient to take drug 1 hour before anticipated sexual activity.

• **WARNING** Warn patient not to take vardenafil if he also takes an organic nitrate continuously or intermittently, or within 4 hours of taking alpha blockers because profound hypotension and death could result.

• Caution against taking vardenafil more than once a day or exceeding 20 mg daily.

• Tell patient to stop taking vardenafil and notify prescriber if he has a sudden loss of vision in one or both eyes, sudden hearing loss, seizures, or trouble remembering.

• Advise patient to seek sexual counseling to enhance drug's effects.

• To avoid possible penile damage and permanent loss of erectile function, urge patient to notify prescriber immediately if erection is painful or lasts longer than 4 hours.

varenicline

Chantix

Class and Category

Chemical class: Tartrate salt

Therapeutic class: Nicotinic blocker
Pregnancy classification: C

Indications and Dosages

➤ *As adjunct to smoking cessation treatment*

TABLETS

Adults. *Initial:* 0.5 mg daily for 3 days, then increased to 0.5 mg b.i.d. for 4 days, and then increased to 1 mg b.i.d. for a total of 12 wk of therapy. If effective, an additional 12 wk of therapy may be given.

DOSAGE ADJUSTMENT If patient has severe renal impairment, maximum dosage should not exceed 0.5 mg b.i.d. If patient is undergoing hemodialysis for end-stage renal disease, maximum dosage should not exceed 0.5 mg daily.

Mechanism of Action

Blocks nicotine from activating alpha$_4$beta$_2$ receptors by binding to them. This inhibits nicotine stimulation of the central nervous mesolimbic dopamine system, which probably is the area that produces pleasure in and reinforcement of smoking.

Contraindications

Hypersensitivity to varenicline or its components

Interactions

DRUGS

nicotine (transdermal): Increased adverse reactions

Adverse Reactions

CNS: Abnormal dreams, agitation, anxiety, asthenia, attention difficulties, behavior changes, depression, dizziness, dysgeusia, fatigue, headache, insomnia, irritability, lethargy, malaise, mental impairment, restlessness, sensory disturbances, seizures, somnolence, stroke, suicidal ideation, thirst

CV: Angina, chest pain, edema, hypertension, MI, peripheral ischemia, thrombosis, ventricular extrasystoles

EENT: Dry mouth, epistaxis, gingivitis, rhinorrhea

ENDO: Hot flashes

GI: Abdominal pain, acute pancreatitis, anorexia, constipation, diarrhea, dyspepsia, flatuence, gastroesophageal reflux disease,

GI hemorrhage, increased appetite, liver enzyme abnormalities, nausea, vomiting
GU: Acute renal failure, polyuria, urine retention
HEME: Leukocytosis, lymphadenopathy, splenomegaly, thrombocytopenia
RESP: Asthma, dyspnea, pulmonary embolism
MS: Arthralgia, back pain, muscle cramp, musculoskeletal pain, myalgia
SKIN: Diaphoresis, pruritus, rash, urticaria
Other: Flulike syndrome, hyperkalemia, hypersensitivity, hypokalemia

Nursing Considerations
•Use cautiously in patients with renal disease because varenicline is substantially excreted by the kidneys.
•Review patient's medication history before starting varenicline because smoking cessation may require dosage adjustments to such drugs as theophylline, warfarin, and insulin.
•If patient has nausea, the most common adverse reaction to varenicline, notify prescriber. Dosage reduction may help.
•Be aware that nicotine withdrawal symptoms and worsening of underlying psychiatric illness may occur with smoking cessation, even with varenicline therapy.
•Watch patient closely for suicidal tendencies, particularly when therapy starts and dosage changes, because depression may worsen temporarily during these times, possibly leading to suicidal ideation.

PATIENT TEACHING
•Explain that using nicotine patches while taking varenicline won't increase its effectiveness and may increase adverse reactions such as dizziness, nausea, and vomiting.
•Instruct patient to set a date to quit smoking and then start taking varenicline 1 week before the quit date.
•Tell patient to take drug after eating and with a full glass of water.
•Encourage patient to continue trying to stop smoking even if an early relapse occurs during varenicline therapy.
•Inform patient that the most common adverse reactions to varenicline therapy are nausea and insomnia, usually transient. If they persist, patient should notify prescriber; dosage reduction may help.
•Caution patient to avoid hazardous activities until CNS effects of drug are known.
•Explain that vivid, unusual, or strange dreams may occur during therapy.
•Urge family or caregiver to watch patient closely for suicidal tendencies, especially when therapy starts or dosage changes.
•Tell patient that nicotine withdrawal can occur even with varenicline use and pre-existing psychiatric illness may worsen during smoking cessation. Advise patient or family to notify prescriber about abnormal thinking or behavior.

vasopressin
(antidiuretic hormone [ADH])
Pitressin, Pressyn (CAN)

Class and Category
Chemical class: Polypeptide hormone
Therapeutic class: Antidiuretic
Pregnancy category: C

Indications and Dosages
➤ *To prevent or control symptoms of central diabetes insipidus caused by insufficient ADH*
I.M. OR SUBCUTANEOUS INJECTION
Adults. 5 to 10 units b.i.d. or t.i.d., as needed.
Children. 2.5 to 10 units t.i.d. or q.i.d., as needed.

➤ *To prevent or treat abdominal distention*
I.M. INJECTION
Adults. 5 units, increased to 10 units every 3 to 4 hr, as needed.

Route	Onset	Peak	Duration
I.M., SubQ	Unknown	Unknown	2 to 8 hr

Contraindications
Chronic nephritis with nitrogen retention, hypersensitivity to vasopressin or its components

Interactions
DRUGS
carbamazepine, chlorpropamide, clofibrate, fludrocortisone, tricyclic antidepressants: Increased antidiuretic effect
demeclocycline, lithium, norepinephrine: Decreased antidiuretic effect

Adverse Reactions
CNS: Dizziness, headache, light-headedness, tremor

Mechanism of Action

Vasopressin, a synthetic form of antidiuretic hormone, treats diabetes insipidus by decreasing urine output and raising urine osmolality. When vasopressin attaches to vaso-pressin$_2$ (V$_2$) receptors on cell membranes in the nephron's collecting duct, it activates the enzyme adenyl cyclase to convert adenosine triphos-phate (ATP) to cyclic adeno-sine monophosphate (cAMP). This action increases the col-lecting duct's permeability and enhances water reabsorp-tion into the blood.

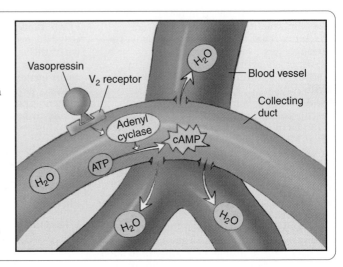

CV: Angina, MI
EENT: Circumoral pallor
ENDO: Water intoxication
GI: Abdominal cramps, diarrhea, eructation, flatulence, intestinal hypermotility, nausea, vomiting
SKIN: Diaphoresis, pallor
Other: Allergic reaction

Nursing Considerations

•Use vasopressin with extreme caution in patients with coronary artery disease because it may cause angina or MI; in those with hy-pertension because it may increase blood pressure; and in those with asthma, epilepsy, heart failure, or migraine headache because extracellular fluid may increase rapidly.
•Monitor fluid and electrolyte balance dur-ing therapy. Monitor intake and output at least every 8 hours, and assess for signs and symptoms of water intoxication and hypona-tremia, including anuria, confusion, drowsi-ness, headache, listlessness, and weight gain.

PATIENT TEACHING

•Teach patient how to administer vasopres-sin; emphasize the need to rotate injection sites.
•Urge patient to notify prescriber immedi-ately if he experiences signs of possible water intoxication, including anuria, confu-sion, drowsiness, headache, listlessness, and unexplained weight gain.
•Inform patient that abdominal cramps,

nausea, and skin blanching will subside after a few minutes and can be minimized by drinking one or two glasses of water.

venlafaxine hydrochloride

Effexor, Effexor XR

desvenlafaxine succinate

Pristiq

Class and Category

Chemical class: Phenylethylamine derivative
Therapeutic class: Antidepressant
Pregnancy category: C

Indications and Dosages

➤ *To treat and prevent relapse of major depression*

E.R. CAPSULES (EFFEXOR XR)
Adults. 75 mg daily with a meal same time each day morning or evening (for some pa-tients, 37.5 mg daily for 4 to 7 days before increasing to 75 mg daily), then increased by 75 mg daily every 4 days, as prescribed. *Maximum:* 225 mg daily.
DOSAGE ADJUSTMENT Initial daily dose de-creased by 25% to 50% for patients with mild to moderate renal impairment and by 50% for patients with hepatic impairment.
E.R. TABLETS (PRISTIQ)
Adults. 50 mg daily, with a meal, at the same

time each day morning or evening
DOSAGE ADJUSTMENT For patient with severe renal impairment, 50 mg every other day.

TABLETS (EFFEXOR)

Adults. 75 mg daily in divided doses b.i.d. or t.i.d., increased by 75 mg daily every 4 days, as prescribed. *Maximum:* 375 mg daily (225 mg/day for outpatients).

➤ *To treat generalized anxiety disorder or social anxiety disorder*

E.R. CAPSULES (EFFEXOR XR)

Adults. 75 mg daily with a meal at same time each day morning or evening (for some patients, 37.5 mg daily for 4 to 7 days before increasing to 75 mg daily), and then increased by 75 mg daily every 4 days, as prescribed. *Maximum:* 225 mg daily.
DOSAGE ADJUSTMENT Initial daily dose decreased by 25% to 50% for patients with mild to moderate renal impairment and by 50% for patients with hepatic impairment.

Route	Onset	Peak	Duration
P.O.	2 wk	Unknown	Unknown

Mechanism of Action

Inhibits neuronal reuptake of serotonin and norepinephrine, along with its active metabolite, O-desmethylvenlafaxine. These actions raise serotonin and norepinephrine levels at nerve synapses, elevating mood and reducing depression.

Contraindications

Hypersensitivity to desvenlafaxine, venlafaxine, or their components; use of an MAO inhibitor within 14 days

Interactions

DRUGS

amitriptyline, clomipramine, desipramine, doxepin, haloperidol, imipramine, linezolid, lithium, nortriptyline, protriptyline, St. John's wort, tramadol, trazodone, triptans: Possibly serotonin syndrome
aspirin, NSAIDs, warfarin: Increased risk of bleeding
cimetidine: Decreased clearance and increased levels of desvenlafaxine and venlafaxine
clozapine: Possibly increased blood clozapine levels and serious adverse reactions, including seizures
CYP3A4 inhibitors, ketoconazole: Increased plasma venlafaxine level and risk of adverse reactions
MAO inhibitors: Increased risk of hypertension; hyperthermia; mental status changes, including coma and delirium; muscle rigidity; and severe myoclonus
metoprolol: Increased plasma metoprolol level but decreased effectiveness in lowering blood pressure
warfarin: Possibly increased PT, partial thromboplastin time, and INR

Adverse Reactions

CNS: Abnormal dreams, agitation, amnesia, anxiety, asthenia, cerebral ischemia, chills, confusion, delusions, depersonalization, depression, dizziness, dream disturbances, drowsiness, dyskinesia, fever, headache, hypesthesia, hypomania, impaired balance and coordination, insomnia, mania, migraine, mood changes, nervousness, neuroleptic malignant syndrome, paresthesia, seizures, somnolence, suicidal ideation, syncope, tremor, vertigo
CV: Arrhythmias, AV block, chest pain, congestive heart failure, elevated cholesterol and triglyceride levels, edema, extrasystoles, hypertension, hypotension, MI, palpitations, sinus tachycardia, thrombophlebitis, vasodilation, worsening of peripheral vascular disease
EENT: Abnormal vision, accommodation abnormality, angle-closure glaucoma, blurred vision, dry mouth, mydriasis, pharyngitis, rhinitis, taste alteration, tinnitus
ENDO: Hyperglycemia, syndrome of inappropriate ADH secretion
GI: Abdominal pain, anorexia, colitis, constipation, diarrhea, elevated liver enzymes, flatulence, GI hemorrhage, indigestion, nausea, vomiting
GU: Anorgasmia (women), decreased libido, ejaculation disorder, impotence, urinary incontinence or urgency, urine retention
HEME: Anemia, leukocytosis, leukopenia, lymphadenopathy, thrombocytopenia
MS: Neck pain, rhabdomyolysis
RESP: Cough, eosinophilic pneumonia, increased dyspnea, interstitial lung disease
SKIN: Diaphoresis, ecchymosis, pruritus, Stevens-Johnson syndrome, toxic epidermal necrolysis

U
V
W

Other: Angioedema, hyponatremia, weight loss

Nursing Considerations
• Use cautiously in patients with a history of mania because desvenlafaxine and venlafaxine therapy may worsen condition. Also use cautiously in patients with a history of seizures, and expect to discontinue drug, as ordered, if seizures occur.
• Use cautiously in patients who have medical conditions that might be made worse by an increased heart rate, as in hyperthyroidism, heart failure, or recent MI.
• WARNING Be aware that serotonin syndrome in its most severe form may resemble neuroleptic malignant syndrome, which includes hyperthermia, muscle rigidity, autonomic instability with possibly rapid changes in vital signs, and mental status changes. Stop drug immediately and provide supportive care.
• Monitor blood pressure often during therapy because it may cause dose-related sustained increase in supine diastolic pressure. Expect to reduce or stop drug, as prescribed, if increase develops.
• Assess patient's electrolyte balance, as ordered, because drug can cause hyponatremia, especially in elderly patients and in patients who take diuretics or are volume-depleted. If patient has evidence of hyponatremia (headache, trouble concentrating, confusion, weakness, unsteadiness), notify prescriber. If imbalance is confirmed, expect to stop drug and give appropriate care.
• Watch patient for suicidal tendencies, especially when therapy starts and dosage changes.
• WARNING Be aware that drug shouldn't be discontinued abruptly because doing so may cause multiple adverse effects, including asthenia, dizziness, headache, insomnia, and nervousness.

PATIENT TEACHING
• Instruct patient not to crush or chew E.R. capsules or tablets. However, if she has difficulty swallowing capsules, tell her to open capsule, sprinkle contents on a spoonful of applesauce, and swallow immediately without chewing, followed by a glass of water.
• Advise patient to avoid alcohol during venlafaxine therapy.
• Advise patient not to stop taking desvenlafaxine or venlafaxine abruptly.

• Caution patient to notify prescriber if she becomes pregnant during therapy because she'll need a different antidepressant. Taking desvenlafaxine or venlafaxine during third trimester of pregnancy increases the risk of complications in the infant after birth.
• Advise patient to tell prescriber about all other prescribed drugs or OTC products she takes because of the risk of interactions.
• Urge caregivers to monitor patient closely for suicidal tendencies, especially when therapy starts or dosage changes.
• Caution patient to avoid aspirin and NSAIDs, if possible, while taking desvenlafaxine or venlafaxine.

verapamil
Apo-Verap (CAN), Calan, Isoptin, Novo-Veramil (CAN), Nu-Verap (CAN)

verapamil hydrochloride
Calan SR, Isoptin SR, Verelan

Class and Category
Chemical class: Phenylalkylamine derivative
Therapeutic class: Antianginal, antiarrhythmic, antihypertensive
Pregnancy category: C

Indications and Dosages
➤ *To treat chronic angina pectoris*
TABLETS (VERAPAMIL)
Adults and adolescents age 15 and over. *Initial:* 80 to 120 mg t.i.d., increased every day or wk, as needed and prescribed. *Maximum:* 480 mg daily in divided doses.
Infants and children up to age 15. 4 to 8 mg/kg daily in divided doses.
➤ *To manage hypertension*
E.R. CAPSULES (VERAPAMIL HYDROCHLORIDE)
Adults and adolescents. *Initial:* 240 mg daily, increased every day or wk, as needed and prescribed. *Maximum:* 480 mg daily.
E.R. TABLETS (VERAPAMIL HYDROCHLORIDE)
Adults and adolescents. *Initial:* 180 mg daily, increased every day or wk, as needed and prescribed, according to following schedule: 240 mg daily in the morning; 180 mg every 12 hr or 240 mg in the morning and 120 mg in the evening; then 240 mg every 12 hr. *Maximum:* 480 mg daily in divided doses.
TABLETS (VERAPAMIL)
Adults and adolescents age 15 and over. *Ini-*

tial: 80 to 120 mg t.i.d., increased every day or wk, as needed and prescribed. *Maximum:* 480 mg daily in divided doses.

Infants and children up to age 15. 4 to 8 mg/kg daily in divided doses.

➤ *To prevent or treat supraventricular tachycardia*

TABLETS (VERAPAMIL)

Adults and adolescents age 15 and over. *Initial:* 80 to 120 mg t.i.d., increased every day or wk, as needed and prescribed. *Maximum:* 480 mg daily in divided doses.

DOSAGE ADJUSTMENT Initial P.O. dosage possibly reduced to 40 mg t.i.d. (120 mg daily for E.R. tablets or capsules) for elderly patients and those with impaired hepatic or left ventricular function.

I.V. INJECTION (VERAPAMIL HYDROCHLORIDE)

Adults and adolescents age 15 and over. *Initial:* 5 to 10 mg slowly over 2 min; then 10 mg, as prescribed, if response isn't adequate after 30 min.

Children ages 1 to 15. *Initial:* 100 to 300 mcg/kg slowly over 2 min, up to maximum of 5 mg; then 10 mg, as prescribed, if response isn't adequate after 30 min.

Infants up to age 1. *Initial:* 100 to 200 mcg/kg slowly over 2 min.

DOSAGE ADJUSTMENT I.V. drug administered over 3 minutes in elderly patients.

Route	Onset	Peak	Duration
P.O.	1 to 2 hr	30 to 90 min	6 to 8 hr
P.O. (E.R.)	1 to 2 hr	30 to 90 min	Unknown
I.V.	1 to 5 min	3 to 5 min	10 min to 6 hr

Incompatibilities

Don't mix I.V. verapamil with albumin, amphotericin B injection, hydralazine hydrochloride injection, nafcillin, or sulfamethoxazole and trimethoprim injection. Solutions with pH above 6.0 cause precipitation.

Contraindications

Cardiogenic shock, concomitant use of beta blockers (with I.V. verapamil), hypersensitivity to verapamil or its components, hypotension, severe heart failure unless secondary to supraventricular tachycardia that responds to verapamil, severe left ventricular dysfunc-tion, sick sinus syndrome or second- or third-degree heart block unless artificial pacemaker is in place, ventricular tachycardia (with I.V. verapamil)

Mechanism of Action

Inhibits calcium movement into coronary and vascular smooth-muscle cells by blocking slow calcium channels in cell membranes. The resulting decrease in the intracellular calcium level has the following effects:

• inhibits smooth-muscle cell contractions
• decreases myocardial oxygen demand by relaxing coronary and vascular smooth muscle, reducing peripheral vascular resistance, and decreasing systolic and diastolic pressures
• slows AV conduction time and prolongs AV nodal refractoriness
• interrupts reentry circuit in AV nodal reentrant tachycardias.

Interactions

DRUGS

alpha blockers, antihypertensives, general anesthetics (hydrocarbon), prazosin: Hypotensive effects

aspirin: Increased bleeding time

beta blockers: Increased risk of heart failure, hypotension, and severe bradycardia

calcium supplements: Decreased response to verapamil

carbamazepine, cyclosporine, theophylline, valproate: Increased risk of toxicity from these drugs

cimetidine: Decreased metabolism and increased blood level of verapamil

dantrolene: Increased risk of hyperkalemia and myocardial depression

digoxin: Increased blood digoxin level and risk of digitalis toxicity

disopyramide, flecainide: Additive negative inotropic effects

erythromycin, ritonavir: Increased blood verapamil level

lithium: Increased risk of neurotoxicity

neuromuscular blockers: Prolonged recovery from neuromuscular blockade

NSAIDs, sympathomimetics: Decreased antihypertensive effect of verapamil

phenobarbital: Increased verapamil clearance

U
V
W

procainamide: Increased Q-T interval, additive negative inotropic effects
protein-bound drugs (hydantoins, salicylates, sulfonamides, sulfonylureas, and warfarin and other oral anticoagulants): Altered blood levels of these drugs
quinidine: Increased risk of quinidine toxicity, increased Q-T interval, additive negative inotropic effects
rifampin: Decreased bioavailability of oral verapamil
telithromycin: Increased risk of bradyarrhythmias, hypotension, and lactic acidosis

FOODS
grapefruit juice: Increased concentrations of verapamil

ACTIVITIES
alcohol use: Increased blood alcohol level and prolonged CNS effects

Adverse Reactions

CNS: Confusion, CVA, disequilibrium, dizziness, extrapyramidal reactions, fatigue, headache, insomnia, paresthesia, psychosis, shakiness, somnolence
CV: Angina, AV conduction disorders, bradycardia, claudication, heart failure, hypotension, peripheral edema, tachycardia
GI: Constipation, elevated liver function test results, nausea
GU: Galactorrhea, menstrual irregularities
MS: Muscle spasms
RESP: Dyspnea, pulmonary edema, wheezing
SKIN: Flushing, rash

Nursing Considerations

•Administer I.V. verapamil with compatible solutions, including Ringer's injection, D₅W, or normal saline solution.
•Maintain continuous ECG monitoring and keep emergency resuscitative equipment and drugs readily available during I.V. therapy.
•Assess patient with hypertrophic cardiomyopathy for early development of hypotension and pulmonary edema because second-degree AV block and sinus arrest can result.
•Assess for bradycardia and hypotension, and notify prescriber if heart rate or blood pressure declines significantly.
•Be aware that disopyramide or flecainide shouldn't be given within 48 hours before or 24 hours after verapamil because additive negative inotropic effects can result.
•Institute measures to prevent constipation, including a high-fiber diet and a stool softener, as prescribed.

PATIENT TEACHING
•Instruct patient not to crush or chew verapamil E.R. tablets or capsules. Inform her that she may break E.R. tablets in half if necessary to aid swallowing.
•Direct patient to check her pulse rate before taking verapamil and to notify prescriber if it's below 50 beats/minute or as instructed by prescriber.
•Caution patient about possible dizziness and the need to avoid potentially hazardous activities until drug's CNS effects are known.
•Inform patient that adverse skin reactions may subside with continued use. Advise her to notify prescriber if rash persists.
•Encourage patient to increase dietary fiber intake to help prevent constipation. Advise her to notify prescriber if problem becomes persistent or severe.

voriconazole

Vfend

Class and Category

Chemical class: Triazole
Therapeutic class: Antifungal
Pregnancy category: D

Indications and Dosages

➤ *To treat invasive aspergillosis; to treat serious fungal infections caused by* Scedosporium apiospermum *and* Fusarium *species, including* Fusarium solani, *in patients intolerant of or refractory to other therapy*

I.V. INFUSION
Adults and children age 12 and over. *Initial:* 6 mg/kg over 1 to 2 hr at a rate not to exceed 3 mg/kg/hr every 12 hr for 2 doses. *Maintenance:* 4 mg/kg over 1 to 2 hr at a rate not to exceed 3 mg/kg/hr every 12 hr.

TABLETS
Adults and children age 12 and over weighing 40 kg (88 lb) or more. *Maintenance:* 200 mg every 12 hr, increased to 300 mg every 12 hr, as needed, and taken at least 1 hr before or after a meal.
Adults and children age 12 and over weighing less than 40 kg. *Maintenance:* 100 mg every 12 hr, increased to 150 mg every 12 hr, as needed, and taken at least 1 hr before or after a meal.

▶ *To treat candidemia in nonneutropenic patients and other deep-tissue disseminated candida infections involving the abdomen, kidney, bladder wall, skin, or a wound*

I.V. INFUSION

Adults. *Initial:* 6 mg/kg over 1 to 2 hr at a rate not to exceed 3 mg/kg/hr every 12 hr for 2 doses. *Maintenance:* 3 to 4 mg/kg over 1 to 2 hr at a rate not to exceed 3 mg/kg/hr every 12 hr for at least 14 days after symptoms resolve or last positive culture, whichever takes longer.

TABLETS

Adults. *Maintenance:* 200 mg every 12 hr taken at least 1 hr before or after a meal.

▶ *To treat esophageal candidiasis*

TABLETS

Adults. 200 mg every 12 hr taken at least 1 hr before or after a meal for at least 14 days and at least 7 days after signs and symptoms resolve.

DOSAGE ADJUSTMENT If patient can't tolerate drug, I.V. maintenance dose may be reduced to 3 mg/kg every 12 hr and oral maintenance dose by 50-mg decrements to at least 200 mg every 12 hr (or to 100 mg every 12 hr for patients weighing less than 40 kg). For use with phenytoin, maintenance dose may be increased to 5 mg/kg I.V. every 12 hr or from 200 mg to 400 mg P.O. every 12 hr (100 mg to 200 mg every 12 hr for patients weighing less than 40 kg). For patients with mild to moderate hepatic cirrhosis, standard loading dose should be used but maintenance dose halved for I.V. or P.O. use. For patients with moderate to severe renal insufficiency (creatinine clearance greater than 50 ml/min), only the oral form should be given, if possible.

Mechanism of Action

Prevents fungal ergosterol biosynthesis by inhibiting fungal cytochrome P450–mediated 14 alpha-lanosterol demethylation. The loss of ergosterol in the fungal cell wall renders the fungal cell inactive.

Incompatibilities

Don't infuse into the same line or cannula with other drugs, including parenteral nutrition, to prevent an increase in subvisible particulate matter. Avoid infusion with blood products and any electrolyte supplements. Don't dilute with 4.2% sodium bicarbonate infusion because the mildly alkaline nature of the diluent causes slight degradation of voriconazole after 24 hours of storage at room temperature.

Contraindications

Coadministration with long-acting barbiturates, carbamazepine, CYP3A4 substrates (astemizole, cisapride, pimozide, quinidine, or terfenadine), efavirenz, ergot alkaloids, rifabutin, rifampin, ritonavir, sirolimus, or St. John's wort; hypersensitivity to voriconazole or its components; galactose intolerance, glucose-galactose malabsorption, or Lapp lactase deficiency (oral form only contains lactose)

Interactions

DRUGS

alfentanil: Increased plasma alfentanil level and increased risk of adverse reactions
benzodiazepines: Possibly prolonged sedative effect of benzodiazepines
calcium channel blockers; HMG-CoA reductase inhibitors, such as lovastatin; omeprazole; sirolimus: Possibly increased plasma concentrations of these drugs, leading to increased risk of adverse reactions and toxicity
carbamazepine, long-acting barbiturates, phenytoin, rifampin: Decreased plasma voriconazole concentration
coumarin, warfarin: Possibly increased PTT
cyclosporine, sirolimus, tacrolimus: Increased serum concentrations of these drugs and risk of toxicity, especially nephrotoxicity
CYP3A4 substrates (astemizole, cisapride, pimozide, quinidine, terfenadine): Increased plasma concentrations of these drugs, which may lead to prolonged QT interval and, rarely, torsades de pointes
ergot alkaloids (ergotamine, dihydroergotamine): May increase plasma concentration of ergot alkaloids leading to ergotism
HIV protease inhibitors (amprenavir, nelfinavir, ritonavir, saquinavir), non-nucleoside reverse transcriptase inhibitors (delavirdine, efavirenz): Possibly inhibited metabolism of these drugs and voriconazole
methadone: Increased plasma concentration of methadone, possibly leading to toxicity, including QT-interval prolongation
oral contraceptives: Increased plasma

voriconazole level and risk of toxicity
rifabutin: Increased rifabutin plasma concentration; decreased voriconazole plasma concentrations
St. John's wort: Decreased plasma voriconazole level
sulfonylureas: Possibly increased plasma concentrations of sulfonylureas and increased risk of hypoglycemia
vinca alkaloids: Possibly increased risk of neurotoxicity

Adverse Reactions
CNS: Chills, dizziness, fever, hallucinations, headache
CV: Chest pain, hypertension, hypotension, peripheral edema, tachycardia, vasodilation
EENT: Abnormal or blurred vision, altered or enhanced visual perception, change in color perception, chromatopsia, dry mouth, eye hemorrhage, photophobia, visual disturbances
GI: Abdominal pain, diarrhea, elevated liver function test results, nausea, pancreatitis, vomiting
GU: Abnormal kidney function, acute renal failure, elevated serum creatinine level
HEME: Anemia, leukopenia, pancytopenia, thrombocytopenia
RESP: Respiratory disorders
SKIN: Cholestatic jaundice, erythema multiforme, jaundice, maculopapular rash, photosensitivity, pruritus, rash, Stevens-Johnson syndrome, toxic epidermal necrolysis
Other: Anaphylaxis (I.V. form), elevated alkaline phosphatase, hypokalemia, hypomagnesemia, sepsis

Nursing Considerations
• Use voriconazole cautiously in patients with known hypersensitivity to other azoles and in patients at risk for proarrhythmic events (such as those receiving cardiotoxic chemotherapy or those who have cardiomyopathy or hypokalemia) because some azoles may cause prolong QT interval.
• Determine if patient has any problems with galactose intolerance, Lapp lactase deficiency, or glucose-galactose malabsorption before starting therapy because voriconazole tablets contain lactose and shouldn't be given to patients with these conditions.
• Obtain specimens for fungal culture and other relevant laboratory studies (including histopathology), as ordered, before giving

first dose. Expect to begin drug before test results are known.
• Assess patient's liver function, including bilirubin, as ordered, at the start of voriconazole therapy and periodically thereafter. Be aware that drug may be discontinued if liver abnormalities occur.
• Check patient's electrolyte levels before start of therapy, as ordered, and correct any imbalances, as prescribed, before administering voriconazole because electrolyte imbalances increase the risk of adverse reactions.
• For I.V. infusion, reconstitute powder with 19 ml of water for injection to obtain 20 ml of concentrate containing 10 mg/ml voriconazole. To make sure exact amount of water is injected into vial, use a standard 10-ml non-automated syringe. Shake the vial until all powder is dissolved. Further dilute so that final concentration is not less than 0.5 mg/ml nor more than 5 mg/ml. This requires withdrawing and discarding at least an equal volume of diluent from the infusion bag or bottle before instillation of concentrate.
• Discard partially used vials after mixing. If infusion isn't administered immediately, store at 2° to 8° C (37° to 46° F) for no longer than 24 hours.
• Administer I.V. infusion over 1 to 2 hours at a rate that doesn't exceed 3 mg/kg/hr.
• Monitor renal function, especially serum creatinine level, when administering I.V. form of voriconazole because drug may accumulate in body when creatinine clearance is less than 50 ml/min, increasing the risk of adverse reactions.
• **WARNING** Observe patient receiving I.V. voriconazole closely for anaphylactoid-type reactions—such as flushing, fever, sweating, tachycardia, chest tightness, dyspnea, faintness, nausea, pruritus and rash—which may occur immediately after starting the infusion. Stop the infusion if these reactions occur, and notify prescriber immediately.
• Monitor patient closely throughout therapy for skin rash, which may indicate a serious cutaneous reaction, such as Stevens-Johnson syndrome. If a rash occurs, notify prescriber, and expect that voriconazole may be discontinued.
• Monitor cyclosporine, tacrolimus, and warfarin closely for elevated levels when voriconazole is coadministered with any of these drugs.

•Monitor diabetic patients also taking sulfonylureas closely for hypoglycemia, and check blood glucose levels regularly.

•Be aware that voriconazole dosage will need to be adjusted when co-administered with phenytoin. Expect to monitor plasma phenytoin levels and observe patient closely for phenytoin-related adverse reactions.

•Assess patient's visual function, including visual acuity, visual field, and color perception, if voriconazole therapy continues longer than 28 days.

•Monitor patient closely for pancreatitis, especially patient with risk factors for acute pancreatitis, such as having had recent chemotherapy or hematopoietic stem cell transplantation or children.

PATIENT TEACHING

•Instruct patient taking oral voriconazole to take the tablets at least 1 hour before or 1 hour after a meal.

•Inform female patient of possible fetal risk, and stress the need to avoid pregnancy. Tell her to use effective contraception throughout therapy and to notify the prescriber immediately if pregnancy is suspected.

•Caution patient not to drive at night and to avoid potentially hazardous activities because drug may cause visual disturbances, including blurring or photophobia.

•Advise patient to avoid exposure to direct sunlight or UV light and to wear sunscreen when outdoors.

warfarin sodium

Coumadin

Class and Category

Chemical class: Coumarin derivative
Therapeutic class: Anticoagulant
Pregnancy category: X

Indications and Dosages

➤ *To prevent or treat pulmonary embolism; recurrent MI; thromboembolic complications from atrial fibrillation, heart valve replacement, or MI; and venous thrombosis (and its extension)*

TABLETS

Adults. *Initial:* 2 to 5 mg daily for 2 to 4 days. *Usual:* 2 to 10 mg daily based on target PT and INR results. *Maximum:* Determined by target PT and INR results, as pre-

scribed.

I.V. INJECTION

Adults. *Initial:* 2 to 5 mg daily infused over 1 to 2 min. *Usual:* 2 to 10 mg daily infused over 1 to 2 min. *Maximum:* Determined by target PT and INR results, as prescribed. **DOSAGE ADJUSTMENT** For patients with hepatic dysfunction, dosage reduced to 0.1 mg/kg, as prescribed. For elderly patients, dosage possibly reduced based on PT and INR results.

Route	Onset	Peak	Duration
P.O	24 hr	3 to 4 days	2 to 5 days
I.V.	Unknown	3 to 4 days	2 to 5 days

Mechanism of Action

Interferes with the liver's ability to synthesize vitamin K–dependent clotting factors, depleting clotting factors II (prothrombin), VII, IX, and X. This action, in turn, interferes with the clotting cascade. By depleting vitamin K-dependent clotting factors and interfering with the clotting cascade, warfarin prevents coagulation.

Incompatibilities

Don't mix warfarin in solution with amikacin sulfate, epinephrine hydrochloride, metaraminol tartrate, oxytocin, promazine hydrochloride, tetracycline hydrochloride, or vancomycin hydrochloride.

Contraindications

Bleeding or bleeding tendencies; blood dyscrasias; cerebral or dissecting aneurysm; cerebrovascular hemorrhage; diverticulitis; eclampsia or preeclampsia; history of warfarin-induced necrosis; hypersensitivity to warfarin or its components; malignant or severe uncontrolled hypertension; malnutrition and emaciation; mental state or condition that leads to lack of patient cooperation; pericardial effusion; pericarditis; polyarthritis; pregnancy; prostatectomy; recent or planned neurosurgery, ophthalmic surgery, or spinal puncture; severe hepatic or renal disease

Interactions

DRUGS

acetaminophen, agrimony, aminoglycosides,

U
V
W

amiodarone, androgens, argatroban, beta blockers, bivalirudin, capecitabine, cephalosporins, chloral hydrate, chloramphenicol, chlorpropamide, cimetidine, clofibrate, corticosteroids, cyclophosphamide, dextrothyroxine, diflunisal, disulfiram, erythromycin, ezetimibe, fluconazole, gemfibrozil, glucagon, hydantoins, ifosfamide, influenza virus vaccine, isoniazid, ketoconazole, lepirudin, loop diuretics, lovastatin, metronidazole, miconazole, mineral oil, moricizine, nalidixic acid, NSAIDs, omeprazole, penicillins, phenylbutazones, propafenone, propoxyphene, quinidine, quinine, quinolones, salicylates, streptokinase, sulfamethoxazole-trimethoprim, sulfinpyrazone, sulfonamides, tamoxifen, tetracyclines, thyroid hormones, urokinase, valdecoxib, vitamin E: Increased anticoagulant effect of warfarin, increased risk of bleeding
aminoglutethimide, barbiturates, carbamazepine, cholestyramine, dicloxacillin, estrogens, ethchlorvynol, etretinate, glutethimide, griseofulvin, nafcillin, oral contraceptives, rifampin, spironolactone, sucralfate, thiazide diuretics, trazodone, vitamin C, vitamin K: Decreased anticoagulant effect of warfarin
atorvastatin, pravastatin: Increased or decreased anticoagulant effect of warfarin
herbal remedies (including bromelains, danshen, dong quai, garlic, ginkgo biloba, and ginseng): Increased anticoagulant effect of warfarin, increased risk of bleeding
I.V. lipid emulsion, other medical products that contain soybean oil: Possibly decreased vitamin K absorption and increased anticoagulant effect of warfarin
nicotine patch: Altered response to warfarin

FOODS
certain multivitamins, enteral feedings, vitamin–K-rich foods: Decreased effects of warfarin

ACTIVITIES
alcohol use: Increased risk of hypoprothrombinemia
smoking, smoking cessation: Altered response to warfarin

Adverse Reactions
CNS: Coma, intracranial hemorrhage, loss of consciousness, syncope, weakness
CV: Angina, chest pain, hypotension
EENT: Epistaxis, intraocular hemorrhage
GI: Abdominal cramps and pain, diarrhea, hepatitis, nausea, vomiting
GU: Hematuria, vaginal bleeding (abnormal)

HEME: Anemia, potentially fatal hemorrhage (from any tissue or organ)
SKIN: Alopecia, ecchymosis, jaundice, petechiae, pruritus, purple-toe syndrome, tissue necrosis
Other: Anaphylaxis

Nursing Considerations
•Reconstitute parenteral warfarin just before administration with 2.7 ml of sterile water for injection to yield 2 mg/ml. Then administer slowly over 1 to 2 minutes through peripheral I.V.
•Expect to administer another parenteral anticoagulant, such as heparin or enoxaparin, with oral warfarin for at least 3 days, or until desired response occurs, before giving warfarin only.
•Avoid I.M. injections during warfarin therapy, if possible, because they can result in bleeding, bruising, and hematoma.
•Monitor INR (daily in acute care setting) and assess for therapeutic effects, as prescribed. Therapeutic INR levels are 2.0 to 3.0 for bioprosthetic heart valve, nonvalvular atrial fibrillation, and venous thromboembolism, and 2.5 to 3.5 after MI and for mechanical heart valve.
•Expect treatment to last up to 12 weeks for bioprosthetic heart valve, 1 to 3 months for nonvalvular atrial fibrillation or venous thromboembolism, and for rest of life after MI and for mechanical heart valve replacement.
•**WARNING** Be aware of the increased risk for intracranial hemorrhage if patient has cerebral ischemia (such as recent transient ischemic attack or minor ischemic CVA) and INR of 3 to 4.5. As prescribed, withhold next warfarin dose and give vitamin K if INR exceeds 4 because of the risk of bleeding.
•Assess for occult bleeding if patient receives I.V. lipid emulsion or other medical product that contains soybean oil. Such products can decrease vitamin K absorption and increase warfarin's anticoagulant effect.

PATIENT TEACHING
•Explain that warfarin therapy aims to prevent thrombosis by decreasing clotting ability while avoiding the risk of spontaneous bleeding.
•Instruct patient to take drug exactly as prescribed at the same time each evening.

•Urge patient to keep weekly follow-up appointments for blood tests after discharge until PT and INR levels are stabilized.

•Advise patient to avoid alcohol during warfarin therapy.

•Urge patient to take precautions against bleeding, such as using an electric shaver and a soft-bristled toothbrush. Advise him to continue these precautions for 2 to 5 days after therapy stops, as directed, because anticoagulant effect may persist during this time.

•Caution patient to avoid activities that could cause traumatic injury and bleeding.

•Advise patient to eat consistent amounts of vitamin K–rich foods, such as dark green, leafy vegetables.

•Urge patient to notify prescriber immediately about unusual bleeding and any unexplained symptoms, such as abnormal vaginal bleeding; dizziness; easy bruising; gum bleeding; headache; nosebleeds; prolonged bleeding from cuts; red, black, or tarry stool; red or dark brown urine; swelling; and weakness.

•Advise patient to consult prescriber before taking other drugs—including OTC drugs and herbal remedies—during therapy.

•Instruct female patient of childbearing age to stop taking warfarin and notify prescriber immediately about known or suspected pregnancy.

•Explain that drug may cause reversible purple-toe syndrome and that this syndrome isn't harmful.

•Urge patient to carry medical identification that reveals he's taking warfarin therapy.

U
V
W

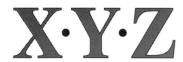

zafirlukast

Accolate

Class and Category

Chemical class: Peptide leukotriene receptor antagonist
Therapeutic class: Antiasthmatic
Pregnancy category: B

Indications and Dosages

➤ *To treat chronic asthma*

TABLETS

Adults and children over age 11. 20 mg b.i.d.
Children ages 5 to 11. 10 mg b.i.d.

Route	Onset	Peak	Duration
P.O.	1 wk	Unknown	Unknown

Mechanism of Action

Inhibits the selective binding of cysteinyl leukotrienes (arachidonic acid derivatives that usually mediate inflammation in asthma and other inflammatory disorders) by competitively blocking receptor sites. This action causes bronchial relaxation and decreases vascular leakage and edema, mucus secretion, eosinophil movement, and bronchial hyperresponsiveness.

Contraindications

Hypersensitivity to zafirlukast or its components

Interactions

DRUGS

alprazolam, amitriptyline, calcium channel blockers, carbamazepine, citalopram, corticosteroids, cyclosporine, diazepam, diclofenac, ibuprofen, imipramine, irbesartan, lidocaine, lovastatin, midazolam, phenytoin, quinidine, simvastatin, tolbutamide, tolterodine, triazolam: Inhibited metabolism and, possibly, additive adverse effects of these drugs
aspirin: Increased blood zafirlukast level
erythromycin, terfenadine: Decreased response to zafirlukast
sildenafil: Increased adverse effects of sildenafil
theophylline: Decreased blood zafirlukast level
warfarin: Prolonged PT

FOODS

any food: Possibly decreased bioavailability of zafirlukast

Adverse Reactions

CNS: Asthenia, dizziness, fever, headache, insomnia, malaise
GI: Abdominal pain, diarrhea, elevated liver function test results, hepatic failure, indigestion, nausea, vomiting
MS: Back pain, myalgia
SKIN: Pruritus
Other: Generalized pain

Nursing Considerations

• Be aware that zafirlukast shouldn't be used to treat bronchospasm during an acute asthma attack or status asthmaticus; it can't relieve symptoms quickly enough.
• Assess patient's respiratory rate, depth, and quality as well as breath sounds before and during treatment to evaluate response to therapy.
• If patient is being weaned from corticosteroids while taking zafirlukast, monitor her for Churg-Strauss syndrome, a rare allergic reaction characterized by eosinophilia, fever, myalgia, and weight loss as well as cardiac complications, neuropathy, and worsening pulmonary symptoms.

PATIENT TEACHING

• Instruct patient to take drug exactly as prescribed, in evenly spaced doses, every day. Stress the need to take drug even during symptom-free periods and acute exacerbations.
• Instruct patient to take drug on an empty stomach at least 1 hour before or 2 hours after meals.
• Advise patient to continue using rescue inhalants, as prescribed, for acute asthma attacks.
• Teach patient how to use peak-flow meter to monitor pulmonary function.
• Tell patient to immediately report evidence of liver dysfunction, such as right upper-quadrant abdominal pain, nausea, fatigue, lethargy, pruritus, jaundice, flulike symptoms, and anorexia.

X
Y
Z

zaleplon

Sonata

Class, Category, and Schedule
Chemical class: Imidazopyridine derivative
Therapeutic class: Sedative-hypnotic
Pregnancy category: C
Controlled substance schedule: IV

Indications and Dosages
➤ *Short-term treatment of insomnia*
CAPSULES
Adults up to age 65. 10 mg daily at bedtime, as prescribed, for up to 35 days. *Usual:* 10 mg daily at bedtime for 7 to 10 days. *Maximum:* 20 mg daily.
DOSAGE ADJUSTMENT For patients who are elderly, have hepatic impairment, or take cimetidine, dosage possibly reduced to 5 mg daily.

Route	Onset	Peak	Duration
P.O.	30 min	Unknown	4 hr

Mechanism of Action
Selectively binds with type 1 benzodiazepine (BZ1 or omega$_1$) receptors on the gamma-aminobutyric acid-A receptor complex. This binding produces muscle relaxation and sedation as well as antianxiety and anticonvulsant effects.

Contraindications
Hypersensitivity to zaleplon or its components

Interactions
DRUGS
amitriptyline; amoxapine; azatadine; benzodiazepines; brompheniramine; chlorpheniramine; clemastine; clomipramine; clozapine; cyproheptadine; dexchlorpheniramine; diphenhydramine; doxepin; entacapone; haloperidol; hydroxyzine; imipramine; maprotiline; mirtazapine; molindone; nefazodone; nortriptyline; olanzapine; opioid analgesics; other anxiolytics, sedatives, and hypnotics; phenindamine; phenothiazines; pimozide; pramipexole; promethazine; quetiapine; risperidone; ropinirole; thioridazine; trazodone; trimipramine; tripelennamine: Possibly additive CNS depression

carbamazepine, phenobarbital, phenytoin, rifampin: Reduced zaleplon effects
cimetidine: Increased blood zaleplon level
flumazenil: Reversal of zaleplon's sedation
FOODS
high-fat foods: Prolonged absorption time and reduced effectiveness of zaleplon
ACTIVITIES
alcohol use: Increased CNS depression

Adverse Reactions
CNS: Amnesia, anxiety, complex behaviors (such as sleep driving), depression, dizziness, drowsiness, fever, hallucinations, hypertonia, insomnia, paresthesia, seizures, suicidal ideation, tremor, vertigo
EENT: Dry mouth, gingivitis, glossitis, mouth ulcers, stomatitis, throat tightness
GI: Anorexia, colitis, constipation, eructation, esophagitis, flatulence, gastritis, gastroenteritis, increased appetite, indigestion, melena, nausea, rectal bleeding, vomiting
MS: Back pain
RESP: Dyspnea
SKIN: Photosensitivity, pruritus, rash
Other: Anaphylaxis, angioedema, physical and psychological dependence

Nursing Considerations
•Give zaleplon just before bedtime because its onset of action is rapid.
•Avoid giving drug with or after a heavy, high-fat meal because decreased absorption may reduce drug's effects.
•Watch patient closely for suicidal tendencies, particularly when therapy starts and dosage changes, because depression may worsen temporarily during these times, possibly leading to suicidal ideation.
•Monitor patient for signs of drug abuse because zaleplon has an abuse potential similar to that of benzodiazepines and benzodiazepine-like hypnotics.
•**WARNING** Monitor patient closely for hypersensitivity reactions, such as dyspnea, throat tightness, nausea, vomiting, and swelling. If present, discontinue zaleplon immediately, notify prescriber, and provide supportive care.
PATIENT TEACHING
•Inform patient that zaleplon is intended for short-term use. Advise her not to use this drug for any condition other than insomnia.
•Caution patient against exceeding prescribed dosage.
•Instruct patient to take zaleplon immedi-

ately before bedtime or right after having trouble falling asleep because of the rapid onset of drug's action.
•Teach patient alternative measures for relaxation and sleep induction.
•Advise patient to consult prescriber before taking other CNS depressants.
•Urge patient to avoid alcohol during zaleplon therapy because alcohol increases the risk of abnormal behaviors, such as sleep driving.
•Warn patient that zaleplon contains FD & C Yellow No. 5 (tartrazine), which can cause an allergic reaction, especially in those with an aspirin sensitivity. Instruct patient to report any allergic reactions, such as rash or difficulty breathing, to prescriber.
•Instruct patient to notify prescriber if inability to sleep continues. Dosage may need to be adjusted.
•Instruct patient to stop taking zaleplon and seek emergency care if she has trouble breathing, throat tightness, nausea, vomiting, or abnormal swelling.
•Advise patient that drug may cause abnormal behaviors during sleep, such as driving a car, eating, talking on the phone, or having sex without any recall of the event. If family notices any such behavior or patient sees evidence of such behavior upon awakening, the prescriber should be notified.
•Urge family or caregiver to watch patient closely for suicidal tendencies, especially when zaleplon therapy starts or dosage changes.

ziconotide

Prialt

Class and Category

Chemical class: 25 amino acid polybasic peptide
Therapeutic class: Analgesic
Pregnancy category: C

Indications and Dosages

➤ *To manage severe chronic pain in patients who are intolerant of or refractory to other pain management measures*

INTRATHECAL

Adults. *Initial:* 2.4 mcg daily (0.1 mcg/hr), increased as needed by 2.4 mcg daily but no more than 3 times/wk. *Maximum:* 19.2 mcg/

day (0.8 mcg/hr) by day 21.

Contraindications

History of psychosis; hypersensitivity to ziconotide or its components; conditions or treatment that make intrathecal use hazardous (infection at microinfusion site, uncontrolled bleeding diathesis, spinal canal obstruction that impairs circulation of CSF).

Interactions

DRUGS

CNS depressants: Increased risk of adverse CNS reactions

Adverse Reactions

CNS: Abnormal gait, agitation, anxiety, aphasia, asthenia, ataxia, chills, confusion, CSF abnormality, CVA, decreased reflexes, depression, difficulty concentrating, dizziness, dysesthesia, emotional lability, fever, hallucinations, headache, hostility, hyperesthesia, hypertonia, incoordination, insomnia, malaise, memory loss, meningitis, nervousness, neuralgia, paranoia, paresthesia, psychosis, seizures, somnolence, speech disorder, stupor, suicidal ideation, syncope, tremor, twitching, unusual dreams, vertigo
CV: Atrial fibrillation, bradycardia, chest pain, edema, hypertension, hypotension, orthostatic hypotension, peripheral edema, tachycardia, T-wave changes on ECG, vasodilation
EENT: Abnormal vision, diplopia, dry mouth, nystagmus, pharyngitis, photophobia, rhinitis, sinusitis, taste perversion, tinnitus
GI: Abdominal pain, anorexia, constipation, diarrhea, indigestion, nausea, vomiting
GU: Acute renal failure, dysuria, urinary hesitancy or incontinence, urine retention, UTI
HEME: Anemia
MS: Arthralgia, arthritis, back pain, leg cramps, muscle spasms or weakness, myalgia, myasthenia, neck pain or rigidity, rhabdomyolysis
RESP: Aspiration pneumonia, bronchitis, cough, dyspnea, lung disorder, pneumonia, respiratory distress
SKIN: Cellulitis, diaphoresis, dry skin, ecchymosis, pruritus, rash
Other: Catheter site infection or pain, dehydration, elevated CK level, flulike symptoms, generalized pain, hypokalemia, sepsis, viral

Mechanism of Action

Pain sensations are transmitted by sensory neurons that travel through N-type calcium channels in the dorsal horn of the spinal cord and ascend to the brain.

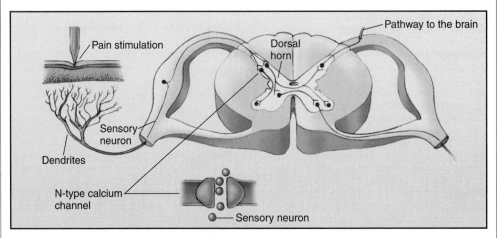

Ziconotide binds to N-type calcium channels on primary nociceptive afferent nerves in superficial layers of the dorsal horn. The channels then become blocked, preventing excitatory neurotransmitter release in the primary afferent nerve terminals and relieving pain.

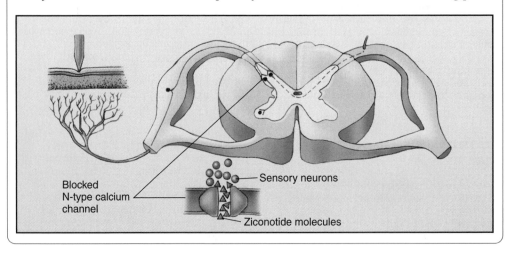

infection, weight loss

Nursing Considerations

•Determine if patient will receive ziconotide therapy via an implanted variable-rate microinfusion device or an external microinfusion device and catheter. Then, follow manufacturer guidelines for programming the microinfusion devise and doing an initial pump fill, including priming using only undiluted 25-mcg/ml solution and rinsing internal surfaces of pump with 2 ml of drug three times.
•Use strict aseptic technique when preparing the ziconotide solution and filling, refilling, or

otherwise handling the microinfusion device.
•Be aware that initial ziconotide dosage
shouldn't exceed 2.4 mcg daily.
•Know that refills can use diluted or undiluted ziconotide solutions. If diluting ziconotide, use only normal saline solution
without preservatives, following manufacturer guidelines. Refrigerate solution up to
24 hours if it isn't used immediately. Expect
the device to need refilling about every
40 days if ziconotide is given diluted or
about 60 days if given undiluted.
•Assess patient's response to ziconotide therapy regularly. Notify prescriber if pain relief
is not adequate, and expect dosage to be increased.
•Check infusion site regularly, and be aware
that meningitis can occur within 24 hours
after contamination of the delivery system; a
disconnected catheter is the most common
problem with external devices.
•Monitor patient closely for signs and symptoms of meningitis, such as headache, stiff
neck, altered mental status, nausea, vomiting, and occasionally seizures caused by inadvertent contamination of the microinfusion
device or catheter tract used to deliver ziconotide. Notify prescriber immediately if
you suspect meningitis.
•Monitor patient closely for cognitive impairment, hallucinations, or changes in mood
or consciousness because ziconotide may
cause severe psychiatric symptoms and neurologic impairment. If present, notify prescriber and expect to decrease dosage or stop
ziconotide. Provide appropriate supportive
care, as prescribed, to relieve adverse effects.
Tell prescriber again if adverse effects are
still present after 2 weeks.
•Expect to stop ziconotide temporarily if patient becomes unresponsive or stuporous
during therapy; drug may be continued when
patient reverts to previous mental status.
•Ziconotide can be stopped abruptly without
causing withdrawal symptoms.
•Monitor patient's serum CK level every
other week for first month of therapy and
monthly thereafter, as ordered. If levels become elevated, notify prescriber and expect
to decrease ziconotide dosage or stop drug
until levels return to normal.

PATIENT TEACHING
•Teach caregiver how to care for external
device, if present. Stress need for strict aseptic technique with microinfusion device and
connections and need to check site often for
problems, such as a disconnected catheter,
which increase the risk of meningitis.
•Review evidence of meningitis with caregiver, and tell her to contact prescriber immediately if she suspects meningitis.
•Advise patient to notify prescriber if pain
relief isn't adequate.
•Tell patient and caregiver to notify prescriber immediately about muscle pain, soreness, and weakness with or without dark
urine or a change in mental status or mood,
including depression or suicidal ideation.
•Advise patient to avoid hazardous activities
that require mental alertness or motor coordination while receiving ziconotide.
•Caution patient to avoid taking OTC preparations that contain CNS depressants because of the risk of adverse CNS effects.

zileuton

Zyflo CR

Class and Category
Chemical class: Leukotriene inhibitor
Therapeutic class: Antiasthmatic
Pregnancy category: C

Indications and Dosages
➤ *To prevent or treat chronic asthma*
E.R. TABLETS
Adults and adolescents. 600 mg b.i.d. *Maximum:* 2,400 mg daily.

Route	Onset	Peak	Duration
P.O.	2 hr	Unknown	Unknown

Mechanism of Action
Inhibits the formation of leukotrienes
found mainly in neutrophils, eosinophils,
monocytes, macrophages, and mast cells.
Normally, leukotrienes augment neutrophil
and eosinophil migration, neutrophil and
monocyte aggregation, leukocyte adhesion,
capillary permeability, and smooth-muscle
contraction. By inhibiting leukotriene formation, zileuton causes bronchial relaxation and decreases vascular leakage and
edema, mucus secretion, eosinophil movement, and bronchial hyperresponsiveness.

X
Y
Z

Contraindications
Hepatic impairment, hypersensitivity to zileuton or its components

Interactions
DRUGS
propranolol, terfenadine: Increased effects of these drugs
theophylline: Doubled blood theophylline level
warfarin: Prolonged PT and INR

Adverse Reactions
CNS: Asthenia, dizziness, fever, headache, hypertonia, insomnia, malaise, nervousness, somnolence
CV: Chest pain
EENT: Conjunctivitis
GI: Abdominal pain, constipation, flatulence, indigestion, nausea, vomiting
GU: UTI, vaginitis
MS: Arthralgia, myalgia, neck pain or rigidity
SKIN: Pruritus
Other: Lymphadenopathy

Nursing Considerations
•Be aware that zileuton shouldn't be used to treat bronchospasm during an acute asthma attack or status asthmaticus; it can't relieve symptoms quickly enough.
•Monitor serum ALT level, as ordered, usually before treatment starts, once a month for 3 months, every 2 to 3 months for remainder of first year, and periodically thereafter during therapy.
•Monitor results of liver and pulmonary function tests and CBC during therapy.
PATIENT TEACHING
•Advise patient to take drug exactly as prescribed, in evenly spaced doses, every day. Stress the importance of taking drug even during symptom-free periods and acute exacerbations.
•Urge patient not to chew, cut, or crush capsule but to swallow it whole.
•Instruct patient to continue using rescue inhalants, as prescribed, for acute attacks.
•Teach patient how to use peak-flow meter to assess and monitor pulmonary function.

zinc acetate

(contains 25 or 50 mg of elemental zinc per capsule)
Galzin

zinc chloride

(contains 1 mg of elemental zinc per ml for I.V. infusion)

zinc gluconate

(contains 1.4 mg of elemental zinc per lozenge; 1.4, 2, 4, 7, 8, 10, 11, 13, 31, 50, or 52 mg of elemental zinc per tablet)
Orazinc

zinc sulfate

(contains 25 or 50 mg of elemental zinc per capsule; 15, 25, 45, or 50 mg of elemental zinc per tablet; 50 mg of elemental zinc per E.R. tablet; and 1 or 5 mg of elemental zinc per ml for I.V. infusion)
Orazinc, Verazinc, Zinc 15, Zinc-220, Zinca-Pak, Zincate

Class and Category
Chemical class: Trace element, mineral
Therapeutic class: Copper absorption inhibitor, nutritional supplement
Pregnancy category: A (oral), C (I.V.)

Indications and Dosages
➤ *To prevent zinc deficiency based on U.S. and Canadian recommended daily allowances*
CAPSULES, E.R. TABLETS, LOZENGES, TABLETS
Men and boys age 11 and over. 15 mg (9 to 12 mg Canadian) of elemental zinc daily.
Women and girls age 11 and over. 12 mg (9 mg Canadian) of elemental zinc daily.
Pregnant women. 15 mg (15 mg Canadian) of elemental zinc daily.
Breast-feeding women. 16 to 19 mg (15 mg Canadian) of elemental zinc daily.
Children ages 7 to 10. 10 mg (7 to 9 mg Canadian) of elemental zinc daily.
Children ages 4 to 6. 10 mg (5 mg Canadian) of elemental zinc daily.
Children from birth to age 3. 5 to 10 mg (2 to 4 mg Canadian) of elemental zinc daily.
I.V. INFUSION
Adults and children. 2.5 to 4 mg daily added to total parenteral nutrition (TPN) solution. *Maximum:* 12 mg daily.
Children from birth to age 5. 100 mcg/kg daily added to TPN solution.
Premature infants weighing up to 3 kg. 300 mcg/kg daily added to TPN solution.
➤ *To treat zinc deficiency*

CAPSULES, E.R. TABLETS, LOZENGES, TABLETS
Adults and children. Dosage individualized based on severity of deficiency.
I.V. INFUSION
Adults and adolescents. 2.5 to 4 mg daily added to TPN solution. *Maximum:* 12 mg daily.
Children from birth to age 5. 100 mcg/kg daily added to TPN solution.
Premature infants weighing up to 3 kg. 300 mcg/kg daily added to TPN solution.
➤ *As adjunct maintenance therapy for patients previously treated for Wilson's disease*
CAPSULES
Adults. 50 mg t.i.d.
Pregnant women. 25 mg t.i.d., increased to 50 mg t.i.d. if drug effectiveness decreases.
Children age 10 and over. 25 mg t.i.d., increased to 50 mg t.i.d. if drug effectiveness decreases.

Mechanism of Action
Necessary for proper functioning of more than 200 metalloenzymes (enzymes containing tightly bound zinc atoms as an integral part of their structure), including carbonic anhydrase, carboxypeptidase A, alcohol dehydrogenase, alkaline phosphatase, and RNA polymerase. Zinc also helps maintain nucleic acid, protein, and cell membrane structure and is essential for certain physiologic functions, including cell growth and division, sexual maturation and reproduction, dark adaptation and night vision, wound healing, host immunity, and taste acuity. This mineral also provides cellular antioxidant protection by scavenging free radicals.

In addition, zinc acetate interferes with intestinal absorption of copper and produces a protein that binds with copper, preventing its transfer to the blood. Bound copper is then excreted in stools, thus decreasing copper toxicity in Wilson's disease.

Contraindications
Hypersensitivity to zinc or its components

Interactions
DRUGS
copper supplements: Impaired copper absorption (with large doses of zinc)
oral iron supplements, oral phosphate salts, penicillamine, phosphorus-containing drugs: Decreased zinc absorption
quinolones, tetracyclines: Decreased absorption and possibly decreased effectiveness of these antibiotics
thiazide diuretics: Increased urinary excretion of zinc
zinc-containing preparations: Increased blood zinc level
FOODS
fiber- or phylate-containing foods (such as bran, whole-grain breads, cereal), phosphorus-containing foods (including milk, poultry): Decreased zinc absorption

Adverse Reactions
None with usual dosages

Nursing Considerations
•**WARNING** Don't administer I.V. zinc preparations that contain benzyl alcohol to neonates or premature infants because this preservative may cause a fatal toxic syndrome characterized by metabolic acidosis and CNS, respiratory, circulatory, and renal function impairment.
•Administer oral zinc supplements 1 hour before or 2 to 3 hours after meals; at least 2 hours after administering oral iron supplements (to prevent decreased zinc absorption) or copper supplements (to prevent decreased copper absorption); and at least 6 hours before or 2 hours after administering quinolone or tetracycline antibiotics (to prevent decreased absorption of these drugs).
•Monitor patient receiving long-term zinc therapy for sideroblastic anemia, which may result from zinc-induced copper deficiency and is characterized by anemia, leukopenia, neutropenia, granulocytopenia, and bone marrow problems. Be aware that these effects are reversible after zinc is discontinued.
•Monitor patient with preexisting copper deficiency for exacerbation of this condition; zinc can decrease serum copper level.
•Assess for signs and symptoms of zinc deficiency, such as growth retardation, hypogonadism, delayed sexual maturation, alopecia, impaired wound healing, skin lesions, immune deficiencies, behavioral disturbances, night blindness, and impaired sense of taste.

X
Y
Z

•Monitor blood alkaline phosphatase (ALP) level monthly, as ordered; it may increase.
•Be aware that zinc chloride contains aluminum, which may accumulate to the point of toxicity if the patient's kidney function is impaired. Assess kidney function regularly.

PATIENT TEACHING
•Explain the need for a zinc supplement.
•Instruct patient to take zinc on an empty stomach, at least 1 hour before or 2 hours after meals. Caution her not to take zinc within 2 hours of iron or copper supplements or phosphorus-containing drugs.
•Instruct patient to let zinc lozenge dissolve in mouth slowly and completely and not to swallow it whole or chew it. Advise her not to take zinc lozenges more often than directed.

ziprasidone hydrochloride

Geodon

ziprasidone mesylate

Geodon for Injection

Class and Category

Chemical class: Benzisoxazole derivative
Therapeutic class: Antipsychotic
Pregnancy category: C

Indications and Dosages

➤ *To treat schizophrenia*

CAPSULES

Adults. *Initial:* 20 mg b.i.d. Dosage increased as indicated q 2 or more days. *Usual:* 20 to 80 mg b.i.d. *Maximum:* 100 mg b.i.d.

I.M. INJECTION

Adults. *Initial:* 10 to 20 mg. 10 mg dose may be administered every 2 hr up to maximum dose; 20 mg dose may be administered every 4 hr up to maximum dose. *Maximum:* 40 mg daily.

➤ *To treat acute manic or mixed episodes of bipolar disorder*

CAPSULES

Adults. *Initial:* 40 mg b.i.d. with food on day 1; then increased to 60 or 80 mg on day 2 with further adjustments as needed.

Incompatibilities

Don't mix injection form with drugs or solvents other than sterile water for injection.

Mechanism of Action

Selectively blocks serotonin and dopamine receptors in the mesocortical tract of the CNS, thereby suppressing psychotic symptoms.

Contraindications

Concomitant use of other drugs that prolong QT interval, history of arrhythmia, hypersensitivity to ziprasidone or its components, known history of QT-interval prolongation, recent acute MI, uncompensated heart failure

Interactions

DRUGS
antihypertensives: Additive antihypertensive effects
carbamazepine: Possibly decreased blood ziprasidone level
CNS depressants: Increased CNS depression
dopamine agonists, levodopa: Decreased therapeutic effects of these drugs
drugs that prolong QT interval (including quinidine, dofetilide, pimozide, sotalol, thioridazine, and sparfloxacin): Increased risk of prolonged QT or QTc interval, torsades de pointes, and sudden death
ketoconazole: Possibly increased blood ziprasidone level

FOODS
all foods: Increased ziprasidone absorption

Adverse Reactions

CNS: Agitation, akathisia, amnesia, anxiety, asthenia, CVA, depression, dizziness, dystonia, extrapyramidal reactions, headache, hypertonia, hypomania, insomnia, mania, neuroleptic malignant syndrome, paresthesia, personality or speech disorder, serotonin syndrome, somnolence, syncope, tardive dyskinesia, tremor
CV: Bradycardia, chest pain, hypercholesterolemia, hypertension, orthostatic hypotension, prolonged QT or QTc interval, tachycardia, thrombophlebitis, vasodilation
EENT: Abnormal vision, dry mouth, increased salivation, rhinitis, tongue swelling
ENDO: Dysmenorrhea, hyperglycemia
GI: Abdominal pain, anorexia, constipation, diarrhea, dysphagia, indigestion, nausea, rectal bleeding, vomiting
GU: Priapism, urinary incontinence
MS: Arthralgia, back pain, dysarthria, myalgia

RESP: Cough, pulmonary embolism, upper respiratory tract infection
SKIN: Allergic dermatitis, diaphoresis, furunculosis, rash, urticaria
Other: Accidental injury, angioedema, flulike symptoms, injection site pain, weight gain

Nursing Considerations

•**WARNING** Ziprasidone shouldn't be used to treat elderly patients with dementia-related psychosis because drug increases the risk of death in these patients.
•Protect ziprasidone vials from light. Reconstitute by adding 1.2 ml of sterile water for injection to vial and shaking vigorously until drug is dissolved. Each ml of reconstituted solution contains 20 mg ziprasidone. Discard any unused portion.
•Give only by I.M. route.
•Reconstituted drug may be stored 24 hours protected from light or up to 7 days if refrigerated and protected from light.
•Administer I.M. form cautiously to patients with impaired renal function.
•**WARNING** Assess cardiac rhythm in patients with hypokalemia or hypomagnesemia. Be aware that dizziness, palpitations, and syncope may indicate life-threatening torsades de pointes. Be prepared to stop ziprasidone if QTc interval is greater than 500 msec.
•Monitor patient, especially elderly woman, for involuntary movements, which may become irreversible tardive dyskinesia. If symptoms develop, notify prescriber immediately and be prepared to stop drug.
•Immediately report evidence of neuroleptic malignant syndrome, a rare but potentially fatal adverse reaction including hyperpyrexia, muscle rigidity, altered mental status, irregular pulse, blood pressure changes, tachycardia, diaphoresis, arrhythmia, myoglobinuria (rhabdomyolysis), and acute renal failure.
•Monitor patient's blood glucose and lipid levels routinely, as ordered, because drug increases the risk of hyperglycemia and hypercholesterolemia.

PATIENT TEACHING

•Instruct patient to take ziprasidone with food to increase drug's absorption.
•Advise patient to avoid hazardous activities until drug's CNS effects are known.
•Tell family to monitor patient closely for suicidal tendencies; patients with psychotic illness or bipolar disorder are at greater risk.
•Urge patient to rise slowly from seated or lying position to minimize orthostatic hypotension.

zoledronic acid

Reclast, Zometa

Class and Category
Chemical class: Bisphosphonate
Therapeutic class: Antihypercalcemic, bone resorption inhibitor
Pregnancy category: D

Indications and Dosages

➤ *To treat hypercalcemia caused by cancer*
I.V. INFUSION (ZOMETA)
Adults. 4 mg infused over at least 15 min. After 7 days, retreatment with 4 mg if serum calcium level doesn't remain at or return to normal. *Maximum:* 4 mg/dose.

➤ *As adjunct treatment for patients with multiple myeloma or bony metastasis who are receiving standard antineoplastic therapy and have a creatinine clearance above 60 ml/min/1.73 m²*
I.V. INFUSION (ZOMETA)
Adults. 4 mg infused over at least 15 min every 3 to 4 wk.
DOSAGE ADJUSTMENT If creatinine clearance is 50 to 60 ml/min/1.73 m², dosage decreased to 3.5 mg; if it's 40 to 49 ml/min/1.73 m², dosage decreased to 3.3 mg; and if it's 30 to 39 ml/min/1.73 m², dosage decreased to 3 mg.

➤ *To treat postmenopausal osteoporosis in women; to treat osteoporosis in men; to treat and prevent glucocorticoid-induced osteoporosis in patients receiving daily prednisone doses of 7.5 mg or greater for at least 12 months*
I.V. INFUSION (RECLAST)
Adults. 5 mg infused over at least 15 min once yearly.

➤ *To treat Paget's disease of the bone*
I.V. INFUSION (RECLAST)
Adults. 5 mg infused over at least 15 min after 2 wk of receiving 1,500 mg elemental calcium daily in divided doses and 800 international units vitamin D daily.

Incompatibilities
Don't mix zoledronic acid with calcium-

X
Y
Z

containing I.V. solutions, such as lactated Ringer's solution.

Contraindications

Hypersensitivity to zoledronic acid, other bisphosphonates, or their components

---

Mechanism of Action

Inhibits resorption of mineralized bone and cartilage by osteoclasts and induces osteoclast breakdown. In cancer-related hypercalcemia, hyperactive osteoclasts cause bone resorption and release of calcium into the blood, which causes polyuria, GI disruption, progressive dehydration, and decreasing GFR. This, in turn, increases renal calcium resorption and worsens hypercalcemia. Zoledronic acid interrupts this process.

Interactions

DRUGS

aminoglycosides: Possibly additive serum calcium–lowering effect
loop diuretics, such as furosemide: Possibly increased risk of hypocalcemia
NSAIDs: Increased risk of nephrotoxicity

Adverse Reactions

CNS: Anxiety, asthenia, chills, confusion, depression, dizziness, fatigue, fever, headache, hyperesthesia, hypoesthesia, insomnia, malaise, paresthesia, tremor, vertigo, weakness
CV: Atrial fibrillation, bradycardia, chest pain, hypertension, hypotension, peripheral edema
EENT: Blurred vision, conjunctivitis, episcleritis, iritis, sore throat, stomatitis, taste disturbance, uveitis
GI: Abdominal pain, anorexia, constipation, diarrhea, dyspepsia, nausea, vomiting
GU: Elevated serum creatinine level, hematuria, proteinuria, renal insufficiency or failure, UTI
HEME: Anemia, neutropenia, thrombocytopenia
MS: Arthralgia; incapacitating bone, joint, or muscle pain; muscle spasms; myalgia; osteonecrosis of the jaw
RESP: Bronchospasm, cough, dyspnea, upper respiratory tract infection
SKIN: Alopecia, dermatitis, flushing, urticaria

Other: Aggravated malignant neoplasm, anaphylaxis, angioedema, flulike illness, hypersensitivity reaction, hyperkalemia, hypernatremia, hypocalcemia, hypomagnesemia, hypophosphatemia, infusion site redness and swelling, weight gain

Nursing Considerations

- Be aware that zoledronic acid isn't indicated for hypercalcemia from hyperparathyroidism or other non–tumor conditions.
- Use cautiously in patients with aspirin sensitivity because biphosphonates such as zoledronic acid have caused bronchoconstriction in these patients.
- Make sure patient has had a dental checkup before zoledronic acid starts, especially if patient has cancer; is receiving chemotherapy, head or neck radiation, or a corticosteroid; or has poor oral hygiene because the risk of osteonecrosis is increased in these patients, and invasive dental procedures during zoledronic acid therapy may worsen osteonecrosis.
- Expect to aggressively hydrate hypercalcemic patient with I.V. normal saline solution before and throughout zoledronic acid therapy, as prescribed, to achieve and maintain a urine output of about 2 L daily.
- **WARNING** During hydration, monitor fluid intake and output often and assess patient, especially one with heart failure, for signs and symptoms of life-threatening overhydration.
- Hypocalcemia and mineral metabolism disorders must be treated before zoledronic acid therapy begins.
- Be aware that Reclast doesn't need reconstitution. Reconstitute Zometa by adding 5 ml of sterile water for injection to drug vial to yield a solution that contains 4 mg of zoledronic acid. Make sure drug is completely dissolved before withdrawing prescribed dose. Further dilute in 100 ml of normal saline solution or 5% dextrose injection, and infuse over no less than 15 minutes.
- Before giving zoledronic acid, inspect the reconstituted and diluted solution and discard it if particles or discoloration are present.
- Expect to administer acetaminophen, if not contraindicated, before giving zoledronic acid to reduce adverse reactions, such as

fever, headache, myalgia and flulike symptoms. These reactions usually occur within the first 3 days after zoledronic acid administration and resolve within 3 days (although for some patients the resolution may take up to 14 days).
•Refrigerate reconstituted drug at 2° to 8° C (36° to 46° F) and discard it after 24 hours.
•Give drug as a single I.V. solution in a separate I.V. line.
•WARNING Be aware that a single dose of Zometa shouldn't exceed 4 mg and that neither Zometa nor Reclast should be infused over less than 15 minutes because exceeding these limits may lead to significant renal function deterioration, which may progress to renal failure.
•WARNING Assess patient's renal function, as ordered, before and during zoledronic acid therapy to detect renal deterioration. For patient with a normal serum creatinine level who develops an increase of 0.5 mg/dl within 2 weeks of receiving zoledronic acid, expect to withhold next dose until serum creatinine level is within 10% of patient's baseline value. For patient with an abnormal serum creatinine level who develops an increase of 1.0 mg/dl within 2 weeks of receiving drug, expect to withhold next dose until serum creatinine level is within 10% of baseline value.
•Monitor patient's serum calcium, magnesium, and phosphate levels, as ordered, during zoledronic acid therapy. If hypocalcemia, hypomagnesemia, or hypophosphatemia occurs, expect to give short-term supplemental therapy.
•Assess aspirin-sensitive asthma patients for worsening of respiratory symptoms during zoledronic acid therapy because other bisphosphonates have caused bronchoconstriction in these patients.
•Store drug at 25° C (77° F).

PATIENT TEACHING
•Teach patient the importance of consuming a nutritious diet, including adequate amounts of calcium and vitamin D.
•Advise patient to alert prescriber about muscle or bone pain.
•Instruct patient on proper oral hygiene and on need to notify prescriber before undergoing invasive dental procedures.
•Advise women of childbearing age to notify prescriber immediately if they are or could be pregnant because drug will need to be stopped.

zolmitriptan

Zomig, Zomig ZMT

Class and Category
Chemical class: Selective 5-hydroxytryptamine agonist
Therapeutic class: Antimigraine
Pregnancy category: C

Indications and Dosages
➤ *To treat acute migraine headache with or without aura*
DISINTEGRATING TABLETS
Adults. 2.5 mg, repeated every 2 hr p.r.n. *Maximum:* 10 mg in 24 hr or three headaches/mo.
TABLETS
Adults. 2.5 mg or less, repeated every 2 hr p.r.n. *Maximum:* 10 mg in 24 hr or three head-aches/mo.
NASAL SPRAY
Adults. 5 mg, repeated in 2 hr if needed. *Maximum:* 10 mg/24 hr.
DOSAGE ADJUSTMENT Dosage reduced to less than 2.5 mg for patients with hepatic impairment.

Mechanism of Action
Constricts inflamed and dilated cranial blood vessels in the carotid circulation and inhibits production of proinflammatory neuropeptides by binding to receptors on intracranial blood vessels and sensory nerves in the trigeminal-vascular system to stimulate negative feedback, which halts the release of serotonin.

Contraindications
Basilar or hemiplegic migraine, cardiovascular disease, concurrent use of ergotamine-containing drugs, hypersensitivity to zolmitriptan or its components, ischemic heart disease, peripheral vascular disease, Prinzmetal's angina, symptomatic Wolff-Parkinson-White syndrome or other accessory pathway conduction disorder, use of another 5-hydroxytryptamine agonist within past 24 hours, use of an MAO inhibitor within 14 days

X
Y
Z

Interactions

DRUGS

acetaminophen: Delayed peak effect of acetaminophen (by 1 hour)
cimetidine: Prolonged zolmitriptan half-life
ergot alkaloids: Prolonged vasoconstriction effects
fluoxetine, fluvoxamine, paroxetine, sertraline: Hyperreflexia, lack of coordination, and weakness
MAO inhibitors: Increased zolmitriptan effects
naratriptan, rizatriptan, sumatriptan: Prolonged zolmitriptan effects
oral contraceptives, propranolol: Increased blood zolmitriptan level
serotonin and norepinephrine reuptake inhibitors: Increased risk of developing serotonin syndrome

Adverse Reactions

CNS: Asthenia, dizziness, hyperesthesia, paresthesia, somnolence, vertigo
CV: Angina, coronary artery vasospasm, hypertension, MI, palpitations, transient myocardial ischemia, ventricular fibrillation or tachycardia
EENT: Dry mouth, vision disturbance
GI: Abdominal pain, bloody diarrhea, dysphagia, GI or splenic infarction, indigestion, ischemic colitis, nausea, vomiting
MS: Myalgia; myasthenia; pain, pressure, or tightness in jaw, neck, or throat
SKIN: Diaphoresis, flushing
Other: Anaphylaxis, anaphylactoid reaction, angioedema

Nursing Considerations

•**WARNING** Monitor patient for signs and symptoms of vasoconstriction, which may lead to vascular and colonic ischemia with abdominal pain and bloody diarrhea, especially if patient has peripheral vascular disease (including Raynaud's phenomenon) or ischemic bowel disease.
•Monitor elderly patients and those with hepatic impairment for increased blood pressure, and notify prescriber immediately if it occurs.
•Monitor patient closely for signs and symptoms of angina. If patient develops chest pain, notify prescriber.
•**WARNING** Monitor patient closely for signs and symptoms of serotonin syndrome, which

may include agitation, hallucinations, coma, tachycardia, labile blood pressure, hyperthermia, hyperreflexia, incoordination, nausea, vomiting, and diarrhea. Notify prescriber immediately because serotonin syndrome may be life-threatening. Be prepared to provide supportive care and discontinue zolmitriptan.

PATIENT TEACHING

•Urge patient to consult prescriber before treating more than three headaches in 30 days.
•Advise patient not to remove disintegrating tablet from blister pack until just before taking the tablet. Instruct her to peel open pack, let tablet dissolve on her tongue, and then swallow.
•Urge patient to notify prescriber about unusual or severe adverse reactions.
•Caution patient using nasal spray to avoid spraying drug into her eyes.
•Instruct patient not to take zolmitriptan within 24 hours of other drugs in the same class.

zolpidem tartrate

Ambien, Ambien CR, Tovalt

Class, Category, and Schedule

Chemical class: Imidazopyridine derivative
Therapeutic class: Antianxiety, sedative-hypnotic
Pregnancy category: B
Controlled substance schedule: IV

Indications and Dosages

➤ *To provide short-term treatment of insomnia*

TABLETS, ORALLY DISINTEGRATING TABLETS

Adults. 10 mg at bedtime for 7 to 10 days. *Maximum:* 10 mg daily.
DOSAGE ADJUSTMENT For elderly or debilitated patients and those with hepatic impairment, dosage possibly reduced to 5 mg at bedtime, with a maximum of 5 mg daily for nursing facility residents

E.R. TABLETS

Adults. 12.5 mg immediately before at bedtime.
DOSAGE ADJUSTMENT For elderly or debilitated patients and those with hepatic impairment, dosage reduced to 6.25 mg immediately before at bedtime.

Mechanism of Action

May potentiate the effects of gamma-aminobutyric acid (GABA) and other inhibitory neurotransmitters. By binding to specific benzodiazepine receptors in the limbic and cortical areas of the CNS, zolpidem increases GABA's inhibitory effects, blocks cortical and limbic arousal, and preserves deep sleep (stages 3 and 4).

Contraindications

Hypersensitivity to zolpidem or its components, ritonavir therapy

Interactions

DRUGS

azole antifungals: Increased CNS activity and additive adverse effects of zolpidem
barbiturates, chlorpromazine, general anesthetics, opioid agonists, other CNS depressants, phenothiazines, tramadol, tricyclic antidepressants: Possibly increased CNS depression and reduced psychomotor function
bupropion: Increased blood zolpidem level, possibly visual hallucinations, loss of alertness
desipramine, imipramine: Increased risk of visual hallucinations and reduced alertness
flumazenil: Antagonized sedative effect
haloperidol: Increased CNS depression
nevirapine: Decreased blood zolpidem level
rifabutin, rifampin: Increased zolpidem clearance
selective serotonin-reuptake inhibitors: Increased risk of delusions, disorientation, and hallucinations

FOODS

all foods: Increased time to peak blood zolpidem level, decreased effects of zolpidem

ACTIVITIES

alcohol use: Increased CNS depression

Adverse Reactions

CNS: Amnesia, asthenia, ataxia, complex behaviors (such as sleep driving), confusion, dizziness, drowsiness, euphoria, hallucinations, headache, insomnia, lethargy, paradoxical CNS stimulation (including agitation, euphoria, hallucinations, hyperactivity, and nightmares), vertigo
EENT: Diplopia, throat tightness, visual abnormality
GI: Constipation, diarrhea, hiccups, indigestion, nausea, vomiting
GU: UTI
MS: Arthralgia, myalgia
RESP: Dyspnea, upper respiratory infection
Other: Anaphylaxis, angioedema, withdrawal symptoms

Nursing Considerations

•Use zolpidem cautiously in patients with additional disorders because it isn't known if zolpidem therapy might aggravate these conditions.
•Administer zolpidem just before patient's bedtime because drug has a rapid onset of action.
•Expect patient to receive no more than a 1-month supply of zolpidem for outpatient therapy.
•**WARNING** If zolpidem is withdrawn abruptly (especially after prolonged therapy), monitor patient for withdrawal symptoms, such as abdominal cramps or discomfort, fatigue, flushing, inconsolable crying, light-headedness, nausea, nervousness, panic attack, rebound insomnia, and vomiting.
•Expect that zolpidem will produce anticonvulsant and muscle relaxant effects at high doses.
•If patient takes other CNS depressants, expect to reduce zolpidem dosage, as prescribed.
•**WARNING** Monitor patient closely for hypersensitivity reactions such as dyspnea, throat tightness, nausea, vomiting, and swelling. If present, discontinue zolpidem immediately, notify prescriber, and provide supportive care.

PATIENT TEACHING

•Caution patient to take drug exactly as prescribed and not to increase dosage unless directed by prescriber.
•Advise patient taking extended-release form to swallow tablet whole and not to break, crush, or chew it.
•Advise patient taking orally disintegrating form to place tablet on tongue, let it dissolve, and then swallow with saliva or, if patient prefers, with water.
•Instruct patient to take zolpidem immediately before going to bed, on an empty stomach.
•Advise patient to notify prescriber immedi-

X
Y
Z

ately about abdominal cramps or discomfort, fatigue, flushing, inconsolable crying, light-headedness, nausea, nervousness, panic attack, and vomiting.

•Instruct patient to stop taking zolpidem and seek emergency care if she has trouble breathing, throat tightness, nausea, vomiting, or abnormally swelling.

•Advise patient that zolpidem may produce abnormal behaviors during sleep, such as driving a car, eating, talking on the phone, or having sex without any recall of the event. If patient's family notices any such behavior or if patient sees evidence of such behavior upon awakening, the prescriber should be notified.

zonisamide

Zonegran

Class and Category

Chemical class: Benzisoxazole derivative, sulfonamide
Therapeutic class: Anticonvulsant
Pregnancy category: C

Indications and Dosages

➤ *As adjunct to treat partial seizures*
CAPSULES
Adults. *Initial:* 100 mg daily. Dosage increased by 100 mg daily every 2 wk, as needed. *Usual:* 200 to 400 mg daily. *Maximum:* 600 mg daily.

Mechanism of Action

May stop seizures and suppress their foci by blocking sodium channels and reducing voltage-dependent, inward currents from calcium channels. This action stabilizes neuronal membranes and suppresses synchronized neuronal hyperactivity.

Contraindications

Hypersensitivity to sulfonamides, zonisamide, or their components

Interactions

DRUGS
carbamazepine, phenobarbital, phenytoin, valproate: Possibly decreased blood zonisamide level

CNS depressants: Additive CNS depressant effects
FOODS
grapefruit juice: Possibly decreased metabolism of zonisamide

Adverse Reactions

CNS: Agitation, ataxia, dizziness, irritability, somnolence
GI: Anorexia

Nursing Considerations

•WARNING Monitor results of patient's CBC and other laboratory tests for signs of blood dyscrasias because zonisamide is a sulfonamide and can be absorbed systemically. Systemic absorption may result in life-threatening reactions, including toxic epidermal necrolysis, Stevens-Johnson syndrome, fulminant hepatic necrosis, agranulocytosis, aplastic anemia, and other blood dyscrasias.

•Be aware that patients receiving doses of 300 mg daily or more are at increased risk for adverse CNS reactions, including decreased concentration, fatigue, drowsiness, and impaired speech.

•Monitor serum creatinine and BUN levels for signs of abnormally decreased glomerular filtration rate (GFR). Expect some decrease in GFR during first 4 weeks of treatment and a return to baseline within 2 to 3 weeks after drug is discontinued.

•Monitor patient for signs and symptoms of renal calculi.

•Be aware that zonisamide should not be discontinued abruptly because doing so may increase the frequency of seizures.
PATIENT TEACHING
•Inform patient that zonisamide is usually prescribed with other anticonvulsants and that she should continue to take all drugs as prescribed.

•Instruct patient to swallow zonisamide capsules whole, and not to chew them or break them open.

•Inform patient that the prescriber may have to adjust zonisamide dosage over several weeks or months before a stable dose is achieved.

•Advise patient to use caution when driving or performing other activities that are hazardous or require mental alertness because zonisamide commonly causes somnolence, dizziness, and decreased concentration, particularly during first month of therapy.

•Advise patient to wear a medical identification bracelet or necklace or carry medical identification with information about her seizure disorder.

•Unless contraindicated, encourage patient to drink 6 to 8 glasses of water each day to prevent kidney stones.

•Advise patient to rise slowly from a lying or seated position to reduce the risk of dizziness.

Appendices

Insulin Preparations

For each category of insulin, the following chart lists the species; common trade names; onset, peak, and duration; and key nursing considerations.

CATEGORY, SPECIES, AND TRADE NAMES	KEY NURSING CONSIDERATIONS
Rapid-acting insulin	
Onset: 15 min **Peak:** 30 to 90 min **Duration:** In 6 hr	
Human •Apidra (insulin glulisine) •Humalog (insulin lispro) •NovoLog (insulin aspart)	•Mix Humalog or NovoLog with other insulin types, but mix Apidra only with NPH insulin, if needed. Administer immediately after mixing. •When mixing rapid-acting insulin with a longer-acting insulin, always draw the rapid-acting insulin into the syringe first to avoid dosage errors. •Give Humalog only SubQ, up to 15 minutes before a meal. Give NovoLog only SubQ 5 to 10 minutes before a meal or via external insulin pump. Give Apidra SubQ up to 15 to 20 minutes before a meal or via insulin pump. If using a pump, NovoLog and Apidra shouldn't be diluted or mixed with any other insulin. •Be aware that 1 unit of rapid-acting insulin has the same glucose-lowering ability as 1 unit of short-acting insulin. •Rapid-acting insulin is available as a cartridge. Make sure to use the correct device for the brand of insulin prescribed, and don't add any other insulin to the cartridge. •Absorption rate of rapid-acting insulin may slow when this type of insulin is mixed in a syringe with human isophane insulin (NPH). Monitor blood glucose level often.
Short-acting insulin	
Onset: 30 min **Peak:** 2 to 5 hr **Duration:** 6 to 8 hr	
Human •Humulin-R •Novolin ge Toronto (CAN) •Novolin ge Toronto Penfill (CAN) •Novolin R •Novolin R PenFill •Novolin R Prefilled •Velosulin BR •Velosulin Human (CAN) Pork •Regular (concentrated), Iletin II, U-500 •Regular Insulin (pork) •Regular Insulin (purified pork)	•Don't use short-acting insulin if it's cloudy, discolored, or unusually viscous. •Use the U-500 strength to treat insulin resistance, as prescribed. •Mix short-acting insulin with other insulin types, if needed. However, don't mix phosphate-buffered insulin with a zinc-containing insulin because the short-acting insulin's effectiveness may be reduced. •Administer SubQ, I.M., or I.V., as prescribed. Use a continuous SubQ infusion pump, if ordered. For an insulin pump, phosphate-buffered insulin is preferred over nonphosphate-buffered insulin. The catheter tubing and reservoir insulin should be changed every 48 hours or as specified by the pump manufacturer. •When giving SubQ or I.M. injections, give the short-acting insulin 15 to 30 minutes before a meal or bedtime snack. •Consider religious restrictions when choosing insulin type.

(continued)

Insulin Preparations (continued)

CATEGORY, SPECIES, AND TRADE NAMES	KEY NURSING CONSIDERATIONS

Intermediate-acting insulin

Onset: 1 to 3 hr **Peak:** 4 to 15 hr **Duration:** 18 to 24 hr

Human
- Humulin N
- Novolin ge Lente (CAN)
- Novolin ge NPH (CAN)
- Novolin ge NPH Penfill (CAN)
- Novolin N
- Novolin N PenFill
- Novolin N Prefilled

Pork
- Lente
- Lente Iletin II

Beef and pork
- Lente Iletin (CAN)
- NPH Iletin I (CAN)

- Don't use intermediate-acting insulin if it contains precipitate that is clumped or granular or that clings to the sides of the vial.
- Roll the vial gently between your palms to mix; don't shake it. Also gently turn the prefilled syringe up and down several times before using to achieve a uniform mixture.
- Administer by SubQ injection only, 30 minutes before a meal or bedtime snack.
- Be aware that intermediate-acting insulin rarely produces a blood glucose level that's as close to normal as possible. So expect to mix it with a short-acting insulin, as prescribed, for optimum blood glucose control.
- Consider religious restrictions when choosing insulin.

Long-acting insulin

Onset: 4 to 6 hr **Peak:** 8 to 20 hr **Duration:** 24 to 28 hr

Human
- Humulin-U (CAN)
- Lantus (insulin glargine)
- Levemir (insulin detemir)
- Novolin ge Ultralente (CAN)

- Don't use long-acting insulin if it contains precipitate that is clumped or granular or that clings to the sides of the vial.
- Mix Humulin-U or Novolin ge Ultralente with other insulin types—usually a short-acting insulin—if needed. Do not mix Lantus or Levemir with another insulin or solution.
- Roll the vial gently between your palms to obtain a uniform mixture; don't shake it.
- Administer by the SubQ route only. Inject Humulin-U or Novolin ge Ultralente 30 to 60 minutes before a meal or bedtime snack. Inject Lantus once daily at any time, keeping the daily injection time consistent. Inject Levemir prescribed once daily with the evening meal or at bedtime; inject Levemir prescribed twice daily with the morning meal and with the evening meal, at bedtime, or 12 hours after the morning dose.
- Give Lentus at bedtime, if possible, so that additional insulin can be given while patient is awake if Lentus effects decline before 24 hours pass. If Lentus is given in the morning and its effects don't last 24 hours, hyperglycemia may occur while patient sleeps.

Insulin Preparations (continued)

CATEGORY, SPECIES, AND TRADE NAMES	KEY NURSING CONSIDERATIONS

Combination insulins

Onset: 30 min **Peak:** 2 to 12 hr **Duration:** 18 to 24 hr

Human
•Humalog Mix 75/25
•Humalog Mix 50/50
•Humulin 10/90 (CAN)
•Humulin 20/80 (CAN)
•Humulin 30/70 (CAN)
•Humulin 40/60 (CAN)
•Humulin 50/50
•Humulin 70/30
•Novolin 70/30
•Novolin ge 10/90 (CAN)
•Novolin ge 20/80 (CAN)
•Novolin ge 30/70 (CAN)
•Novolin ge 40/60 (CAN)
•Novolin ge 50/50 (CAN)
•NovoLog Mix 70/30
•NovoLog Mix 50/50

•Don't use combination insulin if it contains precipitate that is clumped or granular.
•Roll the vial gently between your palms to mix; don't shake it. Also gently turn the prefilled syringe up and down several times before using to achieve a uniform mixture.
•Administer combination insulin by the SubQ route only, 30 minutes before a meal.
•Be aware that Canadian and American products contain the same insulin ratio but express it differently. For example, the Canadian Humulin 30/70 and the American Humulin 70/30 both contain 30 units of a short-acting insulin and 70 units of an intermediate-acting insulin. Canadian products list the short-acting insulin first; American products list it second.

Ophthalmic Drugs

Although less commonly prescribed than oral drugs, drugs instilled into the eyes are frequently brought into the clinical setting by patients with chronic conditions. In most cases, the patient or a family member has administered these preparations at home. Your patient teaching should include a review of proper administration and storage of these drugs. Have the patient or a family member demonstrate proper use of the drug to make sure it will be administered correctly at home. Use this time to reassess the patient's ability to continue self-medication. Also, instruct him to report any changes in the condition being treated, either negative or positive. A properly educated patient not only ensures safe drug administration, but also is more likely to detect adverse reactions that require a dosage reduction or drug discontinuation, thus preventing the development of more serious health problems.

The following chart lists the generic and trade names, FDA-approved indications, and usual adult dosages for those ophthalmic preparations you're most likely to see in your practice setting. The drugs are divided according to therapeutic use.

GENERIC AND TRADE NAMES	INDICATIONS	USUAL ADULT DOSAGES
Ophthalmic antibiotics		
bacitracin AK-Tracin	To treat surface bacterial infections affecting the conjunctiva and cornea	Small amount of ointment applied to conjunctival sac p.r.n.
chloramphenicol Diochloram, Dioptic (CAN), Pentamycetin (CAN), Sopamycetin (CAN)	To treat surface bacterial infections affecting the conjunctiva and cornea	Apply small amount of ointment to lower conjunctival sac every 3 to 6 hr and p.r.n. for at least 48 hr after eye resumes normal appearance
ciprofloxacin hydrochloride 0.3% Ciloxan	To treat corneal ulcers due to *Pseudomonas aeruginosa, Staphylococcus aureus, Staphylococcus epidermidis, Streptococcus pneumoniae,* and possibly *Serratia marcescens* and *Streptococcus viridans*	2 gtt in affected eye every 15 min for first 6 hr, then 2 gtt every 30 min for rest of first day; on day 2, 2 gtt in affected eye every hr; on days 3 to 14, 2 gtt in affected eye every 4 hr
	To treat bacterial conjunctivitis due to *Haemophilus influenzae, S. aureus, S. epidermidis,* and possibly *S. pneumoniae*	1 or 2 gtt in conjunctival sac of affected eye every 2 hr while awake for first 2 days and then 1 or 2 gtt every 4 hr while awake for next 5 days; or ½-inch strip of ointment in affected eye t.i.d. for 2 days, then b.i.d. for next 5 days
erythromycin Ilotycin	To treat acute or chronic conjunctivitis and other eye infections	1 cm (0.39 in) of ointment applied in infected eye up to 6 times/day, depending on severity of infection
	To treat chlamydial ophthalmic infections (trachoma)	Small amount applied in each eye b.i.d. for 2 mo; or b.i.d. on first 5 days of each month for 6 mo

Ophthalmic Drugs (continued)

GENERIC AND TRADE NAMES	INDICATIONS	USUAL ADULT DOSAGES
Ophthalmic antibiotics *(continued)*		
gatifloxacin 0.3% Zymar	To treat bacterial conjunctivitis due to *Corynebacterium propinquum, Staphylococcus aureus, Staphylococcus epidermidis, Streptococcus mitis, Streptococcus pneumoniae,* and *Haemophilus influenzae*	1 gtt every 2 hr while awake, up to 8 times daily on days 1 and 2; then 1 gtt up to q.i.d. while awake on days 3 to 7
gentamicin sulfate Garamycin, Genoptic, Gentacidin, Gentak	To treat blepharitis, blepharoconjunctivitis, conjunctivitis, corneal ulcers, dacryocystitis, keratoconjunctivitis, or meibomianitis due to susceptible organisms	1 or 2 gtt every 4 hr or, for severe infection, up to 2 gtt/hr; alternatively, 1 cm (.39 in) of ointment applied to lower conjunctival sac b.i.d. or t.i.d.
levofloxacin 0.5% Quixin	To treat bacterial conjunctivitis	On days 1 and 2: 1 or 2 gtt every 2 hr while awake, up to 8 times/day; on days 3 to 7: 1 or 2 gtt every 4 hr while awake, up to 4 times/day
moxifloxacin 0.5% Vigamox	To treat bacterial conjunctivitis due to *Staphylococcus aureus, Staphylococcus epidermidis, Staphylococcus haemolyticus, Staphylococcus hominis, Streptococcus pneumoniae,* Streptococcus viridans group, *Haemophilus influenzae, Chlamydia trachomatis*	1 gtt t.i.d. for 7 days
ofloxacin 0.3% Ocuflox	To treat conjunctivitis due to *Staphylococcus aureus, Staphylococcus epidermidis, Streptococcus pneumoniae, Enterobacter cloacae, Haemophilus influenzae, Proteus mirabilis, Pseudomonas aeruginosa,* and *Propionibacterium acnes*	1 or 2 gtt in conjunctival sac every 2 to 4 hr while awake for first 2 days; then 1 gtt q.i.d. for up to 5 more days
	To treat bacterial corneal ulcers due to *S. aureus, S. epidermidis, S. pneumoniae, E. cloacae, H. influenzae, P. mirabilis, P. aeruginosa, Serratia marcescens,* and *P. acnes*	1 or 2 gtt every 30 min while awake and 1 or 2 gtt every 4 to 6 hr after retiring for 2 days; then 1 or 2 gtt/hr while awake for up to 7 more days; then 1 gtt q.i.d. until end of treatment

(continued)

Ophthalmic Drugs (continued)

GENERIC AND TRADE NAMES	INDICATIONS	USUAL ADULT DOSAGES
Ophthalmic antibiotics (continued)		
polymyxin B sulfate	To treat superficial eye infections involving the conjunctiva or cornea caused by *Pseudomonas* or other gram-negative organisms	1 to 3 gtt of 0.1% to 0.25% (10,000 to 25,000 units/ml) every hr; or up to 10,000 units in lower conjunctival sac daily.
sulfacetamide sodium 10% AK-Sulf, Bleph-10, Ocusulf-10, Sodium Sulamyd 10% (CAN), Sulf-10 **sulfacetamide sodium 15%** Isopto Cetamide	To treat inclusion conjunctivitis, corneal ulcers, and chlamydial infections	1 or 2 gtt solution (10%) in lower conjunctival sac every 2 to 3 hr during day, less often at night; or 1 or 2 gtt (15%) in conjunctival sac every 1 to 2 hr; or 1 gtt (30%) in conjunctival sac every 2 hr; or 1.25 to 2.5 cm ointment (10%) in conjunctival sac q.i.d. and bedtime.
sulfacetamide sodium 30%	To treat trachoma	2 gtt (30%) in lower conjunctival sac every 2 hr in combination with systemic sulfonamide or tetracycline
tobramycin AKTob, Tobrex	To treat superficial ocular infections involving the conjunctiva or cornea	1 to 2 gtt every 1 to 4 hr, depending on severity of infection; or 1 cm (.39 in) of ointment applied to lower conjunctival sac every 8 to 12 hr for mild to moderate infections or every 3 to 4 hr for severe infections
tobramycin 0.3% (3 mg) and dexamethasone 0.1% (1 mg) TobraDex	To treat steroid-responsive inflammatory ocular conditions for which a corticosteroid is indicated and where superficial bacterial ocular infection or a risk of bacterial ocular infection exists	1 to 2 gtt every 4 to 6 hr; during first 24 to 48 hrs, dosage may be increased to 1 to 2 gtt every 2 hr; or apply 1 cm (.39 inch) of ointment into the conjunctival sac up to q.i.d.
Ophthalmic anti-inflammatory drugs		
dexamethasone Maxidex **dexamethasone sodium phosphate** AK-Dex, Boldex, R.O. Dexasone (CAN)	To treat allergic conjunctivitis; corneal injury from chemical or thermal burns or from penetration of foreign bodies; inflammatory conditions of the anterior segment of globe, conjunctiva, cornea, or eyelids; iridocyclitis; suppression of graft rejection after keratoplasty; and uveitis	1 or 2 gtt of suspension or solution or 1.25 to 2.5 cm of ointment in conjunctival sac from every hr (in severe disease) to 6 times/day; or ointment may be applied t.i.d. or q.i.d., then tapered to b.i.d., and then daily.

Ophthalmic Drugs (continued)

Ophthalmic anti-inflammatory drugs (continued)

GENERIC AND TRADE NAMES	INDICATIONS	USUAL ADULT DOSAGES
diclofenac sodium 0.1% Voltaren, Voltaren Ophtha (CAN)	To treat postoperative inflammation after removal of cataract	1 gtt in conjunctival sac q.i.d., starting 24 hr after surgery through first 2 postoperative wk
	To treat photophobia in incisional refractive surgery	1 or 2 gtt in operative eye 1 hr before surgery. Then 1 or 2 gtt 15 min after surgery. Then 1 gtt q.i.d. starting 4 to 6 hr after surgery for up to 3 days, p.r.n.
difluprednate Durezol	To treat inflammation and pain associated with ocular surgery	1 gtt in conjunctival sac of affected eye(s) q.i.d. for 2 wk starting 24 hr after surgery. Then 1 gtt b.i.d. for 1 wk.
fluorometholone Fluor-Op, FML Forte, FML Liquifilm, FML S.O.P. **fluorometholone acetate** Eflone, Flarex	To treat inflammatory and allergic conditions of the anterior uvea, conjunctiva, cornea, or sclera	1 or 2 gtt suspension in conjunctival sac b.i.d. to q.i.d. or, in severe conditions, up to every 2 hr during first 1 to 2 days p.r.n.; or 1 cm (.39 in) ointment in conjunctival sac once daily to t.i.d.
flurbiprofen sodium Ocufen	To inhibit intraoperative miosis	1 gtt in affected eye every 30 min, beginning 2 hr before surgery, up to total of 4 gtt
ketorolac tromethamine Acular	To relieve ocular itching due to seasonal allergic conjunctivitis	1 gtt in conjunctival sac of each eye q.i.d.
	To treat postoperative inflammation in patients who have undergone cataract extraction	1 gtt in operative eye q.i.d., starting 24 hr after surgery through first 2 postoperative wk
loteprednol etabonate Alrex, Lotemax	To relieve seasonal allergic conjunctivitis and to treat steroid-responsive inflammatory conditions of the palpebral and bulbar conjunctiva, cornea, and anterior segment of the globe	1 gtt of 0.2% suspension in affected eyes q.i.d.; or 1 or 2 gtt of 0.5% suspension in conjunctival sac of affected eye q.i.d. up to 1 gtt/hr
	To treat postoperative inflammation following ocular surgery	1 or 2 gtt in conjunctival sac of operated eye q.i.d., beginning 24 hr after surgery and continuing through first 2 wk of postoperative period
medrysone HMS Liquifilm	To treat allergic conjunctivitis, episcleritis, ephinephrine sensitivity, and vernal conjunctivitis	1 gtt into conjunctival sac up to every 4 hr

(continued)

Ophthalmic Drugs (continued)

GENERIC AND TRADE NAMES	INDICATIONS	USUAL ADULT DOSAGES
Ophthalmic anti-inflammatory drugs (continued)		
olopatadine hydrochloride 0.1% Patanol	To treat signs and symptoms of allergic conjunctivitis	1 gtt b.i.d. at 6- to 8-hr intervals
prednisolone acetate suspension Econopred Plus, Pred Forte, Pred Mild **prednisolone sodium phosphate solution** AK-Pred, Inflamase Forte, Inflamase Mild	To treat inflammation of the anterior segment of globe, cornea, and palpebral and bulbar conjunctiva	1 or 2 gtt in conjunctival sac b.i.d. to q.i.d. (suspension) or up to 6 times/day (solution)
rimexolone Vexol	To treat anterior uveitis	1 or 2 gtt in conjunctival sac every hr while awake in first week; 1 gtt every 2 hr while awake in second week; then tapered until uveitis resolves
	To treat postoperative inflammation after ocular surgery	1 or 2 gtt in conjunctival sac of affected eye q.i.d., beginning 24 hr after surgery and continuing through first 2 wk of postoperative period
Ophthalmic cycloplegic mydriatics		
atropine sulfate Atropisol, Isopto Atropine, Minims Atropine (CAN)	To treat acute iritis or uveitis	1 gtt up to q.i.d.; or small strip of ointment applied to conjunctival sac up to b.i.d.
	To produce dilation for cycloplegic refraction	1 or 2 gtt of 1% solution 1 hr before refraction
cyclopentolate hydrochloride AK-Pentolate, Cyclogyl, Minims Cyclopentolate (CAN), Pentolair	To produce mydriasis and cycloplegia required in specific diagnostic procedures	1 gtt of 0.5%, 1%, or 2% solution in each eye; then 1 or 2 gtt in 5 to 10 min p.r.n.
homatropine hydrobromide Isopto Homatropine, Minims Homatropine (CAN)	To dilate pupils for cycloplegic refraction	1 or 2 gtt in each eye, repeated in 5 to 10 min for 2 or 3 doses p.r.n.
	To treat uveitis	1 or 2 gtt in each eye every 3 to 4 hr
scopolamine hydrobromide Isopto Hyoscine	To dilate pupils for cycloplegic refraction	1 or 2 gtt of 0.25% solution 1 hr before refraction
	To treat iritis or uveitis	1 or 2 gtt of 0.25% solution once daily to q.i.d.

Ophthalmic Drugs (continued)

GENERIC AND TRADE NAMES	INDICATIONS	USUAL ADULT DOSAGES
Ophthalmic cycloplegic mydriatics *(continued)*		
tropicamide Mydriacyl, Opticyl, Tropicacyl	To dilate pupils for cycloplegic refraction	1 gtt of 1% solution, repeated in 5 min; additional 1 gtt in 20 to 30 min p.r.n.
Ophthalmic miotics		
acetylcholine chloride Miochol-E	To produce papillary miosis in anterior segment surgery	0.5 to 2 ml gently into anterior chamber before or after sutures secured
carbachol 0.01% Carbastat, Miostat **carbachol 0.75%, 1.5%, 2.25%, 3%** Carboptic, Isopto Carbachol	To produce papillary miosis in ocular surgery To treat open-angle glaucoma	0.5 ml (solution) into anterior chamber before or after sutures secured 1 or 2 gtt up to t.i.d.
pilocarpine Ocusert Pilo-20, Ocusert Pilo-40	To treat primary open-angle glaucoma	1 or 2 gtt up to q.i.d.; or 1-cm (.39 cm) ribbon of 4% gel at bedtime; or 1 Ocusert Pilo (20 or 40 mcg/hr) every 7 days
pilocarpine hydrochloride Adsorbocarpine, Akarpine, Isopto Carpine, Miocarpine (CAN), Pilocar, Pilopine HS, Pilostat	To treat acute angle-closure glaucoma as emergency therapy	1 gtt of 2% solution every 5 to 10 min for 3 to 6 doses; then 1 gtt every 1 to 3 hr until pressure is controlled
pilocarpine nitrate Pilagan, P.V. Carpine Liquifilm (CAN), Minims Pilocarpine (CAN)	To treat mydriasis due to mydriatic or cycloplegic drug therapy	1 gtt of 1% solution
Ophthalmic vasoconstrictors		
naphazoline hydrochloride Ak-Con, Albalon Liquifilm, Allerest, Clear Eyes, Comfort Eye Drops, Degest 2, Vasocon Regular	To treat ocular congestion, irritation, or itching	1 gtt of 0.1% solution every 3 to 4 hr; or 1 gtt of 0.012% to 0.03% solution up to q.i.d. for no more than 72 hr
oxymetazoline hydrochloride OcuClear, Visine L.R.	To provide relief from eye redness due to minor eye irritations	1 or 2 gtt in conjunctival sac b.i.d. to q.i.d. (at least 6 hr apart)

(continued)

Ophthalmic Drugs (continued)

GENERIC AND TRADE NAMES	INDICATIONS	USUAL ADULT DOSAGES
Ophthalmic vasoconstrictors *(continued)*		
phenylephrine hydrochloride Ak-Dilate, Ak-Nefrin, Isopto Frin, Mydfrin, Phenoptic, Relief Eye Drops for Red Eyes	To produce mydriasis without cycloplegia	1 gtt of 2.5% or 10% solution before eye exam, then repeated in 1 hr p.r.n.
	To produce mydriasis and vaso-constriction	1 gtt of 2.5% or 10% solution as single dose
	To treat chronic mydriasis	1 gtt of 2.5% or 10% solution b.i.d. or t.i.d.
	To treat posterior adhesion of iris	1 gtt of 2.5% or 10% solution as single dose
proparacaine hydrochloride Alcaine, Ophthaine, Ophthetic	To provide deep anesthesia dur-ing cataract extraction	1 gtt every 5 to 10 min for 5 to 7 doses
	To provide anesthesia during re-moval of eye sutures	1 or 2 gtt 2 to 3 min before pro-cedure
	To provide anesthesia during re-moval of foreign bodies	1 or 2 gtt in affected eye before surgery
	To provide anesthesia during tonometry	1 or 2 gtt immediately before measurement
tetracaine Pontocaine	To provide eye anesthesia (short term)	1 or 2 gtt p.r.n.
tetrahydrozoline hydrochloride Collyrium Fresh Eye Drops, Eyesine, Murine Plus, Optigene 3, Tetrasine, Visine Moisturizing, Visine Extra	To treat conjunctival congestion, irritation, and allergic conditions	1 or 2 gtt of 0.05% solution up to q.i.d. or as directed
Miscellaneous ophthalmic drugs		
apraclonidine hydrochloride Iopidine	To prevent or control elevated in-traocular pressure (IOP) before and after ocular laser surgery	1 gtt of 1% solution 1 hr before laser surgery on anterior seg-ment; then 1 drop immediately after surgery
azelastine hydrochloride 0.05% Optivar	To treat itching of the eye asso-ciated with allergic conjunctivitis	1 gtt in affected eye b.i.d.
betaxolol hydrochloride Betoptic, Betoptic S	To treat chronic open-angle glaucoma or ocular hypertension	1 or 2 gtt of 0.5% solution or 0.25% suspension b.i.d.

Ophthalmic Drugs (continued)

GENERIC AND TRADE NAMES	INDICATIONS	USUAL ADULT DOSAGES
Miscellaneous ophthalmic drugs (continued)		
bimatoprost 0.03% Lumigan	To reduce elevated IOP in patients with open-angle glaucoma or ocular hypertension who can't tolerate or have insufficiently responded to other IOP-lowering medications	1 gtt in affected eye daily in evening
brimonidine tartrate Alphagan, Alphagan P	To reduce IOP in open-angle glaucoma or ocular hypertension	1 gtt in affected eye t.i.d., about 8 hr apart
brinzolamide 1% Azopt	To reduce IOP in ocular hypertension or open-angle glaucoma	1 gtt t.i.d.
carteolol hydrochloride Ocupress	To treat chronic open-angle glaucoma or intraocular hypertension	1 gtt in conjunctival sac of affected eye b.i.d.
cyclosporine emulsion 0.05% Restasis	To increase tear production in keratoconjunctivitis sicca	1 gtt every 12 hr
dipivefrin hydrochloride Ophto-Dipivefrin (CAN), Propine	To reduce IOP in chronic open-angle glaucoma	1 gtt of 0.1% solution every 12 hr
dorzolamide hydrochloride Trusopt	To treat increased IOP in ocular hypertension or open-angle glaucoma	1 gtt in conjunctival sac of affected eye t.i.d.
emedastine difumarate Emadine	To treat allergic conjunctivitis	1 gtt in affected eye up to q.i.d.
fluorescein sodium AK-Fluor, Fluorescite, Fluor-I-Strip, Fluor-I-Strip-A.T., Ful-Glo, Funduscein-10, Funduscein-25, Ophthifluor	To diagnose corneal abrasions and foreign bodies, fit hard contact lenses, determine lacrimal patency, and assist in fundus photography and applanation tonometry	1 or 2 gtt of 2% solution followed by irrigation; or moisten strip with sterile water, then touch conjunctiva or fornix with moistened tip, and flush with irrigating solution; have patient blink several times after application
ketotifen fumarate Zaditor	To treat allergic conjunctivitis	1 gtt in affected eye b.i.d. every 8 to 12 hr
latanoprost Xalatan	To reduce IOP in ocular hypertension or open-angle glaucoma	1 gtt in conjunctival sac of affected eye daily in evening

(continued)

Ophthalmic Drugs (continued)

GENERIC AND TRADE NAMES	INDICATIONS	USUAL ADULT DOSAGES
Miscellaneous ophthalmic drugs *(continued)*		
levobunolol hydrochloride AKBeta, Betagan, Novo-Levobunolol (CAN)	To treat chronic open-angle glaucoma or ocular hypertension	1 or 2 gtt of 0.5% solution once daily or 0.25% solution b.i.d.
levocabastine hydrochloride 0.05% Livostin	To treat signs and symptoms of seasonal allergic conjunctivitis	1 gtt q.i.d.
metipranolol hydrochloride OptiPranolol	To reduce IOP in ocular hypertension or chronic open-angle glaucoma	1 gtt in affected eye b.i.d.
nedocromil sodium 2% Alocril	To treat itching associated with both seasonal and perennial allergic conjunctivitis	1 or 2 gtt b.i.d.
sodium chloride, hypertonic Adsorbonac, AK-NaCl, Muro-128, Muroptic-5	To provide temporary relief from corneal edema	1 or 2 gtt every 3 to 4 hr; or 6 mm (1/4 in) of ointment applied every 3 to 4 hr
timolol hemihydrate Betimol **timolol maleate** Apo-Timop (CAN), Timoptic **timolol maleate extended-release solution** Timoptic-XE	To reduce IOP in ocular hypertension or open-angle glaucoma	1 gtt of 0.25% or 0.5% solution in affected eye b.i.d., then 1 gtt daily; or 1 gtt extended-release solution in affected eye daily
travoprost 0.004% Travatan	To reduce elevated IOP in patients with open-angle glaucoma or ocular hypertension who can't tolerate or have insufficiently responded to other IOP-lowering medications	1 gtt in affected eye daily in evening
unoprostone isopropyl 0.15% Rescula	To reduce elevated IOP in patients with open-angle glaucoma or ocular hypertension who can't tolerate or have insufficiently responded to other IOP-lowering medications	1 gtt in affected eye b.i.d.

Antihistamines

Antihistamines are usually used to relieve immediate hypersensitivity reactions. They're also used as sedatives, antiemetics (especially in motion sickness), antitussives, antidyskinetics, and adjuncts to preoperative or postoperative analgesia.

Antihistamines are contraindicated in patients taking drugs that prolong the QT interval (including some macrolide antibiotics, quinidine, itraconazole, ketoconazole, mibefradil, and zileuton). They're also contraindicated in patients hypersensitive to antihistamines or their components.

The table below includes trade names; usual dosages; and onset, peak, and duration for antihistamines your patient is most likely to use daily or intermittently to control symptoms of allergic rhinitis. When caring for a patient who takes an antihistamine, individualize your plan of care but be sure to include these general interventions:

•Use antihistamines cautiously in patients with a history of glaucoma, peptic ulcer, or urine retention because anticholinergic effects may worsen these conditions.

•Before antihistamine therapy, assess the patient for hypokalemia and correct the imbalance, as prescribed, to reduce the risk of arrhythmias.

•Before antihistamine therapy, obtain a detailed medication history to help prevent drug interactions.

•Give antihistamines with food if GI distress occurs.

•Urge patient to avoid alcohol and other CNS depressants during antihistamine use because the combination can cause additive CNS depression.

•Monitor blood pressure because these drugs' anticholinergic effects may cause hypertension.

•Be aware that short- and long-acting antihistamines may be combined and H_2 blockers added to increase antihistamine effects.

•Be aware that products containing pseudoephedrine should be used for less than 7 days.

GENERIC AND TRADE NAMES	USUAL ADULT DOSAGE	ONSET, PEAK, AND DURATION
acrivastine Semprex-D (also includes pseudoephedrine)	8 mg P.O. every 4 to 6 hr	**Onset:** 30 min **Peak:** Unknown **Duration:** 6 to 8 hr
azatadine Optimine Trinalin Repetabs (also includes pseudoephedrine)	1 to 2 mg P.O. every 8 to 12 hr 1 tablet P.O. every 12 hr	**Onset:** 15 to 60 min **Peak:** 4 hr **Duration:** 12 hr
azelastine Astelin	2 sprays (137 mcg/spray) in each nostril b.i.d.	**Onset:** In 3 hr **Peak:** Unknown **Duration:** 12 hr
cetirizine Zyrtec Zyrtec D (also includes pseudoephedrine)	5 to 10 mg P.O. daily 5 mg/120 mg b.i.d.	**Onset:** 30 to 60 min **Peak:** 1 hr **Duration:** Up to 24 hr
desloratadine Clarinex Clarinex Reditabs	5 mg P.O. daily 5 mg P.O. daily	**Onset:** Unknown **Peak:** Unknown (Clarinex); 3 hr (Clarinex Reditabs) **Duration:** Unknown

(continued)

Antihistamines (continued)

GENERIC AND TRADE NAMES	USUAL ADULT DOSAGE	ONSET, PEAK, AND DURATION
fexofenadine Allegra Allegra-D (also includes pseudoephedrine)	60 mg P.O. b.i.d. or 180 mg P.O. daily 1 tablet P.O. every 12 hr	**Onset:** 1 hr **Peak:** 2 to 3 hr **Duration:** 12 hr
levocetirizine Xyzal	2.5 to 5 mg P.O. daily in evening	**Onset:** Less than 1 hr **Peak:** 0.9 hr **Duration:** 24 hr
loratadine Claritin Claritin-D12 (also includes pseudoephedrine) Claritin-D24 (also includes pseudoephedrine)	10 mg P.O. daily 1 tablet P.O. every 12 hr 1 tablet P.O. every 24 hr	**Onset:** 1 to 3 hr **Peak:** 8 to 12 hr **Duration:** At least 24 hr
olopatadine Patanase	2 sprays (665 mcg/spray) in each nostril b.i.d.	**Onset:** Unknown **Peak:** 15 to 120 minutes **Duration:** Unknown

Topical Drugs

Topical preparations consist of an active drug prepared in a specified medium that promotes absorption through the skin. Media are commonly chosen based on drug solubility; rate of drug release; ability to hydrate the outer skin layer; ability to enhance penetration; drug stability; and interactions between the chosen medium, skin, and active ingredient. Topical media include aerosols, creams, gels, lotions, ointments, powders, tinctures, and wet dressings. Aerosols, gels, lotions, and tinctures are convenient for applications to the scalp and hairy areas. Acutely inflamed areas are best treated with drying preparations, such as lotions, tinctures, and wet dressings. Chronic inflammations do well with applications of lubricating preparations, including creams and ointments.

Because of its physical properties, the skin can act as a holding area for many drugs, allowing for slow penetration and prolonged duration of action. (This characteristic makes it important to understand the patient's allergies.) However, when administering topical or transdermal drugs that aren't prescribed for a specific location, keep in mind that penetration properties may vary in different areas of the skin. For example, the scrotum, face, axillae, and scalp are more permeable than the extremities, and ventral surfaces are generally more permeable than dorsal surfaces.

Topical agents are classified as antibacterials, antifungals (the largest group), antivirals, corticosteroids, retinoids, and other miscellaneous preparations.

•*Antibacterials* may be useful in the early treatment of minor skin infections and wounds. Minor skin infections may respond well to topical drugs applied at the infection site. Minor wounds should be treated at the site and in the immediately surrounding area to prevent other pathogens from colonizing the area.

•*Antifungals* are usually used to treat mucocutaneous infections, such as tineas, primarily ringworm and athlete's foot. Systemic use of antifungals is limited by their potentially toxic adverse effects, most commonly renal or hepatic damage. All fungi are completely resistant to conventional antibacterial drugs.

•*Antivirals* are used to inhibit viral replication. They work by targeting any one of the steps involved in viral replication: penetration into susceptible host cells; uncoating of the virus nucleic acid; synthesis of regulatory proteins, RNA and DNA, and structural proteins; assembly of viral particles; and release of the virus from the cell. Topical antivirals such as penciclovir can shorten the duration of herpetic lesions, lessen lesion pain, and minimize viral shedding.

•*Corticosteroids* reduce the signs and symptoms of inflammation. Topical corticosteroids cause vasoconstriction, probably by suppressing cell degranulation. They also cause decreased cell permeability by reducing histamine release from basal and mast cells.

•*Retinoids,* typically derivatives of vitamin A, are very effective in treating acne vulgaris, although the acne may appear to worsen before it improves. Retinoids are also useful for reducing wrinkles. When applied to the skin, retinoids remain primarily in the dermis; less than 10% of the drug is absorbed into the circulation. Prolonged use of retinoids promotes new dermal growth, new blood vessel formation, and thickening of the epidermis. Because these drugs are absorbed systemically and may have teratogenic effects, they shoudln't be used by pregnant women.

•*Miscellaneous topical drugs* are used to treat a variety of topical skin conditions, including dry skin, ichthyosis, parasitic infestations, psoriasis, and unwanted hair growth.

Before you apply a topical preparation, clean the site and let it dry. Use gloves or a finger cot during application to prevent the drug from being absorbed through your own skin. Inform your patient of any expected discomfort, such as temporary stinging or burning. After application, cover the site only if required; some topical drugs shouldn't be covered with an occlusive dressing. Be sure to teach the patient and a family member correct administration technique. Also, review possible adverse reactions, highlighting those that should be reported to the prescriber. Stress the importance of compliance with the drug regimen because some topical drugs require weeks or months of therapy to eradicate the underlying condition.

The following table includes the generic and trade names of many commonly prescribed topical drugs as well as their FDA-approved indications and usual adult dosage.

(continued)

Topical Drugs (continued)

GENERIC AND TRADE NAMES	INDICATIONS	USUAL ADULT DOSAGES
Antibacterials		
azelaic acid cream Azelex, Finacea, Finevin	To treat mild to moderate inflammatory acne vulgaris	Gently massage thin film into affected area b.i.d., morning and evening.
bacitracin	To treat topical infections, abrasions, cuts, and minor burns or wounds	Apply thin film to affected area once daily to t.i.d. up to 3 wk.
benzoyl peroxide Benzac AC Wash, Clearasil Maximum Strength, Desquam-E 2.5 Gel, Fostex 10 BPO Gel, Triaz	To treat mild to moderate inflammatory acne vulgaris	Apply to affected area once daily, gradually increasing to b.i.d. or t.i.d.
clindamycin phosphate Cleocin, Cleocin T Gel, Cleocin T Lotion, Clinda-Derm, Dalacin, Dalacin T Topical Solution (CAN)	To treat inflammatory acne vulgaris To treat bacterial vaginosis	Apply to affected area b.i.d., morning and evening. 1 applicatorful (100 mg) intravaginally at bedtime for 7 days.
clindamycin 1% and benzoyl peroxide 5% Benzaclin gel DUAC	To treat acne vulgaris	Apply once or twice daily (morning and/or evening) to affected areas
erythromycin Akne-Mycin, A/T/S, Erycette, EryDerm, Erygel, Erymax, Ery-Sol (CAN), Erythrogel, ETS (CAN), Sans-Acne (CAN), Staticin, T-Stat (CAN)	To treat inflammatory acne vulgaris	Apply to affected areas b.i.d., morning and evening.
erythromycin 3% and benzoyl peroxide 5% Benzamycin	To treat moderate inflammatory acne	Apply to affected areas b.i.d., morning and evening.
gentamicin sulfate Garamycin, G-myticin	To prevent or treat superficial skin infections due to susceptible bacteria; to treat superficial burns	Rub small amount gently into skin t.i.d. or q.i.d.
mafenide gel 1% Sulfamylon	As adjunct to treat second- and third-degree burns	Apply $\frac{1}{16}$-inch layer aseptically to affected areas once or twice daily

Topical Drugs (continued)

GENERIC AND TRADE NAMES	INDICATIONS	USUAL ADULT DOSAGES
Antibacterials *(continued)*		
metronidazole MetroCream, MetroGel, MetroGel-Vaginal	To treat inflammatory papules and pustules of acne rosacea	Apply thin film to affected area b.i.d., morning and evening.
	To treat bacterial vaginosis	1 applicatorful (37.5 mg) intravaginally at bedtime or b.i.d. for 5 days.
mupirocin 2% Bactroban, Bactroban Cream, Bactroban Nasal	To treat impetigo	Apply to affected areas t.i.d. for 1 to 2 wk.
	To treat secondary infections of traumatic skin lesions due to *Staphylococcus aureus* and *Streptococcus pyogenes*	Apply thin film and cover with an occlusive dressing t.i.d. for 10 days.
	To eradicate nasal colonization of methicillin-resistant *S. aureus*	Apply half of the contents of a unit-dose tube to each nostril b.i.d. for 5 days.
neomycin sulfate Myciguent	To prevent or treat superficial bacterial infections	Rub fingertip-size dose into affected area once daily to t.i.d.
nitrofurazone Furacin	As adjunct to treat third-degree burns and to treat infection in skin grafts	Apply aseptically, directly to lesions or on gauze; repeat p.r.n.
povidone-iodine Betadine, Betadine Cream, Betadine Spray	To disinfect wounds and burns	Apply or spray to affected area p.r.n.
silver sulfadiazine Flamazine (CAN), Silvadene, Thermazine	To prevent and treat bacterial and fungal infection in second- and third-degree burns	Apply ¹⁄₁₆-inch layer aseptically once to twice daily to clean debrided burns; reapply promptly if removed.
sulfacetamide sodium 10% Klaron	To treat acne vulgaris	Apply thin film b.i.d.
sulfacetamide sodium 10% and sulfur 5% Sulfacet-R	To treat acne rosacea, acne vulgaris, and seborrheic dermatitis	Apply thin film, and massage into affected area once daily to t.i.d.
tetracycline hydrochloride Achromycin, Topicycline	To treat acne vulgaris	Rub solution into affected area b.i.d.
	To prevent or treat superficial skin infections due to susceptible bacteria	Apply to affected area b.i.d. (morning and evening) or t.i.d.

(continued)

Topical Drugs (continued)

GENERIC AND TRADE NAMES	INDICATIONS	USUAL ADULT DOSAGES
Antifungals		
butenafine hydrochloride 1% Lotrimin Ultra, Mentax	To treat tinea corporis, tinea cruris, or tinea versicolor	Apply to affected surrounding area once daily for 2 wk.
	To treat interdigital tinea pedis due to *Epidermophyton floccosum, Trychophyton mentagrophytes,* or *T. rubrum*	Apply to affected and immediately surrounding area once daily for 4 wk or b.i.d. for 1 wk.
butoconazole nitrate Femstat, Femstat One, Mycelex 3	To treat vulvovaginal mycotic infections caused by *Candida* species	1 applicatorful (100 mg) intravaginally at bedtime for 3 days; may repeat course for total of 6 days.
Gynazole-1	To treat vulvovaginal infections caused by *Candida albicans*	1 applicatorful (100 mg) intravaginally once anytime day or night.
ciclopirox olamine 1% Loprox 0.77%	To treat candidiasis due to *Candida albicans;* tinea corporis, tinea cruris, and tinea pedis due to *E. floccosum, T. mentagrophytes, T. rubrum,* or *Microsporum canis;* tinea versicolor due to *Malassezia furfur;* onychomycosis due to *T. rubrum;* and seborrheic dermatitis	Massage gently into affected and surrounding area b.i.d., morning and evening.
ciclopirox olamine 8% Penlac	To treat onychomycosis of the fingernails and toenails	Apply evenly to entire nail surface and surrounding 5 mm of skin at bedtime for up to 48 wk.
clotrimazole Canesten (CAN), Gyne-Lotrimin, Gyne-Lotrimin 3, Lotrimin, Lotrimin Antifungal, Mycelex, Mycelex-7, Mycelex-G, Mycelex OTC, Trivagizole 3	To treat superficial fungal infections (tinea corporis, tinea cruris, tinea pedis, tinea versicolor, candidiasis)	Apply thin film and massage into affected and surrounding area b.i.d., morning and evening, for 2 to 4 wk.
	To treat vulvovaginal candidiasis	Insert 100-mg vaginal tablet at bedtime for 7 days; or 500-mg vaginal tablet at bedtime for 1 day; or 1 applicatorful intravaginally at bedtime for 7 days (or 3 days if using Trivagizole 3).

Topical Drugs (continued)

Topical Drugs (continued)

GENERIC AND TRADE NAMES	INDICATIONS	USUAL ADULT DOSAGES
Antifungals (continued)		
clotrimazole (continued)	To treat oropharyngeal candidiasis	Dissolve oral troche over 15 to 30 min 5 times/day for 14 days.
	To prevent oropharyngeal candidiasis	Dissolve oral troche over 15 to 30 min t.i.d. for duration of chemotherapy or until corticosteroid dosage is reduced to maintenance levels.
econazole nitrate Ecostatin (CAN), Spectazole	To treat tinea corporis, tinea cruris, tinea pedis, tinea versicolor, cutaneous candidiasis	Rub into affected area once or twice daily for at least 2 wk.
	To treat cutaneous candidiasis	Rub into affected area b.i.d. for 2 wk.
gentian violet Genapax	To treat candidiasis	Insert 1 intravaginal tampon t.i.d. to q.i.d. for 12 days; or apply 1% or 2% solution to affected area once or twice daily for 3 days.
haloprogin Halotex	To treat tinea corporis, tinea cruris, tinea manuum, and tinea pedis due to *E. floccosum, M. canis, T. mentagrophytes, T. rubrum,* or *T. tonsurans;* to treat tinea versicolor due to *M. furfur*	Apply liberally to affected area b.i.d. for 2 to 3 wk or, for intertriginous lesions, up to 4 wk.
ketoconazole 2% Nizoral	To treat tinea corporis, tinea cruris, and tinea versicolor due to susceptible organisms; to treat cutaneous candidiasis	Apply thin film to affected and immediately surrounding area and cover with occlusive dressing daily for at least 2 wk.
	To treat tinea pedis	Apply to affected and immediately surrounding area daily for 6 wk; or apply shampoo to wet hair, lather, massage for 1 min, leave drug on scalp for 3 min, then rinse and repeat 2 times/wk for 4 weeks (with at least 3 days between shampoos), then intermittently p.r.n.
	To treat seborrheic dermatitis	Apply to affected and immediately surrounding area b.i.d. for 4 wk.

(continued)

Topical Drugs (continued)

GENERIC AND TRADE NAMES	INDICATIONS	USUAL ADULT DOSAGES
miconazole nitrate Femizol-M, Fungoid, M-Zole 3, Micatin, Monistat-Derm, Monistat 3, Monistat 7, Ony-Clear Nail	To treat tinea corporis, tinea cruris, tinea pedis; cutaneous candidiasis; and common dermatophyte infections	Apply cream sparingly (or powder or spray liberally) over affected area. b.i.d. for 2 to 4 wk.
	To treat tinea versicolor	Apply sparingly to affected area daily for 2 wk.
	To treat vulvovaginal candidiasis	1 applicatorful (100 mg) or vaginal suppository (100 mg) at bedtime for 7 days, repeated p.r.n.; or insert vaginal suppository (200 mg) at bedtime for 3 days.
	To treat onychomycosis	Brush tincture on affected areas of nail surface, beds, and edges and under nail surface b.i.d. for up to several mo; or spray on clean, dry, affected nails, holding actuator down for 1 or 2 sec.
naftifine hydrochloride Naftin	To treat tinea corporis, tinea cruris, and tinea pedis	Apply cream to affected area daily; or apply gel to affected area b.i.d., morning and evening.
nystatin Mycostatin, Nadostine (CAN), Nilstat	To treat cutaneous and mucocutaneous infections due to *C. albicans*	Apply cream to affected area b.i.d. or as indicated; or apply powder b.i.d. or t.i.d.; or insert 1 or 2 lozenges (200,000 to 400,000 units) 4 to 5 times/day for up to 48 hr after symptoms have subsided or 14 days; or insert 4 to 6 ml (400,000 to 600,000 units) of oral suspension in mouth q.i.d. (one-half of dose in each side of mouth) and retain as long as possible before swallowing.
	To treat vulvovaginal candidiasis	Insert 1 intravaginal tablet (100,000 units) or 1 applicatorful (100,000 to 500,000 units) once or twice daily for 14 days.
oxiconazole nitrate Oxistat, Oxizold (CAN)	To treat tinea corporis, tinea cruris, and tinea pedis caused by *E. floccosum, T. mentagrophytes,* or *T. rubrum*	Apply to affected and surrounding area once or twice daily for 2 wk (tinea corporis and tinea cruris) or for 4 wk (tinea pedis).
	To treat tinea versicolor caused by *M. furfur*	Apply cream to affected and surrounding area daily for 2 wk.

Topical Drugs *(continued)*

GENERIC AND TRADE NAMES	INDICATIONS	USUAL ADULT DOSAGES
Antifungals *(continued)*		
selenium sulfide Selsun	To treat tinea versicolor	Apply to scalp, lather with small amount of water, wait 10 min, then rinse, every 7 days.
	To treat dandruff and seborrheic scalp dermatitis	Massage into wet scalp, wait 2 to 3 min, rinse, and repeat 2 times/wk for 2 wk, then p.r.n.
sulconazole nitrate Exelderm	To treat tinea corporis, tinea cruris, and tinea pedis (cream only) caused by *E. floccosum, M. canis, T. mentagrophytes,* or *T. rubrum;* to treat tinea versicolor	Massage small amount gently into affected and surrounding areas once or twice daily (tinea pedis) for up to 6 wk.
terbinafine hydrochloride Lamisil DermGel, Lamisil Solution	To treat tinea versicolor	Apply to affected area b.i.d. for 1 wk.
Lamisil AT Cream	To treat tinea corporis, tinea cruris, and tinea pedis	Apply thin film to affected area b.i.d. for 1 wk or 2 wk (plantar tinea pedis).
Lamisil AT Solution	To treat interdigital tinea pedis, tinea corporis, and tinea cruris	Apply between the toes b.i.d. for 1 wk (interdigital tinea pedis) or to affected area daily for 1 wk (tinea corporis and tinea cruris).
terconazole Terazol 3, Terazol 7	To treat vulvovaginal candidiasis	1 applicatorful (20 mg) intravaginally at bedtime for 3 days (0.4%) or 1 applicatorful (40 mg) for 7 days (0.8%); or insert 80-mg vaginal suppository at bedtime for 3 consecutive days.
tioconazole GyneCure Ovules (CAN), Vagistat-1	To treat vulvovaginal candidiasis	Insert 1 applicatorful (300 mg) or 1 suppository (300 mg) intravaginally at bedtime as a single dose.

(continued)

Topical Drugs (continued)

GENERIC AND TRADE NAMES	INDICATIONS	USUAL ADULT DOSAGES
Antifungals *(continued)*		
tolnaftate Absorbine Footcare, Aftate for Athlete's Foot, Aftate for Jock Itch, Dr. Scholl's Athlete's Foot, Genaspore, NP-27, Pitrex, Quinsana Plus, Tinactin, Ting, Zeasorb-AF	To treat tinea capitis, corporis, cruris, manuum, pedis, and versicolor	Apply 1% aerosol, cream, gel, powder, or solution to affected and surrounding areas b.i.d.; continue for 2 wk after symptoms subside or up to 6 wk.
Antivirals		
acyclovir Zovirax	To treat mucocutaneous herpes simplex in immunocompromised patients	Apply cream to affected area 4 to 6 times daily for 10 days. Apply ointment every 3 hr (6 times/day) for 7 days. Use finger cot, rubber glove, or applicator stick for both forms to prevent herpetic whitlow.
docosanol Abreva	To treat recurrent oral-facial herpes simplex	Apply cream gently and completely to affected area 5 times daily, starting with first visible sign of lesion and continuing until lesion is healed.
penciclovir Denavir	To treat recurrent herpes labialis of lips and face	Apply every 2 hr while awake for 4 days.
Corticosteroids		
alclometasone dipropionate Aclovate	To treat corticosteroid-responsive dermatoses	Apply thin film to affected area and massage b.i.d. to t.i.d.
amcinonide Cyclocort	To treat corticosteroid-responsive dermatoses	Apply thin film to affected area and massage b.i.d. (ointment, lotion) or b.i.d. to t.i.d. (cream).
betamethasone benzoate Beben (CAN), Uticort	To treat corticosteroid-responsive dermatoses	Apply thin film or a few drops to affected area once or twice daily up to 45 g/wk (ointment, cream), 50 g/wk (gel), or 50 ml (lotion).
betamethasone dipropionate Diprolene, Diprolene AF, Diprosone, Topilene (CAN)	To treat corticosteroid-responsive dermatoses	Apply thin film or a few drops to affected area once or twice daily up to 45 g/wk (ointment, cream), 50 g/wk (gel), or 50 ml (lotion).

Topical Drugs (continued)

GENERIC AND TRADE NAMES	INDICATIONS	USUAL ADULT DOSAGES
Corticosteroids *(continued)*		
betamethasome valerate Luxiq, Valisone	To treat corticosteroid-responsive dermatoses	Apply foam to scalp, and massage until foam disappears, b.i.d. Apply thin film of ointment b.i.d.
clobetasol propionate Dermovate (CAN), Embeline, Temovate	To treat corticosteroid-responsive dermatoses	Apply thin film to affected area and rub in gently b.i.d. to t.i.d., up to 50 g/wk, for 2 wk.
Olux	To treat corticosteroid-responsive dermatoses of scalp	Apply to affected area of scalp b.i.d., once in morning and once at night, for 2 wk.
desonide Desowen, Tridesilon	To treat corticosteroid-responsive dermatoses	Apply thin film to affected area b.i.d. to q.i.d.
diflorasone diacetate Florone, Maxiflor, Psorcon	To treat corticosteroid-responsive dermatoses	Apply thin film to affected area once daily to q.i.d.
fluocinolone acetonide Bio-Syn, Derma Smooth FS, Fluocet, Fluoderm (CAN), Fluolar (CAN), Fluonid (CAN), Fluonide (CAN), Flurosyn, Synalar, Synalar-HP, Synamol (CAN), Synemol	To treat corticosteroid-responsive dermatoses	Apply thin film to affected area b.i.d. to q.i.d.
fluocinonide Lidemol (CAN), Lidex	To treat corticosteroid-responsive dermatoses	Apply thin film to affected area b.i.d. to q.i.d.
flurandrenolide Cordran, Cordran Tape, Drenison (CAN)	To treat corticosteroid-responsive dermatoses	Apply thin film to affected area and massage b.i.d. to t.i.d.; or apply tape every 12 to 24 hr.
fluticasone propionate Cutivate	To treat atopic dermatitis and corticosteroid-responsive dermatoses	Apply thin film daily (atopic dermatitis) or b.i.d. (dermatoses).
halcinonide Halog	To treat corticosteroid-responsive dermatoses	Apply sparingly and massage once daily to t.i.d.
halobetasol propionate Ultravate	To treat corticosteroid-responsive dermatoses	Apply thin film to affected area and rub in gently once or twice daily, up to 50 g/wk, for 2 wk.

(continued)

Topical Drugs (continued)

GENERIC AND TRADE NAMES	INDICATIONS	USUAL ADULT DOSAGES
Corticosteroids *(continued)*		
hydrocortisone 0.25% Cetacort, Cort-Dome **hydrocortisone 0.5%** Bactine, Cetacort, Cortate (CAN), Cort-Dome, Cortifair, Delacort, DermiCort, Dermtex HC, Emo-Cort (CAN), Hydro-Tex, Hytone, MyCort, Sential (CAN), S-T Cort **hydrocortisone 1%** Ala-Cort, Allercort, Alphaderm, Acticort 100, Barriere-HC (CAN), Beta-HC, Cetacort, Cort-Dome, Cortifair, Cortril, Dermacort, Emo-Cort (CAN), Gly-Cort, Hi-Cor 1.0, Hydro-Tex, Hytone, LactiCare-HC, Lemoderm, Nutracort, Penecort, Prevex-HC (CAN), Rederm, Sarna HC (CAN), Synacort, Unicort (CAN) **hydrocortisone 2%** Ala-Scalp HP **hydrocortisone 2.5%** Allercort, Anusol-HC, Emo-Cort (CAN), Hi-Cor 2.5, Hytone, LactiCare-HC, Lemoderm, Nutracort, Penecort, Synacort **hydrocortisone acetate 0.1%** Corticreme (CAN) **hydrocortisone acetate 0.5%** 9-1-1, Corticaine, Cortacet (CAN), Cortaid, Cortoderm (CAN), FoilleCort, Gynecort, Hyderm (CAN), Lanacort, Novohydrocort (CAN), Pharma-Cort	To treat corticosteroid-responsive dermatoses	Apply thin film (aerosol foam, cream, lotion, ointment, solution) to affected area once daily to q.i.d.

Topical Drugs (continued)

GENERIC AND TRADE NAMES	INDICATIONS	USUAL ADULT DOSAGES
Corticosteroids *(continued)*		
hydrocortisone acetate 1%, 2%, 2.5% Cortaid, Cortef Feminine Itch, Corticreme (CAN), Cortoderm (CAN), Hyderm (CAN), Maximum Strength Cortaid, Micort HC-Lipocream, Novohydrocort (CAN) **hydrocortisone acetate topical aerosol foam** Epifoam	To treat corticosteroid-responsive dermatoses	Apply thin film (aerosol foam, cream, lotion, ointment, solution) to affected area once daily to q.i.d.
hydrocortisone acetate dental paste Orabase-HCA	To treat inflamed oral mucosa	Apply to oral mucosa b.i.d. to t.i.d. after meals and at bedtime.
hydrocortisone butyrate Locoid **hydrocortisone valerate** Westcort	To treat corticosteroid-responsive dermatoses	Apply to affected area b.i.d. to t.i.d.
hydrocortisone acetate, polymyxin B sulfate, and neomycin sulfate Cortisporin	To treat corticosteroid-responsive dermatoses (short term) with mild bacterial infection	Apply sparingly and massage b.i.d. to q.i.d.
hydrocortisone and iodoquinol Vytone	To treat corticosteroid-responsive dermatoses with mild bacterial or fungal infection (short term)	Apply to affected area once daily to t.i.d.
mometasone furoate Elocom (CAN), Elocon	To treat corticosteroid-responsive dermatoses	Apply thin film or a few drops to affected area daily.
prednicarbate Dermatop	To treat corticosteroid-responsive dermatoses	Apply thin film to affected area b.i.d.
triamcinolone acetonide 0.025%, 0.5% Aristocort, Aristocort A, Aristocort D (CAN), Flutex, Kenac, Kenalog, Kenonel, Triacet, Triaderm (CAN), Trianide Mild (CAN)	To treat corticosteroid-responsive dermatoses	Apply thin film (cream) to affected area b.i.d. to q.i.d.; 0.025% lotion or ointment once or twice daily; 0.1% lotion or ointment once daily; or 0.5% ointment once daily.

(continued)

Topical Drugs (continued)

GENERIC AND TRADE NAMES	INDICATIONS	USUAL ADULT DOSAGES
Corticosteroids *(continued)*		
triamcinolone acetonide 0.1% Aristocort, Aristocort A, Aristocort R (CAN), Delta-Tritex, Flutex, Kenac, Kenalog, Kenalog-H, Kenonel, Triacet, Triaderm (CAN), Trianide Regular (CAN) **triamcinolone acetonide 0.5%** Aristocort, Aristocort A, Aristocort C (CAN), Flutex, Kenalog, Kenonel, Triacet	To treat corticosteroid-responsive dermatoses	Apply thin film (cream) to affected area b.i.d. to q.i.d.; 0.025% lotion or ointment once or twice daily; 0.1% lotion or ointment once daily; or 0.5% ointment once daily.
triamcinolone acetonide dental paste Kenalog in Orabase, Oracort, Oralone	To treat inflammatory or ulcerative oral lesions	Apply to oral mucosa b.i.d. to t.i.d. after meals and at bedtime.
triamcinolone acetonide topical aerosol Kenalog	To treat corticosteroid-responsive dermatoses	Spray affected area t.i.d. to q.i.d.
Retinoids		
adapalene Differin	To treat acne vulgaris	Apply to affected area at bedtime.
tazarotene 0.05%, 0.1% Avage, Tazorac	To treat plaque psoriasis	Apply thin film to affected area at bedtime.
tazarotene 0.1% Avage, Tazorac	To treat facial acne vulgaris or plaque psoriasis	Apply thin film to affected area at bedtime.
tretinoin Avita, Renova, Retin-A, Retin-A Micro, Stieva-A (CAN)	To treat acne vulgaris	Apply sparingly to clean, dry affected area at bedtime.

Topical Drugs (continued)

GENERIC AND TRADE NAMES	INDICATIONS	USUAL ADULT DOSAGES
Miscellaneous topical drugs		
ammonium lactate, 12% Lac-Hydrin	To treat dry skin and ichthyosis	Apply to affected area, and rub in b.i.d.
anthralin Anthranol 1 (CAN), Drithocreme, Dritho-Scalp	To treat chronic psoriasis To treat chronic scalp psoriasis	Apply sparingly and massage into affected lesions daily, Apply to lesions daily for 1 wk.
becaplermin Regranex	To treat lower-extremity diabetic neuropathic ulcers that extend into the subcutaneous tissue or beyond and that have an adequate blood supply	Apply to ulcers daily.
calcipotriene Dovonex	To treat plaque psoriasis	Apply cream or scalp lotion in a thin layer b.i.d. up to 8 wk. Apply thin layer of ointment once or twice daily up to 8 wk.
calcipotriene hydrate 0.005% and betamethasone dipropionate 0.064% Taclonex, Taclonex Scalp	To treat psoriasis vulgaris To treat moderate to severe psoriasis vulgaris of the scalp	Apply ointment to affected skin; rub in gently and completely once daily for up to 4 wk. Apply suspension to affected scalp areas and rub in gently once daily for 2 to 8 wk or until skin clears.
capsaicin Zostrix Capsin Capzacin-P	To provide temporary pain relief from rheumatoid arthritis and osteoarthritis; to relieve neuralgias from pain following shingles (herpes zoster) infection	Apply to affected area no more than q.i.d.
chlorhexidine Hibiclens	To clean skin wounds	Rinse area, apply minimal amount to cover, then wash and rinse thoroughly.
chloroxine Capitrol	To treat dandruff and seborrheic dermatitis	Massage into wet scalp, wait 3 min, rinse, and repeat 2 times/wk.
clotrimazole and betamethasone dipropionate 0.05%, 1% Lotrisone	To treat symptomatic inflammatory tinea corporis, tinea cruris, and tinea pedis	Massage cream gently into affected and surrounding skin areas b.i.d. for 2 wk (tinea corporis, tinea cruris) or for 4 wk (tinea pedis).

(continued)

Topical Drugs (continued)

GENERIC AND TRADE NAMES	INDICATIONS	USUAL ADULT DOSAGES
Miscellaneous topical drugs *(continued)*		
coal tar Zetar, Zetar Shampoo	To treat psoriasis	Add 15 to 20 ml to lukewarm bath, immerse affected area for 15 to 20 min, and rinse thoroughly 3 to 7 times/wk.
	To treat dandruff or scalp seborrhea	Massage into wet scalp, rinse, repeat application and wait 5 min, then rinse again.
crotamiton 10% Eurax	To treat scabies	Massage into cleansed body from chin to soles of feet, and reapply after 24 hr; change bed linens next day, and bathe 48 hr after second dose; repeat in 7 to 10 days if new lesions appear.
desoximetasone Topicort	To relieve inflammatory and pruritic manifestations of corticosteroid-responsive dermatoses, including psoriasis, atopic dermatitis, and eczema	Apply thin film b.i.d. to affected areas; occlusive dressings may be added for severe dermatoses.
diclofenac sodium 3% Solaraze	To treat actinic keratoses	Massage gel gently onto affected lesion areas b.i.d. for 60 to 90 days.
doxepin hydrochloride Zonalon	To treat pruritus associated with dermatitis and chronic lichen simplex	Apply thin film to affected area q.i.d. (every 3 to 4 hr) for up to 8 days.
eflornithine Vaniqa	To retard unwanted hair growth	Apply thin film to affected area of face and chin b.i.d. (at least 8 hr apart); don't wash treated area for at least 4 hr.
fluocinolone acetonide 0.01%, hydroquinone 4%, tretinoin 0.05% TRI-LUMA Cream	To treat severe facial melasma	Apply a thin film lightly and uniformly to hyperpigmented areas of melasma including about ½ in of skin surrounding each lesion daily at least 30 min before bedtime.
fluorouracil cream Carac, Efudex, Fluoroplex	To treat actinic and solar keratoses	Apply to lesions b.i.d. for 2 to 6 weeks.

Topical Drugs (continued)

GENERIC AND TRADE NAMES	INDICATIONS	USUAL ADULT DOSAGES
Miscellaneous topical drugs (continued)		
hexachlorophene pHisoHex	To treat skin preoperatively	Rinse area, apply minimal amount to cover; then wash and rinse thoroughly.
hydrocortisone acetate, polymyxin B sulfate, and neomycin sulfate Cortisporin	To treat dermatoses associated with secondary bacterial infection	Apply small amount to affected areas b.i.d. to q.i.d.
hydroquinone Alustra, Claripel, Eldopaque, Eldoquin, Glyquin, Melanex	To treat hyperpigmentation and melanin	Apply b.i.d. to the affected areas for no longer than 2 months
imiquimod 5% Aldara	To treat external genital and perianal warts	Apply thin layer to affected area and rub in 3 times/wk ay bedtime for up to 16 wk; remove with soap and water after 6 to 10 hr.
lidocaine and prilocaine EMLA	For local anesthesia	Apply 1 disk or thick layer of 2.5-g cream occlusively for at least 1 hr.
malathion lotion 0.5% Ovide	To treat pediculus humanus capitis	Apply to dry hair in amount just sufficient to thoroughly wet the hair and scalp; then let hair dry naturally. After 8 to 12 hr, shampoo and rinse hair to remove dead lice and eggs. If lice are still present after 7 to 9 days, repeat application.
mequinol 2%, retinol 0.01% Solage	To treat solar lentigines	Apply solution b.i.d. morning and evening at least 8 hours apart. Avoid application to surrounding skin, and do not bathe for 6 hr after application.
minoxidil Rogaine 2% and 5%	To treat alopecia and androgenetica	Apply 1 ml to affected areas b.i.d.
monobenzone 20% Benoquin	To treat final depigmentation in extensive vitiligo	Apply b.i.d. to t.i.d. for 1 to 4 months, then b.i.d. weekly for maintenance

(continued)

Topical Drugs (continued)

GENERIC AND TRADE NAMES	INDICATIONS	USUAL ADULT DOSAGES
Miscellaneous topical drugs *(continued)*		
permethrin 1% Nix	To prevent or treat head lice	Wash and dry hair, saturate scalp with 1% cream, leave on hair for 10 min, then rinse; remove nits with provided comb; repeat in 7 days if living mites are still present.
permethrin 5% Acticin, Elimite	To treat scabies	Massage 5% cream into skin from head to soles of feet, and remove after 8 to 10 hr; repeat in 14 days if living mites are still present.
pimecrolimus 1% Elidel	To treat mild-to-moderate atopic dermatitis	Apply to affected areas b.i.d.
podofilox Condylox	To treat anogenital warts (gel); to treat external genital warts (gel or solution)	Apply 0.5% gel to anogenital warts for 3 days, then withhold for 4 days; repeat cycle up to 4 times. Apply 0.5% solution or gel to external genital warts every 12 hr in the morning and evening for 3 days, then withhold for 4 days; repeat cycle up to 4 times
pyrethrum extract and piperonyl butoxide RID, End Lice, Tegrin-LT	To treat head, pubic, and body lice	Apply to dry hair or affected body area. Massage through all hairy areas until hair is wet. Leave on hair for 10 min; then wash with warm water and soap or shampoo. Repeat in 7 to 10 days.
tacrolimus Protopic	To treat moderate to severe atopic dermatitis in patients unresponsive to other therapies	Apply thin layer to affected areas b.i.d., rubbing in gently and completely. Continue for 1 wk after signs and symptoms have disappeared.

Selected Antivirals

Antivirals are used for viral infections, such as influenza, human immunodeficiency virus (HIV), herpes simplex virus (HSV) I and II, herpes zoster, and cytomegalovirus (CMV) infections.

The following chart lists the generic and trade names, indications, and usual adult dosages for some commonly used antivirals. Although you must individualize your care for a patient who receives an antiviral, be sure to include these general interventions in your plan of care:

•Avoid administering HIV drugs all at once.
•If patient takes an antacid, administer it 1 hour before or 2 hours after an antiviral because ant-acids may reduce antiviral absorption.
•Monitor hepatic enzyme levels to detect elevations and help prevent hepatotoxicity.
•Monitor BUN and serum creatinine levels to detect signs of impaired renal function.
•Monitor I.V. injection site for pain or phlebitis, which may result from the high pH of reconstituted solutions.
•Assess immunosuppressed patient for opportunistic infections during antiviral therapy.
•Inform female patient that oral contraceptives may be ineffective when taken with HIV drugs. Suggest alternate contraceptive methods.

GENERIC AND TRADE NAMES	INDICATIONS	USUAL ADULT DOSAGES
Antivirals used for HIV infection		
abacavir sulfate Ziagen	To treat HIV infection	300 mg P.O. b.i.d. or 600 mg P.O. once daily
abacavir sulfate and lamivudine Epzicom	To treat HIV-1 infection	600 mg abacavir and 300 mg lamivudine (1 tablet) P.O. daily
abacavir sulfate, lamivudine, and zidovudine Trizivir	To treat HIV infection	300 mg abacavir, 150 mg lamivudine, and 300 mg zidovudine (1 tablet) b.i.d.
atazanavir sulfate Reyataz	To treat HIV infection in patients not previously treated	400 mg P.O. daily
	To treat HIV infection in patients previously treated	300 mg P.O. daily with ritonavir 100 mg P.O. daily
darunavir Prezista	To treat HIV infection	600 mg P.O. b.i.d. with ritonavir 100 mg P.O. b.i.d.
delavirdine Rescriptor	To treat HIV infection	400 mg P.O. t.i.d.
efavirenz Sustiva	To treat HIV infection	600 mg P.O. daily
emtricitabine Emtriva	To treat HIV infection	200 mg daily (capsules) or 240 mg daily (oral solution)
enfuvirtide Fuzeon	To treat HIV infection	90 mg b.i.d. SubQ

(continued)

Selected Antivirals (continued)

GENERIC AND TRADE NAMES	INDICATIONS	USUAL ADULT DOSAGES
Antivirals used for HIV infection *(continued)*		
etravirine Intelence	To treat HIV-1 infection	200 mg P.O. b.i.d.
fosamprenavir calcium Lexiva	To treat HIV infection in patients who don't take ritonavir	1,400 mg b.i.d.
	To treat HIV infection in patients who take ritonavir but don't take a protease inhibitor	1,400 mg once daily or 700 mg b.i.d.
	To treat HIV infection in patients who take ritonavir and a protease inhibitor	700 mg b.i.d.
indinavir Crixivan	To treat HIV infection	800 mg P.O. every 8 hr.
lamivudine (3TC, lamivudine triphosphate) Epivir	To treat HIV infection in patients who weigh 50 kg (110 lb) or more	150 mg P.O. b.i.d. or 300 mg once daily
	To treat HIV infection in patients who weigh less than 50 kg	2 mg/kg P.O. b.i.d.
lamivudine and zidovudine (3TC/AZT, 3TC/ZDV) Combivir	To treat HIV infection in patients who weigh 50 kg or more	150 mg of lamivudine and 300 mg of zidovudine P.O. b.i.d.
lopinavir and ritonavir Kaletra	To treat HIV infection in patients who weigh more than 40 kg (88 lb) and don't take nevirapine or efavirenz	400 mg lopinavir and 100 mg ritonavir b.i.d.
	As adjunct to treat HIV infection in patients who weigh more than 50 kg and take nevirapine or efavirenz	533 mg lopinavir and 133 mg ritonavir b.i.d.
	To treat HIV infection in patients with no previous treatment	800 mg lopinavir and 200 mg ritonavir daily
maraviroc Selzentry	To treat HIV infection	150 mg P.O. b.i.d. with CYP3A inhibitor; 600 mg P.O. b.i.d. with CYP3A inducers; 300 mg P.O. b.i.d. with all other drugs
nelfinavir Viracept	To treat HIV infection	750 mg P.O. t.i.d.
nelfinavir mesylate Viracept	To treat HIV infection	1,250 mg b.i.d. or 750 mg t.i.d.

Selected Antivirals (continued)

GENERIC AND TRADE NAMES	INDICATIONS	USUAL ADULT DOSAGES
Antivirals used for HIV infection (continued)		
nevirapine Viramune	To treat HIV infection	200 mg P.O. daily
raltegravir Isentress	To treat HIV-1 infection	400 mg P.O. b.i.d. 800 mg P.O. b.i.d. during rifampin therapy
ritonavir Norvir	To treat HIV infection	600 mg P.O. b.i.d.
saquinavir Fortovase, Invirase	To treat HIV infection	1,200 mg P.O. t.i.d. (Fortovase) or 1,000 mg (Invirase or Fortovase) and 100 mg ritonavir b.i.d.
stavudine Zerit, Zerit XR	To treat HIV infection in patients who weigh 60 kg or more	40 mg P.O. every 12 hr (Zerit) or 100 mg P.O. daily (Zerit XR).
	To treat HIV infection in patients who weigh less than 60 kg	30 mg P.O. every 12 hr (Zerit) or 75 mg P.O. daily (Zerit XR).
tenofovir Viread	To treat HIV infection	300 mg P.O. daily
tenofovir and emtricitabine Truvada	To treat HIV-1 infection	300 mg tenofovir and 200 mg emtricitabine (1 tablet) P.O. daily
tipranavir Aptivus	To treat HIV infection	500 mg tipranavir and 200 mg ritonavir P.O. b.i.d.
zidovudine (AZT, ZDV) Apo-Zidovudine (CAN), Novo-AZT (CAN), Retrovir	To treat HIV infection	100 mg P.O. every 4 hr while awake, up to 600 mg/day; or 1 to 2 mg/kg I.V. over 1 hr every 4 hr, up to 6 times/day or 6 mg/kg/day.
	To prevent maternal-fetal HIV transmission	100 mg P.O. 5 times daily after 14 wk of pregnancy and continued until labor. During labor and delivery, 2 mg/kg I.V. over 1 hr followed by continuous infusion of 1 mg/kg/hr until umbilical cord clamped. Starting within 12 hr after birth, neonate given 2 mg/kg P.O. every 6 hr for 6 wk.

(continued)

Selected Antivirals (continued)

GENERIC AND TRADE NAMES	INDICATIONS	USUAL ADULT DOSAGES
Antivirals used for herpes virus infection		
acyclovir Zovirax	To treat HSV encephalitis	10 mg/kg I.V. over 1 hr every 8 hr for 21 days.
	To treat HSV genitalis	200 mg P.O. every 4 hr while awake, up to 5 times/day, for 10 days.
	To treat herpes zoster infection	800 mg P.O. every 4 hr while awake, up to 5 times/day, for 7 to 10 days; or 10 mg/kg I.V. over 1 hr every 8 hr for 7 days.
famciclovir Famvir	To treat HSV genitalis	125 mg P.O. b.i.d. for 5 days.
	To treat herpes zoster infection	500 mg P.O. every 8 hr for 7 days.
foscarnet Foscavir	To treat acyclovir-resistant HSV I and II infections	40 mg/kg I.V. every hr every 8 to 12 hr for 2 to 3 wk or until healed.
idoxuridine Herplex Liquifilm, Stoxil	To treat HSV keratitis	1 cm applied to conjunctiva every 4 hr while awake, up to 5 times/day; or 1 gtt of 0.1% solution every hr during daytime and every 2 hr during nighttime for 7 to 10 days.
penciclovir Denavir	To treat HSV labialis	1% cream applied to lips every 2 hr while awake for 4 days.
valacyclovir Valtrex	To treat HSV genitalis	1 g P.O. b.i.d. for 10 days for initial episode; 500 mg P.O. b.i.d. for 3 days for recurrent episodes.
	To suppress recurrent HSV genitalis	1 g P.O. daily; or, 500 mg P.O. daily for patients with a history of nine or fewer recurrences/year or who have HIV.
	To reduce transmission of genital herpes	500 mg daily for source partner with a history of nine or fewer recurrences/year
	To treat herpes zoster infection	1 g P.O. t.i.d. for 7 days.
	To treat herpes labialis (cold sores)	2 g P.O. b.i.d. for 1 day taken 12 hr apart.

Selected Antivirals (continued)

GENERIC AND TRADE NAMES	INDICATIONS	USUAL ADULT DOSAGES
Antivirals used for herpes virus infections (continued)		
vidarabine Vira-A	To treat acute viral conjunctivitis and recurrent epithelial keratitis caused by HSV infection	1.25 cm applied to conjunctiva every 3 hr until re-epithelialized; then 1.25 cm b.i.d. for 7 days.
Antivirals used for CMV infections		
cidofovir Vistide	To treat CMV retinitis	5 mg/kg I.V. over 1 hr every wk for 2 wk.
foscarnet FoscaviR	To treat CMV infection	*Induction:* 90 mg/kg I.V. over 1.5 to 2 hr every 12 hr; or, 60 mg/kg I.V. over 1 hr every 8 hr for 2 to 3 wk. *Maintenance:* 90 to 120 mg/kg I.V. over 2 hr every 24 hr
ganciclovir Cytovene	To treat CMV infection	5 mg/kg I.V. over 1 hr every 12 hr for 14 to 21 days. *Maintenance:* 1,000 mg P.O. t.i.d.
valganciclovir hydrochloride Valcyte	To treat CMV retinitis	900 mg P.O. b.i.d. for 21 days. Then 900 mg P.O. daily
	To prevent CMV infection in high-risk kidney, heart, and kidney-pancreas transplant patients	900 mg P.O. daily, starting within 10 days of transplantation and continuing until 100 days after transplantation
Antivirals used for influenza infections		
oseltamivir phosphate Tamiflu	To treat uncomplicated, acute infections caused by influenza virus A or B in adults who have had symptoms for no more than 2 days	75 mg P.O. b.i.d. for 5 days, starting within 2 days after symptoms begin. *Maximum:* 75 mg b.i.d. for 5 days.
	To prevent influenza following close contact with infected individual	75 mg P.O. daily for 7 days; start within 2 days of exposure
	To prevent influenza during a community outbreak	75 mg P.O. daily during period of potential exposure
zanamivir Relenza	To treat infections caused by influenza virus A or B	2 inhalations (10 mg) every 12 hr for 5 days.

(continued)

Selected Antivirals (continued)

GENERIC AND TRADE NAMES	INDICATIONS	USUAL ADULT DOSAGES
Antivirals used for hepatitis B infection		
adefovir dipivoxil Hepsera	To treat chronic hepatitis B	10 mg P.O. daily For patients with creatinine clearance of 20 to 49 ml/min, dosage interval changed to every 48 hr; for 10 to 19 ml/min, dosage interval changed to every 72 hr; for patients receiving hemodialysis, drug given every 7 days following dialysis.
lamivudine Epivir HBV	To treat chronic hepatitis B	100 mg P.O. daily
Antivirals used for hepatitis C infection		
ribavirin Copegus, Rebetol, Ribasphere	To treat chronic hepatitis C in combination with interferon alfa-2b in patients who weigh more than 75 kg (165 lb)	400 mg in the morning and 600 mg in the evening daily
	To treat chronic hepatitis C in combination with interferon alfa-2b in patients who weigh 75 kg (165 lb) or less	600 mg b.i.d.
	To treat chronic hepatitis C in combination with peginterferon alfa-2b	400 mg b.i.d.
	To treat chronic hepatitis C in combination with interferon alfa-2a in patients with compensated liver disease who have never received interferon alfa	400 to 600 mg b.i.d.

Antineoplastic Drugs

Antineoplastic drugs have become the standard of treatment for most types of cancer today. Most of these drugs work by inhibiting cell proliferation, thereby leading to cell death. They're most effective at killing cells that are actively dividing. Cell-specific antineoplastics exert their actions during one or more phases of the cell cycle. S-phase antineoplastics interfere with deoxyribonucleic acid (DNA) synthesis; M-phase drugs interfere with the formation of microtubules and disrupt mitosis. Most antineoplastics impair DNA in one of the following four ways:
•preventing separation of DNA strands
•inhibiting DNA repair
•mimicking DNA bases
•disrupting the triplicate codons or producing oxygen free radicals that damage the DNA.

Antineoplastic drugs are cytotoxic, which means that they affect both neoplastic cells and normal cells. As a result, they may cause serious and sometimes life-threatening adverse reactions. Antineoplastics are most harmful to normal cells that exhibit rapid activity and growth, such as bone marrow tissue, the epithelium of the GI mucosa, and hair follicles. When they suppress bone marrow activity, the patient may develop leukopenia, thrombocytopenia, or anemia. When the drugs affect the GI mucosa, the patient may experience nausea, vomiting, anorexia, bowel dysfunction, and mucosal ulcerations. When they affect the hair follicles, the result is hair loss (alopecia), one of the most common adverse reactions; although not life-threatening, hair loss can be emotionally traumatic for patients, especially women.

Drug Classification
Antineoplastics are classified according to their mechanism of action.
•*Alkylating drugs,* the first drugs developed to fight cancer, are most effective against slow-growing tumors. These agents can damage tissue at the injection site and produce systemic toxicity. They can damage cells during all stages of growth, causing mitotic arrest. Because their actions are not limited to neoplastic cells, they also cause myelosuppression, a predictable adverse reaction. They can also result in secondary tumor de-

velopment, even years after the initial therapy.
•*Antibiotic antineoplastics* originated from a genus of fungus-like bacteria called *Streptomyces.* Their classification is based on their origin, not on mechanism of action, toxicity, pharmacokinetics, or varying clinical indications. Many of these drugs bind to specific bases and block DNA synthesis to interfere with cell replication.
•*Antimetabolites* are cell-cycle-specific drugs that act by preventing synthesis of nucleotides or inhibiting enzymes by mimicking nucleotides. These drugs are often more effective when used in combination.
•*Antimitotic antineoplastics* disrupt the formation of microtubule structures within the cell during mitosis. This breakdown of microtubule production stops the formation of the mitotic spindle, inhibiting cellular reproduction.
•*Biological response modifiers* alter tumor-host metabolic and immunologic relationships.
•*Antineoplastic enzymes* interfere with the breakdown of extracellular asparagine, an endogenous enzyme that leukemic cells depend on for their survival. The rapid depletion of asparagine eventually kills leukemic cells by fragmenting them into membrane-bound particles that are eliminated by phagocytosis.
•*Hormonal antineoplastics* act as agonists to inhibit tumor cell growth or as antagonists to compete with endogenous growth-promoting hormones. Steroid hormones form specific receptor complexes that bind to certain nuclear proteins necessary for DNA transcription.
•*Miscellaneous antineoplastics* act in a variety of ways, such as by destroying microtubules that are essential for tumor cell structure before mitosis and by inhibiting topoisomerase, the enzyme that affects the degree of supercoiling in DNA by cutting one or both strands. This inhibition causes DNA strands to break and synthesizes toxic compounds that inhibit DNA strand repair.

The following chart lists the generic and common trade names of common antineoplastic drugs, which are grouped according to mechanism of action. It also includes FDA-approved indications and the usual adult dosage for each drug.

Antineoplastic Drugs (continued)

GENERIC AND TRADE NAMES	INDICATIONS	USUAL ADULT DOSAGES
Alkylating drugs		
bendamustine Treanda	To treat chronic lymphocytic leukemia (CLL)	100 mg/m^2 I.V. infused over 30 minutes on days 1 and 2 of a 28-day cycle for up to 6 cycles
	To treat indolent B-cell non-Hodgkin's lymphoma (NHL) that has progressed within 6 months of treatment with rituximab or a rituximab-containing regimen	120 mg/m^2 I.V. infused over 60 minutes on days 1 and 2 of a 21-day cycle for up to 8 cycles
busulfan Busulfex, Myleran	To provide palliative treatment of chronic myelocytic leukemia (CML)	*Initial:* 0.06 mg/kg P.O. daily until WBC count falls below 15,000/mm^3. *Usual:* 4 to 8 mg P.O. daily (but may range from 1 to 12 mg P.O. daily) *Maintenance:* 1 to 3 mg daily. During remission, treatment resumed when WBC count reaches 50,000/mm^3
	To prepare for hematopoietic progenitor cell transplantation for CML	0.8 mg/kg I.V. over 2 hr every 6 hr for 4 days for a total of 16 doses as an adjunct with cyclophosphamide
carmustine (BCNU) BiCNU, Gliadel Wafer	To treat primary brain tumors and glioblastoma multiforme	Up to 8 implants per surgical procedure
	To treat primary brain tumors, Hodgkin's disease, non-Hodgkin's lymphoma, and multiple myeloma	150 to 200 mg/m^2 by slow I.V. infusion as a single dose every 6 to 8 wk; or 75 to 100 mg/m^2 by slow I.V. infusion daily for 2 days every 6 wk
chlorambucil Leukeran	To provide palliative treatment of chronic lymphocytic leukemia, Hodgkin's disease, malignant lymphomas (including lymphosarcoma and giant follicular lymphoma), and non-Hodgkin's lymphoma	0.1 to 0.2 mg/kg/day as a single dose or in divided doses for 3 to 6 wk. *Usual:* 4 to 10 mg/day as a single dose or in divided doses for 3 to 6 wk
cyclophosphamide Cytoxan, Neosar, Procytox (CAN)	To treat acute lymphocytic leukemia, acute nonlymphocytic leukemia, chronic lymphocytic leukemia, chronic myelocytic leukemia, breast cancer, epithelial ovarian cancer, Hodgkin's disease, multiple myeloma, neuroblastoma, non-Hodgkin's lymphoma, and retinoblastoma	1 to 5 mg/kg P.O. daily; or 40 to 50 mg/kg I.V. in divided doses over 2 to 5 days; or 10 to 15 mg/kg I.V. every 7 to 10 days; or 3 to 5 mg/kg I.V. 2 times/wk; or 1.5 to 3 mg/kg I.V. daily

Antineoplastic Drugs (continued)

GENERIC AND TRADE NAMES	INDICATIONS	USUAL ADULT DOSAGES
Alkylating drugs (continued)		
ifosfamide IFEX	To treat germ cell testicular tumors	1.2 g/m^2/day by I.V. infusion for 5 days every 3 wk
lomustine (CCNU) CeeNU	To treat primary brain tumors and Hodgkin's disease	100 to 130 mg/m^2 P.O. as a single dose every 6 wk
mechlorethamine hydrochloride (nitrogen mustard) Mustargen	To treat bronchiogenic carcinoma, CML, Hodgkin's disease, lymphosarcoma, and mycosis fungoides	0.4 mg/kg I.V. as a single dose or in divided doses over 2 to 4 days
	To treat malignant pericardial, peritoneal, or pleural effusions	0.4 mg/kg (peritoneal or pleural effusion); 0.2 mg/kg into affected cavity (pericardial effusion)
melphalan (L-phenylalanine mustard) Alkeran **melphalan hydrochloride** Alkeran	To treat multiple myeloma	0.15 mg/kg P.O. daily for 7 days; then 0.05 mg/kg daily after 3 wk of no drug. Or, 0.1 to 0.15 mg/kg daily for 2 to 3 wk or 0.25 mg/kg for 4 days; then 2 to 4 mg daily after 2 to 4 wk of no drug 16 mg/m^2/I.V. over 15 min every 2 wk for 4 doses, then at 4 wk
	To treat epithelial ovarian cancer	0.2 mg/kg P.O. daily for 5 days, repeated every 4 to 5 wk
streptozocin Zanosar	To treat islet cell or pancreatic carcinoma	500 mg/m^2 I.V. for 5 days every 6 wk, or 1,000 mg/m^2 I.V. every wk for 2 wk
temozolomide Temodar	To treat astrocytoma	150 mg/m^2 P.O. daily for first 5 days of 28-day cycle, followed by 200 mg/m^2, if tolerated, P.O. daily for first 5 days of subsequent 28-day cycles
thiotepa (TESPA, triethylenethiophosphoramide, TSPA) Thioplex	To treat malignant pericardial or pleural effusions	0.6 to 0.8 mg/kg into affected cavity
	To treat breast cancer, epithelial ovarian cancer, and Hodgkin's disease	0.3 to 0.4 mg/kg I.V. every 1 to 4 wk, or 0.2 mg/kg for 4 to 5 days every 2 to 3 wk
	To treat bladder tumors	30 to 60 mg mixed in 30 to 60 ml of normal saline, instilled into bladder every wk for 4 wk

(continued)

Antineoplastic Drugs (continued)

GENERIC AND TRADE NAMES	INDICATIONS	USUAL ADULT DOSAGES
Antibiotic antineoplastics		
bleomycin sulfate Blenoxane	To treat non-Hodgkin's lymphoma, squamous cell carcinoma, and testicular cancer	0.25 to 0.5 unit/kg or 10 to 20 units/m^2 1 to 2 times/wk I.V., I.M., or SubQ; or 0.25 unit/kg or 15 units/m^2 daily by I.V. infusion over 24 hr
	To treat Hodgkin's disease	0.25 to 0.5 unit/kg I.V., I.M., or SubQ, or 10 to 20 units/m^2 1 to 2 times/wk
	To treat malignant pleural effusions	60 units intrapleural single bolus dissolved in 50–100 ml of normal saline
	To treat squamous cell carcinoma of the cervix, head and neck, penis, or vulva	30 to 60 units by arterial infusion over 1 to 24 hr
cisplatin Platinol, Platinol-AQ	To treat bladder cancer	50 to 70 mg/m^2 by I.V. infusion as a single dose every 3 to 4 wk with other agents
	To treat advanced ovarian cancer	75 to 100 mg/m^2 by I.V. infusion as a single dose every 21 days with paclitaxel
	To treat testicular cancer	20 mg/m^2 by I.V. infusion daily for 5 days with bleomycin and etoposide; repeated every 3 wk for two or more cycles
dactinomycin (actinomycin-D) Cosmegen	To treat Ewing's sarcoma, gestational trophoblastic or Wilms' tumors, rhabdomyosarcoma, sarcoma botryoides, and testicular cancer or tumors	0.15 to 500 mcg/kg/day I.V. daily for 5 days; may repeat after 3 wk
	To treat Ewing's sarcoma and sarcoma botryoides	0.05 mg/kg for lower extremity or pelvis; 0.035 mg/kg for upper extremity as an isolation-perfusion
daunorubicin hydrochloride Cerubidine	To treat acute lymphocytic leukemia	45 mg/m^2 daily for first 3 days of a 32-day course of vincristine, prednisone, and asparaginase combination therapy
	To treat acute nonlymphocytic leukemia	45 mg/m^2 daily for first 3 days of first course of cytarabine combination therapy and first 2 days of second course of cytarabine combination therapy

Antineoplastic Drugs (continued)

GENERIC AND TRADE NAMES	INDICATIONS	USUAL ADULT DOSAGES
Antibiotic antineoplastics (continued)		
daunorubicin, liposomal DaunoXome	To treat AIDS-related Kaposi's sarcoma	40 mg/m² I.V. over 60 min every 2 wk
doxorubicin hydrochloride Adriamycin PFS, Adriamycin RDF, Rubex	To treat acute lymphocytic leukemia, acute nonlymphocytic leukemia; bladder, breast, gastric, epithelial ovarian, or thyroid cancer; Hodgkin's disease; neuroblastoma or Wilms' tumor; non-Hodgkin's lymphoma; small-cell lung carcinoma; and soft-tissue sarcoma or osteosarcoma	60 to 75 mg/m² I.V. as single dose every 21 days; or 25 to 30 mg/m² I.V. daily for 2 to 3 days every 3 to 4 wk; or 20 mg/m² every wk; or 40 to 60 mg/m² every 21 to 28 days in combination with other chemotherapeutic drugs
doxorubicin, liposomal Caelyx (CAN), Doxil	To treat AIDS-related Kaposi's sarcoma	20 mg/m² I.V. over 30 min every 3 wk as tolerated
epirubicin hydrochloride Ellence	To treat breast cancer	100 to 120 mg/m² by I.V. infusion over 3 to 5 min via a free-flowing I.V. solution as a single dose on day 1 or in divided doses on days 1 and 8, repeated every 3 to 4 wk for 6 cycles in combination with other chemotherapy agents
idarubicin hydrochloride Idamycin	To treat acute nonlymphocytic leukemia	12 mg/m²/day I.V. over 10 to 15 min for 3 days in combination with cytarabine therapy
mitomycin (mitomycin-C) Mutamycin	To treat gastric or pancreatic cancer	20 mg/m² as a single dose every 6 to 8 wk
pentostatin (2′-deoxycoformycin) Nipent	To treat hairy cell leukemia	4 mg/m² by rapid I.V. injection or diluted for infusion over 20 to 30 min as a single dose every other wk
plicamycin (mithramycin) Mithracin	To treat testicular cancer	0.025 to 0.03 mg/kg I.V. daily over 4 to 6 hr for 8 to 10 days
	To treat hypercalcemia and hypercalciuria	0.015 to 0.025 mg/kg I.V. daily over 4 to 6 hr for 3 to 4 days; may repeat dose every wk as needed

(continued)

Antineoplastic Drugs (continued)

GENERIC AND TRADE NAMES	INDICATIONS	USUAL ADULT DOSAGES
Antibiotic antineoplastics (continued)		
valrubicin Valstar	To treat bladder cancer	800 mg every wk for 6 wk into affected cavity
Antimetabolites		
capecitabine Xeloda	To treat locally advanced or metastatic breast cancer or metastatic colorectal cancer	1,250 mg/m² P.O. after a meal b.i.d. (morning and evening) for 2 wk, followed by 1-wk rest period; dose repeated in 3-wk cycles
cladribine (2-CdA, 2-chlorodeoxy-adenosine) Leustatin	To treat hairy cell leukemia	0.1 mg/kg/day by continuous I.V. infusion for 7 days
cytarabine (ARA-C, cytosine arabinoside) Cytosar, Cytosar-U	To treat acute nonlympho-cytic leukemia	Initially, 100 mg/m²/day by continuous I.V. infusion for 7 days, alone or with other agents; or 100 mg/m² I.V. every 12 hr on days 1 to 7, then consult manufacturer's literature for specific dosing; or high-dose therapy of 2 to 3 g/m² I.V over 1 to 3 hr for 2 to 6 days, then consult manufacturer's literature for specific dosing
	To treat meningeal leukemia	30 mg/m² intrathecally as a single dose every 4 days
	To prevent or treat acute lymphocytic leukemia and chronic myelocytic leukemia	Consult manufacturer's literature for specific dosage.
cytarabine, liposomal DepoCyt, Depro Tech	To treat lymphomatous meningitis	Initially, 50 mg intrathecally (intraventricular or lumbar puncture) over 1 to 5 min every 14 days for two doses (wk 1 and 3); then 50 mg intrathecally every 14 days for three doses (wk 5, 7, and 9), followed by 1 50-mg dose at wk 13; then 50 mg intrathecally every 28 days for four doses (wk 17, 21, 25, and 29) in combination with dexamethasone 4 mg P.O. or I.V. b.i.d. for 5 days
floxuridine (fluorodeoxyuridine) FUDR	To treat colorectal or hepatic cancer	0.1 to 0.6 mg/kg/day by continuous intra-arterial infusion for 14 to 21 days, followed by 2 wk of no drug; dose repeated in 5-wk cycles

Antineoplastic Drugs (continued)

GENERIC AND TRADE NAMES	INDICATIONS	USUAL ADULT DOSAGES
Antimetabolites (continued)		
fludarabine phosphate Fludara	To treat chronic lymphocytic leukemia	25 mg/m^2 I.V. infused over 30 min for 5 days; cycle repeated every 28 days
fluorouracil (5-fluorouracil, 5-FU) Adrucil, Carac, Efudex, Fluoroplex	To treat colorectal, breast, gastric, or pancreatic cancer	7 to 12 mg/kg/day I.V. for 4 days, followed by no drug for 3 days, then 7 to 10 mg/kg every 3 to 4 days for total of 2 wk; or 12 mg/kg/day for 4 days, followed by 1 day of no drug, then 6 mg/kg every other day for 4 or 5 days, for total of 12 days; thereafter, 7 to 12 mg/kg/day I.V. every 7 to 10 days
	To treat multiple actinic (solar) keratoses	0.5% cream (face, anterior scalp), 1% cream (head, neck, chest), or 2% to 5% cream (hands) applied to skin once or twice daily to cover lesions
	To treat superficial basal cell carcinoma	5% cream applied to skin b.i.d. for up to 12 wk to cover lesions
hydroxyurea Droxia, Hydrea	To treat epithelial ovarian cancer	60 to 80 mg/kg P.O. as a single dose every 3 days alone or with radiation therapy; or 20 to 30 mg/kg P.O. daily
	To treat resistant chronic myelocytic leukemia	20 to 30 mg/kg P.O. once daily or in divided doses b.i.d.
mercaptopurine (6-mercaptopurine, 6-MP) Purinethol	To treat acute lymphocytic leukemia or acute nonlymphocytic leukemia	2.5 mg/kg/day or 80 to 100 mg/m^2/day (rounded to nearest 25 mg) P.O. as a single dose or in divided doses, followed by 1.5 to 2.5 mg/kg/day P.O. or 50 to 100 mg/m^2/day
methotrexate (amethopterin) methotrexate sodium	To treat chorioadenoma destruens, choriocarcinoma, or hydatidiform mole	15 to 30 mg/day P.O. or I.M. for 5 days; repeat three to five times with 2 to 3 wk between courses
	To treat acute lymphocytic leukemia or meningeal leukemia	Initially, 3.3 mg/m^2/day P.O., I.M., or I.V. in combination with prednisone or other drug; as maintenance dose, 30 mg/m^2/ wk P.O. or I.M. in two divided doses or 2.5 mg/kg I.V. every 14 days
	To treat Burkitt's lymphoma (stage I or II)	10 to 25 mg/day P.O. for 4 to 8 days, followed by no drug for 7 to 10 days; course repeated as needed

(continued)

Antineoplastic Drugs (continued)

GENERIC AND TRADE NAMES	INDICATIONS	USUAL ADULT DOSAGES
Antimetabolites *(continued)*		
methotrexate (amethopterin) methotrexate sodium *(continued)*	To treat Burkitt's lymphoma (stage III)	Same as for stage I or II in combination with other drug
	To treat lymphosarcoma (stage III)	0.625 to 2.5 mg/kg/day P.O.
	To treat mycosis fungoides	2.5 to 10 mg/day P.O. for weeks or months; or 50 mg I.M. every wk or 25 mg I.M. 2 times/wk
	To treat osteosarcoma	12 g/m^2 by I.V. infusion over 12 hr, followed by leucovorin rescue on weeks 4, 5, 6, 7, 11, 12, 15, 16, 29, 30, 44, and 45 after surgery in combination with bleomycin, cisplatin, cyclophosphamide, dactinomycin, and doxorubicin
	To treat breast or head and neck cancer and non–small-cell or small-cell lung carcinoma	Consult manufacturer's literature for specific dosing.
pemetrexed disodium Alimta	To treat nonsquamous non–small-cell lung cancer	500 mg/m^2 I.V. on day 1 of each 21-day cycle
	To treat nonsquamous non–small-cell lung cancer in combination with cisplatin; to treat mesothelioma in combination with cisplatin	500 mg/m^2 I.V. followed in 30 minutes by 75 mg/m2 of cisplatin I.V. on day 1 of each 21-day cycle
thioguanine (6-TG, 6-thioguanine) Lanvis (CAN), Tabloid	To treat acute nonlymphocytic leukemia	2 mg/kg/day P.O. as a single dose; if no improvement after 4 wk, increase to 3 mg/kg/day
Antimitotic antineoplastics		
docetaxel Taxotere	To treat breast cancer	60 to 100 mg/m^2 by I.V. infusion over 1 hr every 3 wk
	To treat non–small-cell lung carcinoma	75 mg/m^2 by I.V. infusion over 1 hr every 3 wk

Antineoplastic Drugs (continued)

GENERIC AND TRADE NAMES	INDICATIONS	USUAL ADULT DOSAGES
Antimitotic antineoplastics *(continued)*		
paclitaxel Taxol	To treat ovarian cancer	135 or 175 mg/m^2 by I.V. infusion over 3 or 24 hr every 21 days
	To treat breast cancer	175 mg/m^2 by I.V. infusion over 3 or 24 hr every 21 days
	To treat AIDS-related Kaposi's sarcoma	135 mg/m^2 by I.V. infusion over 3 or 24 hr every 21 days; or 100 mg/m^2 by I.V. infusion over 3 or 24 hr every 14 days
	To treat non–small-cell lung carcinoma	135 mg/m^2 by I.V. infusion over 3 or 24 hr, followed by cisplatin 75 mg/m^2 I.V. every 21 days
vinblastine sulfate (VLB) Velban, Velbe (CAN)	To treat breast cancer, Hodgkin's disease, lymphomas, Kaposi's sarcoma, Letterer-Siwe disease, mycosis fungoides, non-Hodgkin's lymphoma, testicular cancer, and trophoblastic gestational tumors	0.15 to 0.2 mg/kg I.V. every wk
vincristine sulfate (VCR) Oncovin, Vincasar PFS	To treat acute lymphocytic leukemia, Hodgkin's disease, lymphomas, non-Hodgkin's lymphoma, rhabdomyosarcoma, and Wilms' tumor	0.01 to 0.03 mg/kg I.V.; or 0.4 to 1.4 mg/m^2 I.V. every wk as a single dose (maximum of 2 mg)
vinorelbine tartrate Navelbine	To treat non–small-cell lung carcinoma	30 mg/m^2 I.V. over 6 to 10 min every wk alone, or 25 mg/m^2 I.V. over 6 to 10 min every wk with cisplatin 100 mg/m^2 every 4 wk
Biological response modifiers		
aldesleukin (IL-2, interleukin-2) Proleukin	To treat renal cancer and metastatic melanoma	600,000 international units/kg by I.V. infusion over 15 min every 8 hr for 14 doses; then 9 days of no drug; then repeat course of 14 doses for total of 28 doses
alemtuzumab Campath	To treat B-cell chronic lymphocytic leukemia	*Initial:* 3 mg I.V. over 2 hr daily, then increased to 10 mg I.V. over 2 hr daily. *Maintenance:* 30 mg I.V. over 2 hr 3 times/wk on alternate days for up to 12 wk

(continued)

Antineoplastic Drugs (continued)

GENERIC AND TRADE NAMES	INDICATIONS	USUAL ADULT DOSAGES
Biological response modifiers *(continued)*		
bacillus Calmette-Guérin (BCG) live, Connaught strain ImmuCyst (CAN), TheraCys	To treat bladder cancer	81 mg (reconstitute and dilute with 50 ml preservative-free normal saline solution to 53 ml or less) instilled into bladder for 1 to 2 hr every wk for 6 wk, then as a single-dose treatment at 3, 6, 12, 18, and 24 mo
bacillus Calmette-Guérin, Tice strain TICE BCG		50 mg (reconstitute and dilute with 50 ml preservative-free normal saline to 50 ml or less) for 1 to 2 hr every 6 wk; may repeat once, followed by single-dose treatment every mo for 6 to 12 mo
denileukin diftitox Ontak	To treat cutaneous or T-cell lymphomas, including mycosis fungoides	9 or 18 mcg/kg/day by I.V. infusion over at least 15 min for 5 days; repeated every 21 days
interferon alfa-2a, recombinant Roferon-A	To treat hairy cell leukemia	3 million units/day I.M. or SubQ for 16 to 24 wk, followed by 3 million units 3 times/wk
	To treat AIDS-related Kaposi's sarcoma	36 million units/day I.M. or SubQ for 10 to 12 wk; or 3 million units/day I.M. or SubQ on days 1 to 3, 9 million units/day on days 4 to 6, 18 million units/day on days 7 to 9, and 36 million units/day from day 10 until completion of 10- to 12-wk course; maintenance dose, 36 million units 3 times/wk
interferon alfa-2b, recombinant Intron A	To treat hairy cell leukemia	2 million units/m^2 I.M. or SubQ 3 times/wk
	To treat AIDS-related Kaposi's sarcoma	30 million units/m^2 I.M. or SubQ 3 times/wk
	To treat malignant melanoma	20 million units/m^2 by I.V. infusion on days 1 to 5 every wk for 4 wk, followed by 10 million units/m^2 I.V. 3 times/wk for 48 wk
levamisole hydrochloride Ergamisol	To treat colorectal cancer	Beginning 7 to 30 days after surgery, 50 mg P.O. every 8 hr for 3 days, repeated every 2 wk for 1 yr, with fluorouracil 450 mg/m^2 by rapid I.V. infusion daily for 5 days, starting with first or second course of levamisole

Antineoplastic Drugs (continued)

GENERIC AND TRADE NAMES	INDICATIONS	USUAL ADULT DOSAGES
Antineoplastic enzymes		
asparaginase Colaspase, Elspar, Kidrolase (CAN)	To treat acute lymphocytic leukemia	200 international units/kg I.V. daily for 28 days
pegaspargase (PEG-L-asparaginase) Oncaspar	To treat acute lymphoblastic leukemia in adults up to age 21	2,500 international uits/m^2 I.M. or I.V. every 14 days
Hormonal antineoplastics		
anastrozole Arimidex	To treat breast cancer	1 mg P.O. daily
bicalutamide Casodex	To treat prostate cancer	50 mg P.O. daily in combination with luteinizing hormone-releasing hormone (LHRH) analog or after surgical castration
estramustine phosphate sodium Emcyt	To treat prostate cancer To treat postmenopausal breast cancer	14 mg/kg/day P.O. in three or four divided doses 1 hr before or 2 hr after meals
exemestane Aromasin	To treat prostate cancer	25 mg P.O. daily after a meal
flutamide Euflex (CAN), Eulexin	To treat breast cancer	250 mg P.O. every 8 hr
goserelin acetate Zoladex, Zoladex LA, Zoladex 3-Month	To treat prostate cancer	3.6 mg SubQ into upper abdominal wall every 28 days 3.6 mg SubQ into upper abdominal wall every 28 days; or 10.8 mg SubQ every 12 wk
letrozole Femara	To treat breast cancer	2.5 mg P.O. daily
leuprolide acetate Lupron, Lupron Depot, Lupron Depot-3 Month, Lupron Depot-4 Month, Viadur	To treat prostate cancer	*Regular:* 1 mg SubQ daily; *depot:* 7.5 mg every mo; or 22.5 mg every 3 mo; or 30 mg every 4 mo; *implant:* 1 every 12 mo

(continued)

Antineoplastic Drugs (continued)

GENERIC AND TRADE NAMES	INDICATIONS	USUAL ADULT DOSAGES
Hormonal antineoplastics *(continued)*		
medroxyprogesterone acetate Depo-Provera	To treat endometrial or renal cancer	400 to 1,000 mg every wk until stable, then 400 mg or more every mo
megestrol acetate Megace	To treat breast cancer	160 mg/day P.O. daily or in divided doses
	To treat endometrial cancer	40 to 320 mg P.O. daily or in divided doses
nilutamide Anandron (CAN), Nilandron	To treat prostate cancer	300 mg P.O. daily up to 30 days, then 150 mg P.O. daily
tamoxifen citrate Apo-Tamox (CAN), Gen-Tamoxifen (CAN), Nolvadex, Nolvadex-D (CAN), NovoTamoxifen (CAN), Tamofen (CAN), Tamone (CAN)	To prevent breast cancer or reduce the risk of invasive breast cancer in women with ductal carcinoma in situ	20 mg P.O. daily for 5 yr
	To treat breast cancer (node-negative or node-positive)	10 mg P.O. b.i.d. or, in metastatic disease, 10 to 20 mg P.O. b.i.d.
testolactone Teslac	To treat breast cancer	250 mg P.O. q.i.d.
toremifene citrate Fareston	To treat breast cancer	60 mg P.O. daily
triptorelin pamoate Trelstar LA	To provide palliative treatment of advanced prostate cancer	11.25 mg I.M. every 84 days
Miscellaneous antineoplastics		
arsenic trioxide Trisenox	To treat acute promyelocytic leukemia	*Induction:* 0.15 mg/kg I.V. daily until bone marrow remission occurs. *Maximum:* 60 doses. *Consolidation:* Begun 3 to 6 wk after completion of induction, 0.15 mg/kg I.V. daily for 25 doses over up to 5 wk

Antineoplastic Drugs (continued)

GENERIC AND TRADE NAMES	INDICATIONS	USUAL ADULT DOSAGES
Miscellaneous antineoplastics *(continued)*		
bexarotene Targretin	To treat cutaneous manifestations of cutaneous T-cell lymphoma	300 mg/m^2 P.O. daily with food; after 8 wk, may increase to 400 mg/m^2 P.O. daily with food, as needed and tolerated.
Targretin Gel	To treat cutaneous lesions of cutaneous T-cell lymphoma (stages IA and IB)	Apply generously to cover only lesions every other day on 1st wk; then increased as tolerated to once daily on 2nd wk, b.i.d. on 3rd wk, t.i.d on 4th wk and, finally, q.i.d. on 5th wk
dacarbazine DTIC (CAN), DTIC-Dome	To treat Hodgkin's disease	150 mg/m^2 I.V. daily for 5 days in combination with other drugs; may repeat every 28 days; or 375 mg/m^2 every 15 days in combination with other drugs
	To treat malignant melanoma	2 to 4.5 mg/kg I.V. daily for 10 days and every 28 days thereafter; or 250 mg/m^2 I.V. daily for 5 days and every 21 days thereafter
etoposide (VP-16) Toposar, VePesid	To treat germ-cell testicular tumors	50 to 100 mg/m^2/day I.V. on days 1 through 5 up to 100 mg/m^2 I.V. on days 1, 3, and 5; course repeated every 3 to 4 wk
	To treat small-cell lung carcinoma	35 mg/m^2/day I.V. for 4 days up to 50 mg/m^2/day I.V. for 5 days, repeated every 3 to 4 wk; or 70 mg/m^2/day P.O. for 4 days to 100 mg/m^2/day P.O. for 5 days, repeated every 3 to 4 wk
etoposide phosphate Etopophos	To treat germ-cell testicular tumors	50 to 100 mg/m^2/day by I.V. infusion on days 1 through 5 to 100 mg/m^2/day by I.V. infusion on days 1, 3, and 5; course repeated every 3 to 4 wk
	To treat small-cell lung carcinoma	35 mg/m^2/day by I.V. infusion for 4 days to 50 mg/m^2/day by I.V. infusion for 5 days, repeated every 3 to 4 wk
gemcitabine hydrochloride Gemzar	To treat non–small-cell lung carcinoma	1,000 mg/m^2 by I.V. infusion over 30 min daily on days 1, 8, and 15 every 28 days with cisplatin 100 mg/m^2 on day 28; or 1,250 mg/m^2 I.V. daily on days 1 and 8 every 21 days in combination with cisplatin 100 mg/m^2 I.V. on day 21

(continued)

Antineoplastic Drugs (continued)

GENERIC AND TRADE NAMES	INDICATIONS	USUAL ADULT DOSAGES
Miscellaneous antineoplastics *(continued)*		
gemcitabine hydrochloride Gemzar *(continued)*	To treat pancreatic cancer	1,000 mg/m² by I.V. infusion over 30 min every wk for 7 wk, followed by 1 wk of no drug; then every wk for 3 wk, followed by 1 wk of no drug; then repeat 4-wk cycle
gemtuzumab ozogamicin Mylotarg	To treat first relapse in patients with CD33-positive acute myeloid leukemia who are age 60 or over and who are not candidates for cytotoxic therapy	9 mg/m² by I.V. infusion over 2 hr; repeated in 14 days
imatinib mesylate Gleevec	To treat chronic myeloid leukemia in accelerated phase or blast crisis, or in chronic phase after failure of interferon-alpha therapy	400 mg P.O. daily with food (chronic phase) or 600 mg P.O. daily with food (accelerated phase or blast crisis); after 3 mo, dosage may be increased to 600 mg P.O. daily (chronic phase) or 800 mg P.O. given in 2 divided doses of 400 mg (accelerated phase or blast crisis), as needed.
	To treat GI stromal tumor	400 mg/day P.O. or 600 mg/day P.O.
irinotecan hydrochloride Camptosar	To treat colorectal cancer	125 mg/m² I.V. over 90 min every wk for 4 wk, followed by 2 wk of no drug, then repeat 6-wk cycle; or 350 mg/m² I.V. over 90 min every 3 wk
iressa Gefitinib	To treat refractory metastatic non–small-cell lung cancer	250 mg P.O. daily
ixabepilone Ixempra	To treat metastatic or locally advanced breast cancer in combination with capecitabine after failure with an anthracycline and a taxane; to treat metastatic or locally advanced breast cancer after failure with an anthracycline, a taxane, and capecitabine	40 mg/m² I.V. infused over 3 hr every 3 wk
mitotane (o,p′-DDD) Lysodren	To treat adrenocortical carcinoma	2 to 6 g P.O. daily in divided doses t.i.d. or q.i.d.

Antineoplastic Drugs (continued)

GENERIC AND TRADE NAMES	INDICATIONS	USUAL ADULT DOSAGES
Miscellaneous antineoplastics *(continued)*		
mitoxantrone hydrochloride Novantrone	To treat hormone-refractory prostate cancer	12 to 14 mg/m^2 I.V. every 21 days
	To treat acute nonlymphocytic leukemia	12 mg/m^2 by I.V. infusion in free-flowing normal saline or D$_5$W solution over 3 min daily on days 1 to 3, with cytarabine 100 mg/m^2/day by continuous I.V. infusion on days 1 to 7; if response is inadequate, second course at same dosage may be given
nilotinib Tasigna	To treat Philadelphia chromosome positive chronic myelogenous leukemia	400 mg P.O. b.i.d.
porfimer sodium Photofrin	To treat esophageal cancer and non–small-cell lung carcinoma	2 mg/kg I.V. over 3 to 5 min, followed by laser light illumination and debridement of tumor; may repeat course every 30 days three times
procarbazine hydrochloride Matulane, Natulan (CAN)	To treat Hodgkin's disease	2 to 4 mg/kg/day (rounded to nearest 50 mg) P.O. as a single dose or in divided doses for 1 wk, followed by 4 to 6 mg/kg/day until leukopenia, thrombocytopenia, or maximal response
rituximab Rituxan	To treat non-Hodgkin's lymphomas	375 mg/m^2/day by I.V. infusion every wk for 4 or 8 doses
sorafenib Nexavar	To treat unresectable hepatocellular carcinoma; to treat advanced renal cell carcinoma	400 mg P.O. b.i.d.
topotecan hydrochloride Hycamtin	To treat ovarian cancer and small-cell lung carcinoma	1.5 mg/m^2 I.V. over 30 min daily for 5 days, repeated every 21 days
trastuzumab Herceptin	To treat breast cancer	4 mg/kg I.V. over 90 min, followed by 2 mg/kg I.V. over 30 min every 7 days
velcade Bortezomib	To treat multiple myeloma	1.3 mg/m^2 I.V. bolus on days 1, 4, 8, and 11 for 2 wk, followed by rest on days 12–21; then repeat 3-wk cycle

Selected Antihypertensive Combinations

Antihypertensive drugs are used along with lifestyle changes to manage hypertension. Antihypertensive combinations, which commonly include one or two antihypertensives and a diuretic, are used to simplify patients' drug regimens and, in some cases, to enhance drug actions.

The chart below lists the generic and trade names; functional classes; usual adult dosages;

ANTIHYPERTENSIVE COMBINATION TRADE NAMES	ANTIHYPERTENSIVE GENERIC NAMES	DIURETIC GENERIC NAMES
Aldoril-15	methyldopa 250 mg	hydrochlorothiazide (HCTZ) 15 mg
Aldoril-25	methyldopa 250 mg	HCTZ 25 mg
Aldoril D30	methyldopa 500 mg	HCTZ 30 mg
Aldoril D50	methyldopa 500 mg	HCTZ 50 mg
Apresazide 25/25	hydralazine hydrochloride (HCl) 25 mg	HCTZ 25 mg
Apresazide 50/50	hydralazine HCl 50 mg	HCTZ 50 mg
Apresazide 100/50	hydralazine HCl 100 mg	HCTZ 50 mg
Atacand HCT 16/12.5	candesartan cilexetil 16 mg	HCTZ 12.5 mg
Atacand HCT 32/12.5	candesartan cilexetil 32 mg	HCTZ 12.5 mg
Avalide-150	irbesartan 150 mg	HCTZ 12.5 mg
Avalide-300	irbesartan 300 mg	HCTZ 12.5 mg
Benicar HCT 20/12.5	olmesartan medoxomil 20 mg	HCTZ 12.5 mg
Benicar HCT 40/12.5	olmesartan medoxomil 40 mg	HCTZ 12.5 mg
Benicar HCT 40/25	olmesartan medoxomil 40 mg	HCTZ 25 mg
Capozide 25/15	captopril 25 mg	HCTZ 15 mg
Capozide 25/25	captopril 25 mg	HCTZ 25 mg
Capozide 50/15	captopril 50 mg	HCTZ 15 mg
Capozide 50/25	captopril 50 mg	HCTZ 25 mg
Diovan HCT 80/12.5	valsartan 80 mg	HCTZ 12.5 mg
Diovan HCT 160/12.5	valsartan 160 mg	HCTZ 12.5 mg
Diovan HCT 160/25	valsartan 160 mg	HCTZ 25 mg
Diovan HCT 320/12.5	valsartan 320 mg	HCTZ 12.5 mg
Diovan HCT 320/25	valsartan 320 mg	HCTZ 25 mg
Dyazide	triamterene 37.5 mg	HCTZ 25 mg
Exforge	amlodipine 5 mg valsartan 160 mg	None

and onset, peak, and duration for commonly used antihypertensive combinations. For information about the mechanisms of action, interactions, adverse reactions, and nursing considerations related to antihypertensive combinations, review the entries for the specific antihypertensives and diuretics that they contain.

FUNCTIONAL CLASSES	USUAL ADULT DOSAGES	ONSET, PEAK, AND DURATION
Centrally acting antiadrenergic and thiazide diuretic	1 tab b.i.d or t.i.d 1 tab b.i.d. 1 tab daily 1 tab daily	**Onset:** Unknown **Peak:** 4 to 6 hr **Duration:** 12 to 24 hr
Peripherally acting arterial dilator and thiazide diuretic	1 cap once or twice daily 1 cap once or twice daily 1 cap once or twice daily	**Onset:** 20 to 30 min **Peak:** 1 to 2 hr **Duration:** 2 to 4 hr
Angiotensin II receptor antagonist and thiazide diuretic	1 tab once or twice daily 1 tab daily	**Onset:** 1 to 2 wk **Peak:** Within 4 wk **Duration:** Unknown
ACE inhibitor and thiazide diuretic	1 tab daily 1 tab daily	**Onset:** Unknown **Peak:** Unknown **Duration:** Unknown
Angiotensin II receptor antagonist and thiazide diuretic	1 tab daily 1 tab daily 1 tab daily	**Onset:** Unknown **Peak:** Unknown **Duration:** Unknown
ACE inhibitor and thiazide diuretic	1 tab daily to t.i.d. 1 tab once or twice daily 1 tab once daily to t.i.d. 1 tab once or twice daily	**Onset:** 15 to 60 min **Peak:** 60 to 90 min **Duration:** 6 to 12 hr
ACE inhibitor and thiazide diuretic	1 or 2 tabs daily 1 tab daily 1 tab daily 1 tab daily 1 tab daily	**Onset:** 2 hr **Peak:** 6 hr **Duration:** 24 hr
Potassium-sparing diuretic and thiazide diuretic	1 or 2 caps or tabs daily	**Onset:** 2 to 4 hr **Peak:** 1 day **Duration:** 7 to 9 hr
Dihydropyridine and tetrazole	1 or 2 tabs daily	**Onset:** Unknown **Peak:** 6 to 12 hr **Duration:** 24 hr

(continued)

Selected Antihypertensive Combinations (continued)

ANTIHYPERTENSIVE COMBINATION TRADE NAMES	ANTIHYPERTENSIVE GENERIC NAMES	DIURETIC GENERIC NAMES
Hyzaar 50/12.5	losartan potassium 50 mg	HCTZ 12.5 mg
Hyzaar 100/25	losartan potassium 100 mg	HCTZ 25 mg
Inderide 80/25	propranolol HCl 80 mg	HCTZ 25 mg
Inderide LA 80/50	propranolol HCl 80 mg	HCTZ 50 mg
Inderide LA 120/50	propranolol HCl 120 mg	HCTZ 50 mg
Inderide LA 160/50	propranolol HCl 160 mg	HCTZ 50 mg
Lopressor HCT 50/25	metoprolol tartrate 50 mg	HCTZ 25 mg
Lopressor HCT 100/25	metoprolol tartrate 100 mg	HCTZ 25 mg
Lopressor HCT 100/50	metoprolol tartrate 100 mg	HCTZ 50 mg
Lotensin HCT 5/6.25	benazepril HCl 5 mg	HCTZ 6.25 mg
Lotensin HCT 10/12.5	benazepril HCl 10 mg	HCTZ 12.5 mg
Lotensin HCT 20/12.5	benazepril HCl 20 mg	HCTZ 12.5 mg
Lotensin HCT 20/25	benazepril HCl 20 mg	HCTZ 25 mg
Lotrel 2.5/10	amlodipine 2.5 mg, benazepril HCl 10 mg	none
Lotrel 5/10	amlodipine 5 mg, benazepril HCl 10 mg	none
Lotrel 5/20	amlodipine 5 mg, benazepril HCl 10 mg	none
Lotrel 10/20	amlodipine 10 mg, benazepril HCl 20 mg	none
Maxzide 37.5/25	triamterene 37.5 mg	HCTZ 25 mg
Maxzide 75/50	triamterene 75 mg	HCTZ 50 mg
Micardis HCT 40/12.5	telmisartan 40 mg	HCTZ 12.5 mg
Micardis HCT 80/12.5	telmisartan 80 mg	HCTZ 12.5 mg
Moduretic	amiloride 5 mg	HCTZ 50 mg
Prinzide 10/12.5	lisinopril 10 mg	HCTZ 12.5 mg
Prinzide 20/12.5	lisinopril 20 mg	HCTZ 12.5 mg
Prinzide 20/25	lisinopril 20 mg	HCTZ 25 mg
Tekturna	aliskiren 150 mg	HCTZ 12.5 mg

FUNCTIONAL CLASSES	USUAL ADULT DOSAGES	ONSET, PEAK, AND DURATION
ACE inhibitor and thiazide diuretic	1 or 2 tabs daily 1 tab daily	**Onset:** Unknown **Peak:** 6 hr **Duration:** 24 hr or more
Beta blocker and thiazide diuretic	1 or 2 tabs b.i.d. 1 cap daily 1 cap daily 1 cap daily	**Onset:** Unknown **Peak:** 1 to 1.5 hr **Duration:** Unknown
Beta blocker and thiazide diuretic	1 or 2 tabs daily or 1 tab b.i.d. 1 or 2 tabs daily or 1 tab b.i.d. 1 or 2 tabs daily or 1 tab b.i.d.	**Onset:** 1 hr **Peak:** 1 to 2 hr **Duration:** Unknown
ACE inhibitor and thiazide diuretic	1 tab daily 1 tab daily 1 tab daily 1 tab daily	**Onset:** 1 hr **Peak:** 2 to 4 hr **Duration:** 24 hr
ACE inhibitor and calcium channel blocker	1 or 2 caps daily 1 cap daily 1 cap daily 1 cap daily	**Onset:** Unknown **Peak:** Unknown **Duration:** 24 hr
Potassium-sparing diuretic and thiazide diuretic	1 tab daily 1 tab daily	**Onset:** 2 to 4 hr **Peak:** 1 day **Duration:** 7 to 9 hr
Angiotensin II receptor antagonist and thiazide diuretic	1 tab once or twice daily 1 tab once or twice daily	**Onset:** Within 3 hr **Peak:** In 4 wk **Duration:** Several days to 1 wk
Potassium-sparing diuretic and thiazide diuretic	1 or 2 tabs daily	**Onset:** 2 hr **Peak:** 6 to 10 hr **Duration:** 24 hr
ACE inhibitor and thiazide diuretic	1 or 2 tabs daily 1 or 2 tabs daily 1 or 2 tabs daily	**Onset:** 1 hr **Peak:** 6 hr **Duration:** 24 hr
Hemifumarate salt and thiazide diuretic	1 tab daily	**Onset:** Unknown **Peak:** 1 to 3 hr **Duration:** Unknown

(continued)

Selected Antihypertensive Combinations (continued)

ANTIHYPERTENSIVE COMBINATION TRADE NAMES	ANTIHYPERTENSIVE GENERIC NAMES	DIURETIC GENERIC NAMES
Timolide 10/25	timolol maleate 10 mg	HCTZ 25 mg
Uniretic 15/25	moexipril HCl 15 mg	HCTZ 25 mg
Vaseretic 5/12.5	enalapril maleate 5 mg	HCTZ 12.5 mg
Vaseretic 10/25	enalapril maleate 10 mg	HCTZ 25 mg
Zestoretic 10/12.5	lisinopril 10 mg	HCTZ 12.5 mg
Zestoretic 20/12.5	lisinopril 20 mg	HCTZ 12.5 mg
Zestoretic 20/25	lisinopril 20 mg	HCTZ 25 mg
Ziac 2.5/6.25	bisoprolol fumarate 2.5 mg	HCTZ 6.25 mg
Ziac 5/6.25	bisoprolol fumarate 5 mg	HCTZ 6.25 mg
Ziac 10/6.25	bisoprolol fumarate 10 mg	HCTZ 6.25 mg

FUNCTIONAL CLASSES	USUAL ADULT DOSAGES	ONSET, PEAK, AND DURATION
Beta blocker and thiazide diuretic	1 tab b.i.d. or 2 tabs daily	**Onset:** Unknown **Peak:** 1 to 2 hr **Duration:** Unknown
Potassium-sparing diuretic and thiazide diuretic	1 or 2 tabs daily	**Onset:** 1 hr **Peak:** 3 to 6 hr **Duration:** 24 hr
ACE inhibitor and thiazide diuretic	1 tab once or twice daily 1 tab once or twice daily	**Onset:** 1 hr **Peak:** 4 to 6 hr **Duration:** 24 hr
ACE inhibitor and thiazide diuretic	1 or 2 tabs daily 1 or 2 tabs daily 1 or 2 tabs daily	**Onset:** 1 hr **Peak:** 6 hr **Duration:** 24 hr
Beta blocker and thiazide diuretic	1 or 2 tabs daily 1 or 2 tabs daily 1 or 2 tabs daily	**Onset:** Unknown **Peak:** Unknown **Duration:** Unknown

Recommended Immunizations Up To Age 6

This schedule shows basic recommendations from the Centers for Disease Control and Prevention (CDC) for routine administration of vaccines for **children up to age 6,** except for certain high-risk groups. Doses not given at the recommended age can be given at a later visit, as prescribed. Combination vaccines may be used when one component is indicated and the others are FDA-approved for that dose in the series and not contraindicated. Report any significant adverse reactions to the Vaccine Adverse Event Reporting System. For compete information, consult the CDC at www.cdc.gov or the appropriate Advisory Committee on Immunization Practices statement.

	Birth	1 mo	2 mo	4 mo	6 mo	12 mo	15 mo	18 mo	19–23 mo	2–3 yr	4–6 yr
Hepatitis B[1]	1st dose	2nd dose			3rd dose						
Rotavirus[2]			1st dose	2nd dose	Final dose						
Diphtheria, tetanus, pertussis[3]			1st dose	2nd, 3rd doses 4 wk apart			4th dose				Final dose
Haemophilus influenzae **type b**[4]			1st yearly								
Pneumococcal[5]			1st dose	2nd dose	3rd dose	Final dose					
Inactivated poliovirus			1st dose	2nd dose	Last 2 doses, 4 wk apart						
Influenza[6]					1st yearly dose						
Measles, mumps, rubella[7]						1st dose					2nd dose
Varicella[8]						1st dose					2nd dose
Hepatitis A[9]						1st dose					

Range of recommended ages

See official CDC guidelines for administering all vaccines.

1. Hepatitis B (HepB)
•Give monovalent HepB to all newborns before hospital discharge in keeping with mother's hepatitis surface antigen status. Give second dose at 1 to 2 months and final dose after 24 weeks. Some children may receive a fourth dose.

2. Rotavirus (Rota)
•Minimum age 6 weeks. Give first dose at 6 to 12 weeks. Don't start series after age 12 weeks, and give final dose by age 32 weeks.

3. Diphtheria and tetanus toxoids and acellular pertussis vaccine (DTap)
•Minimum age 6 weeks. Fourth dose may be given as early as 12 months if 6 months have passed since last dose. Give final dose in series at age 4 to 6 years.

4. *Haemophilus influenzae* type b conjugate vaccine (Hib)
•Minimum age 6 weeks. If PedvaxHIB or ComVax is given at ages 2 and 4 months, a dose isn't needed at 6 months. Tri-HiBit shouldn't be used for primary vaccination but can be used as booster.

5. Pneumococcal vaccine (PCV)
•Minimum age 6 weeks for pneumococcal conjugate vaccine (PCV), 2 years for pneumococcal polysaccharide vaccine.

6. Influenza vaccine
•Minimum age 6 months for trivalent inactivated vaccine, 5 years for live attenuated vaccine. All children ages 6 months to 59 months and close contacts of childern under 59 months should receive vaccine.

7. Measles, mumps, and rubella vaccine (MMR)
•Minimum age 12 months. Give second dose at age 4 to 6.

8. Varicella vaccine (Vari)
•Minimum age 12 months. Give second dose at age 4 to 6. May be given before age 4 to 6 as long as 3 or more months have elapsed since first dose and both doses are given after age 12 months.

9. Hepatitis A vaccine (HepA)
•Minimum age 12 months. Recommended for all children age 1 year. Give 2 doses at least 6 months apart.

Recommended Immunizations for Ages 7 to 18

This schedule shows basic recommendations from the Centers for Disease Control and Prevention (CDC) for routine administration of vaccines for **children ages 7 to 18,** except for certain high-risk groups. Doses not given at the recommended age can be given at a later visit, as prescribed. Combination vaccines may be used when one component is indicated and the others are FDA-approved for that dose in the series and not contraindicated. Report any significant adverse reactions to the Vaccine Adverse Event Reporting System. For compete information, consult the CDC at www.cdc.gov or the appropriate Advisory Committee on Immunization Practices statement.

	7–10 yr	11–12 yr	13–14 yr	15 yr	16–18 yr
Tetanus, diphtheria, pertussis[1]		1st dose; 2nd in 4 wk	Single Tdap booster if missed earlier		
Human papillomavirus[2]		3-dose series	As needed if missed earlier		
Meningococcal[3]		Single dose	High school or college entry if missed earlier		
Hepatitis B[4]	2- or 3-dose series if not given previously				
Inactivated poliovirus[5]	4 doses if not given by age 4				
Measles, mumps, rubella[6]	2 doses 4 wk apart if not given previously				
Varicella[7]	2 doses if not given previously				

Range of recommended ages   Catch-up immunizations

1. Tetanus and diphtheria toxoids and acellular pertussis vaccine (Tdap)
•Minimum age 10 for Boostrix and 11 for Adacel.
•Give at age 11 to 12 if patient has completed recommended DTP/DTaP vaccination series and hasn't received tetanus and diphtheria booster.
•Teens ages 13 to 18 who completed the DTP/DTaP series but missed the Td/Tdap booster at age 11 to 12 should have a single dose of Tdap.

2. Human papillomavirus vaccine (HPV)
•Give first HPV dose to girls age 11 to 12.
•Give second dose 2 months after first dose and third dose 6 months after first dose.

3. Meningococcal conjugate vaccine (MCV4)
•Give at age 11 to 12. If missed, give at entry to high school or at entry to college if living in dormitory.
•Certain high-risk groups receive meningococcal polysaccharide vaccine (MPSV4).

4. Hepatitis B vaccine (HepB)
•Give 3-dose series to anyone not previously vaccinated.
•A 2-dose series of Recombinvax HB is available for children ages 11 to 15.

5. Inactivated poliovirus vaccine (IPV)
•Minimum age 6 weeks.
•For children who received an all-IPV or all-oral poliovirus (OPV) series, a fourth dose isn't needed if third dose was given at age 4 or older.
•If patient received both OPV and IPV as part of a series, give a total of 4 doses, regardless of child's current age.

6. Measles, mumps, and rubella vaccine (MMR)
•Minimum age 12 months.
•If not previously vaccinated, give 2 doses of MMR with 4 weeks or more between doses.

7. Varicella vaccine
•Minimum age 12 months.
•Give 2 doses to anyone without evidence of immunity.
•For patients under age 13, give 2 doses at least 3 months apart. Don't repeat second dose if given 28 days or more after first dose.
•For patients age 13 or over, give 2 doses at least 4 weeks apart.

Recommended Catch-Up Immunizations

The vaccination schedule on this page shows basic catch-up recommendations and minimum intervals between doses from the Centers for Disease Control and Prevention (CDC) for **children ages 4 months to 6 years** whose vaccinations have been delayed. The schedule on the facing page shows similar information for **children ages 7 to 18 years.** Use the section appropriate for the child's age. A vaccine schedule need not be restarted, regardless of the time that has elapsed between doses.

	Children ages 4 months to 6 years				
	Minimum age for dose 1	**Minimum interval between doses**			
		Dose 1 to dose 2	**Dose 2 to dose 3**	**Dose 3 to dose 4**	**Dose 4 to dose 5**
Hepatitis B	Birth	4 wk	8 wk (and 16 wk after first dose)		
Rotavirus	6 wk	4 wk	4 wk		
Diphtheria, tetanus, pertussis	6 wk	4 wk	4 wk	6 mo	6 mo
Haemophilus influenzae **type b**	6 wk	4 wk if first dose at less than 12 mo 8 wk (as final dose) if first dose at 12 to 14 mo No more doses needed if first dose at over 15 mo	4 wk if current age less than 12 mo 8 wk (as final dose) if current age 12 or over and second dose at less than 15 mo No more doses needed if last dose at 15 mo or over	8 wk (as final dose)*	
Pneumococcal	6 wk	4 wk if first dose at less than 12 mo and current age under 24 mo 8 wk (as final dose) if first dose at 12 mo or more or current age 24 mo or over No more doses needed if first dose at over 24 mo	4 wk if first current age less than 12 mo 8 wk (as final dose) if current age 12 or over No more doses needed if last dose at 24 mo or over	8 wk (as final dose)*	
Inactivated poliovirus	6 wk	4 wk	4 wk	4 wk	
Measles, mumps, rubella	12 mo	4 wk			
Varicella	12 mo	3 mo			
Hepatitis A	12 mo	6 mo			

* This dose only needed for children ages 12 mo to 5 yr who received 3 doses before age 12 mo.

Report any significant adverse reactions to the Vaccine Adverse Event Reporting System. For compete information, consult the CDC at www.cdc.gov or the appropriate Advisory Committee on Immunization Practices statement.

	Minimum age for dose 1	Children ages 7 to18 years			
		Minimum interval between doses			
		Dose 1 to dose 2	Dose 2 to dose 3	Dose 3 to dose 4	Dose 4 to dose 5
Tetanus, diphtheria/ Tetanus, diphtheria, pertussis	7 yr	4 wk	8 wk if first dose at under 12 mo 6 mo if first dose at 12 mo or over	6 mo if first dose at under 12 mo	
Human papillomavirus	9 yr	4 wk	12 wk*		
Hepatitis A	12 mo	6 mo			
Hepatitis B	Birth	4 wk	8 wk (and 16 wk after first dose)		
Inactivated poliovirus	6 wk	4 wk	4 wk	4 wk	
Measles, mumps, rubella	12 mo	4 wk			
Varicella	12 mo	4 wk if first dose at age 13 or over 3 mo if first dose at under age 13			

* Dose 3 no earlier than 24 wk after dose 2.

Recommended Immunizations for Adults

This schedule shows basic recommendations from the Centers for Disease Control and Prevention (CDC) for routine administration of vaccines for **adults**. These recommendations must be supplemented with information available from the CDC at www.cdc.gov. Combination vaccines may be used when one component is indicated and the others are FDA-approved for that dose in the series and not contraindicated. Report any significant adverse reactions to the Vaccine Adverse Event Reporting System. For full information, visit www.cdc.gov or consult the appropriate Advisory Committee on Immunization Practices statement.

	19–49 yr	50–64 yr	65 yr and over
Tetanus, diphtheria, pertussis	1-dose booster every 10 yr		
Human papillomavirus	3 doses*		
Measles, mumps, rubella	2 doses; 2nd in 4–8 wk	1 dose	
Varicella	2 doses; 2nd in 4–8 wk	2 doses; 2nd in 4–8 wk	
Influenza	1 dose yearly	1 dose yearly	
Pneumococcal	1–2 doses		1 dose
Hepatitis A	2 doses; 2nd dose 6–12 mo or 6–18 mo after 1st dose		
Hepatitis B	3 doses; 2nd dose 1–2 mo after 1st dose and 3rd dose 4–6 mo after 1st dose		
Meningococcal	1 or more doses		
Zoster			1 dose age 60 or older

For all of appropriate age if no immunity   Only if warranted by increased risk

* 2nd dose in 2 mo and 3rd dose 6 mo after 1st dose.

Recommended Immunizations in Health Conditions

This schedule shows basic recommendations from the Centers for Disease Control and Prevention (CDC) for administration of vaccines for **adults with certain health conditions**. These recommendations must be supplemented with information available from the CDC at www.cdc.gov. Combination vaccines may be used when one component is indicated and the others are FDA-approved for that dose in the series and not contraindicated. Report any significant adverse reactions to the Vaccine Adverse Event Reporting System. For full information, visit www.cdc.gov or consult the appropriate Advisory Committee on Immunization Practices statement.

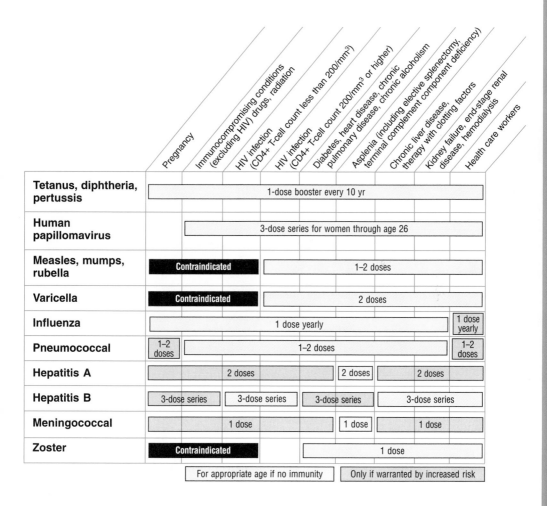

	Pregnancy	Immunocompromising conditions (excluding HIV) drugs, radiation	HIV infection (CD4+ T-cell count less than 200/mm³)	HIV infection (CD4+ T-cell count 200/mm³ or higher)	Diabetes, heart disease, chronic pulmonary disease, chronic alcoholism	Asplenia (including elective splenectomy; terminal complement component deficiency)	Chronic liver disease; therapy with clotting factors	Kidney failure, end-stage renal disease, hemodialysis	Health care workers
Tetanus, diphtheria, pertussis	1-dose booster every 10 yr								
Human papillomavirus		3-dose series for women through age 26							
Measles, mumps, rubella	Contraindicated			1–2 doses					
Varicella	Contraindicated			2 doses					
Influenza	1 dose yearly								1 dose yearly
Pneumococcal	1–2 doses	1–2 doses							1–2 doses
Hepatitis A	2 doses				2 doses		2 doses		
Hepatitis B	3-dose series	3-dose series			3-dose series		3-dose series		
Meningococcal	1 dose				1 dose		1 dose		
Zoster	Contraindicated			1 dose					

For appropriate age if no immunity   Only if warranted by increased risk

Vitamins

As you know, an adequate daily intake of vitamins is essential to vital bodily functions, such as embryonic development (vitamin A), regulation of serum calcium and phosphate (vitamin D), and blood clotting (vitamin K).

Vitamins are classified as one of two types: fat soluble (vitamins A, D, E, and K) and water soluble (vitamin C and all forms of vitamin B). Fat-soluble vitamins can accumulate in body tissue over time; when excessive amounts are ingested through diet or sup-

GENERIC AND TRADE NAMES	RECOMMENDED DAILY INTAKE
vitamin A **(retinol)** Aquasol A	**Adult men and boys over age 10.** 1,000 mcg/day. **Adult women and girls over age 10.** 800 mcg/day. **Pregnant women.** 800 mcg/day. (900 mcg/day [CAN].) **Breast-feeding women.** 1,200 to 1,300 mcg/day. (1,200 mcg/day [CAN].) **Children ages 7 to 10.** 700 mcg/day. (700 to 800 mcg/day [CAN].) **Children ages 4 to 7.** 500 mcg/day. **Neonates and children to age 4.** 375 to 400 mcg/day. (400 mcg/day [CAN].)
vitamin B₁ **(thiamine hydrochloride)** Betaxin (CAN), Bewon (CAN), Biamine	**Adult men and boys over age 10.** 1.2 to 1.5 mg/day. (0.8 to 1.3 mg/day [CAN].) **Adult women and girls over age 10.** 1 to 1.1 mg/day. (0.8 to 0.9 mg/day [CAN].) **Pregnant women.** 1.5 mg/day. (0.9 to 1 mg/day. [CAN].) **Breast-feeding women.** 1.6 mg/day. (1 to 1.2 mg/day [CAN].)

plementation, severe and life-threatening toxicity can develop. Water-soluble vitamins don't accumulate in the body; they are excreted daily so that toxicity is not usually a concern with excessive intake.

The following chart lists the generic and trade names of fat-soluble and water-soluble vitamins, the recommended daily intake to prevent vitamin deficiency, dosages when deficiency occurs, other indications and dosages for vitamin therapy, and guidelines for parenteral administration of vitamins.

OTHER INDICATIONS AND DOSAGES

To treat vitamin A deficiency
CAPSULES, ORAL SOLUTION, TABLETS
Adults and adolescents. Dosage individualized based on severity of deficiency, as prescribed.
I.M. INJECTION
Adults and children age 8 and over. 15,000 to 30,000 retinol equivalent (RE)/day (50,000 to 100,000 international units (IU)/day) for 3 days, followed by 15,000 RE/day (50,000 IU/day) for 2 wk.
Children ages 1 to 8. 1,500 to 4,500 RE/day (5,000 to 15,000 IU/day) for 10 days; for severe deficiency, 5,250 to 10,500 RE/day (17,500 to 35,000 IU/day) for 10 days.
Infants to age 1 year. 1,500 to 3,000 RE/day (5,000 to 10,000 IU/day) for 10 days; for severe deficiency, 2,250 to 4,500 RE/day (7,500 to 15,000 IU/day) for 10 days.
I.V. INFUSION
Adults and children. Dosage individualized as part of total parenteral nutrition solution, as prescribed.

To treat xerophthalmia
CAPSULES, ORAL SOLUTION, TABLETS
Children age 1 and over. 60,000 RE (200,000 IU) as a single dose. Dose repeated on day 2 and again in 4 wk.
Children ages 6 months to 1 year. 30,000 RE (100,000 IU) as a single dose. Dose repeated on day 2 and again in 4 wk.

As an adjunct to treat measles
CAPSULES, ORAL SOLUTION, TABLETS
Children age 1 and over. 60,000 RE (200,000 IU) as a single dose when measles are diagnosed.
Children ages 6 months to 1 year. 30,000 RE (100,000 IU) as a single dose when measles are diagnosed.

To treat vitamin B$_1$ deficiency (beriberi)
ELIXIR, TABLETS
Adults. 5 to 10 mg t.i.d.
Children and infants. 10 mg/day.
I.V. OR I.M. INJECTION
Adults. *Initial:* 5 to 100 mg every 8 hr, switched to P.O. vitamin B$_1$ therapy as soon as possible and continued for total of 1 mo.

PARENTERAL ADMINISTRATION GUIDELINES

•Be aware that anaphylaxis and death have occurred after I.V. administration of vitamin A; I.V. administration is restricted to special solutions, such as in total parenteral nutrition solution. Typically, parenteral administration of vitamin A is by I.M. injection.
•Take precautions to protect vitamin A solution from exposure to light because it's light sensitive.

•Be aware that I.V. administration of vitamin B$_1$ has caused severe and life-threatening reactions, especially with repeat administration. Monitor patient closely for angioedema, GI bleeding, respiratory distress, throat tightness, urticaria, vascular collapse, and weakness during and after administration.

(continued)

Vitamins (continued)

GENERIC AND TRADE NAMES	RECOMMENDED DAILY INTAKE
vitamin B$_1$ *(continued)*	**Children ages 7 to 10.** 1 mg/day. (0.8 to 1 mg/day [CAN].) **Children ages 4 to 7.** 0.9 mg/day. (0.7 mg/day [CAN].) **Children ages 1 to 4.** 0.3 to 0.7 mg/day. (0.3 to 0.6 mg/day [CAN].)
vitamin B$_3$ **(niacin)** Endur-Acin, Nia-Bid, Niac, Niacels, Niacor, Nico-400, Nicobid Tempules, Nicolar, Nicotinex Elixir, Novo-Niacin (CAN), Slo-Niacin	**Adult men and boys age 11 and over.** 15 to 20 mg/day. (14 to 23 mg/day [CAN].) **Adult women and girls age 11 and over.** 13 to 15 mg/day. (14 to 16 mg/day [CAN].) **Pregnant women.** 17 mg/day. (14 to 16 mg/day [CAN].) **Breast-feeding women.** 20 mg/day. (14 to 16 mg/day [CAN].) **Children ages 7 to 11.** 13 mg/day. (14 to 18 mg/day [CAN].) **Children ages 4 to 7.** 12 mg/day. (13 mg/day [CAN].) **Neonates and children to age 4.** 5 to 9 mg/day. (4 to 9 mg/day [CAN].)
vitamin B$_6$ **(pyridoxine hydrochloride)** Beesix, Doxine, Nestrex, Pyri, Rodex, Vita-bee 6	**Adult men and boys age 11 and over.** 1.7 to 2 mg/day. **Adult women and girls age 11 and over.** 1.4 to 1.6 mg/day. **Pregnant women.** 2.2 mg/day. **Breast-feeding women.** 2.1 mg/day. **Children ages 7 to 10.** 1.4 mg/day. **Children ages 4 to 6.** 1.1 mg/day. **Neonates and children to age 3.** 0.3 to 1 mg/day.

OTHER INDICATIONS AND DOSAGES	PARENTERAL ADMINISTRATION GUIDELINES

To treat Wernicke's encephalopathy
I.V. OR I.M. INJECTION
Adults. *Initial:* 100 mg I.V. *Maintenance:* 50 to 100 mg I.V. or I.M. daily until normal recommended daily intake is achieved.

- Rotate sites for I.M. administration of vitamin B_1 to help prevent tenderness and induration that may occur following administration.
- I.M. administration may be painful; use the Z-track method of administration
- Because of incompatibilities, don't add parenteral vitamin B_1 to alkaline or neutral solutions; also, don't mix it with oxidizing and reducing agents, including barbiturates, carbonates, citrates, and copper
- Take precautions to protect vitamin B_1 solution from exposure to light because it's light sensitive.

To treat vitamin B_3 deficiency
E.R. CAPSULES, E.R. TABLETS, ORAL SOLUTION, TABLETS
Adults and children age 11 and over. Dosage individualized based on severity of deficiency, as prescribed. *Maximum:* 6 g/day.
I.V. INJECTION
Adults and children age 11 and over. 25 to 100 mg at least b.i.d.
Children to age 11. Up to 300 mg daily
I.M. INJECTION
Adults and children age 11 and over. 50 to 100 mg at least 5 times/day.
Children to age 11. Dosage individualized based on severity of deficiency.

To treat hyperlipidemia (niacin only)
E.R. CAPSULES, E.R. TABLETS, ORAL SOLUTION, TABLETS
Adults. *Initial:* 1,000 mg t.i.d. Dosage increased by 500 mg/day every 2 to 4 wk, as needed. *Maintenance:* 1 to 2 g t.i.d. *Maximum:* 6 g/day.
DOSAGE ADJUSTMENT To reduce or prevent facial flushing, initial dosage reduced to 100 mg/day (tab) or 500 mg/day (E.R. tab), and then gradually increased to 3 to 4 g/day.

- Be aware that I.V. administration of vitamin B_3 may cause CNS or CV adverse reactions, such as arrhythmias, dizziness, headache, peripheral vasodilation, and syncope. Rate of I.V. administration shouldn't exceed 2 mg/min, regardless of method of I.V. administration.
- Vitamin B_3 must be diluted for I.V. use. For direct injection, dilute to 2 mg/ml; for intermittent or continuous infusion, dilute dose in 500 ml of normal saline or other compatible solution
- Give I.M. injection following routine I.M. administration guidelines. Vitamin B_3 doesn't need to be diluted for I.M. injection.
- Be aware that parenteral administration shouldn't be used to treat hyperlipidemia.

To treat vitamin B_6 deficiency
E.R. CAPSULES, TABLETS
Adults and children. Dosage individualized based on severity of deficiency, as prescribed.
E.R. TABLETS
Adults. Dosage individualized based on severity of deficiency, as prescribed.
I.V. INFUSION
Adults and children. Dosage individualized as part of total parenteral nutrition.

- Be aware that SubQ or I.M. administration of vitamin B_6 may cause injection site burning or stinging. Before giving injection, alert patient that this adverse effect may occur.
- Know that I.V. administration is given as part of a multivitamin solution; follow the guidelines for administering an I.V. multivitamin solution as recommended for the product being used.

(continued)

Vitamins (continued)

GENERIC AND TRADE NAMES	RECOMMENDED DAILY INTAKE
vitamin B$_6$ *(continued)*	**Adult men and boys age 11 and over.** 1.7 to 2 mg/day. **Adult women and girls age 11 and over.** 1.4 to 1.6 mg/day. **Pregnant women.** 2.2 mg/day. **Breast-feeding women.** 2.1 mg/day. **Children ages 7 to 10.** 1.4 mg/day. **Children ages 4 to 6.** 1.1 mg/day. **Neonates and children to age 3.** 0.3 to 1 mg/day.
vitamin B$_9$ (folic acid) Apo-Folic (CAN), Folvite, Novo-Folacid (CAN)	**Adult men and boys age 11 and over.** 150 to 400 mcg/day. (150 to 220 mcg/day [CAN].) **Adult women and girls age 11 and over.** 150 to 400 mcg/day. (145 to 190 mcg/day [CAN].) **Pregnant women.** 400 to 800 mcg/day. (445 to 475 mcg/day [CAN].) **Breast-feeding women.** 260 to 800 mcg/day. (245 to 275 mcg/day [CAN].) **Children ages 7 to 11.** 100 to 400 mcg/day. (125 to 180 mcg/day [CAN].) **Children ages 4 to 7.** 75 to 400 mcg/day. (90 mcg/day [CAN].) **Neonates and children to age 4.** 25 mcg/day. (50 to 80 mcg/day [CAN].)
vitamin B$_{12}$ (cyanocobalamin, hydroxycobalamin)	**Adults age 19 and over.** 2.4 mcg/day. **Pregnant women.** 2.6 mcg/day. **Breast-feeding women.** 2.8 mcg/day. **Adolescents ages 14 to 19.** 2.4 mcg/day. **Children ages 9 to 14.** 1.8 mcg/day. **Children ages 4 to 9.** 1.2 mcg/day. **Children ages 1 to 4.** 0.9 mcg/day. **Infants ages 6 to 12 months.** 0.4 mcg/day. **Neonates and infants to 6 months.** 0.5 mcg/day.

OTHER INDICATIONS AND DOSAGES

To treat pyridoxine dependency syndrome
I.V. OR I.M. INJECTION
Adults and children age 11 and over. 30 to 600 mg daily.
Infants with seizures. *Initial:* 10 to 100 mg, then individualized based on severity of deficiency, as prescribed.

To treat drug-induced pyridoxine deficiency
I.V. OR I.M. INJECTION
Adults and children age 11 and over. 50 to 200 mg/day for 3 wk, then 25 to 100 mg/day, as needed.

To treat vitamin B_9 deficiency
TABLETS
Adults and children. Dosage individualized based on severity of deficiency, as prescribed.
I.V. INFUSION, I.M. OR SUBQ INJECTION
Adults and children. 0.25 to 1 mg daily until hematologic response occurs.

To treat vitamin B_{12} deficiency caused by nutritional intake imbalance (not for use to treat pernicious anemia)
LOZENGES, TABLETS
Adults and children. Dosage individualized based on severity of deficiency, as prescribed.

To treat vitamin B_{12} deficiency caused by pernicious anemia; malabsorption disorders (tropical or nontropical sprue, partial or total gastrectomy, regional enteritis, gastroenterostomy, ileal resection); or malignancies, granulomas, strictures, or anastomoses involving the ileum.
SUBQ INJECTION (CYANOCOBALAMIN)
Adults. *Initial:* 30 mcg daily for 5 to 10 days, then switched to I.M. administration for maintenance therapy.

PARENTERAL ADMINISTRATION GUIDELINES

•Vitamin B_6 may increase AST (SGOT) levels. Be aware that at least one manufacturer warns against I.V. administration of vitamin B_6 to patients with heart disease.
•Take precautions to protect vitamin B_6 solution from exposure to light because it's light sensitive.

•Be aware that some vitamin B_9 solutions contain benzyl alcohol. Don't administer these solutions to neonates or immature infants because of a risk of fatal toxic syndrome, which may include CNS, respiratory, circulatory, and renal impairment and metabolic acidosis.
•Unless ordered otherwise, dilute 5 mg/ml of vitamin B_9 with with 49 ml of sterile water for injection to provide a solution containing 0.1 mg of vitamin/ml.
•Know that parenteral administration may cause anaphylaxis. Parenteral administration should be used only in patients with severe vitamin deficiency or in those with severely impaired GI absorption.
•Be aware that SubQ administration should be injected deeply.
•Take precautions to protect vitamin B_9 solution from exposure to light because it's light sensitive.

•Be aware that parenteral vitamin B_{12} solution is incompatible with many drugs, including ascorbic acid, chlorpromazine hydrochloride, dextrose, heavy metals, phytonadione, prochlorperazine edisylate, warfarin sodium, oxidizing or reducing agents, and alkaline or strongly acidic solutions. Do not administer vitamin with other drugs.
•Know that both cyanocobalamin and hydroxycobalamin may be administered by I.M. injection, but only cyanocobalamin may be administered as an SubQ injection. Be alert to which form is being administered to ensure correct route of administration.

(continued)

Vitamins (continued)

GENERIC AND TRADE NAMES	RECOMMENDED DAILY INTAKE
vitamin B$_{12}$ *(continued)*	**Adults age 19 and over.** 2.4 mcg/day. **Pregnant women.** 2.6 mcg/day. **Breast-feeding women.** 2.8 mcg/day. **Adolescents ages 14 to 19.** 2.4 mcg/day. **Children ages 9 to 14.** 1.8 mcg/day. **Children ages 4 to 9.** 1.2 mcg/day. **Children ages 1 to 4.** 0.9 mcg/day. **Infants ages 6 to 12 months.** 0.4 mcg/day. **Neonates and infants to 6 months.** 0.5 mcg/day.
vitamin C **(ascorbic acid)** Ascorbic Acid, Cecon Drops, Cenolate, Cevi-Bid, Vicks Vitamin C Drops	**Adult men.** 90 mg/day. **Adult women.** 75 mg/day. **Pregnant women age 19 and over.** 85 mg/day. **Breast-feeding women age 19 and over.** 120 mg/day. **Adolescent boys ages 14 to 19.** 75 mg/day. **Adolescent girls ages 14 to 19.** 65 mg/day. **Pregnant girls ages 14 to 19.** 80 mg/day. **Breast-feeding girls ages 14 to 19.** 115 mg/day. **Children ages 9 to 14.** 45 mg/day. **Children ages 4 to 9.** 25 mg/day. **Children ages 1 to 4.** 15 mg/day. **Infants ages 7 to 12 months.** 50 mg/day. **Neonates and infants to age 7 months.** 40 mg/day. DOSAGE ADJUSTMENT Recommended daily intake for people who smoke is 100 mg/day because of an increased utilization of vitamin C. Recommended daily intake should be increased to promote wound healing and for those with a chronic illness, fever, hemovascular disorder, or infection; the amount of vitamin C increase depends on the severity of the underlying condition.

OTHER INDICATIONS AND DOSAGES

Children. *Initial:* 1,000 to 5,000 mcg given in single daily doses of 100 mcg over 2 or more wk. *Maintenance:* 60 or more mcg/mo.
I.M. INJECTION (CYANOCOBALAMIN OR HYDROXYCOBALAMIN)
Adults. *Initial:* 30 mcg daily for 5 to 10 days. *Maintenance:* 100 to 200 mcg every mo.
Children. *Initial:* 1,000 to 5,000 mcg, given in single daily doses of 100 mcg over 2 or more wk. *Maintenance:* 60 or more mcg/mo.
DOSAGE ADJUSTMENT Dosage adjusted, as needed, to maintain normal hematologic morphology and an erythrocyte count greater than 4.5 million/mm^3.

To treat familial selective B$_{12}$ malabsorption
I.M. INJECTION (CYANOCOBALAMIN)
Adults. *Initial.* 1 mg/wk for 3 wk. *Maintenance:* 250 mcg/mo.

To treat hereditary deficiency of transcobalamin II
I.M. INJECTION (CYANOCOBALAMIN)
Adults. 1 to 2 mg/wk.

To treat vitamin C deficiency (scurvy)
E.R. CAPSULES; LOZENGES; ORAL SOLUTION; E.R. TABLETS; TABLETS; SubQ, I.M., OR I.V. INJECTION
Adults. 100 to 250 mg once or twice daily until skeletal changes and signs and symptoms of hemorrhagic disorder are reversed (usually within 2 to 21 days).
ORAL SOLUTION; TABLETS; SubQ, I.M., OR I.V. INJECTION
Infants and children. 100 to 300 mg/day in divided doses until skeletal changes and signs and symptoms of hemorrhagic disorder are reversed (usually within days).

PARENTERAL ADMINISTRATION GUIDELINES

•Be aware that SubQ administration of cyanocobalamin should be injected deeply.
•Know that vitamin B$_{12}$ is excreted more rapidly after I.V. injection; I.V. administration isn't recommended.
•Take precautions to protect vitamin B$_{12}$ solution from exposure to light because it's light sensitive.

•Be aware that I.M. injection is the preferred parenteral route for administering vitamin C, although it may be administered I.V. or SubQ when necessary.
•Rotate sites for I.M. and SubQ administration to help prevent transient mild soreness that may occur following administration. Inform patient that this adverse effect may occur.
•If giving I.V. vitamin C, avoid rapid administration to prevent faintness or dizziness.
•Administer vitamin C solution by itself because it's incompatible with many drugs.
•Be aware that vitamin C solution rapidly oxidizes in air and in alkaline solutions. Take precautions to protect vitamin solution from exposure to air and light.
•Open vitamin C ampules carefully because increased pressure may develop after prolonged storage.

(continued)

Vitamins (continued)

GENERIC AND TRADE NAMES	RECOMMENDED DAILY INTAKE
vitamin D$_2$ **(ergocalciferol)** Calciferol, Calciferol Drops, Drisdol, Drisdol Drops, Ostoforte (CAN), Radiostol Forte (CAN)	**Adults and children ages 11 and over.** 200 to 400 international units (IU)/day. (100 to 200 IU/day [CAN].) **Pregnant and breast-feeding women.** 400 IU/day. (200 to 300 IU/day [CAN].) **Children ages 7 to 11.** 400 IU/day. (100 to 200 IU/day [CAN].) **Children ages 4 to 7.** 400 IU/day. (200 IU/day [CAN].) **Neonates and children to age 4.** 300 to 400 IU/day. (200 to 400 IU/day [CAN].)
vitamin E **(alpha tocopherol)** Amino-Opti-E, Aquasol E, E-Complex 600, E-Vitamin succinate, Liqui-E, Pheryl E, Vita-Plus E, Webber Vitamin E (CAN)	**Adult men and adolescent boys.** 16.7 international units (IU)/day. (10 to 16.7 IU/day [CAN].) **Adult women and adolescent girls.** 13 IU/day. (8.3 to 11.7 IU/day [CAN].) **Pregnant women.** 16.7 IU/day. (13 to 15 IU/day [CAN].) **Breast-feeding women.** 18 to 20 IU/day. (15 to 16.7 IU/day [CAN].) **Children ages 7 to 10.** 11.7 IU/day. (10 to 13 IU/day [CAN].) **Children ages 4 to 7.** 11.7 IU/day. (8.3 IU/day [CAN].) **Infants and children to age 4.** 5 to 10 IU/day. (5 to 6.7 IU/day [CAN].)

OTHER INDICATIONS AND DOSAGES

To treat vitamin D₂ deficiency
CAPSULES, ORAL SOLUTION, TABLETS
Adults and children. Dosage individualized based on severity of deficiency, as prescribed.

To treat vitamin D-resistant rickets
CAPSULES, ORAL SOLUTION, TABLETS
Adults. 12,000 to 150,000 international units daily

To treat vitamin D-dependent rickets
CAPSULES, ORAL SOLUTION, TABLETS
Adults. 10,000 to 60,000 international units daily *Maximum:* 150,000 international units daily.
Children. 3,000 to 10,000 international units daily. *Maximum:* 50,000 international units daily.

To treat osteomalacia caused by long-term anticonvulsant use
CAPSULES, ORAL SOLUTION, TABLETS
Adults. 1,000 to 4,000 international units daily.
Children. 1,000 international units daily.

To treat familial hypophosphatemia
CAPSULES
Adults. 50,000 to 100,000 international units daily.

To treat hypoparathyroidism
CAPSULES
Adults. 50,000 to 150,000 international units daily.
Children. 50,000 to 200,000 international units daily.

To treat intestinal malabsorption
I.M. INJECTION
Adults and children. 10,000 international units daily.

To treat vitamin E deficiency
CAPSULES (ADULTS ONLY), ORAL SOLUTION, TABLETS
Adults and children. Dosage individualized based on severity of deficiency, as prescribed.

PARENTERAL ADMINISTRATION GUIDELINES

•Be aware that vitamin D₂ is usually given orally. However, I.M. injection may be required for patients with GI, liver, or biliary disease associated with malabsorption of vitamin D analogues.
Take precautions to protect parenteral vitamin D₂ solution from exposure to light because light causes it to decompose.

Vitamin E isn't administered parenterally.

(continued)

Vitamins (continued)

GENERIC AND TRADE NAMES	RECOMMENDED DAILY INTAKE
vitamin K₁ **(phytonadione)** AquaMEPHYTON, Mephyton	*Recommended daily intake hasn't been established for vitamin K_1. However, adequate intake is suggested as follows:* **Adult men age 19 and over.** 120 mcg/day. **Adult women age 19 and over, pregnant and breast-feeding women.** 90 mcg/day. **Adolescents ages 14 to 19.** 75 mcg/day. **Children ages 9 to 14.** 60 mcg/day. **Children ages 4 to 9.** 55 mcg/day. **Children ages 1 to 4.** 30 mcg/day. **Infants ages 7 to 12 months.** 2.5 mcg/day. **Neonates and infants to age 7 months.** 2 mcg/day.

OTHER INDICATIONS AND DOSAGES

To prevent hypoprothrombinemia during prolonged use of total parenteral nutrition
I.M. INJECTION
Adults. 5 to 10 mg/wk.
Children. 2 to 5 mg/wk.

To prevent hypoprothrombinemia in infants with diets deficient in vitamin K (less than 100 mcg/L)
I.M. INJECTION
Infants. 1 mg/mo.

To treat anticoagulant-induced hypoprothrombinemia
TABLETS, I.M. OR SUBQ INJECTION
Adults. 2.5 to 25 mg, repeated 12 to 48 hr after P.O. dose or 6 to 8 hr after SubQ or I.M. dose, as prescribed. *Maximum:* 50 mg/dose.
Children. 2.5 to 10 mg SubQ or I.M., repeated in 6 to 8 hr, as prescribed.
Infants. 1 to 2 mg SubQ or I.M., repeated in 4 to 8 hr, as prescribed.

To treat hypoprothrombinemia from other causes
TABLETS, I.M. OR SUBQ INJECTION
Adults. 2 to 25 mg. *Usual:* 25 mg. *Maximum:* 50 mg/dose.
Children. 5 to 10 mg SubQ or I.M.
Infants. 2 mg SubQ or I.M.

To prevent hemorrhagic disease in neonates
I.M. OR SUBQ INJECTION
Neonates. 0.5 to 1 mg within 1 hr after birth, repeated in 6 to 8 hr, as prescribed.

To treat hemorrhagic disease in neonates
I.M. OR SUBQ INJECTION
Neonates. 1 mg (or higher dose if mother took an oral anticoagulant or anticonvulsant during pregnancy).

PARENTERAL ADMINISTRATION GUIDELINES

•Be aware that severe adverse reactions, including anaphylaxis, cardiac and respiratory arrest, hypersensitivity, and shock, may occur during or immediately after I.M. or I.V. administration of vitamin K_1, even if it's diluted to avoid rapid infusion. Administer vitamin by SubQ route whenever possible.
•If vitamin K_1 must be administered I.V., do not exceed rate of 1 mg/min, as prescribed.
•Be aware that some vitamin K_1 solutions contain benzyl alcohol. Don't administer these solutions to neonates or immature infants because of a risk of fatal toxic syndrome, which may include CNS, respiratory, circulatory, and renal impairment and metabolic acidosis.
•Take precautions to protect vitamin K_1 solution from exposure to light because it's light sensitive.

Interferons

Interferons are classified as biological response modifiers or antineoplastics. They fall into three major categories—alpha, beta, and gamma—which are described below.

The chart on the following pages lists the trade names, indications, usual adult dosages, adverse reactions, and nursing considerations for these interferons.

Interferon alpha

Highly purified proteins produced by a recombinant DNA process, drugs in this category exhibit antiviral and antitumor activity. Antiviral activity depends on their inhibition of viral protein synthesis. Antitumor activity results from their ability to exert a cytostatic effect, reducing the rate of cell proliferation by delaying RNA and protein production.

This delay induces cells to enter a resting stage. These drugs also increase the activity of human natural killer (NK) cells, which have the ability to lyse certain tumor cells and normal targets. They also selectively increase the number of cytotoxic T-cells, thereby affecting tumor growth. Phagocytic activity of macrophages also is increased.

INTERFERON ALFACON

This specific form of interferon is produced by fermentation of genetically engineered *Escherichia coli*. It's structurally and functionally related to interferon beta and has greater biological activity than other interferon alfas.

Interferon beta

Produced by fibroblasts and epithelial cells, drugs in this category neutralize the activity of endoge-

GENERIC AND TRADE NAMES	INDICATIONS AND USUAL ADULT DOSAGES
Interferon alpha drugs	
interferon alfa-n3 Alferon N	*To treat condyloma acuminatum:* 250,000 units intralesionally at base of wart 2 times/wk for up to 8 wk.
peginterferon alfa-2a PEGASYS	*As monotherapy to treat patients with chronic heptatitis C who have compensated liver disease and have never received an interferon alpha:* 180 mcg/wk SubQ for 48 wk. *As adjunct to treat patients with chronic hepatitis C who have compensated liver disease and have never received an interferon alpha:* 180 mcg/wk SubQ with ribavirin (Copegus) 800 to 1,200 mg/day P.O. in 2 divided doses with food for 48 wk.
peginterferon alfa-2b PEG-Intron	*To treat patients with chronic hepatitis C:* 1 mcg/kg/wk SubQ every wk on the same day of the wk for 1 year. *To treat patients with chronic hepatitis C in combination with ribvarin* 1.5 mcg/kg SubQ every wk on the same day of the wk for 48 wk.
recombinant interferon alfa-2b Intron A	*To treat hairy cell leukemia:* 2 million units/m^2 I.M. or SubQ 3 times/wk.

nous interferon gamma (IFNG), the substance believed to be responsible for triggering the autoimmune process that leads to multiple sclerosis. In multiple sclerosis, an initial viral infection may stimulate IFNG production by T cells. Then IFNG induces macrophages to produce proteinases that degrade the myelin sheath around the nerves and spinal cord. Cytotoxic T cells then move to the site of inflammation, recognizing antigens as receptor sites, where they attack the tissue affected by IFNG, resulting in progressive neurologic dysfunction. Interferon beta drugs interfere with IFNG production by lymphocytes and the mRNA transcription caused by IFNG. As a result, cytotoxic T cells can't locate receptor sites and cause further damage in the CNS.

Interferon gamma

Produced from genetically engineered *Escherichia coli,* this type of interferon is chemically and therapeutically distinct from interferon alpha. Drugs in this category have potent phagocyte-activating properties. By enhancing oxidative metabolism, they produce toxic oxygen metabolites in phagocytes, which permits more efficient killing of certain fungi, bacteria, and protozoal microbes. Enhanced antibody-dependent cellular cytotoxicity and NK-cell activity reduce the risk of developing a serious infection in patients with chronic disease. These drugs also stimulate production of cytokines, such as interleukin-1-beta, and regulate the immune system by suppressing the IgE level and inhibiting collagen production.

ADVERSE REACTIONS	NURSING CONSIDERATIONS
CNS: Dizziness, fatigue, headache, psychosis **CV:** Hypotension **EENT:** Dry mouth **GI:** Anorexia, diarrhea, hepatotoxicity, nausea, vomiting **HEME:** Anemia, leukopenia, thrombocytopenia **SKIN:** Alopecia, rash **Other:** Flulike symptoms	•Use interferon alpha drugs cautiously in patients with renal impairment and in elderly patients. •Be aware that cross-sensitivity may occur among interferon alpha drugs. •Be aware that interferon alpha drugs aren't interchangeable. •Be aware that patients who are sensitive to mouse immunoglobulin also may be sensitive to recombinant interferon alfa-2a. •Unless contraindicated, ensure that patient is well hydrated at the start of and throughout therapy to reduce the risk of hypotension. •Reconstitute by adding 3 ml of diluent provided by manufacturer and swirling gently to dissolve. •Be aware that reconstitution of peginterferon alfa-2a and interferon alfa-n3 is not necessary. •Don't shake vial. •Be aware that cross-sensitivity with interferon alfa-n3 to mouse immunoglobulin, egg protein, or neomycin may occur. •WARNING Because interferon alpha drugs may cause or aggravate fatal or life-threatening autoimmune, ischemic, infectious, or neuropsychiatric disorders, monitor patient periodically with clinical and laboratory evaluations and expect drug to be discontinued if he develops severe or worsening signs and symptoms of these conditions.

(continued)

Interferons (continued)

GENERIC AND TRADE NAMES	INDICATIONS AND USUAL ADULT DOSAGES

Interferon alpha drugs (continued)

recombinant interferon alfa-2b
Intron A
(continued)

To treat condyloma acuminatum: 1 million units (using only the 10-million units/ml strength) intralesionally at base of wart (up to 5 warts/course) 3 times/wk on alternate days for 3 wk. If response is inadequate 12 to 16 wk after initial treatment, repeat course, as prescribed.

To treat AIDS-related Kaposi's sarcoma: 30 million units/m^2 (using 50 million units/ml) I.M. or SubQ 3 times/wk.

To treat chronic, active hepatitis B and C: 3 million units I.M. or SubQ 3 times/wk. *To treat chronic hepatitis B:* 5 million units/day or 10 million units 3 times/wk I.M. or SubQ for 16 wk.

To treat malignant melanoma: 20 million units/m^2 as I.V. infusion for 5 consecutive days/wk for 4 wk, followed by 10 million units/m^2 SubQ 3 times/wk for 48 wk.

Interferon alfacon drugs

interferon alfacon-1
Infergen

To treat chronic, active hepatitis C: 9 mcg SubQ 3 times/wk, at intervals of at least 48 hours, for 24 wk. If inadequate response or relapse occurs, 15 mcg 3 times/wk for 6 mo.

Interferon beta drugs

interferon beta-1a
Avonex

To treat initial attack or relapsing forms of multiple sclerosis: 30 mcg I.M. once/wk.

Rebif

To treat relapsing forms of multiple sclerosis: 44 mcg SubQ 3 times/wk.

interferon beta-1b
Betaseron

To treat relapsing forms of multiple sclerosis: 0.25 mg SubQ every other day.

ADVERSE REACTIONS	NURSING CONSIDERATIONS
	•Obtain CBC before and regularly during treatment, as ordered, because interferon alpha drugs may cause bone marrow suppression. Expect drug to be discontinued if patient develops severe decreases in platelet or neutrophil count. •Implement bleeding and infection-control measures, according to facility policy. •Use gamma interferon cautiously in patients previously exposed to cytotoxic drugs or radiation therapy. •Be aware that cross-sensitivity may occur with *Escherichia coli*–derived products. •Discard vial if left at room temperature for more than 12 hours. •Implement bleeding and infection-control measures, according to facility policy. •Administer acetaminophen, as prescribed, to prevent or treat headache and fever.
CNS: Anxiety, confusion, decreased concentration, depression, insomnia, nervousness **EENT:** Abnormal vision **HEME:** Leukopenia, thrombocytopenia	•Be aware that use of interferon alfacon-1 isn't recommended for patients with autoimmune hepatitis or psychiatric disorders. •Be aware that cross-sensitivity may occur with other interferon alfa drugs or *Escherichia coli*–derived products. •Don't shake vial. •Implement bleeding and infection-control measures, according to facility policy. •Monitor patient for signs and symptoms of vision abnormalities.
CNS: Fatigue, headache, weakness **GI:** Diarrhea, nausea **HEME:** Anemia, unusual bleeding or bruising **Other:** Flulike symptoms, infection	•Use beta interferons with extreme caution in patients with depression or seizure disorder. •Be aware that cross-sensitivity may occur with natural or recombinant interferon beta or human albumin. •Reconstitute following manufacturer's directions and refrigerate. Use interferon beta-1a within 6 hours of reconstitution. Use interferon beta-1b within 3 hours of reconstitution. •Implement bleeding and infection-control measures, according to facility policy.

(continued)

Interferons (continued)

GENERIC AND TRADE NAMES	INDICATIONS AND USUAL ADULT DOSAGES
Interferon gamma drugs	
interferon gamma-1b Actimmune	*To treat chronic granulomatous disease or to delay progression of severe, malignant osteopetrosis in patients with body surface area greater than 0.5 m²:* 50 mcg/m² (1 million international units/m²) SubQ 3 times/wk. *To treat chronic granulomatous disease or to delay progression of severe, malignant osteopetrosis in patients with body surface area of 0.5 m² or less:* 1.5 mcg/kg/dose SubQ 3 times/wk.

ADVERSE REACTIONS	NURSING CONSIDERATIONS
CNS: Fatigue, headache **GI:** Diarrhea, nausea, vomiting **HEME:** Leukopenia **SKIN:** Rash **Other:** Flulike symptoms	•Use gamma interferon cautiously in patients previously exposed to cytotoxic drugs or radiation therapy. •Be aware that cross-sensitivity may occur with *Escherichia coli–*derived products. •Discard vial if left at room temperature for more than 12 hours. •Implement bleeding and infection-control measures, according to facility policy. •Administer acetaminophen, as prescribed, to prevent or treat headache and fever.

Compatible Drugs in a Syringe

The chart below lets you know at a glance whether particular drugs are compatible for at least 15 minutes when mixed together in a syringe for immediate administration. However, keep in mind that drugs listed as compatible when mixed in a syringe may not be compatible when prepared for other routes of administration. Drug combinations prepared for immediate administration usually require a more concentrated solution than those prepared for infusion.

(**Key:** C = Compatible; I = Incompatible; n/a = Compatibility information not available; no recommendations can be given.)

	atropine	chlorpromazine	dexamethasone	diazepam	diphenhydramine	droperidol	furosemide	glycopyrrolate	haloperidol	heparin	hydromorphone
atropine		C	n/a	n/a	C	C	n/a	C	I	n/a	C
chlorpromazine	C		n/a	n/a	C	C	n/a	C	n/a	I	C
dexamethasone	n/a	n/a		n/a	I	n/a	n/a	n/a	n/a	n/a	C
diazepam	n/a	n/a	n/a		n/a	n/a	n/a	I	n/a	I	n/a
diphenhydramine	C	C	I	n/a		C	n/a	C	I	n/a	C
droperidol	C	C	n/a	n/a	C		I	C	n/a	I	n/a
furosemide	n/a	n/a	n/a	n/a	n/a	I		n/a	n/a	C	n/a
glycopyrrolate	C	C	I	C	C	C	n/a		C	n/a	C
haloperidol	n/a	n/a	n/a	n/a	C	n/a	n/a	n/a		I	C
heparin	C	I	n/a	I	n/a	I	C	n/a	I		n/a
hydromorphone	C	C	n/a	n/a	C	n/a	n/a	C	C	n/a	
hydroxyzine	C	C	n/a	n/a	C	C	n/a	C	I	n/a	C
ketorolac	n/a	n/a	n/a	I	n/a	n/a	n/a	n/a	I	n/a	I
lidocaine	n/a	n/a	n/a	n/a	n/a	n/a	n/a	C	n/a	C	n/a
lorazepam	n/a	n/a	n/a	n/a	n/a	n/a	n/a	n/a	n/a	n/a	C
meperidine	C	C	n/a	C	C	C	n/a	C	n/a	I	n/a
metoclopramide	C	C	n/a	n/a	C	C	I	n/a	n/a	C	C
midazolam	C	C	n/a	n/a	C	n/a	n/a	C	C	n/a	C
morphine	C	C	n/a	n/a	C	C	n/a	C	I	C*	n/a
pentobarbital	C	I	n/a	n/a	I	I	n/a	I	n/a	n/a	C
prochlorperazine	C	n/a	n/a	n/a	C	C	n/a	C	n/a	n/a	I
ranitidine	C	I	C	n/a	C	n/a	n/a	C	n/a	n/a	C
scopolamine	C	C	n/a	n/a	C	C	n/a	C	n/a	n/a	C

* Compatible only with morphine doses of 1 mg, 2 mg, and 5 mg.

hydroxyzine	ketorolac	lidocaine	lorazepam	meperidine	metoclopramide	midazolam	morphine	pentobarbital	prochlorperazine	ranitidine	scopolamine
C	n/a	n/a	n/a	C	C	C	C	C	C	C	C
C	n/a	n/a	n/a	C	C	C	I	I	C	C	C
n/a	n/a	n/a	n/a	n/a	C	n/a	n/a	n/a	n/a	C	n/a
n/a	I	n/a	n/a	n/a	n/a	n/a	n/a	n/a	n/a	I	n/a
C	n/a	n/a	n/a	C	C	C	C	I	C	C	C
C	n/a	n/a	n/a	C	C	C	C	I	C	n/a	C
n/a	n/a	n/a	n/a	n/a	I	n/a	n/a	n/a	n/a	n	n/a
C	n/a	C	n/a	C	n/a	C	C	I	C	C	C
I	I	n/a	n/a	n/a	n/a	n/a	I	n/a	n/a	n/a	n/a
n/a	n/a	C	n/a	I	C	n/a	C	n/a	n/a	n	n/a
C	I	n/a	C	n/a	n/a	C	n/a	C	I	C	C
	I	C	n/a	C	C	C	C	I	C	C	C
I		n/a	n/a	n/a	n/a	n/a	n/a	n/a	I	n/a	n/a
C	n/a		n/a	n/a	C	n/a	n/a	n/a	n/a	n/a	n/a
n/a	n/a	n/a		n/a	n/a	n/a	n/a	n/a	n/a	I	n/a
C	n/a	n/a	n/a		C	C	I	I	C	C	C
n/a	n/a	C	n/a	C		C	C	n/a	C	C	C
C	n/a	n/a	n/a	C	C		C	I	I	I	C
C	n/a	n/a	n/a	n/a	C	C		I	C	C	C
I	n/a	n/a	n/a	I	I	I	I		I	I	C
C	I	n/a	n/a	C	C	I	C	I		C	C
I	n/a	n/a	I	C	C	I	C	I	C		C
C	n/a	n/a	n/a	C	C	C	C	C	C	C	

Drug Formulas and Calculations

When administering drugs, you must be familiar with drug formulas and calculation methods to ensure that your patient receives the prescribed drug in the correct dosage, strength, or flow rate. This appendix will provide you with a quick review of how to calculate the strength of a solution, drug dosages, and I.V. flow rates.

Calculating the Strength of a Solution

Most solutions come prepared in the required strength by the pharmacy or medical supply source. But sometimes only the concentrated form is available, and you'll need to dilute the solution or solid to administer the prescribed strength.

When a solid form of a drug is used to prepare a solution, the drug must be completely dissolved. Solid drug forms, such as tablets, crystals, and powders, are considered 100% strength. (An exception to this is boric acid, which is only 5% at full strength.) The final diluted solution is stated in terms of liquid measurement. To prepare a solution, you'll need to add the prescribed solid or liquid form of the drug (the solute) to the prescribed amount of diluent (the solvent). Two of the most common diluents used in the clinical setting are normal saline solution and sterile water.

You can use two formulas to calculate the strength of a solution, as shown in the examples below.

Method 1: Calculating percentage and volume
Use the following formula:

$$\frac{\text{Weaker solution}}{\text{Stronger solution}} = \frac{\text{Solute}}{\text{Solvent}}$$

Example: You need to dilute a stock solution of 100% strength to a 5% solution. How much solute will you need to add to obtain 500 ml of the 5% solution?

Calculate as follows:

$$\frac{5 \ (\%) \ (\text{weaker solution})}{100 \ (\%) \ (\text{stronger solution})} = \frac{X \ (g) \ (\text{solute})}{500 \ ml \ (\text{solvent})}$$

$$100 \ X = (500)(5) \text{ or } 2{,}500$$

$$X = 25 \ g$$

Answer: You'll need to add 25 g of solute to each 500 ml of solvent to prepare a 5% solution.

Method 2: Calculating percentage and volume
Use the following formula:

$$\frac{(\text{Desired strength})}{(\text{Available strength})} \times \frac{\text{Total amount of}}{\text{desired solution}} = X \frac{(\text{amount of undiluted drug}}{\text{needed to make solution})}$$

Example: You need to make 100 ml of a 20% solution, using an 80% solution. How much of the 80% solution must you add to the sterile water to yield a final volume of 100 ml of a 20% solution?

Calculate as follows:

$$\frac{20 \ (\%) \ (\text{Desired strength})}{80 \ (\%) \ (\text{Available strength})} \times \frac{100 \ ml \ (\text{Total amount}}{\text{of desired solution})} = X$$

$$\frac{0.20}{0.80} = 0.25$$

$$0.25 \times 100 \ (ml) = X$$

$$X = 25 \ ml \text{ of } 80\% \text{ solution}$$

Answer: You'll need to add 25 ml of the 80% solution to the water to make a final volume of 100 ml of a 20% solution.

Drug Formulas and Calculations (continued)

Calculating Drug Dosages

You may be required to calculate drug dosages when you need to administer a drug that's available only in one measure, but prescribed in another. You should also be prepared to convert various units of measure, such as milligrams (mg) to grains (gr), and dry measurements to liquid. You can use three common methods of ratio and proportion to calculate drug dosages, as shown in the examples below.

CALCULATING ORAL DRUG DOSAGES

Example: You need to give a patient 0.25 mg of digoxin, which comes only in 0.125-mg tablets. How many tablets will you need to give him to attain the proper dosage?

Method 1: Using labeled amount of drug
In this method, true proportions between the drug label and the prescribed dose are used to determine ratio and proportion. The drug label, which states the amount of drug in one unit of measurement—in this case, 0.125-mg in each tablet of digoxin—is the first ratio, expressed as follows:

$$\text{milligrams : tablets} = \text{milligrams : tablets}$$

$$\text{0.125 mg (amount of drug) : 1 tablet (unit of measure)}$$

The prescribed dose—in this case, 0.25-mg—is the second ratio; it must be stated in the same order and units of measure as the first, as follows:

$$\text{0.125 mg : 1 tablet} = \text{0.25 mg : X (tablets)}$$

Calculate as follows:

$$0.125 \, X = 0.25$$
$$X = \frac{0.25}{0.125}$$
$$X = 2$$

Answer: You'll need to give the patient 2 tablets of digoxin 0.125 mg.

Be sure to use critical thinking to assess whether your answer is correct. Because the amount of drug prescribed is greater than the amount of drug in one tablet, it's reasonable to expect the required number of tablets to be greater than one.

Method 2: Using an established formula
To determine the correct number of digoxin tablets to give using this method, use the following formula:

$$\frac{\text{Prescribed dose}}{\text{Dose available}} \times \text{Quantity (unit of measure)} = \text{X (unknown quantity to be given)}$$

Calculate as follows:

$$\frac{0.25 \, \text{mg}}{0.125 \, \text{mg}} \times 1 \, \text{tablet} = \text{X (number of 0.125-mg tablets)}$$

$$\frac{0.25}{0.125} = 2X$$

$$2 = X$$

Answer: You'll need to give the patient 2 tablets of digoxin 0.125 mg.

(continued)

Drug Formulas and Calculations (continued)

Method 3: Calculating according to proportion size

This method uses the same components as method #1, but the ratio is based on proportions according to size. To determine the correct number of digoxin tablets to give using this method, use the following formula:

$$\frac{\text{smaller}}{\text{larger}} = \frac{\text{smaller}}{\text{larger}}$$

Substitute 0.125 into the smaller part and 0.25 into the greater part of the first ratio. Critical thinking leads us to believe that you'll need more than 1 tablet of the weaker 0.125-mg strength to equal the stronger 0.25 mg. Set up the proportion as follows:

$$\frac{0.125\ \text{mg}}{0.25\ \text{mg}} = \frac{1\ \text{(tablet)}}{X\ \text{(tablets)}}$$

Calculate as follows:

$$0.125\ X = 0.25$$
$$X = \frac{0.25}{0.125}$$
$$X = 2\ \text{tablets}$$

Answer: You'll need to give the patient 2 tablets of digoxin 0.125 mg.

CALCULATING PARENTERAL DRUG DOSAGES

The same methods used for calculating oral drugs and solutions can be used for preparing parenteral injections.

Example: You need to administer a prescribed dose of 1 mg morphine sulfate from a unit-dose cartridge containing 4 mg per 2 ml. How many milliliters will you need to give to equal the prescribed dose of 1 mg?

Method 1: Using labeled amount of drug

Using the same ratio as for oral drugs, the drug label—in this case, 4 mg—is the first ratio, and the prescribed dose—in this case, 1 mg—is the second ratio, expressed as follows:

4 mg (the amount of drug) : 2 ml (the unit of measure)

Calculate as follows:

$$4\ \text{mg} : 2\ \text{ml} = 1\ \text{mg} : X\ \text{ml}$$
$$4X = 2$$
$$X = \frac{2}{4}$$
$$X = 0.5\ \text{ml}$$

Answer: You'll need to give 0.5 ml of morphine sulfate to equal the prescribed dose of 1 mg.

Method 2: Using an established formula

Use this formula:

$$\frac{\text{Prescribed dose}}{\text{Dose available}} \times \text{Quantity (unit of measure)} = X\ \text{(unknown quantity to be given)}$$

Drug Formulas and Calculations (continued)

Calculate as follows:

$$\frac{1 \text{ mg}}{4 \text{ mg}} \times 2 \text{ ml} = X \text{ (number of ml)}$$

$$\frac{4}{2} = 0.5$$

Answer: You'll need to give 0.5 ml of morphine sulfate to equal the prescribed dose of 1 mg.

Method 3: Calculating according to proportion size
To determine the correct amount of morphine sulfate to give using this method, use the following formula:

$$\text{smaller : greater} = \text{smaller : greater}$$

$$\text{milligrams : milligrams} = \text{milliliters : milliliters}$$

Critical thinking leads us to believe that 1 mg is less than 4 mg and that you'll need less than 2 ml to give 1 mg of the drug; therefore, 1 mg goes into the smaller part of the first ratio, and X goes into the smaller part of the second ratio. Set up the proportion as follows:

$$1 \text{ mg} : 4 \text{ mg} = X \text{ (ml)} : 2 \text{ ml}$$

$$4X = 2$$

$$X = \frac{2}{4}$$

$$X = 0.5$$

Answer: You'll need to give 0.5 ml of morphine sulfate to equal the prescribed dose of 1 mg.

Calculating I.V. Flow Rates

When an I.V. solution is delivered by gravity, you must calculate the number of drops needed per minute for proper infusion. To calculate I.V. flow rates, you need to know three things:
•the drip factor—or the number of drops contained in 1 ml for the type of I.V. set you'll be using. This information is provided on the individual package label.
•the amount and type of fluid that you'll infuse as prescribed on the physician's order sheet
•the infusion duration time in minutes.
   Once you've gathered this information, you can calculate the I.V. flow rate using the following equation:

$$\frac{\text{Total number of ml}}{\text{Total number of minutes}} \times \text{drip factor (gtt/ml)} = \text{flow rate (gtt/min)}$$

Example 1: If the physician prescribes 1,000 ml of D_5W to infuse over 10 hours, and the drip rate for your administration set delivers 15 drops (gtt) per ml, calculate as follows:

$$\frac{1,000 \text{ ml}}{10 \text{ hours} \times 60 \text{ minutes}} \times 15 \text{ gtt/ml} = X \text{ gtt/minute}$$

$$\frac{1,000 \text{ ml}}{600 \text{ minutes}} \times 15 \text{ gtt/ml} = X \text{ gtt/minute}$$

(continued)

Drug Formulas and Calculations (continued)

$$1.67 \text{ ml/minute} \times 15 \text{ gtt/ml} = X \text{ gtt/minute}$$
$$25.05 \text{ gtt/minute} = X$$

Answer: To infuse, round off 25.05 to 25 gtt/minute or according to your institution's policy.

Example 2: If the physician prescribes 500 ml of half-normal (0.45%) saline solution to infuse over 2 hours, and the drip rate for your administration set delivers 10 gtt/ml, calculate as follows:

$$\frac{500 \text{ ml}}{2 \text{ hours} \times 60 \text{ minutes}} \times 10 \text{ gtt/ml} = X \text{ gtt/minute}$$

$$\frac{500 \text{ ml}}{120 \text{ minutes}} \times 10 \text{ gtt/ml} = X \text{ gtt/minute}$$

$$4.17 \text{ ml/minute} \times 10 \text{ gtt/ml} = X \text{ gtt/minute}$$

$$41.7 \text{ gtt/minute} = X$$

Answer: To infuse, round off 41.7 to 42 gtt/minute or according to your institution's policy.

Note: When preparing for I.V. administration using a controlled infusion device, the electronic flow-regulator will either count drops using an electronic eye or use a controlled pumping action to deliver the fluid in milliliters. Your final calculation will be based on the unit of measure used by the device: drops per minute, or ml per hour.

Weights and Equivalents

The following three tables show approximate equivalents among the various systems of measurement.

Table 1: Liquid Equivalents Among Household, Apothecaries', and Metric Systems

HOUSEHOLD	APOTHECARIES'	METRIC
1 teaspoon (tsp)	1 fluid dram	5 milliliters (ml)
1 tablespoon (tbs)	0.5 fluid ounce	15 ml
2 tbs (1 ounce [1 oz])	1 fluid ounce	30 ml
1 cupful	8 fluid ounces	240 ml
1 pint (pt)	16 fluid ounces	473 ml
1 quart (qt)	32 fluid ounces	946 ml (1 liter)

Table 2: Solid Equivalents Among Apothecaries' and Metric Systems

APOTHECARIES'	METRIC
15 grains (gr)	1 gram (g) (1,000 milligrams [mg])
10 gr	0.6 g (600 mg)
7.5 gr	0.5 g (500 mg)
5 gr	0.3 g (300 mg)
3 gr	0.2 g (200 mg)
1.5 gr	0.1 g (100 mg)
1 gr	0.06 g (60 mg) or 0.065 g (65 mg)
0.75 gr	0.05 g (50 mg)
0.5 gr	0.03 g (30 mg)
0.25 gr	0.015 g (15 mg)
1/60 gr	0.001 g (1 mg)
1/100 gr	0.6 mg
1/120 gr	0.5 mg
1/150 gr	0.4 mg

(continued)

Weights and Equivalents (continued)

Table 3: Solid Equivalents Among Avoirdupois, Apothecaries', and Metric Systems

AVOIRDUPOIS	APOTHECARIES'	METRIC
1 gr	1 gr	0.065 g
15.4 gr	15 gr	1 g
1 ounce (1 oz)	480 gr	28.35 g
437.5 gr	1 oz	31 g
1 pound (lb)	1.33 lb	454 g
0.75 lb	1 lb	373 g
2.2 lb	2.7 lb	1 kilogram (kg)

Equianalgesic Doses for Opioid Agonists

An equianalgesic dose of a synthetic opioid agonist is the dose that produces the same level of analgesia as 10 mg of I.M. or SubQ morphine, the prinicipal opioid obtained from opium poppies. If your patient is switched from one opioid to another, expect to use the equianalgesic dose to decrease the risk of adverse reactions while increasing the likelihood of adequate pain relief. The chart below compares equianalgesic doses (oral and parenteral) for adults and children who weigh 50 kg (110 lb) or more.

OPIOID	ORAL DOSE	PARENTERAL DOSE
codeine	200 mg (not recommended dose)	120 to 130 mg
hydrocodone	30 mg	Not applicable
hydromorphone	7.5 mg	1.5 mg
levorphanol	4 mg	2 mg
meperidine	300 mg	75 to 100 mg
morphine (around-the-clock dosing)	30 mg	10 mg
morphine (single or intermittent dosing)	60 mg	10 mg
oxycodone	30 mg	Not applicable

Abbreviations

The following abbreviations, which are common to nursing practice, may be used throughout the book.

ABG	arterial blood gas		ECG	electrocardiogram
a.c.	before meals		EEG	electroencephalogram
ACE	angiotensin-converting enzyme		EENT	eyes, ears, nose, and throat
ADH	antidiuretic hormone		ENDO	endocrine
AIDS	acquired immunodeficiency syndrome		E.R.	extended-release
			°F	degrees Fahrenheit
ALT	alanine aminotransferase		FDA	Food and Drug Administration
ANA	antinuclear antibodies		g	gram
APTT	activated partial thromboplastin time		GABA	gamma aminobutyric acid
			GFR	glomerular filtration rate
AST	aspartate aminotransferase		GI	gastrointestinal
ATP	adenosine triphosphate		gtt	drop
AV	atrioventricular		GU	genitourinary
b.i.d.	twice a day		H_1	histamine$_1$
BUN	blood urea nitrogen		H_2	histamine$_2$
°C	degrees Celsius		HDL	high-density lipoprotein
cAMP	cyclic adenosine monophosphate		HEME	hematologic
(CAN)	Canadian drug trade name		HIV	human immunodeficiency virus
cap	capsule		HMG-CoA	hydroxymethylglutaryl-coenzyme A
CBC	complete blood count		HPV	human papilloma virus
cGMP	cyclic guanosine monophosphate		hr	hour
CK	creatine kinase		HSV	herpes simplex virus
Cl	chloride		HZV	herpes zoster virus
cm	centimeter		ICP	intracranial pressure
CMV	cytomegalovirus		I.D.	intradermal
CNS	central nervous system		IgA	immunoglobulin A
COPD	chronic obstructive pulmonary disease		IgE	immunoglobulin E
			I.M.	intramuscular
C.R.	controlled-release		INR	international normalized ratio
CSF	cerebrospinal fluid		I.V.	intravenous
CV	cardiovascular		IVPB	intravenous piggyback
CVA	cerebrovascular accident		kg	kilogram
D$_5$LR	dextrose 5% in lactated Ringer's solution		KIU	kallikrein inactivator units
			L	liter
D$_5$NS	dextrose 5% in normal saline solution		LA	long-acting
			lb	pound
D$_5$/0.2NS	dextrose 5% in quarter-normal saline solution		LD	lactate dehydrogenase
			LDL	low-density lipoprotein
D$_5$/0.45NS	dextrose 5% in half-normal saline solution		LOC	level of consciousness
			LR	lactated Ringer's solution
D$_5$W	dextrose 5% in water		M	molar
D$_{10}$W	dextrose 10% in water		m^2	square meter
D$_{50}$W	dextrose 50% in water		MAO	monoamine oxidase
dl	deciliter		mcg	microgram
DNA	deoxyribonucleic acid		mEq	milliequivalent
DS	double-strength		mg	milligram
EC	enteric-coated		MI	myocardial infarction

Abbreviations (continued)

min	minute	T_4	thyroxine
ml	milliliter	t.i.d.	three times a day
mm	millimeter	USP	United States Pharmacopeia
mm^3	cubic millimeter	UTI	urinary tract infection
mmol	millimole	VLDL	very-low-density lipoprotein
mo	month	WBC	white blood cell
MS	musculoskeletal	wk	week
msec	millisecond		
Na	sodium		
NaCl	sodium chloride		
NG	nasogastric		
ng	nanogram		
NPH	human isophane insulin		
NPO	nothing by mouth		
NS	normal saline solution		
0.225NS	quarter-normal saline (0.225%) solution		
0.45NS	half-normal saline (0.45%) solution		
NSAID	nonsteroidal anti-inflammatory drug		
NYHA	New York Heart Association		
OTC	over the counter		
oz	ounce		
p.c.	after meals		
PCA	patient-controlled analgesia		
P.O.	by mouth		
P.R.	by rectum		
p.r.n.	as needed		
PSVT	paroxysmal supraventricular tachycardia		
PT	prothrombin time		
PTCA	percutaneous transluminal coronary angioplasty		
PTT	partial thromboplastin time		
PVC	premature ventricular contraction		
q.i.d.	four times a day		
RBC	red blood cell		
REM	rapid eye movement		
RESP	respiratory		
RNA	ribonucleic acid		
RSV	respiratory syncytial virus		
SA	sinoatrial		
sec	second		
S.L.	sublingual		
S.R.	sustained-release		
stat	immediately		
SubQ	subcutaneous		
supp	suppository		
tab	tablet		
T_3	triiodothyronine		

Index

Index

- **Generic and alternate names:** lowercase initial letter
- **Trade names:** uppercase initial letter
- **Illustrations:** *i* after page number
- **Tables:** *t* after page number